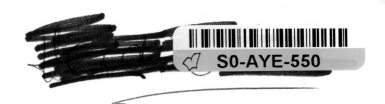

S0-AYE-550

ACUTE & CHRONIC WOUNDS

CURRENT MANAGEMENT CONCEPTS

ACUTE & CHRONIC WOUNDS

CURRENT MANAGEMENT CONCEPTS

RUTH A. BRYANT, RN, MS, CWOCN

Partner, Bryant Rolstad Consultants, LLC
Program Director, webWOC Nursing Education Program
Minneapolis, Minnesota

DENISE P. NIX, MS, RN, CWOCN

President, Nix Consulting, Inc.
WOC Nurse Specialist
Park Nicollet Methodist Hospital
Minneapolis, Minnesota

FOURTH EDITION

ELSEVIER
MOSBY

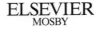

3251 Riverport Drive
St. Louis, Missouri 63043

ACUTE & CHRONIC WOUNDS:
CURRENT MANAGEMENT CONCEPTS, FOURTH EDITION
Copyright © 2012, 2007, 2000, 1992 by Mosby, Inc., an affiliate of Elsevier Inc.

ISBN: 978-0-323-06943-4

Notice

Knowledge and best practice in this field are constantly changing. As new research and experience broaden our understanding, changes in research methods, professional practices, or medical treatment may become necessary.

Practitioners and researchers must always rely on their own experience and knowledge in evaluating and using any information, methods, compounds, or experiments described herein. In using such information or methods they should be mindful of their own safety and the safety of others, including parties for whom they have a professional responsibility.

With respect to any drug or pharmaceutical products identified, readers are advised to check the most current information provided (i) on procedures featured or (ii) by the manufacturer of each product to be administered, to verify the recommended dose or formula, the method and duration of administration, and contraindications. It is the responsibility of practitioners, relying on their own experience and knowledge of their patients, to make diagnoses, to determine dosages and the best treatment for each individual patient, and to take all appropriate safety precautions.

To the fullest extent of the law, neither the Publisher nor the authors, contributors, or editors, assume any liability for any injury and/or damage to persons or property as a matter of products liability, negligence or otherwise, or from any use or operation of any methods, products, instructions, or ideas contained in the material herein.

Library of Congress Cataloging-in-Publication Data

Acute & chronic wounds: current management concepts / [edited by] Ruth A. Bryant, Denise P. Nix. — 4th ed.
   p. ; cm.
  Acute and chronic wounds
  Rev. ed. of: Acute and chronic wounds / [edited by] Ruth A. Bryant, Denise P. Nix. 3rd ed. c2007.
  Includes bibliographical references and index.
  ISBN 978-0-323-06943-4 (hardcover : alk. paper)
1. Surgical wound infections—Nursing. 2. Skin—Ulcers—Nursing. 3. Wound healing. I. Bryant, Ruth A. II. Nix, Denise P. III. Acute and chronic wounds. IV. Title: Acute and chronic wounds.
  [DNLM: 1. Wounds and Injuries—nursing. 2. Enterostomy—nursing. 3. Patient Care Planning. 4. Wound Healing. WY 161]
  RD98.3.A38 2012
  617'.9195—dc22

2010038243

Vice President and Publisher: Loren Wilson
Senior Acquisitions Editor: Sandra Clark
Senior Developmental Editor: Cindi Crismon Jones
Publishing Services Manager: Pat Joiner-Myers
Senior Project Manager: Joy Moore
Design: Teresa McBryan

Printed in the United States of America

Last digit is the print number: 9 8 7 6 5 4 3 2 1

To my mother, Marilyn Elizabeth Cullivan Bryant.
She is an amazing woman who has been my inspiration
and role model throughout my life both professionally
and as a Christian woman and mother.
My mom is always there for me, guiding
and counseling me through the ups and downs of life;
I love you, Mom. Thanks for everything.

Ruth Ann Bryant

To my boys: John, Ian, and Adam Nix.
You are a dream come true.
Having a wife and mom that is a nurse and an author
is not without sacrifice. I am so grateful for your patience with my
long days at the hospital or long nights in front of the computer.
Thank you for cheering me on for all of these years.
I love you with all of my heart.

Denise Patricia Henry Nix

Contributors

Joyce M. Black, PhD, RN, CPSN, CWCN
Associate Professor of Nursing
University of Nebraska Medical Center
College of Nursing
Adult Health and Illness Department
Omaha, Nebraska
Chapter 33. Reconstructive Surgery

Steven B. Black, MD, FACS
Medical Director
Wound and Ostomy Services
The Nebraska Medical Center
Omaha, Nebraska
Chapter 33. Reconstructive Surgery

Craig L. Broussard, PhD, RN, CNS, CHRNC, CWS
President
Clinical Consultants
Port Arthur, Texas
Chapter 22. Hyperbaric Oxygenation

Ruth A. Bryant, RN, MS, CWOCN
Partner, Bryant Rolstad Consultants, LLC
Program Director, webWOC Nursing Education
    Program
Minneapolis, Minnesota
Chapter 1. Principles for Practice Development;
Chapter 2. Billing, Reimbursement, and Setting Up a Clinic;
Chapter 5. Types of Skin Damage and Differential Diagnosis;
Chapter 8. Developing and Maintaining a Pressure Ulcer
Prevention Program;
Chapter 15. Foot and Nail Care;
Chapter 18. Topical Management;
Chapter 30. Intrinsic Diseases and Uncommon Cutaneous
Wounds;
Chapter 36. Skin Care Needs of the Pediatric and Neonatal
Patient: Part II. The Neonate;
Chapter 37. Managing Wounds in Palliative Care;
Chapter 38. Management of Draining Wounds and Fistulas;
Chapter 39. Percutaneous Tube Management

Susan Gallagher Camden, PhD, MSN, MA, CBN,
    CWOCN, RN
Clinical Advisor
Celebration Institute, Inc.
Conroe, Texas
Chapter 35. Skin Care Needs of the Obese Patient

Jane E. Carmel, MSN, RN, CWOCN
Program Co-Director
Harrisburg Area Wound Ostomy Continence Nursing
    Education Program
Mechanicsburg, Pennsylvania
Chapter 12. Venous Ulcers

Teri Coha, RN, APN, CWOCN
Children's Memorial Hospital
Chicago, Illinois
Chapter 36. Skin Care Needs of the Pediatric and Neonatal
Patient: Part I. The Pediatric Patient

Renee Cordrey, PT, MSPT, MPH, CWS
Visiting Professor
Doctor of Physical Therapy Program
School of Medicine and Health Sciences
The George Washington University
Washington, DC
Chapter 24. Ultraviolet Light and Ultrasound

CDR David R. Crumbley, MSN, CWCN
Division Officer, Complex Wound and Limb Salvage Clinic
National Naval Medical Center/Walter Reed Army
    Medical Center
Bethesda, Maryland
Chapter 31. Traumatic Wounds: Bullets, Blasts, and Vehicle
Crashes

Dorothy B. Doughty, MN, RN, CWOCN, FAAN
Director
Wound Ostomy Continence Nursing Education Center
Emory University
Atlanta, Georgia
Chapter 4. Wound-Healing Physiology; Chapter 11. Arterial
Ulcers

Vickie R. Driver, MS, DPM, FACFAS, FAPWCA
Associate Professor of Surgery
Director, Clinical Research Foot Care, Endovascular
    and Vascular Services
Director, Research Fellowship Program
Medical Director, Wound Care and Limb Preservation
    Center
Boston University School of Medicine and Boston
    Medical Center
Boston, Massachusetts
Chapter 14. Neuropathic Wounds: The Diabetic Wound

Eric Elster, MD, FACS
Commander, Medical Corps, United States Navy
Operational and Undersea Medicine
Naval Medical Research Center
Department of Surgery
Associate Professor of Surgery
Uniformed Services University of Health Sciences
Bethesda, Maryland
Chapter 31. Traumatic Wounds: Bullets, Blasts, and Vehicle Crashes

JoAnn Ermer-Seltun, RN, MS, ARNP, CWOCN
Family Nurse Practitioner, Certified Wound Ostomy
   and Continence Nurse
Bladder Control Solutions, LLC
Wound Clinic, Continence Clinic
Mercy Medical Center–North Iowa
Mason City, Iowa
Associate Program Director and Faculty,
   webWOC Nursing Education Program
Minneapolis, Minnesota
Chapter 10. Lower Extremity Assessment

Jill Evans, RN, MSN
Coordinator, Pediatric Burn Services
Medical University of South Carolina Children's
   Hospital
Charleston, South Carolina
Chapter 32. Burns

Rita A. Frantz, PhD, RN, FAAN
Kelting Dean and Professor
College of Nursing
The University of Iowa
Iowa City, Iowa
Chapter 23. Electrical Stimulation

Margaret T. Goldberg, MSN, RN, CWOCN
Wound Care Specialist
Delray Wound Treatment Center
Delray Beach, Florida
Chapter 37. Managing Wounds in Palliative Care

John Christopher Graybill, MD
Captain, Medical Corps, United States Army
Resident, General Surgery
Walter Reed Army Medical Center
Washington, DC
Chapter 31. Traumatic Wounds: Bullets, Blasts, and Vehicle Crashes

Harriet W. Hopf, MD
Professor, Department of Anesthesiology
Adjunct Professor, Department of Bioengineering
University of Utah School of Medicine
Salt Lake City, Utah
Chapter 26. Managing Wound Pain

Sheila Howes-Trammel, MSN, CFNP, CLNC, CCCN, CWCN, CFCN
Family Nurse Practitioner
Hennepin County Medical Center
Faculty, webWOC Nursing Education Program
Minneapolis, Minnesota
Chapter 15. Foot and Nail Care

Scott Junkins, MD
Assistant Professor
Department of Anesthesiology
School of Medicine
University of Utah
Salt Lake City, Utah
Chapter 26. Managing Wound Pain

Diane L. Krasner, PhD, RN, CWCN, CWS, BCLNC, FAAN
Wound and Skin Care Consultant
WOCN/Special Projects Nurse
Rest Haven–York
York, Pennsylvania
Chapter 25. Wound Pain: Impact and Assessment

Mary Anne Landowski, MSN, RN, CWCN, CFCN
Director of the Wound Care Clinic
Madigan Army Medical Center
Tacoma, Washington
Chapter 14. Neuropathic Wounds: The Diabetic Wound

Jonathan M. LeBretton, RN, BSN
Clinical Research Nurse Coordinator
Clinical Research, Foot Care
Endovascular and Vascular Services
Department of Surgery
Boston Medical Center and Boston University School
   of Medicine
Boston, Massachusetts
Chapter 14. Neuropathic Wounds: The Diabetic Wound

Dianne M. Mackey, RN, BSN, CWOCN
Wound/Skin Coordinator
Kaiser Permanente
San Diego, California
Chapter 9. Support Surfaces

J. L. Madsen
Madigan Army Medical Center
Fort Lewis, Louisiana
Chapter 14. Neuropathic Wounds: The Diabetic Wound

Debra S. Netsch, DNP, APRN, FNP-BC, CWOCN
Family Nurse Practitioner/Advanced Practice WOC
  Nurse
Mankato Clinic, Ltd.
Owner, Continence Consulting, LLC
Mankato, Minnesota
Associate Director and Faculty
webWOC Nurse Education Program
Metropolitan State University
Minneapolis, Minnesota
Chapter 21. Negative Pressure Wound Therapy

Denise P. Nix, MS, RN, CWOCN
President, Nix Consulting, Inc.
WOC Nurse Specialist
Park Nicollet Methodist Hospital
Minneapolis, Minnesota
Chapter 1. Principles for Practice Development;
Chapter 6. Skin and Wound Inspection and Assessment;
Chapter 8. Developing and Maintaining a Pressure Ulcer
Prevention Program;
Chapter 9. Support Surfaces;
Chapter 15. Foot and Nail Care;
Chapter 18. Topical Management;
Chapter 29. Noncompliance, Nonadherence, or Barriers to a
Sustainable Plan?;
Chapter 36. Skin Care Needs of the Pediatric and Neonatal
Patient: Part II. The Neonate

Ben Peirce, RN, CWOCN, COS-C
Assistant Vice President, Clinical Practice
Gentiva Health Services
Fort Lauderdale, Florida
Chapter 29. Noncompliance, Nonadherence, or Barriers to a
Sustainable Plan?

Barbara Pieper, PhD, RN, ACNS-BC, CWOCN, FAAN
Professor/Nurse Practitioner
Wayne State University
Detroit, Michigan
Chapter 7. Pressure Ulcers: Impact, Etiology, and
Classification

Janet M. Ramundo, MSN, RN, CWOCN
Special Projects Director
Distance Learning Program
Emory University Wound Ostomy and Continence
  Nursing Education Program
Atlanta, Georgia
Chapter 17. Wound Debridement

Catherine Ratliff, PhD, RN
Nurse Practitioner/Associate Professor
University of Virginia Health System
Charlottesville, Virginia
Chapter 13. Lymphedema

Bonnie Sue Rolstad, RN, MS, CWOCN
Program Administrator
webWOC Nursing Education Program
College of Nursing and Health Sciences
Metropolitan State University
Minneapolis, Minnesota
Chapter 18. Topical Management; Chapter 38. Management
of Draining Wounds and Fistulas

Gregory Schultz, PhD
Professor
Obstetrics and Gynecology
Director
Institute for Wound Research
University of Florida
Gainesville, Florida
Chapter 20. Molecular and Cellular Regulators

Susie Seaman, MSN, NP, CWOCN
Nurse Practitioner
Sharp Rees-Stealy Wound Clinic
San Diego, California
Chapter 19. Skin Substitutes and Extracellular Matrix
Scaffolds

Dag Shapshak, MD
Assistant Professor
Department of Medicine, Section of Emergency
  Medicine
Medical University of South Carolina
Charleston, South Carolina
Chapter 26. Managing Wound Pain

Bonnie Sparks-DeFriese, PT, RN, CWS, CWOCN
WOC Nurse Clinician/Instructor
Emory Wound Ostomy Continence Nursing Education
  Center
Emory University
Atlanta, Georgia
Chapter 4. Wound-Healing Physiology

COL Alexander Stojadinovic, MD
General Surgery Department
Walter Reed Army Medical Center
Washington, DC
Chapter 31. Traumatic Wounds: Bullets, Blasts, and Vehicle
Crashes

Nancy A. Stotts, RN, CNS, EdD, FAAN
Professor
School of Nursing
University of California, San Francisco
San Francisco, California
Chapter 16. Wound Infection: Diagnosis and Management;
Chapter 27. Nutritional Assessment and Support

Deanna Vargo, RN, BSN, CWS, FCCWS, DAPWCA, CWON
Territory Manager
MPM Medical
Cuyahoga Falls, Ohio
Wound Care Specialist
Acute/Outpatient Services
Summa Barberton Hospital
Barberton, Ohio
Chapter 2. Billing, Reimbursement, and Setting Up a Clinic

JoAnne D. Whitney, PhD, RN, CWCN, FAAN
Professor
Harborview Medical Center Endowed Professor in
   Critical Care Nursing
University of Washington, School of Nursing
Nurse Scientist
Harborview Medical Center
Seattle, Washington
Chapter 28. Perfusion and Oxygenation; Chapter 34. Surgical Wounds and Incision Care

Annette B. Wysocki, PhD, RN, FAAN
Professor
University of Mississippi Medical Center
Jackson, Mississippi
Chapter 3. Anatomy and Physiology of Skin and Soft Tissue; Chapter 36. Skin Care Needs of the Pediatric and Neonatal Patient: Part II. The Neonate

Reviewers

Phyllis Bonham, PhD, RN, MSN, CWOCN
Associate Professor
Director, Wound Care Education Program
Medical University of South Carolina
College of Nursing
Charleston, South Carolina

Carrie Carls, RN, BSN, CWOCN
Pelvic Floor Retraining & Urodynamics
West Central UOAA Support Group
Passavant Area Hospital
Jacksonville, Illinois

Lea Crestodina, MSN, RN, GNP, CWOCN, CDE
Wound, Ostomy, Continence Nurse Specialist
Memorial Regional Hospital
Hollywood, California

Janet M. Davis, MSN, RN, GNP-BC, CWOCN
Past Program Director, WOC Nurse Education
 Program
The University of Texas
MD Anderson Cancer Center
Houston, Texas
3M Clinical Nurse Consultant
Proherant
Overland Park, Kansas

Mary Walden, DNP, RN, CWOCN
Wound Care Consultant
Gilmore Memorial Regional Medical Center
Amory, Mississippi
Faculty, Itawamba Community College
Fulton, Mississippi

Preface

The volume of literature on the many facets concerning wound healing, wound care, and risk reduction/prevention is extensive. Since the last edition was published in the fall of 2007, national guidelines for wound management have been published by the WOCN Society, Wound Healing Society, EPUAP/NPUAP, RNAO (Registered Nurses Association of Ontario), AWHONN (Association of Women's Health, Obstetric and Neonatal Nurses), and the Association of periOperative Registered Nurses. The Wound Healing Society has also published prevention guidelines for the acute wound; venous, arterial, and neuropathic wound; and pressure ulcer. Further evidence of the growing thirst to conquer the dilemmas and unknowns in wound care are the increased number of annual national and international conferences dedicated to wound management (at least eight), the number of peer-reviewed journals that publish predominantly or solely wound-related manuscripts (at least seven), and the variety of professional designations and certifications in wound care that are currently available. The third edition of this textbook was also translated into Japanese, which further underscores the fact that wound healing and chronic wounds are worldwide concerns!

As our knowledge about the prevention and treatment of wounds deepens, regulations and expectations also change. The responsibility of the wound care professional is to integrate the new evidence into policies and procedures, decision-making processes, programs for staff education and competency assessment, formulary modifications, and outcomes management. This fourth edition of *Acute & Chronic Wounds: Current Management Concepts* introduces many new findings in wound research and incorporates guideline recommendations. In light of the vast amount of material in the literature, the book is physically larger to accommodate more content, formularies, figures, and color plates. To facilitate a better learning experience, the format for this edition has been modified so that the content is organized into sections with similar themes. Many of the chapters that in previous editions were quite lengthy have been separated into more than one chapter in this edition. "Checklists" have been introduced in this edition and are used to provide a list of actions or steps necessary to achieve or satisfy a particular objective.

Self-assessment exercises (Appendix A) have been organized according to the content categories of the WOCNCB wound certification exam. This should provide additional guidance to the reader in preparation for the CWCN certification exam.

Appendix B has been expanded to include additional assessment tools and documentation forms commonly used in the care of the patient with a wound. These can be used by the reader as needed in their practice. Appendix C contains convenient documents for infrastructure support: sample policies procedures and protocols and decision-making tools that can be used as an example or as is by readers to enhance their wound care programs.

Section I: Foundations contains six chapters that lay the foundation for wound care, both in the professional structure of a wound care practice (inpatient or clinic based) and the underlying concepts and principles of wound care that pertain to all wounds. New in this section is a chapter dedicated to the economic aspects of creating and maintaining wound care services: specifically, structural and procedural components of a wound care service, staffing and roles, documentation needed for billing, and business plan development.

Section II: Pressure Ulcers is now subdivided into three chapters. The chapter on prevention and risk assessment is discussed within the context of creating a pressure ulcer prevention program (PUPP), including creating a best practice bundle, risk assessment and pressure prevention in special settings (operating room, emergency room, etc). Concepts such as "present on admission" and avoidable/unavoidable pressure ulcers are explored. Most unique, however, is the discussion of the integration of the PUPP into the culture and infrastructure of the health care system and barriers to integration. Concurrent daily reporting of nosocomial pressure ulcers and root cause analysis are strategies described in the discussion of quality tracking.

In **Section III: Lower Extremity Wounds**, the common lower extremity wounds are each addressed within individual chapters. Unique to this section are chapters dedicated to lower extremity assessment and foot and nail care.

Section IV: Wound Bed Preparation contains three chapters: infection, debridement, and topical management. The concepts of bioburden, planktonic bacteria, and biofilm and their symptoms and management are described.

In **Section V: Biophysical and Biologic Agents**, content is divided into six chapters, each presenting a unique wound care method: skin substitutes, molecular regulation, negative pressure wound therapy, hyperbaric oxygenation, electrical stimulation, and ultrasound.

In **Section VI: Critical Cofactors**, conditions that impair wound repair, such as pain and nutrition are presented. Unique in this edition, the significance of tissue perfusion and oxygenation has been highlighted by drawing it out of various locations in the textbook and consolidating it into one chapter. The final chapter in this section, "Noncompliance, Nonadherence, or Barriers to a Sustainable Plan?", is the thought-provoking chapter that challenges the health care provider to work with the patient to create a realistic, achievable plan for self care.

Section VII: Acute and Traumatic Wounds has five chapters, each of which addresses wounds that occur as an acute event, disease process, or surgery. New chapters include intrinsic skin diseases and atypical wounds, traumatic wounds, and management of the surgical incision. The chapter on traumatic wounds is a special contribution to this edition and was inspired by the current issues in clinical practice as a result of the wars in Iraq and Afghanistan. This chapter discusses the pathology and management of wounds caused by gunshots and explosions.

Section VIII: Special Patient Populations is an exciting new collection of five chapters that describe the unique skin and wound care needs of special patient populations. A particular highlight of this section is the chapter on the skin care needs of the pediatric patient. In the palliative care chapter, the philosophy of palliative care versus hospice care is described. Palliative wound care is addressed for both malignant and nonmalignant wounds, including cutaneous malignant wounds (e.g., fungating wounds).

We had several goals in editing the fourth edition of this textbook. Of course, we wanted to provide a coherent yet succinct and somewhat directive resource on the broad topic of wound management that any health care professional could either read cover to cover or simply pick up and reference specific questions. In addition, we wanted to provide a resource that could guide the reader through the process of program development and quality management planning and implementation. We wanted to provide tools and sample documents that readers could use at least as a template of what should be incorporated into their wound care program. We also wanted to provide guidance to the reader when making decisions about staffing or credentials or certifications. We trust you will find the information we have compiled in the fourth edition of *Acute & Chronic Wounds: Current Management Concepts* beneficial to you personally as well as professionally.

ACKNOWLEDGMENTS

We would like to acknowledge the women in our lives who have contributed in a variety of ways to our accomplishments during the creation of this book: Sandra Maureen, Cassie, and Cindi (our amazing editors), Liza, Dorna, Roxanne, Mary, Joy, Bonnie, Dorothy, the webWOC sisters, the game day girls, Shelly and Maria, and our Moms, Barbara Henry and Marilyn Bryant.

Ruth and DeeDee

Contents

SECTION VII
ACUTE AND TRAUMATIC WOUNDS

SECTION VIII
SPECIAL PATIENT POPULATIONS

SECTION I

Foundations

1

Principles for Practice Development

Ruth A. Bryant and Denise P. Nix

OBJECTIVES

1. Describe the services provided by the wound specialist.
2. Identify a certification process that is legally defensible.
3. Distinguish between prevalence and incidence, addressing how each is calculated and the clinical utility of each measure.
4. Describe the data that are collected and used to drive practice and justify the wound specialist position.
5. Provide an example of two stakeholders and why they hold that position in a skin and wound care practice.
6. Cite three examples of how the wound specialist can affect cost savings within an institution.

A comprehensive wound care program is essential to any organization, agency, or health care system offering a full scope of services to its clientele. The wound specialist can provide a multitude of valuable services: state-of-the-art, evidence-based wound management; staff education; control of wound-related costs; quality improvement activities; protocol and formulary development; pressure ulcer risk reduction; and insight into efficient use of personnel and resources. The wound specialist is instrumental in bringing together many departments to more fully appreciate and manage the condition of the patient with a wound. In addition, the wound specialist can affect the quality of care in an organization or agency through administrative activities, collaboration with materials management personnel, establishment of a skin/wound care team, and provision of direct patient care and indirect patient care through consultation and staff education.

Many factors contribute to a successful practice as a wound specialist. Obviously the specialist must have a strong knowledge base in wound care and the relevant pathologies. In addition, the specialist must establish credibility, which is earned by demonstrating clinical competence, critical thinking, organization, self-confidence, and an eagerness to collaborate and share information with colleagues. However, a successful practice also requires the wound specialist to integrate business skills to develop goals that reflect the organization's mission and goals, effectively define services, identify benefits of services,

outline a marketing approach to potential referral sources, and draft a conservative but realistic budget. Many decision-making tools and clinical resources are needed in a wound management program. The wound specialist would be wise to assemble a business plan for new skin and wound-related programs. Components of a business plan are listed in Chapter 2, Box 2-1. This chapter discusses the application of business skills in terms of qualifications, role development, time management, data collection, marketing, value-added services, and outcomes measurement.

EDUCATIONAL PREPARATION OF THE WOUND SPECIALIST

When an organization is developing a skin and wound management program, it is incumbent upon the administration to demand appropriate educational preparation, qualifications, and credentialing of the health care professional who will function as the wound specialist. Appropriate education and certification should not be confused with attendance at individual seminars or continuing education courses. Upon completion of a continuing education course, the attendee receives a certificate of completion. However, in no way should this certificate of completion be misconstrued as an indication of the attendee's expertise, mastery, or competence. The certificate simply denotes the individual's attendance at the educational event.

NATIONAL CERTIFICATION: VALUE AND ROUTES

National certification yields many benefits to the individual, the employer, and the patient (Box 1-1) (Bonham, 2009; Cary, 2001; Fleck, 2008; Gray, 2008; Woods, 2002). National certification is the formal recognition of an individual's knowledge and expertise in a defined functional or clinical area of care. National certification is intended to protect the public and should validate an individual's specialty knowledge, experience, and clinical judgment. Table 1-1 presents a comparison of wound certification programs (WOCNCB, 2009). Because not all programs are legally defensible or psychometrically sound, the following critical components of the organization providing the certification are important to assess: national accreditation, eligibility criteria (educational degree, formal wound care education, structured clinical practicum in wound care, prior clinical experience), and recertification requirements. Collectively, these components influence the extent to which the certification designation is legally defensible (Hess, 2005). Checklist 1-1 presents questions to ask when comparing certifying organizations and certifications.

National Accreditation and Testing Standards

Accreditation of the certifying organization by an independent national certifying body is important because accreditation denotes the certifying organization's compliance with national standards relevant to all aspects of the certification process. Additionally,

> **CHECKLIST 1-1**
> *Questions to Ask when Comparing Certifications*
>
> ✓ Is the credentialing organization accredited by an independent, national certifying body?
> ✓ Was a job analysis or role delineation study performed?
> ✓ Is the examination created by an individual or by a committee of content experts?
> ✓ Does the certifying organization's mission agree with the mission of your work environment?
> ✓ Does the certifying organization provide self-assessment (or practice) to measure your professional knowledge and prepare you for the actual credentialing examination? (It must not teach the answers to the test.)
> ✓ Does the certifying organization require that the coursework be completed by an outside, accredited program focusing on wound care?

accreditation ensures that the certification credential meets specific criteria consistent with a testing process that is psychometrically sound (i.e., accuracy and effectiveness of each test item). A strong psychometric foundation underlying the certifying process assures candidates of fairness and accuracy of content in the testing process.

Eligibility Criteria

A key distinction among the certification designations is the education and clinical experience criterion for eligibility. Eligible disciplines and their educational preparation differ among certifying organizations. For example, the designation CWOCN (Certified Wound, Ostomy, Continence Nurse) is bestowed only upon eligible baccalaureate prepared nurses, whereas other certifications are available to licensed practical nurses. Table 1-1 lists additional examples.

Preexamination wound-specific coursework and clinical practicum requirements vary among certifying organizations. Coursework requirements can range from 0 to 5 days to many weeks. Similarly, required clinical experience varies among certifying bodies. Only one certification route requires a competency-based precepted clinical practicum following the coursework, thus facilitating integration of new knowledge into an actual patient care setting in the presence of a qualified, experienced expert.

Recertification Requirements

In the ever changing world of wound care and the need to stay current, recertification requirements must be considered and vary among credentialing organizations. Required frequency of recertification is 5 or 10 years, depending on the organization. Methods of recertification vary significantly and include self-assessment, proof of experience, and retesting.

> **BOX 1-1 | Value of Certification**
>
> **Consumer's (Patient's) Perspective**
> - Patients are aware that specialty certifications exist
> - Patients want to receive care from certified staff
> - Patients are more confident when they are cared for by certified staff
>
> **Administrator's Perspective**
> - Certification is associated with job satisfaction and retention
> - Certified staff have greater skill competence and less risk for error or harm
> - Certified staff have better skill-related knowledge and skill performance than noncertified staff
>
> **Certified Individual's Perspective**
> - Colleagues recognize certified staff as experts
> - Certified staff have job satisfaction
> - Certified staff have significant positive impact on patient care and safety
> - Managers express preference for hiring certified staff
> - Certified staff have advancement potential
> - Certification provides more effective resource to staff

TABLE 1-1 | **Comparison of Wound Certification Programs**

	WOCNCB®	NAWC®	AAWM	
	Wound, Ostomy, and Continence Nursing Certification Board	**National Alliance of Wound Care**	**American Academy of Wound Management**	
Credential(s) Offered	**CWCN®—Certified Wound Care Nurse** CWOCN®, COCN®, CCCN®, CWON™, plus advanced practice credentialing in wound, ostomy, or continence nursing. Foot care certification offered for registered nurses at all levels (CFCN®). Credentials are offered to registered nurses with a minimum of a bachelor's degree. Established: 1978 Term of Certification: 5 years	**WCC®—Wound Care Certified** Credentials are offered to registered nurses, licensed practical/vocational nurses, nurse practitioners, physical therapists, physical therapy assistants, occupational therapists, physicians, or physician's assistants with active, unrestricted licenses. Established: 2002 Term of Certification: 5 years	**CWS®—Certified Wound Specialist** Credentials are offered to any licensed health care professional with a bachelor's, master's, or doctoral degree in life sciences-related field. Established: 1995 Term of Certification: 10 years	**CWCA™—Certified Wound Care Associate** Credentials are offered to any licensed health care professional with at least 3 years' clinical experience. Established: 1995 Term of Certification: 10 years
Accreditation	**American Board of Nursing Specialties (ABNS),** the only national body to independently accredit nursing specialty certification programs (CWOCN®, CWCN®, COCN®, CCCN®). **National Commission for Certifying Agencies (NCCA),** an administratively independent resource recognized as the authority on accreditation standards for professional certification organizations/programs (CWOCN®, CWCN®, COCN®, CCCN®)	**National Commission for Certifying Agencies (NCCA),** an administratively independent resource recognized as the authority on accreditation standards for professional certification organizations/programs	**National Commission for Certifying Agencies (NCCA),** an administratively independent resource recognized as the authority on accreditation standards for professional certification organizations or programs	**No independent accreditation** of certification program

Entry-level Eligibility for Credential(s): Didactic Education and Clinical Training	• RN licensure AND
	• Bachelor's degree or higher AND
	• 40 hours of didactic wound specialty education in a WOCN Society-accredited single specialty wound care program and 20 additional hours dedicated to meet student learning needs AND
	• 40 hours of precepted clinical practice in a WOCN Society accredited single- or tri-specialty wound care program
	An experiential pathway is available for nurses that cannot attend a WOCN Society-accredited program
		• Professions listed above AND
		• Currently active in care of wound patients, or in management, education, or research directly related to wound care while actively licensed for at least 2 years full-time/4 years part-time within the past 5 years AND
		• Must meet ONE of the following:
		  o 4-day training program consisting of classroom training and lab practice
		  o Current certification through AAWM or WOCNCB
		  o Experiential option
		  o No additional supervised practicum required
			• Occupations listed above AND
			• Must have a Bachelors Degree or higher in a life sciences related field AND
			• Must have three (3) years of clinical experience in wound care
			No additional supervised practicum required
				• Occupations listed above AND
				• Must have 3 years of clinical experience in wound care
				No additional didactic education required
				No additional supervised practicum required

Exam Fees	$300 examination fee. No annual maintenance fees.	$330 examination fee. No annual maintenance fees. For those taking the course, exam fee is included in course fee of $2,497.	$550 examination fee with $150 annual fee to maintain certification ($1,900 total).	$300 examination fee with $150 annual fee to maintain ($1,650 total).
	<u>Recertification Fee: $300</u>	<u>Recertification Fee: $330</u>	<u>Recertification Fee: $400</u>	<u>Recertification Fee: $300</u>
Recertification Requirements	Successful completion of one of the following: a. Examination b. Portfolio submission (minimum of 10 CE credits (contact hours) plus professional activities or projects related to specialty focus)	Successful completion of one of the following: a. Examination b. Wound management training course $530 (no exam required) c. Continuing education (60 hours) d. Continuing education and outreach program (30 hours plus community outreach, publication, research, or leadership)	Minimum of (6) hours of CEUs annually. Self-assessment examination every 10 years.	Minimum of (6) hours of CEUs annually. Self-assessment examination every 10 years.

From Wound, Ostomy, and Continence Nursing Certification Board (WOCNCB): *WOCNCB comparison of wound certification programs,* 2009, available at www.wocncb.org/become-certified/how_to_choose.pdf, accessed July 12, 2009.
CEU, Continuing education unit.

ROLES, FUNCTIONS, AND RESPONSIBILITIES OF A WOUND SPECIALIST

The wound specialist is not responsible for conducting every wound assessment or dressing change. Clarity in terms of expectations of the wound specialist, staff nurse, and physical therapist (PT) is essential to promote collaboration and deliver comprehensive and effective skin and wound care. This clear delineation of roles is important to foster an empowering environment, avoid duplication of efforts, and maximize the efficient use of resources, including personnel. Table 1-2 provides examples of role delineation of a wound specialist and a staff nurse.

Participation in staff orientation programs is a key strategy to communicate roles, functions, and responsibilities. This setting offers an opportunity to orient new staff members to their role in maintaining skin health, providing wound care, skin assessment and surveillance, risk assessment, and pressure ulcer prevention. The wound specialist should take the time to instruct personnel on when and how to access the wound specialist. Key stakeholders (e.g., physicians, information technology personnel, purchasing director, materials management, director of nursing) should be contacted and the role of the wound specialist discussed and clarified. Stakeholders, by definition, may affect or be affected by the skin and wound program; thus, keeping them involved and informed can minimize or eliminate negative ramifications. As with all discussions, emphasizing the benefits of the skin and wound care program to the success of the facility or patient practice is important. The support and confidence of key stakeholders are so critical that the extra effort and time taken to nurture these relationships are well worth it. Ultimately, however, the wound specialist will need to demonstrate competence and confidence in his or her practice. Regardless of the health care setting in which the wound specialist will practice, role implementation will share common components: clinical consultant/expert, educator, integrator of research and quality improvement, and leader/coordinator (Box 1-2).

Consultant

Although many wound specialists provide direct patient care for the most complex wounds, in most settings the wound specialist serves primarily as a consultant. As a consultant, the specialist can better meet the majority of the patients' needs by coordinating a skin and wound care program implemented by a multidisciplinary team of health care providers. The consultant role builds on the foundations of the wound specialist's clinical expertise in wound-related pathophysiology, physical assessment, wound assessment, appropriate use of interventions, and documentation. A successful consultant must effectively communicate, collaborate, and educate. Clinical decision-making tools and resources, such as protocols, product formularies, and standardized care plans, pave the way for the specialist to adopt a consultative approach within the organization (Pasek et al, 2008).

Educator

Knowledge about skin inspection, pressure ulcer prevention, basic wound care, and comprehensive, accurate documentation is essential to maintaining and restoring skin integrity. Information about wound and skin care is increasingly available from the literature and from

TABLE 1-2	Delineation of Roles of Wound Specialist and Staff Nurse	
Wound and Skin Specialist	**Staff Nurse**
Facilitate creation and implementation of pressure ulcer risk assessment protocol.	Conduct risk assessment per protocol.
Establish protocol for prevention guidelines to correlate with risk assessment.	Implement appropriate risk reduction interventions.
Establish protocol for management of minor skin lesions (candidiasis, skin tears, incontinence-associated dermatitis, Stage I and II pressure ulcers).	Implement appropriate care of minor skin lesions.
Formulate skin and wound care product formulary to specify indications and parameters for use of products.	Use wound products per formulary. Notify wound specialist if product performs poorly or if expected outcome is not achieved.
Conduct comprehensive assessment, establish plan of care for complex patients (e.g., leg ulcers, stages III and IV pressure ulcers), conduct regular reevaluation of healing.	Notify wound specialist of complex patients. Conduct focused wound assessment. Implement appropriate care per wound specialist's direction and facility protocols.
Provide competency-based staff education for new employees and annual competency-based education for existing employees.	Identify and recommend topics of interest for staff education and updates.
Track outcomes and identify skin and wound care issues. Initiate quality improvement activities.	Participate in quality improvement activities.

BOX 1-2 | **Roles of the Wound Specialist**

Consultant/Expert
- Evaluates patient response to treatment and the progress of wound healing, making adjustments and modifications as indicated
- Where qualified and appropriate, provides conservative sharp debridement of devitalized tissue and applies silver nitrate to epibole, granulation tissue, and areas with minor bleeding
- Provides consultation and follow-up for patients with draining or chronic wounds, fistulas, or percutaneous tubes through outpatient clinic visits and/or phone consultations; initiates appropriate referrals for medical or surgical intervention

Educator
- Provides appropriate education to patient, caregiver, and staff regarding skin care, wound management, percutaneous tubes, and draining wound/fistula management
- Assists staff to maintain current knowledge and competence in the areas of skin and wound care through orientation and regularly scheduled education
- Attends continuing education programs related to skin and wound management

Change Agent (see Tables 1-3 and 1-4)
- Identifies barriers to change
- Provides evidence that persuades staff that change will achieve desired outcome
- Considers all stakeholders when planning change
- Communicates aspects of practice changes that will positively affect key stakeholders (especially the staff expected to implement the change)

Program Coordinator
- Provides consultation and assistance to staff in developing and implementing protocols used in the identification and management of patients with potential or actual alteration in skin integrity
- Provides guidance to staff in implementation of protocols to identify, control, or eliminate etiologic factors for skin breakdown, including selection of appropriate support surface
- Establishes protocols and guidelines for appropriate and cost-effective use of therapeutic support surfaces
- Maintains records and statistics and submits reports to employer
- Analyzes inventory and recommends appropriate additions and deletions to ensure quality and cost-effectiveness of products used for skin and wound care
- Serves on agency-wide committees and participates in agency-wide projects as requested
- Coordinates wound management teams or committees

Integrator of Research and Quality Improvement
- Assists staff to maintain current state-of-the-art practice by reviewing and revising policies and procedures to be consistent with national guidelines and other sources of evidence-based literature
- Provides leadership with prevalence and incidence studies
- Conducts product evaluations or contributes to research studies related to skin and wound care when indicated; submits reports and recommendations based on results

---

commercial sources. Reimbursement restrictions provide greater incentive for staff to familiarize themselves with basic skin care and pressure ulcer prevention. However, the wound specialist needs to organize the information into retrievable and clinically useful formats so that a formulary of wound and skin care products is available, the process for selecting and ordering an appropriate support surface is specified, and the documentation is comprehensive, easily accomplished, and not repetitive. As an educator, the wound specialist will develop routine orientation sessions to introduce new staff to the pressure ulcer prevention program, covering, for example, basic wound assessment, support surface selection, and the essential nature of skin inspection and risk assessment.

By auditing chart documentation or surveying the staff's knowledge about specific areas of wound care, the specialist can identify additional needs and target follow-up educational activities to satisfy those needs. Beitz, Fey, and O'Brien (1999) warn that "professional staff who perceive little need for additional wound care education may 'tune out' opportunities for increasing their knowledge base because they consider themselves 'competent.'" The information underscores the importance of using pretests and other means of educational needs assessments; however, education does not guarantee practice change.

Change Agent

Although education is an important role and tool for the wound specialist, it can be viewed as a burden that will increase workload rather than an innovation that eventually will decrease workload and improve patient outcomes (Landrum, 1998b). The organization will need to integrate principles for innovation adaptation to increase the likelihood of success with the educational efforts. An individual's reaction to and decision about new information, ideas, or practice (i.e., innovations) develops over time and seldom is spontaneous. The Diffusion of Innovations Theory (Rogers, 1995) provides a framework for changing practices in a group, individual, or organization (Dobbins et al, 2005; Landrum, 1998a). This theory describes how people adopt innovations using five stages: knowledge, persuasion, decision, implementation, and confirmation. Whether the innovation is implementing a new product or improving upon an existing product, and whether the innovation is preventive or has immediate observable results, a failure to consider these stages can spell disaster and frustration. Table 1-3 outlines these stages, defines each stage, and discusses considerations relative to skin and wound care.

Innovation is more likely to be adopted and behaviors changed when the innovation is perceived as relevant

TABLE 1-3	Five Stages of Rogers's Innovation-Decision Process
Stage	**Description**
1. Knowledge	Individual becomes aware of an innovation and of how it functions. May occur with reading, reviewing posted flyers, attending lectures.
2. Persuasion	Favorable or unfavorable attitude toward an innovation forms. To form a favorable attitude, the individual must be convinced that the innovation has greater value than current practice (e.g., identify patients at risk for pressure ulcers or target appropriate interventions).
3. Decision	Individual receives enough information to form an opinion about innovation. Individual pursues activities that lead to adoption or rejection of the innovation.
4. Implementation	Once an individual makes a decision to adopt the innovation, barriers (structural, process, psychological) to implementation must be overcome (e.g., adequate number of forms is available).
5. Confirmation	Individual seeks to reinforce his or her decision. Observable and positive results are critical at this stage to prevent a reversal in decision. Careful monitoring is required, and information validating positive effects is important (e.g., decrease in incidence of pressure ulcers after adoption of new risk assessment tool).

Data from Landrum BJ: Marketing innovations to nurses, part I. How people adopt innovations, *JWOCN* 25:194, 1998.

and consistent with the individual's attitudes and the perceived attitudes of colleagues within the organization (Dobbins et al, 2005). Generally, an individual will seek like-minded peers who already have embraced the innovation to discuss the consequences of adopting the innovation, and an individual's motivation to embrace the innovation is increased when these colleagues are supportive and positive about the innovation. Five attributes of an innovation significantly influence the rate at which the innovation is adopted: relative advantage, compatibility, complexity, trialability, and observability (Table 1-4). These attributes should be considered before the persuasion stage so that adjustments can be made to enhance the likelihood of success with the education efforts.

Integrator of Research and Quality Improvement

The wound specialist serves a pivotal role in integrating research findings into practice and coordinating quality improvement related to skin and wound care.

Evidence-based Care. Integrating research results into practice (i.e., research utilization) is a fundamental expectation of the wound specialist and a key component of an evidence-based practice. Defined as "the integration of best research evidence with clinical expertise and patient values to facilitate clinical decision making" (Sackett et al, 2000), evidence-based practice acknowledges that the care provided patients should not be based on habit but rather supported by the best possible evidence of effectiveness. Best research evidence is further defined as care decisions deriving from sources that are methodologically sound and clinically relevant (DiCenso, Ciliska, and Guyatt, 2005).

Many individual and organizational barriers exist to research utilization and evidence-based care (DiCenso, Ciliska, and Guyatt, 2005; Webb, 2008). One individual barrier is a wound specialist who may feel inadequately prepared to evaluate the quality of research and lacks knowledgeable colleagues with whom to discuss research. In addition, the wound specialist's access to the literature may be a hardship because of workload and time limitations. On an organizational level, barriers may arise from

TABLE 1-4	Attributes that Influence Adoption of Innovation
Attributes of Innovation	**Description**
Relative advantage	Is this better than an existing practice (e.g., potential decrease in costs, decrease in staff time, ease of use)?
Compatibility	Is this consistent with the individual's existing values, experiences, and needs?
Complexity	Is this innovation difficult to understand or use? For example, when a protocol is developed that links risk assessment scores with nursing interventions, the decision about which preventive nursing intervention to use may be perceived as less complex than before the protocol; therefore, the protocol may be more likely to be adopted.
Trialability	Can the individual experiment with the innovation on a limited basis?
Observability	Are the results of an innovation visible to others? Subtle outcomes are harder to communicate to others, so the innovation often is slower to be adopted.

Adapted from Landrum BJ: Marketing innovations to nurses, part 1. How people adopt innovations, *J Wound Ostomy Continence Nurs* 25:194, 1998.

a lack of interest, motivation, vision, and strategy on the part of managers. Organizational barriers also may be related to library access, the extent of library holdings, and Internet access. Recognizing and overcoming these barriers is important in order to positively impact research utilization.

To embark on the path of evidence-based care, the specialist must keep abreast of relevant health care literature to "find the evidence." In the face of a constantly growing body of health care literature, remaining current in the literature may seem impossible or all-consuming. However, practical information sources, referred to as *preprocessed resources,* are available that expedite access to evidence (Collins et al, 2005).

Preprocessed resources are products that have been developed by an individual or group that has reviewed the literature, filtered out the flawed studies, and included only the methodologically strongest studies. A hierarchy of preprocessed information sources with

relevant examples is given in Table 1-5. Such sources include practice guidelines, clinical pathways, evidence-based abstract journals, and systematic reviews. For example, guidelines pertinent to skin and wound care have been published by the Wound, Ostomy and Continence Nurses Society (WOCN Society, 2002, 2003, 2004a, 2005a, 2010), the Wound Healing Society (Hopf et al, 2006; Robson et al, 2006; Steed et al, 2006; Whitney et al, 2006), the National Guideline Clearinghouse (www.guideline.gov), the National Medical Directors Association, and the Cochrane Collaboration (www.cochrane.org).

When preprocessed information resources relative to a particular clinical issue are not available, unprocessed resources are necessary. Unprocessed resources are databases (e.g., CINAHL, MEDLINE, EMBASE) that contain millions of primarily original study citations (Table 1-6). The World Wide Web also is an unprocessed resource, although its potential for inaccurate information is

TABLE 1-5 Hierarchy of Preprocessed Information Sources

	Hierarchy Levels	Examples
(Highest-Level Resource)	Systems	Clinical practice guidelines Evidence-based textbook summaries *Clinical Evidence* (BMJ Publishing Group)
	Synopses of syntheses	Evidence-based abstract journals (e.g., *Evidence-Based Nursing*) Systematic reviews
	Syntheses	*Cochrane Reviews* Cochrane Library (www.cochrane.org)
	Synopses of single studies	Evidence-based abstract journals
(Lowest-Level Resource)	Single studies	PubMed clinical queries

TABLE 1-6 Unprocessed Databases

Database	Maintained by	Unique Features	Contents
CINAHL	Information systems and updated quarterly	Largest bibliographic database specifically related to nursing, allied health disciplines, and consumer health	Full text articles Clinical practice guidelines Bibliographies of major articles Research instruments Government publications Comments Book reviews Evaluations of multimedia and computer software and systems Patient education materials
MEDLINE	United States National Library of Medicine	Readily accessible Searching effectively requires thorough knowledge of how database is structured and publications are indexed	Comprehensive coverage of health care journals
EMBASE	Elsevier Science	Comprehensive bibliographic database of worldwide literature Requires thorough knowledge of how database is structured and publications are indexed	Biomedical and pharmaceutical literature fields Indexes large proportion of European biomedical and science literature

substantial. Seven criteria have been developed (Table 1-7) that can be used to assess the quality of health care information obtained from the Internet (AHCPR, 1999; Holloway et al, 2000).

Because the methodologic quality of studies obtained using unprocessed sources will vary, each study or report will require a critical appraisal to differentiate misleading research reports from valid reports. Many sources that discuss the critical appraisal of research are available (Callihan, 2008; Webb, 2008). However, many providers are not comfortable with their research appraisal skills. To simplify the process, Cullum and Guyatt (2005) propose asking three discrete, sequential questions, as discussed in Table 1-8.

The value of research-based care to the organization and the patient is significant. Results of a meta-analysis of studies have demonstrated that research-based care offers patients better outcomes than does routine procedural care. However, the wound specialist not only should *apply* evidence to practice but also should *generate* evidence from practice (Ehrenberg, Fraser, and Gunningberg, 2004). Evidence can be generated by publishing individual case studies or by partnering with doctoral prepared researchers to design and conduct basic research that answers clinically relevant questions.

Historically, a gap in health care has existed between what is known and what is practiced. The wound specialist has a critical leadership role in making evidence-based practice a reality. When leaders not only expect but also promote evidence-based practice to staff, research utilization is enhanced (Cummings, Mallidou,

and Scott-Findlay, 2004). Caregivers are most effective at integrating research into practice when the leader is clinically based, has specific clinical expertise and knowledge, and expresses a positive attitude toward research (Ferguson, Milner, and Snelgrove-Clarke, 2004).

Hierarchy of evidence. Evidence for an apparent relationship between health care events comes from many sources. The unsystematic clinical observations of an individual practitioner and the physiology-based opinion of the clinical expert constitute two very basic sources of evidence. Systematic studies, such as clinical trials, prospective studies, and case studies, are additional sources of evidence. The more structured and systematic the source of evidence, the more reliable the conclusion and results will be. In general, unsystematic clinical observations and expert opinion provide important insights that can further define a clinical problem or an intervention from which a systematic study can be designed. Therefore, there exists a hierarchy of evidence largely defined by the source of the evidence and the process used to gather it (Table 1-9). Clinical observations, expert opinions, and generalizations from physiology constitute the weakest forms of evidence. The strongest evidence results from randomized clinical trials (RCTs). However, not all clinical questions can be researched using an RCT design (e.g., rare conditions and ethical concerns); therefore, RCTs cannot be the expected standard applied to all research questions (Collins et al, 2005).

Quality Improvement. Quality improvement activities incorporate elements of research and are a high priority for the wound specialist. Quality improvement initiatives often are generated from noted deficiencies (e.g., nosocomial pressure ulcers) or are generated proactively as opportunities are identified that decrease cost, save time, or improve patient or staff satisfaction (Orsted et al, 2009). Such activities often consist of simple chart audits designed to ascertain the adequacy of documentation of assessment parameters, interventions, and effects or outcomes. Without a quality improvement process, delays, inefficiencies, or harmful interventions may go undetected and thus contribute to staff or patient dissatisfaction, delayed discharge, or increased costs of care. Quality improvement activities that should be central to all wound care programs are prevalence and incidence studies (discussed later in this chapter) and pressure ulcer prevention programs (Chicano and Drolshagen, 2009; Hiser et al, 2006; Orsted et al, 2009).

Program Coordinator

A fundamental need of any practice is a skin and wound care program consisting of skin and wound care policies, dressing change procedures, decision support tools, skin and wound care product formularies, support surface algorithms, and treatment protocols. Decision support tools enhance the clinician's decision-making capacity (Ehrenberg et al, 2004), thus

TABLE 1-7	Criteria for Evaluating Internet Health Information
Criteria	**Description**
Credibility	Includes source, currency, relevance/utility, and editorial review process for the information
Content	Must be accurate, complete, and provide an appropriate disclaimer
Disclosure	Includes informing the user of the purpose of the site as well as any profiling or collection of information associated with site use
Links	Evaluated according to selection, architecture, content, and back-linkages
Design	Encompasses accessibility, logical organization (navigability), and internal search capability
Interactivity	Includes feedback mechanisms and means for information exchange among users
Caveats	Clarifies whether site functions as marketer of products and services or as provider of primary information content

Data from Agency for Health Care Policy and Research (AHCPR): *Assessing the quality of Internet health information,* 1999, available at http://www.AHRQ.Gov/Data/Infoqual.htm, accessed July 6, 2009, and Mitretek Systems, McLean, Va.

TABLE 1-8	Guide for Evaluating Intervention-based Research	
Steps	**Description**	**Related Study Design Questions**
1. Are the results valid?	The study must be designed and conducted in a valid manner so that the results are believable and credible. A study design that is less than rigorous and contains sources of bias will generate skewed and false conclusions. Only when the study methods are valid and rigorous should the reader continue on to further assess the study results.	Did intervention and control groups begin the study with a similar prognosis? Were patients randomized? Was randomization concealed? Were patients analyzed in the groups to which they were randomized? Were groups shown to be similar in all known determinants of outcome, or were analyses adjusted for differences? Did intervention and control groups retain a similar prognosis after the study started? Were patients aware of group allocation? Were clinicians aware of group allocation? Were outcome assessors aware of group allocation? Was follow-up complete?
2. What are the results?	Any difference between the groups in the study will be expressed in terms of a risk measure, such as risk reduction or benefit increase. The accuracy of the risk measure (the effect of the intervention) will be expressed in terms of a confidence interval or p-value. In general, a narrow confidence interval, which does not include zero, suggests more precision and, therefore, greater confidence in the results.	How large was the intervention effect? How precise was the estimate of the intervention effect?
3. How can results be applied to patient care?	The patients in the wound care specialist's practice should be similar to the patient population that participated in the study if the research results are to be applied to them.	Were the study patients similar to the patients in my clinical setting? Were all of the important outcomes considered? Are the likely intervention benefits worth the potential harm and costs?

TABLE 1-9	Hierarchy of Strength of Evidence	
Strength of Evidence	**Rating**	**Definition**
(Highest Level)	Level 1	More than one RCT supports safety and efficacy of intervention (greatest strength)
	Level 2	Majority of RCTs support safety and efficacy of intervention, but others are equivocal or fail to support efficacy
	Level 3	Quasi-experimental studies (nonrandomized trials) support safety and efficacy
	Level 4	Case series or case studies suggest potential for safety and efficacy
(Lowest Level)	Level 5	Consensus or expert opinion (best practice)

Adapted from Gray M, Bliss DZ, Bookout K et al: Evidence-based nursing practice: a primer for the WOC nurse, *JWOCN* 29(6):283-286, 2002.

RCT, Randomized controlled trial.

empowering caregivers to act independently and wisely in a consistent fashion. Specifically, treatment protocols guide staff to (1) address critical assessment parameters, (2) perform steps of assessment and treatment procedures in a proper sequence, (3) learn proper application and utilization of specific products, and (4) assess the effectiveness of interventions (Pasek et al, 2008).

Policies and procedures are essential for guiding the delivery of care and meeting standards required by The Joint Commission and state health departments. Relative to skin and wound care, each facility or health care organization should develop policies for skin assessment, pressure ulcer risk assessment, wound cleansing, wound assessment, treatment of wounds, documentation and staging, compression therapy, debridement, and culturing. In addition, a policy should exist to delineate appropriate interventions for different levels of pressure ulcer risk as well as for high-risk patients. Examples of policies, procedures, and decision-making tools are given in Appendix C.

Skin and wound assessment parameters (see Chapter 6) should be incorporated into the admission database to ensure that the data are collected. Such data can also be incorporated into daily documentation flow sheets. Flow sheets that are dedicated to wound assessment and wound care interventions are particularly useful because they will best reflect changes in wound status over time at a glance. Documentation in multiple places increases the risk of errors, inconsistencies, and omissions and should be avoided. Examples of documentation forms are given in Appendix B. Electronic medical records are becoming more common in the health care setting but may not necessarily facilitate appropriate documentation or effective integration of wound and skin-related evidence-based practice guidelines (Milne et al, 2009). Therefore, it is critical that the wound specialist serve as content expert when choosing or building an electronic documentation system so that wound and skin-specific data can be aggregated into relevant clinical information (Golinko et al, 2009).

Skin and Wound Care Committees and Teams. As a leader and program coordinator, the wound specialist will develop programs and projects that reflect the needs of the patient population, are consistent with the priorities of the corporation, and are fiscally responsible, evidence based, and educationally and professionally valuable to the staff. A skin and wound care program is basic and essential to all care settings and facilities. In the United States, the gold standard for a comprehensive wound care program is a system-wide skin and wound care committee with unit-based skin care teams. Such programs consistently demonstrate enhanced clinical outcomes, reduced liability, increased staff satisfaction, and reduced costs (Andriessen, Polignano, and Abel, 2009; Chicano and Drolshagen, 2009; Hiser et al, 2006; Lloyd-Vossen, 2009; McIsaac, 2007; Orsted et al, 2009). Keys to the success of a skin and wound care program are dissemination of information, involvement of all stakeholders, and consistent, intuitive documentation.

From a structural aspect, the program will need a mechanism for oversight of the program and for operationalizing the program at the bedside. Program oversight is provided by a system-wide committee (e.g., skin and wound care committee) that is responsible for creating policies and procedures, formularies, decision-making guides, documentation tools, and educational resources. This group also facilitates transfer of knowledge and guidelines to the unit and bedside (Lloyd-Vossen, 2009). Members of the skin and wound care committee providing oversight of the program are representative of all stakeholders and key decision-makers, including administration, pharmacy, purchasing, and utilization review (UR).

Operationalizing or implementing the skin and wound care program will be dictated by the size of the facility or agency, the magnitude of the existing skin and wound care needs, and the available personnel. The mechanism created for operationalizing the skin and wound care program requires identifying who will implement the program at the bedside. In large facilities or agencies, a unit-based core group of staff nurses with a special interest in skin health and wound management should be identified. The program oversight committee is responsible for providing the unit-based staff with the information, tools, and resources they will need to provide patient consultation, conduct staff education, and lead the initiative for skin and wound care. Often referred to as *skin care champions,* this group of nurses become the "eyes and ears" of the program oversight committee and are responsible to the program oversight committee. In addition, these unit-based skin care members are empowered to identify and problem-solve adverse clinical findings, such as Stage I pressure ulcers and incontinence-associated dermatitis. For small agencies or facilities, the skin and wound care committee often provides operationalization of the program as well as oversight. The certified wound care nurse or designated staff nurse with additional education in skin and wound care will generally be responsible for providing direct care, conducting staff education, implementing and promoting policy, and leading the skin care initiative.

The process by which the unit-based skin team member functions is dictated by census, patient acuity, length of stay, and realistic staff expectations. In one scenario, the unit-based skin team members makes rounds of all patients with a skin-related issue or a Braden score less than 15 once or twice weekly, based on a list of patients to be seen provided by the charge nurse. Between rounds, any Stage I or II pressure ulcers would be reported immediately to a member of the unit-based skin team so that a root cause analysis can be performed to identify the source and to take corrective action. This information is taken back to the program oversight committee to further evaluate and make modifications to the infrastructure (policies, procedures, decision-making tools) as needed so that the situation does not recur.

Responsibilities and membership. Responsibilities and membership will vary according to the needs of the patient population, community laws, and the regulating bodies of the various disciplines involved. Skin and wound care committees and teams may fulfill many functions (Boxes 1-3 and 1-4).

CWOCN or certified wound specialist. At least one member of the skin and wound management team should possess a legally defensible certification in wound care issued by an independent national certification organization that validates specialty knowledge, experience, and clinical judgment. As previously stated, this is particularly important for the delivery of quality outcomes as well as the ability to legally defend the validity of the certification (see Table 1-1 and Checklist 1-2). This member will serve as content expert specifically related to pressure ulcer prevention and wound care.

When this member is a certified wound, ostomy, continence (WOC) nurse, the committee reaps additional benefits because of the nurse's expertise in a full range of skin issues (e.g., incontinence-associated dermatitis, tube site care, ostomy skin issues, complex fistula care) and the nurse's multifaceted role (Bonham, 2009). Given the

---

BOX 1-3	Skin and Wound Care Committee Oversight Responsibilities

Protocols and Decision-Making Tools
- Decision-making tools linking risk assessment with preventive interventions
- Offloading (specialty beds, heels, chair cushions)
- Policies or guidelines for pressure ulcer prevention, assessment and treatment
- Protocols for care of common clinical conditions (e.g., incontinence, incontinence-associated dermatitis, skin tears)

Formulary
- Skin care and continence products
- Wound care products
- Offloading products

Documentation
- Admission database to incorporate wound and skin assessment
- Ongoing documentation methods for prevention, assessment, and treatment
- Patient education

Education
- Patient education materials
- Staff educational needs assessment
- Staff orientation
- Annual education and competency
- Newsletter for just-in-time updates, announcements, learnings

Quality Management
- Review AHEs and RCA
- Implement infrastructure changes based on AHE and RCA findings
- Analyze unit-based reports for outcomes and trends

Research
- Clinical trials of products using standard evaluation protocols
- Prevalence and incidence studies
- Ongoing review of literature to maintain evidence-based practice

AHE, Adverse health event; *RCA,* root cause analysis.

BOX 1-4	Potential Members of a Skin and Wound Care Oversight Committee

- Medical director
- Certified wound specialist
- Certified wound, ostomy, and continence (WOC) nurse
- Physical therapist
- Nurse
- Dietician
- Occupational therapist
- Speech therapist
- Quality management representative
- Consultants/ad hoc members
  - Infection control specialist
  - Dermatologist
  - Podiatrist
  - Orthotics specialist
  - Diabetologist
  - Gerontologist
  - Plastic surgeon
  - Information technologist
  - Vascular surgeon
  - Pharmacist

Medical director. The medical director of the skin and wound management team is a physician. The medical director oversees ongoing treatment and overall management of patients with complex wounds. The medical director interacts as needed with primary and consulting physicians to facilitate consistent and effective skin and wound management that is in alignment with overall patient goals. Responsibilities include, but are not limited to, assisting the facility in the development and implementation of policies and procedures for prevention

---

CHECKLIST 1-2
Maintenance of Infrastructure

✓ Ensure time and staff are available to convert policies, procedures, and formulary with every change in contract, documentation, or technology. New initiatives (e.g., revised documentation forms, conversion to electronic medical records) require adaptations to existing processes and procedures, reorientation of staff.
✓ Network with key stakeholders and committees that can affect infrastructure; be visible and "in the loop" so that decisions that may impact on the skin and wound care program are recognized and addressed.
✓ Include the patient as a key stakeholder; conduct patient satisfaction surveys, customized patient education to reflect patient demographics.
✓ Report to a director or vice president, not unit manager.
✓ Ensure program is sustainable regardless of new technology, changes in staffing, changes in care delivery model.
✓ Position wound specialist as a high profile change agent, not a technician.
✓ Generate data and reports that justify sufficient staffing without compromise.
✓ Utilize operation reports as tools for monitoring and driving change, not as tasks to complete (Box 1-6).

---

increased incidence of device-related pressure ulcers (see Chapter 8), the nurse with this broader skill set is invaluable to the wound and skin care committee. The certified WOC nurse has been prepared at the baccalaureate level, and the nurse practitioner WOC has been prepared at the master's degree level. The certified WOC nurse often serves as the skin and wound care program coordinator by (1) organizing outcomes measurement studies as well as prevalence and incidence studies, (2) providing individualized holistic patient assessments, (3) making recommendations for wound care products, adjunctive therapies, and specialty beds or equipment, (4) performing debridements, if within the individual's skill level and scope of practice, (5) providing ongoing assessment and evaluation of healing for patients with complex wounds, and (6) educating staff in the prevention, assessment, and treatment of skin and wound problems. Research has demonstrated faster healing when a WOC nurse is involved in the care of a patient with a wound (Bonham, 2009; Harris and Shannon, 2008).

and treatment of skin breakdown that are consistent with national guidelines. Ideally, the medical director of a skin and wound management program is a certified wound specialist. However, when supported by qualified and competent team members, a physician without certification can be very effective as a medical director of a skin and wound management team.

Nursing. The registered nurse directs the development and implementation of an individualized plan of care based on the needs and goals assessed for the patient. Nursing focuses on risk assessment, early problem identification, preventive measures to promote skin integrity, and responses to treatments. The nurse documents and reports condition changes and revises the plan of care as necessary. In the United States, several training pathways for nurses are available, ranging from licensed practical nurses to registered nurse to advanced practice and nurses with doctoral degrees. The nurse is instrumental in providing valuable patient-centered input to the committee. The success of the skin and wound program ultimately lies with the ability and commitment of the nurse to operationalize the program at the unit level and on to the bedside.

Physical therapy. The role of the physical therapist (PT) can differ widely among care settings and facilities. If involved in wound care, the role of the PT may appear to overlap with that of the certified wound nurse or the WOC nurse. PTs may collaborate during evaluation and care planning, or they may coordinate a team. PTs often are involved throughout the process of care, from preventing breakdown to facilitating healing. PT interventions address range of motion, strength training, seating and positioning, support surfaces, and functional mobility training. PTs may offer therapeutic intervention for contractures, edema, motor control, muscle weakness, and pain. Other interventions, such as electrical stimulation, pulsed lavage, and sharp debridement, may be within the scope of practice for some PTs. As with nurses, PTs should function within their scope of practice, be regulated by accredited educational programs and curricula, and have certifications with sound practicum experience.

Occupational therapy. The occupational therapist (OT) plays a rehabilitative role, assessing cognitive and functional capabilities and then introducing patient-specific adaptive techniques and equipment. Patient-specific adaptive techniques and equipment promote the patient's optimal performance of activities of daily living, including the patient's ability to take an active role in wound care. The patient with a slow-healing or nonhealing wound may benefit from the expertise of the OT in promoting the patient's overall health maintenance and quality of life by incorporating skin and wound care into the patient and family's daily routine.

Speech therapy. The speech therapist helps promote optimal nutrition by ensuring that the patient is able to safely swallow. Speech therapy may include strengthening oral and/or pharyngeal musculature, performing swallow-

ing trials for diet advancement, and/or providing compensatory techniques with oral intake to improve the safety of the patient's swallowing and reduce aspiration risk. The speech therapist focuses on improving the patient's ability to effectively communicate to his or her maximum functional level. Cognitively, speech therapy works to improve cognitive-linguistic skills for safe and effective communication upon the patient's transition to the least restrictive environment possible.

Dietician or nutritionist. The dietician promotes optimal nutrition through nutritional assessment and intervention. The dietician monitors nutritionally related laboratory values, anthropometric measurements, and food intake or nutrition support parameters. The dietician collaborates with the team in making recommendations that optimally meet the nutritional needs and goals of the patient.

Social services. The social worker is a key member of the skin and wound management team. The patient with a wound often is vulnerable and requires astute assessment of the home situation, particularly as it relates to the patient's safety, support, and ability to realistically adhere to wound management goals. The social worker is knowledgeable about financial resources and the barriers to follow-up care that are unique to each individual situation. The social worker obtains prior authorization for supplies and other services needed upon discharge to prevent unexpected costs to the patient. As the key liaison between care settings, the social worker coordinates and leads discharge planning conferences, which include the patient, skin and wound management team members, and the family. Representatives from facilities and agencies responsible for future care often are included in discharge planning meetings for patients having complex management issues. This collaboration among the patient, the family, and the health care team members from both settings helps to establish mutual goals and continuity in care.

Utilization review. In the United States, the utilization review (UR) specialist functions as a critical link among the patient, the physician, and the payer (insurance company, health maintenance organization, state or federal provider). Both nurses and social workers may hold UR positions. In many care settings, UR responsibilities have become incorporated into the case management role. The UR specialist provides information to payers to ensure funding for the most appropriate and cost-effective care.

PREVALENCE/INCIDENCE STUDIES

Prevalence and incidence measures are the primary measures of how frequently a condition, such as a pressure ulcer, develops. Incidence can be reflected as cumulative incidence or incidence density. These terms are not interchangeable. Box 1-5 provides the formula for calculating each measure.

Prevalence

Prevalence is the number of individuals who have a specific condition at a particular moment in time. Expressed as a percentage or proportion (or a ratio, not a rate), prevalence is a cross-sectional measure. As a snapshot in time, prevalence reflects how many people in a target population (e.g., patients in the orthopedic unit) have a condition (e.g., a pressure ulcer) at a point in time (e.g., during the month of July). For example, the prevalence of pressure ulcers in the orthopedic unit for the month of July may be five out of a unit census of 50 (5/50, or 10%). The issue of whether the condition is "new" or ongoing is irrelevant when calculating prevalence; all patients with the condition at that point in time are counted. Generally considered to be a stable measure, prevalence should not vary significantly over time unless changes in practice patterns, referral bases, or marketing have occurred or the average duration of the disease has changed. As a measure of disease frequency (or burden of disease), prevalence is a useful tool for health care planning. Because it is a reflection of the general norm, prevalence provides a means of identifying workload needs, staff needs, or resource allocation needs to satisfy the demands of a particular disease burden or volume. Prevalence should never be misconstrued as a measure of quality of care or a measure of risk. An institution or agency that specializes in wound care is expected to have a high volume or prevalence of wounds because marketing strategies are geared toward recruiting or enrolling patients with wounds.

Incidence

Incidence is the proportion of patients who *acquire* the condition over a given period of time. The term *nosocomial* refers to hospital acquired. In the case of pressure ulcers, for example, the incidence is the number of patients in a defined population (e.g., patients in the intensive care unit) who initially were ulcer-free but then developed a pressure ulcer within a particular time (e.g., during their hospital stay). Incidence is calculated as a cumulative incidence (expressed as a percentage) or as incidence density (expressed as a rate).

Cumulative Incidence. *Cumulative incidence* is the number of new patients in a group who develop a condition over a period of time. The denominator for cumulative incidence is the total number of people in the population being observed at the beginning of the designated time period. Cumulative incidence is a measure of risk and provides an estimate of the probability (risk) of developing a condition or disease over a specific period of time (Kelsey et al, 1996). Therefore, cumulative incidence can be used to gauge the effects of risk factors and prevention efforts. Characteristics of cumulative incidence include the following (Gordis, 1996):

1. Cumulative incidence is a measure of *new* (not existing) cases of a particular condition.
2. The denominator must include only those individuals *at risk* for developing the condition.
3. Cumulative incidence always refers to a specific time period (e.g., 1 day, 1 week, 1 month, 1 year).
4. As with prevalence, cumulative incidence is a proportion (not a rate) and ranges from 0% to 100%.
5. All individuals in the group at risk (represented by the denominator) are followed or observed for the entire time period specified.

To calculate cumulative incidence, consider the following situation. The number of patients on an orthopedic unit on July 1 is 50 (the population at risk); five were admitted with an existing pressure ulcer, and five developed a pressure ulcer after admission. The cumulative incidence of pressure ulcers on the orthopedic unit is calculated as follows. A total of 50 patients are at risk (the denominator), and five of the 50 patients developed a pressure ulcer, so the cumulative incidence of pressure ulcers in patients on the orthopedic unit on July 1 is 5/50, or 10%.

Incidence Density. Incidence density differs from cumulative incidence in that the denominator used to calculate incidence density is the aggregate duration of exposure. Thus, incidence density is a rate that can be reported as patient-days or device-days (Streed and Loehne, 2007; WOCN Society, 2004b). For example, when the incidence density rate of pressure ulcers on an orthopedic unit in the month of July is calculated, the length of time that each patient remains on the unit will vary. Some

---

BOX 1-5	Formulas for Prevalence, Cumulative Incidence, and Incidence Density

$$\text{Prevalence*} = \frac{\text{No. of persons with a condition (e.g., pressure ulcer)}}{\text{No. of persons in the target population at a particular point in time}} \times 100$$

$$\text{Cumulative Incidence*} = \frac{\text{No. of persons}}{\text{No. of persons in the population at the beginning of the time period}} \times 100$$

$$\text{Incidence Density\dagger} = \frac{\text{No. of persons developing the condition (e.g., new pressure ulcer)}}{\text{Total time (patient-days or patient-years) persons were free of the condition or observed}} \times 1,000$$

*Expressed as a percentage.
†Expressed as a rate.

patients may be on the unit 3 days before being discharged, whereas others may be on the unit for 2 weeks. Consequently, these individuals will be observed (and at risk) for different periods of time. The first patient is at risk for pressure ulcer formation for only 3 days, whereas the second patient is at risk for 2 weeks. If these two patients developed a pressure ulcer during their time on the unit, the incidence density rate would be 2 per 17 patient days. A formula for calculating incidence density per 1,000 patient-days is provided in Box 1-5.

A more feasible technique for calculating incidence density uses the number of patient-days available from the agency or facility. The formula for this technique is as follows: number of pressure ulcers divided by number of patient days, multiplied by 1,000 to give a rate. For example, during 1 month, eight incident pressure ulcers are reported with 8,000 patient days. The incidence density then is 1 per 1,000 patient days, or a rate of 1.0.

Benchmarks and Generalizability of Results

Cumulative incidence is commonly reported in the literature; however, using the data for benchmarking and comparisons has limitations. The groups from which the cumulative incidence is drawn must be comparable with regard to key risk factors, such as acuity and patient mix as well as data collection methods. The National Database of Nursing Quality Indicators (NDNQI) can provide realistic benchmarks by enrolling large numbers of facilities and breaking down data according to level of risk so that similar facilities can be compared. Furthermore, NDNQI provides pressure ulcer education (available at www.nursingquality.org) to promote consistent techniques for data collection throughout participating facilities.

Reliance on cumulative incidence measure alone has limitations. Because cumulative incidence is generally obtained through a 1-day study performed annually or quarterly, it reflects adverse events discovered on 1 day. However, from a quality-of-care perspective, all adverse events need to be reported and tracked 24 hours per day, 7 days per week, so that root cause analysis can be determined and corrective action implemented in a timely fashion. For this purpose, an incidence density process using concurrent real-time data collection is critical. The success of concurrent real-time data collection is dependent on the infrastructure in place. The reporting process must be clear (i.e., what exactly to report), simple (e.g., a 1-minute process rather than a 15-minute report), and accessible 24/7. Data should be sent to a central location for immediate analysis and action by qualified staff (Kartes, 1996).

Methodology

Prevalence and incidence studies can be an onerous undertaking but yield considerable information if the objective is clear from the onset. *Prevalence and Incidence: A Toolkit for Clinicians* (WOCN Society, 2004b) and the NDNQI pressure ulcer education site (www.nursingquality.org) outline the specific steps required to prepare for and conduct a prevalence and incidence study. They also provide documentation forms generally required of such a process and education for data collectors.

A key decision in planning the study is determining the staffing mix and the numbers for data collection. Data were analyzed from pressure ulcer prevalence studies conducted in nursing homes between 2004 and 2006 on differences in observed rates when one nurse compared to two nurses conducted skin inspections. Results revealed that the number of raters did not influence the observed rate, leading researchers to conclude that adequate preparation and training of staff nurses for data collection were sufficient to achieve reliable data (Kottner et al, 2009).

Another important decision in planning the study is determining which population to study, or the at-risk population. The term *at risk* implies, from an epidemiologic standpoint, those individuals who have the potential for developing a condition; *at risk* does *not* refer to the pressure ulcer risk assessment score obtained by using the Braden scale, for example. With this broader interpretation of the concept of at risk, all patients in the hospital may be assumed to be at risk for pressure ulcer formation, for example. However, whether the assumption holds that all patients who are hospitalized are at risk is arguable. When studies report the incidence for hospital-wide populations, they often exclude pediatric, obstetric, or mental health patient populations. For this reason, conducting incidence and prevalence studies on targeted patient populations may be more meaningful as well as more feasible (Aronovitch, 1999; Grous, Reilly, and Gift, 1997; Jacksich, 1997).

For example, a study could examine all patients undergoing an operation lasting 3 hours or longer, all patients with a specific diagnosis such as hip fracture, patients who have diabetes and are admitted to home care from Hospital Z, or all patients on a specific hospital unit. Allman et al (1995) reported a 12.9% cumulative incidence of pressure ulcers after a median of 9 days from admission to final skin examination in a very specific patient population: patients were 55 years or older, had a hip fracture or were confined to a bed or chair for at least 5 days, and did not have a Stage III or greater pressure ulcer.

MARKETING, JUSTIFYING, AND SECURING THE WOUND SPECIALIST ROLE

A key factor to a successful skin and wound care practice is effective communication and marketing of the role and the service. Measuring productivity and outcomes and communicating benefits are critical in securing and maintaining the role. Demonstrating and communicating the impact are essential so that the specialist and the services provided remain visible and the administration can justify the budget required to fund the wound specialist's position and program. This goal is accomplished not only through outstanding outcomes but, more importantly, by tracking and communicating outcomes through routine operations reports to key stakeholders and committees. These reports will help remind the administration that a low incidence of wound and skin-related problems is a result of having a qualified wound specialist; it is not an indication that staffing for the wound specialist should be reduced. This section outlines the benefits of having a wound specialist and the operations reports that are necessary to market, justify, and secure the role of the wound specialist. Checklist 1-2 on page 13 provides tips for maintaining program infrastructure and securing the specialist's role. Appendix C contains an example of a patient satisfaction survey.

Benefits of the Wound Specialist Role

Employing a wound specialist yields many benefits to the organization, the value of which are more dramatic in the current climate of cost constraints. Through efficient use of materials, accurate and thorough documentation, prompt reassessment and revisions to the plan of care, and adherence to a formulary, the wound specialist has the potential to positively impact on staff retention, physician satisfaction, facility reimbursements, infection rates, and patient satisfaction.

Increased Accountability. One benefit of the services of a wound specialist is increased accountability for national guidelines and compliance with regulatory statutes. The Centers for Medicare & Medicaid Services (CMS) and the Joint Commission are clear in their intent to encourage all facilities to adopt evidenced-based pressure ulcer protocols. The surveyor community has a common language that should be used in the medical record when referring to pressure ulcers. For example, CMS recognition and definition of the *avoidable* and *unavoidable* pressure ulcer in long-term care and *Present on Admission (POA)* criteria (see Chapter 8) highlight the need for incorporation of regulatory updates into practice (van Rijswijk and Lyder, 2005). Wound specialists are in a position to implement the requisite pressure ulcer prevention and treatment components. In addition to performing implementation, the wound specialist can facilitate documentation that is clear and appropriate and accurately reflects appropriate prevention, assessment, and treatment of pressure ulcers.

Improved Financial Outcomes. Cost-effectiveness is a significant method for acquiring the administration's support. The costs of caring for a patient with a wound ranges widely across the world, from approximately $3,000 to $30,000 per wound (Gruen, Chang, and Maclellan, 1994). When a major amputation is required,

the cost will increase by a factor of seven because of the need to make home improvements to accommodate a wheelchair (Appelquist et al, 1994). When patients at risk are identified and interventions are put in place before the wound develops or progresses, morbidity and health care costs are decreased (Granick, McGowan, and Long, 1998; Long and Granick, 1998).

The wound specialist has the opportunity and the ability to use resources more efficiently and, in some situations, to generate revenue. Through ongoing continuing education opportunities, the wound specialist can foster state-of-the-art patient care and evidence-based practice by using products that have scientific evidence of their effectiveness. Again, not only do the patients benefit from this expertise, but the facility benefits financially by cutting expenditures. The wound specialist can work with quality improvement team members to identify select aspects of care that can be monitored and tracked over time and thus obtain outcomes data and clinical effectiveness information.

Efficient Use of Resources. The wound specialist must become cognizant of the implications of the efficient use of resources (both materials and personnel). Information on the cost implications of the skin and wound care practice or the cost savings that have been generated must be gathered and specifically communicated routinely to the supervisor. Wound management is costly; in most situations, wound management is more costly than prevention (Lapsley and Vogels, 1996). Effective wound management reduces costs by allowing use of fewer supplies and providing more efficient and effective use of dressings. In addition, cost savings can be realized when preventive interventions are linked to risk level (Richardson, Gardner, and Frantz, 1998). This practice could result in a significant decrease in annual expenditures for materials used. Cost-effectiveness is a positive way of acquiring the support of the nursing administration, which is essential to obtaining institutional support.

The wound specialist should become involved with the establishment of supply contracts in order to sort through the maze of different products and their indications. A successful means of proven cost-effectiveness is limiting the number of similar supplies stocked by the facility. When a formulary for skin and wound care products and support surfaces is created, use of these products can be standardized and simplified. Furthermore, the wound specialist can serve as a resource to materials management, providing clarification on product use. Collaboration with materials management can increase the success of contractual arrangements with manufacturers and increase the facility's ability to maintain compliance with contracts.

Another area with potential for cost savings is standardizing the use of support surfaces. A policy that describes patient indicators for the use of specialty beds should be developed, and compliance with contracts for these specialty beds should be supported. A procedure for "stepping down" from a specialty bed as the patient's condition warrants should be established. In addition, units with a high prevalence of at-risk patient populations might benefit from the implementation of replacement mattresses. Standardizing the products and providing indicators or patient characteristics that guide use of these products can reduce overuse and enhance appropriate use.

Finally, by incorporating appropriate use of skin and wound care products and state-of-the-art wound care, the wound specialist affects the use of personnel. Decreased frequency of dressing changes, expedient access to the correct dressing supplies, and printed directions for dressing changes will reduce staff frustration and time required for wound care.

Revenue Generation. Depending on payer sources, the level of education of the wound specialist, and whether or not the specialist is employed by the institution, the services that are provided may be billable. Working closely with the billing department and fiscal intermediaries may be productive with regard to revenues. Chapter 2 provides specific details about the development of an outpatient clinical practice and reimbursement.

The skin and wound care program, like all departments, must have a means for tracking productivity. A mechanism for documenting visits and referrals can be formulated with the assistance of the billing department. One possible method is a system of "charge codes" for skin and wound care services based on increments of time or services provided. This is an excellent way to track, document, and justify the value of a wound specialist. However, the specialist should avoid providing services that are considered basic nursing care in order to inflate the number of charges. The specialist should not focus solely on the number of patients or charges but rather on the types of patients and services provided. This charging system also may assist with the compilation of workload and time management data for the department. Another consideration is whether the wound specialist's interventions are affecting outcomes.

Depending on payer sources, the services that are provided through the skin and wound care program might be billable. If the services are classified as a therapy rather than a nursing service, the services may be billable. The availability of skin and wound care services may enable the institution to market itself for managed care contracts. This again defines the value of a skin and wound care program. However, inpatient skin and wound care services will seldom, if ever, be a revenue-producing area. Working closely with the billing department and fiscal intermediaries may be productive with regard to revenues.

The value of a skin and wound care program is not limited to just providing care to inpatients. The wound specialist can serve as a link to community and outreach programs and provide education that draws attention to the wound care program and the facility. The wound specialist can provide education within his or her facility in collaboration with colleagues, such as PTs and occupational therapists. Grants to conduct some of these programs may be available from manufacturers. The manufacturers often have established programs that have been approved by licensing boards for continuing education hours, and these programs may be a cost-effective way to provide continuing education to staff. Continuing medical education programs also may be attractive, for example, well-recognized speakers may be invited to conduct an educational session at a dinner program.

When starting the skin and wound care program, the specialist initially may conduct a series of chart audits or a prevalence and incidence study (Chicano and Drolshagen, 2009; Orsted et al, 2009). These activities may provide information that would be helpful in determining whether a certain problem (e.g., pressure ulcers, inadequate documentation) exists. From this information, the continuous improvement process can be initiated with involved departments and personnel so that problems can be discussed and possible solutions identified. As the wound specialist begins an inpatient practice, visibility is essential. Being open to new ideas and opportunities will assist the wound specialist in creating and maintaining a successful program. Maintaining visibility and an alliance with physicians and staff will reinforce the message that the skin and wound care program is an indispensable service.

Staff Retention. A key role of the wound specialist is establishing decision-making tools to expedite and standardize delivery of care. These tools help the staff to develop their comfort level in skin and wound care, facilitate utilization of products, and implement appropriate preventive interventions. Recognition and rewards can be provided for program contributions or accomplishments. Establishing skill competencies in wound care can provide a professional objective that the staff can strive for, again targeting the individual's personal satisfaction.

Critical features of a successful, enduring skin and wound care program are routine and regular operations reports, analysis of clinical practice data, and sharing of these data (Box 1-6). Clinical practice data become the tool by which workload is measured, trends are identified, outcomes are quantified, and the valuable contribution of the wound specialist is recorded and measured. Data collection should be purposeful and outcomes oriented. In fact, data collection and practice improvement are inseparable because improvement requires measurement (Nelson et al, 1998). Clinical practice data should include time management and outcomes reports.

Operations and Outcomes Reports

When cost containment, efficient use of resources, and managed care dominate discussions, information concerning time use is invaluable. This type of data can validate any subjective perception of an increase or change in workload and communicates a strong objective message. Data should be recorded daily and tabulated weekly, monthly, quarterly, and annually. Summary data (e.g., number of patient referrals, number of visits, average length of visits, average number of visits per patient or wound type, reason for referral, number of projects/activities, and time per project) should be submitted to the wound specialist's supervisor on a monthly basis, with trends highlighted. Plots can graphically display time or volume by month. Data collection can be maintained by hand on paper or by computer through one of the many commercially available software packages. Reports can be generated from an electronic medical record system through collaboration with the information technology department. Appendix C contains an example of a simple database created using the Windows Excel program.

Benefits of services to the organization become tangible and coherent when they are phrased in terms of outcomes. Outcomes should include specific patient population outcomes and organizational outcomes. Potential outcomes should be discussed relative to behaviors or physical conditions that can be affected by the wound specialist. For example, an outcome of shortened length of stay in the hospital may not be realistic because many variables impact an individual's length of stay and are not necessarily under the control of the wound specialist. However, the outcome could be rephrased to more precisely define the patient population or type of wound for which length of stay will be decreased. Another outcome could address the control of wound care products. However, in order for this outcome to be feasible, tools that will assist the staff in appropriate product use, such as protocols and a formulary, would be required.

SUMMARY

Establishing a skin and wound care practice in any setting requires the skills of an entrepreneur and a strong foundation in pathophysiology and clinical management. The wound specialist must determine how his or her role will be implemented, how his or her relationship with colleagues will be defined, what quality management processes can be implemented, and what type of data is needed. Data should describe how time is spent and what outcomes are being achieved. The wound specialist must stay current in the art and science of wound management by adopting lifelong learning strategies, such as regularly attending continuing education programs, critically reading journals, and monitoring select websites. The time and energy spent in initial and ongoing practice development are critical to a successful, satisfying, and effective skin and wound care practice.

REFERENCES

Agency for Health Care Policy and Research (AHCPR): *Assessing the quality of Internet health information,* 1999, available at http://www.AHRQ.Gov/Data/Infoqual.htm, accessed July 6, 2009.

Allman RM et al: Pressure ulcer risk factors among hospitalized patients with activity limitation, *JAMA* 273(11):865, 1995.

Andriessen AE, Polignano R, Abel M: Development and implementation of a clinical pathway to improve venous leg ulcer treatment, *Wounds* 21(5):127, 2009.

Appelquist J et al: Diabetic foot ulcers in a multidisciplinary setting. An economic analysis of primary healing and healing with amputation, *J Intern Med* 235:463, 1994.

Aronovitch S: Intraoperatively acquired pressure ulcer prevalence: a national study, *J Wound Ostomy Continence Nurs* 26(3):130, 1999.

Beitz JM, Fey J, O'Brien D: Perceived need for education vs actual knowledge of pressure ulcer care in a hospital nursing staff, *Dermatol Nurs* 11(2):125, 1999.

Bonham P: The role of Wound, Ostomy and Continence (WOC) specialty nurses in managing complex cases, *The Remington Report* 17:10, 2009.

Callihan D: Simplifying the process of research review for the novice researcher. *J Wound Ostomy Continence Nurs* 35(1):30, 2008.

Cary AH: Certified registered nurses: results of the Study of the Certified Workforce, *Am J Nurs* 101(1):44, 2001.

Chicano SG, Drolshagen C: Reducing hospital-acquired pressure ulcers, *J Wound Ostomy Continence Nurs* 36(1):45, 2009.

Collins S et al: Finding the evidence. In DiCenso A, Guyatt G, Chiliska D, editors: *Evidence-based nursing: a guide to clinical practice,* Philadelphia, 2005, Mosby.

Cullum N, Guyatt G: Health care interventions and harm: an introduction. In DiCenso A, Guyatt G, Chiliska D, editors: *Evidence-based nursing: a guide to clinical practice,* Philadelphia, 2005, Mosby.

Cummings GG, Mallidou AA, Scott-Findlay S: Does the workplace influence nurses' use of research? *J Wound Ostomy Continence Nurs* 31(3):106, 2004.

DiCenso A, Ciliska D, Guyatt G: Introduction to evidence-based nursing. In DiCenso A, Guyatt G, Chiliska D, editors: *Evidence-based nursing: a guide to clinical practice,* Philadelphia, 2005, Mosby.

Dobbins M et al: Changing nursing practice in an organization. In DiCenso A, Guyatt G, Chiliska D, editors: *Evidence-based nursing: a guide to clinical practice,* Philadelphia, 2005, Mosby.

Ehrenberg A, Fraser KD, Gunningberg L: Can decision support improve nurses' use of knowledge? *J Wound Ostomy Continence Nurs* 31(5):256, 2004.

Ferguson L, Milner M, Snelgrove-Clarke E: The role of intermediaries: getting evidence into practice, *J Wound Ostomy Continence Nurs* 31(6):325, 2004.

Fleck C: To certify or not to certify; that is the question, *Today's Wound Clinic,* 2(3):26, 2008.

Golinko MS et al: Wound emergencies: the importance of assessment, documentation, and early treatment using a wound electronic medical record, *Ostomy Wound Manage* 55(5):54, 2009.

Gordis L: *Epidemiology*, Philadelphia, 1996, W.B. Saunders.

Granick MS, McGowan E, Long CD: Outcome assessment of an in-hospital cross-functional wound care team, *Plast Reconstr Surg* 101(5):1243, 1998.

Gray M: Market your certification. Presented at the 2008. WOCN Society 40th Annual Conference, *Marketing the gold standard: educating others about WOCNCB certification,* 2008, available at http://www.wocncb.org/resources/marketing-resources/market-your-certification.php, accessed July 12, 2009.

Grous CA, Reilly NJ, Gift AG: Skin integrity in patients undergoing prolonged operations, *J Wound Ostomy Continence Nurs* 24:86, 1997.

Gruen RL, Chang S, Maclellan DG: The real costs of leg ulcers: a hospital based audit, In *Proceedings of the Australian International Wound Management Conference,* March 1994, Melbourne, Australia.

Harris C, Shannon R: An innovative enterostomal therapy nurse model of community wound care delivery: a retrospective cost-effectiveness analysis, *J Wound Ostomy Continence Nurs* 35(2):169, 2008.

Hess CT: *WOC credentials: a legally defensible process,* WOCNCB, 2005, available at www.wocncb.org/pdf/value_of_certification.pdf, accessed July 13, 2009.

Hiser B et al: Implementing a pressure ulcer prevention program and enhancing the role of the CWOCN impact and outcomes, *Ostomy Wound Manage* 52(2):48, 2006.

Holloway N et al: Evaluating health care information on the Internet. In Fitzpatrick JJ, Montgomery KS, editors: *Internet resources for nurses,* New York, 2000, Springer.

Hopf HW et al: Guidelines for the treatment of arterial insufficiency ulcers, *Wound Repair Regen* 14(6):693, 2006.

Jacksich BB: Pressure ulcer prevalence and prevention of nosocomial development: one hospital's experience, *Ostomy Wound Manage* 43(3):32, 1997.

Kartes SK: A team approach for risk assessment, prevention, and treatment of pressure ulcers in nursing home patients, *J Nurse Care Qual* 10(3):34, 1996.

Kelsey JL et al: *Methods in observational epidemiology,* ed 2, New York, 1996, Oxford University Press.

Kottner J et al: Does the number of raters influence the pressure ulcer prevalence rate? *Appl Nurs Res* 22(1):68, 2009.

Landrum BJ: Marketing innovations to nurses, part 1. How people adopt innovations, *J Wound Ostomy Continence Nurs* 25:194, 1998a.

Landrum BJ: Marketing innovations to nurses, part 2. Marketing's role in the adoption of innovations, *J Wound Ostomy Continence Nurs* 25:227, 1998b.

Lapsley HM, Vogels R: Cost and prevention of pressure ulcers in an acute teaching hospital, *Int J Qual Health Care* 8(1):61, 1996.

Lloyd-Vossen J: Implementing wound care guidelines: observations and recommendations from the bedside, *Ostomy Wound Management* 55(6):50, 2009.

Long C, Granick M: A multidisciplinary approach to wound care in the hospitalized patient, *Clin Plast Surg* 25(3):425, 1998.

McIsaac C: Closing the gap between evidence and action: How outcome measurement informs the implementation of evidence-based wound care practice in home care, *Wounds* 19(11):299, 2007.

Milne CT et al: Reducing pressure ulcer prevalence rates in the long-term acute care setting, *Ostomy Wound Manage* 55(4):50, 2009.

Nelson EC et al: Building measurement and data collection in to medical practice, *Ann Intern Med* 128:460, 1998.

Orsted HL, Rosenthal S, Woodbury MG: Pressure ulcer awareness and prevention program: A quality improvement program through the Canadian association of wound care, *J Wound Ostomy Continence Nurs* 36(2):178-183, 2009.

Pasek TA et al: Skin care team in the pediatric intensive care unit: a model for excellence, *Crit Care Nurse* 28(2):125, 2008.

Richardson GM, Gardner S, Frantz RA: Nursing assessment: impact on type and cost of interventions to prevent pressure ulcer, *J Wound Ostomy Continence Nurs* 25(6):273, 1998.

Robson MC et al: Guidelines for the treatment of venous ulcers, *Wound Repair Regen* 14(6):649, 2006.

Rogers EM: *Diffusion of innovations,* ed 4, New York, 1995, Free Press.

Sackett DL et al: *Evidence-based medicine: how to practice and teach EBM,* London, 2000, Churchill Livingstone.

Steed DL et al: Guidelines for the treatment of diabetic ulcers, *Wound Repair Regen* 14(6):680, 2006.

Streed SA, Loehne HB: Preventing infections to improve wound care outcomes: an epidemiological approach, *Wounds* 19(11):320, 2007.

van Rijswijk L, Lyder CH:. Pressure ulcer prevention and care: implementing the revised guidance to surveyors for long-term care facilities, *Ostomy Wound Manage* 51(4 Suppl):7, 2005.

Webb JJ: Nursing research and evidence-based practice. In Cherry B, Jacob SR, editors: *Contemporary nursing: issues, trends, & management,* ed 4, St. Louis, 2008, Mosby.

Whitney J et al: Guidelines for the treatment of pressure ulcers, *Wound Repair Regen* 14(6):663, 2006.

Woods DK: Realizing your marketing influence, part 3: professional certification as a marketing tool, *J Nurs Admin* 32(7-8):379, 2002.

Wound, Ostomy and Continence Nurses Society (WOCN): *Guideline for management of patients with lower extremity arterial disease, WOCN clinical practice guideline series #1,* Glenview, IL, 2002, Author.

Wound, Ostomy and Continence Nurses Society (WOCN): *Guideline for management of pressure ulcers, WOCN clinical practice guideline series #2,* Glenview, IL, 2003, Author.

Wound, Ostomy and Continence Nurses Society (WOCN): *Guideline for management of patients with lower extremity neuropathic disease, WOCN clinical practice guideline series #1,* Glenview IL, 2004a, Author.

Wound, Ostomy and Continence Nurses Society (WOCN): *Prevalence and incidence: a toolkit for clinicians, Glenview, IL,* 2004b, Author.

Wound, Ostomy and Continence Nurses Society (WOCN): *Guideline for management of patients with lower extremity venous disease, WOCN clinical practice guideline series #1,* Glenview, IL, 2005a, Author.

Wound, Ostomy and Continence Nurses Society (WOCN): *Guideline for management of pressure ulcers, WOCN clinical practice guideline series #2,* Glenview, IL, 2010, Author.

Wound, Ostomy and Continence Nursing Certification Board (WOCNCB): *WOCNCB comparison of wound certification programs,* 2009, available at www.wocncb.org/become-certified/how_to_choose.pdf, accessed July 12, 2009.

Billing, Reimbursement, and Setting Up a Clinic

Deanna Vargo and Ruth A. Bryant

OBJECTIVES

1. Describe how wound clinics may differ with regard to their management, location, and services offered.
2. List key components of a wound clinic.
3. List documentation that must be in the medical record to meet Medicare and billing requirements.

4. Distinguish among the different Medicare and insurance programs, including how they relate to billing for clinic services.

Patients come to wound care clinics expecting state-of-the art wound care treatments. Many patients have exhausted options for treating their wound prior to arrival at the wound clinic, and they are anticipating rapid healing by people knowledgeable about wound care. In general, outpatient wound clinics treat chronic wounds and difficult-to-heal wounds, including pressure ulcers, venous, arterial, and diabetic wounds, as well as skin disorders and unusual wound types. The common goal of outpatient wound clinics is to improve and standardize wound care while addressing many medical problems and teaching prevention of further wounds. This chapter outlines the essential components of the operation and structure of an outpatient wound clinic and the impact of various regulatory issues and reimbursement requirements.

CREATING THE BUSINESS PLAN

The first step in creating a new clinic is to establish a business plan (Box 2-1). The goal of a business plan is to provide a step-by-step guide to follow when creating a new program or project. A well-constructed business plan is an important tool to use when obtaining administrative support because the plan will enumerate the benefits of the service and summarize existing internal and external competitors. The business plan should include a pro forma or projected operating budget for the next 5 years. Getting started requires consideration of several topics that should be covered in the business plan: local health care environment, referral sources, customers, competitors, regulators, and revenue sources. The business plan

must emphasize the product or service being proposed as well as the marketing plan. A key element of the business plan is often referred to as the *unique service advantage,* which is what this business will do that no other business currently does, or how this new business will do it better than the competition does.

The benefits of a wound care clinic to a hospital or organization are numerous (Box 2-2) and should be outlined in the business plan. A completed sample business plan is available through the Wound Ostomy and Continence Nurses Society's *Professional Practice Manual* (Wound Ostomy and Continence Nurses Society, 2005).

CLINIC MANAGEMENT

Although wound clinics offer similar services, they differ in their management arrangements and structure. Management can be overseen externally by a managed contract or proprietor or they may be self-directed (internal), similar to a physician office. Table 2-1 lists advantages of both types of management. Available resources are a key consideration in determining the type of management needed. Resources include guidelines for care, policies, and forms, materials for staff and patient education, and quality improvement processes. Another essential consideration is access to the staff with expertise in developing these resources. External management often has these resources ready for use. However, such an arrangement could conservatively commit more than half of the wound center revenue to the management contract. Decision-makers should be aware of the type and extent

---

BOX 2-1   Components of a Business Plan

I. Executive Summary
  - Summarizes the entire business plan, giving administration a "quick read": a 1- to 1.5-page overview of the plan summarizing mission, purpose, competitive edge, evidence supporting the need, potential services provided, financial and resource requirements, and benefits including financial and patient outcomes.

II. Present Situation
  - Describes factors and demographic information that support the need for this venture; includes external analysis, competitive analysis, and internal analysis.

III. Goals and Objectives
  - Provides a step-by-step guide as to what has to be done and how; includes realistic time frames.

IV. Product/Service Descriptions
  - Describes the service to be provided and the benefits of that service to the patient, the facility, and the community.

V. Market Analysis/Strategy
  - Identifies customers, competitors, and the service's position in the market.

VI. Critical Success Factors/Key Assumptions
  - Identifies the conditions that must be met to achieve success.

VII. Qualifications
  - Specifies the education, experience, and certification of the staff. What makes this staff or individual so well qualified to care for patients with a wound?

VIII. Financial Projections
  - Articulates a pro forma budget that projects the expected revenues and expenses for 3 to 5 years. A pro forma is an operating budget for the next 3 to 5 years and indicates a break-even point.

IX. Appendix
  - Includes all backup documents that support the data provided in the plan, curricula vitae of the staff, and staff job descriptions.

---

of support that the management company can provide before choosing that company as a partner.

CLINIC STRUCTURE

Structurally, the physical space of a wound clinic can be attached to a hospital (a hospital-*based* clinic or hospital outpatient clinic) or freestanding (clinic

---

BOX 2-2   Benefits of a Wound Clinic to an Organization

- Addresses a significant need in the community
- Provides a competitive edge through a unique offering
- Is a convenient referral source for physicians
- Keeps patient and revenue within the organization
- Allows continuity of care:
  - Decrease in lead time from inpatient to outpatient treatment
  - Patient, medical record, referral are already in the system
  - Patient does not have to search for a clinic

---

without any physical attachment to a hospital). The hospital-based clinic is a portion of a hospital that provides diagnostic, therapeutic, and rehabilitation services to sick or injured persons who do not require hospitalization. When determining the physical location of the clinic, particularly of the hospital-based clinic, it is important to consider ease of patient access to the clinic and ease of parking. Within the clinic space itself, a variety of issues must be considered in the design of the individual treatment rooms, the floor plan, the location of stocked equipment, lighting, and the need for stretcher access or lounge chair space (Checklist 2-1). Consultation with qualified individuals early in the planning to assist with these unique clinic space issues may be beneficial.

Billing Differences

The billing of clinic services is one of the consistent differentiations between the hospital-based clinic and the freestanding clinic. At a hospital-based clinic, services billed to Medicare or Medicaid patients will be reimbursed at the Medicare facility rate (facility submits a facility rate for the overhead cost and physician submits a separate bill for professional services). At a freestanding clinic, services billed to Medicare or Medicaid patients will be reimbursed at the Medicare nonfacility rate (a higher reimbursed dollar amount compared to the facility rate because the overhead cost is not billed separately).

Additional Means of Financial Viability

The survival of any wound clinic will depend upon more than desire and quality outcomes. No wound center can continue to provide care unless the costs of providing care are covered. Wound care is a volume business, that is, the center must see a certain number of patients in order to create a positive cash flow. The bottom line number of patients who must be seen will depend on the center's overhead: salaries, rent, utilities, cost of supplies, and other expenses. Financial success is difficult to attain if professional charges are the sole source of income, such as with the freestanding clinic.

A hospital-based clinic can offer additional referrals to the hospital for laboratory, radiology, nuclear medicine, magnetic resonance imaging, arteriogram, and surgical procedures and even for admissions, all of which add to the clinic's financial viability. The clinic should record these referrals and communicate to administrators in regular reports to reinforce the financial contributions of the wound center (Trendwell, 2007). Hospital outpatient clinics have the ability to obtain the facility fee for services provided by charging the facility rate when procedures are performed; this will assist in capturing some of the overhead.

TABLE 2-1	Advantages of External versus Internal Clinic Management
External (Outside) Management	**Internal (Self-directed) Management**
Policy and documentation forms already developed	Able to create policy and forms that flow with current hospital tools already in place
Education and resources available via managed company	Establish and seek education via both national and local conferences based on clinic focus
Able to compare productivity and outcome numbers with other management facility to gauge quality outcomes	Quality care program based on internal data or nationally available data
Established evidence-based pathway provided	Create clinic pathway to fit patient population and current hospital protocols using available evidence-based resources
Decisions and goals made at the corporate level and can be implemented with corporate support	Decisions and goals made at local level with flexibility to respond based on internal assessment and preferences
Audits by oversight to determine compliance, alert to national changes	Verify changes to payment rate, make local coverage determinations at least quarterly, make policy/form changes as prompted from data to fit local changes
Database system to assist with reports and documentation	If database desired, may choose from many available for reports and documentation; this option may offer benchmarking with other sites for outcome comparisons
Potential for faster startup/growth due to already created tool and knowledge	Potential to add services other than wound care if clinic desires (e.g., nail care, ostomy clinic, lymphedema, continence clinic)
Staffing needs determined by job descriptions	Less outgoing expense, increased clinic revenue potential

In contrast, the freestanding clinic needs to increase financial stability by performing supplementary procedures in the center. Vascular evaluations with Doppler, transcutaneous oxygen pressure (TcPO2) studies, and measurements of ankle-brachial index (ABI) can generate charges for the center and enhance the bottom line. Clinics may choose to provide outpatient intravenous antibiotic therapy, ostomy care/education, lymphedema therapy, or foot and nail services, allowing patients to come to a familiar location for multiple services. In turn, these visits provide the staff with an opportunity to keep a close eye on the patient's wound while offering one-stop convenience to the patient.

CLINIC OPERATIONS

Numerous operations-related issues must be addressed: regulatory compliance, consents, infection control, national guidelines, laboratory and radiology needs, staff education, documentation, billing guidelines, and much more. Many of these issues are common to all outpatient clinics regardless of their location.

Hours of Operation and Scheduling

Hours of operation need to accommodate the population served and be compatible with staff availability and support services, such as transportation, laboratory, and radiology departments. The schedule should include time allocated for follow-up communication, emergency visits, staff education and meetings, quality reviews, and audits.

Special scheduling considerations include a longer time slot for new patients and anticipated procedures, teaching sessions, and review of test results. As the clinic volume grows, it will be prudent to establish predetermined time slots for these types of visits. A communication process should be established so that the scheduling staff is aware of these special needs. This can be accomplished with a notation on the medical record or on the scheduling book to remind scheduling staff to consider this information prior to scheduling the appointment.

Another consideration for scheduling is staff and skill mix needs. For example, a plastic surgeon with many immobile individuals may require higher numbers of staff to help position and hold patients versus a podiatry clinic, where the majority of patients can self-ambulate and remove/replace their shoes.

Chart Preparation and Storage

Prior to the appointment, the clerical staff should prepare the chart with necessary forms and verification of insurance authorization. New and returning patient visits require different paperwork. New patients will need to provide a history and sign consent forms and the documentation forms necessary for return visits. Locked file storage within the clinic will be necessary, with potential for offsite storage if space is limited. However, it is important to consider how accessible these charts will be if a request is made to retrieve these records. A master list for storage boxes should be maintained to assist with retrieval, sign-out, and replacement.

CHECKLIST 2-1
Clinic Space and Supply Needs

Space-Related
- ✓ Individual treatment rooms with sinks
- ✓ Adequate front office space
- ✓ Offices
- ✓ Waiting area (include bariatric friendly furniture)
- ✓ Clinic workspace
- ✓ Dictation area
- ✓ Storage areas
- ✓ Clean and dirty utility rooms

Hyperbaric-Related (If Applicable)
- ✓ Patient changing rooms
- ✓ Oxygen supply
- ✓ Fire safety
- ✓ Floor weight loading with consideration to wax on floor and types of lights in ceiling

Nail Care-Related (If Applicable) (see Chapter 15)

Debridement-Related
- ✓ Forceps (toothed and/or smooth)
- ✓ Scalpels with blade (no. 10, 11, 15)
- ✓ Clamps or hemostats
- ✓ Curettes of several sizes
- ✓ Scissors or tissue nippers (various types: bandage removal, sharp for cutting tissue or dressings)
- ✓ Rongeurs
- ✓ Punch biopsy
- ✓ Sterile drapes
- ✓ Dressings

Wound Management-Related
- ✓ Normal saline
- ✓ Dressings
- ✓ Tube stabilizers
- ✓ Ostomy and wound pouches
- ✓ Wound measuring guides
- ✓ Camera
- ✓ Monofilaments
- ✓ Doppler
- ✓ Pulsate lavage supplies/ Non Contact Low Frequency Ultrasound (if applicable)
- ✓ Durable equipment that accommodates bariatric and spinal cord-injured population
- ✓ Transfer devices (e.g., hover mat, Hoyer lift)
- ✓ Examination tables and chairs
- ✓ Offloading overlay surface
- ✓ Scales
- ✓ Full range of blood pressure cuff sizes

Lists specify items other than routine examination room-related supplies, such as gloves, gowns, masks, and drapes.

Obtaining Consents

Preprinted consent forms (treatment, photography, surgical/biopsy) should be available and signed prior to the visit. Consents can be mailed or faxed to the appropriate authority prior to the appointment to prevent delay in treatment when the patient is unable to sign independently. A protocol for the frequency of renewing consents should be established. Some facility registration cycles require monthly consents with each new registration; others refer to this as a reoccurring series and require annual updates if the patient has continued uninterrupted visits during the course of treatment. All consents should be maintained in the legal chart.

Compliance Program

With the numerous rules and regulations existing today that ultimately impact on quality of care, reputation, and payment for services, most organizations have a compliance program to oversee both corporate and regulatory issues. The objective of a compliance program is to identify potential sources of risk and implement policy and process modifications to reduce risk (Hess, 2008). Corporate compliance addresses employee behaviors and ethical issues in an attempt to protect the corporation from criminal and civil liability. This is accomplished through corporate-sponsored training activities on topics such as code of conduct (e.g., sexual harassment, interaction with vendors, ethics, publication, involvement with media), grievance without retribution procedures, and disciplinary processes.

Regulatory issues are dictated by whether the clinic is freestanding or hospital based. Most hospital-based clinics are included in annual hospital audits/surveys and are required to follow standard hospital policies; freestanding clinics may not have the same requirements. During the planning process, regulatory requirements within the geographical area need to be addressed as established by The Joint Commission, the Department of Health, and the Certificate of Need (Fusaro et al, 2008). Compliance with National Patient Safety Goals (including patient identification, appropriate hand-off communication, and medication safety) and with coding and billing guidelines is essential to the financial health of a clinic. Coding experts should be used in setting up the "charge master" (clinic billing charges linking codes and dollar amounts), training staff in coding visits and procedures, and ensuring accurate documentation that reflects compliance and maximizes payment.

The clinic staff should be familiar with and in compliance with the Health Insurance Portability and Accountability Act of 1996 (HIPAA) privacy rule. HIPAA was enacted for many reasons, including improving the portability and continuity of health insurance coverage and combating waste, fraud, and abuse in health insurance and delivery of health care (US Department Health and Human Services, 2009). The HIPAA privacy rule also established national standards to protect the privacy of a patient's health information from health plans, health care clearinghouses, and most health care providers. Further information and guidance on implementing the HIPAA privacy rule are available on the websites listed in Table 2-2.

TABLE 2-2	Website Addresses Relevant to Clinic Function, Structure, and Operations
Information Available	**Website Url**
Directory and information	http://www.cms.hhs.gov
Guidance on HIPAA privacy rules and teaching materials	http://www.hhs.gov/ocr/privacy/hipaa/understanding/index.html
Local information regarding coverage	http://www.cms.hhs.gov/mcd/search.asp?from2=search.asp&
Fee schedules	http://www.cms.hhs.gov/FeeScheduleGenInfo/
CPT codes	http://www.cms.hhs.gov/PFSlookup/02_PFSSearch.asp#TopOfPage
Directory of fiscal intermediaries and intermediary carriers	http://www.cms.hhs.gov/apps/contacts/incardir.asp
Most current information regarding Medicare contractors	http://www.cms.hhs.gov/MedicareContractingReform
Medicare Coverage Database with current NCDs and draft and final LCDs	http://www.cms.gov/mcd/overview.asp
NCCI edits	http://www.cms.hhs.gov/NationalCorrectCodInitEd/NCCIEHOPPS/list.asp#TopOfPage http://www.cms.hhs.gov/NationalCorrectCodInitEd/01_overview.asp#TopOfPage

CPT, Current Procedural Terminology; *HIPAA,* Health Insurance Portability and Accountability Act of 1996; *LCD,* local coverage determination; *NCCI,* National Correct Coding Initiative; *NCD,* national coverage determination.

Insurance Authorization. Generally, Medicare policy requires providers to update beneficiary payer information for every admission, outpatient encounter, or start of care prior to submitting a bill to Medicare. The provider should retain a copy of the completed questionnaire on file or online for audit purposes. It is prudent for providers to retain these records. When a provider believes Medicare may not cover his or her services as medically reasonable and necessary, the provider should give the patient an acceptable Advance Beneficiary Notice (ABN); otherwise, the provider generally cannot hold the patient liable if Medicare denies payment. Managed care contracts and some group health care plans may require prior authorization for care at the wound clinic. Authorizations may come open-ended or may have restricted time frames and visit numbers. A tracking system needs to be created so that staff is alerted when reauthorization is required.

Some wound treatment orders require authorization prior to implementation (e.g., biologic skin grafts, negative pressure wound treatments, noncontact low-frequency ultrasound); therefore the provider and staff should be aware of these requirements to prevent loss of reimbursement. In addition, the office staff should verify that the physician or nonphysician provider is covered by the insurance plan.

Treatment Orders. Nonphysician-driven clinics may require a written physician's order to treat the patient. A copy of this order must remain in the patient's record. In most wound clinics when a physician is present to see the patient at each visit, a physician referral or a prior physician order to treat is not required. The office staff should be familiar with this requirement so that they can obtain the necessary authorization.

Documentation. Payment sources mandate appropriate documentation of the care provided. However, documentation alone will not guarantee reimbursement. To ensure optimal payment and compliance, documentation must meet the following criteria:

- Appropriate and accurate diagnoses are documented by clinic staff and physician treating the patient.
- The exact anatomic locations of all wounds treated are denoted, including specific and consistent measurements.
- Clinic and physician documentation support each other.
- Physician documentation is present, supports the necessity of treatment, and is linked to the diagnosis code (Fife and Weir, 2007).
- Treatments including the dressing specifics are recorded. Many treatment modalities and dressings (e.g., dermal substitutes, negative pressure wound therapy, debridement) are reimbursed based on the size of the affected area (Sullivan, 2007).

Additional documentation needed to complete the clinic chart is listed in Table 2-3. Documentation requirements are extensive. Compliance is easier to ensure by using checklists or template electronic documentation systems, which will prompt staff to include all necessary data, rather than handwritten notes. Appendix B provides numerous examples of clinic documentation forms.

Debridement. Wound debridement is an integral part of the day-to-day care provided in wound clinics. As required by Medicare, documentation of debridement must communicate exactly what was done and why specifically: type of tissue removed, depth of removal, instrument used (type of instrument, dressing, drug), wound size, condition of wound/bleeding stopped, and how the wound was redressed after debridement (Fife, 2007). A clear picture must be presented given the Office of the Inspector General (OIG) report revealing that 64% of claims for debridement did not meet Medicare requirements (OIG, 2007). Chapter 17 provides critical information related to debridement.

Contractor or Payer Audits. Occasionally the contractor or payer will request that the wound clinic or

TABLE 2-3	Items in an Outpatient Clinic Chart
Comprehensive admission assessment	Patient's name, gender, race, ethnicity, primary language spoken, address, phone number, date of birth, height/weight, name and phone of any legally authorized representative, past and present diagnoses, wound history, reason for visit, barriers to care, allergies, current mediations, advanced directive, family history
Wound assessment, compliance/teaching record	Vital signs, any medicine changes, procedure or hospitalizations since last visit, reason for visit, complete wound description and photography (if applicable); compliance to treatment plan, pain, any teaching reviewed at visit and response to teaching, treatment applied prior to discharge, vascular assessment if lower extremity wounds
Physician progress notes	Reason for visit and relevant history, physician examination findings and prior diagnostic test results, assessment, clinical impression or diagnosis, plan of care, rationale for ordering any test, patient's progress and response to changes in treatment plan; codes reported on billing statement should be supported in the documentation; any consult advice provided or received acknowledges as reviewed
Discharge orders	Any new test or medications ordered, wound treatment orders, next follow-up appointment or consult appointment, compression or offloading directions
Acuity	Used by hospital-based clinic if no procedure was completed to bill evaluation and management of services based on facility resources acuity score; all resources considered should be supported in the medical record (consider acuity form a permanent documentation form to prevent charges not documented; use as a documentation and scoring tool)
Billing form	Complete listing of any diagnoses codes or procedure codes used for billing; supporting documentation must be in the medical record
Consents, insurance information, HIPAA documents	Consent for treatment, consent for photography, insurance information or copy of insurance card, HIPAA notification

provider furnish specific documentation demonstrating compliance. Common issues reviewed by auditors include the following:

- Every service billed must be documented because the patient's record must contain clear evidence that the service, procedure, or supply actually was performed or supplied.
- The medical necessity for choosing the procedure, service, or medical supply must be substantiated.
- Every service must be coded correctly. Diagnoses must be coded to the highest level of specificity, and procedure codes must be current.
- Documentation must clearly indicate who performed the procedure or supplied the equipment.
- Legible documentation, which may be dictated and transcribed, is required. Existing documentation may not be embellished; however, additional documentation that supports a claim may be submitted.
- Voluntary disclosure of information by the provider is encouraged. When an error is discovered, any overpayment should be returned to Medicare (Centers for Medicare & Medicaid Services, 2004).

Checklist 2-2 lists examples of typical documentation that the contractor may request from the clinic.

Clinic Composition: Staffing with a Multidisciplinary Team

A wound outpatient clinic requires a variety of individuals and professionals and an extensive referral network. All staff will require some level of education about the types of patients the clinic will see and the range of the patients' physical needs. The education should be tailored to each employee's job and role expectations so that all staff members are best prepared to fulfill their roles.

Because wound etiology often is multidimensional, the solution often requires a multidisciplinary team approach, which in turn requires coordination among many areas. Many clinics are considered multidisciplinary, referring to the variety of physician provider specialties available as well as the range of the staff assisting with patient care. Other clinics may be nurse (Certified Wound, Ostomy, Continence Nurse [CWOCN], Certified Wound Care Nurse [CWCN]) or physical therapy (physical therapist [PT], certified wound specialist [CWS]) driven

CHECKLIST 2-2
Typical Documentation Items Requested by Audit Contractor or Payer

- ✓ Office records (progress notes, current history and physical, treatment plan)
- ✓ Documentation of identity and professional status of clinician
- ✓ Laboratory and radiology reports
- ✓ Comprehensive problem list
- ✓ Current list of prescribed medications
- ✓ Progress notes for each visit indicating patient's response to prescribed treatment
- ✓ Documentation supporting time spent with patient when time-based codes are used
- ✓ Required referrals or prescriptions (for many nonphysician services/supplies)
- ✓ Required Certificates of Medical Necessity

and work off physician orders and/or treatment plans. The patient must obtain a referral to an outside multidisciplinary specialist from the primary care provider. Table 2-4 lists the variety of health care professionals who should be available, some on site and some with part-time schedules or as consultants, to a wound clinic. In general, the wound clinic staff and their responsibilities will primarily be dictated by the types of wound patients who attend the clinic, the patients' wound care needs, and the regulating bodies of the various disciplines involved.

Communication with the primary care provider is essential for maintaining collegial relationships; physicians want to trust that the patient will be returned to the primary physician's care after healing. Thorough and frequent communication between the wound center and the referring physician cannot be overemphasized, regardless of the clinic structure.

Medical Director. The medical director of the clinic is extremely relevant to the success of the clinic in that he or she can influence physician colleagues and potential referral sources. The medical director of the clinic may be a generalist or specialist but should also bring some degree of knowledge specific to wound care. Communication skills, organizational skills, and the ability to be a team player are key attributes of the wound clinic medical director. The medical director's responsibilities can be divided into clinical and administrative issues. The

extent to which the medical director is involved in these issues on a day-to-day basis will depend upon the type of clinic structure. For some clinics, the medical director serves as a resource for the wound specialist in the clinic and oversees policies developed by the wound specialist. In other clinic settings, the medical director works closely with the wound specialist, seeing patients, making policy decisions, coordinating research studies, and overseeing outcomes, data collection, and analysis. Representation of the hospital-based outpatient wound clinic to relevant hospital medical committees may be instrumental in increasing the existence of wound care services and can be a responsibility the medical director shares with the wound specialist and/or clinic director.

Clinic Director. The clinic director provides administrative oversight of the clinic, including staffing, scheduling, materials management, staff preparation/education, regulatory compliance, and profitability. The clinic director may a certified wound care specialist. Routine and frequent contact of the clinic director with insurance, billing, and coding personnel will facilitate early identification of any problems in reimbursement or documentation so that corrective steps can be taken promptly. The clinic director also focuses on representing the clinic within nursing administrative structures. The clinic director can use educational outreach programs to become acquainted with possible referral sources, such as home health care agencies, nursing homes, physician offices, urgent care centers, and emergency rooms.

Certified Wound Specialist. At least one member of the wound clinic should be certified in wound care by an independent national certification organization that validates specialty knowledge, experience, and clinical judgment. The value and contributions of a certified wound specialist are described in detail in Chapter 1. The primary roles of the wound care specialist in the outpatient clinic are expert clinician and consultant. The wound specialist collaborates with the medical director in overseeing the holistic care of patients and their wounds. The wound care specialist creates policies and procedures to facilitate the standardization of care and delivery of evidence-based care. The wound care nurse, either alone or in collaboration with the clinic director, may be responsible for establishing referral networks with home care, durable equipment providers, etc. Development of staff education as well as resources for patient education is a vital component of the wound specialist's role so that staff are well prepared and reliable. The wound specialist establishes and monitors competencies in assessment, basic wound dressing change technique, and care. The wound care specialist also works closely with the physician in monitoring and tracking patients' progress and outcomes. When the wound specialist is also an advanced practice nurse (APN), the clinic benefits from the APN's broader base of knowledge as well as the APN's ability to bill for charges. When the wound specialist is a wound, ostomy,

TABLE 2-4	Wound Clinic Multidisciplinary Team Members	
Position	Onsite	Available as Consultant
Medical director	X	
General surgeon		X
Peripheral vascular surgeon		X
Orthopedic surgeon		X
Dermatologist		X
Reconstructive surgeon		X
Podiatry		X
Infectious disease		X
Geriatrician		X
Occupational therapist		X
Certified wound care nurse (CWCN, CWOCN, CWON)	X	
Registered nurse	X	
Physical therapist (may be certified wound specialist)	X	
Medical or surgical assistant	X	
Office staff (e.g., receptionist)	X	
Diabetes educator	X	
Dietitian	X	
Billing/coder	X	

and continence (WOC) nurse, patients benefit from the APN's additional expertise related to skin and wound care associated with tube site, incontinence, ostomy, and complex fistula management.

Nurse Coordinator. The nurse coordinator assists with the daily clinic flow of patients, implement treatments according to policy, and works closely with the wound specialist to promote consistently efficient and effective patient care. The nurse coordinator often interviews the patient, removes dressings, assesses the wound, and consults with the wound specialist in developing a plan, providing patient education, and implementing referrals as needed. Basic competencies in wound care and skin assessment are essential to optimal functioning of the nursing staff in the wound clinic (Morrison, 2007).

Insurance and Billing Coder. The value and expertise of insurance and billing coders cannot be understated. Close collaboration with the coding department will secure optimal regulatory compliance and reimbursement. In addition, insurance coordinators may assist with pre-approvals from various private insurance companies.

Ancillary Staff. Ancillary clinic staff may include schedulers, medical assistants, and surgical assistants, who may work in the clinic and assist with office duties. Ancillary staff should assist with chart preparation, patient registration, placing appointment reminder calls, scheduling tests, and data entry for billing and supplies. Training ancillary staff to work in the clinical area (within their job scope and reporting significant findings to clinic nurses and physicians) and to cover the office allows for flexibility in scheduling during slow clinic times and vacation schedules.

Utilizing the ancillary staff while scrutinizing staffing ratios (nursing hours versus ancillary hours and all hours worked versus patient visits) will assist with monitoring worked hours per patient visit. Closely watching this ratio may show the need to bring on new staff as clinic visits increase, alter staff hours during slower days during the week, and shift staff hours to busier work days.

Referral Network

Outpatient care in large part requires referrals to, and use of, community services: local transportation companies, durable medical equipment (DME) companies, orthotics and prosthetics suppliers, physician offices, home care agencies, laboratories, and radiology and other hospital departments. Everyone in the clinic should be familiar with how to access these resources and the requirements that must be fulfilled in order to complete a referral. This kind of detail when providing care to the clinic patient will convey a sense of calmness and confidence to the patient and facilitate the patient's ability to follow through, which ultimately will enhance outcomes.

Hospital facilities likely have access to onsite laboratory, radiology, vascular laboratory, surgical suite, and emergency rooms. The place or site to which the patient

is referred must always be the patient's choice rather than a mandate that the patient be sent to a particular facility. The insurance company often drives this decision. When referred sites are freestanding, it may be beneficial to have a list of local sites where such tests can be obtained, along with their hours of business, address, and phone number.

DME supplies will be a common need of the wound clinic patient. Most patients are unaware of where to obtain supplies and what products may be equivalent substitutes. Therefore, the patient will need a list of local DME providers as well as mail order companies to facilitate accessing supplies. The patient who has limited mobility cannot easily pick up supplies and will need either free home delivery or mail delivery. Providing patients with written instructions detailing their wound care supplies and the wound care procedure will facilitate continuity in their care. In many situations, wound care orders can be sent directly to the DME.

Clinic Space and Equipment

Equipment needed for the wound clinic is similar to that needed in many routine outpatient clinics; however, additional equipment items unique to the care of the patient with a wound are necessary to provide the patient with efficient care (see Checklist 2-1).

Room Equipment. At a minimum, multipatient rooms should have privacy curtains separating patients. Individual rooms are preferred to facilitate privacy. From an infection control perspective, rooms in which treatments with potential for generating aerosolization are conducted should be separated by walls rather than curtains to prevent the spread of microorganisms. Considering how the patient will arrive may be critical to determining what equipment to place in a room. Carts and large wheelchair transports may be cumbersome when turning corners, so considering this early in the planning phase will be important in deciding needed clinic room space.

The type of clinic room equipment may vary depending on the type of patients expected. Spinal cord injury or reconstructive surgery clinics may require space to accommodate patients arriving on stretchers with pneumatic treatment tables and additional staff or adaptive equipment to assist with transfers. An offloading overlay surface should be added to the examination table to reduce pressure and provide comfort; it also can be used for educational purposes when teaching positioning and hand checks. Examination chairs (e.g., podiatry chairs) are preferable for the ambulatory patient with a lower extremity ulcer. The positioning made available with this type of chair will facilitate patient comfort, allow for better visualization of lower extremity wounds, promote ergonomic movements by the staff, thus reducing their risk of musculoskeletal injury, and maintain a good distance from the floor so that the risk of cross-contamination from microorganisms on the floor is minimized.

A Mayo stand (a stand for treatment supplies with wheels that can be positioned within reach of patient and caregiver) or similar stand for each patient as well as a place for the chart and documentation is necessary. Additional items needed include a stool for the clinician, a visitor chair, and good lighting. Basic equipment includes items such as thermometers, sphygmomanometers, needle boxes, gloves boxes, dirty linen containers, trash cans, and hazardous waste receptacles.

Wound centers may want to purchase a bariatric treatment chair. Many treatment chairs have a weight limit between 275 and 400 pounds; however, a certain patient population will require a treatment chair that can hold between 500 and 800 pounds.

Another important piece of equipment for wound centers is a scale to help monitor (1) nutrition and (2) fluid balance, especially when diuretics are used with compression wraps. Patient safety should be considered when purchasing a scale. A scale with handrails provides a stable base for patients to step onto. A wheelchair scale may be necessary, or one with a weight limit up to 850 pounds.

Wound Care Supplies. A formulary of wound care supplies for the wound clinic will need to be developed. The formulary should be selected with a knowledge of the most common wound needs seen in the clinic and the function of the various dressings. A basic formulary should include transparent dressing, hydrogel, alginate, foam, impregnated gauze strips, nonadhering wrap, hydrocolloid, collagen, compression wrap, and silver-impregnated dressings. The range of products included in the formulary should be kept narrow to reduce the potential for confusion on utilization, ordering, or storage. Due to product expiration times, supplies used less often or for specific procedures (e.g., biologic graft) may need to be special ordered.

Pharmaceuticals (topical anesthetics and topical creams) should be kept locked and made available for minor procedures such as debridement. Medications should not be administered in a nurse-run clinic without a physician's order, unless the nurse is an APN with prescriptive authority. Patients attending a clinic where medications cannot be administered should be encouraged to take a pain medication prior to their visit.

Many wound care visits will require conservative sharp debridement, so appropriate tools should be available. However, no package should be opened (during room setup) in anticipation of debridement; rather, package materials should be opened only after the need for the tools is confirmed. Basic sharp debridement tools can be disposable or resterilized; consider patient volumes when determining the number of tools needed and the time allotment for resterilizing equipment.

Education

Education of patient and staff is a vital component of any wound care program in any setting and is addressed throughout this textbook. In the outpatient setting, documentation of the education and handouts provided and their understanding is important not only in providing quality wound care but also can be used to justify additional clinic visits as well as potential referrals (e.g., psychiatrist, cognitive evaluation, home care). When setting up a clinic, planners should consider the variety of electronic media that can be used and made available to the patient, either in a separately designated "education" room or from a library, from which the patient can access the material, review it at home, and then return it (Armstrong et al, 2008).

Staff education should be mandatory and competency based for a variety of reasons, such as patient safety, appropriate use of resources, improved patient care, standardization of care, and compliance with facility policy; education also can facilitate staff enthusiasm and support for changes (Wallin et al, 2005). Checklist 2-3 provides a listing of competencies to be considered for staff education in a wound clinic.

Policies, Procedures, and Guidelines

As described in Chapter 1, the wound specialist plays a pivotal role in integrating research findings into policies, procedures, and guidelines for the clinic. Evidence-based policies, procedures, and guidelines for care must be readily available to clinic personnel. Familiarity with these documents should be addressed through competency-based staff education programs as already described. See Checklist 2-3 for a list of possible wound clinic policies.

Continuous Quality Improvement Plan

Quality outcome data are necessary to evaluate compliance with evidence-based wound care and progress of the overall treatment plan. The data may be shared with the patient to encourage continued treatment, shared with insurance companies to demonstrate medical necessity, and compared locally or nationally to display the cost benefit of treatment. Although economic factors in wound care are common measures in product evaluation, ultimately the bottom line is efficacy. An inexpensive product that makes up for its low cost with increased clinic visits due to delayed healing time quickly loses its product price advantage; additional costs will be incurred if infection develops (Jacobs and Tomazak, 2008). Healing times in relation to cost is another valuable piece of outcome data. Stratification of data by etiology, providers, and clinic days provides additional information about efficiency, effectiveness, and best practice. Further analysis includes measuring the impact of clinic-based care on the number of home care visits, use of wound care-related medications, acute care readmissions, emergency room visits, number of surgical procedures, limb salvage, and healing times. These data are useful for substantiating best practice and for marketing the clinic.

CHECKLIST 2-3
Examples of Wound Clinic Policies and Competencies

Policies	Competencies
✓ Wound measurement	✓ Wound measurement
✓ Wound photo	✓ Wound photography
✓ Nurse visits/"incident-to" visits	✓ Wound culture
✓ Quality program	✓ Compression wraps
✓ Conservative care designation	✓ Negative pressure dressing
✓ Chart order	✓ Low-frequency ultrasound treatments
✓ Billing guidelines	✓ Skin inspections
✓ Form completion guidelines	✓ Room cleaning between patients
✓ Clinic scheduling	✓ Isolation/infection control
✓ RN case manager responsibilities	✓ Offloading techniques
✓ Insurance authorization process	✓ Ankle-brachial index
	✓ Monofilament/sensory testing
	✓ Conservative sharp debridement
	✓ Chemical cautery with silver nitrate
	✓ Pulsate lavage

RN, Registered nurse.

DESCRIPTION OF PAYMENT SYSTEMS

Successful wound management is a culmination of quality wound care practices and knowledge of coverage and payment polices. Reimbursement is based on what is done and documented at the clinic visit. Knowing the type of insurance and whether authorization is required, keeping track of visits, and knowing whether the patient has Medicare/Medicaid and how this coverage affects billing is essential.

The Centers for Medicare & Medicaid Services (CMS) is responsible for establishing the payment system for Medicare and Medicaid beneficiaries. It pays the majority of the health care dollars in the United States. Billing principles are similar for other insurance types using the billing codes established by the American Medical Association (AMA) known as *diagnosis codes,* also known as International Classification of Diseases, 9th Revision (ICD-9) codes, to support the disease/reason for visit. Acronyms are common in the billing process, and a directory of acronyms related to the billing process is provided in Box 2-3.

Medicare

Title XVIII of the Social Security Act, designated "Health Insurance for the Aged and Disabled," is more commonly known as *Medicare.* The Social Security Amendments of 1965 created a health insurance program for aged persons to complement retirement, survivor, and disability insurance benefits. When first implemented in 1966, Medicare covered most persons aged 65 years and over. In 1973, additions made to Medicare benefits included (1) persons entitled to Social Security or Railroad Retirement disability cash benefits for at least 24 months, (2) most persons with end-stage renal disease, and (3) certain otherwise noncovered aged persons who elected to pay a premium for Medicare coverage.

Medicare traditionally has consisted of two parts: Part A and Part B (Original Medicare). A third part, Part C or the Medicare Advantage program (also known as Medicare + Choice), is available to individuals who qualify for Original Medicare. The drug coverage, known as Medicare Part D, is provided by private health plans; this coverage can be drug only or can be provided through a Medicare Advantage plan that offers comprehensive benefits.

Medicare Part A. Medicare Part A, referred to as "Hospital Insurance," helps cover services and supplies related to inpatient hospital stays. In addition, Part A covers care in a skilled nursing facility (SNF) if the care follows a Medicare Part A–covered 3-day hospital stay. Finally, Part A covers hospice and, in some situations, home health care. When the beneficiary is entitled to Part A benefits, the beneficiary's red, white, and blue Medicare identification card will indicate "Hospital (Part A)."

Medicare Part B. Medicare Part B, commonly known as "Medical Insurance," essentially helps cover doctors' services, certain medical items, and outpatient care when such services are provided under a doctor's care and are documented to be medically necessary. Specifically, clinical laboratory services, some home health care, outpatient hospital services, blood transfusions (after the first three pints), some preventive services, ambulance services (when other transportation would endanger health), and medical social services are provided under Part B. Physical therapy and some home health care furnished by hospitals, SNFs, and other institutional providers likewise are eligible for Part B coverage. When the beneficiary has Part B benefits, the Medicare card will stipulate "Medicare (Part B)." Part B requires payment of a

BOX 2-3	Acronyms Related to Billing and Reimbursement Process

APC: Ambulatory Payment Classification—System used for outpatient services, attached to assigned CPT code for payment

CPT: Current Procedural Terminology—Codes that describe the procedure performed, such as debridement

DME: Durable Medical Equipment—Supplies ordered by physician for use in the home (item must be reusable)

DMERC: Durable Medical Equipment Regional Carrier—Contractor for CMS who provides claims processing and payment for DME

E&M: Evaluation and Management— CPT code used to obtain the fee for the corresponding services provided

FI: Fiscal Intermediary—Contractor for CMS who processes claims for services covered under Medicare

HCPCS: Healthcare Common Procedure Coding System—Uniform method used by providers and suppliers to report professional services, procedures, and supplies (codes describe dressing supply) assigned and maintained by local Medicare contractors

ICD-9: International Classification of Diseases, 9th Revision—National coding method designed to enable providers to effectively document the medical condition, symptom, or complaint that forms the basis for rendering a specific service

LCD: Local Coverage Determination—Formal statement developed through a specifically defined process that defines the service, provides information about when the service is considered reasonable and necessary, outlines any coverage criteria and/or documentation requirements, and provides coding information

Level II HCPCS—Method for obtaining reimbursement for products, supplies, or procedures not covered in the CPT codes

MAC: Medicare Administrative Contractor—A single authority consisting of integrated Fiscal Intermediaries and carriers responsible for the receipt, processing, and payment of Medicare claims. MAC will perform functions related to the beneficiary and provider service, appeals, provider outreach and education, financial management, program evaluation, reimbursement, payment safeguards, and information systems security.

NCCI: National Correct Coding Initiative—Developed to promote correct coding by providers and supplies (to prevent payment for noncovered and/or incorrectly coded services)

NCD: National Coverage Determination—Developed by CMS to describe the circumstances for Medicare coverage for a specific medical service procedure or device

OPPS: Outpatient Prospective Payment System—a prospective payment system (fee schedule) that sets payments for individual services as identified by the HCPCS codes and used for hospital outpatient services, certain Part B services furnished to hospital inpatients who have no Part A coverage, and partial hospitalization services furnished by hospitals and community mental health centers

PPS: Prospective Payment System—Method of reimbursement in which Medicare payment is made based on a predetermined, fixed amount

monthly premium that usually is taken out of the beneficiary's Social Security, Railroad Retirement, or Office of Personnel Management Retirement payment. Otherwise, Medicare will bill for the premium every 3 months. In addition to the premium, the beneficiary must meet an annual deductible and pay all coinsurance amounts unless he or she has other supplemental insurances.

Providers who submit Part B claims should always refer to their carrier's local coverage determinations (LCDs) and other billing guidance for specific coverage and payment criteria. Box 2-4 gives a list of services and supplies covered under Part B, when medically necessary.

Medicare Advantage Plan, Part C. The Medicare Advantage program was established by the Balanced Budget Act of 1997 (BBA). This program consists of a set of options created by the BBA to provide care under contract to Medicare, to possibly reduce the beneficiary's out-of-pocket expenses, and to offer more health care and contractor choices. The Medicare Advantage plan must provide the same services a beneficiary would be eligible to receive from Medicare if he or she were in Original Medicare. However, the beneficiary technically still is "on Medicare" but has selected a different contractor and is required to receive services according to that contractor's arrangements.

Providers, suppliers, and their billing personnel must be aware that Medicare Advantage plans do not operate under the same coverage and payment policy for claims processing as Original Medicare. If a beneficiary is a member of a Medicare Advantage plan, the local Part B carrier cannot process claims for that beneficiary. When claims are submitted the local Medicare Part B carrier will deny payment (except for dialysis services). After the denial, the carrier will automatically transfer the claim to the appropriate Medicare Advantage plan. The medical managed care plan is not responsible for paying Medicare Advantage claims, except when (1) the physician or supplier is affiliated with the Medicare Advantage plan or (2) the physician or supplier furnishes emergency services, urgently needed services, or other

BOX 2-4	Services and Supplies Covered under Medicare Part B, When Medically Necessary

Medical Care and Other Services
- Doctor's services
- Outpatient medical and surgical services and supplies
- Diagnostic examinations and tests
- Ambulatory surgery center facility fees for approved procedures
- DME such as wheelchairs, hospital beds, oxygen, walkers
- Second surgical opinions
- Outpatient mental health care
- Outpatient physical and occupational therapy, including speech/language therapy

Clinical Laboratory Services
- Blood tests
- Urinalysis
- Other tests requested by provider

Home Health Care
- Part-time skilled nursing care
- Physical therapy
- Occupational therapy
- Speech/language therapy
- Home health aide services
- Medical social services
- DME such as wheelchairs, hospital beds, oxygen, walkers
- Medical supplies and other services

Additional Coverage Related to Wound Care
- Ambulance services when other transportation would endanger the patient's health
- Artificial limbs that are prosthetic devices and their replacement parts
- Braces (arm, leg, back, neck)
- Emergency care
- Medical nutrition therapy services for people who have diabetes or kidney disease (unless currently on dialysis), with doctor's referral
- Medical supplies, such as ostomy pouches, surgical dressings, splints, casts, some diabetic supplies
- Second surgical opinion by a doctor (in some cases)
- Services of a practitioner, such as clinical social worker, physician's assistant, nurse practitioner
- Telemedicine services in some rural areas
- Therapeutic shoes for people with diabetes (in some cases)
- X-ray films, magnetic resonance imaging, computed tomographic scanning, electrocardiography, and some other purchased diagnostic tests

DME, Durable medical equipment.

covered services not reasonable available through the Medicare Advantage plan.

A provider may be reimbursed when filing a claim to a Medicare Advantage plan if he or she is an in-network provider. An out-of-network provider may be covered if specific criteria are met as stipulated by the Medicare Advantage plan, such as prior authorization. If the plan denies the claim, the provider has the right to appeal the claim. An out-of-plan provider may also collect the full fee directly from the patient for services provided if the patient did not receive prior authorization. Before rendering services, a provider who is an affiliate with a Medicare Advantage plan should emphasize to his or her patients what their financial liability will be if they did not receive prior authorization to see the out-of-plan provider.

Medicaid

Title XIX of the Social Security Act is a federal/state entitlement program that pays for medical assistance for certain individuals and families with low incomes and resources. The program, known as Medicaid, became law in 1965 as a cooperative venture jointly funded by the federal and state governments for furnishing medical assistance to eligible needy persons. Medicaid is the largest source of funding of medical and health-related services for America's poorest individuals.

Each state (1) establishes its own eligibility standards; (2) determines the type, amount, duration, and scope of services; (3) sets the rate of payment for services; and (4) administers its own program. Medicaid eligibility and/or services within a state can change during the year.

Medicare beneficiaries who have low incomes and limited resources may also receive help from the Medicaid program. For persons who are eligible for full Medicaid coverage, Medicare health care coverage is supplemented by services that are available under their state's Medicaid program, according to eligibility category. For persons enrolled in both programs, any services that are covered by Medicare are paid for by the Medicare program before any payments are made by the Medicaid program, as Medicaid is always the "payer of last resort."

Group Health Plans, Medicare Secondary Payer Program, and Medicare Coordination of Benefits

Until 1980 Medicare was the primary payer in all situations except those involving Workers' Compensation (WC). Since 1980, changes in the Medicare law have resulted in Medicare being the secondary payer in situations. The Medicare Secondary Payer (MSP) program protects Medicare funds and ensures that Medicare does not pay for services reimbursable under private insurance plans or other government programs.

The MSP program precludes Medicare from making primary claims payment when a beneficiary has other insurance that should pay first. If a beneficiary is covered by a group health plan as a benefit of current employment, charges for medical services must first be submitted to the group health plan (Centers for Medicare & Medicaid Services, 2004).

The Medicare Coordination of Benefits (COB) program works to identify health care coverage that beneficiaries may have that pays primary to Medicare and to coordinate the payment process to prevent mistaken Medicare primary payments. Although the various insurance programs may set separate guidelines, they generally follow similar guidelines as established by the Medicare and/or Medicare Advantage Programs. Verification monthly for services and specific procedures may be necessary to gather payment.

Medigap (Supplemental Insurance)

A Medigap policy is a health insurance policy sold by private insurance companies to fill "gaps" in the Original Medicare plan. The Medigap policy must clearly identify it as "Medicare Supplemental Insurance."

FACTORS THAT INFLUENCE PROVIDER REIMBURSEMENT

When implemented in 1966, Medicare was a fee-for-service insurance plan. Part B providers were paid on a reasonable charge basis for most services. Since then Congress has mandated several changes to the Medicare reimbursement models that vary depending on the care setting and services provided. Today most payments are based on federally established predetermined payments per procedure or item rather than randomly created clinic or hospital fees. Several factors influence the amount of payment the provider is reimbursed: the care setting, the payer or payment plan, and the type of provider.

Care Setting: Nonfacility/Freestanding Sites (Part B)

Part B providers include physicians, nurse practitioners, physical therapists in private practice, and suppliers of durable medical equipment, prosthetics, orthotics, or supplies (DMEPOS). A Part B provider will always accept assignment on claims submitted on behalf of the Medicare beneficiary. When a Part B provider accepts assignment, the Part B provider agrees to bill the beneficiary only for any coinsurance or deductible that may be applicable and accepts the Medicare payment as full payment.

Physician services are paid by the carrier based on the Medicare Physician's Fee Schedule (MPFS). A fee schedule is a complete listing of fees used by Medicare to pay doctors or other providers/suppliers. This comprehensive listing of "fee maximums" is used to reimburse a physician and/or other providers on a fee-for-service basis. CMS develops fee schedules for physicians, ambulance services, clinical laboratory services, and DMEPOS. These fee schedules are used with the nonfacility rate when services are provided in a standard office setting/nonfacility site.

Care Setting: Hospital Outpatient Facility Settings (Part B)

Reimbursement is limited to a facility fee rate when services are performed in one of the following settings: (1) an inpatient or outpatient hospital setting, (2) a hospital emergency room, (3) an SNF, (4) a comprehensive inpatient or outpatient rehabilitation facility, (5) an inpatient psychiatric facility, or (6) an ambulatory surgical center (ASC). Medicare pays less for services provided in these settings because Medicare assumes the physician's overhead and other related expenses are lower than they would have been in a standard office setting. Physicians are not allowed to bill the beneficiary for the difference. The fee schedule is updated annually on January 1 and available online (Table 2-2).

Care Setting: Hospital-based Clinic (Part A)

Part A providers include comprehensive outpatient rehabilitation facilities (CORFs); end-stage renal disease (ESRD) facilities; home health agencies (HHAs), including hospital subunits; hospitals (including freestanding facilities or units of a medical complex, such as critical access hospitals [CAHs]); and outpatient rehabilitation facilities (ORFs).

Today most Part A providers, including hospitals, SNFs, and HHAs, receive payments through a prospective payment system (PPS), which is designed to cover the costs of all items and services furnished to beneficiaries while they are under the care of that facility. PPS is a method of reimbursement in which Medicare payment is made based on a predetermined, fixed amount. The payment amount for a particular service is derived based on the classification system of that service (e.g., diagnosis-related groups [DRGs] for inpatient hospital services and ambulatory payment classifications [APCs] for outpatient services).

Many items and services that once were billable now are covered under the "Consolidated Billing" provisions of the Part A PPS system. Under this coverage, many dressing supplies and services (e.g., physical therapy) must be billed by the facility even if the services were furnished by a Part B provider (in which the payment would generally fall within the PPS). Part B suppliers should contact their local carrier to learn what "Consolidated Billing" provisions may apply to their provider type or services they furnish.

All services paid under the new PPS to the outpatient clinic are classified into APCs. Services in each APC are similar clinically in terms of the resources they require. A payment rate is established for each APC. Depending on the services provided, hospital clinics may be paid for more than one APC per encounter. The APC codes are attached to the assigned Current Procedural Terminology (CPT) code as further described in the Procedure Codes (CPT) section and in Table 2-5.

Medicare Managed Care Plan

A beneficiary can select a managed care plan to provide Medicare services. CMS will pay a fixed amount (i.e., a capitated rate) to the managed care plan selected by the beneficiary. CMS pays the plan, which then reimburses the provider for services. However, enrollment as a Part B provider does not ensure payment from a Medicare managed care plan. Provider reimbursement in a managed care plan is based solely upon the terms of the provider's agreement with the plan, regardless of the amount Medicare pays for the services.

Nonphysician Practitioners and Incident-to Services

Medicare allows payment for services furnished by nonphysician practitioners, which include APNs (e.g., nurse practitioner, clinical nurse specialist, nurse anesthetist) and physician's assistants (PAs). Therapeutic services and supplies that a hospital provides on an outpatient basis that are incident to the services of the physician are referred to as *incident-to services*. To be covered as incident-to-physician's services, the services and supplies must be furnished by the hospital and must be an integral, although incidental, part of the physician's professional service in the course of treatment. The services must be furnished under the order of a physician or other practitioner and under the direct supervision of a physician. "Direct supervision" means the physician must be present and on the premises of the location (the provider-based department of the hospital) and immediately available to furnish assistance and direction throughout the performance of the procedure. It does not mean that the physician must be present in the room when the procedure is performed (Vargo, 2009). A hospital service or supply would not be considered incident to a physician's service if the attending physician merely wrote an order for the services or supplies and referred the patient to the hospital without being involved in the management of that course of treatment (Centers for Medicare & Medicaid Services, 2009). During any course of treatment rendered by the nonphysician practitioner, the physician must personally see the patient periodically and sufficiently often to assess the course of treatment and the patient's progress and, where necessary, to change the treatment regimen.

In general, Medicare requires that practices bill services under the provider number of the individual clinician performing the service. However, Medicare rules allow "incident-to" billing (i.e., submitting bills under a physician's provider number for services provided by a supervised employee). For services billed as "incident to," practices may be reimbursed at 100% of

TABLE 2-5	Types of Codes Necessary for Provider Billing		
Code	Description	Caveat	Example
ICD-9	Describes the diagnosis or problem/reason for visit	Identified as 2-3 numbers with decimal followed by 2 numbers	707.05: pressure ulcer of buttock 998.83: nonhealing surgical wound
CPT	Describes the procedure or service provided	Identified as a 5-digit code	11041: debride skin full-thickness 97597: active wound care/20 cm or under
HCPCS	Describes dressing, supplies, drugs, or procedures that do not have a CPT code	Identified as a letter and numbers	A6234: hydrocolloid dressing 4×4 with adhesive A6257: transparent film, 4×4 size

CPT, Current Procedural Terminology; *HCPCS,* Healthcare Common Procedure Coding System; *ICD-9,* International Classification of Diseases, 9th Revision.

the Physician Fee schedule rate and must follow certain rules. When the APN or PA renders services that are integral but incidental to a physician's services and therefore are "incidental to" services, the physician's provider number must be submitted on the claim. In this situation, the APN or PA provider number is not needed.

The APN may provide physician services and bill as the provider with the APN's provider number when the APN is not following the "incidental to" service. Medicare reimburses the APN at a rate of 85% of the physician rate. Medicare will pay 80% of the patient's bill for the services, and the patient will pay 20% (Buppert, 2007). A service that does not meet Medicare's definition of a "physician service" will not be reimbursed. For example, health services that are within the realm of nursing but are not "physician services" are not covered under Medicare Part B. Medicare defines physician services as diagnosis, therapy, surgery consultation, and care plan oversight (Buppert, 2007). Box 2-5 lists Medicare rules for nurse practitioner (NP) payment. No separate payment may be made to the nonphysician practitioner if a facility or other physician payment is also made for such professional services (Centers for Medicare & Medicaid Services, 2004). For more information, refer to the incident-to policy of the carrier (Centers for Medicare & Medicaid Services, 2006).

Fiscal Intermediaries, Carriers, and Medicare Administrative Contractors

Medicare Part A and Part B claims are processed by nongovernmental organizations or agencies that contract to serve as fiscal agents between providers and suppliers and the federal government. Historically these claims processors were known as fiscal intermediaries (FIs) and carriers. These contractors apply Medicare coverage rules to determine appropriateness of claims. Currently, Medicare FIs process Part A claims for institutional services, including inpatient hospital claims, SNFs, HHAs, and hospice services. FIs also process

Part B claims submitted by institutional providers, including hospital outpatient services. Providers who submit claims to FIs should always refer to their FI's local LCD policy and other billing guidance for specific coverage and payment criteria.

Currently, Medicare carriers handle Part B claims for services provided by physicians and medical suppliers. Carriers can process only Part B claims. Conversely, institutional providers that have claims processed by FIs are considered Part A providers. This situation can cause confusion because FIs process Medicare claims for both Part A and Part B benefits. Part B providers (physicians and suppliers) can bill for services only under the Part B benefit. Part A providers can bill for services under the Part A benefit, the Part B benefit, or both. To view a current directory of FIs and carriers, see the Directory of Fiscal Intermediaries and Intermediary Carriers website listed in Table 2-2.

From October 2004 through October 2011, all existing FIs and carriers will be integrated into entities called *Medicare administrative contractors* (MACs). As a single authority, MAC will be responsible for the receipt, processing, and payment of Medicare claims. In addition to providing core claims processing operations for both Medicare Part A and Part B, MAC will perform functions related to the beneficiary and provider service, appeals, provider outreach and education (also referred to as provider education and training), financial management, program evaluation, reimbursement, payment safeguards, and information systems security. To access the most current information on Medicare contractors, see the website reference listed in Table 2-2.

National Coverage Determinations and Local Coverage Determinations

National coverage determinations (NCDs) were developed by CMS to describe the circumstances for Medicare coverage for a specific medical service procedure or device. NCDs outline the conditions for which a service is considered to be covered or not covered. Once published by the CMS, an NCD is binding on all Medicare contractors and providers or suppliers. A list of current NCDs available on the CMS website is given in Table 2-2. Box 2-6 gives a list of Medicare NCDs pertaining to wound care.

The LCD is a formal statement developed through a specifically defined process that (1) defines the service, (2) provides information about when the service is considered reasonable and necessary, (3) outlines any coverage criteria and/or specific documentation requirements, (4) provides specific coding and/or modifier information, and (5) provides references upon which the policy is based. Copies of draft and final LCDs are available with the Medicare Coverage Database (see Table 2-2 for the CMS website).

BOX 2-5	Medicare Rules for Nurse Practitioner (NP) Reimbursement

The NP meets Medicare qualification requirements;

The practice or facility accepts Medicare's payment, which is 85% of the physician fee schedule rate for bills submitted under the NP's provider number;

The services performed are "physician services" or those for which a physician can bill Medicare;

The services are performed in collaboration with a physician;

The services are within the NP's scope of practice as defined in state law; and

No facility or other provider charges are paid with respect to the furnishing of the services.

BOX 2-6	Medicare National Coverage Determinations Pertaining to Wound Dressings and Modalities

- Porcine skin and gradient pressure dressings
- Treatment of decubitus ulcers
- Hyperbaric oxygen therapy for hypoxic wounds and diabetic wounds of the lower extremities
- Electrical stimulation and electromagnetic therapy for treatment of wounds
- Noncontact normothermic wound therapy
- Nonautologous blood-derived products for chronic nonhealing wounds

Generally the LCD is an administrative and education tool used to assist providers and suppliers in completing claims for payments correctly and to guide medical reviewers. These documents specify the clinical circumstances that qualify for select service and the correct coding. The contractor shall ensure that all LCDs are consistent with all regulations and national coverage payment and coding policies. If a contractor develops an LCD, this LCD applies only within the geographic area in which that contractor services.

Clinic personnel who are primarily responsible for ensuring fiscal success in the wound clinic should be aware of any NCD and LCD pertaining to the wound care services provided in the clinic. A mechanism should be in place for this information to be shared with the practitioners, who are expected to read and know the information. In the event both an NCD and an LCD address the same procedure or service, the NCD will always take precedence. In the absence of an NCD addressing a specific procedure or service, local Medicare contractors may establish a LCD that summarizes medical necessity, criteria for coverage, codes for novel procedures or supplies, and references upon which a temporary coverage policy is based.

CODING AND BILLING FOR SERVICES AND SUPPLIES

Prospective payment billing (for the hospital outpatient department) and fee-for-services billing (for provider services) each requires identifying the diagnosis and services provided via the coding methods described in the following section. Table 2-5 lists the types of codes necessary for provider billing.

Medical Condition Codes (ICD-9)

The national coding method designed to enable providers to effectively document the medical condition, symptom, or complaint that forms the basis for rendering a specific service is known as the ICD-9.

Wound types and presenting signs and symptoms must be attached to the appropriate (most similar) diagnosis code. The appropriate diagnosis must be identified in order to obtain reimbursement for services. Common wound care ICD-9 codes include pressure ulcer, buttock 707.05; pressure ulcer, heel 707.07; nonhealing surgical wound 998.83; and varicose veins of lower extremities with ulcer 454.0. A list of all common visit diagnoses assembled as a billing sheet will benefit the clinic in capturing charges.

Some ICD-9 codes are unspecified, referred to as *Not Otherwise Specified (NOS)*. These codes lack sufficient detail in the statement of diagnosis to be able to assign it to a more specific subdivision within the classification. *Not Elsewhere Classified (NEC)* codes are used when the coder lacks the information necessary to code the term to a more specific category. These codes do not justify the medical necessity for most work performed and should be avoided when more specific codes that pertain to the diagnoses of patients can be used (Schaum, 2008).

Procedure Codes (CPT)

Procedures provided in the clinic are billed using CPT codes that describe the procedures performed, such as debridement, strapping, biopsy, chemical cautery, application of negative pressure, and application of biologic skin substitutes. These codes are derived from a standardized numeric coding system developed and maintained by the AMA.

It is essential to match the CPT codes to the services performed during the wound clinic visit in order to bill both CMS and private health insurance programs. A created list of all services provided should be reviewed with the billing/coding department to find the most closely related code to the service provided, with frequent reviews to incorporate any changes to the frequently used codes. The physician-reported procedure code and the facility-reported procedure codes should match and be supported via documentation in the medical record.

When no procedure is completed and the patient receives care, the visit is billed using an evaluation and management (E&M) service code. The E&M code is also a CPT code used to obtain the fee for the corresponding services provided. E&M codes are based on the complexity of the service rendered to the patient. Unlike procedure codes, the E&M code level of the physician service and the clinic services may not always match. The physician will utilize this code to describe how the information about the patient's illness-related condition was gathered and analyzed and the course of treatment devised. The facility will base the E&M level on the acuity scoring tool.

E&M codes 99211 through 99215 describe varying levels of complexity for an "established patient" visit. E&M codes 99201 through 99205 describe varying levels of complexity for the "new patient" visit. Taken collectively, when visit levels are graphed, the majority of visits would be expected to be in the middle level of complexity and present as a bell curve. An example of an acuity tool is provided in Appendix B.

Supply Codes (Healthcare Common Procedure Coding System)

Medicare does not allow for reimbursement of routine dressing supplies provided during a clinic visit. Under the outpatient prospective payment system (OPPS), the cost of routine dressing supplies considered integral to the visit are bundled into the visit codes and costs of many procedures; thus, supplies are included in the payment for the service (i.e., packaged services). No separate payment is made for packaged services. Although supplies may be marked on the bill to show the cost of the visit, most insurance providers will not reimburse for wound care supplies used during an outpatient clinic visit and tend to follow the Medicare guidelines on packaged codes. For example, routine supplies, anesthesia, recovery room use, and most drugs are considered an integral part of a surgical procedure, so payment for these items is packaged into the APC payment for the surgical procedure (Centers for Medicare & Medicaid Services, 2008).

Unless a facility is also a DME provider, the ability for an outpatient clinic to provide and bill supplies for use at home is cost prohibitive. The patient may qualify for home dressing supplies per Medicare guidelines if home care is not providing the wound care. Medicaid may reimburse for supplies if home care is active, and group health plans may offer coverage at times with a possible copayment. Understanding how to assist patients obtain home supplies is integral to successful patient outcomes. Patients will need information about suppliers in their area as well as those that do business by mail (electronic and postal) and by phone. The wound specialist should be aware of additional services provided by suppliers, such as billing insurance directly, offering free delivery, obtaining physician prescriptions for supplies, and making reminder phone calls for reorders. Box 2-7 lists Medicare guidelines for DME orders.

Knowledge of coverage limits and criteria will assist with the ordering of products that are readily available in the community and reimbursed by Medicare. This valuable information on coverage can be obtained from the CMS website (see Table 2-2).

A complete list of supplies frequently used in the clinic, such as hydrocolloid, alginates, or compression wraps, should be developed and matched to the corresponding Healthcare Common Procedure Coding System (HCPCS). These codes describe the dressing supply assigned and maintained by local Medicare contractors. Level II HCPCS provides a method for obtaining reimbursement for products, supplies, or procedures not covered in CPT codes.

BOX 2-7 | **Medicare Guidelines for DME Arrangements for the Home**

1. Written orders for DME can be submitted as a photocopy, facsimile image, electronic file, or original "pen-and-ink" order.
2. For dressing supplies that will be provided on a periodic basis, the written order should include
   A. the start date of the order, and
   B. a detailed description listing all options or additional features that will be separately billed or that will require an upgraded code.
3. Medical necessity information (diagnosis code) is not considered part of the order, although it may be included within the same document.
4. Someone other than the physician may complete the detailed description of the item or service; however, the treating physician must review the detailed description and personally sign and date the order to indicate agreement.
   Example: One 4×4 hydrocolloid dressing changed two times per week for 1 month, or until the ulcer is healed.

DME, Durable medical equipment.

In the OPPS, outpatient clinics are encouraged to mark on the bill all supplies used at each visit, regardless of expected reimbursement. The total cost of the visit will help ensure future reimbursement of clinic CPT and E&M services by showing the average cost of visits over time.

National Correct Coding Initiative Edits

CMS developed the National Correct Coding Initiative (NCCI) to promote correct coding by providers and suppliers. NCCI edits apply to claims that contain more than one procedure on the same patient, on the same date, and by the same provider or supplier. Payment edits are designed and put in place to prevent payment for noncovered and/or incorrectly coded services. These edits are also used to select targeted claims for review prior to payment (Vargo, 2008). NCCI edits can be located online at the CMS website listed in Table 2-2. Wound debridement codes include the wound debridement, the dressing placed after the debridement, and the assessment and documentation of the wound; therefore, E&M would not be added to the bill along with the debridement because E&M is a necessary part of the debridement and is already captured in the debridement code.

Modifier 59: Distinct Procedural Service

Under certain circumstances, the physician may need to indicate that a procedure or service was distinct or independent from other services performed on the same day. Multiple procedures involving one wound site are almost always billed under one code. The code modifier 59 policy only applies when multiple procedures involving multiple anatomic sites or different patient encounters are performed. In this situation, it is appropriate to bill for additional procedures, adding the modifier 59 to indicate that the various procedures involved were at different wound sites even though they were performed on the same day.

Understanding the edits for bundled services and the code modifier for multiple services is essential to comprehending expected reimbursement.

Status Indicator

CPT codes are assigned a status indicator (SI). A T indicates that reimbursement will be adjusted downward to a discount for multiple procedures. An S indicates that no downward adjustment will be made, that is, no discount for multiple procedures. This adjustment reflects a situation where multiple services are provided with the understanding that resources (e.g., room setup, registration) for multiple procedures will not be duplicated for each of the additional procedures. For example, if three debridements are done to three different anatomic sites on the same patient on the same day, the first debridement is paid in full and the additional debridements are paid at a discounted rate.

Wavier of Deductible and Coinsurance

Routinely waiving the collection of deductible or coinsurance from a beneficiary constitutes a violation of the law pertaining to false claims and kickbacks. Where a physician/supplier makes a reasonable collection effort for the payment of coinsurance/deductibles, failure to collect payment is not considered a reduction in the charges. To be considered reasonable collection efforts, the efforts must be similar to those made to collect from non-Medicare patients. This may include actions such as subsequent billings, collection letters, and telephone calls or personal contacts that constitute a genuine, rather than token, collection effort (Centers for Medicare & Medicaid Services, 2008b).

SUMMARY

Clinics will obtain reimbursement differently depending on the clinic structure (i.e., hospital-based clinic, freestanding clinic). The freestanding clinic will mirror the physician office in utilizing the physician fee schedule for reimbursement, whereas the hospital outpatient department will utilize the hospital outpatient prospective payment system (HOPPS). In the hospital outpatient clinic, when a physician sees a patient while utilizing the hospital staff, a bill is submitted by the physician (at a lower reimbursement rate than if the patient were seen in his or her private office) and a bill is submitted by the facility (to capture hospital resources of room, staff, and supplies based on the HOPPS). Further differences between clinics consist of

determining who the practitioners will be: physician, non-physician practitioner (reimbursed at 85% of physician rate when billing physician services), nurse, PT, or a combination, while also considering which multidiscipline programs will be attached to the clinic. Checklist 2-4 summarizes steps to consider for establishing a successful outpatient clinic.

CHECKLIST 2-4
Establishing an Outpatient Clinic

✓ Determine services to be provided
✓ Create business plan
✓ Gain support and approval from administration and medical colleagues
✓ Decide clinic structure and staffing needs
  o Management/clinic director
  o Medical director
  o Wound specialist nationally certified as CWCN or CWS
  o Nurse
  o Physical therapist
  o Insurance and billing coders
  o Ancillary staff
✓ Determine clinic location and space needs
✓ Develop compliance program
  o HIPAA privacy rule
  o Centers for Medicare & Medicaid Services
  o The Joint Commission
  o Department of Health Certificate of Need
  o National Patient Safety Goals
  o Billing codes
  o Corporate compliance
✓ Meet with coders and create charge master
  o Establish policies
  o Documentation
  o Photography
  o Frequency of visits
  o Referrals for tests and consults
  o Infection control
  o Treatment orders
  o Obtaining consents
  o Debridement
  o Staffing
  o Staff education
  o Wound care outcomes
  o Insurance authorization
✓ Create patient and staff education and competencies
✓ Determine equipment needs and formulary of supplies
✓ Create/gather teaching documents including list of durable medical equipment contacts
✓ Establish operations
  o Hours
  o Scheduling
  o Documentation forms
  o Chart storage and retrieval
  o Room cleaning
✓ Develop marketing plan

HIPAA, Health Insurance Portability and Accountability Act of 1996.

REFERENCES

Armstrong DG et al: New opportunities to improve pressure ulcer prevention and treatment: implications of the CMS inpatient hospital care present on admission (POA) indicators/hospital-acquired conditions (HAC) policy, *Adv Skin Wound Care* 21:469-478, 2008.

Buppert C: *Billing for nurse practitioners services—update3 2007: guidelines for NPs, physicians, employers, and insurers,* 2007, available at http://www.medscape.com/viewprogram/7767_pnt, accessed September 24, 2007.

Centers for Medicare & Medicaid Services, US Department of Health and Human Services: *A reference guide for Medicare physicians and supplier billers,* 2004, ICN006209.

Centers for Medicare & Medicaid Services, US Department of Health and Human Services: *A resource for residents, practicing physician, and other health care professionals,* 2006, ICN005933

Centers for Medicare & Medicaid Services, Department of Health & Human Services: *Medicare claims processing manual: fee schedule administration and coding requirements,* 2008b, available at http://www.cms.hhs.gov/manuals/downloads/clm104c23.pdf, accessed September 27, 2008.

Centers for Medicare & Medicaid Services, Department of Health & Human Services: *CMS Manual System Publication 100-02: Medicare benefits policy transmittal 101,* 2009, available at http://www.cms.hhs.gov/transmittals/downloads/R101BP.pdf, accessed January 16, 2009.

Fife C: The debridement dilemma, *Today's Wound Clinic* Fall: 24-27, 2007.

Fife C, Weir D: Getting started, *Today's Wound Clinic* Spring: 22-26, 2007.

Fusaro ME et al: *Principles to initiate and maintain a successful wound care center: a white paper by the APWCA,* version 1.1, 2008, available at http://www.apwca.org/initiatives/APWCA-Wound-Cntr-Priniciples-061508.pdf, accessed March 10, 2009.

Hess CT: Developing a wound care compliance program (part I), *Adv Skin Wound Care* 21(10):496, 2008.

Jacobs AM, Tomczak R: Evaluation of bensal HP for the treatment of diabetic foot ulcers, *Adv Skin Wound Care* 21:461-465, 2008.

Morrison CA: If you build it, they will come: marketing your wound clinic to its fullest potential, *Today's Wound Clinic* Spring:32-33, 2007.

Office of Inspector General (OIG): Medicare payments for surgical debridement services in 2004, OEI-02-05-00390, May 2007.

Schaum K: New/revised wound care ICD-9-CM codes will be implemented, *Adv Skin Wound Care* 21(9):413-414, 2008.

Sullivan V: Educating staff—what wound clinic clinicians need to know, *Today's Wound Clinic* Spring:14-17, 2007.

Trendwell, T: How are we doing? Evaluating your wound clinic operations, *Today's Wound Clinic* Spring:29-31, 2007.

US Department Health and Human Services: *Health information privacy,* 2009, available at http://hhs.gov/ocr/privacy/hipaa/understanding/index.html, accessed March 21, 2009.

Vargo D: Make sense of wound care billing, turn your cents into reimbursement dollars, *J Wound Ostomy Continence Nurs* 35(2):186-198, 2008.

Vargo D: Direct supervision requirements and incident to services a primer for the WOC nurse, *J Wound Ostomy Continence Nurs* 37(2):148-151, 2009.

Wallin L et al: Implementing nursing practice guidelines: a complex undertaking *J Wound Ostomy Continence Nurs* 32(5):294-300, 2005.

Wound, Ostomy and Continence Nurses (WOCN) Society: Professional practice manual, ed 3, Mt. Laurel, NJ, 2005, Author.

3

Anatomy and Physiology of Skin and Soft Tissue

Annette B. Wysocki

The skin is the one organ of the body that is constantly exposed to a changing environment. Maintaining its integrity is a complex process, and without appropriate treatment, assaults from surgical incisions, injuries, or burns can lead to life-threatening consequences.

The skin of the average adult covers approximately 3,000 in², or an area almost equivalent to 2 m². From birth to maturity the skin covering will undergo a sevenfold expansion. It weighs about 6 lb (or up to 15% of total adult body weight), is the largest organ of the body, and receives one third of the body's circulating blood volume. The skin forms a protective barrier against the external environment while maintaining a homeostatic internal environment. Epidermal appendages (nails, hair follicles, sweat or sebaceous glands) that are lined with epidermal cells are also present in the skin. During healing of partial-thickness wounds, these epidermal cells migrate to resurface the wound. This organ is capable of self-regeneration and can withstand limited mechanical and chemical assaults. The skin varies in thickness from 0.5 mm in the tympanic membrane to 6 mm in the soles of the feet and the palms of the hands. Variations are attributable to differences in the thickness of the skin layers covering underlying organs, bones, muscle, and cartilage. Diseases of the skin can result from genetic causes, so-called genodermatoses, infection, immune dysfunction, and trauma. Skin diseases can involve some or all skin layers and, in the case of various skin cancers, metastasize to other organs and/or tissues.

Population projections indicate that changing demographics will occur over the next decades, and that by 2042 a majority of the US population will be composed of people with skin of color: Hispanic (30%), African American (15%), Asian (9.2%), American Indian and Native Alaskan (2%), and Native Hawaiian and other Pacific Islanders (0.6%) (US Census Bureau, 2008). Unique characteristics of darker versus lighter pigmented skin (Box 3-1) are described throughout the chapter.

SKIN LAYERS

Human skin is divided into two primary layers: epidermis (outermost layer) and dermis (innermost layer) (Figure 3-1). These two layers are separated by a structure called the *basement membrane.* Beneath the dermis is a layer of loose connective tissue called the *hypodermis,* or *subcutis.*

Epidermis

The epidermis, the outermost skin layer, is avascular and derived from embryonic ectoderm. This layer is relatively uniform in thickness over the body, between 75 and 150 μm, except on the soles and palms, where thickness is between 0.4 and 0.6 mm. The epidermal layer is

BOX 3-1	**Unique Characteristics of Darker Pigmented Skin**

- Higher lipid content in stratum corneum
- Increased junctional integrity
- Stratum corneum contains melanosomes (light skin has no melanosomes in stratum corneum)
- Inflammatory reactions (i.e., reddened areas) can be masked
- Inflammation may appear violet-black or black
- Vitiligo and keloids more common
- More blood vessels and dilated lymph channels
- Less abundant distribution of elastic fibers
- Greater protection against photoaging or dermatoheliosis due to no obvious signs of damage to elastic fibers upon exposure to sun light
- Increase in hair breakage and higher prevalence of traumatic alopecia
- More prone to pseudofolliculitis due to spiral configuration and curvature of hair follicles
- Better protection against skin cancer due to increased synthesis, amount, distribution of melanin
- Can mask precancerous and cancerous tumors due to increased melanin content
- Reduced level of vitamin D

constantly being renewed, with turnover time ranging from 26 to 42 days. Complete epidermal renewal occurs over a period lasting between 45 and 75 days, or about every 2 months (Odland, 1991). The epidermal layer is composed of stratified squamous epithelial cells, or keratinocytes, and is divided into five layers (see Figure 3-1). These layers, beginning from the outermost to the innermost, are the stratum corneum, stratum lucidum, stratum granulosum, stratum spinosum, and stratum basale (stratum germinativum or, simply, the basal layer).

Stratum Corneum. The stratum corneum, or horny layer, is the top layer and is composed of dead keratinized cells. These squames, or corneocytes, are the cells that are abraded by the daily mechanical and chemical trauma of handwashing, scratching, bathing, exercising, and changing of clothes. The stratum corneum is composed of layers of thin, stacked, pancake-appearing, anucleate cells. Approximately 80% of these cells are filled with keratin, a tough, fibrous, insoluble protein; hence, they are called *keratinocytes*. Keratinocytes are initially formed in the basal layer and undergo the process of differentiation. The normal stratum corneum is composed of completely differentiated keratinocytes. Keratin is resistant to changes in temperature and pH and to chemical digestion by trypsin and pepsin. This same protein is found in hair and nails; in these

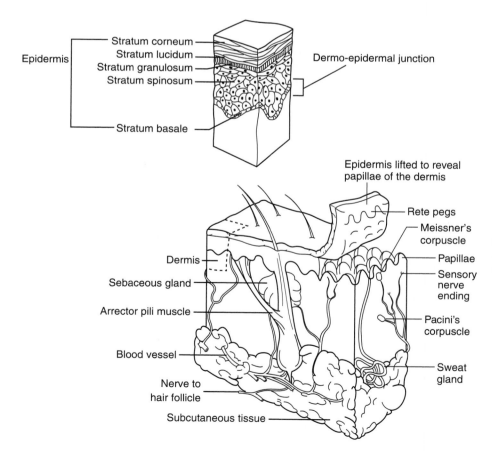

FIGURE 3-1 Schematic diagram of anatomy of skin and subcutaneous tissue. (From Hooper BJ, Goldman MP: *Primary dermatologic care,* St. Louis, 1999, Mosby.)

structures, keratin is referred to as "hard" keratin compared with the "soft" keratin of the skin (Jacob et al, 1982; Solomons, 1983). Stratum corneum thickness varies with age, gender, and disease. In the deeper layer of the stratum corneum, the stratum compactum, the keratin is more densely packed and the cells have a diminished capacity to bind water (Haake, Scott, and Holbrook, 2001). In the upper layer, the stratum dysjunctum, cells are partly shed as a result of proteolytic degradation of the desmosomes.

The stratum corneum is enriched with a lipid matrix that enhances the barrier properties of the skin. Although not universally agreed upon, across the skin color spectrum, differences in the stratum corneum exist as summarized by Taylor (2002). At least two studies (LaRuche and Cesarini, 1992; Rienertson and Wheatley, 1959) report that black stratum corneum has a higher lipid content and this may in part contribute to the conflicting results regarding strateum corneum thickness. The stratum corneum in darkly pigmented skin has been reported to have increased junctional integrity as evidenced by the increased number of tape strippings required to remove the stratum corneum. Whether the stratum corneum is thicker in darkly pigmented skin is unclear (Taylor, 2002).

Stratum Lucidum. The stratum lucidum is directly below the stratum corneum. This layer is found in areas where the epidermis is thicker, such as the palms of the hands and the soles of the feet, but it is absent from thinner skin, such as the eyelids. This layer can be one to five cells thick and is transparent. Cell boundaries often are difficult to identify in histologic sections under a light microscope. The stratum lucidum is a transitional layer where active lysosomal enzymes degrade the nucleus and cellular organelles before they are moved into the stratum corneum (Jacob et al, 1982; Wysocki, 1995).

Stratum Granulosum. The stratum granulosum, or granular layer, is beneath the stratum lucidum when the stratum lucidum is present; otherwise, the stratum granulosum lies beneath the stratum corneum. This layer is one to five cells thick and is so named because of the granules present in the keratinocytes of this layer. The cells of the stratum granulosum have not yet been compressed into a flattened layer and are diamond shaped. The structures contained in these cells are keratohyalin granules, which become intensely stained with the appropriate acid and basic dyes. The proteins contained in these granules (profilaggrin, intermediate keratin filaments, and loricrin) help to organize the keratin filaments in the intracellular space. Profillaggrin is cleaved to form filaggrin, which is further degraded to form urocanic acid and pyrrolidone carboxylic acid. Both urocanic acid and pyrrolidone carboxylic acid provide additional hydration to the stratum corneum and limited filtering against ultraviolet radiation (UVR). The major component of the cornified envelope is loricrin, which is cross-linked to other protein components (involucrin, cystatin A, small proline-rich proteins [SPRR1, SPRR2], elafin, envoplakin) that together form up to 70% of the molecular mass of the cells in this layer. Cells in this layer still have active nuclei (Millington and Wilkinson, 1983; Wheater et al, 1987).

Stratum Spinosum. The stratum spinosum is below the stratum granulosum. This layer often is described as the prickly layer because cytoplasmic structures in these cells take on this morphology. Generally the cells of this layer are polyhedral. A prominent feature of the prickle layer is the desmosome, a type of cell–cell junction. The desmosomes provide adhesion between cells and resistance to mechanical forces. Cells in this layer begin to synthesize involucrin, a soluble precursor of the cornified envelopes (Millington and Wilkinson, 1983). The spinous cells contain large bundles of newly synthesized keratin filaments (K1/K10) in addition to K5/K14 still present from the basal layer (Haake, Scott, and Holbrook, 2001). The identification of various classes of desmosomal proteins (plakoglobin, desmoplakin, plakophilins) and transmembrane glycoproteins (desmogleins, desmocollins) have led to the identification of their roles in various epidermal pathologies, such as bullous impetigo, pemphigus vulgaris, and other genodermatoses.

Stratum Basale or Stratum Germinativum. The stratum basale, or stratum germinativum, is the innermost epidermal layer. It often is referred to simply as the basal layer (see Figure 3-1). It is a single layer of mitotically active cells called *basal keratinocytes,* or *basal cells.* These active cells respond to several factors, such as extracellular matrix, growth factors, hormones, and vitamins. Skin metabolism is mediated by glucose. Glucose utilization in the skin is comparable to that in muscle. Glucose leaving the circulation crosses the basement membrane and forms a concentration gradient that decreases as the glucose moves to the upper layers of the epidermis.

Once cells leave the basal layer they begin an upward migration, which can take 2 to 3 weeks. A cell takes approximately 14 days to move to the stratum corneum and another 14 days to move through the stratum corneum and desquamate (Haake, Scott, and Holbrook, 2001). After leaving the basal layer, the cells begin the process of differentiation. All layers of the epidermis consist of peaks and valleys, but this arrangement is more dramatic in the basal layer such that these protrusions are partly responsible for anchoring the epidermis, thus providing structural integrity. These epidermal protrusions of the basal layer point downward into the dermis and are called *rete ridges,* or *rete pegs.* The basal layer is the primary location of mitotically active cells of the epidermis and has been noted to have increased proliferative capacity compared with cells at the top of the ridges (Briggamann, 1982).

Epidermal stem cells compose about 10% of the basal cell population. These stem cells have a slow cell cycle. When labeled with a radiolabeled DNA precursor, epidermal stem cells retain the label for long periods, thus they are identified as label-retaining cells (Bickenbach 1981). Once cell division occurs, daughter cells that will undergo differentiation as they move toward the stratum corneum are called *transient amplifying cells*. These transient amplifying cells make up approximately 50% of the basal keratinocyte population. Transient amplifying cells progress to become postmitotic cells that then terminally differentiate. A portion of the stem cell population is found in the epidermal crypts of the rete pegs and in the bulge region of hair follicles. Dividing cells go through the cell cycle, and the G_1 phase is shortened in states such as wound healing. The normal keratinocyte cell cycle time is 300 hours but may be as short as 36 hours when psoriasis is present. These stem cell compartments and the transient amplifying cells both are capable of limited or continuing cell division and thus are the cells most likely to reside long enough in the skin to undergo genetic modifications that lead to the development of skin cancers. The use of stem cells alone and in combination with tissue engineering approaches is an area of active research and development in wound care (Griffith and Naughton, 2002).

Melanocytes, the cells responsible for skin pigmentation as a result of melanin synthesis, also are distributed in the basal layer. Melanocytes are dendritic cells that arise from melanoblasts, which derive from the neural crest. During development, they migrate to other locations, including the bulge region of hair follicles, the choroid of the eye, the heart, and the brain (Goding, 2007). Melanocytes are also required for hearing; genetic mutations resulting in a loss of melanocytes are a major cause of deafness (Steel and Barkway, 1989). Melanin is packaged inside the cell into melanosomes, which are transported via the cytoskeletal network of microfilaments and microtubules to the dendritic processes of the melanocyte, where they are then transferred to keratinocytes. Incorporation into the keratinocytes is thought to occur via one or more of the following processes: release and endocytosis, engulfment, active transport, or passage through channels or pores between the melanocyte and neighboring keratinocytes (Boissy, 2003). Melanocytes can be detected by 50 days' gestation in fetal development (Holbrook, 1998). Under normal conditions, melanocytes rarely divide. In normal skin, the number of melanocytes present is nearly the same regardless of skin color. There is approximately one melanocyte for every 36 basal cells. Dendritic melanocyte structures are responsible for the transfer of pigment to a large number of keratinocytes. The primary difference between light- and dark-skinned individuals is the size, number, and distribution of melanosomes, the structures containing the melanin pigment, and the activity of the melanocytes. Carotene or carotenoids are responsible for imparting the yellow hue to the skin of some individuals (Jacob et al, 1982; Sams, 1990; Solomons, 1983).

Melanin pigment is a complex polymer that is synthesized from tyrosine by activity of the tyrosinase gene pathway. Melanin is difficult to study because it is relatively insoluble (Boissy, 2003). The two primary types of melanin are brown/black eumelanin and red/yellow pheomelanin (Lin and Fisher, 2007). Pheomelanin is more photolabile, and damage leads to release of oxygen radicals such as hydrogen peroxide, superoxide, and hydroxyl radicals, resulting in oxidative stress and DNA damage (Lin and Fisher, 2007). Constitutive synthesis, or the synthesis that occurs at basal levels, results primarily from genetic regulation. Facultative synthesis is the additional up- or down-regulation of melanin synthesis in response to UVR, hormones, cytokines, immune regulation, chemical exposure, or other agents (Boissy, 2003). Interestingly, once delivered to the keratinocytes, melanosomes are preferentially, although not exclusively, clustered around the apical side of the nucleus, where they can more effectively provide protection from UVR to prevent DNA damage leading to mutations (Boissy, 2003). In addition to its photoprotective effect, melanin is thought to act as a sink for highly reactive oxygen species that can also lead to DNA damage (Goding, 2007). Pathologies associated with melanocytes or pigmentation are melanoma, dyschromias such as vitiligo and melasma, xeroderma pigmentosa, and albinism.

As a result of genetics, genetic recombination, and selective environmental pressures (e.g., UVR intensity and exposure, age, hormonal influences), skin pigmentation demonstrates considerable variation across the human population. Presently more than 150 genes have been identified that either directly or indirectly affect skin color (Yamaguchi and Hearing, 2009). Key proteins and receptors identified with the synthesis and transport of melanin or melanosomes include melanocyte-stimulating hormone, melanocortin-1 receptor (MC1R), keratinocyte growth factor, and protease-activated receptor-2. The red hair/light skin phenotype is associated with mutations found in the residues of MC1R, which lead to increased risk for skin cancer (Miyamura et al, 2006). Thus, the skin color spectrum ranges from dense black, with the highest level and distribution of melanosomes, to various shades of brown to white and finally to albino, or the complete absence of pigment (but not an absence of melanocytes). In general, Caucasian and Asian skin has smaller melanosomes that form small clusters or aggregates, whereas dense African skin has larger melanosomes that are distributed primarily as single units (Montagna et al, 1993; Szabo et al, 1969; Szabo et al, 1972). In darkly pigmented skin, despite the hydrolytic degradation that occurs with keratinocyte differentiation, some melanosomes can still be seen in the stratum corneum, whereas in light skin no melanosomes are seen in the stratum corneum (Boissy, 2003). Various shades of brown skin occur across African, African American, Hispanic, Asian, Caucasian, and Native American peoples; these shades are influenced by the number, size, and distribution of melanosomes. The range of variation can even occur in the same individual, depending on skin location and sun exposure (Szabo, 1954). In general, the density of melanocytes is slightly higher in skin covering the upper dorsal surfaces compared to skin on the lower dorsal surfaces, and the amount of melanin present in the skin correlates well with visible skin pigmentation seen on physical examination (Miyamura et al, 2006).

Intensely pigmented skin can mask the detection of skin inflammatory reactions, which normally are seen as reddened areas that may appear in response to conditions such as contact dermatitis, pressure, or folliculitis. Inflammation may appear as darker areas in black skin, violet-black in intensely black skin, or black in brown skin. Other signs of inflammation may include the detection of heat or warmth to touch or induration detected as skin tightening or hardening over areas where there is skin damage. Dermatologic disorders accompanied by inflammation can result in postinflammatory hypopigmentation or hyperpigmentation that can be especially distressing to individuals with more darkly pigmented skin in which the color contrast can be dramatically evident. Other dermatologic disorders more commonly associated with darkly pigmented skin include vitiligo and keloids. Keloids occur 3 to 18 times more frequently in darkly pigmented skin, and the incidence has been reported as between 4.5% to 16% in Chinese, Hispanic, and African American individuals (Oluwasanmi, 1974; Robles and Berg, 2007; Taylor, 2002; Taylor, 2003).

Universal agreement concerning comparative differences, if any, across the skin color spectrum for transepidermal water loss (TEWL), stratum corneum structure, epidermal thickness, and sweat and sebaceous gland number or distribution, are fraught with numerous points of criticism that include low numbers of subjects, variation in age, sex, circadian rhythms, use of emollients, relative temperature and humidity, geographic location, location of skin sample, sun exposed versus sun protected areas, nutrition, validity and reliability of instrumentation, and accurate indexing to skin color (McDonald, 1988; Taylor, 2002). It has been noted that there are 31 climate zones around the globe subject to the adaptation, lifestyle, and conditions of people with various customs and resources and climate can influence birth weight, body shape, and cranial morphology (Lambert et al, 2008), Thus, definitive studies of skin biology across the range of the skin color spectrum relative to age and gender await more exhaustive and comprehensive research studies and may require more precise instrumentation for some measures.

Basement Membrane Zone

The basement membrane zone (BMZ), or dermal–epidermal junction, is the area that separates the epidermis from the dermis. Closer examination of the BMZ in the past decade has revealed the BMZ to be more complex than previously believed. Basal keratinocytes use hemidesmosomes to structurally and functionally attach to the BMZ. The BMZ is subdivided into two distinct zones, the lamina lucida and the lamina densa. The lamina lucida is so named because it is an electron-translucent zone compared with the electron-dense zone of the lamina densa. The major proteins found in the BMZ are fibronectin, an adhesive glycoprotein; laminin, a glycoprotein; type IV collagen, a non–fiber-forming collagen; and heparin sulfate proteoglycan, a glycosaminoglycan. A lesser amount of type VII collagen has also been detected. The BMZ anchors the epidermis to the dermis and is the layer that is affected in blister formation associated with dermatologic diseases, second-degree burns, full-thickness wounds, and mechanical trauma. During wound healing the BMZ is disrupted and must be re-formed (Sams, 1990).

Dermis

The dermis, or corium, is the thickest tissue layer of the skin. Compared with the cellular epidermal layer, the dermis is sparsely populated (primarily by fibroblast cells) and is vascularized and innervated. The dermal layer is derived from the middle embryonic germ layer, the mesoderm. Dermal thickness ranges from 2 to 4 mm but on average is 2 mm. Variations in dermal thickness account for differences in total skin thickness that have been measured throughout the body. The dermis of the back is thicker than the dermis covering the scalp, forehead, abdomen, thigh, wrist, and palm.

The dermal vasculature consists of a network of papillary loops, supported by a deep horizontal plexus. The vasculature functions to provide nutritional support, immune surveillance, wound healing, thermal regulation, hemostasis, and the inflammatory response. Formation of the vascular system involves vasculogenesis and angiogenesis. *Vasculogenesis* is the process that occurs de novo during embryonic development and is mediated by angioblasts derived from the mesoderm. *Angiogenesis* is the process whereby new vessels are formed from preexisting vessels. It is involved in wound healing, tumor growth and metastasis, hemangiomas, telangiectasia, psoriasis, and scleroderma. Vascular endothelial growth factor (VEGF), or vascular permeability factor, is secreted by keratinocytes in response to hypoxia. It is increased in wound healing and is responsible for stimulating angiogenesis. Other factors that stimulate angiogenesis include acidic and basic fibroblast growth factor, interleukin-8, platelet-derived endothelial growth factor, placental growth factor, transforming growth factor-α and transforming growth factor-β, oncostatin M, angiogenin, and heparin-binding epidermal growth factor. Inhibitors of angiogenesis include angiostatin, thrombospondin, endostatin, interferon-γ, interleukin-12, and platelet factor-4.

The major proteins found in the dermis are collagen and elastin. The other category of proteins found occupying the space between collagen and elastin fibers is referred to as the *ground substance*. The ground substance in black skin is distinctly more abundant in both the papillary and reticular layers than in white skin (Montagna and Carlisle, 1991). This category of proteins is largely composed of proteoglycans and glycosaminoglycans. Included in this category of proteins are chondroitin sulfates and dermatan sulfate (versican, decorin, biglycan), heparan and heparan sulfate proteoglycans (syndecan, perlecan), and chondroitin-6 sulfate proteoglycans. Although these proteins account for only approximately 0.2% of the dry weight of the dermis, these large molecules are capable of binding up to 1,000 times their volume. Thus, proteoglycans and glycosaminoglycans play a role in regulating the water-binding capacity of the dermis, which can determine dermal volume and compressibility. Hyaluronan is also found in the dermis and in higher abundance in fetal skin, where it forms a watery, less stable matrix that allows greater cell movement; it also is a critical factor in scarless healing (Longaker et al, 1990). Hyaluronan can bind growth factors and provide cellular linkages with other matrix materials that together function to regulate cell migration, adhesion, proliferation, differentiation, morphogenesis, and tissue repair (Haake and Holbrook, 1999). Other glycoproteins found in the dermis include fibronectin, thrombospondin, laminin, vitronectin, and tenascin. These glycoproteins are synthesized and secreted by fibroblasts in the dermis.

Data indicate that skin fibroblasts from different anatomic locations contain different transcriptional patterns that can indicate position and can be differentiated from fibroblasts in other locations using microarray analysis (Chang et al, 2002). Fibroblasts present in the dermis range in size and number. It has been reported that fibroblasts in black facial skin were larger, occurred in greater numbers, and were more likely to be binucleated or multinucleated compared to white skin. Overall, the dermis in black skin was thick and compact compared to thinner and less compact in white skin (Montagna and Carlisle, 1991). In this same study, collagen fiber bundles were observed to be smaller, more tightly packed and were oriented parallel to the epidermis in black skin and had more fiber fragments. Somewhat in contrast, white skin was noted to have larger collagen fiber bundles with some degraded collagen fragments, which may have resulted from sun exposure, but had greater variability in the number of fibroblasts. No differences in mast cells were observed. However, black skin did have more binucleated and multinucleated macrophages in the papillary dermis, and the accompanying melanophages in black skin contained melanosomes both singly and in complexes, whereas in white skin the melanophages were almost exclusively in complexes (Montagna and Carlisle, 1991). Again, these findings should be viewed with caution given the lack of comprehensive studies across the skin color spectrum. The dermis is a matrix

that supports the epidermis. It can be divided into two areas: papillary dermis and reticular dermis (see Figure 3-1). The papillary and reticular layers appear more distinct in white skin and less distinct in black skin (Montagna and Carlisle, 1991).

Papillary Dermis. The papillary dermis lies immediately below the BMZ and forms interdigitating structures with the rete ridges of the epidermis called *dermal papillae*. The dermal papillae contain papillary loops (Figure 3-2), which supply the necessary oxygen and nutrients to the overlying epidermis via the BMZ. The collagen fibers contained in the papillary dermis are much smaller in diameter and form smaller, wavy, cable-like structures compared with the reticular dermis. This portion of the dermis also contains small elastic fibers and has a greater proportion of ground substance than the reticular dermis. The superficial subepidermis in darkly pigmented skin contains more numerous blood vessels along with many more dilated lymph channels (Montagna and Carlisle, 1991). The papillary dermis also contains lymphatic vessels that play a role in controlling interstitial fluid pressure by resorption of fluid and assist in clearing the tissues of cells, lipids, bacteria, proteins, and other degraded substances. The papillary lymph vessels drain into the horizontal plexus of larger lymph vessels located in the deep subpapillary venous plexus. This system is further connected to the lymph system in the reticular dermis. Fluid flow through this system is partially controlled through arterial pulsations, muscle contractions, and body movement. Renewed interest in the skin lymphatic system has resulted from the identification of markers such as VEGF-C, VEGFR-3, and lymphatic vessel endothelial receptor-1 (LYVE-1) and the findings of the role of these lymphatic vessels in tumor promotion (Chu, 2008).

Reticular Dermis. The reticular dermis (the area below the papillary dermis) forms the base of the dermis. The collagen fibers in the reticular dermis are thicker in diameter and form larger cablelike structures than in the papillary dermis. There is no clear separation of papillary and reticular dermis because the collagen fibers change in size gradually between the two layers. Thicker elastic fibers are found in the reticular dermis, but substantially less ground substance is present. A complex of cutaneous blood vessels is found in this part of the dermis.

Dermal Proteins. *Collagen,* the protein that gives the skin its tensile strength, is the major structural protein found in the dermis and accounts for 25% of the skin's total weight (Stryer, 1995). The primary constituents of collagen are proline, glycine, hydroxyproline, and hydroxylysine. Collagen is secreted by dermal fibroblasts as tropocollagen, which undergoes additional extracellular processing so that mature collagen fibers are formed. Normal human dermis is primarily composed of type I collagen, a fiber-forming collagen. Type I collagen represents 77% to 85% of the collagen present; type III

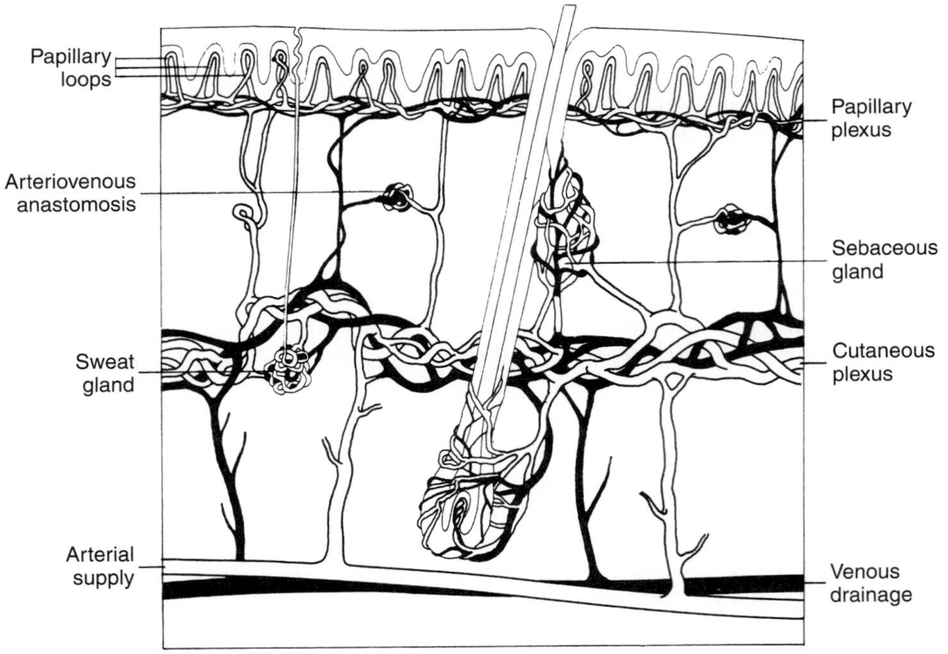

FIGURE 3-2 Blood circulation in the skin with papillary loops, which supply oxygen and nutrients to the epidermis, and dermal cutaneous plexuses, which arise from the deeper blood supply located in the hypodermis. (From Young B et al: *Wheater's functional histology: a text and colour atlas,* ed 5, Edinburgh, 2006, Churchill Livingstone.)

collagen, also a fiber-forming collagen, represents the remaining 15% to 23% (Gay and Miller, 1978; Wysocki et al, 2005). Very small amounts of type V collagen (less than 5%) and type VI collagen also are present.

Elastin, another protein found in the dermis, provides the skin's elastic recoil, a feature that prevents the skin from being permanently reshaped. It is a fiber-forming protein, like collagen. Elastin has a high amount of proline and glycine. However, unlike collagen, elastin lacks large amounts of hydroxyproline. Elastin fibers form structures, similar to coils, that allow this protein to be stretched and, when released, to return to its inherent configuration. Elastin accounts for less than 2% of the skin's dry weight (Millington and Wilkinson, 1983; Sams, 1990; Wysocki, 1995). Elastin is distributed with collagen but in smaller amounts. Large concentrations of elastin are found in blood vessels (especially the aortic arch near the heart) and lymphatic vessels. The distribution of elastic fibers ranges from less abundant in darkly pigmented skin to more abundant in light skin. Upon exposure to sunlight, elastic fibers in darkly pigmented skin show no obvious signs of damage, whereas elastic fibers in light skin show obvious signs of elastosis (Montagna et al, 1993). The lower distribution of elastic fibers in darkly pigmented skin also extends to the anchorage of hair follicles, leading to an increase in hair breakage and a higher prevalence of traumatic alopecia in both men and women (Taylor, 2002). Furthermore, the curvature of hair follicles and the spiral configuration seen in Africans and African Americans lead to pseudofolliculitis, especially in men who shave.

Other cells found in the dermis are mast cells, macrophages, and lymphocytes. All of these cells are involved with immune surveillance of the skin, often referred to as the *skin immune system*. The dermis also contains dermal appendages that include hair follicles, sebaceous glands, and eccrine and apocrine sweat glands.

Hypodermis

Hypodermis, or superficial fascia, forms a subcutaneous layer below the dermis. It is an adipose layer containing a subdermal plexus of blood vessels giving rise to the cutaneous plexus in the dermis, which in turn gives rise to the papillary plexus and loops of the papillary dermis (see Figure 3-2). The hypodermis attaches the dermis to underlying structures. This layer provides insulation for the body, a ready reserve of energy, and additional cushioning; it also adds to the mobility of the skin over underlying structures (Haake and Holbrook, 1999). Growing hair follicles and apocrine and eccrine sweat glands can extend into this layer. The hypodermis is largely absent in certain pathologic disease states, such as Werner syndrome and scleroderma. Adipocytes form the primary cells in this tissue layer, and their activity is regulated by leptin.

SKIN FUNCTIONS

The skin provides several functions: protection, immunity, thermoregulation, sensation, metabolism, and communication (Jacob et al, 1982; Millington and Wilkinson, 1983; Woodburne and Burkel, 1988).

Protection

The skin protects the body against aqueous, chemical, and mechanical assaults; bacterial and viral pathogens; and UVR. It also prevents excessive loss of fluids and electrolytes in order to maintain the homeostatic environment. The effectiveness of the skin in preventing excessive fluid loss can be seen in patients with burns. Patients with burns involving 30% of their body can lose up to 4.1 L of fluid compared with 710 ml for normal adults (Rudowski, 1976). The skin maintains the internal milieu, and a progressive decrease in water content across the epidermal layers helps to prevent excessive transepidermal water loss under basal conditions. Water constitutes 65% to 70% of the basal layer, and decreases to 40% in the granular layer and 15% in the stratum corneum (Warner et al, 1988). The skin's barrier function is so effective that percutaneous drug delivery is limited except in premature babies and in newborns. In general, compounds are restricted to those with a molecular mass of 500 daltons or less with a daily dose of 10 mg or less. Protection against mechanical assaults is mainly provided by the tough fibroelastic tissue of the dermis, collagen, and elastin.

Protection Against Pathogens. Protection against aqueous, chemical, bacterial, and viral pathogens is provided by the stratum corneum, secretions from the sebaceous glands, and the skin immune system. The primary line of defense against all of these agents is an intact stratum corneum (Roth and James, 1988). The insoluble protein keratin, found in the horny layer, provides good resistance. In addition, the constant shedding of squames from the stratum corneum prevents the entrenchment of microorganisms.

Sebum, a lipid-rich, oily substance secreted by the sebaceous glands onto the skin surface, usually via hair follicles and shafts, provides an acidic coating with a pH ranging from 4 to 6.8 (Spince and Mason, 1987) and a mean pH of 5.5 (Roth and James, 1988; Wysocki et al, 2005). This acidity, together with natural antibacterial substances found in sebum, retards the growth of microorganisms. These glands are stimulated by sex hormones (androgens) and become very active during adolescence. Sebum, along with keratin, provides resistance to aqueous and chemical solutions. When sebaceous glands occur in association with hair follicles, they are called a *pilosebaceous unit*. Sebaceous glands are not found on palms or soles; they occur in areas that lack hair, such as lips. These glands are largest when they are located on the face and when associated with hair follicles. Sebaceous glands may increase in size by 100 to 150 times as sebum accumulates. Maximum secretion occurs in persons in their late teens to early twenties. Rates of secretion are higher in men and decline 32% per decade in females compared with 23% per decade in males.

Resistance to pathogenic microorganisms is also provided by normal skin flora through bacterial interference (Noble, 2004; Weinberg and Swartz, 1987). Conceptually, the two categories of skin flora are (1) resident (bacteria normally found on a person) and (2) transient (bacteria not normally found on a person and usually shed by daily hygienic practices, such as bathing and hand washing). Resident bacteria are found on exposed skin; moist areas such as the axillae, perineum, and toe webs; and covered skin. Bacterial microcolonies are found in hair follicles and at the edges of squames as halos in the upper loose surface layers. The following species of bacteria are found on human skin: *Staphylococcus, Micrococcus, Peptococcus, Corynebacterium, Brevibacterium, Propionibacterium, Streptococcus, Neisseria,* and *Acinetobacter*. The yeast *Pityrosporum* and the mite *Demodex* are also found. Not all species are found on any one individual, but most individuals have at least five of these genera. Normal viral florae are not known to exist (Noble, 2004). However, viruses have been detected in compromised skin and in individuals who are not immunocompetent.

An association exists between skin pH and bacteria. For example, *Propionibacterium acnes* grows well at pH values of 6 and 6.5, but its growth is markedly decreased at pH 5.5 (Korting and Braun-Falco, 1996). However, this association can vary depending on the specific bacterial species involved and the body location. The formation of bacterial biofilms has been scrutinized (Wysocki, 2002), and the role of normal skin flora in the formation of these biofilms is an area of active investigation. Biofilms are essentially an extracellular polysaccharide matrix, or glycocalyx, in which microorganisms are embedded. Biofilms are composed of mixed bacterial species living in their own microniche in a complex, metabolically cooperative microbial community that maintains its own form of homeostasis and rudimentary circulatory system (Costerton et al, 1995). Biofilms are resistant to host immune responses and are markedly more resistant to antibiotic and topical bactericidals (Xu et al, 2000). Reports indicate that biofilm cells can be at least 500 times more resistant to antibacterial agents (Costerton et al, 1995). Biofilm formation is familiar to clinicians and can be identified on endotracheal tubes, Hickman catheters, central venous catheters, contact lenses, and orthopedic devices. *Pseudomonas aeruginosa* forms biofilms in conjunction with other bacterial species. Quorum sensing by bacteria is a feature in biofilm formation. These biofilms complicate the eradication of infections because they give rise to sessile and planktonic bacteria. Planktonic bacteria can be cleared by phagocytosis, antibodies, and antibiotics (Costerton et al, 1999). Sessile bacteria in biofilms can evade antibiotics by giving rise to planktonic bacteria, which respond to antibiotics and host immune responses, but the sessile bacteria remain. Cycles of antibiotic treatment often are administered without success, and the symptoms of infection recur. In these situations, biofilm formation should be suspected, and surgical removal of the sessile population most likely will be required to eliminate the pathogenic bacteria. Moist skin areas, such as the axillae, perineum, toe webs, hair follicles, nail beds, and sweat glands, are especially prone to an increased presence of bacteria. Protection from bacterial invasion is mediated in part by proteins called *defensins* (Hoffman et al, 1999). Findings show that β-defensin is abundant in skin and may be important for wound healing. Defensins act in conjunction with phagocytosing neutrophils and the membrane attack complex of complement. Thus, optimal skin and wound care is a cornerstone of clinical practice in preventing the progression from bacterial colonization to infection (Wysocki, 2002).

Protection Against UVR. Protection against UVR is provided by skin pigmentation, which results from synthesis of the pigment melanin. Harmful effects are primarily attributable to UVA, the long-wave form of UVR, which ranges spectrally from 320 to 400 nm, and UVB, the short-wave ultraviolet form, which ranges from 290 to 320 nm (Council on Scientific Affairs, 1989). The shorter the waves, the more dangerous they are. UVC is effectively blocked by an intact ozone layer. Holes appearing in the ozone layer have raised concern over the effects of UVR in causing skin diseases. Because darker-skinned individuals have increased synthesis, amount, and distribution of melanin, they are better protected against skin cancer. More melanin is distributed in all layers of the epidermis in dark skin than in light skin (Spince and Mason, 1987).

Darkly pigmented black skin provides more efficient protection from both UVB and UVA. The mean transmission of UVB is approximately 7.4% and that of UVA is 17.5% in darkly pigmented skin compared to 29.4% and 55.5%, respectively, in white skin. The mechanism for the more efficient absorption and scattering of UVB and UVA in darkly pigmented skin is attributed to the larger size and number of melanosomes in black skin. The superior UVB/UVA efficiency in black skin can provide a skin protection factor of approximately 13.4 compared to 3.4 for white skin (Montagna et al, 1993), with a range from 10- to 15-fold that seen in the absence of melanin when the minimal erythematous dose is used as a measure (Lin and Fisher, 2007). However, in terms of protection against various types of skin cancer, highly pigmented skin affords a 500 to 1,000 times reduction in risk (Lin and Fisher, 2007). An inverse relationship exists between melanin levels and DNA damage, with darker skin having less DNA damage. Higher melanin levels also decrease damage to basal stem cells and melanocytes in the deep epidermis. Thus, DNA damage in darkly pigmented skin is largely restricted to the upper layers of the epidermis, whereas DNA damage in lightly pigmented skin occurs throughout all layers of the epidermis (Miyamura et al, 2006). Melanocytes in darkly pigmented skin are more efficient than melanocytes in lighter skin in their response to the same UVR challenge (Miyamura et al, 2006). The immediate response in darkly pigmented skin leads to a more efficient distribution and trafficking of melanosomes to the upper epidermis. An actual increase in melanin synthesis is largely a delayed response (Tadokoro et al, 2005). Finally, UV-induced apoptosis leading to removal of damaged cells is

higher in darkly pigmented skin, resulting in an overall lower incidence of skin carcinogenesis (Yamaguchi et al, 2008). However, even individuals with darkly pigmented skin can develop skin cancers, and the increased melanin content often can mask precancerous and cancerous lesions, leading to poorer outcomes when the lesions eventually are detected and treated.

Clinically, the skin phototype system (SPT) was developed as a valid and practical tool to characterize the reactivity of human skin to ultrviolet radiation based on the minimal errythmatous dose and the ability to tan upon sun exposure (Fitzpatrick, 1988; Pathak, Nghiem, and Fitzpatrick, 1999). It is one of the most widely used systems to classify skin pigmentation by dermatologists and the Food and Drug Administration (Fitzpatrick, 1988; Taylor, 2002). Originally this system was developed to guide the exposure of indidividuals receiving PUVA for psoraisis when it was found that hair and eye color were not sufficient to determine the level of exposure (Fitzpatrick, 1988). Over time the system was expanded from primarily one that defined various light skinned individuals to include darkly pigmented skin. The SPT system ranges from I (ivory, white) to VI (dark brown or black) and is now defined based on 1) constitutive or unexposed skin color, 2) minimal erythmatous dose and minimal melanogenic dose for UVB ad UVA, 3) reactivity to ultraviolet light, 4) sunburn and tanning history, 5) immediate pigment darkening, 6) delayed tanning, 7) extent of photoaging, and 8) susceptibility to skin cancer (Pathak, Nghiem, and Fitzpatrick, 1999).

Exposure to UVR can lead to skin cancer, sunburn (first- or second-degree burns), compromised immunity, and long-term skin damage. Sun-exposed epidermal skin is thicker and rougher than unexposed skin, is more prone to benign and malignant growths, and tends to have a greater decrease in Langerhans cells (which seems to occur independent of skin color) (Scheibner et al, 1986). And the increase in skin pigmentation that occurs in sun-exposed skin also leads to an increase in pigmentation in sun-protected skin (Stierner et al, 1989). Infrequent sun exposure may be more harmful than regular exposure (Miyamura et al, 2006). Sun-exposed dermis has increased elastogenesis and a greater decrease in mature collagen with fragmented collagen fibrils compared to unexposed dermis.

Skin Immune System. The skin immune system also provides protection against invading microorganisms and antigens. The cells of the skin that provide immune protection are the Langerhans cells, which are antigen-presenting cells found in the epidermis; tissue macrophages, which ingest and digest bacteria and other substances; mast cells, which contain histamine (released in inflammatory reactions); and dendrocytes. Both macrophages and mast cells are found in the dermis (Auger, 1989; Benyon, 1989; Wolff and Stingl, 1983). Using a standard panel of 41 allergens, allergic contact dermatitis and irritant contact dermatitis overall do not appear to be different in white compared to black individuals, although their response to specific allergens is different (DeLeo et al, 2002)

Langerhans cells are responsible for the recognition, uptake, processing, and presentation of soluble antigens and haptens to sensitized T lymphocytes. This occurs through binding of T cells to Langerhans cells. Exposure to UVB light decreases the functional capability of Langerhans cells (Bergstresser et al, 1980).

Tissue macrophages are derived from monocytes, which arise from bone marrow precursor cells. Macrophages are among the most important cells of the skin's immune system because they are versatile. Once monocytes migrate into the tissue, they differentiate and become macrophages. Cells in the dermis that are not completely differentiated are difficult to distinguish, and much effort has been made in the last decade to recognize the various cells in the dermis. Macrophages, in addition to their antibacterial activity, can process and present antigen to immunocompetent lymphoid cells, are tumoricidal, and can secrete growth factors, cytokines, and other immunomodulatory molecules. Macrophages are involved in coagulation, atherogenesis, wound healing, and tissue remodeling (Haake and Holbrook, 1999).

Mast cells usually distributed in the papillary dermis, around epidermal appendages, blood vessels, and nerves in the subpapillary plexus, and in subcutaneous fat. These cells are distributed in connective tissue throughout the body in places where organs interface with the environment. Mast cells contain or secrete, on demand, a host of proteins. Thus, mast cells are the primary effector cells in allergic reactions. They also are involved in conditions of subacute and chronic inflammatory disease. Increased numbers of mast cells have been detected in tissues affected by chronic eczema, psoriasis, scleroderma, porphyria cutanea tarda, lichen simplex chronicus, and lichen planus, and in healing wounds. As a part of the skin immune system, mast cells play a role in protecting against parasites, stimulating chemotaxis, and promoting phagocytosis, are involved in the activation and proliferation of eosinophils, are capable of altering vasotension and vascular permeability, and can promote connective tissue repair and angiogenesis (Haake and Holbrook, 1999).

Dermal dendrocytes are highly phagocytic cells found in the papillary and upper reticular dermis. They also are distributed near vessels in the subpapillary plexus, reticular dermis, and subcutaneous fat. These immunologically competent cells are highly phagocytic and can be recognized as melanophages. Their numbers are increased in fetal, infant, and photoaged skin and in pathologic skin conditions such as psoriasis and eczema (Headington, 1986). Their numbers are decreased in malignant fibrotic tumors and fibroproliferative lesions, such as keloids, scars, and scleroderma (Headington and Cerio, 1990).

Thermoregulation

Thermoregulation of the body is provided by the skin forming a barrier between the outside and inside environments, thus maintaining the body's temperature. The two primary thermoregulatory mechanisms are circulation and sweating. Blood vessels can either dilate to dissipate heat or constrict to shunt heat to underlying body organs. When dilated, these vessels have increased blood flow and release heat by conduction, convection, radiation, and evaporation. Vasoconstriction is often accompanied by the action of arrector pili muscle attached to hair follicles. This action results in the hair standing vertically. In mammals that depend on hair for warmth, this action fluffs up the fur to increase thermal capacity. The resulting visible bulge around hair shafts is commonly referred to as *goose bumps*. In humans, shivering is more important than the vertical orientation of hair for maintaining body temperature when the outside environment is cold (Jacob et al, 1982; Sams, 1990). In cold weather the "core" body temperature encompasses a smaller zone, whereas in warm weather the "core" is expanded. Sensations of cold and warm are generally detected below 30°C and above 37°C, respectively. Clinically it has been estimated that for each 1°C (1.8°F) increase in fever, a patient's fluid and calorie needs increase by 13%. At rest, the trunk, viscera, and brain account for 70% of heat production but compose only 36% of body mass. However, during exercise, muscle and skin account for 90% of heat production but represent 56% of body mass (Wenger, 1999).

Unlike other skin structures, hair follicles have a repeated cycle of growth and regression. Follicle development begins in month 4 of gestation. The hair growth cycle consists of anagen (growth phase), catagen (follicle involution), and telogen (dormant or resting phase) phases. In addition, a population of epidermal stem cells in the bulge region of the hair follicle contributes to reepithelialization in partial-thickness wounds. Hair shape varies depending on ethnicity and location. Asians have the largest diameter scalp hair and Caucasians the smallest. In the scalp, approximately 85% of hair is in anagen phase and 15% in telogen phase. The anagen phase lasts from 2 to 5 years. On the extremities, anagen lasts from 22 to 28 days (Freinkel, 2001).

Sweating occurs when the activity of the sweat glands is increased. It has been estimated that the human body has from two to five million sweat glands ranging in size from 0.05 to 0.1 mm. Sweat glands are of two types—eccrine and apocrine. Eccrine glands arise from epidermal invagination and are found abundantly on the palms of the hands and the soles of the feet. These glands are largely under the control of the nervous system, responding to temperature differences and emotional stimulation. Their secretory activity also is influenced by muscular activity. These sweat glands, located in the dermis as a coil, secrete fluid that is 99% to 99.5% water; the remainder consists of sodium chloride, urea, sulfates, and phosphates (Solomons, 1983; Spince and Mason, 1987). The pH is slightly acidic. Thermoregulatory control occurs as a result of cooling when fluid evaporates from the skin surface, as evaporation requires heat. The odor associated with sweat is largely a result of bacterial action. Eccrine sweat glands are capable of producing 1 to 4 L of sweat per hour, resulting in a 75% to 90% reduction in body heat. Man is capable of losing heat more rapidly and for longer periods than is any other animal (Quinton, 1983).

Apocrine sweat glands usually are found in association with hair follicles; they do not play a significant role in thermoregulation. These coiled, tubular glands are present in the axillae and in the anogenital area; modifications of these glands are found in the ear and secrete ear wax, or cerumen (Spince and Mason, 1987). There are approximately 100,000 apocrine glands, each 2 to 3 mm in diameter. Apocrine glands produce secretions in small amounts. The secretions are turbid, and they contain iron, carbohydrates, and lipids.

In general, no differences in the quantity, structure, or function of eccrine or apocrine sweat glands between individuals have been identified (Badreshia-Bansal and Taylor, 2009). However, scant data on functional activity indicate that white individuals have a higher degree of sweating with physical labor than do black Africans or Asian Indians and that eccrine gland activity for Hispanic individuals falls between that of white and black individuals (Badreshia-Bansal and Taylor, 2009). Other data indicate that the sodium content in sweat is lower in Africans, indicating the existence of a more efficient electrolyte conservation system in Africans (Badreshia-Bansal and Taylor, 2009). It has been reported that apocrine glands, sweat glands that are a combination of apocrine and eccrine glands, are more abundant in the facial skin of blacks compared to whites (Montagna and Carlisle, 1991). The significance of these findings, if any, awaits more comprehensive study.

Sensation

Nerve receptors located in the skin are sensitive to pain, touch, temperature, and pressure. Nerve fibers are located in the dermis and throughout the epidermis. Nerve structures in the skin originate from the neural crest and are detectable in the developing embryo at approximately 5 weeks' gestation. When stimulated, these receptors transmit impulses to the cerebral cortex where they are interpreted. Combinations of the four basic types of sensations result in burning, tickling, and itching (Jacob et al, 1982). These sensations are propagated by unmyelinated free nerve endings, Merkel cells, Meissner corpuscles, Krause end bulbs, Ruffini terminals, and pacinian corpuscles. Identification of particular responses with specific nerve structures has not been successful, in part because some receptors seem to respond to a variety of stimuli. However, Meissner corpuscles are involved in touch reception; pacinian corpuscles (see Figure 3-1) respond to pressure, coarse touch, vibration, and tension; and free nerve endings respond to touch, pain, and temperature (Wheater et al, 1987). Merkel cells are instrumental in propagating light sensory touch in the skin (Maricich et al, 2009) and are distributed in the rete ridges among basal keratinocytes. They can be identified in association with hair follicles, digits, lips, and regions of the oral cavity.

Skin sensation is a part of the body's integrative response to protect itself from the surrounding environment. Sensation assists with the skin's regulatory function and can signal sweating, shivering, weight shifts (Parish et al, 2007), laughter, and scratching.

Merkel cells function as mechanoreceptors. In the epidermis these cells produce nerve growth factor, whereas in the dermis, Merkel cells express receptors for nerve growth factor (Narasawa et al, 1992). Merkel cells are found around the arrector pili muscle in the bulge region of hair follicles and contribute to the development of eccrine sweat glands, nails, and nerves of the skin (Boulais and Misery, 2008; Kim and Holbrook, 1995; Narasawa et al, 1996).

Sensation also moderates the psychobiologic phenomena made famous by Harlow, (Harlow and Zimmermann, 1959; van der Horst et al, 2008) who demonstrated the preference of young animals for objects that were warm and those that provided better tactile sensitivity. In addition, early studies by Spitz (1947) point to the importance of touch in mediating social interactions with children and infants. Deprivation of touch can lead to psychomotor retardation and increased risk of death (Ottenbacher et al, 1987). Stroking, handling, talking, and playing resulted in a 60% decrease in aortic atherosclerotic lesions (Nerem et al, 1980), even though study groups had the same cholesterol-containing diet, blood pressures, heart rates, and serum cholesterol levels.

In healing wounds, sensory nerves sprout abundantly for about the first 3 weeks, then return to their normal density. The role of neuropeptides in stimulating growth of connective tissue is increasingly being recognized. This includes a role for these neuropeptides in modulating matrix production by fibroblasts and in acting as growth factors for keratinocytes (Baraniuk, 1997; Kiss et al, 1995; Metze and Luger, 2001).

Metabolism

Synthesis of vitamin D in the skin occurs in the presence of sunlight. UVR converts a sterol (7-dehydrocholesterol) to cholecalciferol (vitamin D). Vitamin D participates in calcium and phosphate metabolism and is important in the mineralization of bone. Because vitamin D is synthesized in the skin but then transmitted to other parts of the body, it is considered an active hormone when converted to calcitriol (1,25-dihydroxycholecalciferol) (Lehninger,

1982; Stryer, 1995). Synthesis of vitamin D is higher in lightly pigmented skin and lower in darkly pigmented skin (Badreshia-Bansal and Taylor, 2009; Wilkins et al, 2009), a condition that may have implications for mood and cognitive status (Wilkins et al, 2009) and for protection against cardiovascular disease, diabetes, and some cancers (Harris, 2006). On the other hand, the reduced level of vitamin D in darkly pigmented skin does not seem to be associated with a higher level of osteoporotic fractures (Harris, 2006). Consequently, clinicians are being encouraged to promote an increased level of vitamin D intake, especially among individuals with darkly pigmented skin (Harris, 2006; Wilkins et al, 2009).

Communication

In addition to its biologic, structural, functional, and physiologic functions, human skin functions as an organ of communication and identification. The skin over the face is especially important for identification of a person and plays a role in internal and external assessments of beauty. Injury to the skin can result not only in functional and physiologic consequences but also in changes in body image. Scarring from trauma, surgery, or incisions can lead to changes in clothing choices, avoidance of public exposure, and decreased self-esteem. Research (Koblenzer, 2005; Shuster et al, 1978) indicates that self-image is progressively reduced with increased scarring from facial acne. Adolescents are especially sensitive to physical appearance (Bernstein, 1976; Van Loey and Van Son, 2003). As an organ of communication, facial skin along with underlying muscles is capable of expressions such as smiling, frowning, and pouting. The sensation of touching can convey feelings of comfort, concern, friendship, and love.

FACTORS ALTERING SKIN CHARACTERISTICS

Many factors alter the normal characteristics of the skin: age, sun, hydration, soaps, nutrition, smoking, and medications. Although normal age-related changes in the skin cannot yet be changed, the effects of the other variables that impact the skin can be modified or prevented.

Age

The aging process is associated with numerous morphologic and functional changes in the skin (Tables 3-1 and 3-2). Distinctive differences exist in fetuses, premature infants (23 to 32 weeks' gestation), full-term newborns, adults, and older adults. By the midcentury of 2030, approximately one in five Americans will be 65 years or older (US Census Bureau, 2008); therefore, understanding age-related changes in the skin is important for all

health care providers in any health care setting so that complications can be averted.

At birth the skin and nails are thinner in the newborn than in the adult, but with aging they gradually increase in thickness. Formation of the epidermal and dermal layers occurs within the first 2 weeks of embryonic development. Epidermal development is complete by the end of the second trimester, and at birth epidermal thickness is almost that of adult skin, although newborn skin is not as effective as adult skin in providing a barrier to transcutaneous water loss. On the other hand, development of the dermis lags behind and does not take on the characteristics of adult dermis until after birth (Chang and Orlow, 2008).

A key feature of fetal tissue that has come under more intense investigation is its ability for scarless healing (Longaker et al, 1990; Siebert et al, 1990). Until 120 days of gestation, wounds in the fetal lamb heal without scarring. Differences in chemical composition and growth factor concentrations of fetal skin contribute to its capacity for scarless healing and are summarized in Box 3-2 (Bullard et al, 2003; Longaker et al, 1990). An understanding of the factors that contribute to the phenomenon may lead to the achievement of scarless healing in adults. For example, in the laboratory setting, topical application of hyaluronic acid has been associated with a reduction in scar formation in postnatal wounds.

At birth the skin and nails are thinner than those in an adult, but with aging they will gradually increase in thickness. Formation of the epidermal and dermal layers occurs within the first 2 weeks of embryonic development. Epidermal development is complete by the end of the second trimester, and at birth, epidermal thickness is almost that of adult skin, although newborn skin is not as effective as adult skin in providing a barrier to transcutaneous water loss. On the other hand, development of the dermis lags behind and does not take on the characteristics of adult dermis until after birth. Until about 6 months of age, the ratio of type I to type III collagen is similar to that in the fetus; soluble collagen is approximately 24%, compared with 1% in the adult.

Immature skin, or skin from premature infants between 23 or 24 weeks' and up to 32 weeks' gestation, requires special attention compared with that of infants beyond 32 weeks' gestation. In particular, before 28 weeks' gestation the skin is thin and poorly keratinized and functions weakly as a barrier. An article appearing in Lancet (Immature skin, 1989) has characterized the skin of infants born at the limits of viability as more suitable to an "aquatic environment" than to atmospheric conditions. Transepidermal water loss is high, and application of adhesives to the outer immature epidermal layer can leave behind raw, damaged skin prone to infection and occasional scarring. At 24 weeks' gestation, transepidermal water loss can be 10 times greater per unit area compared with an infant born at term (Rutter, 1996).

(Text continues on page 56.)

TABLE 3-1 Morphologic Differences in Skin at Various Ages

	Premature Newborn	Term Newborn	Adult	Aged
Skin thickness (total)	Approximately 50% of adult Higher surface to weight ratio Approximately 13% of body weight	Approximately 70% of adult Higher surface to weight ratio	Full thickness Approximately 3% of body weight	Approximately 65%–70% of adult
Periderm	Present up to approximately 120 days	Absent	Absent	Absent
Epidermis	Thinner (2–3 cells thick) Stratum corneum absent until 2–4 weeks after air exposure Melanin production absent/low Immature junctional integrity Fewer desmosomes Immature keratin filament bundles	Equivalent to smaller adult, more uniform cell size Reduced melanin production Vernix caseosa present Immature melanin granule formation	Mature stratum corneum Junctional integrity Immune cells and melanin production relative to skin phototype	Epidermal thinning is minimal (10%–50%) Increased corneocyte surface area Decreased number of active melanocytes by 10%–20% each decade Increased time for epidermal turnover Loss of epidermal stem cell population Progressive reduction in moles from 15–40 in the 30s to 4 at 60–80 years Increase in apoptosis below granular layer
Dermal-epidermal junction	Flat Absent to few rete pegs/dermal papillae before 34 weeks with immature hemidesmosomes	Rete ridges only weakly developed at birth	Mature with full junctional integrity	Flat with loss of rete pegs/dermal papillae
Dermis	Thin Higher type I to type III collagen ratio Approximately 24% soluble collagen compared to 1% in the adult Smaller, more uniform collagen fibers/fiber bundles in both papillary and reticular dermis High amount of hyaluronic acid Higher water content More immature elastin fiber bundles Fibroblasts more abundant in reticular dermis	Thinner (approximately 60% of adult) Much higher cellular component compared with mature adult skin Higher type I to type III collagen ratio persists Collagen development continues up to 3–6 months postnatally Smaller, finer collagen fiber bundles Some immature elastin fiber bundles become mature at approximately 3 years Fibroblasts more abundant in reticular dermis	Mature array of collagen and elastin fibers Larger, denser collagen fiber bundles in reticular dermis 1% of collagen is soluble Elastin fibers mature in size, distribution Fibroblasts more abundant in papillary dermis Level of advanced glycation end-products begins to increase around age 35 years	Approximately 20% loss of dermal thickness (1% reduction each year) Increase in size, number, diameter of elastic fibers Decrease in elastin synthesis Decrease in number of fibroblasts Decrease in synthesis and turnover of collagen types I and III Increase in collagen cross-linking Slight decrease in levels of hyaluronic acid, glycosaminoglycans, proteoglycans Increased matrix metalloproteinase expression Increase in advanced glycation end-products

Subcutaneous	No/little subcutaneous tissue	Thinner subcutaneous tissue	Mature subcutaneous tissue	Contraction of septae in subcutaneous fat; Loss of subcutaneous fat; Changes more dramatic in papillary than reticular dermis
Vasculature	Capillary beds not organized; Poor/reduced vasoconstriction/vasodilation of cutaneous vessels	Capillary beds not completely organized, continues up to 14–17 weeks postnatally	Mature organization of cutaneous vessels in papillary and reticular dermis	Approximately 30% reduction in venular cross-sections; Approximately 60% reduction in peak cutaneous blood circulation; Reduced vascular response; Up to 50% reduction in vascular wall thickness at age 80 years; Decreased vasoconstriction/vasodilation arteriole response; Decrease in vascular endothelial growth factor; Decreased endothelial cell permeability response
Innervation/sensation	Meissner corpuscles not fully developed; Nervous network not as organized; Axon flare response attenuated	Meissner corpuscles not fully developed; Axon reflex muted	Mature complement of Meissner and pacinian corpuscles	Reduced number of pacinian and Meissner corpuscles to one third that in adult; Pain threshold increases up to 20%
Apocrine glands	Present	Present	Present and active	Reduction in gland size, function
Immune cells	Decreased immune function	Reduced immune function	Mature immune function	Langerhans cells reduced by 20%–50%; Up to 50% reduction in mast cells; Increase in autoantibodies (bullous pemphigoid, antinuclear antibodies, antithyroglobulin, rheumatoid factor)
Eccrine glands	Structure present by 24–29 weeks but not responsive until 36 weeks, with cells more undifferentiated	Structure present but not responsive for 1 to several days after birth, with complete neural control by age 2–3 years		15% reduction in number of glands, with 70% reduction in sweating

Continued

TABLE 3-1	Morphologic Differences in Skin at Various Ages—cont'd			
	Premature Newborn	Term Newborn	Adult	Aged
Sebaceous glands	Large and active	Large and active but decreased in size, activity Sebum composition different from adult	Increased estrogen and androgens at puberty Increase activity of pilosebaceous glands	Decreased sebum production by approximately 65%, but number and size remain similar to adult
Hair	Lanugo hair may be present	Vellus and terminal hair present	Axillary and pubic hair appear at puberty	Reduced hair follicle density Reduced/absent hair follicle melanocyte activity Increased time for hair growth Up to approximately 50% gray/white hair by age 50 years 20% decrease in number of hair follicles by 60 years Reduction in hair diameter Bitemporal hair line recession in both genders Increased baldness in at-risk individuals

Ig, Immunoglobulin; *TEWL,* transepidermal water loss.

Data for this chart compiled from the following resources; complete references provided at end of chapter.
Braverman, 1986; Bullard et al, 2003; Evans and Rutter, 1986; Gilchrest, 1989; Gilchrest, 1991; Gilchrest et al, 1982; Harpin and Rutter, 1983; Holbrook, 1991; Kalia et al, 1998; Lavker et al, 1986; Lin and Carter, 1986; Longaker et al, 1990; Metze and Luger, 2001; Nordlund, 1986; Rutter, 1988; Sauder, 1986; Silverberg and Silverberg, 1989; Varani et al, 2006; Yaar and Gilchrest, 2007; Yanagishita, 1994

TABLE 3-2	Functional Differences in Skin Among Premature Newborn, Term Newborn, Adult, and Aged			
	Premature Newborn	**Newborn**	**Adult**	**Aged**
Protection	Highly permeable TEWL 10 times higher at 24 weeks of prematurity TEWL up to 100 g/m²/hr Skin maturation may require up to 5–7 weeks Higher surface to body weight ratio leading to greater absorption and toxicity from topical agents Excessive fluid loss and risk of hypernatremia Low melanin production leading to increased sunburn risk Increased risk of bacterial invasion Increased risk of trauma up to 15% or more of body surface area from monitor probes, rubbing, tape stripping Higher pH becomes more acidic over time (up to 8 days or more) Stratum corneum hydration higher than newborn or adult	Somewhat permeable leading to increased risk of toxicity from topical agents TEWL 6–8 g/m²/hr More readily sunburns Active sebaceous glands due to maternal hormone exposure Sebum secretion higher at birth than at 6 months Slightly higher pH compared to adult that stabilizes over 2 days Reduced stratum corneum hydration initially	Mature barrier function with good resistance to penetration Protection from UV radiation related to skin phototype	Decreased barrier function Delayed barrier recovery of stratum corneum Dry, flaky stratum corneum Higher pH (≈5.0 vs 4.5) at 80+ years (increased risk of infection) Decline in lipid content Decline in sebum production Loss of UV protection due to decrease in melanocyte activity Delayed wound healing Increased risk of mechanical injury (i.e., skin tears) Decrease in skin turgor Higher risk of premalignant and malignant lesions
Immune	Antimicrobial peptides (dermcidin, LL-37) in sweat absent Decreased IgG, IgM Reduced neutrophil chemotaxis and neutrophil phagocytosis Decreased T lymphocytes			Muted allergic and contact reactions Decreased inflammatory reaction Sun-protected skin more reactive than sun-exposed skin Impaired humoral/cell-mediated immunity Decreased DNA repair capacity Increased oncogene activation
Sensation	Sensory nerve endings present and functioning			Decreased/delayed sensory perception Increased risk of burn injury 20% increase in radiant pain threshold
Metabolism	Immature metabolism Oxygen absorption and carbon dioxide excretion 6–11 times higher before 30 weeks but upon air exposure for 2–3 weeks approaches that of adult		Vitamin D production peaks with decreased synthesis depending on skin phototype	Decreased metabolism Reduced vitamin D production contributing to osteoporosis, diabetes, hypertension, tumor formation Decreased clearance of transepidermal substances Increased UV-induced reactive oxygen species damage
Thermoregulation	High risk of hypothermia Reduced/no sweating for up to 24 days Compromised ability to regulate body temperature requires humidified thermal incubator Evaporative heat loss can exceed resting heat production	Reduced sweating for up to 5 days	Full sweating capability	Loss of ability to control/maintain body temperature when exposed to cold or excessive heat by vasoconstriction, vasodilation, shunting

TEWL, Transepidermal water loss; *UV,* ultraviolet.

BOX 3-2	Unique Characteristics of Fetal Skin

- Collagen deposition occurs more rapidly (Longaker et al, 1990)
- Collagen deposition follows normal dermal pattern (Longaker et al, 1990)
- Approximately 30%–60% of collagen is type III (10%–15% in adult skin) (Bullard et al, 2003)
- Higher concentrations of hyaluronic acid than in adult (Siebert et al, 1990)
- Less TGF-β1 in fetal wounds (Roberts and Sporn, 1996)
- Differential patterns of expression of various isoforms of TGF-β in fetal wounds
- Difference in cell responses
  - Decrease in inflammatory cells, particularly polymorphonuclear leukocytes and macrophage
  - Platelets do not aggregate in response to collagen
  - Platelets do not release same amount of TGF-β1 and platelet-derived endothelial growth factor-AB as adult cells
  - Fibroblasts can migrate at faster rate
  - Fibroblasts synthesize more total collagen
- Differences in protease and inhibitor activity, level of growth factors, and expression of homeobox genes detected (Bullard et al, 2003)

TGF, Transforming growth factor.

Infants born between 22 and 25 weeks' gestation may require up to 4 weeks to develop a functional stratum corneum (Evans and Rutter, 1986; Harpin and Rutter, 1983; Kalia et al, 1998; Rutter, 1996). In addition, premature infants have high evaporative heat losses that result in increased risk for hypothermia.

Because premature infants have a greater surface-area-to-volume ratio compared with full-term infants, they are at an increased risk for skin complications and systemic toxicity from topically applied agents. These infants may also have alterations in metabolism, excretion, distribution, and protein binding of chemical agents, placing them at increased risk for local or systemic toxicity from soaps, lotions, or other topical agents (Weston and Lane, 1999). Other dangers are percutaneous absorption of topical agents, including antiseptics. Hemorrhagic necrosis of the dermis from alcohol absorption has been reported, if the alcohol does not quickly evaporate, and is sometimes mistaken for bruising. The use of topical antibiotic sprays containing neomycin should be avoided since it is an ototoxic aminoglycoside. Thus water-based topical antiseptics are preferred but should be used sparingly. Cleaning should be done with care, using normal saline or water. Chlorhexidine, a commonly used antiseptic, is not known to have any adverse effects, but it is probably absorbed from the skin and should be used judiciously. Likewise iodine has been reported to be absorbed, leading to goiter and hypothyroidism (Rutter, 1988). If required, moisturizing creams or ointments may be applied to dry, flaking, or fissured skin, and the best agents appear to be those with few or no preservatives since these offer the greatest benefit with decreased risk (Weston and Lane, 1999). Other topical agents that can place the premature or neonate at risk are aniline dyes (methemoglobinemia), hexachlorophene (neurotoxicity), corticosteroids (adrenal suppression), lidocaine-prilocaine cream or EMLA (methemoglobinemia, seizures, petechiae), N,N-dimethyl-meta-toluamide or DEET (neurotoxicity), salicylates (salicylism, metabolic acidosis, encephalopathy), and silver sulfadiazine (kernicterus, agranulocytosis) (Mancini, 2004).

The next period of change occurs in adolescence, when hormonal stimulation results in increased activity of sebaceous glands and hair follicles. Sebaceous glands increase their secretory rate, and hair follicles become activated, giving rise to secondary sexual characteristics. From adolescence to adulthood there is a gradual change in skin characteristics. By the time the skin reaches mature adulthood, several changes become apparent. The dermis decreases in thickness by about 20%, whereas the epidermis remains relatively unchanged. Epidermal turnover time is increased; this means that wound healing may take longer. For instance, in young adults, epidermal turnover takes about 21 days, but by 35 years of age this turnover time is doubled. Barrier function is reduced, and such reduction may increase the risk of irritation. The number of active melanocytes per unit body surface area decreases with aging, which means that protection against UVR is diminished. However, across the lifespan, darker skin offers greater protection against photoaging or dermatoheliosis (Miyamura et al, 2006). Skin dryness is also associated with aging and an increase in wrinkles. Sensory receptors are diminished in capacity, meaning that the skin is more likely to be burned or traumatized without perception. Vitamin D production is decreased and may be a factor in osteomalacia.

With aging there is a decrease in the number of Langerhans' cells, which affects the immunocompetence of the skin and can lead to an increased risk of skin cancer and infection by invading microorganisms. The density of Langerhans' cells changes from 10 per 3 mm cross-section of unexposed skin in 22- to 26-year-old persons to 5.8 per 3 mm cross-section in 62- to 68-year-old persons (Gilchrest et al, 1982). There is also a decrease in the numbers of mast cells and melanocytes. The inflammatory response is decreased, and such a decrease may alter allergic reactions and healing. A decrease in the number of sweat glands, diminished vascularity, and a reduction in the amount of subcutaneous fat compromise the thermoregulatory capacity of the skin. Epidermal-dermal junction changes, such as the flattening of the prominent dermal papillae and of the rete ridges, alter junctional integrity. Consequently, the skin is more easily torn in response to mechanical trauma, especially shearing forces. Because the epidermal rete pegs flatten, the unique microenvironment of the basal keratinocytes changes; it is thought that this explains the decrease in epidermal proliferative capacity that occurs with aging (Lavker et al, 1986).

Skin elasticity decreases with age and is related to a combination of aging and solar damage. Microscopic analysis of collagen and elastin fibers reveals that these are more compact, with a loss of ground substance from the spaces between these cablelike structures. Collagen fibers appear to be unwinding whereas elastin fibers appear to be lysing. The degradation of elastin can be detected at about 30 years of age but becomes marked at 70 years of age (Braverman, 1986). Changes in dermal proteoglycans usually occur after 40 years of age (Yanagishita, 1994). By 70 years of age, most of the elastin network is affected. Changes in collagen content and structure are mediated by an under-expression of procollagen, an over-expression of collagenase (MMP-1), stromelysin (MMP-3), and gelatinase A (MMP-2), and a decreased expression of tissue inhibitors of matrix metalloproteinase-1 (TIMP-1). Fibroblasts in aged skin have a reduced abilty to synthesize collagen Type I and Type III and collagen fragments further reduce the ability of fibroblasts to synthesize new collagen. In addition, fibroblasts in young adult skin have a higher amount of their cell surface in contact with collagen and exhibit more extensive cell spreading compared to fibroblasts in old skin (Varani et al, 2006). There is also a marked reduction in vascular beds in the vertical capillary loops in the dermal papillae. There is an approximately 35% decrease in the cross-sectional area of these loops in aged skin. It is thought that this leads to atrophy of the hair bulbs, the sweat glands, and the sebaceous glands. Because the hypodermis also becomes thinner, mature individuals are more prone to pressure necrosis (Gilchrest, 1989). With aging, a progressive loss of mechanoreceptors to one third of their average density occurs from the second to the ninth decade (Metze and Luger, 2001).

The density of skin melanocytes is relatively constant until about 40 years of age. By about 45 years of age, skin melanocytes have decreased in density to approximately half that seen between 30 and 39 years of age (Nordlund, 1986). Melanocytes decrease 6% to 8% each decade after age 30. It is thought that the loss of skin melanocytes contributes to an increase in the formation of skin cancers. Other overt changes are wrinkling and sagging, which occur as a result of the loss of underlying tissue, in addition to changes seen in collagen and elastin.

Changes in hair color and hair follicles also accompany aging. Age-related changes in active melanocytes result in gray hair. About 50% of the body's hair will be gray by the age of 50 in about 50% of the population. This change is accompanied by a reduction in the number of hair follicles and a decrease in the diameter of the hair. The rate of hair growth is also decreased (Silverberg and Silverberg, 1989). Nail growth rates also decrease by 40% to 50%.

Changes in thermoregulatory capacity occur with age, and older individuals are more prone to hypothermia and heat stroke. This has been attributed to changes in blood capillaries and eccrine sweat glands. In healthy older individuals, sweating may be decreased by up to 70% (Gilchrest, 1991). Sebum secretion also declines with age. Barrier function decreases with aging owing to the decreased level of all the major lipid species, especially ceramides. In addition, corneocytes are larger and less cohesive. In addition to these changes, pain perception is dulled, and there is reduced skin reactivity upon exposure to irritants. Cutaneous immune function also changes with aging, as seen by a reduction in Langerhans' cell density. Skin damaged by sun exposure, or actinically damaged skin, has been found to have a 50% reduction of Langerhans' cell density compared with sun-protected skin (Sauder, 1986). Reduction in immunocompetence of the skin is thought to contribute in part to skin cancer in the elderly.

Other factors that may contribute to the development of skin cancer in aged individuals are cumulative exposure to carcinogens, diminished DNA repair capacity, decreased melanocyte density, and alterations in dermal matrix (Lin and Carter, 1986). Not surprisingly, wound healing in older individuals is delayed compared with that of younger individuals.

Menopausal changes appear to somewhat accelerate skin changes in women where the decreased levels of ciculating levels of estrogen result in a reduction in dermal collagen and elasticity. Other changes include a reduction in dermal hydration, increased dryness and wrinkling. Surface lipids are also reduced due to changes in sebaceous gland function. Changes in estrogen and progesterone affect inflammatory response, keratinocyte prolieration, collagen and hyaluronic acid synthesis, and matrix metalloproteinase activity (Yaar and Gilchrest, 2007).

Sun

Excessive exposure to UVR can have harmful effects that accelerate aging of the skin. For this reason the condition associated with UVR-damaged skin is referred to as *photoaging*. Dermatologically, the condition is called *dermatoheliosis*. Across the lifespan, darker skin offers greater protection against photoaging and dermatoheliosis (Miyamura et al, 2006). Obvious clinical signs of photodamaged skin are dryness, tough and leathery texture, wrinkling as a result of collagen and elastin degeneration, and irregular pigmentation from changes in melanin distribution (Box 3-3) (Silverberg and Silverberg, 1989; Young and Walker, 2008). Excessive exposure to UVR increases the risk of developing skin cancers such as basal or squamous cell carcinoma and malignant melanoma, especially in white or lightly pigmented skin. Damage to the DNA of skin cells leads to transformation of cells and cancer (Council on Scientific Affairs, 1989). Changes also occur in epidermal and dermal cells. Epidermal cells become thickened (Varani et al, 2006) and more numerous, and dermal vessels become dilated

---

BOX 3-3	Photoaging Effects on Skin Characteristics

- Hyperkeratosis
- Atrophy
- Leathery appearance, especially in lighter skin phototypes
- Melanosomes may be increased with increase in dopa-positive melanocytes up to twofold
- Telangiectasia
- Further elastogenesis/degeneration accompanied by mass accumulations
- Increased lysozyme deposition on elastic fibers
- Decreased amounts of mature collagen
- Further increased matrix metalloproteinase activity
- Presence of hyperplastic fibroblasts
- Perivascular infiltrate of lymphocytes, histiocytes, mononuclear cells, mast cells
- Prominent grenz zone (a zone of normal appearing dermis just below the epidermis, but below this normal appearing zone is abnormal dermis)
- Glycosaminoglycans and proteoglycans increase
- Reduction in vascular circulation
- Venule wall thickening
- Further reduction in number of Langerhans cells
- More infiltrating mononuclear cells present
- Increased $CD4^+$ T cells

---

and tortuous. Langerhans cells are reduced in number by approximately 50%, thereby diminishing the immunocompetence of the skin (Lober and Fenske, 1990).

Exposure to excessive UVR results in the production of reactive oxygen species that lead to activation of several cell surface receptors such as interleukin-1, epidermal growth factor, and keratinocyte growth factor, which signal the induction of the nuclear transcription complex AP-1. The AP-1 complex blocks synthesis of collagen I and III by suppressing expression of transforming growth factor-β. These same reactive oxygen species lead to damage of the lipid cell membrane, which results in release of prostaglandins that are responsible for mediating inflammatory reactions (Yaar and Gilchrest, 2007). Together these processes can create a pattern of heightened inflammation that is responsible for the net degradation of collagen tissue by the activation and overexpression of matrix metalloproteinases (MMPs), particularly MMP-1, MMP-3, MMP-8, and MMP-9. Other cell-mediated damage results from damage to mitochondrial DNA, protein oxidation, especially in the upper dermis, and telomere shortening (Yaar and Gilchrest, 2007).

The effects of reactive oxygen species in aged skin are not effectively countered by the presence of the naturally occurring antioxidant enzymes, such as catalase, superoxide dismutase, and glutathione peroxidase, and nonenzymatic molecules such as coenzyme Q10, ascorbate or vitamin C, tocopherol or vitamin E, and carotenoids, which are present at higher levels in young adult skin. Over the last decade the study of the reactive oxygen

species system and its role in skin damage has resulted in use of various antioxidants in topical sunscreens and cosmetics. Among the antioxidants used are tocopherol acetate, stable forms of vitamin C, vitamin E, polyphenolic molecules such as procyanidin and flavonoids, curcumin, genistein (found in soybeans), and resveratrol (found in red wine, nuts, and grapefruit) (Yaar and Gilchrist, 2007). Other agents that have been investigated or are being used to reverse the effects of photodamaged skin include dietary lipids such as omega-3 fatty acids and eicosapentaenoic acid, osmolytes, and α-hydroxy acids derived from fruit, sugar cane, and dairy products. Retinoids have been used since the 1980s to abrogate the effects of sun damage that can be seen visually and histologically. More recently retinoids have been used as a pretreatment approach (Yaar and Gilchrest, 2007).

Exposure to UVR can lead to sunburn. Sunburn is partly the result of a vasodilatory response that increases blood volume. Whether an individual will become sunburned depends on the extent of skin pigmentation. Naturally, those with the least pigmentation are more prone to sunburn and the harmful, long-term effects of UVR. Severe short-term exposure of unprotected, lightly pigmented skin can lead to blistering (a second-degree burn).

There is an association between melanoma and sunburn. An individual who has sustained more than six serious sunburns is at increased risk for melanoma (Green et al, 1985). Exposure to UVR and the rise of malignant melanomas have led to the development of more effective sun-blocking agents. Over time the lifetime risk of malignant melanoma has increased from 1:1,500 people in 1930 to 1:250 in 1980 to 1:62 in 2005, and as of 2010 it is expected to be 1:50 (Potts, 1990; Rigel et al, 2005). Sunscreens should be used on a regular basis, applied at least 30 minutes before sun exposure, and have a sun protection factor (SPF) ranging from 15 to 30 (Pathak et al, 1999). Individuals with moderately pigmented skin require about three to five times more exposure to UVR to induce sunburn inflammation compared with Caucasians; individuals with darker skin require 10 times more exposure (McGregor and Hawk, 1999; Young and Walker, 2008). The age-adjusted incidence rates for melanoma have been reported as 1.0 per 100,000 for blacks versus 4.5 for Hispanics and 21.6 for white non-Hispanics (Rouhani et al, 2008).

Hydration

Adequate skin hydration is normally provided by sebum secretion and an intact stratum corneum with its keratinized cells. Several factors can affect skin hydration, including relative humidity, removal of sebum, and age. Each of these factors increases water loss from the skin, leading to dryness and scaling. Application of emollients to the skin replaces the barrier function of lost sebum or decreased evaporative water loss when the relative humidity is low. Retention of water in the epidermal layers after application of a lotion leads to swelling of the skin, which is perceived as smoothness and softness.

Various products often are promoted with claims of superiority over other products without adequate in vitro, in vivo, or clinical data. The superiority of oil baths over water baths was found to be only marginal (Stender et al, 1990). Twenty minutes after both kinds of bath, skin hydration was increased when measured by water evaporation and electrical conductance and capacitance. A small but significantly greater amount of water was bound in the skin after the oil bath, but no change was seen in evaporation, conductance, or capacitance. Thus, increases in water-holding capacity of the skin after an oil bath may not be of importance. However, a difference in skin-surface lipids was found, and the difference lasted at least 3 hours. This effect is comparable to that seen with application of a traditional moisturizing lotion. The authors of the study concluded that because daily use of bath oil is not practical, application of moisturizing lotions may be more advantageous, and the beneficial effects of bath oils are related to lipidization of the skin surface (Stender et al, 1990).

Soaps

Washing or bathing with an alkaline soap reduces the thickness and number of cell layers in the stratum corneum (White et al, 1987). Generally, soap emulsifies the lipid coating of the skin and removes it, along with resident and transient bacteria. Excessive use of soap or detergents can interfere with the water-holding capacity of the skin and may impair bacterial resistance. Use of alkaline soaps increases skin pH, which may change bacterial resistance. The time for recovery to normal skin pH of 5.5 depends on the length of exposure. Ordinary washing requires 45 minutes to restore skin pH, whereas prolonged exposure can require 19 hours (Bettley, 1960). Other agents that can lead to delipidization or dehydration of skin are alcohol and acetone. Currently, acidic skin cleansers appear to be less irritating than neutral or alkaline cleansers, and some evidence suggests that acidic cleansers decrease the number of acne lesions on the face (Korting and Braun-Falco, 1996).

Nutrition

Normal, healthy skin integrity can be maintained by adequate dietary intake of protein, carbohydrate, fats, vitamins, and minerals. Under normal conditions in healthy persons, supplementary nutrition is not beneficial if dietary intake is adequate. If the skin is damaged, increased dietary intake of some substances, such as vitamin C for collagen formation, may be beneficial. A healthy diet of protein supplies the necessary amino acids for protein synthesis. Fats are broken down into

essential fatty acids, which cells can use to form their lipid bilayer. Carbohydrates are digested to supply energy for cell metabolism. Maintenance of normal, healthy skin requires ingestion of the following: vitamins C, D, and A; the B vitamins pyridoxine and riboflavin; the mineral elements iron, zinc, and copper; and many others. Adequate dietary intake can be ensured by ingestion of amounts consistent with the recommended daily allowances (RDAs) (Boelsma et al, 2001; Roe, 1986).

Smoking

Smoking decreases capillary blood flow and changes the oxygen gradient in skin via its vasoconstrictive effects. Data indicate that the dermis in smokers has a reduced level of collagen and elastin fibers leading to tissue that is less elastic and hardened. Epidermal effects include keratinocyte dysplasia, telangiectasias, roughness, and excessive wrinkling (Kennedy et al, 2003; Leow and Maibach, 1998). Furthermore, a dose–response effect of smoking and wrinkle formation has been identified (Kennedy et al, 2003).

Medications

Various medications affect the skin, and the prevalence rate of skin reactions to medications in hospitalized individuals is 2% to 3% (Ramdial and Naidoo, 2009; Gerson et al, 2008). Some of the best studied medications are the corticosteroids, which interfere with epidermal regeneration and collagen synthesis (Ehrlich and Hunt, 1968; Pollack, 1982; Ramdial and Naidoo, 2009; Wicke et al, 2000). Medications also cause photosensitive and phototoxic reactions. Some categories of medications that can affect the skin are antibacterials, antihypertensives, analgesics, tricyclic antidepressants, antihistamines, antineoplastic agents, antipsychotic drugs, diuretics, hypoglycemic agents, sunscreens, and oral contraceptives (Potts, 1990; Ramdial and Naidoo, 2009). Skin eruptions have been more frequently reported for antibiotics, antiepileptics, antiarrhythmic, and anticoagulants (Gerson et al, 2008). Skin flora can be changed by the use of antibacterials, orally administered steroids, and hormones. Analgesics, antihistamines, and nonsteroidal antiinflammatory drugs can alter inflammatory reactions. Thus, whenever drugs are prescribed and skin reactions occur, medications should always be checked to determine whether they are responsible.

SUMMARY

As the body's largest organ, the skin serves several complex functions: protection, thermoregulation, sensation, metabolism, and communication. Numerous factors that influence the skin's ability to adequately provide these functions are age, UVR exposure, hydration, medications, nutrition, and soaps. The skin's integrity also can be jeopardized by many of these factors.

Wound management and skin care must be grounded in a comprehensive knowledge base of the structure and function of the skin. After reviewing this chapter, the care provider should closely scrutinize many of the skin care practices and bathing routines that are subconsciously engrained in day-to-day patient care activities and that may compromise the function and integrity of the skin.

REFERENCES

Auger MJ: Mononuclear phagocytes, *BMJ* 298:546, 1989.
Badreshia-Bansal S, Taylor SC: The structure and function of skin of color. In Kelly AP, Taylor SC, editors: *Dermatology for skin of color*, New York, 2009, McGraw Hill.
Baraniuk JN: Neuropeptides in the skin. In Bos JD, editor: *The skin immune system*, ed 2, Boca Raton, 1997, CRC Press.
Benyon RC: The human skin mast cell, *Clin Exp Allergy* 19:375, 1989.
Bergstresser PR, Toews GB, Streilein JW: Natural and perturbed distributions of Langerhans cells: responses to ultraviolet light, heterotopic skin grafting, and dinitrofluorobenzene sensitization, *J Invest Dermatol* 75:73, 1980.
Bernstein NR: Appearance: concepts of perception and disfigurement; Body and face images: personality and self-representation; Disfigurement and personality development. In Bernstein NR: *Emotional care of the facially burned and disfigured*, Boston, 1976, Little, Brown.
Bettley FR: Some effects of soap on the skin, *BMJ* 1:1675, 1960.
Bickenbach JR: Identification and behavior of label-retaining cells in oral mucosa and skin, *J Dent Res* 60:1611, 1981.
Boelsma E et al: Nutritional skin care: health effects of micronutrients and fatty acids, *Am J Clin Nutr* 73(5):853-864, 2001.
Boissy RE: Melanosome transfer to and translocation in the keratinocyte, *Exp Dermatol* 12(Suppl 2):5-12, 2003.
Boulais N, Misery L: The epidermis: a sensory tissue, *Eur J Dermatol* 18:119-127, 2008.
Braverman IM: Elastic fiber and microvascular abnormalities in aging skin. In Gilchrest BA, editor: The aging skin, *Dermatol Clin* 4:391, 1986.
Briggamann RA: Epidermal-dermal interaction in adult skin, *J Invest Dermatol* 88:569, 1982.
Bullard KM et al: Fetal wound healing: current biology, *World J Surg* 27:54, 2003.
Chang HY et al: Diversity, topographic differentiation, and positional memory in human fibroblasts, *Proc Natl Acad Sci U S A* 99(20):12877-12882, 2002.
Chang MW, Orlow SJ: Neonatal, pediatric and adolescent dermatology. In Wolff K et al, editors: *Fitzpatrick's dermatology in general medicine*, ed 7, New York, 2008, McGraw-Hill Medical.
Chu DH: Development and structure of skin. In Wolff K et al, editors: *Fitzpatrick's dermatology in general medicine*, ed 7, New York, 2008, McGraw-Hill Medical.
Costerton JW et al: Microbial biofilms, *Annu Rev Microbiol* 49:711, 1995.
Costerton JW et al: Bacterial biofilms: a common cause of persistent infections, *Science* 284:1318, 1999.
Council on Scientific Affairs: Harmful effects of ultraviolet radiation, *JAMA* 262:380, 1989.
DeLeo VA et al: The effect of race and ethnicity on patch test results, *J Am Acad Dermatol* 46:S107, 2002.
Ehrlich HP, Hunt TK: Effects of cortisone and vitamin A on wound healing, *Ann Surg* 167:324, 1968.

Evans NJ, Rutter N: Development of the epidermis in the newborn, *Biol Neonate* 49:74, 1986
Fitzpatrick TB: The validity and practicality of sun-reactive skin types I through IV, *Arch Dermatol* 124:869m 1988.
Freinkel RK: Hair. In Freinkel RK, Woodley DT, editors: *The biology of the skin*, New York, 2001, Parthenon Publishing Group.
Gay S, Miller S: *Collagen in the physiology and pathology of connective tissue*, Stuttgart, Germany, 1978, Gustav Fischer Verlag.
Gerson D et al: Cutaneous drug eruptions: a 5-year experience, *J Am Acad Dermatol* 59:995, 2008.
Gilchrest BA: Skin aging and photoaging, *J Am Acad Dermatol* 21:610, 1989.
Gilchrest BA: Physiology and pathophysiology of aging skin. In Goldsmith LA, editor: *Physiology, biochemistry, and molecular biology of the skin*, ed 2, New York, 1991, Oxford University Press.
Gilchrest BA et al: Effect of chronologic aging and the ultraviolet irradiation on Langerhans cells in human epidermis, *J Invest Dermtol* 79:85, 1982.
Goding CR: Melanocytes: the new Black, *Int J Biochem Cell Biol* 39(2):275-279, 2007.
Graham-Brown R, Burns R: *Lecture notes: dermatology*, ed 9, Oxford, 2007, Blackwell Publishing.
Green A et al: Sunburn and malignant melanoma, *Br J Cancer* 51:393, 1985.
Griffith LG, Naughton G: Tissue engineering—current challenges and expanding opportunities, *Science* 295:1009, 2002.
Haake AR, Holbrook K: The structure and development of skin. In Freedberg IM et al, editors: *Fitzpatrick's dermatology in general medicine*, ed 5, New York, 1999, McGraw-Hill.
Haake A, Scott GA, Holbrook KA: Structure and function of the skin: overview of the epidermis and dermis. In Freinkel RK, Woodley DT, editors: *The biology of the skin*, New York, 2001, Parthenon Publishing Group.
Harlow HF, Zimmermann RR: Affectional responses in the infant monkey, *Science* 130:421-432, 1959.
Harpin VA, Rutter N: Barrier properties of the newborn infant's skin, *J Pediatr* 102:419, 1983.
Harris SS: Vitamin D and African Americans, *J Nutr* 136(4):1126, 2006.
Headington JT: The dermal dendrocyte, *Adv Dermatol* 1:159, 1986.
Headington JT, Cerio R: Dendritic cells and the dermis, *Am J Dermatopathol* 12:217, 1990.
Hoffman JA et al: Phylogenetic perspectives in innate immunity, *Science* 284:1313, 1999.
Holbrook KA: Structure and function of the developing human skin. In Goldsmith LA, editor: *Physiology, biochemistry, and molecular biology of the skin*, ed 2, New York, 1991, Oxford University Press.
Holbrook KA: Melanocytes in human embryonic and fetal skin: a review and new findings, *Pigment Cell Res* 1(Suppl):6, 1998.
Immature skin, *Lancet* 2(8672):1138, 1989.
Jacob SW, Francone CA, Lossow WJ: *Structure and function in man*, ed 5, Philadelphia, 1982, W.B. Saunders.
Kalia VN et al: Development of skin barrier function in premature infants, *J Invest Dermatol* 111:320, 1998.
Kennedy C et al: Effect of smoking and sun on aging skin, *J Invest Dermatol* 120:458, 2003.
Kim DK, Holbrook KA: The appearance, density and distribution of Merkel cells in human embryonic and fetal skin: their relation to sweat glands, and hair follicle development, *J Invest Dermatol* 104:411, 1995.
Kiss M et al: Alpha-melanocyte stimulating hormone induces collagenase/matrix metalloproteinase-1 in human dermal fibroblasts, *Biol Chem Hoppe Seyler* 376:425, 1995.

Koblenzer CS: The emotional impact of chronic and disabling skin disease: a psychoanalytic perspective, *Dermatol Clin* 23(4):619-627, 2005.

Korting HC, Braun-Falco O: The effect of detergents on skin pH and its consequences, *Clin Dermatol* 14(1):23-27, 1996.

La Ruche G, Cesarini JP: [Histology and physiology of black skin], *Annales de Dermatologie et de Venereologie*, 119(8):567-74, 1992.

Lambert MI et al: Ethnicity and temperature regulation, *Med Sport Sci* 53:104, 2008.

Lavker RM, Sun TT: Epidermal stem cells: properties, markers, and location, *Proc Natl Acad Sci U S A* 97(25):13473-13475, 2000.

Lavker RM et al: Morphology of aged skin. In Gilchrest BA, editor: The aging skin, *Dermatol Clin* 4:379, 1986.

Lehninger AL: *Principles of biochemistry*, New York, 1982, Worth Publishers.

Leow YH, Maibach HI: Cigarette smoking, cutaneous vasculature, and tissue oxygen, *Clin Dermatol* 16:579, 1998.

Lin AN, Carter DM: Skin cancer in the elderly, *Dermatol Clin* 4(3):467, 1986.

Lin JY, Fisher DE: Melanocyte biology and skin pigmentation, *Nature* 445:843, 2007.

Lober CW, Fenske NA: Photoaging and the skin: differentiation and clinical response, *Geriatrics* 45:36, 1990.

Longaker MT et al: Studies in fetal wound healing. VI. Second and early third trimester fetal wounds demonstrate rapid collagen deposition without scar formation, *J Pediatr Surg* 25:63, 1990.

Longaker MT et al: Studies in fetal wound healing. VII. Fetal wound healing may be modulated by hyaluronic acid and stimulating activity in amniotic fluid, *J Pediatr Surg* 25:430, 1990.

Mancini AJ: Skin, *Pediatrics* 113:1114, 2004.

Maricich SM et al: Merkel cells are essential for light-touch responses, *Science* 324:1580, 2009.

McDonald CJ: Structure and function of the skin: Are there differences between black and white skin, *Dermatol Clin* 6(3):343, 1988.

McGregor JM, Hawk JLM: Acute effects of ultraviolet radiation on the skin. In Freedberg IM et al, editors: *Fitzpatrick's dermatology in general medicine*, ed 5, New York, 1999, McGraw-Hill.

Metze D, Luger T: Nervous system in the skin. In Freinkel RK, Woodley DT, editors: *The biology of the skin*, New York, 2001, Parthenon Publishing Group.

Millington PF, Wilkinson R: *Skin*, Cambridge, 1983, Cambridge University Press.

Minwalla L et al: Keratinocytes play a role in regulating distribution patterns of recipient melanosomes in vitro, *J Invest Dermatol* 117(2):341-347, 2001.

Miyamura Y et al: Regulation of human skin pigmentation and responses to ultraviolet radiation, *Pigment Cell Res* 20(1):2-13, 2006.

Montagna W, Carlisle K: The architecture of black and white facial skin, *J Am Acad Dermatol* 24:929, 1991.

Montagna W, et al: *Black skin: Structure and function*, San Diego, Academic Press, 1993.

Narasawa Y et al: Biological significance of dermal Merkel cells in development of cutaneous nevus in human fetal skin, *J Histochem Cytochem* 40:65, 1992.

Narasawa Y, Hashimoto K, Kohda H: Merkel cells participate in the induction and alignment of epidermal ends of arrector pili muscles of human fetal skin, *Br J Dermatol* 134:494, 1996.

Nerem RM et al: Social environment as a factor in diet-induced atherosclerosis, *Science* 208:1475, 1980.

Noble WC: *The skin microflora and microbial skin disease*, Cambridge, 2004, Cambridge University Press.

Noble WC: *The skin microflora and microbial skin disease*, London, 1983, Edward Arnold.

Nordlund JJ: The lives of pigment cells. In Gilchrest BA, editor: The aging skin, *Dermatol Clin* 4:407, 1986.

Odland GF: Structure of the skin. In Goldsmith LA, editor: *Physiology, biochemistry, and molecular biology of the skin*, ed 2, New York, 1991, Oxford University Press.

Oluwasanmi JO: Keloids in the African, *Clin Plast Surg* 1:179, 1974.

Ottenbacher KJ et al: The effectiveness of tactile stimulation as a form of early intervention: a quantitative evaluation, *J Dev Behav Pediatr* 8:68, 1987.

Parish LC et al: The decubitus ulcer: many questions but few definitive answers, *Clin Dermatol* 25(1):101-108, 2007.

Pathak MA et al: Sun-protective agents: formulations, effects, and side effects. In Freedberg IM et al, editors: *Fitzpatrick's dermatology in general medicine*, ed 5, New York, 1999, McGraw-Hill.

Pathak MA, Nghiem P, Fitzpatrick TB: Acute and chronic effects of the sun. In Freedberg IM et al, editors: *Fitzpatrick's dermatology in general medicine*, ed 5, New York, 1999, McGraw-Hill.

Pollack SV: Systemic medications and wound healing, *Int J Dermatol* 21:489, 1982.

Potts JF: Sunlight, sunburn, and sunscreens, *Postgrad Med* 87:52, 1990.

Quinton PM: Sweating and its disorders, *Annu Rev Med* 34:429, 1983.

Ramdial PK, Naidoo DK: Drug-induced cutaneous pathology, *J Clin Pathol* 62(6):493-504, 2009.

Rigel DS et al: ABCDE—An evolving concept in the early detection of melanoma, *Arch Dermatol* 141:1032, 2005.

Rienertson RP, Wheatley VR: Studies on the chemical composition of human epidermal lipids, *J Invest Dermatol* 32:49, 1959.

Roberts AB, Sporn MB: Transforming growth factor-B. In Clark RAF (editor): *The molecular and cellular biology of wound repair*, ed 2, New York, 1996, Plenum Press.

Robles DT, Berg D: Abnormal wound healing: keloids, *Clin Dermatol* 25(1):26-32, 2007.

Roe DA: *Nutrition and the skin*, New York, 1986, Alan R. Liss.

Roth RR, James WD: Microbial ecology of the skin, *Annu Rev Microbiol* 42:441, 1988.

Rouhani P et al: Melanoma in Hispanic and black Americans, *Cancer Control* 15:248, 2008.

Rudowski W: *Burn therapy and research*, Baltimore, 1976, Johns Hopkins University Press.

Rutter N: The immature skin, *Eur J Pediatr* 155:S18, 1996.

Scheibner A, Hollis DE, McCarthy WH, Milton GW: Effects of sunlight exposure on Langerhans cells and melanocytes in human epidermis, *Photodermatology* 3:15, 1986.

Sams WM: Structure and function of the skin. In Sams WM, Lynch PJ, editors: *Principles and practice of dermatology*, New York, 1990, Churchill Livingstone.

Sauder DN: Effect of age on epidermal immune function. In Gilchrest BA, editor: The aging skin, *Dermatol Clin* 4:447, 1986.

Shuster S et al: The effect of skin disease on self image, *Br J Dermatol* 90(Suppl 16):18, 1978.

Siebert JW et al: Fetal wound healing: a biochemical study of scarless healing. *Plast Reconstr Surg* 85:495, 1990.

Silverberg N, Silverberg L: Aging and the skin, *Postgrad Med* 86:131, 1989.

Solomons B: *Lecture notes on dermatology*, ed 5, Oxford, 1983, Blackwell Scientific.

Spince AP, Mason EB: *Human anatomy and physiology*, Menlo Park, Calif, 1987, Benjamin/Cummings.

Spitz R: An inquiry into the genesis of psychiatric conditions in early childhood. In Nagera H, editor: *Psychoanalytical studies of the child*, vol 2, London, 1947, International.

Steel KP, Barkway C: Another role for melanocytes: their importance for stria vascularis development in the mammalian inner ear, *Development* 107:453, 1989.

Stender IM et al: Effects of oil and water baths on the hydration state of the epidermis, *Clin Exp Dermatol* 15:206, 1990.

Stierner U, et al: UVB irradiation induces melanocyte increase in both exposed and shielded human skin, *J Invest Dermatol* 92:561, 1989.

Stryer L: *Biochemistry*, ed 4, New York, 1995, WH Freeman.

Szabo G. The number of melanocytes in human epidermis. *Br Med J* i:1016-1017, 1954.

Szabo G et al: Racial differences in the fate of melanosomes in human epidermis. *Nature* 222:1081-1082, 1969.

Szabo G et al:. The ultrastructure of racial color differences in man. In Riley V, editor: *Pigmentation: its genesis and biologic control*, New York, 1972 Appleton Century.

Tadokoro T et al: Mechanisms of skin tanning in different racial/ethnic groups in response to ultraviolet radiation, *J Invest Dermatol* 124:1326, 2005.

Taylor SC: Skin of color: biology, structure, function, and implications for dermatologic disease, *J Am Acad Dermatol* 46(2 Suppl Understanding):S41-S62, 2002.

Taylor SC: Epidemiology of skin diseases in people of color, *Cutis* 71:271, 2003.

US Census Bureau: *US Census Bureau news: an older and more diverse nation by midcentury,* August 14, 2008, available at http://www.census.gov/Press-Release/www/releases/archives/population/012496.html, accessed June 8, 2009.

Van der Horst FCP et al: "When stranger meet": John Bowlby and Harry Harlow on attachment behavior, *Integr Psych Behav* 42:370-388, 2008.

Van Loey NE, Van Son MJ: Psychopathology and psychological problems in patients with burn scars: epidemiology and management, *Am J Clin Dermatol* 4(4):245-272, 2003.

Varani J et al: Decreased collagen production in chronologically aged skin: roles of age-dependent alteration in fibroblast function and defective mechanical stimulation, *Am J Pathol* 168:1861, 2006.

Warner RR et al: Electron probe analysis of human skin: determination of the water concentration profile, *J Invest Dermatol* 90(2):218-224, 1988.

Weinberg AN, Swartz MN: General considerations of bacterial diseases. In Fitzpatrick TB et al, editors: *Dermatology in general medicine: textbook and atlas*, New York, 1987, McGraw-Hill.

Wenger CB: Thermoregulation. In Freedberg IM et al, editors: *Fitzpatrick's dermatology in general medicine*, ed 5, New York, 1999, McGraw-Hill.

Weston WL, Lane AT: Neonatal dermatology. In Wolf K et al, editors: *Fitzpatrick's dermatology in general medicine*, ed 5, New York, 1999, McGraw-Hill Medical.

Wheater PR, et al: *Functional histology*, ed 2, Edinburgh, 1987, Churchill Livingstone.

White MI et al: The effect of washing on the thickness of the stratum corneum in normal and atopic individuals, *Br J Dermatol* 116:525, 1987.

Wicke C et al: Effects of steroids and retinoids on wound healing, *Arch Surg* 135(11):1265-1270, 2000.

Wilkins CH et al: Vitamin D deficiency is associated with worse cognitive performance and lower bone density in older African Americans, *J Natl Med Assoc* 101(4):349, 2009.

Wolff K, Stingl G: The Langerhans' cell, *J Invest Dermatol* 80:17S, 1983.

Woodburne RT, Burkel WE: *Essentials of human anatomy*, New York, 1988, Oxford University Press.

Wysocki AB: A review of the skin and its appendages, *Adv Wound Care* 8(2 Pt 1):53-54, 56-62, 1995.

Wysocki AB: Evaluating and managing open skin wounds: colonization versus infection, *AACN Clin Issues* 13(3):382, 2002.

Wysocki AB et al: Skin, Molecular Cell Biology of. In Robert A. Meyers (Ed.), *Encyclopedia of molecular cell biology and molecular medicine*, (2nd ed., Vol. 13, pp. 217-250), Weinheim, Germany, 2005, Wiley-VCH Verlag GmbH & Co. KgaA.

Xu KD et al: Biofilm resistance to antimicrobial agents, *Microbiol* 146:547, 2000.

Yaar M, Gilchrest FA: Photoageing: mechanism, prevention and therapy, *Br J Dermatol* 157:874, 2007.

Yamaguchi Y, Hearing VJ: Physiological factors that regulate skin pigmentation, *Biofactors* 35(2):193-199, 2009.

Yamaguchi Y et al: Melanin mediated apoptosis of epidermal cells damaged by ultraviolet radiation: factors influencing the incidence of skin cancer, *Arch Dermatol Res* 300(Suppl 1):S43, 2008.

Yanagishita M: A brief history of proteoglycans, *EXS* 70:3, 1994.

Young AR, Walker SL: Acute and chronic effects of ultraviolet radiation on the skin. In Wolff K et al, editors: *Fitzpatrick's dermatology in general medicine*, ed 7, New York, 2008, McGraw-Hill.

4

Wound-Healing Physiology

Dorothy B. Doughty and Bonnie Sparks-DeFriese

OBJECTIVES

1. Compare and contrast wound-healing processes for each type of closure: primary intention, secondary intention, and tertiary intention.
2. Distinguish between partial-thickness wound repair and full-thickness wound repair, addressing the key components, phases, usual time frames, and wound appearance.
3. Explain the difference between acute and chronic full-thickness wounds.
4. Describe four characteristics of a chronic wound.
5. Describe the role of the following cells in the wound repair process: platelets, polymorphonuclear leukocytes, macrophages, fibroblasts, endothelial cells, and keratinocytes.
6. Explain how bioactive agents (e.g., growth factors and cytokines) and extracellular matrix proteins (e.g., matrix metalloproteinases and tissue inhibitors of metalloproteinases) help to regulate the repair process.
7. Describe features and characteristics of scarless healing.
8. Distinguish between keloid and hypertrophic scarring and the treatment of each.
9. Identify conditions and comorbidities that affect the wound-healing process.

For centuries, wound healing was regarded as a mysterious process, with wound management based on practitioner preference as opposed to scientific principles. Research over the past 3 decades has contributed much information regarding the wound-healing process and the factors that facilitate this process. We now know that repair is an extremely complex process involving hundreds, possibly thousands, of overlapping and "linked" processes (Goldman, 2004). It is critical for all wound care clinicians to base their interventions and recommendations on current data and to remain abreast of new findings and their implications for care. This chapter reviews the process of wound healing and discusses the implications for wound management.

MECHANISM OF WOUND HEALING

The ability to repair tissue damage is an important survival tool for any living organism. Regardless of the type or severity of injury, repair occurs by only two mechanisms—*regeneration,* or replacement of the damaged or lost tissue with more of the same, and *scar formation,* replacement of damaged or lost tissue by connective tissue that lacks some of the functions of the original tissue. Regeneration is the preferred mechanism of repair because normal function and appearance are maintained. Scar formation is a less satisfactory alternative and occurs only when the tissues involved are incapable of regeneration. Many invertebrate and amphibian species have the ability to regenerate entire limbs. Humans have only limited capacity for regeneration, and most wounds heal by scar formation (Calvin, 1998; Mast and Schultz, 1996; Wilgus, 2007).

In humans, the mechanism of repair for any specific wound is determined by the tissue layers involved and their capacity for regeneration. Wounds that are confined to the epidermal and superficial dermal layers heal by regeneration because epithelial, endothelial, and connective tissue can be reproduced. In contrast, deep dermal structures (e.g., hair follicles, sebaceous glands, sweat glands), subcutaneous tissue, muscle, tendons, ligaments, and bone lack the capacity to regenerate; therefore loss of these structures is permanent, and wounds involving these structures must heal by scar formation (Martin, 1997; Mast and Schultz, 1996).

The standard repair mechanism for human soft tissue wounds is connective tissue (scar) formation; however, an exception to this rule is the early-gestation fetus. Intrauterine surgical procedures performed during the second trimester result in scarless healing, a phenomenon that has been consistently reproduced in laboratory studies. Interestingly, the fetus loses the ability to heal without scarring at approximately 22 to 24 weeks' gestation. Repair during the third trimester and the postnatal period follows the "usual" rules for repair and results in scar formation. A number of differences in the molecular environment for repair in the early-gestation fetus are thought to contribute to scarless repair and are discussed throughout this chapter (Bullard et al, 2002; Dang et al, 2003; Wilgus, 2007; Yang et al, 2003).

Mechanism of wound healing is dependent upon the tissue layers involved (partial-thickness vs full-thickness), onset and duration (acute vs chronic), and type of wound closure (primary, secondary, or tertiary intention).

Partial Thickness/Full Thickness

Partial-thickness wounds involve only partial loss of the skin layers, that is, they are confined to the epidermal and superficial dermal layers. Full-thickness wounds involve total loss of the skin layers (epidermis and dermis) and frequently involve loss of the deeper tissue layers as well (subcutaneous tissue, muscle, and bone) (see Figure 3-1). The time frame for repair and the repair process itself differ significantly for partial-thickness and full-thickness wounds.

Acute/Chronic

Acute wounds typically are traumatic or surgical in origin. Acute wounds occur suddenly, move rapidly and predictably through the repair process, and result in durable closure. In contrast, chronic wounds fail to proceed normally through the repair process. Chronic wounds frequently are caused by vascular compromise, chronic inflammation, or repetitive insults to the tissue, and they either fail to close in a timely manner or fail to result in durable closure (Brissett and Hom, 2003; Clark, 2002; Pradhan et al, 2009).

Primary, Secondary, Tertiary

Classification of repair as primary-, secondary-, or tertiary-intention healing is based on the ideal of primary surgical closure for all wounds. Primary closure minimizes the volume of connective tissue deposition required for wound repair and restores the epithelial barrier to infection (Figure 4-1, A). Approximated surgical incisions are said to heal by primary intention; they usually heal quickly, with minimal scar formation, as long as infection and secondary breakdown are prevented. Wounds that are left open and allowed to heal by scar formation are classified as healing by secondary intention (Figure 4-1, B). These wounds heal more slowly because of the volume of connective tissue required to fill the defect. They are more subject to infection because they lack the epidermal barrier to microorganisms until late in the repair process. These wounds are characterized by prolongation of the inflammatory and proliferative phases of healing. Chronic wounds such as pressure ulcers and dehisced incisions typically heal by secondary intention. Wounds managed with delayed closure are classified as healing by tertiary intention, or delayed primary closure (Figure 4-1, C). This approach is sometimes required for abdominal incisions complicated by significant infection (Gabriel et al, 2010). Closure and/or

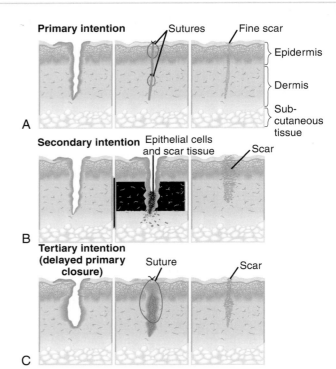

FIGURE 4-1 A, Wound healing by primary intention, such as with a surgical incision. Wound edges are approximated and secured with sutures, staples, or adhesive tapes, and healing occurs by epithelialization and connective tissue deposition. **B,** Wound healing by secondary intention. Wound edges are not approximated, and healing occurs by granulation tissue formation, contraction of the wound edges, and epithelialization. **C,** Wound healing by tertiary (delayed primary) intention. Wound is kept open for several days. The superficial wound edges then are approximated, and the center of the wound heals by granulation tissue formation. (From Black JM, Hawks JH: *Medical surgical nursing, clinical management for positive outcomes,* ed 7, St Louis, 2005, WB Saunders.)

approximation of the wound is delayed until the risk of infection is resolved and the wound is free of debris.

WOUND-HEALING PROCESS

Wound healing is best understood as a cascade of events. Injury sets into motion a series of physiologic responses that are coordinated and sequenced and that, under normal circumstances, result in durable repair. Critical factors in the repair process include the cells that establish a clean wound bed and generate the tissue to fill the defect, the bioactive molecules that control cellular activity (growth factors and cytokines), and the wound-healing environment (extracellular matrix [ECM]). The wound-healing environment (matrix) provides a scaffold that promotes cell migration, and it contains a number of substances that regulate the activity of growth factors and cytokines and promote cell migration (e.g., matrix metalloproteinases) (Cheresh and Stupack, 2008; Gill and Parks, 2008; Macri and Clark, 2009).

Our current understanding of wound repair is based primarily on acute wound-healing models. Therefore, the processes for partial-thickness wound healing and full-thickness wound healing by primary intention are presented first, followed by a discussion of the repair process for wounds that heal by secondary intention.

Partial-Thickness Wound Repair

Partial-thickness wounds are shallow wounds involving epidermal loss and possibly partial loss of the dermal layer (Plate 1). Partial-thickness wounds typically are approximately 0.2 cm in depth. These wounds are moist and painful because of the loss of the epidermal covering and the resultant exposure of nerve endings. When the wound involves loss of the epidermis with exposure of the basement membrane, the wound base appears bright pink or red. In the presence of partial dermal loss, the wound base usually appears pale pink with distinct red "islets." These "islets" represent the basement membrane of the epidermis, which projects deep into the dermis to line the epidermal appendages. These islands of epidermal basement membrane are important in partial-thickness wound healing because all epidermal cells are capable of regeneration, and each islet will serve as a source of new epithelium (Clark, 2002; Winter, 1979).

The major components of partial-thickness repair include an initial inflammatory response to injury, epithelial proliferation and migration (resurfacing), and reestablishment and differentiation of the epidermal layers to restore the barrier function of the skin (Monaco and Lawrence, 2003; Staiano-Coico et al, 2000; Winter, 1979). If the wound involves dermal loss, connective tissue repair (granulation tissue formation) will proceed concurrently with epithelial repair (see Table 4-1) (Jahoda and Reynolds, 2001).

Epidermal Repair. Tissue trauma triggers the processes that result in epidermal repair: an acute inflammatory response followed by epidermal mitosis and migration (Harrison, et al, 2006). The inflammatory response produces erythema, edema, and a serous exudate containing leukocytes. When this exudate is allowed to dry on the wound surface, a dry crust, commonly referred to as a "scab," is formed. In partial-thickness wounds the inflammatory response is limited, typically subsiding in less than 24 hours (Winter, 1979).

Epidermal resurfacing begins as the inflammatory phase subsides and is dependent on two processes: proliferation of epidermal cells throughout the wound bed and lateral migration of the epidermal cells at the leading edge. In order to migrate laterally, the keratinocytes at the wound edge must undergo several changes. First they must acquire a migratory phenotype. This involves breakdown of their attachments to adjacent cells, the basement membrane, and the underlying dermis. These attachments normally prevent lateral migration and provide epithelial stability. The keratinocytes then must undergo cytoskeletal alterations that support lateral movement. These alterations include flattening of the cells at the advancing edge of epithelium and formation of protrusions known as *lamellipodia,* which attach to binding sites in the wound bed. The migratory keratinocytes then move across the wound bed by alternately attaching to the ECM and then detaching and reattaching at a more distal point (Chen and Abatangelo, 1999; Frank et al, 2002; Harrison et al, 2006; Henry and Garner, 2003; Monaco and Lawrence, 2003; Staiano-Coico et al, 2000; Werner and Grose, 2003).

The epithelial cells within the wound bed continue this pattern of lateral migration until they contact epithelial cells migrating from the opposite direction. Once the epithelial cells meet, lateral migration ceases; a phenomenon known as *contact inhibition* (Monaco and Lawrence, 2003; Staiano-Coico et al, 2000).

Epithelial resurfacing is supported by increased production of basal cells just behind the advancing edge and throughout the wound bed. The process typically peaks between 24 and 72 hours after injury. The rate of reepithelialization is affected by a number of factors of clinical significance. For example, resurfacing is promoted by maintenance of a moist wound surface. Winter (1979) found that partial-thickness wounds left open to air required 6 to 7 days to resurface, whereas moist wounds reepithelialized in 4 days. This is because cells can migrate much more rapidly in a moist environment (Figure 4-2). In contrast, when the surface of the wound is covered with a scab, migration is delayed while the epithelial cells secrete enzymes known as matrix metalloproteinases (MMPs). The MMPs lift the scab by cleaving the bonds that attach the scab to the wound bed, creating a moist pathway that supports keratinocyte migration (Clark, 2002; Harrison et al, 2006; Monaco and Lawrence, 2003; Staiano-Coico et al, 2000; Winter, 1979). Interestingly, hypoxic conditions in the wound bed also serve to stimulate keratinocyte migration, probably through increased production of the MMPs that promote lateral migration. This positive response to wound bed hypoxia is lost in the

TABLE 4-1	Partial-Thickness Repair	
Level of Injury (Tissue Layers Involved)	Primary Phases of Repair	Outcomes
Epidermal loss	Inflammation (brief) Epithelial resurfacing Restoration of normal epithelial thickness/ repigmentation	No loss of function No scar No change in skin appearance or color
Possible partial dermal loss	Dermal repair (if dermal loss involved)	Restoration of rete ridges/dermal papillae when dermis involved

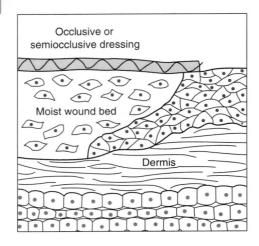
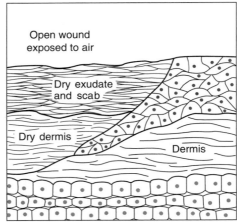

FIGURE 4-2 Migration of epidermal cells in moist environment and dry environment.

elderly, which may be one factor contributing to slower rates of reepithelialization in the aged (O'Toole et al, 2008). In contrast, high bacteria levels may serve as an impediment to reepithelialization. Data indicate that keratinocyte migration is inhibited by bacterial byproducts such as lipopolysaccharide (Loryman and Mansbridge, 2008). In vivo evidence strongly suggests that elevated glucose levels are another major impediment to epidermal proliferation and migration. This may be one factor contributing to delayed healing of superficial wounds in diabetic patients with poorly controlled glucose levels (Lan et al, 2008).

The newly resurfaced epithelium appears pale, pink, and dry in people of all races (see Plate 1). Because it is only a few cell layers thick, the new epithelium is very fragile and requires protection against mechanical forces such as superficial shear and friction.

Once epithelial resurfacing is complete, the epithelial cells resume vertical migration and epidermal differentiation so that normal epidermal thickness and function are restored. The normal anchors to adjacent epidermal cells and to the basement membrane are reestablished (Harrison et al, 2006). The "new" epidermis gradually repigments, matching the individual's normal skin tone (see Plate 1). This is clinically relevant, as the wound is not completely healed until repigmentation has occurred (Monaco and Lawrence, 2003).

Regulatory Factors. The processes of epithelial proliferation and migration are regulated by a complex interplay between various MMPs and selected growth factors. Specifically, lateral migration is dependent on normal levels and function of multiple MMPs, which serve to break the attachments that bind the edge keratinocytes to adjacent cells and the underlying wound bed. In addition to playing a key role in establishment of a migratory phenotype, MMPs facilitate continued resurfacing by assisting the migrating keratinocytes to detach from the wound bed. Repetitive detachment and distal reattachment are critical to the resurfacing process (Gill and Parks, 2008; Lan et al, 2008). Epithelial

proliferation is dependent in part on keratinocyte attachment to the ECM and in part on exposure to growth factors. Keratinocyte attachment is required for the cell to exit from the G_0 phase of mitosis, and growth factors are required to stimulate cellular reproduction. A number of growth factors promote keratinocyte proliferation. They include transforming growth factor-α (TGF-α), keratinocyte growth factor, platelet-derived growth factor (PDGF), and epidermal growth factor (EGF). PDGF and EGF seem to be of particular importance. PDGF promotes keratinocyte migration early postinjury, and EGF seems to play an important role throughout the epithelialization process (Braiman-Wiksman et al, 2007; Myers et al, 2007; Schneider et al, 2008). Insulin-like growth factor may also play a role. An animal study demonstrated that exogenous application of insulin to partial-thickness wounds produced a significant increase in both epithelial proliferation and migration rate (Liu et al, 2009). See Chapter 20 for further discussion of the molecular factors regulating wound repair.

Dermal Repair. In wounds involving both dermal and epidermal loss, dermal repair proceeds concurrently with reepithelialization. By the fifth day after injury, a layer of fluid separates the epidermis from the dermal tissue. New blood vessels begin to sprout, and fibroblasts become plentiful by about the seventh day. Collagen fibers are visible in the wound bed by the ninth day. Collagen synthesis continues to produce new connective tissue until about 10 to 15 days after injury. This new connective tissue grows upward into the fluid layer. At the same time, the flat epidermis falls down around the new vessels and collagen fibers, recreating ridges at the dermal–epidermal junction. As the new connective tissue gradually contracts, the epidermis is drawn close to the dermis (Winter, 1979). Insulin and insulin-like growth factor may contribute to reformation of the dermal–epidermal junction. An animal study by Liu et al (2009) demonstrated more epidermal rete ridges and dermal papillae in wounds treated with exogenous insulin.

Full-Thickness Wound Repair: Wounds Healing By Primary Intention

Full-thickness wounds, by definition, extend at least to the subcutaneous tissue layer and possibly as deep as the fascia–muscle layer or bone (see Plate 2). Full-thickness wounds may be either acute or chronic. This section addresses acute wound healing by primary intention, such as a surgical incision.

Many steps are involved in full-thickness repair, but they are commonly conceptualized as four major phases: hemostasis, inflammation, proliferation, and remodeling. Considerable overlap exists among the phases, and the cells involved in one phase produce the chemical stimuli and substances that serve to move the wound into the next phase. Thus normal repair is a complex and well-orchestrated series of events (Figure 4-3) and is affected by a number of systemic and local factors, including the wound environment/ECM.

Hemostasis. Any acute injury extending beyond the epidermis causes bleeding, which activates a series of overlapping events designed to control blood loss, establish bacterial control, and seal the defect. Immediately upon injury, disruption of blood vessels exposes the subendothelial collagen to platelets, which trigger platelet activation and aggregation. Simultaneously, injured cells in the wound area release clotting factors that activate both the intrinsic and extrinsic coagulation pathways. As part of the coagulation pathway, circulating prothrombin is converted to thrombin, which is used to convert fibrinogen to fibrin. The end result is formation of a clot composed of fibrin, aggregated platelets, and blood cells. Hemostasis is further accomplished by a brief period of vasoconstriction mediated by thromboxane A_2 and prostaglandin 2-α,

substances released by the damaged cells and activated platelets. Clot formation seals the disrupted vessels so that blood loss is controlled. The clot also provides a temporary bacterial barrier, a reservoir of growth factors, and an interim matrix that serves as scaffolding for migrating cells (Brissett and Hom, 2003; Monaco and Lawrence, 2003; Phillips, 2000; Pullar et al, 2008; Werner and Grose, 2003).

Clot formation, followed by fibrinolysis (clot breakdown), is a critical event in the sequence of wound healing (Figure 4-4). The activation and degranulation of platelets cause the α-granules and dense bodies of the platelets to rupture, releasing a potent "cocktail" of energy-producing compounds and cytokines/growth factors (including complement factor C5a). These substances attract the cells needed to begin the repair process. They also provide fuel for the energy-intensive process of wound healing. The platelet-derived substances

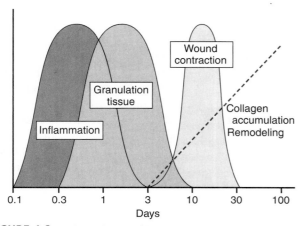

FIGURE 4-3 Orderly phases of healing. Time line (in days) reflects healing trajectory of acute wound healing model. (Modified from Clark RA: Cutaneous wound repair. In Goldsmith LA, editor: *Physiology, biochemistry and molecular biology of the skin,* ed 2, vol 1, New York, 1991, Oxford University Press. In Kumar V, Cotran RS, Robbins ST: *Robbins basic pathology,* ed 7, Philadelphia, 2003, WB Saunders.)

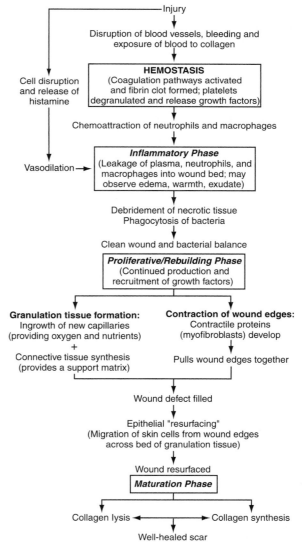

FIGURE 4-4 Cascade of events in wound repair process.

thought to be most critical to repair include PDGF, TGF-β, and fibroblast growth factor-2. Thus hemostasis, which is the body's normal response to tissue injury, actually initiates the entire wound-healing cascade. The importance of hemostasis to wound healing is underscored by the finding that inadequate clot formation is associated with impaired wound healing and that the extrinsic coagulation pathway is critical to repair (Brissett and Hom, 2003; Frank et al, 2002; Monaco and Lawrence, 2003; Pullar et al, 2008; Samuels and Tan, 1999; Staiano-Coico et al, 2000).

Inflammation. Once the bleeding is controlled, the focus becomes control of infection and establishment of a clean wound bed. This process can be compared to the repair of a damaged home or building. Before rebuilding can begin, the damaged components must be removed. Wound "cleanup" involves breakdown of any devitalized tissue and elimination of excess bacteria by a team of white blood cells. Acute wounds, such as sutured lacerations or incisions, typically have limited devitalized tissue and low bacterial loads, so the cleanup phase usually is brief, lasting only hours to a few days (Braiman-Wiksman et al, 2007; Pradhan et al, 2009).

Within 10 to 15 minutes following injury, vasoconstriction subsides, followed by vasodilation and increased capillary permeability. Vasoactive substances released by damaged cells and by clot breakdown (histamine, prostaglandins, complement factor, thrombin) mediate this response. The dilated capillaries permit plasma and blood cells to leak into the wound bed. Clinically, this process is observed as edema, erythema, and exudate. At the same time, the damaged cells and platelets from the injured vessels produce cytokines and growth factors that attract leukocytes (neutrophils, macrophages, lymphocytes) to the wound bed. The twin processes of chemoattraction and vasodilation result in the delivery of multiple phagocytic cells to the wound site within minutes of injury (Gill and Parks, 2008; Rodriguez et al, 2008; Pradhan et al, 2009).

Leukocyte migration out of the vessels and into the wound bed occurs via margination and diapedesis. *Margination* involves adherence of the leukocytes to the endothelial cells lining the capillaries in the wound bed. Integrins on the surface of the leukocytes attach to cell adhesion molecules on the surface of the endothelial cells, causing the leukocytes to "line up" against the vessel wall. Through a process known as *diapedesis,* the leukocytes migrate through the dilated capillaries into the wound bed (Cross and Mustoe, 2003; Monaco and Lawrence, 2003; Wilgus, 2007).

The first leukocytes to arrive in the wound space, the neutrophils, are present in the wound bed within minutes following injury and dominate the scene for the first 2 to 3 days. The primary function of neutrophils is phagocytosis of bacteria and foreign debris. Neutrophils first bind to the damaged tissue or target bacteria via cell adhesion molecules and then engulf and destroy the

target molecules via intracellular enzymes and free oxygen radicals. In addition, growth factors released by the neutrophils attract additional leukocytes to the area (Cross and Mustoe, 2003; Goldman, 2004; Monaco and Lawrence, 2003; Pullar et al, 2008; Schultz et al, 2003).

By days 3 to 4 after injury, the neutrophils begin to spontaneously disappear as a result of apoptosis and are replaced by macrophages (activated monocytes). The macrophages continue to phagocytize bacteria and break down damaged tissues as already described. In addition, the macrophages release a large number of potent growth factors that stimulate angiogenesis, fibroblast migration and proliferation, and connective tissue synthesis (Pullar et al, 2008; Rodriguez et al, 2008).

T lymphocytes are present in the wound tissue in peak quantities between days 5 and 7 after injury. T lymphocytes contribute to the inflammatory phase of wound healing by secreting additional wound-healing cytokines and by destroying viral organisms and foreign cells. The elimination of these cells can delay or compromise the repair process (Monaco and Lawrence, 2003).

Although all leukocytes contribute to elimination of bacteria and establishment of a clean wound bed, macrophages contribute the most significantly to the repair process. Studies indicate that wounds can heal without neutrophils, especially if no bacterial contamination is present. However, elimination of macrophages severely compromises wound repair (Cross and Mustoe, 2003; Gabriel et al, 2010).

The result of the inflammatory phase of wound healing is a clean wound bed. In acute wounds healing by primary intention, the inflammatory phase lasts approximately 3 days. At this point, bacterial levels usually are controlled, and any devitalized tissue has been removed. Elimination of these noxious stimuli allows the wound to transition to the "rebuilding" phase. During this transition, the cells in the wound bed begin to produce growth factors that stimulate proliferation rather than inflammation (Goldman, 2004; Staiano-Coico et al, 2000). However, in wounds complicated by necrosis and/or infection, the inflammatory phase is prolonged and wound healing is delayed (Braiman-Wiksman et al, 2007; Clark, 2002). A prolonged inflammatory phase increases the risk for wound dehiscence because approximation of the incision is totally dependent upon the closure material (sutures, staples, fibrin glue) until sufficient connective tissue has been synthesized to provide tensile strength to the incision. (Tensile strength during the inflammatory phase is 0%.)

Factors Affecting the Duration and Intensity of Inflammation. The intensity and duration of the inflammatory phase appear to be critical factors in the amount of scar tissue produced. Numerous studies support a strong link between prolonged inflammation and hyperproliferative scarring (Dubay and Franz, 2003; Pradhan et al, 2009; Pullar et al, 2008; Rahban and

Garner, 2003; Robson, 2003). Thus the clinician needs to have a clear understanding of both proinflammatory and antiinflammatory factors and the implications for wound management. As noted, local factors such as bacterial loads and presence of devitalized tissue are major proinflammatory factors that should be aggressively managed through debridement and appropriate use of antimicrobial agents. The ECM is another important determinant and can either promote or inhibit inflammation, depending on the types of MMPs produced and their functions. Some MMPs promote inflammation by releasing proinflammatory cytokines from the cells in the wound bed; others inhibit inflammation by degrading proinflammatory cytokines or inhibiting their release (proinflammatory cytokines promote inflammation by continuing to attract inflammatory cells to the wound bed) (Pradhan et al, 2009). For example, tumor necrosis factor-α (TNF-α) is a proinflammatory cytokine that normally is present at high levels during the early inflammatory phase, and levels of TNF-α are controlled by two ECM proteins. One protein, a disintegrin and metalloproteinase (ADAM-17), promotes release of TNF-α. Another protein (tissue inhibitor of metalloproteinase-3 [TIMP-3]) controls ADAM-17, thereby reducing production of TNF-α. Research is ongoing into factors that determine the combination and concentration of ECM proteins and into strategies for measuring and controlling levels of various MMPs to achieve therapeutic outcomes (Gill and Parks, 2008; Macri and Clark, 2009).

Diabetes is a clinical condition associated with prolonged inflammation. Some data suggest that leukocyte migration may be impaired; in addition, the leukocytes that do migrate to the wound bed frequently are dysfunctional, especially in the presence of hyperglycemia. The end result of diminished leukocyte migration and impaired leukocyte function is failure to effectively control bacterial loads. This situation results in a persistent stimulus for proinflammatory cytokines, chronic inflammation, and delayed healing (Pradhan et al, 2009). Conditions resulting in ischemia/hypoxia also produce prolonged inflammation, because oxygen and reactive oxygen species (ROS) are required for oxidative killing of bacteria. The inability to control bacteria that accompanies hypoxia results in chronic inflammation and failure to heal. Hyperbaric oxygen therapy can improve tissue oxygen levels, contribute to bacterial control, and reduce the production of proinflammatory cytokines, thus promoting the repair process (Rodriguez et al, 2008; Thom, 2009).

Conditions and medications that affect the function of autonomic and sensory nerves and their receptors may also affect inflammation. For example, diabetes is associated with diminished production of substance P, a neuropeptide that normally contributes to a healthy inflammatory response by supporting vasodilation and leukocyte migration. Diminished production of substance P may be one factor leading to compromised inflammation and impaired healing in the diabetic population (Pradhan et al, 2009). From a therapeutic perspective, β-adrenergic agents may reduce inflammation by reducing neutrophil recruitment and production of inflammatory cytokines; further research on this topic is needed (Pullar et al, 2008).

Proliferation. The third phase of acute full-thickness wound healing is the proliferative phase. During this phase, the wound surface is covered with new epithelium that restores the bacterial barrier, vascular integrity is restored, and the incisional defect is mended with new connective tissue. The key components of the proliferative phase are epithelialization, neoangiogenesis, and matrix deposition/collagen synthesis. Limited contraction of the newly formed ECM also may occur.

Epithelialization. Epithelialization of a full-thickness wound healing by primary intention begins within hours after injury and typically is complete within 24 to 48 hours. This "neoepithelium" is only a few cells thick but is sufficient to provide a closed wound surface and a bacterial barrier. This process is the basis for the Centers for Disease Control recommendation that new surgical incisions be covered with a sterile dressing for the first 24 to 48 hours postoperatively. Until reepithelialization is complete, the potential for bacterial invasion exists, and the wound should be managed with sterile wound care and a cover dressing that provides a bacterial barrier (Cross and Mustoe, 2003; Mangram et al, 1999; Monaco and Lawrence, 2003). As with partial-thickness wound repair, the processes of lateral migration, vertical migration, and differentiation continue throughout the proliferative phase and gradually reestablish epidermal thickness and function (Braiman-Wiksman et al, 2007; Myers et al, 2007). In full-thickness wounds, the new epidermis is slightly thinner than the original epidermis. Because the neoepidermis rather than normal dermis is covering scar tissue, the rete pegs that normally dip into the dermis are lacking (Monaco and Lawrence, 2003).

Granulation Tissue Formation. A hallmark outcome of the proliferative phase is the formation of granulation tissue, which begins as the inflammatory phase subsides, at 3 to 4 days postinjury (Braiman-Wiksman et al, 2007). Granulation tissue is composed primarily of capillary loops and newly synthesized connective tissue proteins and is often referred to as the *extracellular matrix* (ECM). Fibroblasts and inflammatory cells also are present in this new matrix. Neoangiogenesis and connective tissue synthesis occur simultaneously in a codependent fashion to form the new ECM that will fill the wound defect. Through angiogenesis, new capillaries are formed and joined with existing severed capillaries, thus restoring the delivery of oxygen and nutrients to the wound bed. At the same time, a new "provisional" ECM is formed through the synthesis of connective tissue proteins (Figure 4-5) (Pradhan et al, 2009).

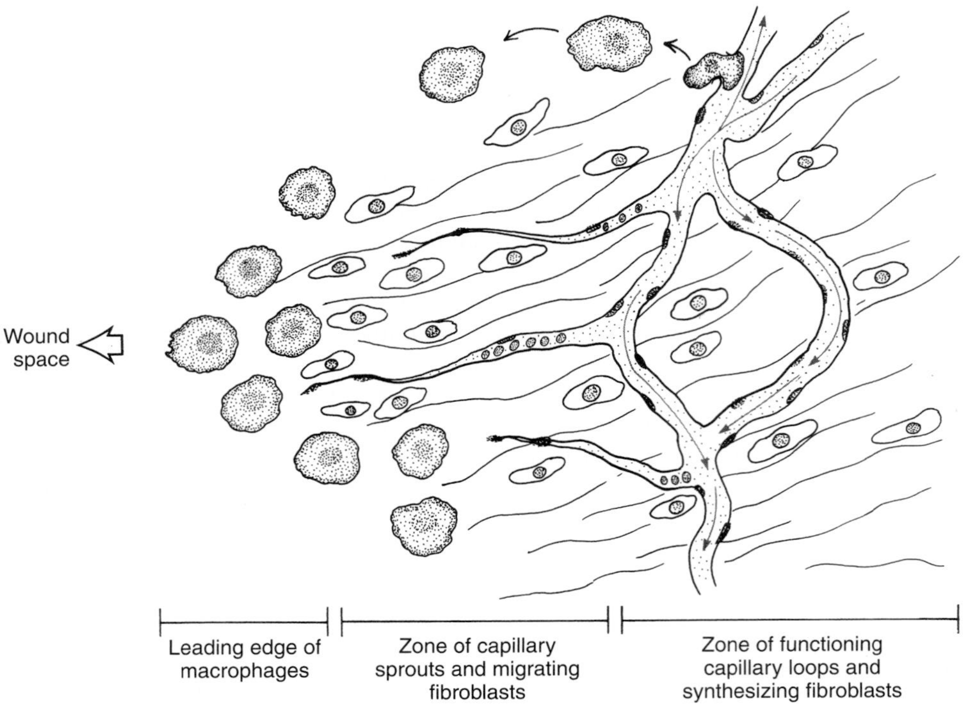

FIGURE 4-5 Advancing module of reparative tissue during proliferative and remodeling phases. (From Whalen GF, Zetter BR: Angiogenesis. In Cohen IK, Dieglemann RF, Lindbald WJ, editors: *Wound healing: biochemical and clinical aspects,* Philadelphia, 1992, WB Saunders.)

Wound space

Leading edge of macrophages

Zone of capillary sprouts and migrating fibroblasts

Zone of functioning capillary loops and synthesizing fibroblasts

Neoangiogenesis. Endothelial cells typically are quiescent. Neoangiogenesis requires stimulation by growth factors, which convert the quiescent cells to actively proliferating cells. Molecules in the ECM also play a critical role by influencing the response of endothelial cells to angiogenic growth factors (Cheresh and Stupack, 2008). Neoangiogenesis occurs by two mechanisms: production of new vessels by local endothelial cells and recruitment of circulating stem progenitor cells to form new vessels de novo (Thom, 2009).

The growth factors that stimulate production of new vessels are produced by the cells in the wound bed (injured endothelial cells, macrophages, fibroblasts, keratinocytes) and include vascular endothelial growth factor (VEGF), basic fibroblast growth factor, and possibly PDGF. The most important angiogenic growth factor is VEGF; in addition to stimulating local endothelial cells to proliferate and migrate, VEGF attracts stem progenitor cells to the wound bed and stimulates them to differentiate into endothelial cells (Braiman-Wiksman et al, 2007; Gill and Parks, 2008; Pullar et al, 2008; Thom, 2009). A number of ECM factors also impact on neoangiogenesis. One is the provisional matrix itself, which affects the migration of endothelial cells (Gill and Parks, 2008). Another is the level of TIMP-3, which has a very negative effect on angiogenesis. TIMP-3 binds to the receptor sites for VEGF and blocks its angiogenic effects (Gill and Parks, 2008). A third factor is the level of nitric oxide, which promotes angiogenesis by activating MMP-13 (Lizarbe et al, 2008).

Clinical factors affecting neoangiogenesis include oxygen levels within the wound bed, patient age, gender,

diabetes, coronary artery disease, radiation therapy, and chemotherapy. Hypoxia acts as an initial stimulus to angiogenesis, but persistent hypoxia interferes with endothelial cell proliferation and new vessel formation. Hyperglycemia and glycolysis are associated with production of substances that are toxic to endothelial cells. Diabetes, aging, female sex, coronary artery disease, radiation therapy, and chemotherapy all interfere with angiogenesis by reducing mobilization of stem progenitor cells, thus compromising the potential for de novo development of new vessels. Aging is also associated with dysfunction and impaired mobilization of local endothelial cells, partly due to impaired expression of VEGF and other angiogenic stimuli. Of interest, some data suggest that exercise can partially reverse these age-related changes (Hoenig et al, 2008; Rodriguez et al, 2008; Thom, 2009). Therapeutic modalities that may promote angiogenesis include exogenous application of basic fibroblast growth factor. Animal studies and limited human case reports indicate potent stimulation of angiogenesis and granulation tissue formation (O'Goshi and Tagami, 2007).

Matrix Deposition/Collagen Synthesis. Fibroblasts are responsible for synthesis of the connective tissue proteins that compose the provisional ECM; therefore fibroblasts are critical to the repair process. Fibroblasts migrate into the wound bed from the surrounding tissues in response to growth factors and interleukins released by degranulating platelets, activated leukocytes (neutrophils and macrophages), and keratinocytes. Migration requires up-regulation of binding sites (integrin receptors) on the cell wall, which is mediated by PDGF and

TGF-β. This up-regulation of binding sites is essential because fibroblasts migrate by maintaining attachment to one binding site while extending lamellipodia in search of another site. Once the fibroblast is able to bind to a new site, it releases the original attachment and "moves" in the direction of the wound bed (Monaco and Lawrence, 2003; Myers et al, 2007).

Fibroblasts begin to appear in the wound bed toward the end of the inflammatory phase, 2 to 3 days after injury. By day 4, fibroblasts are the predominant cells in the wound matrix (Dubay and Franz, 2003). Once fibroblasts arrive at the wound site, growth factors bind to fibroblast receptor sites and trigger intracellular processes that move the fibroblasts into the reproductive phase of the cell cycle, thus stimulating proliferation of the fibroblast. Finally, the fibroblasts are converted into "wound fibroblasts" by TGF-β, a growth factor secreted by macrophages. These wound fibroblasts differ from typical dermal fibroblasts in that they exhibit decreased proliferative behavior but increased synthesis of connective tissue proteins such as collagen (Frank et al, 2002).

Collagen synthesis follows the established process for synthesis of any protein. The collagen molecule is characterized by a glycine-X-Y repeating sequence. The collagen molecule must undergo a series of intracellular modifications before the molecule is secreted into the extracellular environment and becomes part of the ECM. One of the most critical modifications is "cross-linking" of the proline and lysine molecules, a process known as *hydroxylation*. These cross-links are essential for the development of tensile strength. A number of factors are required for normal hydroxylation, including oxygen, ascorbic acid, iron, copper, and selected enzymes. Thus hypoxia, vitamin C deficiency, copper deficiency, and iron deficiency all can compromise hydroxylation and the development of tensile strength. High-dose corticosteroids also can impair tensile strength because corticosteroids suppress the enzymes needed for hydroxylation. Following intracellular modifications, the collagen molecule is secreted into the extracellular environment as the triple helix procollagen. It then undergoes additional steps that culminate in the formation of cross-linked fibrils. The enzyme lysyl oxidase is essential to these processes and to the development of stable collagen fibers (Monaco and Lawrence, 2003).

The early granulation tissue is a provisional matrix characterized by unstructured collagen and high levels of fibronectin. This provisional matrix also includes vibronectin, laminin, and proteoglycans such as hyaluronic acid (Braiman-Wiksman et al, 2007; Gill and Parks, 2008; Schneider et al, 2008). As the ECM matures, collagen becomes the predominant protein, representing a little over 50% of the new ECM. Proteoglycans such as hyaluronic acid are present in small amounts but serve critical functions. For example, hyaluronic acid facilitates cell migration, protects cells against free-radical and proteolytic damage, and contributes viscoelastic properties to the new matrix (Chen and Abatangelo, 1999; Monaco and Lawrence, 2003).

Wounds healing by primary intention, such as sutured incisions, require a limited amount of connective tissue to mend the defect. In these wounds, ECM production is essentially complete within 14 to 21 days (Clark, 2002; Henry and Garner, 2003; Monaco and Lawrence, 2003). Although the granulation tissue is not visible in these wounds, a "healing ridge" can be palpated just under the intact suture line by days 5 to 9. The healing ridge is produced by the newly formed connective tissue proteins. Absence of this healing ridge indicates impaired healing and increased risk for dehiscence (Hunt and Van Winkle, 1997).

Factors Affecting Granulation Tissue Formation. Factors affecting granulation tissue formation include perfusion status, oxygen levels, nutritional status, and glucose levels/diabetes. Granulation tissue formation is very much an oxygen-dependent process. Hypoxia can act as a stimulus to fibroblast proliferation and initial collagen synthesis, but adequate levels of oxygen (30–40 mm Hg) are absolutely essential for the latter steps in collagen synthesis and for the cross-linking that provides tensile strength. Adequate oxygen levels are also required for prevention of infection. Data indicate that infection rates in surgical wounds are inversely proportional to oxygen levels (Rodriguez et al, 2008). Tissue oxygenation of acute wounds is discussed in more detail in Chapters 28 and 34. Nutritional status affects granulation because granulation tissue formation requires adequate levels of protein and micronutrients such as ascorbic acid, iron, and copper. Diabetes is associated with delayed deposition of granulation tissue and insufficient production of collagen to establish a mature matrix (Braiman-Wiksman et al, 2007).

Contraction. Contraction occurs when specialized fibroblasts known as *myofibroblasts* exert tractional forces on the ECM, reducing the size of the wound. Wounds healing by primary intention have limited or no contraction because the wound edges have been surgically approximated (Monaco and Lawrence, 2003).

Maturation/Remodeling. The final phase in full-thickness wound healing is the maturation, or remodeling, phase, which begins around day 21 after wounding and continues beyond 1 year. The early collagen is characterized by poorly organized fibers having limited tensile strength. At 3 weeks after injury, the healing wound exhibits only 20% of the strength of intact dermis. The provisional matrix is gradually converted to a mature scar, a process that involves conversion of the type III collagen in the provisional matrix to type I collagen, the type normally found in dermal tissue. However, even the final form of collagen does not exhibit the normal basket-weave pattern of the collagen in unwounded dermis. Rather, the fibers of "repair collagen" are aligned parallel to the stress lines of the wound. The new ECM also lacks elastin, which provides the uninjured skin with elasticity; thus scar tissue is "stiff" compared to normal tissue (Monaco and Lawrence, 2003; Rodriguez et al, 2008).

Remodeling involves the dual processes of synthesis and degradation of the ECM, and is regulated by fibroblasts and ECM proteins (MMPs). The new collagen that is formed is more orderly and provides more tensile strength to the wound. However, the tensile strength of the remodeled ECM (scar tissue) is never more than 80% of the tensile strength in nonwounded tissue (Clark, 2002; Gill and Parks, 2008; Monaco and Lawrence, 2003; Rodriguez et al, 2008; Schneider et al, 2008).

An imbalance between the dual processes of matrix synthesis and matrix breakdown can complicate wound healing. For example, hypertrophic scarring and keloid formation are believed to be caused in part by an excess of matrix synthesis compared to matrix degradation (Rahban and Garner, 2003; Wilgus, 2007). In contrast, hypoxia, malnutrition, or excess levels of MMPs can interfere with synthesis and deposition of new matrix proteins, resulting in wound breakdown (Monaco and Lawrence, 2003).

Full-Thickness Wound Repair: Wounds Healing By Secondary Intention

Although full-thickness wounds healing by secondary intention (e.g., pressure ulcers) proceed through the same phases as full-thickness wounds healing by primary intention, key differences do exist within each phase. These differences are summarized in Table 4-2 and discussed here.

Absence of Hemostasis. The absence of hemostasis has a tremendous impact on the healing trajectory of wounds. Bleeding and hemostasis do not occur in wounds healing by secondary intention. Failure to bleed and clot compromises the repair process because the wound-healing sequence of events is normally initiated by clot breakdown and the subsequent release of growth factors. One theorized benefit of surgical debridement of chronic wounds is to trigger clot formation and the release of growth factors so that the repair process is reactivated.

Prolonged Inflammatory Phase. The inflammatory phase frequently is prolonged. Because the goal of this phase is to establish a clean wound bed and to obtain bacterial balance, the wound will remain in this phase until necrotic tissue has been eliminated and bacterial loads have been controlled. Wounds healing by secondary

TABLE 4-2	Full-Thickness Repair Process	
	Primary Intention	**Secondary Intention**
Examples	Laceration Surgical incision	Chronic wound (e.g., pressure ulcer, venous ulcer) Wound dehiscence
Hemostasis	Bleeding Platelets rupture and release growth factors Coagulation pathways (intrinsic and extrinsic) activated	No bleeding No coagulation Hemostasis absent
Inflammatory phase	Any necrotic tissue removed Bacterial balance restored Duration usually limited to 1–3 days unless complicated by infection	Necrotic tissue removed Bacterial balance restored Duration prolonged until nonviable tissue eliminated and bacteria controlled; also prolonged by presence of excess proinflammatory cells
Proliferative phase	Epithelialization (first event in proliferative phase) Synthesis of connective tissue Duration typically 14–21 days	Granulation tissue formation Neoangiogenesis Synthesis of connective tissue proteins Contraction of wound edges Epithelialization (last event in proliferative phase) Duration is dependent on size and depth of wound and host's ability to synthesize new extracellular matrix
Maturation (remodeling phase)	Collagen synthesis and lysis Tensile strength partially reestablished	Collagen synthesis and lysis Tensile strength partially reestablished

intention frequently are characterized by large amounts of devitalized tissue and heavy bacterial loads. Thus the inflammatory phase generally lasts considerably longer than the 3 days that are typical in the approximated incision.

Prolonged Proliferative Phase. The proliferative phase is prolonged, and the sequence of events is different. In wounds healing by primary intention, epithelialization occurs first, followed by angiogenesis and formation of a limited volume of connective tissue proteins (ECM); contraction does not occur or is very limited. These processes usually are complete within 14 to 21 days. In secondary-intention wound healing, the proliferative phase begins with granulation tissue formation (to fill in the soft tissue defect), followed by contraction (to minimize the defect); epithelialization is the final phase.

The volume of granulation tissue required to fill the defect (and the time required for this phase of repair) is determined by the size of the wound and the degree to which contraction is able to reduce the size of the defect. Because the wound bed is visible, the clinician is able to assess progress in healing. Healthy granulation tissue presents as a red, vascular, granular wound bed as a result of the numerous capillary loops in combination with the newly synthesized ECM proteins (see Plate 3).

Increased Amount of Contraction. Contraction is much more important in secondary-intention wound healing than in closed wounds because contraction reduces the size of the soft tissue defect and thus reduces the amount of granulation tissue required. The rate of contraction for open wounds averages 0.6 to 0.7 mm/day (Gabbiani, 2003; Monaco and Lawrence, 2003). The degree to which a specific wound will contract is determined partly by the mobility of the surrounding tissue. For example, the tissue surrounding sacral and abdominal wounds is quite mobile and can contract easily. In contrast, the tissue surrounding a wound on the extremity or overlying a bony prominence has limited potential for contraction. Contraction is considered undesirable in some wounds because it can cause cosmetic deformities or flexion contractures of joints (Gabbiani, 2003; Monaco and Lawrence, 2003).

Contraction is mediated by myofibroblasts, modified fibroblasts that contain actin and myosin monofilaments and smooth muscle proteins. Differentiation of fibroblasts into myofibroblasts is stimulated by growth factors such as TGF-β1 and PDGF. Substances within the ECM itself are also thought to contribute to the development of myofibroblasts. Intracellular actin filaments and extracellular fibronectin work jointly to establish a contractile force that compresses and "shrinks" the ECM, thus pulling the wound edges toward each other (Gabbiani 2003; Pullar et al, 2008).

Delayed Epithelialization. Because full-thickness wounds involve loss of the deep dermis and epidermal appendages (along with their epithelial lining), epithelialization in these wounds proceeds from the periphery of the wound inward in a centripetal fashion. Epithelial migration requires an open, proliferative wound edge. Closed, nonproliferative wound edges, also known as *epibole,* are sometimes seen in open wounds healing by secondary intention, probably due to premature keratinization of the wound edges (Figure 4-6 and Plate 4). In these wounds, an open edge must be reestablished, by either surgical excision or chemical cauterization, before epithelial migration can occur (Cross and Mustoe, 2003; Monaco and Lawrence, 2003).

Prolonged Remodeling. The remodeling process for wounds healing by secondary intention is essentially the same as that for wounds healing by primary intention. Clinicians and caregivers must remain acutely aware that newly "healed" wounds initially lack tensile strength, and measures should be initiated to minimize stress on the remodeling wound until tensile strength has developed, which occurs 2 to 3 months after closure. For example, the patient with a newly healed pressure ulcer should remain on a therapeutic support surface and should minimize time spent lying on the involved surface.

WHAT MAKES A CHRONIC WOUND CHRONIC?

An acute wound in a relatively healthy host will heal fairly quickly because of a cascade of growth factors, cytokines, and matrix proteins that tend to keep the acute wound on the "healing track." In clinical practice, however, chronic wounds such as pressure

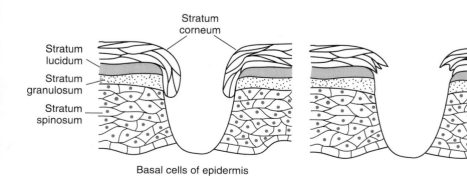

Stratum corneum
Stratum lucidum
Stratum granulosum
Stratum spinosum
Basal cells of epidermis

FIGURE 4-6 *Left,* Closed wound edges in which epidermis of wound edges has rolled under so that epithelial cells cannot migrate. *Right,* Open wound edges from which epithelial cells can migrate.

ulcers, vascular ulcers, and neuropathic wounds behave much differently and may be extremely slow to heal. In order to intervene effectively, the clinician must be knowledgeable regarding the various factors contributing to delayed healing.

Over the past decade, extensive research analyzing the cellular, biochemical, and molecular components of acute and chronic wounds has significantly expanded the understanding of the detailed complexities of normal wound healing and the pathophysiologic mechanisms of chronic wounds. Box 4-1 summarizes the characteristics of a chronic wound.

Underlying Pathology

The nature of the injury differs between acute and chronic wounds. Acute wounds usually begin with a sudden, solitary insult and proceed to heal in an orderly manner. In contrast, chronic wounds are commonly caused by an underlying pathologic process, such as vascular insufficiency, that produces repeated and prolonged insults to the tissues. Failure to correct or control the underlying pathology can result in a persistent cycle of injury that causes repetitive tissue damage. In contrast, correction of the underlying pathology frequently can shift the wound to a healing pathway (Goldman, 2004).

Increased Levels of Inflammatory Substances

Chronic wounds frequently are complicated by impediments to healing, such as ischemia, necrotic tissue, heavy bacterial loads, and high levels of proinflammatory MMPs. These factors prolong the inflammatory phase of wound healing by continuing to recruit macrophages and neutrophils into the wound bed. In addition, high levels of proinflammatory MMPs are associated with ongoing destruction of the ECM (Gill and Parks, 2008; Goldman, 2004). Studies indicate that the levels of inflammatory substances in chronic wounds are 100 times higher than the levels in acute wounds (Berg Vande and Robson, 2003). Fortunately, this cycle can be interrupted by elimination of the noxious stimuli, that is, by debridement of necrotic tissue and control of the bacterial burden (Goldman, 2004).

BOX 4-1	Characteristics of a Chronic Wound

Prolonged inflammatory phase
Cellular senescence
Deficiency of growth factor receptor sites
No initial bleeding event to trigger fibrin production and release of growth factors
High level of proteases

Low Levels of Growth Factors

In addition to high levels of inflammatory proteases, low levels of growth factors commonly characterize the environment of chronic wounds. Normal levels of growth factors are critical to repair, because a "threshold level" of growth factors is required to move target cells out of the quiescent G_0 phase and into the reproductive cycle (Berg Vande and Robson, 2003). The low levels of growth factors commonly found in chronic wounds may be the result of inadequate production by the cells of the wound bed (or insufficient numbers of "producer" cells). Additional potential causes include rapid breakdown of growth factors by the high levels of MMPs or "binding" of the growth factors by the ECM (Berg Vande and Robson, 2003; Henry and Garner, 2003; Steed, 2003). Although this imbalance between inflammatory and proliferative stimuli usually is thought to be the cause of impaired healing, some investigators suggest that the imbalance instead may be a result of chronicity. When the wound begins to heal, the ratio of inflammatory to proliferative stimuli normalizes (Goldman, 2004; Henry and Garner, 2003; Staiano-Coico et al, 2000).

A deficiency of growth factor receptor sites on host target cells and cellular senescence (decrease in proliferative potential and loss of ability to respond to growth factors) also have been identified as characteristics of the chronic wound. Cellular senescence appears to be particularly common among elderly individuals and may contribute to the delayed healing commonly seen in this population (Berg Vande and Robson, 2003; Pittman, 2007). However, optimal wound management may result in successful "recruitment" of nonsenescent cells to the wound bed.

Miscellaneous Host Conditions

Additional "host factors" that trigger chronicity in a wound include ischemia, malnutrition, and comorbidities such as diabetes (Steed, 2003). Malnutrition is a particularly common contributor to wound chronicity. Fibroblasts that lack the requisite raw ingredients cannot synthesize connective tissue proteins. The importance of nutritional status is reflected in studies documenting consistently impaired wound healing in patients whose albumin levels were lower than 2.0 g/L (Burns et al, 2003). In addition, a study on wound fluid as a predictor of healing found the only constituents to reliably predict healing were total protein and albumin, that is, albumin levels greater than 2.0 g/L (James et al, 2000; Schultz et al, 2003).

Pale pink tissue that is smooth rather than granular is indicative of delayed healing and a compromised ability to synthesize collagen and other connective tissue proteins (see Plates 5a and 5b).

Denervation

Denervation is another potential cause of failure to heal. Sensory nerves secrete neuropeptides (e.g., substance P) that are highly chemotactic for inflammatory cells. Therefore denervated wounds are subject to impaired inflammation and compromised healing. Denervation may be one of the factors contributing to chronicity of pressure ulcers in patients with spinal cord injury and neuropathic ulcers in diabetic patients (Macri and Clark, 2009; Richards et al, 1997).

In summary, differences in the healing trajectory for acute and chronic wounds stem from the nature of the injury, the cellular events that follow injury, and miscellaneous host factors. In general, healing wounds are characterized by high mitotic activity, therapeutic levels of inflammatory cytokines, low levels of proteases, and mitotically competent cells. In contrast, chronic wounds exhibit low mitotic activity, excessive levels of inflammatory cytokines, high levels of proteases, and senescent or mitotically incompetent cells.

MEDIATORS OF WOUND HEALING

In order for healing to occur normally, the critical cells must be recruited to the wound bed (at the appropriate time), stimulated to reproduce, and then directed to carry out essential functions, such as neoangiogenesis, connective tissue synthesis, and reepithelialization. This complex process is controlled and coordinated by an equally complex array of regulatory substances; key elements include bioactive molecules, matrix proteins, and the matrix itself. The effect of these regulatory factors is further influenced by "host" factors, such as cell receptor sites, cellular senescence, availability of nutrients, and cofactors required for phagocytosis and collagen synthesis, and comorbid conditions, such as hypoxia and diabetes. This section provides a brief overview of regulatory factors, which are discussed further in Chapter 20.

Bioactive Molecules

Bioactive molecules include growth factors and cytokines. They are produced by the cells in the wound bed (e.g., platelets, neutrophils, macrophages, and fibroblasts) and act as "directors" of cell function and thus of the repair process. They do so by attracting the needed cells to the wound bed, stimulating them to proliferate, and then directing the cells to carry out specific aspects of repair. For example, TNF-α is a proinflammatory cytokine that attracts neutrophils and macrophages to the wound bed and is present in high concentrations during the inflammatory phase, whereas VEGF is a growth factor that supports proliferation and migration of endothelial cells and therefore is important during angiogenesis (Gill and Parks, 2008; Macri and Clark, 2009; Thom, 2009).

Matrix Proteins

Growth factors and cytokines act as "controllers" for the cells critical to the repair process. However, awareness is increasing that the levels and function of growth factors and cytokines are in turn controlled by proteins within the ECM. Key categories of matrix proteins include MMPs, ADAMs, and TIMPs. MMPs and ADAMs can "up-regulate" the levels of growth factors and cytokines by cleaving them from the cell and thus activating them; however, they also can "down-regulate" the levels of growth factors and cytokines by degrading them or by inhibiting their release. TIMPs control the activity of MMPs by binding to them, thus blocking their effects (Gill and Parks, 2008).

Extracellular Matrix

The ECM serves as a scaffold for migrating cells and as a repository for growth factors. It also influences the response of the cells to growth factors. For example, keratinocyte proliferation requires both attachment to the ECM and stimulation by growth factors. Cell migration is another aspect of repair that is dependent on both matrix proteins and integrins within the matrix itself. Matrix proteins promote migration by degrading the bonds between the migrating cells and the underlying wound bed, and the matrix promotes reattachment through the expression of binding sites (integrins) within the matrix. The matrix also supports cell-to-cell communication. The ECM needs to be porous and pliable in order to support the movement of cells, nutrients, and growth factors through the wound environment (Cheresh and Stupack, 2008). From a therapeutic perspective, studies suggest that matrix dressings may promote cell migration, granulation tissue formation, and epithelialization in nonhealing wounds (Chandra et al, 2007; Minke et al, 2007; Nataraj et al, 2007).

Host Factors

A number of host factors influence cells' response to growth factors, cytokines, and matrix proteins. One of these factors is the type of receptors on the cell wall. This is an important factor because all cells within the wound bed are exposed to the same mix of regulatory substances, but only select cells respond. In addition, different cells may exhibit different responses to the same regulatory substance because regulatory substances exert their effects primarily through binding with cell receptors. Therefore only cells with the specific receptor sites respond to the regulatory substance, and the effects of receptor binding vary based on cell type. For example, PDGF stimulates migration of some cells and mitosis in others, but it has no effect on some cells (Martin, 1997; Witte and Barbul, 1997). Furthermore, studies indicate that fibroblasts and keratinocytes in elderly individuals have a decreased number of receptor sites, which may explain why elderly patients tend to exhibit a diminished response to some regulatory substances (Ashcroft et al, 2002).

Another factor that may adversely affect cellular response to regulatory factors is cellular senescence. Senescent cells lack the ability to respond to growth factors and other regulatory factors, so they fail to reproduce and to contribute to the repair process. As noted earlier, cellular senescence is a common impediment to wound healing in the elderly (Pittman, 2007).

Other factors that impact on an individual's ability to heal normally are systemic factors such as nutritional status, perfusion, oxygenation, and comorbidities such as diabetes. These factors are addressed briefly in this chapter and in greater depth in other chapters in this text.

EXTREMES OF REPAIR: SCARLESS HEALING VERSUS EXCESSIVE SCARRING

This chapter has focused on what is currently considered "normal" repair for full-thickness wounds, that is, formation of granulation tissue (scar) to mend the defect, with a covering of new epithelium. This form of repair represents an intermediate point between "ideal" repair, also referred to as *scarless healing,* and "abnormal" repair. Hypertrophic and keloid scars are examples of abnormal repair or excessive scarring. As we learn more about the factors that lead to "normal" and excessive scarring, we hope to be able to optimize repair and minimize scarring for all patients.

Scarless Healing

As mentioned earlier in this chapter, the early-gestation fetus typically heals without scarring, an ability that is lost at 22 to 24 weeks of gestation. Features and characteristics of early-gestation healing are listed in Box 4-2. One significant difference is a markedly diminished inflammatory response. Multiple studies using various models have demonstrated that inflammation is minimal

---

BOX 4-2	Characteristics of Scarless Healing

Decreased amount of platelet-derived growth factor
Decreased amount of proinflammatory proteases and growth factors
Increased levels of fibronectin and hyaluronic acid
Balance of TIMP and MMP
New collagen structure and function indistinguishable from native collagen

MMP, Matrix metalloprotease; *TIMP,* tissue inhibitor of matrix metalloprotease.

---

or essentially absent in early-gestation (scarless) healing. This finding is consistent with other studies showing a strong link between the intensity and duration of the inflammatory response and the subsequent development of scar tissue (Wilgus, 2007). The specific factors thought to contribute to this very minimal inflammatory response include the following:

- Marked reduction in migration of inflammatory cells (neutrophils, macrophages, T cells) to the wound bed. Fetal platelets release much lower levels of proinflammatory growth factors and cytokines, so chemoattraction of inflammatory cells to the wound bed is minimal. In addition, the walls of fetal vessels have fewer adhesion molecules (integrins), so inflammatory cells are much less likely to adhere to the vessel walls and to migrate out into the wound bed.
- Significantly lower levels of inflammatory mediators (e.g., interleukins, prostaglandins) in the fetal ECM.
- Marked reduction in angiogenesis and angiogenic stimuli (VEGF, TGF-β1, PDGF, prostaglandin E$_2$). These angiogenic stimuli have been linked to scar formation.

Another difference in early-gestation healing is the rate at which epithelial resurfacing occurs. Rapid up-regulation of the adhesion molecules within the ECM allows cells to move laterally, which promotes early keratinocyte migration (Wilgus, 2007).

Most importantly, a number of differences in fetal healing contribute to production of a new ECM that retains the characteristics of unwounded tissue. One contributing factor may be the high levels of hyaluronic acid and hyaluronic acid stimulating activity factor. This factor is significant because hyaluronic acid supports rapid cell migration. In addition, high levels of MMPs compared to TIMPs favor degradation of the ECM, which is thought to help prevent overproduction of collagen. Finally, fetal fibroblasts retain the ability to produce new matrix proteins that retain the basketweave configuration characteristic of normal dermis (Wilgus, 2007).

In summary, early-gestation fetal repair is characterized by a significantly reduced inflammatory response and a rapid and balanced proliferative phase that restores the dermal architecture without scarring (see Box 4-2).

Excessive Scarring

Excessive or hyperproliferative scarring is a complication of acute full-thickness wound healing that presently is not well understood. The two types of hyperproliferative scarring are hypertrophic scars and keloid scars (see Plate 7, *C* and *D*). Both types appear raised, are red or pink, and are pruritic. Hypertrophic scars are confined to the original incisional or scar area, whereas keloids expand beyond the incision into the surrounding tissue.

TABLE 4-3   Therapy Options for Hyperproliferative Scarring

Treatment	Indications	Considerations
Surgical excision	Hypertrophic scars Keloid scars	Recurrence rare with hypertrophic Recurrence common (45%–100%) with keloid if surgical excision is done without adjunctive therapies
Radiation (as adjunct to surgical excision)	Hypertrophic scars Keloid scars	Promotion of fibroblast apoptosis (death) Low recurrence rates (1%–35%) Theoretical risk of radiation-induced malignancy (no data)
Corticosteroid therapy (systemic), intralesional injections (triamcinolone)	Hypertrophic scars Keloid scars	Reduces scar overgrowth, pruritus, contractures Pain of repeated injections may limit patient adherence Adverse effects: skin atrophy, depigmentation, telangiectasias
Silicone gel, sheeting	Hypertrophic scars Keloid scars	Increases wound hydration Decreases fibroblast activity Down-regulates fibrogenic isoforms of TGF-β Worn 12–24 hr/day for at least 2–3 months Risk of maceration and skin breakdown with gel (gel use limited to areas where sheeting will not conform)
Laser (CDL, PDL)	Hypertrophic scars Keloid scars	Stimulates regression of keloid Reduces pruritus with hypertrophic (PDL) Variable results if used independently; best if used in conjunction with steroids or silicone gel CDL: recurrence rate as high as 50% PDL: Works best with steroids + silicone No data indicate that laser is more effective than surgery and adjunctive therapy
Retinoids (topical)	Hypertrophic scars Keloid scars	Suppresses collagen synthesis Increases epithelial cell turnover May be applied topically both preoperatively/postoperatively 80% of lesions have favorable short-term outcomes
Intralesional cryotherapy	Hypertrophic scars Keloid scars	Scar regression through reduction of hyperproliferative response
Compression garments	Hypertrophic scars (primary indication) Keloid scars	Hypoxic and thermal effects in compressed areas reduce fibroblast activity Must be worn 8–24 hr/day for first 6 months Must be fit correctly
Antiproliferative agents (5-fluorouracil, bleomycin)	Hypertrophic scars Keloid scars	Induce scar regression 5-Fluorouracil more effective with hypertrophic Provide short-term suppression of small keloids Few small studies support use of bleomycin topically Side effects: pulmonary fibrosis, fever, rash, hyperpigmentation
Intralesional injections of verapamil	Keloid scars	Inhibit inflammation Stimulate production of collagenase and other enzymes to degrade excess extracellular matrix Used for both prevention and treatment
Immunotherapy (immunomodulators, immunosuppressants, antibody therapy [e.g., imiquimod, tacrolimus, sirolimus, tumor necrosis factor-α, interferons, interleukins])	Keloid scars	Suppresses fibroblast activity Promotes fibroblast apoptosis Helps reduce inflammation and regulate cellular activity Significant side effects depending on agent and dose
Suture ligature	Keloid scars Removal of tissue Nutrient deprivation Pressure therapy	Deprives tissue of nutrients and oxygen, thus promoting tissue death Keloid must be amenable to suture ligature Requires weekly office visits and daily maintenance of local wounds
Growth factors (TGF-β1, TGF-β2)	Hypertrophic scars Keloid scars	May abrogate hyperproliferative response Neutralize or abrogate hyperproliferative action of fibrogenic isoforms of TGF-β

Data from Al-Attar et al, 2006; Berman, 2007; D'Andrea, 2002; Franz et al, 2007; Funayama et al, 2003; Gupta and Kumar, 2001; Har-Shai, 2003; Parikh, 2008; Stashower, 2006; Xia et al, 2004.
CDL, Carbon dioxide laser; *PDL,* pulsed dye laser; *TGF,* transforming growth factor.

TABLE 4-4	Factors Affecting Wound Healing	
Factor	**Effects on Repair Process**	**Clinical Implications**
Perfusion/ oxygenation Hypoxia Adequate oxygen levels	Initiates new vessel development, promoting fibroblast proliferation Critical for cellular production of ATP, bacterial killing, collagen synthesis, development of tensile strength Critical oxygen levels ≥30–40 mm Hg (higher for bacterial killing)	Hypovolemia, hypotension, vasoconstriction, vascular impairment, edema, hypoxia all deleterious to repair Intervene to promote perfusion and oxygenation: warmth, hydration, pain control, management of edema, maintenance or restoration of blood flow Supplemental oxygen may be beneficial See Chapter 28
Smoking/ tobacco use	Byproducts (nicotine, carbon monoxide, hydrogen cyanide) reduce oxygenation, impair immune response, reduce fibroblast activity, increase platelet adhesion and thrombus formation Smoking associated with significantly higher infection rates	Counsel patients on negative effects of tobacco use Offer comprehensive program for smoking cessation: support groups, nicotine replacement, medications (No increase in wound infection with nicotine patch) See Chapter 28
Nutritional status	Adequate nutritional status critical for collagen synthesis, tensile strength, immune function Critical nutrients include micronutrients (vitamins, minerals), key amino acids (glutamine, L-arginine), adequate protein	Nutritional assessment and support are critical aspects of effective wound care program and must include attention to micronutrients as well as calorie and protein intake See Chapter 27
Diabetes mellitus	Associated with • Abnormal and prolonged inflammation • Reduced collagen synthesis • Decreased tensile strength • Impaired epithelial migration • Compromised vasculature Hyperglycemia associated with compromised neutrophil function, impaired epithelial migration	Tight glycemic control (glucose levels <130 mg/dl) associated with 10-fold reduction in incidence of postoperative wound infections among cardiac surgery patients See Chapter 14
Obesity	Adipose tissue poorly vascularized Large volumes of adipose tissue put additional stress on incisional lines, increasing risk of dehiscence Associated with higher incidence of infection, seroma formation, wound dehiscence	Monitor intake to ensure adequate intake of protein and micronutrients and appropriate caloric intake Incisional support (binders) beneficial in reducing risk of dehiscence See Chapter 35

Factor	Pathophysiology	Interventions
Medications	Chemotherapeutic agents impair production of white blood cells and fibroblasts, interfering with both inflammatory and proliferative phases of repair and increasing risk of infection. Corticosteroids suppress inflammation and reduce proliferation of keratinocytes and fibroblasts, thereby impairing both granulation and epithelial resurfacing; impact is dose dependent, with greatest effect occurring in patients taking >30–40 mg/day. High doses of NSAIDs may impair healing	Delay chemotherapy when possible to permit healing (delay in healing most significant when chemotherapy given within first weeks following surgery/injury). Limited data suggest that topical vitamin A may partially reverse negative effects of corticosteroids (applied to clean wound bed prior to dressing application). Recommended dose range is 25,000–100,000 international units per day. For patient with impaired healing taking high-dose NSAIDs, collaborate with prescribing provider to reduce dose if possible
Advanced age	Diminished proliferation of cells critical to repair. Hormonal changes. Increased number of senescent cells. Diminished production of growth factors and possible reduction in receptor sites for growth factors. Multiple existing comorbidities	Correct any reversible comorbidities. Optimize nutritional status. Provide evidence-based wound care
Immunosuppression	Increased susceptibility to infection. Compromises body's ability to manifest signs of infection	Provide meticulous wound care to minimize risk of infection. Monitor wound closely for muted signs of infection (faint erythema, mild increase in exudate, pain) and treat appropriately
Stress	Increased production of corticosteroids	Implement strategies to minimize stress: pain control, environmental management, patient education and counseling
Other	Malignancy. Multisystem failure. Failure to maintain clean, moist wound bed	Provide holistic wound management that addresses comorbidities. Implement topical therapy to eliminate necrotic tissue and heavy bacterial loads. Keep wound surface clean and moist

Data from Anstead, 1998; Burns et al, 2003; Ehrlich and Hunt, 1968; Ehrlich and Hunt, 1969; Greenhalgh, 2003; Hardman and Ashcroft, 2008; Manassa et al, 2003; Pittman, 2007; Sorensen et al, 2003; Whitney, 2003; Wicke et al, 2009; Wientjes, 2002; Williams and Barbul, 2003; Wilson and Clark, 2003.
NSAID, Nonsteroidal antiinflammatory drug.

This expansion, sometimes described as a mushroom effect, is the result of continued proliferation of connective tissue proteins that may continue indefinitely (Atiyeh, 2005; Slemp and Kirschner, 2006).

Hypertrophic scars are characterized by increased vasculature, increased numbers of white blood cells and fibroblasts, and a thickened epidermal layer (Atiyeh, 2005). The collagen fibers in hypertrophic scars are organized and oriented parallel to the epidermal layer; however, they contain an abundance of myofibroblasts, which leads to contracture formation. One positive feature of hypertrophic scars (compared to keloids) is their potential to eventually regress during the remodeling phase (Slemp and Kirschner, 2006).

Keloids are a much more serious problem than hypertrophic scars. Keloids may continue to expand, creating both functional and cosmetic deficits. In addition, scars that initially appear to be "normal" may deviate into a pattern of keloid growth over time. Biochemical analysis of keloid scars reveals increased numbers of receptor sites for growth factors (both PDGF and TGF-β), which may partially explain the continued keloid growth. Most importantly, the balance between synthesis and degradation of connective tissue proteins is lost. This loss of balance is theorized to result from abnormalities in cell-to-cell communication and immune function, failure of apoptosis (spontaneous cell death), and the effects of hypoxia and oxygen free radicals. Keloid scars are characterized by disorganized collagen bundles; however, these scars do not contain myofibroblasts and are not associated with contracture formation (Atiyeh, 2005; Slemp and Kirschner, 2006).

Risk factors for hyperproliferative scarring include a strong family history (particularly important with keloid formation), age 10 to 30 years, and darkly pigmented skin. In the United States, individuals of African American descent have a 5% to 15% increased risk compared to Caucasians (Atiyeh, 2005; Slemp and Kirschner, 2006).

Strategies designed to prevent or correct hyperproliferative scarring have provided inconsistent and often suboptimal results. Surgical excision, intralesional steroids, and topical silicone sheeting are the most commonly prescribed therapies. Table 4-3 lists current treatment options and considerations. Research is ongoing, with the goals of accurately identifying the cellular and biochemical abnormalities that produce these scars and designing therapies to prevent and correct them.

FACTORS AFFECTING THE REPAIR PROCESS

By observing a number of similar wounds and tracking their time to healing, it is possible to construct a curve that represents the healing "trajectory" for that type of wound. For example, epithelialization of a surgical wound healing by primary intention typically is complete by 48 hours, a healing ridge should be palpable by days 5 to 9, and initial collagen deposition should be complete by postoperative day 21. Interestingly, it also is possible to plot a "healing trajectory" for neuropathic ulcers, venous ulcers, and pressure ulcers. Studies indicate that the usual "time to healing" is similar for all patients with a particular type of wound (Steed, 2003). Knowledge of the normal healing trajectory for any wound allows the clinician to promptly identify wounds with impaired healing and to intervene accordingly. It also allows investigators to objectively determine the impact of various interventions or impediments on the repair process. For example, any deterrent to healing would shift the healing trajectory to the right, whereas an intervention that enhances healing would shift the trajectory to the left. Whether "normal" healing can be "accelerated" by use of exogenous growth factors or by other interventions is not known at this time. However, accelerated healing would be tremendously beneficial to the many patients undergoing surgical procedures. Factors that can delay the healing process and shift the trajectory to the right are outlined in Table 4-4.

SUMMARY

Wound healing is a complex series of events. Normally wound healing is initiated by an injury that leads to clot formation and platelet degranulation, is controlled by a myriad of cytokines and growth factors, and is affected significantly by systemic factors such as perfusion, nutritional status, and steroid levels. Effective management of any wound requires an understanding of the normal repair process and the factors that may interfere with normal repair. This understanding provides the foundation for comprehensive assessment of the wound and of the patient and for selection of interventions designed to optimize healing.

REFERENCES

Al-Attar A et al: Keloid pathogenesis and wound treatment, *Plastic Reconstr Surg* 117:286-300, 2006.
Anstead G: Steroids, retinoids, and wound healing, *Adv Wound Care* 11:277, 1998.
Ashcroft GS et al: Aging and wound healing, *Biogerontology* 3(6):337, 2002.
Atiyeh B: Keloid or hypertrophic scar: the controversy. Review of the literature, *Ann Plast Surg* 54(6):676-680, 2005.
Berg Vande JS, Robson MC: Arresting cell cycles and the effect on wound healing, *Surg Clin North Am* 83:509, 2003.
Berman B: A review of the biologic effects, clinical efficacy, and safety of silicone elastomer sheeting for hypertrophic and keloid scar treatment and management, *Dermatol Surg* 33(11):1291-1302, 2007.
Braiman-Wiksman L et al: Novel insights into wound healing sequence of events, *Toxicol Pathol* 35:767-779, 2007.
Brissett AE, Hom DB: The effects of tissue sealants, platelet gels, and growth factors on wound healing, *Curr Opin Otolaryngol Head Neck Surg* 11(4):245, 2003.

Bullard KM et al: Fetal wound healing: current biology, *World J Surg* 27:54, 2002.

Burns JL et al: Impairments to wound healing, *Clin Plast Surg* 30:47, 2003.

Calvin M: Cutaneous wound repair, *Wounds* 10(1):12, 1998.

Chandra N et al: Extracellular wound matrices: novel stabilization and sterilization methods for collagen-based wound dressings, *Wounds* 19(6):148-156, 2007.

Chen WYJ, Abatangelo G: Functions of hyaluronan in wound repair, *Wound Repair Regen* 7:79, 1999.

Cheresh D, Stupack D: Regulation of angiogenesis: apoptotic cues from the ECM, *Oncogene* 27:6285-6298, 2008.

Clark JJ: Wound repair and factors influencing healing, *Crit Care Nurs Q* 25(1):1, 2002.

Cross KJ, Mustoe TA: Growth factors in wound healing, *Surg Clin North Am* 83:531, 2003.

D'Andrea F: Prevention and treatment of keloids with intralesional verapamil, *Dermatology* 204(1):60-62, 2002.

Dang C et al: Fetal wound healing: current perspectives, *Clin Plast Surg* 30:13, 2003.

Dubay KA, Franz MG: Acute wound healing: the biology of acute wound failure, *Surg Clin North Am* 83:463, 2003.

Ehrlich P, Hunt T: Effects of cortisone and Vitamin A on wound healing, *Ann Surg* 167(3):324, 1968.

Ehrlich P, Hunt T: The effects of cortisone and anabolic steroids on the tensile strength of healing wounds, *Ann Surg* 170(2):203, 1969.

Frank S et al: Nitric oxide drives skin repair: novel functions of an established mediator, *Kidney Int* 61:882, 2002.

Franz M et al: Optimizing healing of the acute wound by minimizing complications, *Curr Prob Surg* 44(11):684-689, 2007.

Funayama E et al: Keratinocytes promote proliferation and inhibit apoptosis of the underlying fibroblasts: an important role in the pathogenesis of keloid, *J Invest Dermatol* 121(6):1326-1331, 2003.

Gabbiani G: The myofibroblast in wound healing and fibrocontractive diseases, *J Pathol* 200:500, 2003.

Gabriel A et al: *Wound healing, growth factors*, available at http://emedicine.medscape.com/article/1298196-overview, accessed April 26, 2010.

Gill S, Parks W: Metalloproteinases and their inhibitors: regulators of wound healing, *Int J Biochem Cell Biol* 40:1334-1347, 2008.

Goldman R: Growth factors and chronic wound healing: past, present, and future, *Adv Skin Wound Care* 17(1):24, 2004.

Greenhalgh DG: Wound healing and diabetes mellitus, *Clin Plast Surg* 30:37, 2003.

Gupta S, Kumar B: Intralesional cryosurgery using lumbar puncture and/or hypodermic needles for large, bulky, recalcitrant keloids, *Int J Dermatol* 40(5):349-353, 2001.

Hardman M, Ashcroft G: Estrogen, not intrinsic aging, is the major regulator of delayed human wound healing in the elderly, *Genome Biol* 9(5):R80, 2008.

Harrison C et al: Use of an in vitro model of tissue-engineered human skin to study keratinocyte attachment and migration in the process of reepithelialization, *Wound Repair Regen* 14:203-209, 2006.

Har-Shai Y: Intralesional cryotherapy for enhancing the involution of hypertrophic scars and keloids, *Plast Reconstr Surg* 111(6):1841-1852, 2003.

Henry G, Garner WL: Inflammatory mediators in wound healing, *Surg Clin North Am* 83:483, 2003.

Hoenig M et al: Decreased vascular repair and neovascularization with ageing: mechanisms and clinical relevance with an emphasis on hypoxia-inducible factor, *Curr Mol Med* 8(8):754-767, 2008.

Hunt TK, Van Winkle W Jr: Normal repair. In Hunt TK, Dunphy JE, editors: *Fundamentals of wound management*, New York 1997. Appleton-Century-Crofts.

Jahoda CAB, Reynolds AJ: Hair follicle dermal sheath cells: unsung participants in wound healing, *Lancet* 358(9291):1445, 2001.

James TJ et al: Simple biochemical markers to assess chronic wounds, *Wound Repair Regen* 8:264, 2000.

Lan C-CE et al: Hyperglycaemic conditions decrease cultured keratinocyte mobility: implications for impaired wound healing in patients with diabetes, *Br J Dermatol* 159:1103-1115, 2008.

Liu Y et al: Cell and molecular mechanisms of keratinocyte function stimulated by insulin during wound healing, *BMC Cell Biol* 10(1):1-20, 2009.

Lizarbe T et al: Nitric oxide elicits functional MMP-13 protein-tyrosine nitration during wound repair, *FASEB J* 22:3207-3215, 2008.

Loryman C, Mansbridge J: Inhibition of keratinocyte migration by lipopolysaccharide, *Wound Repair Regen* 16:45-51, 2008.

Macri L, Clark R: Tissue engineering for cutaneous wounds: selecting the proper time and space for growth factors, cells, and extracellular matrix, *Skin Pharmacol Physiol* 22(2):83-93, 2009.

Manassa EH et al: Wound healing problems in smokers and non-smokers after 132 abdominoplasties, *Plast Reconstr Surg* 111(6):2082, 2003.

Mangram AJ et al: Guideline for prevention of surgical site infection, *Infect Control Hosp Epidemiol* 20(1):250, 1999.

Martin P: Wound healing: aiming for perfect skin regeneration, *Science* 276:75, 1997.

Mast BA, Schultz G: Interactions of cytokines, growth factors, and proteases in acute and chronic wounds, *Wound Repair Regen* 4:411, 1996.

Minke G et al: Extracellular wound matrix (OASIS): exploring the contraindications and results of 32 consecutive outpatient clinic cases, *Wounds* 19(10):258-263, 2007.

Monaco JL, Lawrence WT: Acute wound healing: an overview, *Clin Plast Surg* 30:1, 2003.

Myers S et al: Epidermal repair results from activation of follicular and epidermal progenitor keratinocytes mediated by a growth factor cascade, *Wound Repair Regen* 15:693-701, 2007.

Nataraj C et al: Extracellular wound matrices: novel stabilization and sterilization method for collagen-based biologic wound dressings, *Wounds* 19(6):148-156, 2007.

O'Goshi K-I, Tagami H: Basic fibroblast growth factor treatment for various types of recalcitrant skin ulcers: reports of nine cases, *J Dermatol Treat* 18:375-381, 2007.

O'Toole E et al: Hypoxia induces epidermal keratinocyte matrix metalloproteinase-9 secretion via the protein kinase C pathway, *J Cell Physiol* 214:47-55, 2008.

Parikh D: Keloid banding using suture ligature: a novel technique and review of literature, *Laryngoscope* 118(11):1960-1965, 2008.

Phillips SJ: Physiology of wound healing and surgical wound care, *ASAIO J* 46(6):S2-S5, 2000.

Pittman J: Effect of aging on wound healing: current concepts, *JWOCN* 34(4):412-417, 2007.

Pradhan L et al: Inflammation and neuropeptides: the connection in diabetic wound healing, *Exp Rev Mol Med* 11:e2, 2009.

Pullar C et al: β-adrenergic receptor modulation of repair, *Pharmacol Res* 58(2):158-164, 2008.

Rahban SR, Garner WL: Fibroproliferative scars, *Clin Plast Surg* 30:77, 2003.

Richards AM et al: Neural innervation and healing, *Lancet* 350(9074):339, 1997.

Robson MC: Proliferative scarring, *Surg Clin North Am* 33:557, 2003.

Rodriguez P et al: The role of oxygen in wound healing: a review of the literature, *Dermatol Surg* 34:1159-1169, 2008.

Samuels P, Tan AKW: Fetal scarless wound healing, *J Otolaryngol* 28(5):296, 1999.

Schneider A et al: Self-assembling peptide nanofiber scaffolds accelerate wound healing, *PLoS ONE* 3(1):e1410, 2008.

Schultz GS et al: Wound bed preparation: a systematic approach to wound management, *Wound Repair Regen* 11(s1):1, 2003.

Slemp A, Kirschner R: Keloids and scars: a review of keloids and scars, their pathogenesis, risk factors, and management, *Curr Opin Pediatr* 18(4):396-402, 2006.

Sorensen LT et al: Abstinence from smoking reduces incisional wound infection: a randomized controlled trial, *Ann Surg* 238(1):1, 2003.

Staiano-Coico L et al: Wound fluids: a reflection of the state of healing, *Ostomy Wound Manage* S46(1A):85, 2000.

Stashower M: Successful treatment of earlobe keloids with imiquimod after tangential shave excision, *Dermatol Surg* 32(3):380-386, 2006.

Steed DL: Wound-healing trajectories, *Surg Clin North Am* 83:547, 2003.

Thom S: Oxidative stress is fundamental to hyperbaric oxygen therapy, *J Appl Physiol* 106:988-995, 2009.

Werner S, Grose R: Regulation of wound healing by growth factors and cytokines, *Physiol Rev* 83:835, 2003.

Whitney JD: Supplemental perioperative oxygen and fluids to improve surgical wound outcomes: translating evidence into practice, *Wound Repair Regen* 11(6):462, 2003.

Wicke C et al: Aging influences wound healing in patients with chronic lower extremity wounds treated in a specialized wound care center, *Wound Repair Regen* 17(1):25-33, 2009.

Wientjes KA: Mind-body techniques in wound healing, *Ostomy Wound Manage* 48(11):62, 2002.

Wilgus T: Regenerative healing in fetal skin: a review of the literature, *Ostomy Wound Manage* 53(6):16-31, 2007.

Williams JZ, Barbul A: Nutrition and wound healing, *Surg Clin North Am* 83:571, 2003.

Wilson JA, Clark JJ: Obesity: impediment to wound healing, *Crit Care Nurs Q* 26(2):119, 2003.

Winter G: Epidermal regeneration studied in the domestic pig. In Hunt T, Dunphy J, editors: *Fundamentals of wound management*, New York, 1979, Appleton-Century-Crofts.

Witte M, Barbul A: General principles of wound healing, *Surg Clin North Am* 77(3):509, 1997.

Xia W et al: Complex epithelial-mesenchymal interactions modulate transforming growth factor-beta expression in keloid-derived cells, *Wound Repair Regen* 12(5):546-556, 2004.

Yang GP et al: From scarless fetal wounds to keloids: molecular studies in wound healing, *Wound Repair Regen* 11(6):411, 2003.

5

Types of Skin Damage and Differential Diagnosis

Ruth A. Bryant

OBJECTIVES

1. Describe the process of at least five factors that contribute to skin damage.
2. Distinguish among the following terms: macule, papule, plaque, nodule, wheal, pustule, vesicle, and bulla.
3. Describe four types of mechanical trauma by the extent of tissue damage associated with each.
4. Discuss at least three interventions for preventing each type of mechanical trauma.
5. Describe three preventive interventions for three common causes of chemical damage.
6. Describe the process of an allergic contact dermatitis.
7. Identify factors that predispose a patient to candidiasis.
8. Describe the types of lesions common to candidiasis, folliculitis, impetigo, and herpes.
9. Discriminate among incontinence-associated dermatitis, candidiasis intertrigo, Stage I pressure ulcer, suspected deep tissue injury (sDTI), perianal herpes, tinea cruris, and inverse psoriasis.
10. Describe the manifestations and care of skin damage due to irradiation.

Skin integrity can be jeopardized or compromised by a multitude of factors: mechanical, moisture, chemical, vascular, infectious, allergy, inflammatory, intrinsic disease, burn, radiation, and miscellaneous assaults. Each type of injury creates a complex set of skin responses, such as erythema, macules, papules, pustules, vesicles/bullae, erosion, and ulcers. Primary lesions of the skin are the first recognizable lesions in the skin. Plate 6 shows the definition and appearance of common primary lesions. Secondary skin lesions evolve from primary lesions due to the natural history of the disease or as a result of scratching/infection. Common secondary lesions are depicted and defined in Plate 7. Because periwound skin can develop skin complications and because many of these conditions provide clues to the etiology of the skin alteration, the health care provider for patients in acute care, home care, outpatient, and long-term care facilities must be familiar with these terms.

ASSESSMENT

A systematic skin assessment and an accurate description of any lesions are essential to obtain a reasonable list of differential diagnoses. Additional assessments and diagnostic tests then can be used to derive the most likely diagnosis. Lesions should be described by five morphologic parameters: distribution, shape or arrangement, border and margins, associated changes within the lesion(s), and pigmentation. These parameters, including options for descriptive terminology, are listed in Table 5-1.

Before a treatment plan for any skin lesion or wound can be initiated, the underlying cause of that condition must be determined. Clues to the cause are derived from the patient's history and physical assessment and specifically by an assessment of the following parameters: location, characteristics, and distribution. These clues can be used to direct subsequent tests that may be necessary to develop a definitive diagnosis. Once the cause of the wound or skin lesion is identified, realistic goals for care can be established and a comprehensive, multidisciplinary treatment plan devised. This chapter introduces a classification system for types of skin damage, briefly describes the pathophysiologic process, and discusses the prevention and treatment of the most common types of skin damage (Box 5-1). The more atypical types of skin lesions, particularly those associated with intrinsic disease, are addressed in Chapter 30.

MECHANICAL FORCES

The forces that are applied externally to the skin, such as pressure, shear, friction, and skin stripping (skin tears), create mechanical skin damage. Each may occur in isolation or in combination with other mechanical insults, such

TABLE 5-1	Morphologic Characteristics of Skin Lesions	
Characteristic	Description	Examples
Distribution		
Localized	Lesion appears in one small area	Impetigo, herpes simplex (e.g., labialis), tinea corporis ("ringworm")
Regional	Lesions involve a specific region of the body	Acne vulgaris (pilosebaceous gland distribution), herpes zoster (nerve dermatomal distribution), psoriasis (flexural surfaces and skin folds)
Generalized	Lesions appear widely distributed or in numerous areas simultaneously	Urticaria, disseminated drug eruptions
Shape/Arrangement		
Round/discoid	Coin or fine shaped (no central clearing)	Nummular eczema
Oval	Ovoid shape	Pityriasis rosea
Annular	Round, active margins with central clearing	Tinea corporis, sarcoidosis
Zosteriform (dermatomal)	Following a nerve or segment of the body	Herpes zoster
Polycyclic	Interlocking or coalesced circles (formed by enlargement of annular lesions)	Psoriasis, urticaria
Linear	In a line	Contact dermatitis
Iris/target lesion	Pink macules with purple central papules	Erythema multiforme
Stellate	Star shaped	Meningococcal septicemia
Serpiginous	Snakelike or wavy line track	Cutanea larva migrans
Reticulate	Netlike or lacy	Polyarteritis nodosa, lichen planus lesions of erythema infectiosum
Morbilliform	Measles-like: maculopapular lesions that become confluent on the face and body	Measles, roseola
Border/Margin		
Discrete	Well demarcated or defined, able to draw a line around it with confidence	Psoriasis
Indistinct	Poorly defined, have borders that merge into normal skin or outlying ill defined papules	Nummular eczema
Active	Margin of lesion shows greater activity than center	*Tinea* spp. eruptions
Irregular	Nonsmooth or notched margin	Malignant melanoma
Border raised above center	Center of lesion is depressed compared to the edge	Basal cell carcinoma
Advancing	Expanding at margins	Cellulitis
Associated Changes within Lesions		
Central clearing	An erythematous border surrounds lighter skin	Tinea eruptions
Desquamation	Peeling or sloughing of skin	Rash of toxic shock syndrome
Keratotic	Hypertrophic stratum corneum	Calluses, warts
Punctation	Central umbilication or dimpling	Basal cell carcinoma
Telangiectasias	Dilated blood vessels within lesion blanch completely, may be markers of systematic disease	Basal cell carcinoma, actinic keratosis
Pigmentation		
Flesh	Same tone as the surrounding skin	Neurofibroma, some nevi
Pink	Light red undertones	Eczema, pityriasis rosea
Erythematous	Dark pink to red	Tinea eruptions, psoriasis
Salmon	Orange-pink	Psoriasis
Tan-brown	Light to dark brown	Most nevi, pityriasis versicolor
Black	Black or blue-black	Malignant melanoma
Pearly	Shiny white, almost iridescent	Basal cell carcinoma
Purple	Dark red-blue-violet	Purpura, Kaposi sarcoma
Violaceous	Light violet	Erysipelas
Yellow	Waxy	Lipoma
White	Absent of color	Lichen planus

From Seidel HM et al: *Mosby's guide to physical examination*, ed 6, St Louis, 2006, Mosby.

BOX 5-1	Classification of Common Types of Skin Damage*

Mechanical
Pressure
Shear
Friction
Skin stripping (skin tears)

Moisture
Urine
Perspiration
Moisture donating wound dressing

Chemical
Feces
Gastrointestinal contents
Drainage from percutaneous tubes
Povidone-iodine complex (Betadine)
Alkaline soaps
Alcohol

Vascular/Neuropathic
Venous
Arterial
Neuropathic

Infectious
Fungal
Candidiasis
Dermatophyte (tinea)

Bacterial
Cellulitis
Erysipelas
Erythrasma
Folliculitis
Impetigo
Bullous impetigo
Nonbullous impetigo

Viral
Herpes simplex
Varicella-zoster virus

Allergic
Radiation

*See Chapter 30 for atypical types of skin damage.

as pressure and shear. This chapter presents shear, friction, and skin stripping. Pressure damage is discussed in detail in Chapter 7. Preventive interventions for pressure are discussed in Chapters 8 and 9.

Shear

Shearing force is the sliding movement of skin and subcutaneous tissue while the underlying muscle and bone are stationary (AORN, 2008). This type of skin damage is created by the interaction of tangential forces and friction (resistance) against the surface of the skin. Friction is always present when shearing force is present. The classic example of a shear injury occurs when the patient

is in a semi-Fowler position. While the bony structures and muscles slide downward to the foot of the bed, the bed surface generates enough resistance that the skin and subcutaneous tissue over the sacrum remain in the same location (Figure 5-1). Ultimately, the skin is held in place while the skeletal structures pull the body (by gravity) toward the foot of the bed. Consequently, blood vessels in the area are stretched and angulated, the vasculature is disrupted, and small-vessel thrombosis and tissue death may develop (Wright and O'Connor, 2007).

Shear may cause shallow or deep ulcers and extends the tissue damage of pressure ulcers. This extension is manifested in the pressure ulcer by the presence of undermining (dissection or separation of tissue parallel to the skin surface; see Figure 6-4). Shear injury is predominantly localized at the sacrum or coccyx and is commonly a consequence of elevating the head of the bed or improper transfer technique. Prevention requires an awareness of those situations in which the skin is subjected to shearing force. For example, the patient with pulmonary distress requires the head of the bed to be elevated to facilitate adequate ventilation; however, the patient is at great risk for shear injury. Likewise, the patient with a cerebrovascular accident may experience shear injury when being transferred from the bed to the wheelchair. In the operating room, shear may be present with lateral transfers of the patient from the stretcher to the operating table (AORN, 2008).

Most strategies for prevention of shear have derived from expert opinion. Because shear is an important contributing factor to pressure ulcer development, strategies to simultaneously prevent shear and pressure are warranted (see Chapter 8). The primary intervention for reducing shear is the use of lift sheets when repositioning the patient; this eliminates drag on the sacral skin. The head of bed should be maintained at less than 30 degrees; elevations higher than 30 degrees may be needed for meals but should be limited to short periods of time. Also, the knee gatch can be used to interrupt gravity's pull on the body toward the foot of the bed. Sheepskin may be used; however, its use should not be confused with pressure-redistribution measures. Many support surfaces have a slick fabric covering, which anecdotally and intuitively seems to reduce shear. A standardized method for measuring the ability of a support surface to reduce shear is not currently available.

Fontaine et al (1998) proposed a calculated pressure/shear factor (PSF), which would quantify support surface efficiency for the combined effect of pressure and shear reduction. PSF is calculated by adding the rounded average interface pressure (in millimeters of mercury) to the rounded average gross shearing force (g) multiplied by the impact factor of 4. The equation is as follows:

$$\text{Pressure} + (4 \times \text{shearing force}) = \text{PSF}$$

or

$$\text{mm Hg} + (4\text{ g}) = \text{PSF}$$

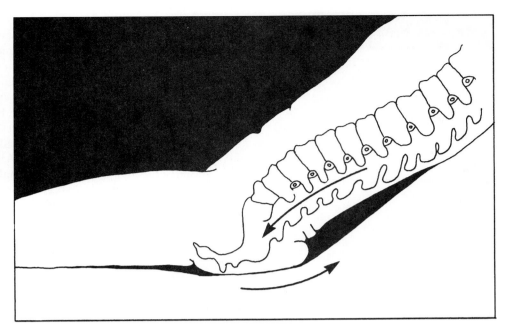

FIGURE 5-1 Shearing force. (From Loeper JM et al: *Therapeutic positioning and skin care,* Minneapolis, 1986, Sister Kenny Institute.)

A pressure sensor and a shear sensor are required to obtain the values to put into the PSF equation. Potentially, PSF could become a tangible support surface measurement. In this way, PSF would provide additional objective information on the potential for the support surface to prevent ulceration. For example, Fontaine et al (1998) studied PSF for three support surfaces classified as group 2 devices according to the Medicare Part B policy (described in Chapter 9). PSF was calculated for a powered, alternating-pressure mattress overlay; a powered, zoned, air-filled mattress replacement device; and a nonpowered fluid overlay. The resulting PSFs were 939, 1,043, and 331, respectively. The implication of this finding is that the nonpowered fluid overlay was more effective in reducing the pressure/shearing force. However, because PSF is a newly defined variable, further research is required to establish the validity of the variable as well as its predictive value and clinical effectiveness.

Friction

The National Pressure Ulcer Advisory Panel (NPUAP) defines friction as the resistance to motion in a parallel direction relative to the common boundary between two surfaces (NPUAP, 2007). Skin injury by friction initially appears as erythema and progresses to an abrasion. As stated previously, shearing force is created by the interaction of tangential forces and friction (resistance) against the surface of the skin. Friction is frequently seen on elbows or heels because the patient easily abrades these surfaces against sheets when repositioning. Injury is characteristically very shallow and limited to the epidermis. Friction primarily affects superficial layers, and thus does not result in tissue necrosis, while shearing forces mainly affect deeper tissue layers (WOCN, 2010).

Interventions to prevent friction and superficial shear involve the use of protective padding over the elbows or heels and moisturizers applied to vulnerable areas to maintain proper hydration of the epidermis. Both maneuvers decrease friction and thereby decrease shear. Transparent adhesive dressings, thin hydrocolloids, low-adhesion foam dressings, and skin sealants are effective at reducing friction. Adhesive dressings are contraindicated if the shear is sufficient to loosen the dressing. Braces, splints, prosthetic devices, and shoes should be assessed frequently for evidence of shear, and modifications (e.g., reshaping, molding, extra padding) should be implemented as needed.

Skin Stripping and Lacerations (Epidermal and Dermal)

Skin stripping is the inadvertent removal of the epidermis, with or without the dermis, by mechanical means. Trauma such as tape removal, electrode removal, or bumping into furniture and assisting with repositioning or mobility can precipitate skin tears (Meuleneire, 2002; Payne and Martin, 1990). For most patients skin tears do not extend hospital stay, but they are painful and distressing in appearance and can be interpreted as being the result of poor care (Ratliff and Fletcher, 2007). In the neonate or premature infant, however, skin tears are a significant portal of entry that can lead to septicemia (Furdon, 2003). Unique considerations concerning skin tears in the neonate or premature infant are addressed in Chapter 36. Data suggest that skin tears heal in 7 to 21 days, depending on the extent of tissue damage (Milne and Corbett, 2005; Meuleneire, 2002).

Although never tested for validity or reliability, the Payne-Martin classification system for skin tears is an instrument commonly used to classify skin tears (Table 5-2). Category I skin tears are distinguished by a resulting skin flap or avulsed skin that can cover the exposed wound (Plates 8-9). Category II wounds (Plates 10-11) are distinguished by the degree of damage to the epidermal avulsed skin. Category III lesions (Plate 12) have no epidermal flap. Typically, skin stripping lesions are irregularly shaped and shallow, involving only the epidermis. Only category IA lesions are full thickness (involve the dermis). The frequency of various locations of skin-stripping injuries is as follows: upper extremities (73%–80%), legs and feet (20%), head (3%–4%), and torso (3%) (Malone et al, 1991; McGough-Csarny and Kopac, 1998; Payne and Martin, 1990). In 2006, the Pennsylvania Patient Safety Reporting System (PA-PSRS) reported similar results and further specified the involved sites on the upper extremities (Pennsylvania Patient Safety Authority, 2006). PA-PSRS reports the most frequent site of injury is the forearm, followed by the arm, hand, and lower extremities (Pennsylvania Patient Safety Authority, 2006).

Risk factors for a skin tear include advanced age, sensory loss, dehydration and malnutrition, history of previous skin tears, cognitive impairment, dependency, poor locomotion, and presence of ecchymosis (McGough-Csarny and Kopac, 1998; Lablanc et al, 2008). However, it is important to remember that even independent, ambulatory patients are at risk for this injury; they experience the second highest number of skin tears (Baranoski, 2001). In this population, patients often have edema, purpura, or ecchymosis, and the skin tears occur primarily on the lower extremities.

Elderly skin and immature skin both are vulnerable to skin tears because the dermal–epidermal junction is not optimally functional. The interlocking dermal papillae and epidermal rete pegs at the dermal–epidermal junction are critical to providing resiliency and the ability to withstand mechanical forces. In the premature infant's skin, the dermal–epidermal junction is undeveloped and weak. As the skin ages the epidermis thins, the dermal–epidermal junction flattens, and cohesion is diminished. In addition, the amounts of collagen and elastin present in the aging skin decrease so that the skin becomes wrinkled, thin, and less compliant. Furthermore, similar connective tissue changes around blood vessels increase the fragility of capillaries. Therefore mechanical stresses can trigger a subcutaneous hemorrhage (e.g., senile purpura) between the skin layers, which results in further separation of the dermis and epidermis. Disease management regimens also can alter the skin's vitality. For example, corticosteroids reduce tissue collagen strength and elasticity and thereby increase the patient's risk of skin tears. Long-term consequences of radiation therapy are epidermal atrophy, microvascular occlusions, reduced fibroblast proliferation, and tissue fibrosis.

Daily care activities, such as bathing, dressing, transfers, and toileting, all require frequent handling of the patient with vulnerable skin. Therefore their potential for inducing a skin tear increases. Use of equipment (e.g., mechanical lifts, wheelchairs, and geriatric chairs) also increases the patient's exposure to potential trauma, which may precipitate a skin tear (McGough-Csarny and Kopac, 1998).

A standardized care plan for patients at high risk for skin tears is given in Box 5-2 (Ayello, 2003; Lablanc et al, 2008; White et al, 1994). Recognizing "at-risk" individuals and implementing key preventive strategies has been shown to decrease the incidence of skin tears (Bank and Nix, 2006; Brillhart, 2005). Extreme care and a gentle touch are critical when touching the patient or performing patient care, because most skin tears occur during the course of providing routine patient care activities (e.g., bathing, dressing, transferring) (Malone et al, 1991; McGough-Csarny and Kopac,

TABLE 5-2	Skin Tears: Definition and Payne-Martin Classification System	
Category	**Subcategory**	**Description**
I: Skin tear can fully approximate wound	A: Linear skin tear	Full-thickness wound that occurs in wrinkle or furrow of skin. Both epidermis and dermis are pulled apart as if an incision has been made, exposing tissue below.
	B: Flap-type skin tear	Partial-thickness wound in which the epidermal flap can be completely approximated or approximated so that no more than 1 mm of dermis is exposed.
II: Skin tear with partial-thickness loss	A: Scant tissue loss	Partial-thickness wound in which 25% or less of the epidermal flap is lost and at least 75% or more of the dermis is covered by the flap.
	B: Moderate to large tissue loss	Partial-thickness wound in which more than 25% of the epidermal flap is lost and more than 25% of the dermis is exposed.
III: Skin tear with complete tissue loss		Partial-thickness wound in which an epidermal flap is absent.

From Payne RL, Martin ML: Defining and classifying skin tears: need for a common language, *Ostomy Wound Manage* 39(5):16, 1993.

BOX 5-2	Standardized Care Plan for Patients at High Risk for Skin Tears

1. Provide a safe environment.
   - Free room of obstacles that obstruct pathway around bed and bathroom.
   - Provide adequate lighting in resident's room.
   - Leave on nightlight in bathroom and leave door open.
   - Leave side rails down at night.
   - Make hourly rounds.
   - Provide safe area for wandering.
   - Implement bed or ankle alarm.
   - Provide well-fitting supportive shoes with skid-free soles.
   - Use protective garments for arms, legs, areas of purpura (e.g., fleece-lined jogging suits, knee-length athletic socks, stockinette doubled, skin sleeves).
   - Pad rough edges of furniture.
   - Relocate or loosen ID band when determined to be cause of skin tears.
2. Maintain nutrition and hydration.
   - Obtain dietary consult.
   - Obtain physician's order for double portions or high-protein snacks between meals.
   - Keep intake and output records.
   - Offer fluids between meals twice every shift.
   - Encourage fluids at every meal.
   - Inspect and moisturize arms and legs twice daily.
3. Protect from self-inflicted injury or injury incurred during routine cares.
   - Keep nails clipped.
   - Use wheelchair for transport only.
   - Use sling around chair legs to prevent feet from falling off footrests.
   - Position with pillows and folded blankets to prevent head and arms from dangling over side of chair.
   - Use palm of hands and lift sheet instead of fingers to position patient.
   - Use mechanical lift for transfers.
   - Obtain occupational or physical therapy consultation if needed for safe positioning.
   - Use appropriate methods for application and removal of adhesives; avoid adhesives if possible (see Box 5-3).

Reprinted with permission from White et al: Skin tears in frail elders: a practical approach to prevention, *Ger Nurs* 15(2):95-99, 1994.

1998; White et al, 1994). Because harsh soaps and frequent bathing can reduce the skin's natural lubrication and lead to dry skin, gentle skin cleansers and frequent moisturizing are important components of skin tear prevention (Bank and Nix, 2006; Birch and Coggins, 2003; Brillhart, 2005; Hunter et al, 2002; Ratliff and Fletcher, 2007). It may be necessary to decrease bathing schedules and use humidifiers to increase environmental moisture (Lablanc and Baranoski, 2009; Lablanc et al, 2008). Rooms should be adequately lit to reduce the risk of bumping into furniture and equipment (Ratliff and Fletcher, 2007; Nazarko, 2005) Beyond these measures, the current focus of prevention is on the application of products and garments that serve as barriers between the skin and potential trauma; such products include commercially available skin sleeves, roll gauze, pants, and long-sleeve shirts (Bank and Nix, 2006).

Unnecessary use of adhesives and tapes should be avoided, particularly on vulnerable, fragile skin. It is important to be creative when securing dressings without applying tape to the skin. For example, tubular stockinette gauze, roll gauze, or self-adhering tape can be used. In general, it is best to avoid applying adhesives in an area receiving radiation.

If adhesives must be used, skin sealants can be placed on the skin before the tape is applied to provide protection from skin tears. Only alcohol-free skin sealants should be used when the skin is denuded or when contact with wound edges is likely because alcohol can cause intense stinging. It is important to allow the skin sealant to dry completely before applying tape. Many central-line dressing kits are prepackaged with a skin sealant.

When frequent tape removal is needed for dressing changes, application of an adhesive barrier (e.g., solid-wafer skin barrier or thin hydrocolloid) can be used on periwound skin to anchor tape and prevent skin stripping. The protocol should clearly indicate that the barrier is not changed routinely. The barrier should be left undisturbed and allowed to fall off. Loose edges should be clipped rather than removing the old barrier and applying a new one. Used in this way, the skin barrier or hydrocolloid dressing can remain in place for several days while caregivers easily apply and reapply the tape without traumatizing the epidermis. Box 5-3 summarizes interventions for preventing skin tears in conjunction with the use of adhesives and tapes.

Ideally, category I skin tears can be treated by repositioning a residual flap over the wound surface to maintain viability and facilitate reattachment (Lablanc et al, 2008; Ratliff and Fletcher, 2007). The skin flap can be approximated and secured with Steri-strips. The strips should be used judiciously because traction on the skin (even from Steri-strips) can cause further damage (Ratliff and Fletcher, 2007). Approximated edges also may be secured with 2-octetyl-cyanoacrylate (also referred to as topical skin bandage or skin glue) (Baranoski, 2003; Fleck, 2007; Lablanc et al, 2008; Roberts, 2007).

For treatment of category II and III skin tears, non-adherent dressings or topical liquid films are recommended to minimize tissue trauma and pain when the dressings are removed (Meuleneire, 2002; Milne and Corbett, 2005; Roberts, 2007). Thomas et al (1999) reported that dressings with a high moisture vapor transmission rate, such as those with a low-adhesive foam dressing, result in complete healing of 94% (16/17) category II and III skin tears within 21 days. This is in comparison with complete healing of only 65% (11/17) of skin tears when film dressings are used. The researchers suggest that film dressings keep the skin tear excessively moist and exacerbate the separation of epidermis from dermal papillae. These results underscore the importance of selecting dressings based on the

BOX 5-3	Prevention of Skin Stripping from Tapes and Adhesives*

1. Secure dressings with roll gauze, tubular stockinette, or self-adhering tape (avoids unnecessary tape on skin).
2. Apply tape without tension (prevents blistering of skin under tape).
3. Use porous tapes (allows moisture to evaporate).
4. Use skin sealants, thin hydrocolloids, or solid-wafer skin barriers under adhesives (provides protective layer over skin for adhering tapes).
5. Secure dressings with Montgomery straps (prevents repeated tape applications).
6. Remove tape slowly, peel away from anchored skin or pull one corner of tape at an angle parallel with skin. Solvents can be used to break bond with skin, although solvents have drying effect on skin. Plain tap water can often serve this purpose effectively (decreases trauma to epidermis and dermal–epidermal junction).

Neonates (See also Chapter 36)
- Solvents and adhesive removers should not be used with the neonate due to reports of skin toxicity.
- Skin sealants should not be used with neonates less than 30 days old. Alcohol free skin sealants may be used for the neonate greater than 30 days old.

*Rationale for intervention is given in parentheses.

"needs" of the wound or the wound characteristics (see Chapter 18).

Skin tears cannot be prevented by one individual. Because the typical individual at risk for skin tears is dependent on caregivers for many aspects of care, preventive interventions must be embraced by all staff members. Therefore staff education is a critical component of a skin tear prevention and treatment program. By using a web-based educational program, McTigue et al (2009) found that acute care registered nurses from two affiliated hospitals (N = 416) had significantly improved their ability to identify, assess, classify, and treat skin tears ($p <.001$) after they had completed the program.

MOISTURE AND CHEMICAL FACTORS

When the skin is exposed to moisture, such as body fluids or cleansers, for extended periods of time or repeatedly (i.e., frequent cleansing), the normal barrier function of the stratum corneum is diminished. As a result, skin pH rises and the risk of bacterial colonization increases, predisposing the patient to development of cutaneous infections. The two most common organisms are *Candida albicans* (from the gastrointestinal tract) and *Staphylococcus* (from the perineal skin).

The nomenclature used to describe and classify skin damage caused by these conditions is extensive and confusing. For example, dermatitis caused by chemical irritants has been referred to as *irritant contact dermatitis*. The term *diaper dermatitis*, familiar to most health care providers, specifically refers to inflammation of the skin in the diaper area (perineal or perigenital areas) of the infant (Zulkowski, 2008). However, when the same condition develops in the perineal area in the adult, it is often called *perineal dermatitis*. The dilemma with both terms is that they do not adequately address the irritant, and the terms exclude locations outside of the diaper or perineum, such as the inner thighs or buttocks.

Recognizing the multiplicity and limitations of terms, a panel of six clinical experts recommended replacing these terms with *incontinence-associated dermatitis* (IAD), defined as a reactive response of the skin to chronic exposure to urine and fecal material, which could be observed as inflammation and erythema with or without erosion or denudation (Gray et al, 2007a). This term describes the response of the skin (dermatitis, which is inflammation and erythema with or without erosion or denudation), specifically identifies the source of the irritant (urine or fecal incontinence), and acknowledges that a larger area of the skin is commonly affected (Plate 13). Coexisting infections may develop with IAD, most often candidiasis. Additional infections that can arise include herpes zoster or herpes simplex virus (HSV), candidal intertrigo, tinea cruris (a dermatophyte infection of the squamous cells and trapped in a skin fold), and inverse psoriasis (Visscher, 2009).

Skin damage due to moisture on the skin is not limited to the etiology of incontinence. During a consensus meeting of four clinicians addressing the problem with adequate terminology for this condition, the term *moisture-associated skin damage* (MASD) was coined as a generic term to refer to skin damage in any location on the body that occurs due to exposure to moisture "and associated irritants" (Gray and Weir, 2007; Gray et al, 2007b). Conditions identified by the group to be associated with MASD included periwound maceration, IAD and candidiasis. However, many more moisture-related skin problems probably can be added to this list, including Stage I and II pressure ulcers, intertrigo, and tinea cruris.

From a practical standpoint, it is helpful to discuss skin damage or dermatitis from the perspective of the agent triggering the response in the skin regardless of the anatomic body location. In this manner, the etiology of the skin damage is identified, and appropriate interventions for prevention and treatment are derived. For example, fecal content has a stronger association with skin damage than does urine, which may impact the choice of preventive interventions (Bliss et al, 2006; Junkin and Lerner-Selekof, 2007). In this textbook, we refer to moisture as a factor that weakens intact skin but does not cause breaks in skin integrity. Moisture (e.g., urine, perspiration) is not caustic; the skin generally does not become eroded when exposed to moisture. Conversely, chemicals (e.g., gastrointestinal secretions, stool, harsh cleansing solutions and solvents) are caustic to the skin due to their acidic pH, or high volume of enzymes, and will erode the top layers of the epidermis.

Moisture

The prolonged presence of moisture (more than 2 hours) on the skin places the skin at risk for overhydration and maceration of the epidermis. Although maceration is a seemingly innocent and common experience for anyone who soaks in the hot tub or washes dishes by hand, the corresponding weakening of the collagen fibers can reduce the skin's resiliency or ability to remain intact in the presence of mechanical action (e.g., friction, tape removal, pressure) or chemical exposure (e.g., gastrointestinal contents). Moisture-related conditions are those in which the skin is exposed to fluid that is neither caustic nor enzymatic. Sources of moisture most commonly include urinary incontinence, perspiration, and moisture-donating wound dressings such as hydrogel and saline-saturated gauze. Moisture can be trapped against the skin by clothing, diapers, gauze, wound dressings, and skin folds.

Clinical manifestations of skin macerated by the presence of excess or prolonged moisture include pale skin color and a wrinkling, swollen appearance of the exposed skin surface (Plate 14). As the length of exposure continues, the skin may become erythematous, and eventually fissures may develop. For example, linear shallow fissures may develop in the cleft between the buttocks and between the toes.

Maceration compromises protective skin mechanisms such as pH and normal flora. Ammonia in urine also raises the skin's pH, and changes in skin flora occur. As irritants penetrate the epidermis, they interact with keratinocytes and fibroblasts stimulating the release of cytokines, which act on the vasculature of the dermis to trigger inflammation. Consequently, the lipid bilayer structure of the stratum corneum is damaged, which may allow microorganisms to enter the epidermis (Visscher, 2009). Prolonged moisture also reduces the ability of the skin to resist additional stresses, such as shear, friction, and pressure, because of a higher frictional coefficient (Visscher, 2009) leading to secondary skin breakdown.

Chemical Factors

When the fluid penetrating the epidermis contains caustic or enzymatic contents, the skin will be further damaged by the chemical exposure. Fluids containing chemicals include, but are not limited to, povidone-iodine complex (Betadine), alkaline soaps, alcohol, gastrointestinal contents, and drainage from percutaneous tubes. Exposure to fecal incontinence (especially liquid to loose consistency) results in chemical dermatitis because of the chemical composition of the fecal material (e.g., enzymes). Skin damage may be evident within only a few hours in the presence of a strong irritant (e.g., small

bowel discharge). In fact, infants may develop a chemical-related skin injury as soon as they pass a loose stool into the diaper. In other situations, skin breakdown may occur only after repeated or prolonged exposure over several days, such as with soft or formed stool.

Chemical dermatitis can be distinguished from maceration by examining the exposure sites. Initially, irritants extract water-binding chemicals and lipids from the stratum corneum, and the skin decompensates so that it becomes dry and erythematous or develops an erythematous macular rash (Habif, 2004) (Plate 13). With continued exposure to chemical irritants, the protective layer of the stratum corneum becomes damaged, resulting in a loss of epidermis in the area of exposure which is described as superficial erosion or moist denudement. In contrast, skin with moisture-related damage most often remains intact. Chemically induced dermatitis is uncomfortable for the patient because the chemicals often stimulate neurocutaneous pain receptors. In differentiating chemical dermatitis from the possible skin conditions in the perineal, perianal, or buttocks region, it is also important to recognize that chemical dermatitis will only appear in the area that is directly in contact with the irritant. To facilitate further distinctions, Table 5-3 lists the typical assessment features of a variety of perineal–perianal skin conditions, such as IAD, candidiasis, HSV, herpes zoster, and pressure ulcers.

Acute fecal incontinence is a common instigator of chemical dermatitis. The etiology of acute fecal incontinence can be the result of a number of factors: nutritional (hyperosmolar enteric solutions, rapid rate of administration of enteric solutions, hypoalbuminemia), medications (antibiotics, cathartics), gastrointestinal function (short bowel syndrome, fat malabsorption, antibiotic-associated diarrhea, incomplete bowel obstruction, fecal impaction), and gastrointestinal disease (inflammatory bowel disease, infection, radiation enteritis). The patient's medical history is helpful in identifying the most likely etiology; additional laboratory tests or radiologic examinations may be indicated for confirmation. A digital rectal examination should be conducted to rule out a fecal impaction causing an incomplete bowel obstruction. When a fecal impaction is present, the stool will be dry and hard, and the patient will not be able to pass the stool unassisted; diarrheal stool will be passed around the impaction (Abeloff et al, 2008). When an impaction is present, a sodium phosphate enema (i.e., fleet enema) and oral cathartics may be indicated.

Antibiotic-associated diarrhea is an increasingly frequent cause of fecal incontinence. Broad-spectrum antibiotics, such as fluoroquinolones, amoxicillin, clindamycin, and cephalosporins, are the most common culprits (Imhoff and Karpa, 2009). Antibiotics alter the gastrointestinal microflora, thus increasing the concentration of pathogenic organisms within the bowel. The predominant pathogens in antibiotic-associated diarrhea are *Clostridium difficile, Staphylococcus aureus,*

TABLE 5-3	Differential Diagnosis of Skin Conditions in Proximity of Perineal/Perianal Region			
	Incontinence-Associated Dermatitis	Candidiasis	Herpes Simplex	Pressure
Location	Perineum Buttocks Inner thighs Groin Low abdominal skin folds	Perineum Buttocks Inner thighs Groin Low abdominal skin folds	Perianal Buttocks Genitals	Near bony prominences Coccyx, sacrum, ischium Under device/tube
Confirmed risk factors	Urinary and/or fecal incontinence	Moisture Antibiotics Immunosuppression	Immunosuppression	Limited mobility or activity Dependent on others for repositioning, transferring, etc.
Blisters	Yes	No	Initially	Sometimes (Stage II)
Distribution pattern	Confluent or patchy Irregular edges with erythema Shallow denudement, and/or maceration	Confluent or patchy rash Small round pustules, plaques, and/or satellite lesions	Clusters or isolated individual shallow lesions or blisters	Isolated individual lesions on or near bony prominence or pressure-causing device Damage ranges from intact discoloration to partial- or full-thickness wounds
Color	Pink/red	Pink/red	Initial: Pink/red Later: Crust	Pink, red, yellow, tan, gray, brown, black
Discomfort	Pain may be mild to severe	Itching, burning	Tingling sometimes noted initially Can become very painful	Pain may be absent to severe
Diagnostic tests	None	Potassium hydroxide preparation scraping (KOH)	Viral culture	None

and *Clostridium perfringens. C. difficile* is the most common of these pathogens and is more severe than *Escherichia coli* and *Salmonella* (Rohde et al, 2009). *C. difficile,* an opportunistic spore-forming, gram-positive bacillus, is transmitted via the fecal–oral route, and the spores remain on surfaces for extended periods of time. Only bleach is effective at killing *C. difficile* on surfaces. *C. difficile*–associated diarrhea (CDAD) has become the most common nosocomial diarrheal pathogen in hospitalized patients; from 20% to as much as 50% of antibiotic-associated diarrhea is attributed to *C. difficile* (Asha et al, 2006).

Antibiotic-associated diarrhea/CDAD often begins 4 to 9 days after the antibiotic is stopped but can develop up to 8 weeks later (Rohde et al, 2009). Symptoms of CDAD include watery diarrhea, abdominal cramping and tenderness, abdominal distention, fever, leukocytosis, nausea, and dehydration. Significant inflammation of the colonic mucosa develops primarily as a consequence of the adverse actions of two toxins: toxin A and toxin B. Both secretory diarrhea and osmotic diarrhea occur with CDAD (Eddins and Gray, 2008). As the mucosal surface is damaged, liquid accumulates in the bowel lumen, resulting in secretory diarrhea. Toxins A and B attract proinflammatory cytokines, which further damage the bowel wall and impair its ability to absorb water, electrolytes, and nutrients, thus precipitating osmotic diarrhea (Eddins and Gray, 2008).

C. difficile infection is confirmed by clinical presentation of symptoms (usually diarrhea), exclusion of other causes of diarrhea, and a culture or positive toxin assay (McFarland, 2009). Toxin assay is the preferred method of detecting *C. difficile.* Most commonly used is the rapid enzyme immunoassay, which detects toxin A or toxin A plus toxin B. Results are available within 2 to 3 hours, although many false-negative results are reported (Bartlett, 2008; McFarland, 2009). The more sensitive tissue culture assay also can be done to detect cytotoxin or toxin B, but results take longer. A direct stool polymerase chain reaction assay provides quick results and reports fewer false-negative results than the enzyme immunoassay (McFarland, 2009). A stool culture for *C. difficile* is possible but results are not available for 3 days. Before *C. difficile* toxin assays were available, colonoscopic examinations were common; a colonic biopsy positive for pseudomembranes in the presence of diarrhea is diagnostic of CDAD (Bartlett, 2008).

Standard treatment of CDAD is (1) prompt discontinuation of the antibiotic, (2) stool toxin assay, (3) oral metronidazole (500mg three times per day for 10 days), (4) correction of fluid and electrolyte imbalance, and (5) discontinuation of antiperistalsis medications. Metronidazole should be started even before the stool culture results are available; the systemic symptoms present create a high level of suspicion of CDAD. If abdominal pain persists or the patient does not respond to metronidazole therapy, oral vancomycin (125 mg four times per day for 10 days) is warranted. After initial antibiotic therapy, almost one fourth of patients with CDAD relapse within 2 months because spores can prevent peristalsis and delay exposure to antibiotics by "hiding" in the mucosal folds (Rohde et al, 2009). A more virulent strain has been discovered and is associated with increased disease severity and death (Redelings et al, 2007).

Prevention and Treatment

In a systematic review of the literature, a structured skin care protocol was demonstrated to reduce the incidence of IAD (Beeckman et al, 2009). A structured skin care protocol is a 3 step process: gentle skin cleansing, moisturization, and the application of a skin protectant; the type of skin protectant used will be dictated by the type of fluid on the skin and frequency of exposure. Box 5-4 lists interventions and products that can be used to prevent and treat moisture and chemical related skin damage. Table 5-4 lists a formulary of products used to prevent and manage moisture- and chemical-related skin damage. Unique considerations concerning the prevention and management of IAD in the neonate or premature infant are addressed in Chapter 36.

Skin cleansers with a pH near the skin's pH are more effective than soap and water at preventing IAD (Beeckman et al, 2009). Moisturizers are an important second step in the perineal skin care regimen and often are incorporated into commercially prepared skin cleansers. The three categories of skin protectants are skin sealant, moisture barrier ointment, and moisture barrier paste. Skin sealant protects the skin from maceration; it has limited effectiveness at protecting the skin from enzymes. Moisture barrier ointment protects the skin from effluent with enzymes but may be inadequate with high-volume output or excessively frequent effluent production or diarrhea. In these situations, moisture barrier paste should be used. Proper use of an ointment or paste consists of applying the product and, when the surface becomes soiled, using a soft pad to gently wipe off the stained surface of the product. The skin should not be scrubbed in an attempt to completely remove the product. When the product must be completely removed, mineral oil can be used to facilitate removal. Commercially available incontinence cleansers also can be used to remove a barrier paste.

Containment devices include external pouches and indwelling catheters. Containment devices may be indicated for containment of contaminated stool for infection control purposes and/or when the frequency or volume of stool overwhelms the moisture barrier ointment or paste. Rectal pouches are adhesive ostomy pouches specifically designed to fit the perianal contours and contain the incontinent stool. By protecting the skin from chemicals and moisture buildup, these products

---

BOX 5-4	Strategies to Prevent Moisture- and Chemical-Related Skin Damage*

Periwound
- Routine hygiene to keep skin clean and dry using skin cleanser and moisturizer.
- Use skin sealant, skin barrier ointment, skin barrier paste, or solid-wafer skin barrier to protect periwound skin.
- Use dressing with adequate absorptive capacity (see also Chapter 18).
- Change dressings before saturation occurs.
- Use low air loss support surface for moisture control of large surface areas that cannot be adequately protected with dressings, absorptive pads, or skin barrier.

Peritube or Drain (see also Chapter 39)
- Collaborate with appropriate service (i.e., intervention radiology) to determine cause of leakage, confirm proper placement, and optimal stabilization.
- Routine mild cleansing with skin cleanser and moisturizer.
- Use skin sealant, skin barrier ointment, skin barrier paste, or solid-wafer skin barrier to protect peritube skin.
- Use dressing with adequate absorptive capacity.
- Change dressings before saturation occurs.

Between Skin Folds
- Routine hygiene to keep skin clean and dry.
- Dust intertriginous skin surfaces with absorbent skin barrier powder.

- Separate intertriginous skin surfaces with skin sealant, barrier, and/or soft cloth or gauze.
- Place commercially available textile in skin fold (do not use emollients with this product).

Incontinence
- Determine and treat etiology.
- Identify patients at risk for skin damage.
- Use absorptive padding (without plastic back) as needed; change after incontinent episodes.
- Cleanse with mild incontinence skin cleanser; repeat after each incontinent episodes.
- Apply moisturizer to skin.
- Apply appropriate skin barrier to keep urine and feces off epidermis.
- Apply condom catheter or external pouch.
- Use indwelling catheters *only* with clear indication, assessment of contraindications, and order; change per manufacturer's instructions.
- *Low risk* of skin breakdown (urine and/or formed, soft stools): Apply skin sealant or moisture barrier ointment; reapply skin sealant per manufacturer's instructions; reapply moisture barrier ointment with each incontinent episode.
- *High risk* of skin breakdown (impaired skin integrity apparent, actual or anticipated loose stools): Apply skin barrier *paste* and repeat per manufacturer's instructions.

*See Table 5-4 for product examples.

TABLE 5-4	Formulary of Products* Used to Prevent and Manage Moisture- and Chemical-Related Skin Damage**		
Product	**Purpose**	**Examples***	**Additional Information**
Perineal cleanser	Perineal skin cleansing	Coloplast CarraFoam, or CarraWash, Medline Soothe & Cool, Smith & Nephew Secura	Liquid, foam, or impregnated cloth products available in rinse or no rinse.
Perineal cleanser and protectant	Combination product for cleansing and protecting perineal skin	Coloplast Baza Cleanse and Protect, Sage Comfort Shield, Medline Remedy	Skin cleanser that does not have to be rinsed off and simultaneously applies a skin protectant. Available in liquid, foam, or impregnated cloth products.
Moisture barrier ointment	Perineal skin protection	Calmoseptine ointment, Lantiseptic skin protectant, Proshield Plus skin protectant, Critic-Aide clear hydrophilic ointment	May impair adhesion if used in combination with perianal pouches.
Moisture barrier paste	Periwound, perifistula, peritube, high-risk perineal skin protection	Critic-Aide skin paste, Ilex skin protectant paste, Remedy Calazime protectant paste	More durable than moisture barrier ointment. Appropriate for open, denuded skin. Only need to remove top soiled layer of ointment prior to reapplication. Do not use force to remove. Mineral oil and selected perineal cleansers. May impair adhesion if used in combination with adhesive dressings and pouches. Some wound care treatments cannot be used with zinc-based pastes.
Solid skin barrier	Peristomal, perifistula, peritube, periwound skin protection	Stomahesive, Eakin, premium skin barrier	More durable than moisture barrier ointments and pastes. Available in multiple sizes and shapes (e.g., wafer, rings, strips). Waterproof; can be worn for several days.
Skin sealant	Perineal, peristomal, perifistula, peritube, periwound skin protection	No Sting Skin Prep protective dressing, Cavilon No Sting barrier film, skin gel wipe	Liquid transparent film delivered by a wipe, wand, or spray. Contains plasticizing agents (e.g., copolymer). Some products contain isopropyl alcohol. Non–alcohol-based products should be used when skin is compromised.
Skin barrier powder	Absorbs and dries weepy denuded skin to improve adherence of ointments, pastes, adhesive barriers	Stomahesive protective powder, Karaya powder, premium powder	Will impair adhesion if used on intact skin or if used in excess. Discontinue when the skin is no longer denuded.
External perianal pouch	Perianal, peristomal skin protection, containment of stool	Hollister fecal incontinence collector, ConvaTec fecal collector	Combines pouch with solid skin barrier for non-ambulatory patients. Comes with spout for use with bedside drain; spout can be cut off and replaced with provided tail closure. Odorproof and waterproof with gas filter option.
External urinary catheter	Perineal skin protection, containment of urine	Mentor-Coloplast Freedom Hollister extended wear, Hollister retracted penis pouch, Kendall Uri-Drain	Products made in variety of sizes and must be properly fit. Available in latex and nonlatex. Application involves self-adhesives or added adhesive strips.
Indwelling fecal containment device	Perianal skin protection, containment of loose stool	Hollister ActiFlo indwelling bowel catheter, ConvaTec Flexi-Seal fecal management system, Bard DigniCare stool management system	Do not use without physician's order. Critical to read manufacturer's instruction for contraindications and safe use. May need additional perianal protection with moisture barrier paste.
Textile	Skin fold protection	InterDry Ag textile with antimicrobial silver complex	Wicks away moisture from skin-to-skin contact areas to manage moisture, odor, and inflammation. Comes in rolls; cut amount needed.

*Examples of product names are not inclusive or intended as an endorsement.
**Some of these products may not be appropriate for neonates; please see Chapter 36 and Box 36-2 specifically for important considerations in selecting skin care products for neonates.

can be extremely cost-effective by reducing linen changes and freeing up nursing time for other types of care. Rectal pouches also preserve the patient's dignity by containing odor and feces. Acceptable wear time for the rectal pouch is 24 hours. Extra care should be used when repositioning the patient to prevent excess shear on the pouch and the surrounding skin. Step-by-step directions for application are provided by the manufacturer and should be followed closely.

Historically, large indwelling urinary catheters or devices called *rectal* or *colon tubes* designed for enema and medication administration have been inserted into the rectum and left in place. This practice is not safe because it has the potential to damage the anal sphincter and/or perforate the bowel. Only indwelling bowel and fecal management systems approved by the US Food and Drug Administration are designed to safely divert, collect, and contain potentially harmful and contaminated gastrointestinal waste without damaging the anal sphincter. It is important to review the manufacturer's instructions for each product to understand differences in features, indications, and contraindications. Researchers have reported efficient evacuation with minimal leakage or anorectal mucosal injury, reduction of perineal skin breakdown and pressure ulcers, and no anorectal mucosal injury (Kim et al, 2001; Kowal-Vern et al, 2009). Reduction of perineal skin injury and pressure ulcers as well as decreased rates of urinary tract, soft tissue, skin, and bloodstream infections also have been reported (Benoit and Watts, 2007; Kowal-Vern et al, 2009). These studies highlight the potential of these devices beyond the scope of skin protection and into the realm of managing infection and cross-contamination.

Drainage around catheters and tubes should be managed such that the drainage is eliminated, when possible, or the skin is not directly exposed to the drainage. For example, when leakage occurs around a gastrostomy tube, the first step is to ascertain proper placement and stabilization of the tube. If drainage persists once this is accomplished, appropriate use of skin barriers (particularly moisture barrier ointments, solid-wafer skin barriers, thin hydrocolloids, or foam dressings) is indicated. A solid-wafer skin barrier, hydrocolloid, or foam dressing can be trimmed to fit around a tube site; it can remain in place for several days and changed only when it loosens at the tube site. When ointment is the selected treatment, it should be reapplied periodically throughout the day to ensure adequate skin protection. However, ointments can never be used under an adhesive dressing. Regardless of the type of skin protection selected, gauze dressings are applied over the barrier to absorb drainage and are changed when damp.

Improper use of skin care products, particularly solvents, adhesives, and skin sealants, can contribute to chemical skin damage. Only pH-neutral skin cleansers should be used. Adhesive solvents must be thoroughly rinsed from the skin to prevent buildup of harmful substances. Soaps should be avoided to prevent disruption of the skin's normal acid pH. Skin sealants and adhesives, such as cements, must be allowed to dry adequately so that solvents evaporate before other products are applied.

VASCULAR DAMAGE

Ulcerations, particularly on the legs or feet, can occur as a result of venous hypertension, arterial insufficiency, neuropathy, or a combination of these factors. Although these types of lesions commonly develop incidental to benign trauma (i.e., by bumping against the leg of a chair), each ulcer has distinct distinguishing features, pathologic processes, and treatment regimens. Arterial ulcers, venous ulcers, and lymphedema wounds are discussed in detail in Chapters 11 through 13. Neuropathic ulcers, such as diabetic ulcers, are discussed in Chapter 14.

INFECTIOUS AGENTS

Many skin rashes or ulcers are indicative of an infectious process and can occur around wounds or be misinterpreted as a pressure, shear, or chemical injury. Infections can be categorized according to infecting organism: fungus, bacteria, virus, or arthropod. The wound care specialist may be the first person to observe some of these infections. In many cases, the wound specialist will be responsible for identifying and managing the infections. The common skin infections are discussed here; the more unusual skin infections are addressed in Chapter 30.

Fungal

Candidiasis. Candidiasis is the most common opportunistic fungal infection (Kauffman, 2008). *Candida* spp., which are yeast-like organisms that reproduce by budding, normally colonize the skin, gastrointestinal tract, genitourinary tract, and vagina. When immunologic defenses are compromised or the normal flora is altered, *Candida* spp. become opportunistic pathogens.

Cutaneous candidiasis is an epidermal infection with *Candida* spp. Although more than 150 species of *Candida* exist, the most common is *C. albicans* (Plates 15, 16). The primary lesion of candidiasis is a pustule or erythematous papules or plaques that may have associated scaling or crusting or a cheesy white exudate. Maceration is common. Lesions typically are beefy red, with satellite erythematous papules and pustules. Satellite lesions (outside the advancing edge of candidiasis) are an important diagnostic feature of candidiasis (Habif, 2004). Intact pustules are not always visible because opposing skin and clothing will unroof the pustule so that the lesion appears to be a macule or papule. Pruritus is the key indicator of candidiasis and may be severe.

A common location for development of candidiasis is in skin folds; *intertrigo* is the term used for an inflammatory condition of skin folds (Plate 17). Intertrigo can be induced by heat, moisture, maceration, and friction. In addition to *Candida* spp., intertrigo can be complicated by other fungal infections (tinea) and by bacterial infection (erythrasma). Candida intertrigo is located in the skin folds (intertriginous areas) and is characterized by an intensely red, macerated, glistening, confluent macular papular rash. The half moon-shaped edge of the rash or plaque often extends just beyond the limits of the opposing skin folds. Satellite lesions usually are present (Brannon, 2009).

Predisposing factors to candidiasis include the presence of a moist environment, a hot and humid environment, tight underclothing, diabetes, and antibiotic therapy. Skin under damp surgical dressings, the perineum, the perineal area, and intertriginous areas (beneath pendulous breasts, overhanging abdominal folds, and inguinal skin folds) are typical moist areas that provide an excellent medium for yeast growth. Diabetes predisposes the patient to development of candidiasis because the associated increase in the amount of glucose in the saliva, sweat, and urine in patients with diabetes prevents bacteria from inhibiting yeast growth (Carpenter and de Sanctis, 2008). Antibiotics predispose the patient to development of candidiasis by removing the competing organisms. An altered skin pH also increases susceptibility to yeast infection. Immunosuppressed patients and patients with irritant contact dermatitis are vulnerable to candidiasis.

Folliculitis and contact dermatitis can be confused with candidiasis. Furthermore, candidiasis can be disguised by being superimposed on irritant contact dermatitis. The distribution and types of lesions are important to identifying the underlying problem. Folliculitis, the inflammation of a hair follicle, is characterized by the presence of pustules pierced in the center by a hair (Plate 18), whereas candidiasis causes nonfollicular pustules. Manifestations of contact dermatitis include erythema with papules, whereas pustules are unusual and warrant culture to rule out superimposed infection. Distribution can help distinguish contact dermatitis from candidiasis because a contact dermatitis conforms to the specific shape of the irritant and therefore has well-defined borders, does not have satellite lesions, and does not have pruritus.

Intertrigo candidiasis is also easily confused with tinea cruris, erythrasma (both discussed later), and inverse psoriasis. Psoriasis is a chronic inflammatory papular skin disease characterized by scaly plaques that may affect skin, nails, and joints. It is attributed to abnormal T-lymphocyte function rather than an infection (Habif et al, 2005). One of the many unique clinical forms is intertriginous psoriasis (also known as *inverse psoriasis*). It is uncommon but can occur in the groin or under the breasts. The skin appears macerated with smooth red, sharply defined plaques. Satellite lesions will not be present unless a candidal infection is superimposed on the psoriasis. The application of a topical

steroid is associated with contributing to the added complication of candidiasis.

Candidiasis is most often determined clinically by signs, symptoms, and predisposing factors. Pruritus and burning at the site are common. The most relevant laboratory test for confirming candidiasis is a potassium hydroxide preparation scraping. Scrapings from an intact pustule and the contents are needed to yield the best results. Budding spores and elongated pseudohyphae are observed. Because the skin can be colonized with *C. albicans* but not infected, swab cultures for *Candida* are not informative, as such cultures cannot distinguish between infection and colonization (Carpenter and de Sanctis, 2008).

Nonpharmacologic treatment includes reduction of predisposing factors, such as humidity, moisture, antibiotics, hyperglycemia, and tight-fitting clothes. Body powders (e.g., Zeasorb-AF) or wide-mesh gauze can be placed in intertriginous areas to absorb moisture. Prevention of moisture buildup is the most important intervention to prevent candidiasis. Box 5-4 lists additional strategies to protect the skin from moisture-related complication. Table 5-4 lists a formulary of products used to prevent moisture- or chemical-related skin damage.

Burow solution soaks followed by air drying are soothing when maceration or severe pruritus is present. Topical antifungal creams can be applied twice daily for limited involvement, and antifungal powders can be used in less severe cases. When creams are used, they should be applied sparingly to reduce moisture entrapment. Recalcitrant or severe fungal infections require orally administered therapy.

Dermatophyte (Tinea). The dermatophyte is a type of fungus that is responsible for the majority of fungal infections on the skin, nails, and hair (Habif et al, 2005). Known as *tinea,* a dermatophyte infection infects only dead keratin, so the stratum corneum on the skin is vulnerable. A tinea infection cannot survive in the mouth or vagina because these sites do not have a keratin layer. As a pruritic superficial fungal infection, tinea can be challenging to diagnose and treat (Wiederkehr and Schwartz, 2008). The manifestations of tinea infections vary according to body site. Box 5-5 lists the types of tinea based on body location. Tinea pedis occurs on the feet and is more familiar as *athlete's foot*. Tinea cruris

BOX 5-5	Tinea Patterns

- Tinea pedis (foot)
- Tinea cruris (jock itch) (groin)
- Tinea corporis (ringworm) (body)
- Tinea faciei (face)
- Tinea manuum (hand)
- Tinea capitis (scalp)
- Tinea of barbae (beard)
- Tinea of onychomycosis (nails)

occurs in the groin skin folds and is more commonly known as *jock itch*. Tinea corporis is present on the body and is also known as *ringworm*, although no worm is involved with this infection.

Fungi live on damp surfaces, and most tinea infections develop on moist surfaces (e.g., skin folds, web between toes, soles of the feet). Dermatophytes can be picked up from the floor of public showers or lockers, from a pet that is infected, or from loaning or borrowing clothing items from other individuals. Some individuals may be genetically predisposed to tinea infections (Habif et al, 2005). The active border of tinea will be scaly, red, and slightly elevated. When inflammation is significant, vesicles may be present along this active border.

Tinea can be diagnosed by directly visualizing the branches of keratinized strands under the microscope. This is done with a potassium hydroxide wet mount preparation where a scale is removed from the active edge of the infection with a no. 15 surgical blade, placed on the microscope slide, and prepared for viewing (Habif et al, 2005). Dermatophytes will appear as translucent, branching, rod-shaped strands (hyphae) with uniform width. A wood's light examination of hair will fluoresce blue to green when infected with *Microsporum* spp. of the dermatophyte fungi. Fungal infections of the skin do not fluoresce.

Box 5-6 lists the interventions for prevention of tinea infections. Treatment varies slightly by body site but primarily consists of topical antifungal medications such as butenafine (Lotrimin Ultra), terbinafine (Lamisil), or sertaconazole (Ertaczo) applied twice daily for 2 to 4 weeks. When interdigital web spaces are severely macerated, the antifungal medication econazole nitrate

(Spectazole) also provides an antibacterial effect that addresses common secondary bacterial infections (Habif et al, 2005; Noble et al, 1998; Wiederkehr and Schwartz, 2009). Moist lesions also can be treated with a Burow dressing for 20 to 30 minutes two to six times daily until the skin is dry.

Topical corticosteroid creams are commonly prescribed for inflammatory skin lesions, particularly in the groin; however, corticosteroids must be avoided when a dermatophyte infection is suspected. Use of these products can alter the clinical presentation of a dermatophyte infection, creating a condition called *tinea incognito*. When topical steroids are applied, they decrease the inflammation, which is interpreted as improvement. However, the dermatophyte fungus will flourish in the localized steroid-induced immunosuppression. When the corticosteroid is discontinued because the inflammation is resolving, the rash will return, but then the appearance will be different (absent scaling at the margins, diffuse erythema, scattered pustules or papules, and brown hyperpigmentation) and the area of involvement greatly expanded. Treatment remains topical antifungal agents; oral antifungal medications may be needed for extensive lesions (red papules and pustules).

Bacterial

Folliculitis, impetigo, and erysipelas are bacterial skin infections caused by coagulase-positive *Staphylococcus (aureus)*, coagulase-negative *Staphylococcus (epidermidis)* or beta hemolytic streptococcus (Bradley, 2008; File and Stevens, 2008). Although *S. aureus* can be recovered from normal intact skin, especially in the nares, axillae, and groin, it is rarely a true member of resident bacterial flora and is considered a highly invasive pathogen. Staphylococci are able to quickly develop resistance to antibiotics; all staphylococci should be considered resistant to penicillins. Methicillin-resistant *Staphylococcus aureus* (MRSA) and methicillin-resistant *Staphylococcus epidermidis* (MRSE) account for up to 50% of *S. aureus*–identified nosocomial infections in some medical centers (Bradley, 2008). Community-associated methicillin-resistant *Staphylococcus aureus* (CA-MRSA) strains also have been reported. Vancomycin-resistant *Staphylococcus aureus* (VRSA) has developed as a consequence of prolonged use of vancomycin as the primary treatment of serious MRSA infections. First-generation cephalosporins and penicillinase-resistant penicillins are the most effective drugs for treating mild to moderate infections.

Cellulitis. Cellulitis is an infection of the dermis and subcutaneous tissue that is most commonly caused by *S. aureus, Staphylococcus pyogenes*, and group A streptococcus (Sachdeva and Tomecki, 2008). Cellulitis is preceded by some type of break in the skin, such as an ulcer, laceration, surgical incision, bite, burn, or body piercing, which becomes the portal of entry for the infecting organism (File and Stevens, 2008). The most frequent sites on the body

---

BOX 5-6 | **Preventing Tinea Infections**

- Expose feet to air whenever home.
- Change socks and underwear daily, especially in warm weather.
- Dry feet carefully (especially between toes) after using locker room or public shower.
- Avoid walking barefoot in public areas; wear flip-flops, sandals, or water shoes.
- Do not wear thick clothing for long periods of time in warm weather; heavy clothes will cause increased sweating, which can encourage growth of fungal infections.
- Discard worn exercise shoes. Never borrow other people's shoes.
- Do not borrow or lend personal towels or clothing to other people.
- Check pets for areas of hair loss and ask veterinarian to check pets as well. Determine if pets are causing patient's fungal infection; otherwise patient may become infected again, even after treatment.
- Make sure shared exercise equipment (e.g. treadmill at gym) is clean before using it.

for occurrence of cellulitis are the posterior legs and hands. The head, abdomen, back, neck, buttocks, perigenital and perineal areas, and inner thighs are uncommon to rare sites for cellulitis (Habif, et al, 2005).

Cellulitis should be differentiated from the erythema associated with venous dermatitis (see Table 12-3) or contact allergic dermatitis (distribution has very precise edges and shape is consistent with outline of offending agent). In the perineal and perigenital areas, cellulitis can be distinguished from the erythema associated with a Stage I pressure ulcer based on the location of the lesion (Stage I pressure ulcer is most often limited to skin overlying bony prominence). Relative to IAD, cellulitis should be distinguished from intertrigo, erythrasma, chemical denudation, and psoriasis.

Assessment findings characteristic of cellulitis include localized erythema with diffuse borders, tenderness upon palpation, warmth, and edema. Crepitus (palpation of gas in the subcutaneous tissue), however, is pathologic for aerobic infections, such as *Clostridia*, most often *Clostridia perfringens*. An elevated white blood cell count and erythrocyte sedimentation rate may be present. Recurrent cellulitis will impair lymphatic drainage and lead to lymphedema, dermal fibrosis, and epidermal thickening. A culture is required to discern the invading organism and the appropriate antibiotic initiated. Empiric treatment may begin before the culture results are obtained but should be effective for both staphylococcal and streptococcal organisms (Habif et al, 2005). Most patients respond to oral antibiotic therapy; reevaluation and consideration of intravenous antibiotics should be considered if the patient does not respond. Clostridial infections will require high-dose intravenous penicillin in addition to prompt debridement and surgical exploration of the cellulitis site (Sachdeva and Tomecki, 2008).

Erysipelas. Erysipelas is an acute inflammatory form of cellulitis that occurs as a complication of a break in skin integrity, as occurs with abrasions or dry skin. Erysipelas differs from other types of cellulitis because it involves the cutaneous lymphatics, in the form of "streaking." This disease has a very high morbidity rate if left undiagnosed (up to 80% in infants and 75% in the elderly) (File and Stevens, 2008).

Erysipelas most commonly occurs in infants, young children, and older adults. Additional risk factors include malnutrition, alcoholism, recent infections, stasis dermatitis, lymphedema, nephrotic syndrome, and diabetes mellitus. Small, seemingly insignificant breaks in the skin can serve as a portal of entry for infection. The extremities and the face are the most common sites (Sachdeva and Tomecki, 2008).

Erysipelas means "red skin," and the involved body part is characterized by well-defined erythema. (In contrast, cellulitis is less demarcated.) The classic primary lesion is a plaque. Prodromal symptoms, such as malaise, myalgias, chills, and high fever, may occur within 4 to 48 hours of infection. The surrounding skin rapidly progress to become erythematous, edematous, and intensely painful. Secondary lesions are vesicles, bullae, and cutaneous hemorrhage. Within 5 to 10 days of onset, desquamation of the affected area occurs (Stevens et al, 2008). Associated lymphangitis is demonstrated by the presence of erythematous streaking over lymphatics draining the area of infection.

Erysipelas usually is diagnosed by clinical findings of sharply defined erythema, edema, and/or streaking. Accompanying systemic complaints of fever, chills, malaise, and localized pain also raise suspicion for the presence of the condition. Although cultures (via needle aspiration) of any drainage from the advancing edge and skin biopsies are appropriate, the organism is difficult to culture, leaving the test uninformative. When septicemia is suspected, a white blood cell count and blood cultures are warranted.

Nonpharmacologic interventions include bed rest, elevation of the affected extremity, and hot packs. Uncomplicated cases of erysipelas can be treated with oral antibiotics. Toxic, debilitated, and elderly patients or children with extensive facial involvement or any patients with rapidly evolving erythema, pain, and swelling require intravenous antibiotics; penicillin, a cephalosporin, or nafcillin is warranted. Symptoms should diminish within 24 hours of treatment. Pain control measures are essential.

Erythrasma. A bacterial infection (corynebacterium) can develop in skin folds (e.g., axilla, groin), resulting in the condition known as *erythrasma*. This chronic condition is mildly pruritic, with a reddish brown pigmentation, well-defined borders, and little scaling. Overweight patients, those with diabetes, and people living in warmer climates are at increased risk for developing erythrasma. This infection can be diagnosed by microscopy or culture. Erythrasma is often confused with candidiasis intertrigo based on clinical presentation but is easily distinguished because the erythrasma rash, when exposed to long-wave ultraviolet radiation, will fluoresce to a coral pink color due to the action of the corynebacterium. The absence of satellite lesions should also help distinguish erythrasma from candidiasis. Treatment of erythrasma consists of washing the area vigorously with antibacterial soap and either applying clotrimazole lotion three times per day for 7 days, administering erythromycin tablets (500 mg) four times per day for 7 to 10 days, or applying erythromycin gel to the affected area. As with tinea infections, erythrasma can be prevented by keeping the skin dry, wearing absorbent clean clothing, and practicing good hygiene (Habif et al, 2005).

Folliculitis. Folliculitis is an inflammation of the hair follicle (Plate 18). It can be mechanical, bacterial, or fungal in origin. Mechanical folliculitis is the result of tight clothing or persistent trauma. Bacterial folliculitis is most commonly caused by *S. aureus*. Fungal folliculitis is associated with tinea (dermatophyte infection) of the skin where hair is present (e.g., beard, head). Fungal folliculitis also can develop in the presence of untreated tinea corporis (Habif et al, 2005). Occlusion of the skin from occlusive ointment or the prolonged presence of oil or grease on the skin also will cause development of folliculitis (occlusion folliculitis). Improperly cleaned hot tubs are also responsible for causing *Pseudomonas* folliculitis. Steroids will trigger steroid folliculitis characterized by multiple small pustules and papules resulting in a neutrophilic inflammation of the hair follicle.

The primary lesions in folliculitis are dome-shaped, 2- to 5-mm erythematous papules that surround the hair follicle and may manifest central pustules; secondary lesions are crusts and erythema (File and Stevens, 2008). Folliculitis may be limited to the superficial area of the hair follicle or progress deeper into the follicle. Although most common on the scalp or the extremities, folliculitis may develop on any hairy body location, particularly under adhesive wound dressings. Folliculitis also may develop as a secondary infection in the presence of excoriations from scratching that accompanies scabies and insect bites.

Risk factors for developing folliculitis are diabetes mellitus, obesity, malnutrition, immunodeficiency, and chronic staphylococcal infections. When treating folliculitis, avoid or reduce heat, friction, and occlusion. Antibacterial soaps should be used and hygiene improved. Potassium hydroxide examination of the hair and surrounding skin is warranted to exclude a dermatophyte infection (i.e., tinea) so that the appropriate oral antifungal medications, such as Lamisil, can be used. When folliculitis is limited and superficial, topical Mupirocin is effective (Habif et al, 2005).

Impetigo. Impetigo, most commonly seen in children, is a highly contagious superficial vesiculopustular skin infection that is caused primarily by the gram-positive bacterium *S. aureus. Streptococcus pyrogenes* occasionally may be the offending pathogen causing a more significant infection. Poor hygiene or malnutrition is typical of patients with impetigo. Lesions develop within 10 to 14 days (Stevens et al, 2008). The initial onset is a vesicle involving the superficial layer of the stratum corneum. The patient may experience itching and mild soreness; systemic symptoms are uncommon. Impetigo most often develops on seemingly intact skin, although it also may develop with minor breaks in the skin, such as inset bites and minor abrasions.

It is important to distinguish impetigo from HSV. HSV can be distinguished from impetigo by culture and by early manifestations. HSV begins with grouped, clear vesicles that are uniform in size, and it recurs at the same site.

Impetigo is often self-limited and resolves spontaneously, although it may also become chronic and/or recurrent. The treatment of choice for impetigo is topically administered 2% mupirocin cream (Bactroban). It has been shown to be as effective as oral erythromycin without the side effects (Habif, 2004). The cream should be applied three times daily until the lesions clear. Oral penicillin is indicated when streptococci are present. Impetigo may present clinically as bullous or nonbullous.

Bullous Impetigo. Bullous impetigo is a primarily staphylococcal disease that develops when certain strains of *S. aureus* produce a specific epidermolytic toxin (File and Stevens, 2008). They may occur anywhere on the body, but the most common location is the face. One or more vesicles enlarge, creating a superficial, fragile, clear fluid-filled bulla that gradually becomes filled with cloudy fluid. When the center of the bulla collapses, a rim of the bulla roof often remains, encircling the lesion. The center of the lesion then develops a thin, honey-colored crust. When this is removed, a red, inflamed, moist base is revealed that is exudative with serous fluid. Eventually the outer edges of the bulla become dry and flaky, and a crust forms. Bullous impetigo lesions have little if any surrounding erythema; they can range in size from 2 to 8 cm and remain for several months. Infants must be monitored for signs and symptoms of serious secondary infections, such as septic arthritis and pneumonia (Habif et al, 2005).

Nonbullous Impetigo. The lesions associated with nonbullous impetigo are asymptomatic, with minimal surrounding erythema. Lesions begin as small vesicles or pustules but soon rupture, exposing a moist, red base that becomes crusted over. The most common sites affected are around the mouth, the nose, and the extremities. In the usual sequence of events, the infectious agent is present on intact skin and, after minor trauma such as scratching, the skin is broken and an infection develops (Habif, 2004). During the early development of the lesions, group A beta-hemolytic streptococci may be isolated; however, the lesions quickly become contaminated with staphylococci. Predisposing factors for streptococcal impetigo are warm, moist climates and poor hygiene.

Viral

Viral infections, particularly HSV and varicella-zoster virus (VZV), are commonly triggered by stress and illness. It is important to recognize these highly contagious infections to facilitate prompt appropriate treatment and prevent spread to other individuals.

Herpes Simplex Virus. HSV infections of the epidermis are highly contagious and can be spread when a susceptible, noninfected person comes into direct contact (via mucous membrane or broken skin) with a person shedding the virus. Viral shedding occurs even in the absence of symptoms. Most transmission of HSV occurs during periods of asymptomatic shedding (Kimberlin and Whitley, 2008). Consequently, HSV infection should be considered a chronic process rather than an intermittent process, and all HSV-infected people should be treated as potentially contagious. Furthermore, because the primary infection often is subclinical, a negative history of vesicles or blisters does not rule out previous HSV infection.

HSV has been divided into two types: HSV-1 (oral herpes) and HSV-2 (genital herpes). HSV-1 is associated with cold sores (fever blisters). HSV-2 causes genital and perianal herpes. However, genital lesions from HSV-1 and oral lesions from HSV-2 are becoming more common, a trend that may be a consequence of sexual freedom and the ease of transmission. Ultimately, HSV lesions are not limited to the lips and genital area and may occur anywhere on the skin.

HSV infections have two phases: primary infection and secondary phase. During the primary infection, the virus becomes established in a nerve ganglion. HSV-1 most often occurs during childhood, whereas HSV-2 commonly occurs after sexual contact in sexually active individuals. Symptoms of the primary infection range from being undetectable to localized pain, headache, generalized aching, malaise, and tender regional adenopathy. A significant inflammatory response develops that extends from the base of the lesions down into the dermis, which results in the classic presentation of uniform, grouped vesicles on an erythematous base; the vesicles contain large numbers of infective viral particles. As more inflammatory cells are recruited to the site, vesicles become pustules that erode, drain, and crust (Plate 19). Primary lesions last for 2 to 6 weeks and heal without scarring. As the lesion heals, the virus enters the skin nerve endings and ascends through peripheral nerves to the dorsal root ganglia, where it remains in a latent stage.

Reactivation of the virus can occur in response to local trauma (abrasion, ultraviolet light) or systemic changes (e.g., stress, illness, fatigue, fever, compromised immune system). The virus then travels back down the peripheral nerve to the site, or in the vicinity, of the initial infection to trigger a recurrence. Prodromal symptoms of burning at the site may precede the recurrence. The reactivated virus presents as vesicles on an erythematous base, or ulcers. Crusts cover the eruptions within 24 to 48 hours and are shed in approximately 12 days, exposing a reepithelialized surface (Hunter et al, 2002).

Clinical presentation of grouped vesicles on an erythematous base is a key indicator of HSV and can be confirmed with a Tzanck smear. However, the Tzanck smear is most reliable when the lesion sampled is a vesicle; the smear becomes less reliable with pustules, crusts, and ulcers.

Primary HSV-1 infections are generally asymptomatic. When symptoms are present, the lesions include painful vesicles or shallow ulcers on the lips or lower face or in the oral cavity, and they last for 2 to 3 weeks. Recurrent HSV-1 infections are foreshadowed by pain and tingling or a burning sensation 2 to 24 hours before the eruption of vesicles (Kimberlin and Whitley, 2008). Recurrent HSV-1 lasts about 2 days as vesicles, which progress to pustules, ulcers, and eventually crusts. Complete healing occurs in 8 to 10 days.

Primary genital herpes (typically HSV-2 infection) lesions initially are macules and papules, followed by vesicles, pustules, and ulcerations. Lesions may occur on the genitalia, the perineum, and the buttocks. The lesions

are extremely painful and persist for 2 to 3 weeks. Spontaneous resolution of the primary infection is common. Recurrent genital herpes is less pronounced and lasts for 8 to 10 days. Ulcers are shallow and may or may not be painful.

Genital herpes lesions are commonly misinterpreted as pressure, chemical damage, or scabies (Plate 20). Therefore the differential diagnosis for ulcers located in the perianal area or on the buttocks must include HSV. Genital herpes can be distinguished from pressure sores in that the lesions are not limited to a bony prominence and are more typical over the fleshy part of the buttocks. Genital herpes in the perianal area also can be distinguished from chemical irritation (such as occurs with diarrhea) by the presence of several isolated ulcers rather than the confluence of superficial denudement or erythema that impinges on the anal opening.

The clinical presentation of grouped vesicles on an erythematous base is highly suggestive of HSV regardless of body site. The most definitive method for confirming the infection is to unroof the intact vesicle so that the vesicular fluid can be cultured. Rapid testing (within a few hours) also can be done with direct fluorescent antibody examination. Commercially available kits can distinguish among HSV-1, HSV-2, and VZV.

Antiviral medications are effective in treating HSV infection and are available for topical, oral, and intravenous administration. Early initiation of oral acyclovir for genital herpes decreases healing time, viral shedding, and duration of pain.

Nursing care should be directed at absorbing excess moisture, avoiding trauma, and providing comfort. Alginate dressings with a secondary dressing, such as a transparent dressing or foam, can be used to absorb exudate (Chacon and Ferreira, 2009). When the lesions are relatively dry yet painful, Burow solution (aluminum acetate) soaks and refrigerated hydrogel dressings can relieve the topical pain. When shedding HSV lesions are present, skin cleansing should be done cautiously to prevent spreading of the virus, particularly when the lesions are present on the buttocks.

Varicella-Zoster Virus. VZV causes varicella (chicken pox) and herpes zoster (shingles). VZV is highly contagious and is transmitted by direct contact with either vesicular fluid or airborne droplets from the infected host's respiratory tract. Airborne transmission as a mode for spreading VZV is very serious. Spread of varicella with no direct contact has been reported; the sole exposure was to air that flowed from the room of the infected individual to another room. Patients with herpes zoster are less contagious than are patients with varicella (American Academy of Dermatology, 2008).

Herpes zoster is an infection within the epidermis that is characteristically unilateral and occurs along one or two adjacent dermatome distributions (Figure 5-2). Eruptions result from the reactivation of VZV in cranial or spinal nerve ganglia that then spread to cutaneous

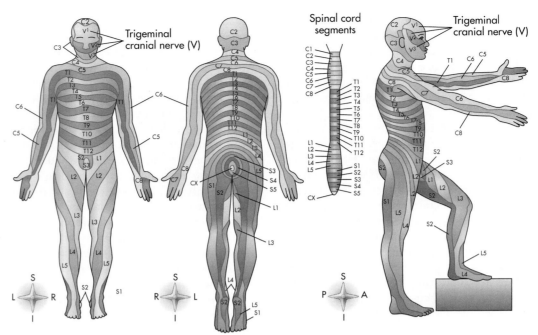

FIGURE 5-2 Segmental dermatome distribution of spinal nerves to the front, back, and side of the body. Dermatomes are specific skin surface areas innervated by a single spinal nerve or group of spinal nerves. *C*, Cervical segments; *CX*, coccygeal segment; *L*, lumbar segments; *S*, sacral segments; *T*, thoracic segments. (From Patton KT, Thibodeau GA: *Anatomy and physiology,* ed 7, St. Louis, 2010, Mosby.)

nerves. Reactivation, which can occur as a result of immunosuppression, fatigue, and emotional trauma, occurs in 15% of people (American Academy of Dermatology, 2008). The elderly may be predisposed to herpes zoster as a consequence of a potential decline in immunologic function. Individuals who are immunocompromised are at risk for developing VZV and experience more severe infections. These patients are more likely to develop disseminated disease with extensive skin lesions, pneumonia, hepatitis, or encephalitis (Zaia, 2008). Diagnosis is most often based on history and clinical appearance. The DNA polymerase chain reaction assay and direct immunofluorescent stain of a skin scraping for VZV antigen are accurate and rapid diagnostic tests for chickenpox and zoster and are preferred over the Tzanck preparation or tissue culture (Zaia, 2008).

Herpes zoster has characteristic manifestations that begin with a burning pain, followed by erythema that evolves into a grouped unilateral vesicular rash along one or two dermatomes (Plate 21). Over the next few days, the clear vesicles become filled with purulent fluid (i.e., pustules form) that then rupture and crust over (Hunter et al, 2002). In some debilitated patients, the eruption becomes more extensive and inflammatory, with necrosis or secondary infections developing. VZV in the immunocompromised patient may last from weeks to months, and the resulting ulcer may develop a black, adherent eschar. Postherpetic neuralgia (pain that persists beyond 1 month after healing) is a major complication of shingles; thus aggressive analgesia is an essential component of treatment.

Treatment of herpes zoster is similar to that of HSV. Early intervention with systemic antiviral medications lessens postherpetic neuralgia and decreases healing time and viral shedding. Burow solution can be applied to act as an astringent on the lesions. Daily soaks with salt solutions may minimize bacterial infection (Zaia, 2008). Lesions should not be occluded because this delays their healing.

ALLERGIC FACTORS

Numerous allergic responses, both local and systemic, can be manifested on the skin. Because the wound specialist is in a likely position to observe such reactions, it is important to be able to describe the manifestations accurately and to report the assessment to the physician in a timely fashion. This section focuses on those allergic responses that are localized reactions to items as adhesives, wound care products, and solutions. These types of skin damage are commonly referred to as *allergic contact dermatitis.*

Allergic contact dermatitis is an immunologic response to an allergen. Contact dermatitis occurs more readily in the presence of a preexisting skin disorder in which the cutaneous barrier is disrupted.

A true allergic dermatitis requires exposure to an allergen and has two phases:

1. The sensitization phase (the skin of a nonsensitized individual is exposed to a substance or chemical) transpires over a 7- to 10-day period. Small molecules

from the allergen pass through the epidermis and attach to an epidermal protein found on the surface of the Langerhans cell. From here these cells migrate through the dermis to the lymph nodes, where they present the allergen to T lymphocytes. Subsequently, effector and memory T lymphocytes proliferate in the lymph node, are released to circulate in the blood, and ultimately return to the skin. Here the body develops the ability to recognize the antigen when it reappears on the skin, and the T lymphocytes are now "primed" (Hunter et al, 2002).

2. When the individual is reexposed to the allergen, the elicitation phase occurs within 48 to 72 hours. Once the Langerhans cell delivers the antigen to memory T cells in the skin, effector T cells begin to produce lymphokines. Inflammatory cells are summoned by the lymphokines, and allergic manifestations can be observed. Suppressor T cells are believed to end the inflammatory reaction.

An acute inflammatory response occurs within 48 hours of reexposure to an allergen. Clinical manifestations begin with erythema, followed by pruritus. Primary lesions are vesicles, bullae, papules, plaques, and wheals. Secondary lesions include moist desquamation (Plate 22), edema, fissure, excoriation, and crust. An acute reaction usually resolves in days to weeks, after the allergen has been removed.

The cause or source of the allergen may be obvious, or it may be obscured by other concurrent processes. A careful, detailed assessment and interview are imperative to identify the skin reaction as an allergic response. Common allergic sensitizers include poison ivy, nickel (used in jewelry), rosins, rubber compounds (used in elastic, gloves), benzocaine (used in antipruritic creams), paraphenylenediamine (dye used to color hair), and preservatives. Topical preparations with one of the following ingredients are other common allergic offenders: aloe vera, fragrances, parabens, quaternium 15, diphenhydramine (Benadryl spray or Caladryl lotion), neomycin (Neosporin), and para-aminobenzoic acid (PABA) (Habif, 2004). Overuse of soaps, cleansers, moisturizers, and cosmetics can produce reactions. Many chemicals with similar structures cross-react, so a person who is sensitive to one product may be sensitive to several other products.

The location and distribution of the skin inflammation is an important clue in identifying the causative agent. Allergic contact dermatitis is localized to the skin where the product is applied, and involved areas typically have sharp margins. For example, an allergic reaction to an adhesive will be in the shape of the adhesive and will have well-defined borders. Allergic contact dermatitis can spread from the original site of application through inadvertent transfer of the allergen by the hands or, as the disease progresses, by the circulating T lymphocytes. However, the skin reaction begins and remains most severe in the area in which contact with the antigen occurred (Hunter et al, 2002).

Patch tests can be conducted to confirm the suspected agent that is causing the allergic reaction; however, these tests must be properly conducted and interpreted. Suspected allergens are applied to the skin and secured with tape. The patient's back usually is the preferred site for patch testing. After 48 hours, the patches are removed and the test site assessed for skin damage, which is graded using a standard scale as listed in Box 5-7. Although the patch test seems simple to apply and read, it is a complicated procedure that requires training and experience to obtain valid results (Rietschel and Fowler, 2001).

Simply avoiding contact with allergens can prevent allergic contact dermatitis. However, recognizing or identifying potential allergens is the key to prevention and may not be an easy task.

When an allergic response is suspected, use of the offending product or chemical should be discontinued. Often a substitute can be used. Use of antiinflammatory medications may be warranted topically or systemically and usually is determined based on the severity of the allergic reaction.

RADIATION

Radiation therapy is an established, common treatment of cancer. It is estimated that as many as half of all patients with cancer will receive radiation therapy as a primary, adjunctive, or palliative intervention (Bolderston et al, 2006). Although the techniques and technologies for radiotherapy have improved, skin reactions and complications continue to be problematic for patients (Wells and MacBride, 2003), and the evidence for the optimal treatments for prevention and management remain inconclusive (Olascoaga et al, 2008; Wickline, 2004).

Etiology

Ionizing radiation exerts direct tissue injury to curtail the growth of neoplastic cells; however, it also generates free radicals and reactive oxygen intermediates that further

BOX 5-7	Scale for Interpretation of Patch Test Results
Score	**Signifies**
+	Weak (nonvesicular) positive reaction: erythema, infiltration, possibly papules
+ +	Strong (edematous or vesicular) positive reaction
+ + +	Extreme (spreading, bullous, ulcerative) positive reaction
−	Negative reaction
IR	Irritant reactions of different types
NT	Not tested
Macular erythema only is a doubtful reaction.	

Adapted from Habif T: *Clinical dermatology: a color guide to diagnosis and therapy*, ed 4, St Louis, 2004, Mosby.

damage cellular components, including DNA, proteins, and cellular membranes. In response to the free radicals, the damaged keratinocytes recruit inflammatory cytokines, specifically interleukin-1 and interleukin-6, tumor necrosis factor-α, and transforming growth factor-β (Bernier et al, 2008). Unfortunately, the effects of radiation therapy are not restricted to malignant cells. Rapidly proliferating tissues, such as intestinal mucosa, bone marrow, and skin, are more susceptible to radiation. In addition, radiosensitization techniques may be used to enhance the effect of radiation on normal and malignant tissues (Camidge and Price, 2001).

The skin is particularly vulnerable to the effects of radiation because it is in a continuous state of cellular renewal. Damage is incurred by rapidly dividing cells, such as keratinocytes, hair follicles, sebaceous glands, epidermal basal cells, endothelial cells, and vascular components. A reduction of Langerhans cells also occurs (Bernier et al, 2008). Because radiation damages the mitotic ability of stem cells in the basal layer, regrowth of new cells is slowed and skin integrity becomes impaired (Maki and Clarey-Sanford, 2007).

Pathophysiologic Characteristics

The onset of radiation dermatitis depends on dose intensity and the individual's normal tissue sensitivity. The spectrum of skin reactions that can occur with radiation therapy (radiation dermatitis) as categorized by the National Cancer Institute is listed in Table 5-5. Treatment effects will be confined to the treatment area. Early effects will generally manifest within 2 to 3 weeks after beginning therapy. Because acute radiation effects are cumulative, the greatest reactions occur toward the end of therapy. However, side effects usually are self-limiting, and most subside 1 to 3 months after therapy has ended (Bernier et al, 2008).

Initially the skin in the treatment field will develop faint, transient erythema, which may become more brisk and persistent. Erythema will appear as a red, macular rash on warm-appearing skin that may feel sensitive and tight. It is an inflammatory response thought to be caused by dilation of the capillaries and increased vascular permeability; therefore edema may accompany erythema.

Dry desquamation may follow and will appear as red or tan pigmented skin that is dry, itchy, and peeling or flakey. This reaction is a result of the decreased ability of the basal cells of the epidermis to replace the surface layer cells and the decreased ability of the sweat and sebaceous gland to produce sweat. As the cumulative dose of radiation increases, the erythema and dry desquamation may evolve into moist desquamation, which is characterized by exposure of the dermis as a result of blisters, peeling, and sloughing. Moist desquamation could occur by the third week of treatment and increases the risk of infection, discomfort, and pain, possibly requiring interruption of the treatment plan to allow for healing (Bernier et al, 2008; Olascoaga et al, 2008). A combination of erythema and dry and moist desquamation may be seen within a single treatment field (Wells and MacBride, 2003).

Long-term, irradiated skin will have epidermal atrophy, so the epidermis is thin, dry, and more translucent. Sweat and sebaceous gland and hair follicles usually are absent. Telangiectasias and blood vessels are easily visible. Subendothelial connective tissue in small arteries proliferates, causing narrowing and thrombosis of the microvasculature (i.e., progressive obliterative endarteritis), and loss of elasticity due to damage to the elastic fibers in the dermis causes fibrosis (Olascoaga et al, 2008). Late effects develop gradually over several months or years and are a function of the total dose, volume of the area irradiated, energy and particles used, interval between fractions, and concomitant chemotherapy or biologic modifier (Olascoaga et al, 2008). Late effects are more likely to be significant when acute reactions are significant. Late radiation damage can be complicated by secondary ulceration, impaired joint mobility, shedding or deformity of the nails, malignancies (basal and squamous cell), and lymphedema caused by fibrosis of the lymph glands. When ulceration and necrosis occur years after radiation therapy, they usually occur in conjunction with trauma or infection. These lesions can become very painful and difficult to manage.

TABLE 5-5	Grading of Radiation Dermatitis		
Grade 1	**Grade 2**	**Grade 3**	**Grade 4**
Faint erythema or dry desquamation	Moderate to brisk erythema; patchy moist desquamation, mostly confined to skin folds and creases; moderate edema	Moist desquamation other than skin folds and creases; bleeding induced by minor trauma or abrasion	Skin necrosis or ulceration of full-thickness dermis; spontaneous bleeding from involved site

Adapted from National Cancer Institute Common Terminology Criteria for Adverse Events v 3.0 (CTCAE) available at http://ctep.cancer.gov/protocoldevelopment/electronic_applications/docs/ctcaev3.pdf. Accessed April 15, 2010.

Another reaction to radiation is termed *radiation recall* which is defined as the "recalling" by skin of previous radiation exposure following the administration of certain chemotherapeutic agents. The medications most commonly associated with radiation recall are docetaxel, doxorubicin, gemcitabine, and paclitaxel (Hird et al, 2008). Most recall reactions occur when less than 2 months separates completion of radiation therapy and resumption of chemotherapy (Azria et al, 2005; Hird et al, 2008). Once recall dermatitis is detected, chemotherapy is withheld until the dermatitis resolves; when it is resumed, premedication with corticosteroids is indicated.

Risk Factors

Substantial variations in the degree of acute and late normal tissue reactions exist even in patients who have received identical treatments. Thus identifying patients at risk for severe radiation-induced skin reactions is difficult. Treatment schedule and total dosage in radiation therapy are based on the tumoricidal doses and the tolerance dose of the perifocal normal tissue.

The quality of the irradiation and its modalities, including total dose, fractionation, and interfractional interval, appear to affect functional and cosmetic outcome the most. Risk factors that appear to influence the severity, onset, and duration of radiation skin reaction include age, general skin condition, and nutritional status. At risk for the highest stages of reaction are body areas within the treatment field, including bony prominences, and moist areas on the body, such as skin folds, under the breast, the axillae, neck, perineum, and groin (Wells and MacBride, 2003). Patients who are receiving combination therapy also are at risk because concomitant use of chemotherapy may sensitize the basal cells to radiation (Bernier et al, 2008).

Care of Irradiated Skin

Skin care before, during, and after radiation is aimed at minimizing the undesirable physiologic effects of radiation. Patients and caregivers are included in planning care and selection of goals and objectives. Intervention choices should be based on the available evidence of effectiveness, the ability to soothe the skin and promote patient comfort, and compatibility with ionizing radiation.

Patient education on skin care is critical when preparing the patient for radiation and during the course of the therapy. Patients should be instructed on the typical effects of radiation on the skin (dry desquamation), measures to promote moisture retention in the treatment area, the potential for radiation recall (when applicable), to protect the area from trauma and potential irritants (i.e., alcohol, perfumes, products containing α-hydroxy acid), and to only use products in the treatment field that have been approved by the health care team.

Several literature reviews on radiation skin care (prevention and management of dermatitis) have been published in the past few years (Aistars, 2006; Bernier et al, 2008; Bolderston et al, 2006; McQuestion, 2006; Nystedt et al, 2005; Olascoaga et al, 2008; Wickline, 2004). The findings from these reviews are quite similar and have been summarized in Table 5-6. A practice guideline for skin care and prevention of acute skin reactions based on these reports is given in Checklist 5-1. Most interventions have extremely limited evidence due to the absence of randomization, lack of controls, small sample size or inconsistent outcome measures. Most recommended skin care interventions are related to bathing, hygiene, and use of topical preparations and creams. Of particular interest are the following findings:

(1) Products containing aluminum, magnesium or zinc do not cause a "bolus effect" (i.e., increased dose and skin reaction) as previously considered (McQuestion, 2006).
(2) There is insufficient evidence to support or refute most topical preparations (see Table 5-6) for the prevention of acute skin reactions (Bolderston et al, 2006; McQuestion, 2006).
(3) There is insufficient evidence to support or refute corticosteroids or sucralfate cream for the management of acute skin reaction (Bolderston et al, 2006; McQuestion, 2006; Olascoaga et al, 2008)
(4) Calendula ointment may decrease radiation dermatitis in breast cancer patients (Bolderston et al, 2006; McQuestion, 2006)

Dressings. Numerous topical dressings have been used to treat acute radiation dermatitis, including transparent film dressings, hydrogels, foams, alginates, slow-released silver hydrofiber dressing, silver sulfadiazine (SSD) cream, and hydrocolloid dressings (Maki and Clarey-Sanford, 2007; Olascoaga et al, 2008; McQuestion, 2006). When a topical dressing is needed to manage a radiation skin injury, the type of dressing selected must be compatible with the priority needs of the skin condition. For example, transparent film dressings absorb little exudate and would be inappropriate for moist desquamation. In contrast, hydrocolloids can be used with minimal to moderate amounts of exudate, such as what occurs with moist desquamation. Given that irradiated skin is characterized by a loss of elasticity, atrophy, and fibrosis, nonadhesive wound dressings are generally preferred to minimize trauma to irradiated skin, avoid skin tears, and prevent pain upon dressing removal (see Chapter 18 for further information about wound care dressings).

Adjunctive Interventions. Hyperbaric oxygen, growth factors, biologic skin substitutes, pentoxifylline, interferon-γ therapy, and surgery have been used for treatment of radiation-induced necrotic wounds (Olascoaga et al, 2008). Hyperbaric oxygen improves collagen formation, neovascularization, epithelialization, and leukocyte bactericidal

TABLE 5-6	Skin Care Products and Radiation Therapy: Summary of Evidence	
Product	**Description**	**Findings**
Evidence for Use or FDA Approved		
Hydrophilic lotions and creams	Moisturizers: Lubriderm, Glaxal base, Eucerin, Keri lotion, Aquaphor	• May be helpful in preventing radiation skin reactions • Product should be unscented, lanolin-free • Gently apply (do not rub) twice per day
Calendula ointment	Pot marigold believed to have antiviral and antiinflammatory effects Has been used to treat acne, control bleeding, soothe irritated tissue	• May decrease occurrence of radiation dermatitis (limited evidence) • When compared to Biafine, reported to provide statistically significant reduction in skin reaction, pain and need for treatment interruption.
Hyaluronic acid cream	Lubricating agent found in the body	• May be radioprotective (limited evidence) • Used to treatment very dry, scaly skin
Aloe vera gel	Extracted from pulp of aloe vera leaves	• May be used to sooth, cool radiated skin for comfort • Lack of evidence supporting or refuting use for prevention or treatment of radiation dermatitis • Product does not moisturize and should be discontinued if skin becomes dry
Miaderm cream (Aiden Industries)	Formulated with aloe vera, calendula, hyaluronic acid	• FDA approved for prevention or treatment of radiation dermatitis of skin (limited evidence)
Biafine emulsion (OrthoNeutrogena)	Water-based emulsion paraffin and avocado oil are among the many ingredients	• FDA approved for treatment of radiation dermatitis, burns, other superficial wounds (limited evidence) • Contraindicated for use on bleeding wounds • Temporary tingling sensation may occur 10–15 minutes after application • Apply three times per day but not within 4 hours of radiation treatment
Topical corticosteroid creams	Used to decrease erythema and pruritus (itching)	• Radioprotective effect may be present with use of mometasone furoate or Bepanthen cream (limited evidence) • Use only temporarily with caution in collaboration with physician's order • Induces vasoconstriction, atrophy of dermal collagen, resulting in thinning of skin • Increases susceptibility to infection, masks superficial infection, delays wound healing
Contraindicated, Off Label, or Lack of Evidence for Use		
α-Hydroxy acid (AHA) cream	Glycolic acid and lactic acid most common AHAs Exfoliates and soothes dry, scaly skin (xerosis)	• Can increase radiation skin reaction • Stinging, burning may occur when applied to irritated skin
Skin sealant wipes, wands, sprays	Protective transparent film containing plasticizing agents such as copolymer Some products contain isopropyl alcohol	• Lack of evidence supporting or refuting use for prevention or treatment of radiation dermatitis • See Table 5-4 for examples of skin sealants • Do not use products with alcohol on radiated skin
Chamomile cream	Extracted from chamomile plant	• Lack of evidence supporting or refuting use for prevention or treatment of radiation dermatitis
Almond ointment	Made with almond oil	• Lack of evidence supporting or refuting use for prevention or treatment of radiation dermatitis
Petrolatum jelly–based products	Hydrophobic/water repelling	• Do not use for prevention or treatment of radiation dermatitis
Aqueous cream	Paraffin-based emulsion containing petroleum jelly, phenoxy ethanol, and purified water	• No evidence supporting use for prevention of radiation skin reactions • Contains petroleum, which is not recommended for prevention or treatment of radiation dermatitis of skin
Sucralfate/Sulcralfate derivatives	Antiulcer drug for many years Protects mucous membranes during radiotherapy and chemotherapy Recently demonstrated in animal model to stimulate regeneration of the skin and accelerate wound healing	• Not FDA approved for topical use for prevention or treatment of radiation dermatitis of skin • Small studies in radiation therapy reported that cream significantly prevented acute skin reactions and damaged skin healed significantly faster (findings not consistent in subsequent studies)

FDA, Food and Drug Administration.
Information compiled from the following sources: Aistars, 2006; Bernier et al, 2008; Bolderston et al, 2006; McQuestion, 2006; Nystedt et al, 2005; Olascoaga et al, 2008; Wickline, 2004.

CHECKLIST 5-1
Prevention and Management of Radiation Skin Reactions

Promote (Do Not Limit) Personal Hygiene Practices
✓ Continue showers and baths.
✓ Use lukewarm water and mild nonalkaline soap (e.g., baby soap, Dove, Ivory, Basis).
✓ Use mild nonmedicated shampoo (i.e., baby shampoo) for scalp in patients receiving radiation therapy to the head.
✓ Use electric razor for shaving.
✓ Apply deodorant as usual to intact skin throughout treatment.

Promote Comfort
✓ Gently apply (do not rub) unscented, lanolin-free hydrophilic moisturizer twice per day (see Table 5-6 for product examples).
✓ Do not use petrolatum-based products, products with irritants such as alcohol, perfumes, or additives, or products containing α-hydroxy acids.
✓ May use aloe vera to sooth and cool the skin (does not moisturize, so discontinue if skin becomes dry).
✓ For burning and itching, apply normal saline compresses as needed or hydrocortisone cream (if ordered).
✓ Wear loose, soft, breathable, nonbinding clothing that protects skin from sun and wind.
✓ Use cool mist humidifier if humidity is needed.

Prevent Trauma
✓ Avoid swimming in chlorinated pools, hot tubs, and lakes to minimize exposure to chemicals and bacteria.
✓ Avoid heating pads and ice packs to prevent thermal injury.
✓ Avoid adhesives and tapes to prevent skin tears.

Manage Radiation Dermatitis
✓ Normal saline soaks to provide cooling sensation and loosen crusting in treatment field.
✓ Plain, non-scented lanolin-free hydrophilic cream for dry desquamation but discontinue when skin breakdown occurs.
✓ Nonadherent dressings may be used for moist desquamation when it occurs during the course of radiation therapy but should be removed during the treatment.
✓ Dressings may be used based on the wound/skin care needs (i.e., absorb moisture) once radiation therapy has concluded.

activity to improve acute radiation injury by reducing tissue hypoxia and edema (see Chapter 22 for further discussion of hyperbaric oxygen therapy).

Growth factors can be used to manipulate the wound environment to stimulate healing of radiation ulcers. Platelet-derived growth factor, epidermal growth factor, and transforming growth factor-β stimulate tissue regeneration, remodeling, and proliferation of capillary endothelial cells, and they chemoattract neutrophils, monocytes, and fibroblasts to the wound site (see Chapter 20 for discussion of growth factors).

Pentoxifylline, used to treat peripheral vascular disease and improve peripheral microcirculation by increasing the flexibility of red blood cells, may reduce the severity of late radiation injury when administered preventively or in the postirradiation period (Aygenc et al, 2004). In addition, time to heal of existing radiation-induced ulcers appears to be decreased (Olascoaga et al, 2008). A few studies have used interferon-γ therapy with radiation-induced ulcers to reduce fibrosis because it inhibits collagen production in normal dermal fibroblasts (Gottlober et al, 2001). Additional studies using comparison groups and larger samples are needed to replicate these findings.

Surgical interventions may be used for treatment of some radiation-induced wounds. These procedures involve extensive surgical debridement and removal of all poor-quality tissue and timely reconstruction with well-vascularized soft tissue flaps (see Chapter 33 for further discussion of surgical interventions for wound closure).

SUMMARY

The intact skin provides the first line of defense against microbial invasion and trauma. Different factors can jeopardize the skin's integrity. It is important to be able to recognize the skin-related signs of these factors so that the factors can be eliminated or their intensity reduced substantially. Most often, the type of skin damage that the wound specialist will encounter is mechanical or vascular. Only with an in-depth skin assessment and history of the skin eruption can the etiology of the skin damage be identified and the negative sequelae arrested through appropriate prevention and treatment interventions.

Because the more rare inflammatory, infectious, or disease-related skin lesions often require prompt treatment to be effective, the wound specialist should also be familiar with these types of lesions. Although the underlying disease is the critical determinant for wound healing in these situations, the wound specialist is an important partner and interdisciplinary team member because he or she can provide valuable recommendations for wound management that will best address the requirements of the wound and the needs of the patient.

REFERENCES

Abeloff MD et al: *Abeloffs clinical oncology*, ed 4, St Louis, 2008, Elsevier.
Aistars J: The validity of skin care protocols followed by women with breast cancer receiving external radiation, *Clin J Oncol Nurs* 10:487-492, 2006.
American Academy of Dermatology: *Herpes zoster*, 2008. available at http://www.aad.org/public/publications/pamphlets/viral_herpes_zoster.html, accessed October 11, 2009.
Asha NJ et al: Comparative analysis of prevalence, risk factors and molecular epidemiology of antibiotic-associated diarrhea due to *Clostridium difficile, Clostridium perfringens,* and *Staphylococcus aureus, J Clin Microbiol* 44:2785-2791, 2006.
Association of periOperative Registered Nurses (AORN): *AORN recommended practices for positioning the patient in the perioperative practice setting. AORN standards, recommended practices, and guidelines,* Denver, 2008, Author.

Ayello EA: Preventing pressure ulcers and skin tears. In Mezey M et al, editors: *Geriatric nursing protocols for best practice,* ed 2, New York, 2003, Springer.

Aygenc E et al: Prophylactic effect of pentoxifylline on radiotherapy complications: a clinical study, *Otolaryngol Head Neck Surg* 130(3):351-356, 2004.

Azria D et al. Radiation recall: a well recognized but neglected phenomenon, *Cancer Treat Rev.* 31:555–570, 2005.

Bank D, Nix D: Preventing skin tears in a nursing and rehabilitation center: an interdisciplinary effort, *Ostomy Wound Manage* 52(9):38-46, 2006.

Baranoski S: Skin tears, *Nurs Manage* 32(8):25, 2001.

Baranoski S: How to prevent and manage skin tears, *Adv Skin Wound Care* 16(5):268-270, 2003.

Bartlett JG: Antibiotic-associated diarrhea, In Schlossberg D, editor: *Clinical infectious disease,* Philadelphia, 2008, Cambridge University Press.

Beeckman D et al: Prevention and treatment of incontinence-associated dermatitis: literature review, *J Adv Nurs* 65(6):1141-1154, 2009.

Benoit RA Jr, Watts C: The effect of a pressure ulcer prevention program and the bowel management system in reducing pressure ulcer prevalence in an ICU setting, *J Wound Ostomy Continence Nurs* 34(2):163-175, 2007.

Bernier J et al: Consensus guidelines for the management of radiation dermatitis and coexisting acne-like rash in patients receiving radiotherapy plus EGFR inhibitors for the treatment of squamous cell carcinoma, *Annals of Oncology* 19(1):142-149, 2008. Also available at http://www.medscape.com/viewarticle/573362_2.

Birch S, Coggins T: No-rinse, one-step bed bath: the effects on the occurrence of skin tears in a long-term care setting, *Ostomy Wound Manage* 49(1):64-67, 2003.

Bliss DZ, et al: Prevalence and correlates of perineal dermatitis in nursing home residents, *Nursing Research* 55(4):243-251, 2006

Bolderston A et al: The prevention and management of acute skin reactions related to radiation therapy: a systematic review and practice guideline, *Support Care Cancer* 14:802-817, 2006.

Bradley SF: Staphylococcus. In Schlossberg D, editor: *Clinical infectious disease,* Philadelphia, 2008, Cambridge University Press

Brannon J: *Intertrigo. Yeast infection in skin folds.* About.com: dermatology, updated November 13, 2004, available at http://dermatology.about.com/od/fungalinfections/a/intertrigo.htm, accessed September 15, 2009.

Brillhart B: Pressure sore and skin tear prevention and treatment during a 10-month program, *Rehabil Nurs* 30(3):85-91, 2005.

Camidge R, Price A: Characterizing the phenomenon of radiation recall dermatitis, *Radiother Oncol* 59:237-245, 2001.

Carpenter CF, de Sanctis J: Candidiasis. In Schlossberg D, editor: *Clinical infectious disease,* Philadelphia, 2008, Cambridge University Press.

Chacon J, Ferreira L: Hemicellulose dressing for skin lesions caused by herpes zoster in a patient with leukemia—an alternative dressing, *Wounds* 21(1):10-14, 2009.

Eddins C, Gray M: Are probiotic or symbiotic preparations effective for the management of clostridium difficile-associated or radiation-induced diarrhea? *JWOCN* 35(1):50-58, 2008.

File TM, Stevens DL: Superficial skin infections (pyodermas). In Tan JS et al, editors: *Expert guide to infectious diseases,* ed 2, Philadelphia, 2008, ACP Press.

Fleck CA: Preventing and treating skin tears, *Adv Skin Wound Care* 20(6):315-320, 2007.

Fontaine R et al A quantitative analysis of pressure and shear in the effectiveness of support surfaces, *J Wound Ostomy Continence Nurs* 25:233, 1998.

Furdon SA: Challenges in neonatal nursing: providing evidence based skin care, *MedScape Nurses,* 2003, available at http://cme.medscape.com/viewarticle/465017, accessed August 24, 2009.

Gottlober P et al: Interferon-gamma in 5 patients with cutaneous radiation syndrome after radiation therapy, *Int J Radiat Oncol Biol Phys* 50:159-166, 2001.

Gray M, Weir D: Prevention and treatment of moisture-associated skin damage (maceration) in the periwound skin, *J Wound Ostomy Continence Nurs* 34(2):153-157, 2007.

Gray M et al: Incontinence associated dermatitis: a consensus, *J Wound Ostomy Continence Nurs* 34(1):45-54, 2007a.

Gray M et al: Moisture vs pressure: making sense out of perineal wounds, *J Wound Ostomy Continence Nurs* 34(2):134-142, 2007b.

Habif TP: *Clinical dermatology: a color guide to diagnosis and therapy,* ed 4, St Louis, 2004, Mosby.

Habif TP et al: *Skin disease: diagnosis and treatment,* ed 2, Philadelphia, 2005, Mosby.

Hird AE et al: Radiation recall dermatitis: case report and review of the literature, *Curr Oncol* 15(1):53-62, 2008.

Hunter JAA et al: *Clinical dermatology,* Oxford, 2002. Blackwell Science.

Hunter S et al: Clinical trial of a prevention and treatment protocol for skin breakdown in two nursing homes, *J Wound Ostomy Continence Nurs* 30(5):250-258, 2003.

Imhoff A, Karpa K: Is there a future for probiotics in preventing *Clostridium difficile*-associated disease and treatment of recurrent episodes? *Nutr Clin Pract* 4(1):15-32, 2009.

Junkin J, Lerner-Selekof J: Prevalence of incontinence and associated skin injury in the acute care inpatient, *J Wound Ostomy Continence Nurs* 34(3):260-269, 2007.

Kauffman CA: Candidiasis. In Tan JS et al, editors: *Expert guide to infectious disease,* ed 2, Philadelphia, 2008, ACP Press.

Kim J et al: Clinical application of continent anal plug in bedridden patients with intractable diarrhea, *Dis Colon Rectum* 44:1162-1167, 2001.

Kimberlin DW, Whitley RJ: Herpes simplex viruses 1 and 2. In Schlossberg D, editor: *Clinical infectious disease,* Philadelphia, 2008, Cambridge University Press.

Kowal-Vern A et al: Fecal containment in bedridden patients: economic impact of 2 commercial bowel catheter systems, *Am J Crit Care* 18:2-14, 2009.

Lablanc K, Baranoski S: Prevention and management of skin tears, *Adv Skin Wound Care* 22:325-332, 2009.

Lablanc et al: Best practice recommendations for the prevention and treatment of skin tears, *Wound Care Canada* 6(1):14-32, 2008.

Loeper JM et al: *Therapeutic positioning and skin care,* Minneapolis, 1986, Sister Kenny Institute.

Maki L, Clarey-Sanford C: Using slow-released silver hydrofiber dressings on a neck radiation burn, *J Wound Ostomy Continence Nurs* 34(5):542-545, 2007.

Malone ML et al: The epidemiology of skin tears in the institutionalized elderly, *J Am Geriatr Soc* 39(6):591, 1991.

McFarland LV: Renewed interest in a difficult disease: *Clostridium difficile* infections—epidemiology and current treatment strategies, *Curr Opinion Gastroenterol* 25(1):24-35, 2009.

McGough-Csarny J, Kopac CA: Skin tears in institutionalized elderly: an epidemiological study, *Ostomy Wound Manage* 44(Suppl 3A):14S, 1998.

McQuestion M: Evidence-based skin care management in radiation therapy, *Sem Onc Nurs* 22(3):163-173, 2006.

McTigue T et al: Efficacy of a skin tear education program: improving the knowledge of nurses practicing in acute care settings, *J WOCN* 36(5):486-492, 2009.

Meuleneire F: Using a soft silicone-coated net dressing to manage skin tears, *J Wound Care* 11(10):365-369, 2002.

Milne CT, Corbett LQ: A new option in the treatment of skin tears for the institutionalized resident: formulated 2-octylcyanoacrylate topical bandage, *Geriatr Nurs* 26(5):321-325, 2005.

National Pressure Ulcer Advisory Panel (NPUAP): *Terms and definitions related to support surfaces*, 2007. Available at http://www.npuap.org/NPUAP_S3I_TD.pdf, accessed September 22, 2009.

Nazarko L: Preventing and treating skin tears, *Nursing & Residential Care* 7(12):549-550, 2005.

Noble SL et al: Diagnosis and management of common tinea infections, *Am Fam Physician* 58(1):163-174, 177-178, 1998, available at http://www.aafp.org/afp/980700ap/noble.html, reviewed/updated March 2009, accessed October 9, 2009.

Nystedt KE et al: The standardization of radiation skin care in British Columbia: a collaborative approach, *Onc Nurs Forum* 32(6):1199-1205, 2005.

Olascoaga AJ et al: Wound healing in radiated skin: pathophysiology and treatment options, *Int Wound J* 5:246-257, 2008.

Patton KT, Thibodeau GA: *Anatomy and physiology*, ed 7, St. Louis, 2010, Mosby.

Payne RL, Martin ML: The epidemiology and management of skin tears in older adults, *Ostomy Wound Manage* 26:26, 1990.

Payne RL, Martin ML: Defining and classifying skin tears: need for a common language, *Ostomy Wound Manage* 39(5):16, 1993.

Pennsylvania Patient Safety Authority: Skin tears: the clinical challenge, September 2006. *Patient Safety Advisory (newsletter)* 3(3):1, 5-10, available at http://www.patientsafetyauthority.org., accessed October 3, 2009.

Ratliff CR, Fletcher KR: Skin tears: a review of the evidence to support prevention and treatment, *Ostomy Wound Manage* 53(3):32-34, 2007.

Redelings MD et al: Increase in *Clostridium difficile*-related mortality rates, United States, 1999-2004, *Emerg Infect Dis* 13 1417-1419, 2007.

Rietschel RL, Fowler JF Jr: *Fisher's contact dermatitis*, ed 5, Philadelphia, 2001, Lippincott, Williams & Wilkins.

Roberts MJ: Preventing and managing skin tears: a review, *J Wound Ostomy Continence Nurs* 34(3):256-259, 2007.

Rohde CL et al: The use of probiotics in the prevention and treatment of antibiotic-associated diarrhea with special interest in *Clostridium difficile*-associated diarrhea, *Nutr Clin Pract* 24(1):33-40, 2009.

Sachdeva MP, Tomecki KJ: Cellulitis and erysipelas. In Schlossberg D, editor: *Clinical infectious disease*, Philadelphia, 2008, Cambridge Press.

Stevens DL et al: Streptococcus groups A, B, C, D, and G. In Schlossberg D, editor: *Clinical infectious disease*, Philadelphia, 2008, Cambridge Press.

Thomas DR, et al: A comparison of an opaque foam dressing versus a transparent film dressing in the management of skin tears in institutionalized subjects, *Ostomy/Wound Management* 45(6):22-28, 1999.

Visscher ML: Recent advances in diaper dermatitis: etiology and treatment, *Pediatric Health* 3(1):81-89, 2009.

Wells M, MacBride S: Radiation skin reactions. In Faithfull S, Wells M, editors: *Supportive care in radiotherapy*, New York, 2003, Churchill Livingstone

White MW, Karam S, Cowell B: Skin tears in frail elders: a practical approach to prevention, *Geriatr Nurs* 15(2):95, 1994.

Wickline MM: Prevention and treatment of acute radiation dermatitis: a literature review, *Oncol Nurs Forum* 31(2):237, 2004.

Wiederkehr M, Schwartz RA: *Tinea cruris: treatment and medication*, updated May 20, 2008, available at http://emedicine.medscape.com/article/1091806-overview, accessed September 15, 2009.

Wound, Ostomy and Continence Nurses Society (WOCN): *Guideline for management of pressure ulcers*, WOCN *clinical practice guideline series #2*, Glenview, IL, 2010, Author.

Wright K, O'Connor AD: Causes and risks of pressure sores, *Nurs Resident Care* 9(11):516-523, 2007.

Zaia JA: Varicella-zoster virus. In Schlossberg D, editor: *Clinical infectious disease*, Philadelphia, 2008, Cambridge Press.

Zulkowski K: Perineal dermatitis versus pressure ulcer: distinguishing characteristics, *Adv Skin Wound Care* 21(8):382-388, 2008.

6

Skin and Wound Inspection and Assessment

Denise P. Nix

OBJECTIVES

1. Differentiate between skin inspection and skin assessment.
2. List six factors to consider when assessing darkly pigmented skin.
3. Distinguish between wound assessment and evaluation of healing.
4. Define partial-thickness and full-thickness tissue loss.
5. Compare and contrast a normal and an abnormal finding for each wound assessment parameter.
6. Describe how to measure the length, width, depth, tunneling, and undermining of a wound.

An initial skin and wound assessment provides the foundation for developing a patient's plan of care. However, ongoing skin and wound assessments also are critical because they provide the mechanism for monitoring the effectiveness of that plan, thus allowing determination of progress or deterioration of the wound. Documentation of assessment findings facilitates communication among caregivers. Because of the myriad etiologic, systemic, and local factors commonly involved in the pathogenesis of a wound, a comprehensive patient assessment is essential to identify cofactors that may impair wound healing and jeopardize skin integrity. Whereas all patients with or without wounds require a skin assessment upon admission, the patient with a wound requires additional assessments, including underlying causes for the wound and healing impediments.

SIGNIFICANCE

In order to adequately convey the condition of a wound or a skin lesion, wound and skin assessment requires access to a unique vocabulary. As with monitoring blood pressure, temperature, and pulse rate, those attending to a wound preferably should use objective parameters to reflect its present status. However, the state of the science is such that both subjective and objective measures are required to adequately capture the condition of the wound. Because subjective measures by definition can vary in interpretation from one user to another, it is essential that accurate use of wound assessment terminology be emphasized in staff education and that competencies for wound and skin assessment be used (Appendix C).

The economics of health care impose additional motivation for conducting and documenting a systematic measurement of wound healing. Without objective criteria of the status or progress of repair, it is difficult to justify treatments or assign appropriate reimbursement for services. The standard of care is to provide accurate and routine skin and wound assessments. Failure to assess the patient systematically also carries a great legal liability risk (Murphy, 1996). Without accurate, consistent, and retrievable documentation, it is very difficult to retrospectively create a clear picture of the patient's condition and of the care that actually was provided.

ASSESSMENT

Assessment is a two-step process that requires inspection and collection of data and then interpretation of that data so that a plan of care can be derived. During the initial encounter an assessment provides the baseline data to which comparisons can be made to determine changes; this is the process of *monitoring*.

The word *assessment* alone as it relates to the prevention and management of wounds can be confusing because a number of assessments are required: risk assessment (see Chapter 8), skin assessment, wound assessment, and physical assessment. For clarity and safety, findings from each type of assessment must be documented using appropriate terms to describe the patient's skin or wound condition. Staff education should include how to conduct the assessments and how to link appropriate interventions to the findings.

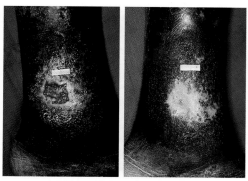

PLATE 1 Partial-thickness venous ulcer healing by epithelialization. Resurfaced venous ulcer lacks normal dark pigmentation because of depth of damage (below basement membrane).

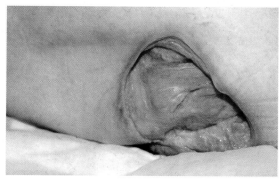

PLATE 2 Stage IV pressure ulcer with exposed muscle.

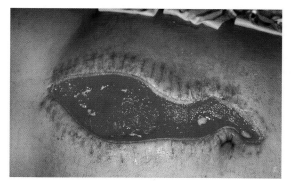

PLATE 3 Full-thickness abdominal wound healing by secondary intention with healthy (red, cobblestone) granulation tissue and attached wound edges.

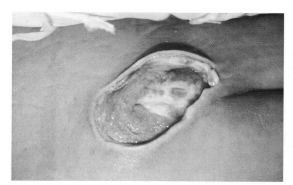

PLATE 4 Stage IV sacral pressure ulcer wound edges are rolled (epibole), which is an impediment to wound healing.

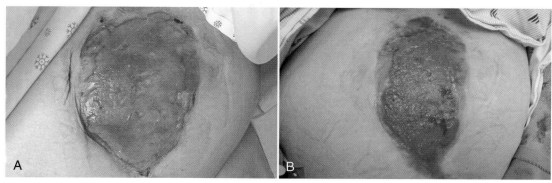

PLATE 5 A, Wound clean, not granulating (note lack of red cobblestone appearance), suggesting heavy bacterial load or other impediment to wound healing. **B,** Same wound after 1 week of topical antimicrobial use (note healthy red cobblestone appearance).

PLATE 6 | **Primary Skin Lesions**

Description	Examples		
A. Macule Flat, circumscribed area that is a change in the color of the skin <1 cm in diameter	Freckle, flat mole (nevus), petechia, measles, scarlet fever	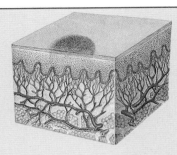	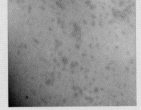 Measles. (From Habif TP: *Clinical dermatology: a color guide to diagnosis and therapy*, ed 5, St. Louis, 2004, Mosby.)
B. Papule Elevated, firm, circumscribed area <1 cm in diameter	Wart (verruca), elevated mole, lichen planus	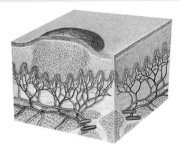	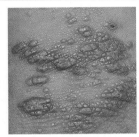 Lichen planus. (From Weston W et al: *Color textbook of pediatric dermatology*, ed 4, Edinburgh, 1996, Mosby.)
C. Patch Flat, nonpalpable, irregular-shaped macule >1 cm in diameter	Vitiligo, port-wine stain, Mongolian spot, café au lait spot	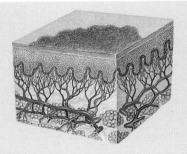	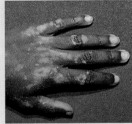 Vitiligo. (From Weston W et al: *Color textbook of pediatric dermatology*, ed 4, Edinburgh, 1991, Mosby.)
D. Plaque Elevated, firm, rough lesion with flat top surface >1 cm in diameter	Psoriasis, seborrheic keratosis, actinic keratosis	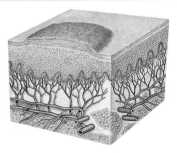	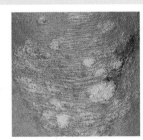 Plaque. (From Habif TP: *Clinical dermatology: a color guide to diagnosis and therapy*, ed 5, St. Louis, 2004, Mosby.)

PLATE 6 **Primary Skin Lesions—cont'd**

Description	Examples

E. Wheal
Elevated, irregular-shaped area of cutaneous edema; solid, transient, variable diameter

Insect bite, urticaria, allergic reaction

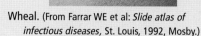
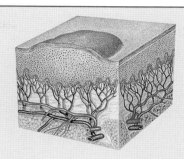

Wheal. (From Farrar WE et al: *Slide atlas of infectious diseases*, St. Louis, 1992, Mosby.)

F. Nodule
Elevated, firm, circumscribed lesion; deeper in dermis than a papule; 1–2 cm in diameter

Erythema nodosum, lipoma

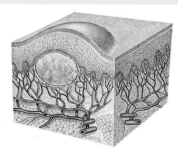
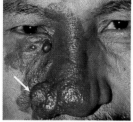

Hypertrophic nodule. (From Goldman MP: *Cutaneous and cosmetic laser surgery*, Edinburgh, 1994, Mosby.)

G. Tumor
Elevated and solid lesion; may or may not be clearly demarcated; deeper in dermis; >2 cm in diameter

Neoplasm, benign tumor, lipoma, hemangioma

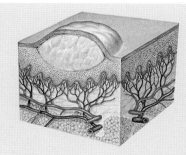
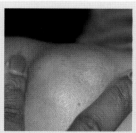

Lipoma. (From Lemmi FO, Lemmi CAE: *Physical assessment findings CD-ROM*, St. Louis, 2000, Saunders.)

H. Vesicle
Elevated, circumscribed, superficial, not into dermis; filled with serous fluid; <1 cm in diameter

Varicella (chicken pox), herpes zoster (shingles)

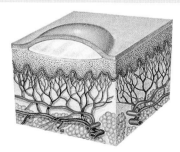
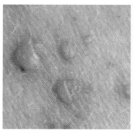

Vesicles caused by varicella. (From Farrar WE et al: *Slide atlas of infectious diseases*, St. Louis, 1992, Mosby.)

Continued

PLATE 6 | Primary Skin Lesions—cont'd

Description	Examples		
I. Bulla Vesicle >1 cm in diameter	Blister, pemphigus vulgaris	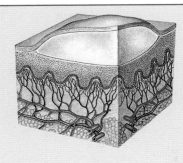	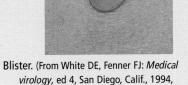 Blister. (From White DE, Fenner FJ: *Medical virology,* ed 4, San Diego, Calif., 1994, Academic Press.)
J. Pustule Elevated, superficial lesion; similar to vesicle but filled with purulent fluid	Impetigo, acne	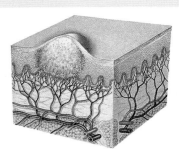	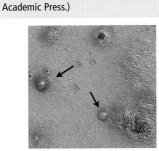 Acne. (From Weston W et al: *Color textbook of pediatric dermatology,* ed 4, Edinburgh, 1996, Mosby.)
K. Cyst Elevated, circumscribed, encapsulated lesion; in dermis or subcutaneous layer; filled with liquid or semisolid material	Sebaceous cyst, cystic acne	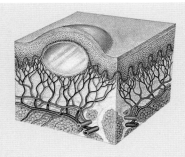	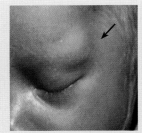 Sebaceous cyst. (From Weston W et al: *Color textbook of pediatric dermatology,* ed 4, Edinburgh, 1996, Mosby.)
L. Telangiectasia Fine, irregular red lines produced by capillary dilation	Telangiectasia in rosacea	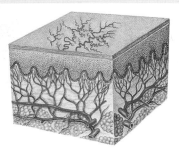	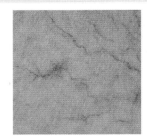 Telangiectasia. (From Lemmi FO, Lemmi CAE: *Physical assessment findings CD-ROM,* St. Louis, 2000, Saunders.)

(Modified from Wilson SF, Giddens JF: *Health assessment for nursing practice,* ed 4, St Louis, 2009, Mosby/Elsevier. In Seidel HM et al: *Mosby's guide to physical examination,* ed 7, St Louis, 2011, Mosby/Elsevier.)

PLATE 7   **Secondary Skin Lesions**

Description	Examples

A. Scale
Heaped-up, keratinized cells; flaky skin; irregular; thick or thin; dry or oily; varies in size

Flaking of skin with seborrheic dermatitis following scarlet fever or flaking of skin following drug reaction, dry skin

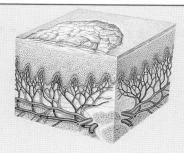

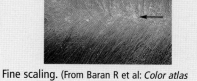

Fine scaling. (From Baran R et al: *Color atlas of the hair, scalp, and nails,* St. Louis, 1991, Mosby.)

B. Lichenification
Rough, thickened epidermis secondary to persistent rubbing; itching, or skin irritation; often involves flexor surface of extremity

Chronic dermatitis

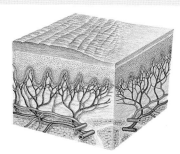

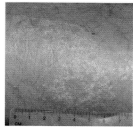

Lichenification. (From Lemmi FO, Lemmi CAE: *Physical assessment findings CD-ROM,* St. Louis, 2000, Saunders.)

C. Keloid
Irregular-shaped, elevated progressively enlarging scar; grows beyond boundaries of wound; caused by excessive collagen formation during healing

Keloid formation following surgery

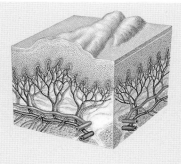

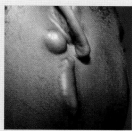

Keloid. (From Weston W et al: *Color textbook of pediatric dermatology,* ed 4, Edinburgh, 1996, Mosby.)

D. Hypertrophic scar
Overproduction of collagen, causing the scar to be raised above skin level but not outside the boundaries of the wound.

Healed wound or surgical incision

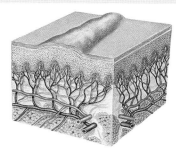

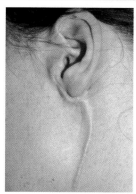

Hypertrophic scar. (From Eisele D, Smith R: *Complications in head and neck surgery,* ed 2, Philadelphia, 2009, Mosby/Elsevier.)

Continued

PLATE 7   **Secondary Skin Lesions—cont'd**

Description	Examples		
E. Excoriation Loss of epidermis; linear hollowed-out, crusted area	Abrasion or scratch	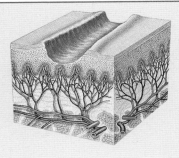	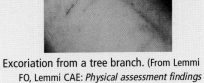Excoriation from a tree branch. (From Lemmi FO, Lemmi CAE: *Physical assessment findings CD-ROM*, St. Louis, 2000, Saunders.)
F. Fissure Linear crack of break from epidermis; may be moist or dry	Athlete's foot, crack at corner of mouth	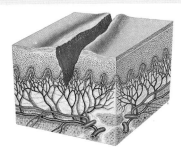	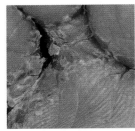Scaling and fissures of tinea pedis. (From Lemmi FO, Lemmi CAE: *Physical assessment findings CD-ROM,* St. Louis, 2000, Saunders.)
G. Erosion Loss of part of epidermis; depressed, moist, glistening; follows rupture of vesicle or bulla	Varicella, variola after rupture	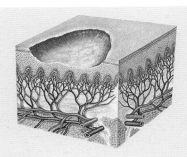	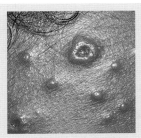Erosion. (From Cohen IK et al: *Wound healing,* Philadelphia, 1993, Saunders.)
H. Ulcer Loss of epidermis and dermis; concave; varies in size	Neuropathic wound ulcer	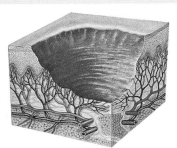	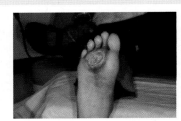Neuropathic foot ulcer. (Courtesy of J. Lebretton and V. Driver.)

PLATE 7 | Secondary Skin Lesions—cont'd

Description	Examples
I. Crust Dried serum, blood, or purulent exudates; slightly elevated; varies in size; brown, red, black, tan, or straw color	Scab on abrasion, eczema Scab.
J. Atrophy Thinning of skin surface and loss of skin markings; skin translucent and paper-like	Striae, aged skin Striae. (Courtesy of Antoinette Hood, MD, Department of Dermatology, School of Medicine, University of Indiana, Indianapolis, IN.)

(Modified from Wilson SF, Giddens JF: *Health assessment for nursing practice,* ed 4, St Louis, 2009, Mosby/Elsevier. In Seidel HM et al: *Mosby's guide to physical examination,* ed 7, St Louis, 2011, Mosby/Elsevier.)

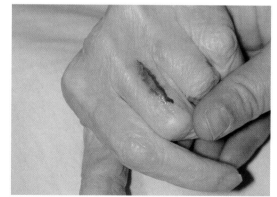

PLATE 8 Category I skin tear without tissue loss: linear type (full thickness). (From LeBlanc K, Christensen D, Orsted HL et al: Best practice recommendations for the prevention and treatment of skin tears, *Wound Care Canada* 6(1):22, 2008. Image courtesy of K. LeBlanc.)

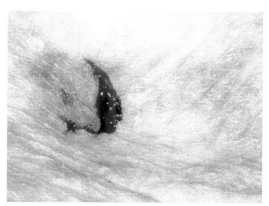

PLATE 9 Category I skin tear without tissue loss: flap type (full thickness). (From LeBlanc K, Christensen D, Orsted HL et al: Best practice recommendations for the prevention and treatment of skin tears, *Wound Care Canada* 6(1):22, 2008. Image courtesy of K. LeBlanc.)

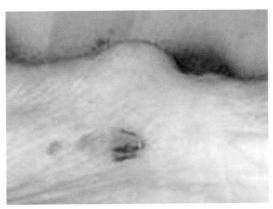

PLATE 10 Category II skin tear with <25% partial tissue loss. (From LeBlanc K, Christensen D, Orsted HL et al: Best practice recommendations for the prevention and treatment of skin tears, *Wound Care Canada* 6(1):22, 2008. Image courtesy of K. LeBlanc.)

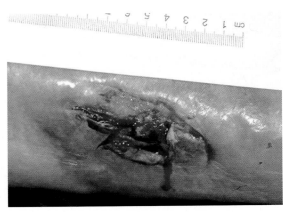

PLATE 11 Category II skin tear with >25% partial tissue loss. (From LeBlanc K, Christensen D, Orsted HL et al: Best practice recommendations for the prevention and treatment of skin tears, *Wound Care Canada* 6(1):22, 2008. Image courtesy of K. LeBlanc.)

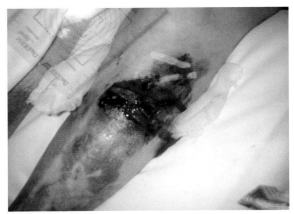

PLATE 12 Category III skin tear with complete tissue loss. (From LeBlanc K, Christensen D, Orsted HL et al: Best practice recommendations for the prevention and treatment of skin tears, *Wound Care Canada* 6(1):22, 2008. Image courtesy of K. LeBlanc.)

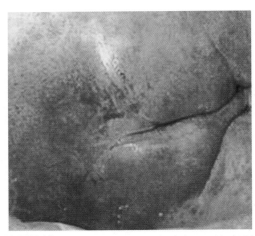

PLATE 13 Incontinence-associated dermatitis (IAD).

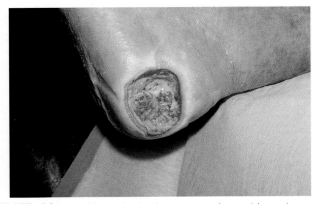

PLATE 14 Unstable right heel pressure ulcer with periwound maceration.

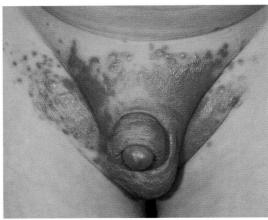

PLATE 15 Candidiasis in moist diaper area with characteristic satellite lesions. (From Habif TP: *Clinical dermatology*, ed 5, London, 2009, Mosby/Elsevier.)

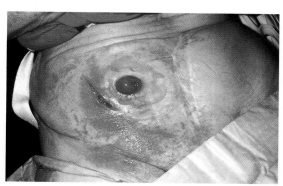

PLATE 16 Patient with an ileostomy who developed peristomal abscess that was incised. Chemical dermatitis present along inferior aspect of incision because of inadequate protection of skin from drainage. Candidiasis also presents as papular satellite lesions and solid plaque-like rash advancing into groin and over suprapubic area.

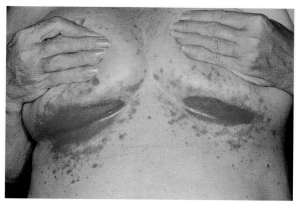

PLATE 17 Intertrigo. (From Habif TP: *Clinical dermatology,* ed 5, London, 2009, Mosby/Elsevier.)

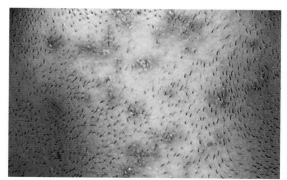

PLATE 18 Folliculitis, an infection of hair follicles resulting from inappropriate hair removal technique. (From Jarvis C: *Physical examination & health assessment,* ed 4, St Louis, 2004, Saunders.)

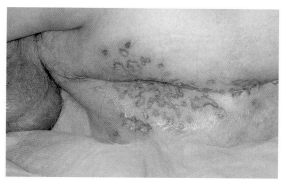

PLATE 19 Herpes simplex virus (HSV) infection. Vesicles become pustules that erode, drain, and crust.

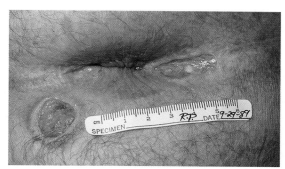

PLATE 20 Perianal herpes simplex ulcer initially misinterpreted as pressure ulcers.

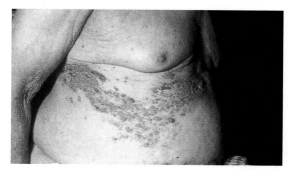

PLATE 21 Herpes zoster involving simple thoracic dermatome. Vesicles are clustered and erythematous.

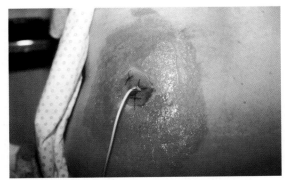

PLATE 22 Moist desquamation after an allergic reaction in response to the second application of benzoin to a percutaneous nephrostomy site.

Wound Assessment: Anatomy of a Wound

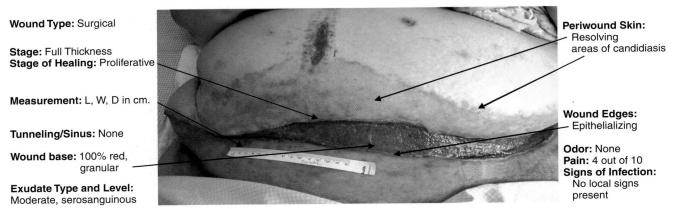

Wound Type: Surgical

Stage: Full Thickness
Stage of Healing: Proliferative

Measurement: L, W, D in cm.

Tunneling/Sinus: None

Wound base: 100% red, granular

Exudate Type and Level: Moderate, serosanguinous

Periwound Skin: Resolving areas of candidiasis

Wound Edges: Epithelializing

Odor: None
Pain: 4 out of 10
Signs of Infection: No local signs present

PLATE 23 Anatomy of a wound.

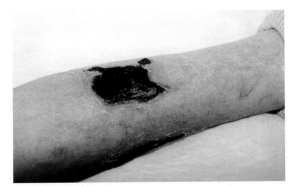

PLATE 24 Arterial ulcer with dry, stable eschar covering. Note dry condition of leg.

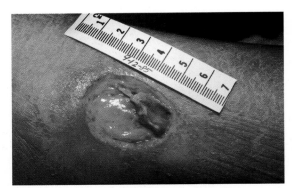

PLATE 25 Arterial ulcer with loose and adherent yellow slough present in wound bed. Mild erythema present along left lateral edge.

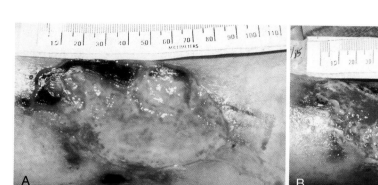

PLATE 26 **A,** Highly exudative venous ulcer with slough present in wound bed and eschar present along superior aspect. **B,** After 1 week of hydrocolloids and compression therapy, autolysis has occurred, and venous ulcer has presence of granulation tissue. Amount of slough and eschar is reduced; remaining eschar is softened.

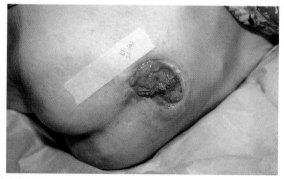

PLATE 27 Stage III pressure ulcer with excess granulation tissue.

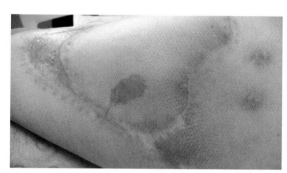

PLATE 28 Right trochanter Stage I pressure ulcer at surgical flap site.

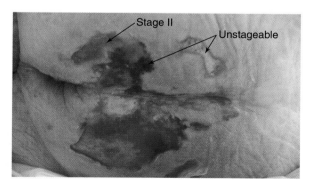

PLATE 29 Sacral pressure ulcer, multiple stages of depth (note classic butterfly shape with additional chemical skin damage from incontinence).

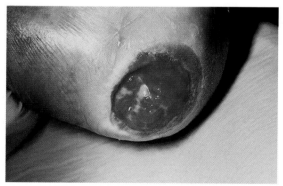

PLATE 30 Stage III pressure ulcer. (From Cain JE: *Mosby's PDQ for wound care,* St. Louis, 2009, Mosby/Elsevier.)

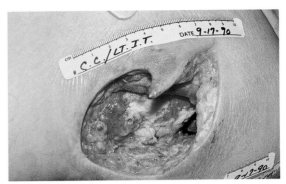

PLATE 31 Left ischial tuberosity, Stage IV pressure ulcer.

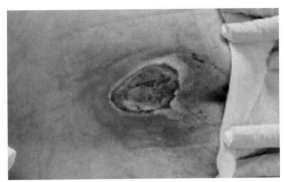

PLATE 32 Sacral pressure ulcer with yellow nonadherent nonviable wound base. Periwound skin shows signs of suspected deep tissue injury (sDTI).

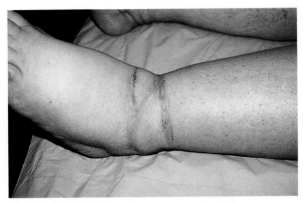

PLATE 33 Pressure ulcer from a poorly fitting compression stocking. (From Morison M et al: *Chronic wound care: a problem-based learning approach,* London, 2004, Mosby, Ltd.)

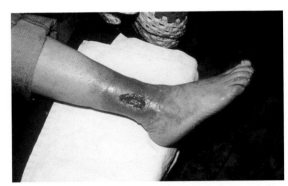

PLATE 34 Typical appearance and location of venous ulcer. Surrounding skin has been moisturized to eliminate dry skin. Note hemosiderin staining of surrounding skin and ruddy red color of wound bed.

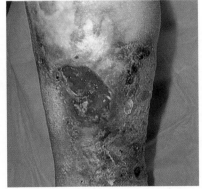

PLATE 35 Atrophie blanche dermal sclerosis with dilated abnormal vasculature and ivory white plaques on the lower extremity and hemosiderin borders.

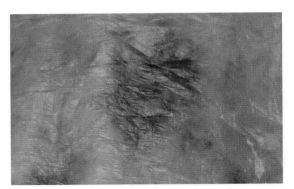

PLATE 36 Senile purpura. Red purpura. Purple nonblanchable discoloration >0.5 cm in diameter. Causes are intravascular defects, infection.

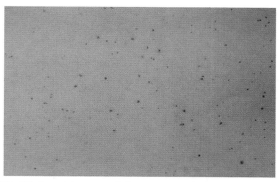

PLATE 37 Petechiae on abdomen. Petechiae red–purple non-blanchable discoloration <0.5 cm in diameter. Causes are intravascular defects, infection.

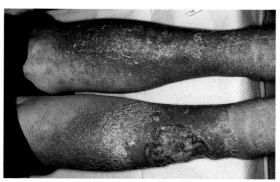

PLATE 38 Venous dermatitis of lower leg. Note extensive hemosiderin staining and lipodermatosclerosis.

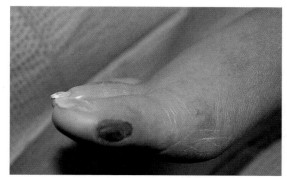

PLATE 39 Arterial ulcer with necrotic base and halo of periwound erythema.

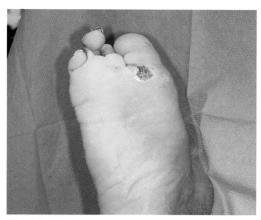

PLATE 40 Diabetic foot ulcer. Charcot foot with neuropathic plantar ulcer on the first metatarsal head. Note callus and foot and toe deformities. (Courtesy of J. Lebretton and V. Driver.)

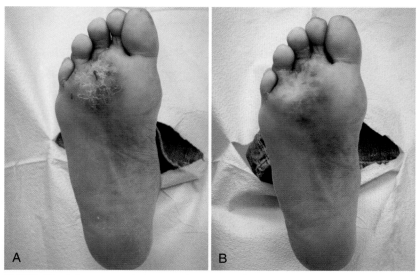

PLATE 41 Callus removal. **A,** Hyperkeratotic callus causing increased plantar pressure. **B,** After rotary debridement, the surface is smooth and conducive to pressure redistribution. (Courtesy of J. Lebretton and V. Driver.)

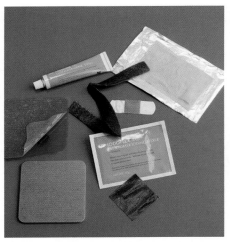

PLATE 42 Antimicrobial dressings are available in a variety of formulations. (Courtesy of Bonnie Sue Rolstad.)

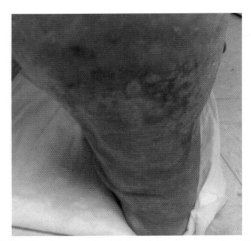

PLATE 43 Silver staining. Epithelialized venous insufficiency ulcer on the periwound aspect of the lower leg. Note periwound staining secondary to the use of silver dressings. (Courtesy of Julie Freyberg.)

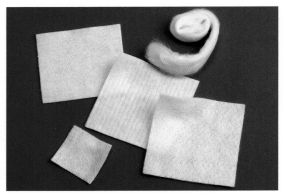

PLATE 44 Variety of alginate dressings. (Courtesy of Bonnie Sue Rolstad.)

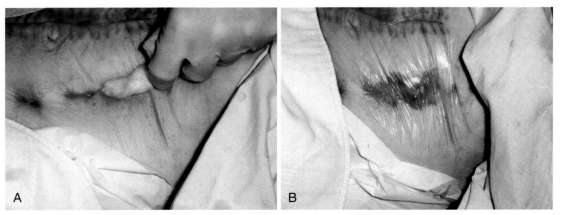

PLATE 45 A, Alginate dressing applied to fill dead space and absorb exudate in a full-thickness abdominal wound. **B,** Alginate dressing secured with a secondary transparent dressing. Note that 2 days later at the scheduled dressing change, the alginate had formed an expected gel-like appearance as the wound fluid was absorbed. The periwound skin has been protected with a liquid skin barrier.

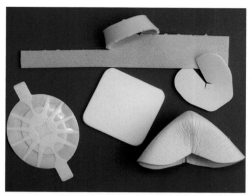

PLATE 46 Variety of foam dressings. (Courtesy of Bonnie Sue Rolstad.)

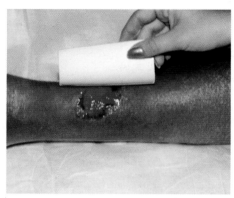

PLATE 47 Application of foam dressing to venous ulcer by family member.

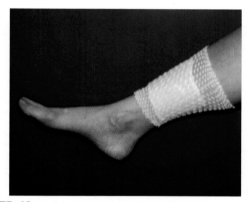

PLATE 48 Foam dressing secured with stretch-net nonadherent secondary dressing.

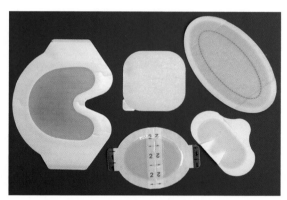

PLATE 49 Variety of sizes and shapes of hydrocolloid dressings. (Courtesy of Bonnie Sue Rolstad.)

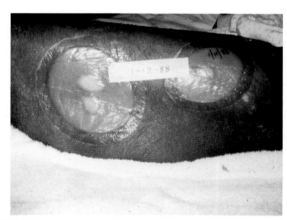

PLATE 50 Hydrocolloid dressing prior to removal. Note the gel developing under the dressing which is expected as the wound exudate is absorbed by the hydrocolloid.

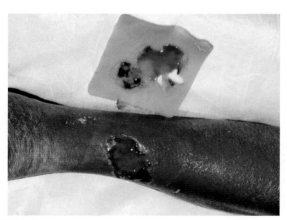

PLATE 51 Hydrocolloid dressing after removal from a venous ulcer. Purulent appearing exudate is present on the dressing and wound. This is expected with autolysis under a hydrocolloid dressing and should not be misinterpreted as evidence of infection. Upon cleansing, the wound bed is clean and granular.

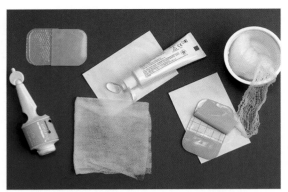

PLATE 52 Variety of hydrogel dressings. (Courtesy of Bonnie Sue Rolstad.)

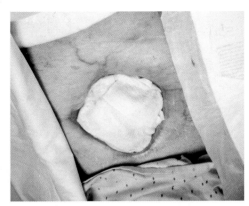

PLATE 53 Hydrogel-impregnated gauze used to maintain a moist wound bed and fill dead space in this deep abdominal wound with undermining present.

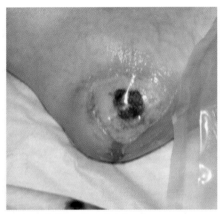

PLATE 54 Hydrogel sheet dressing in place over a granular wound bed on foot ulceration. This dressing overlaps onto intact periwound skin, which is contraindicated with this particular brand of hydrogel dressing because of the risk of periwound maceration.

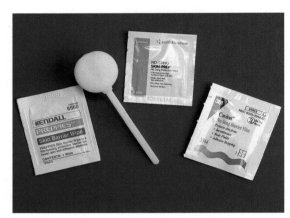

PLATE 55 Liquid skin barrier (skin sealant). (Courtesy of Bonnie Sue Rolstad.)

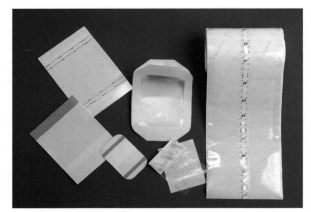

PLATE 56 Variety of transparent film dressings. (Courtesy of Bonnie Sue Rolstad.)

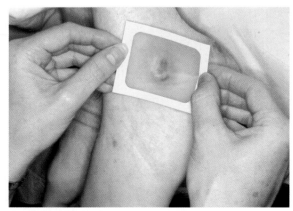

PLATE 57 Application of a transparent dressing by a family member in the home setting.

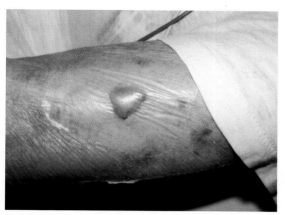

PLATE 58 Transparent dressing prior to removal. Note collection of fluid under the dressing, which is to be expected as autolysis occurs.

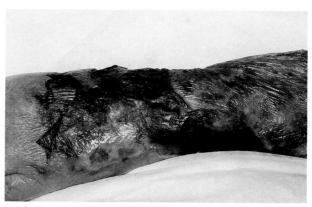

PLATE 59 Necrotizing fasciitis affecting left lower arm and extending distally onto dorsal surface of hand. Note significant amount of eschar distributed over entire surface of lower arm and edema in dorsal surface of hand. (From Bolognia JL et al: *Dermatology,* ed 2, Edinburgh, 2008, Mosby/Elsevier.)

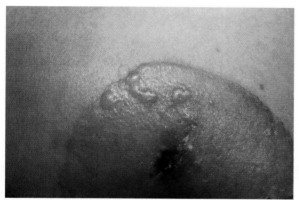

PLATE 60 Brown recluse spider bite. Note central necrosis surrounded by purplish area and blisters. (From Hockenberry M, Wilson D: *Wong's essentials of pediatric nursing,* ed 8, St. Louis, 2009, Mosby/Elsevier.)

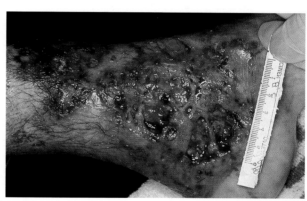

PLATE 61 Classical ulceration form of pyoderma gangrenosum. Note violaceous (purple) color of skin surrounding ulceration.

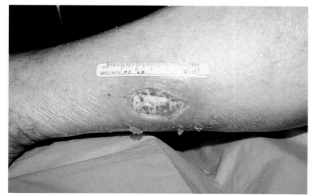

PLATE 62 Vasculitic ulcer that developed in patient with rheumatoid arthritis. Wound bed has attached dry slough present, and surrounding skin is slightly erythematous.

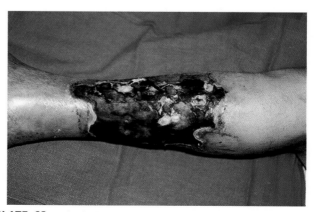

PLATE 63 Calciphylaxis in patient with end-stage renal disease. Appearance can be similar to pyoderma gangrenosum with severe pain, and eschar or loose slough in the wound bed. (From Morison M et al: *Chronic wound care: a problem-based learning approach,* London, 2004, Mosby, Ltd.)

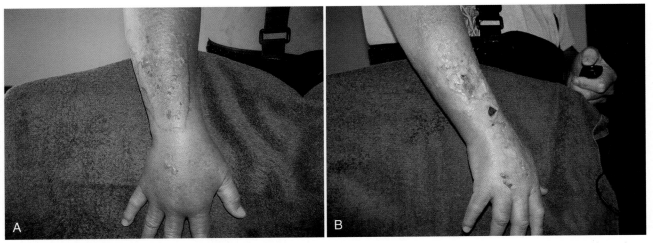

PLATE 64 Untreated doxorubicin (Adriamycin) extravasation of the dorsum of the hand, with tissue damage extending throughout his forearm. **A,** Swelling, redness, and blistering apparent 3 days after the extravasation occurred. **B,** Early stages of tissue necrosis appearing 1 month later. (Copyright © 2008 by Lisa Schulmeister. Reprinted with permission.)

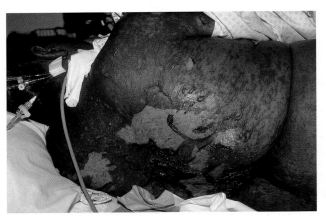

PLATE 65 Clinical features of toxic epidermal necrosis (TEN) apparent with detachment of large sheets of epidermis (>30% of body surface area), leading to extensive areas of denudement. A few intact bullae are still present. Wrinkling and lateral sliding of skin near blisters (positive Nikolsky sign) are apparent. (From Bolognia JL et al: *Dermatology*, ed 2, Edinburgh, 2008, Mosby/Elsevier.)

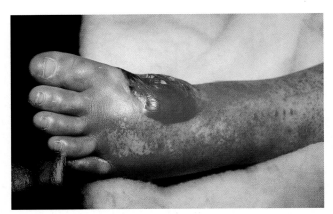

PLATE 66 Graft-versus-host disease (GVHD) in a patient after allogenic bone marrow transplantation. Note macular–papular rash is barely distinguishable and has become confluent. Edema, erythema, and bulla formation are present.

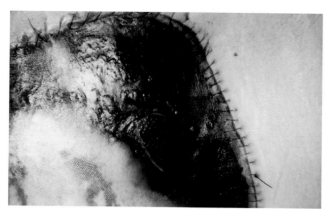

PLATE 67 Edges of incision approximated with sutures. This photograph illustrates the importance of documenting not only the condition of the incision but also the condition of the periwound skin.

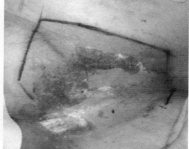

PLATE 68 Abdomen of obese patient with skin breakdown under pannus due to pressure and moisture. (Courtesy of Judith L. Gates.)

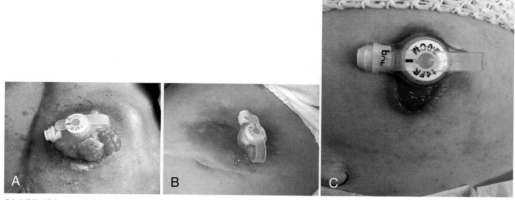

PLATE 69 Complications at the site of the gastrostomy button. **A,** Hyperplasia/hypergranulation. **B,** Cellulitis. **C,** Dehiscence. (Courtesy of Teri Crawley Coha.)

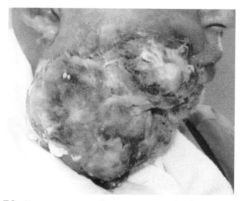

PLATE 70 Cutaneous malignant wound (fungating wound) involving the right side of the face and neck. (From Morison M et al: *Chronic wound care: a problem-based learning approach*, London, 2004, Mosby, Ltd.)

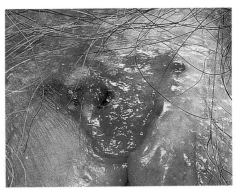

PLATE 71 Basal cell carcinoma may be a primary lesion anywhere on the body. Existing chronic wounds of various etiologies may convert to malignant cutaneous wounds also known as *Marjolin's ulcer.* (From Habif T, Campbell M, Chapman S et al: *Skin disease: diagnosis and treatment*, ed 2, London, 2005, Mosby.)

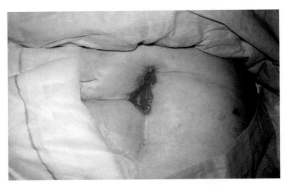

PLATE 72 Patient with enterocutaneous fistula with irregular surrounding skin surfaces and depression along fistula–skin junction at interior aspect and upper left aspect.

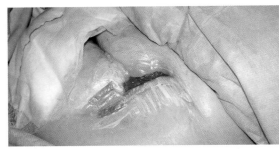

PLATE 73 Tapered layers of solid-wafer skin barrier used to help level skin depression at inferior aspect. Skin barrier paste has been applied to surrounding wound margins and in all three depressions (over skin barrier wafer wedges) to level and protect the skin from effluent. Cement has been painted onto adhesive field (over paste and wedges) to increase adhesion.

Skin Inspection and Monitoring

Skin *inspection* involves data collection related to skin changes based on visual observation. A complete skin inspection must be completed by trained staff upon admission (for baseline data) and daily. It is important to inspect all of the skin from head to toe (WOCN, 2010). An adequate skin inspection requires the removal of garments (including shoes and stockings) and effective positioning for optimal visualization. Staff conducting the inspection will need to gently spread skin folds (including the buttocks), check between the toes, and remove or reposition medical devices to inspect for pressure-related skin damage from devices such as oxygen tubing, nasogastric tubes, urinary tubing, drainage tubing, therapeutic stockings, and splints. Staff performing the skin inspection should be expected to report the overall skin condition, such as change in skin condition (e.g., intact, broken, denuded), skin color (e.g., red, dusky), texture (e.g., pinpoint macular–papular rash, dry skin), and wounds. These findings then are communicated to a registered nurse or a physician for interpretation and additional information collected as needed to further describe and understand the present condition.

The skin and wound condition should be monitored on a routine and regular basis as defined by the facility policy and the severity of the condition. *Monitoring* allows the staff to keep track or "watch" for changes that deviate from the baseline data. For example, 3 days after admission, a reddened area is identified through routine monitoring, while the baseline assessment and documention indicated no redness upon admission. The new finding should prompt further assessment to identify etiology so that modifications to the plan of care can be implemented. Part of the plan of care will include continued monitoring and perhaps more frequent repositioning.

When dressings are in place and do not require changing, the dressing should be monitored for intactness and the surrounding skin inspected for the presence or absence of discoloration (erythema, bruising), rash, break in skin integrity, and pain (van Rijswijk and Lyder, 2005). Narrative documentation can be as simple as "dressing dry and intact, surrounding skin within defined limits," or a flow chart can be used (Appendix B).

Therefore, monitoring can occur independent of dressing change. However, if the dressing is leaking or new observations are made (swelling, pain, erythema), the dressing should be removed and a thorough wound assessment obtained. Monitoring usually occurs more frequently than an assessment or head-to-toe skin inspection, for example, every 8 hours in the acute care setting or every day in the long-term care setting. To conserve staff time and patient energy, monitoring and skin inspection can be conducted at the same time that other routine cares are provided (Table 6-1).

TABLE 6-1	Routine Activities Coordinated with Skin Inspection
Routine Activity	**Skin Inspection Site**
Oxygen application	Back of ears and bridge of nose
Retaping or securing nasogastric tube	Nares
Tracheotomy care	Neck (under ties or strap)
Listening to lung sounds	Occiput, spinous process, scapula, coccyx, and sacrum
Listening to bowel sounds	Between and under skin folds of pannus and groin
Placing pillows under calves	Feet, heels, toes
Application or removal of antiembolism stockings or splints	Feet, heels, toes
Intravenous site care	Elbows and arms
Transferring in or out of chair	Coccyx and sacrum
Repositioning side to side	Feet, heels, toes, coccyx, sacrum, occiput, scapula, spinous process, trochanter

Skin Assessment

The standard of care is to conduct a routine and systematic skin assessment of all patients upon admission. Skin assessment parameters and deviations from normal are listed in Table 6-2. Examples and descriptions of lesions are presented in Chapter 5 (see Table 5-1 and Plates 6 and 7).

Subsequent skin assessments should be performed routinely. Frequency of reassessment is based on baseline data, care setting, and risk for skin breakdown. For example, patients require daily skin assessments when they (1) are at increased risk for skin breakdown, (2) have impaired skin integrity, or (3) are in an acute care or long-term acute care setting.

Skin assessments require good lighting for optimal visualization. Alterations including dry skin or xerosis should be noted. Skin palpation is used to assess skin temperature and texture in all patients but is of particular importance when assessing darkly pigmented skin. Skin with deviations from normal (e.g., firm to touch, boggy, pain, itching, warmth, coolness) should be compared with the adjacent skin or contralateral body part and documented (NPUAP and EPUAP, 2009).

Darker Skin Tones. Health care in the United States and Europe has experienced a shift in racial and ethnic demographics, with black and Latino/Hispanic populations being the fastest growing among patients 85 years and older (ONS 2002; Salcido, 2002). Therefore accurate assessment of patients with darker skin pigmentation is an essential skill for all health care providers, and particularly wound care providers. The unique characteristics of darker versus lighter pigmented skin are summarized in

TABLE 6-2	Skin Assessment Parameters: Findings and Interpretation		
Parameter	**Technique and Tips**	**Findings**	**Interpretation**
Color	Conduct inspection in good light; artificial light often distorts colors and masks jaundice Ask patients/family if they have noticed any skin color changes	Pallor	Anemia, decreased blood flow, or arterial insufficiency Advanced lung disease Congestive heart failure Anemia
		Central cyanosis (lips, oral mucosa or tongue)	Venous obstruction
		Yellow	Jaundice in sclera and skin with liver disease or excessive hemolysis of red blood cells
		Brown discoloration in lower extremities	Hemosiderin staining from venous insufficiency
		Redness	Erythema, an inflammatory response or pressure ulcer
Moisture	Visual inspection in good light	Dry skin	Xerosis Hypothyroidism
		Dermatitis or macular–papular rash in skin folds, perineum, thighs, groin	Intertrigo, tinea or psoriasis
Temperature	Palpate using the back of fingers Infrared thermography	Generalized increased warmth	Fever Hyperthyroidism
		Local increased warmth	Inflammation
		Coolness	Hypothyroidism or poor vascularization
Olfaction	Note odor	Present	Bacteria, metabolic acidosis, hygiene issues
Texture	Palpate using back of fingers	Roughness	Hypothyroidism
Turgor	Pinch fold of skin and note speed with which it returns (normally, skin returns quickly to baseline state)	Decreased turgor	Dehydration
Lesions	Observe any lesions of the skin, noting characteristics such as type, location, color, distribution, arrangement	Primary or secondary skin lesions (macule, papule, pustule)	See Plates 6 and 7 and Chapter 5
Skin injury	Skin should be intact If skin is open, assess for type of injury	Denuded	Chemical damage, fecal incontinence
		Ulcerated	Unrelieved pressure
		Excoriated	Pruritus, xerosis
Nails (see Chapter 15 for nail abnormalities)	Inspect and palpate fingernails and toenails Note color, shape, and presence of lesions	Clubbing of the fingers	Lung problems
		Onycholysis	Painless separation of nails from nail bed beginning distally
Hair	Inspect and palpate Note quantity, distribution, texture	Alopecia	Hair loss (diffuse)
		Hirsutism	Excessive body hair (may be patchy or total)

Box 3-1. Teaching points and unique considerations when assessing darkly pigmented skin are provided in Checklist 6-1 (Bennett, 1995).

Unfortunately, detection and accurate identification of erythema and Stage I pressure ulcers with standard visual inspection are unreliable in persons with darkly pigmented skin (Bates-Jensen et al, 2009; Rosen et al, 2006; WOCN Society, 2010). This inability to detect and diagnose erythema in people with highly pigmented skin is evidenced by the incongruity between the prevalence of Stage I pressure ulcers in Caucasians (48%) versus African Americans (20%) (Baumgarten et al, 2004). Another study found that 32% of pressure ulcers detected in Caucasian residents were Stage I, whereas no Stage I pressure ulcers were detected in African American residents (Rosen et al, 2006).

CHECKLIST 6-1

Assessing Pressure Ulcers on Darkly Pigmented Skin

✓ Color remains unchanged when pressure is applied.

✓ Color changes occur at site of pressure which differ from the patient's usual skin color.

✓ Circumscribed area of intact skin may be warm to touch. As tissue changes color, intact skin will feel cool to touch. Note gloves may diminish sensitivity to changes in skin temperature.

✓ If patient previously had a pressure ulcer, that area of skin may be lighter than original color.

✓ Localized area of skin may be purple/blue or violet (eggplant) instead of red.

✓ Localized heat (inflammation) is detected by making comparisons to surrounding skin. Localized area of warmth eventually will be replaced by area of coolness, which is a sign of tissue devitalization.

✓ Edema (nonpitting swelling) may occur with induration and may appear taut and shiny.

✓ Patient complains of discomfort at a site that is predisposed to pressure ulcer development.

CHECKLIST 6-2

Physical Assessment Parameters

✓ Wound etiology and differential diagnosis

✓ Duration of wound

✓ Cofactors that impede healing:

• Comorbid conditions (malignancy; diabetes; cardiac, respiratory, renal issues)

• Medications (corticosteroids, cancer medications, immunosuppressants)

• Host infection

• Pressure ulcer risk factors

• Decreased oxygenation and tissue perfusion

• Alteration in nutrition and hydration

• Psychosocial barriers; family support; impaired access to appropriate resources, financial limitations

• Past therapies (e.g., radiation near the site of the wound)

A handheld dermal phase meter measuring subepidermal moisture has been studied in an attempt to identify early pressure ulcer damage (Bates-Jensen et al, 2009). Findings from a descriptive cohort study of 66 nursing home residents showed that subepidermal moisture provided a more accurate method of detecting early pressure ulcer damage than did visual assessment. If these findings are supported in larger studies, subepidermal moisture may emerge to be a useful clinical technique for detecting early damage in persons with darker skin tones.

Focused Physical Assessment

Healing is a phenomenon composed of multiple processes (see Chapter 4), each of which must function properly and sequentially. Whereas all patients require a physical assessment, the patient with a wound requires particular attention to systemic, psychosocial, and local factors that affect wound healing. A wound specialist is specifically educated to conduct this type of focused physical assessment and to interpret the results. The focused physical assessment should be obtained upon admission and with a change of condition. Components of a wound focused physical assessment are listed in Checklist 6-2.

Etiology and Differential Diagnosis. Based on the wound-focused physical assessment, a differential diagnosis and likely etiology of the wound will be determined, which will drive intervention choices and treatment strategies. The completed physical assessment should help to exclude many possible etiologies

for the wound but also will exclude treatment options. For example, compression is a critical intervention for successful management of the patient with venous insufficiency, but compression is contraindicated in the presence of arterial disease (see Chapter 11). Offloading is needed for management of a pressure ulcer (see Chapters 8 and 9), and glucose must be managed when the patient has diabetes (see Chapter 14). Wound etiology will also provide clues regarding the type of healing to anticipate. For example, a venous ulcer generally has little depth, so it often heals by epithelialization rather than wound contraction, which is in contrast to the deeper Stage III or IV pressure ulcer, which requires contraction for healing to occur. Measuring wound depth in the pressure ulcer clearly is an important piece of information but may be of little relevance in venous ulcers. Various types of skin damage are discussed in Chapter 5 and throughout this text. Interpretation of the data gathered through the focused physical assessment will guide the plan of care so that wound etiology and existing cofactors can be addressed.

Duration of Wound and Critical Cofactors that Impair Healing. A 4-week-old pressure ulcer that has not improved suggests the presence of cofactors that have not been adequately addressed, such as unresolved pressure, malnutrition, osteomyelitis, critical colonization, squamous cell cancer, or infection. Guidelines for pressure ulcers and arterial wounds recommend consideration of referral and biopsy for wounds that are unresponsive to 2 to 4 weeks of appropriate therapies (WOCN Society 2002, 2003).

Given a clear understanding of healing, these wounds must be considered out of synchronization and require reevaluation to identify factors that impede healing. Factors that impede healing are described in chapters throughout the text and listed in Checklist 6-2. Approaches used to assess systemic cofactors that affect wound healing along with the chapters that describe them in detail are listed in Table 6-3.

Wound Assessment

Wound assessment is the collection of subjective data that characterize the status of the wound specifically as well as the periwound skin (see Plate 23). Parameters that compose a wound assessment are listed in Checklist 6-3 and described in this section. Conducting a wound assessment is a skill and requires precision and appropriate use of unique terms; use of appropriate terms is critically important. Therefore competency-based education for wound assessment is essential. Prior to assessment, the wound must be cleansed of loose debris, particulate matter, and dressing residue so that the normal architecture and color of the wound bed and surrounding skin can be fully appreciated.

Anatomic Location. The anatomic location of the wound is important to record using proper terminology that will also provide clues about the etiology. Anatomic locations such as the sacrum and the coccyx must be clearly delineated (Figure 6-1). The location of a wound on the plantar surface of the foot can be accurately specified by terms such as metatarsal head. Anatomic location will also convey plan of care needs. For example, a wound on the ischial tuberosity should prompt caregivers to explore the patient's sitting surface. A typical venous ulcer commonly appears on the medial aspect of the lower leg and will require compression. A patient with diabetes and a plantar surface foot ulcer typically has neuropathy and will need adequate blood glucose control and offloading.

Extent of Tissue Involvement. The extent of tissue damage guides the selection of appropriate interventions to restore tissue integrity; it also provides some information about the length of time required for the healing process. Extent of tissue involvement can be described as partial thickness or full thickness, or "staged" if indicated. Numerous staging and classification systems exist that are primarily based on wound etiology and therefore are precise and descriptive for that type of wound.

Partial Thickness and Full Thickness. A partial-thickness wound is confined to the skin layers; damage does not penetrate below the dermis and may be limited to the epidermal layers only. These wounds heal primarily by reepithelialization (see Table 4-1 and Plate 1). A full-thickness wound indicates that the epidermis and dermis have been damaged into the subcutaneous tissue or beyond; tissue loss extends below the dermis (see Table 4-2 and Plates 2–5). Wound repair will occur by neovascularization, fibroplasia, contraction, and then epithelial migration from the wound edges. Partial thickness and full thickness can be used to describe most wounds but are not precise terms for specific types of tissue loss and depths of the wound. For example, a full-thickness wound can expose subcutaneous tissue, or it may extend to bone.

Classification Systems. Accurate classification requires knowledge of the anatomy of skin and deeper tissue layers, the ability to recognize these tissues, and the ability to differentiate between them. Classification systems for vascular and diabetic wounds assign a "grade" to the wound based on levels of tissue involvement, history of previous ulceration, presence of bony deformity, presence and severity of ischemia, and presence and severity of infection (Crawford and Fields-Varnado, 2004). Careful evaluation of the wound bed facilitates accurate classification, a complex skill that can take time to develop. Additional classification systems include skin tears (see Chapter 5), pressure ulcers (see Chapter 7), vascular wounds (see Chapter 11), diabetic wounds (see Chapter 14), and burns (see Chapter 32). However, as with all classification systems, these additional classification systems tell only a small part of the story and

TABLE 6-3	Assessment of Cofactors	
Cofactor	**Diagnostic Test**	**Chapter**
Tissue oxygenation	Transcutaneous oxygen	28
Bacterial load	Culture	16
	Biopsy	
Circulation	Ankle–brachial index	14
	Toe–brachial index	
Nutrition	Weight	27
	Body mass index	
	Albumin	
	Prealbumin	
	Total lymphocyte count	
Glycemic control	Blood glucose, hemoglobin A_{1c}	14

CHECKLIST 6-3
Wound Assessment Parameters

✓ Anatomic location of wound
✓ Extent of tissue loss (i.e., stage)
✓ Characteristics of wound base
✓ Type of tissue
✓ Percentage of wound containing each type of tissue observed
✓ Dimensions of wound in cm (length, width, depth, tunneling, undermining)
✓ Exudate (amount, type)
✓ Odor
✓ Wound edges
✓ Periwound skin
✓ Presence or absence of local signs of infection
✓ Wound pain

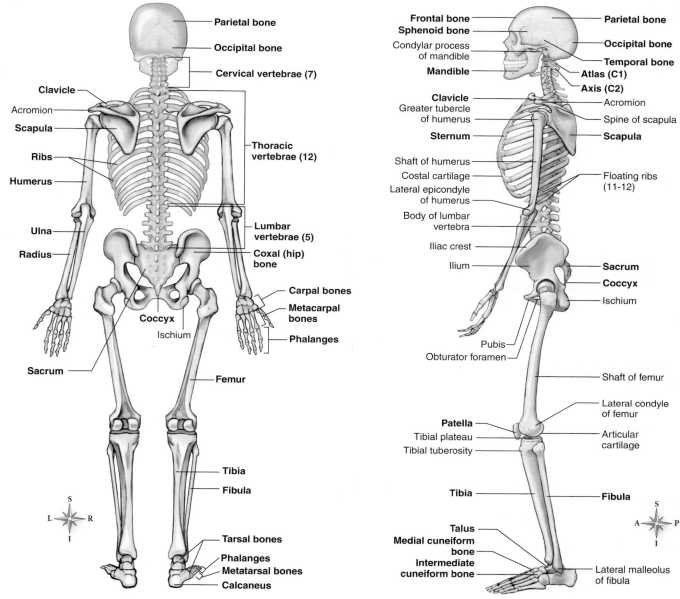

FIGURE 6-1 Bony structures of human body; note delineation of sacrum and coccyx. (From Patton KT, Thibodeau GA: *Anatomy and physiology,* ed 7, St Louis 2010, Mosby.)

therefore should be used in conjunction with additional wound descriptors.

Type of Tissue in Wound Base. The amount and type of tissue in the wound bed provide insight into the severity and duration of the wound, the extent to which the wound is progressing toward healing, and the effectiveness of current interventions. Healing wounds are characterized by increasing amounts of viable tissue (e.g., granulation tissue) and decreasing amounts of nonviable tissue (e.g., eschar or slough). When the wound bed contains a combination of tissue types, each type of tissue should be described in percentages. For example "50% of the wound bed contains eschar and 50% contains granulation tissue." Terms used to describe tissue and the wound bed as well as other

descriptions used for wound assessment are listed in Table 6-4 and the glossary.

Viable Tissue. Viable tissue is healthy tissue, such as granulation, epithelialization, muscle, or subcutaneous tissue. Healthy granulation tissue is characteristically described as beefy, red, moist, and cobblestone-like or berry-like in appearance (see Plate 3). New epithelial tissue is light pink and dry (see Plate 1). Deviations from an optimal state should be described carefully and correlated with conditions that may account for the abnormality, such as the patient's fluid status, serum hemoglobin level, nutrition, or colonization.

Nonviable Tissue. Color, texture, moisture, and adherence of necrotic tissue to the wound bed should be noted. As with viable tissue, nonviable tissue can provide

TABLE 6-4	Wound Bed Descriptors
Necrotic, nonviable, or devitalized	Tissue that has died and therefore has lost its physical properties and biologic activity
Eschar	Black or brown necrotic, devitalized tissue; tissue can be loose or firmly adherent; hard, soft, or boggy
Slough	Soft, moist, avascular (necrotic/ devitalized) tissue; may be white, yellow, tan, or green; may be loose or firmly adherent
Scab	Crust of hardened blood and serum over the wound
Granulation tissue	Pink/red moist tissue composed of new blood vessels, connective tissue, fibroblasts, and inflammatory cells fills an open wound when it starts to heal; typically appears deep pink or red; surface is granular, berry-like, or cobblestone
Clean, nongranulating	Absence of granulation wound; surface appears smooth and red but not granular, and berry-like or cobblestone
Epithelial	Regenerated epidermis across the wound surface; pink and dry

information related to wound status. The presence of nonviable tissue (or necrotic tissue) in the wound often is associated with altered tissue oxygenation, wound desiccation, or increased bacterial burden. In addition, a wound initially described as dry adherent eschar will progress to moist softening brown necrotic tissue that is lifting, loosening, or demarcating from the wound base. It then progresses to yellow slough, which can be firm and adherent or moist and stringy. This transformation in the color, moisture, and texture of nonviable tissue is evidence that the natural autolysis process is occurring as desired. This process of autolysis is facilitated by appropriate topical care and a moist wound environment. Chapters 17 and 18 provide details of the significance and process for debridement and moist wound healing.

Tissue Color. A myriad of color often can be found in the wound bed: red, pink, yellow, tan, black, green, etc. It is helpful to record the color of the tissue in the wound bed because the color gives a general indication of healing status. For example, if the wound bed is red and granulation tissue is present, these are considered a positive sign that conditions for healing are right. Eschar is black (see Plate 24); as it softens (thus moving closer to being debrided through autolysis), the color will transition to yellow (see Plate 25) or yellow tan, then small red islets develop in the wound bed among the nonviable yellow slough. More granulation tissue is revealed as the wound progresses (see Plates 26a and 26b).

Color can be used to differentiate normal structures from the wound bed. However, color alone does not sufficiently describe viable or nonviable tissue and trivializes the complexities of the healing process. For example, nonviable tissue could be yellow however, viable tendon is also yellow. A wound base may be red but with an unhealthy smooth surface (lacking the cobblestone or berry-like appearance) in which case the wound should be described as "clean, nongranulating" (see Plate 5A). In contrast, healthy granulation tissue will have a red color with a cobblestone appearance as shown in Plate 5b. A pale red color can be indicative of anemia or hypoxia. Hypergranulation tissue is also red or pink in color but is not considered healthy. Hypergranulation tissue is the overproduction of granulation tissue generally caused by excess moisture (see Plate 27).

Wound Size. Several approaches to wound measurement are described in the literature, each with their own advantages and disadvantages and some more appropriate for research than the clinical setting. These techniques have been summarized in Table 6-5. For massive tissue loss, calculation of the percentage of body surface area wounded with the Lund-Browder Chart is the most common and realistic measure (see Chapter 32, Figure 32-2).

Linear two-dimensional (length and width) and three-dimensional (length, width, and depth) measurement techniques using disposable plastic/acetate or paper rulers are most common in the clinical setting. Three-dimensional measurements are required with full-thickness wounds because, by definition, full-thickness wounds are below the dermis and therefore should have measurable depth. Measurements should be recorded in centimeters or millimeters and include the extent and location of undermining and tunneling when present. From these dimensions, the area of the wound can be estimated by multiplying length by width by depth. To strengthen the accuracy of wound measurement, a uniform approach among staff should be used. This can be facilitated by consistent patient positioning and identifying specific wound landmarks from which to align the measuring instrument (NPUAP and EPUAP, 2009). Documentation requirements for consistency should be described in policies, procedures, and flow sheets.

Unfortunately, numerous potential reliability problems exist when measuring a wound. Because the perimeter of open wounds often is irregular, it can be difficult to determine the best position on the wound surface from which to obtain the readings (Langemo et al, 2008). Even defining the edge of the wound from which measurements should be taken will vary among providers and will introduce inconsistencies in dimensions. In addition, the rigor with which the measurement is obtained influences the results (Langemo et al, 2008). However, serial

TABLE 6-5	Methods of Wound Measurement
Measurement Methods	**Description**
Ruler-based linear method	Disposable, three-dimensional. Should include length, width, and depth; and extent and location of undermining and tunneling with consistent approach. Estimated wound area = length × width × depth.
Kundin Wound Gauge	Disposable, three-dimensional, plastic-coated paper wound gauge. Rarely used in clinical practice.
Computerized wound-measurement through digital photography	Two-dimensional, noncontact method requires uploading to computer software program.
Planimetry	Two-dimensional technique where wound is traced onto a transparency and a metric grid used to count the number of square centimeters within the wound perimeter. High reliability except when estimating partial squares.
Wound tracings	Two-dimensional technique where wound is traced, providing a pattern against which subsequent tracings can be compared.
Stereophotogrammetry	Two-dimensional. Combines video camera and software to videotape, download onto computer, and trace with a mouse; software calculates measurement. High reliability.
Wound molds	Three-dimensional. Foam or alginate substance placed into wound and retained for serial reviews. Impractical in clinical settings.
Fluid instillation	Fluid instilled into the wound, extracted, and measured. Difficult to fill wound completely. Impractical in clinical settings.
Structured light	Three-dimensional. Wound is illuminated with set of parallel lights via projector. Image is picked up by camera connected to computer. Not applicable for very large or undermining wounds. Impractical in clinical settings.

measurements repeated over time can at least be used to reveal a trend in the presence or absence of healing in the wound.

As with each wound assessment parameter, wound size should be interpreted within the context of the other parameters enumerated in Checklist 6-3. For example, as an eschar-covered ulcer undergoes autolysis, the percent of eschar will decrease, and consequently wound dimensions will predictably increase. Looking only at wound dimensions as an assessment parameter may lead to misinterpretation of the increase as an indication of delayed or absent wound healing. However, because wound dimensions are changing at the same time that the type and volume of tissue in the wound bed are evolving from eschar to slough to granulation tissue, the increase in size that accompanies the removal of nonviable tissue is considered desirable and indicative of a positive trend in the wound healing process.

Measuring Length, Width, and Depth. Length is measured by placing the ruler at the point of greatest length (or head to toe). Width is measured by placing the ruler at the point of greatest width (or side to side) (Figure 6-2) (Bryant et al, 2001; Doughty, 2004; Langemo et al, 2008). The most common method of obtaining wound depth is by inserting a cotton-tipped applicator into the wound bed at the greatest depth and placing a mark on the applicator at the level of the skin (Figure 6-3). This mark may simply be the examiner's thumb and index finger, but an ink mark applied to the applicator at skin level should provide more accuracy in the measurement. The cotton-tipped applicator then is

held against a metric ruler to determine the depth of the wound. Unfortunately, this technique is inherently imprecise (particularly with an irregularly shaped wound bed), but it does provide a method of at least detecting a trend.

Measuring Tunneling and Undermining. The terms *tunnel* and *sinus tract* are often used interchangeably. A tunnel is a channel that extends from any part of the

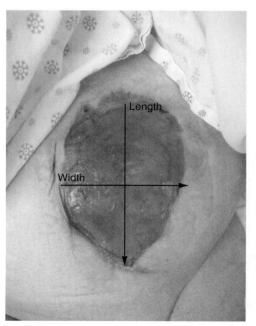

FIGURE 6-2 Measuring wound length and width.

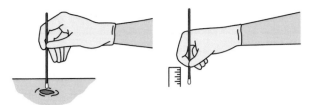

FIGURE 6-3 Measuring wound depth.

wound through subcutaneous tissue or muscle (Figure 6-4). Undermining is tissue destruction that occurs under intact skin around the wound perimeter. Pressure ulcers that have been subjected to shear often are first seen with undermining. Undermining and tunneling can be documented by measuring depth and noting the location using the face of the clock as a model. The superior aspect of the wound (12 o'clock position) points toward the patient's head, whereas the inferior aspect of the wound (6 o'clock position) points toward the patient's feet. Examples are shown in Figures 6-4 and 6-5.

Wound Shape. Terms used to describe the shape of the wound includes adjectives such as round, oval, triangular, irregular, and butterfly shaped. Documenting the shape of the wound provides not only a more accurate clinical description but also clues to wound etiology. For example, device-related pressure ulcers will be apparent because they will replicate the shape of the device, such as tubing, telemetry cable, or needle cap. Similarly, acute onset of a butterfly-shaped area of erythema over the upper buttocks and coccyx is consistent with unrelieved pressure while the patient is in the supine position.

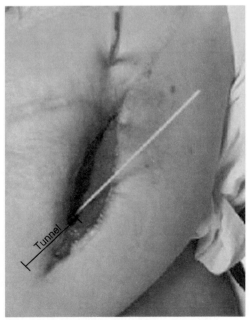

FIGURE 6-4 Wound tunneling. Tunneling is present in this abdominal wound at the 7 o'clock position and measures 2 cm in length. Tunnel and sinus tract are often used interchangeably.

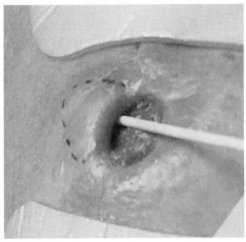

FIGURE 6-5 Undermining extends 2 cm from 7 to 11 o'clock.

Wound Exudate. The characteristics of wound exudate should be assessed in terms of volume (none, light, moderate, or heavy) and type (clear, serosanguineous, sanguinous, purulent). Exudate quantity generally varies with the type of wound. For example, a venous ulcer is more exudative than an arterial ulcer. An increase in wound exudate may coincide with hyperplasia, critical colonization, biofilm, or wound infection. Subjective indicators used to quantify the volume of wound exudate include frequency of dressing change and persistent presence of periwound maceration. The type of dressing used will also provide an indication of the volume of exudate, as hydrofiber and alginate dressings are much more absorbent than hydrocolloid dressings. Sodium-impregnated gauze also can be expected to contain more exudate than plain gauze. Objective measurement of the volume of wound exudate can be obtained by using a wound containment system, such as a wound pouch or closed suction.

Odor. Odor can be described as absent, faint, moderate, or strong and often varies according to wound moisture, the type and density of microorganisms present, and the amount of nonviable tissue present. Extremely odorous, purulent exudate is suggestive of an infection. However, it is important to note that most wounds have a slight odor. The type of dressing used as well as personal and wound-related hygiene also can affect wound odor (Keast et al, 2004).

Wound Edge. The rim of the wound or wound edge provides information regarding epithelialization, chronicity, and even etiology. Ideally, the wound edges should be attached, moist, and flush with the wound base so that epithelial cells can migrate from the wound edges across the surface of the wound bed. Unattached wound edges are those in which undermining is present between the dermis and subcutaneous tissue. Closed wound edges are characterized as dry with a loss of the intervening moist red reproductive epithelium. In some situations, closed wound edges are also thickened and "rolled." This premature closure of the wound edge is a common complication of chronic wounds and is referred to as *epibole* (Doughty, 2004). Epibole results when squamous cells migrate along base, wall, and edge of the wound, thus preventing migration of epithelial cells and wound closure (see Plate 4). Cautery or surgical debridement of epibole is needed to "open" the wound edges.

Periwound Skin. The periwound skin should be described in terms of color (erythema, pale, white, blue), texture (moist, dry, indurated, boggy, macerated), skin temperature (warm, cool), integrity (denudement, maceration, excoriation, stripping, erosion, papules, pustules), and presence or absence of lesions.

The periwound assessment can give clues to the effectiveness of the treatment plan and the technique used for dressing application or removal. For example, maceration (see Plate 14), dermatitis, or denudement of periwound skin occurs when exudate pools on intact skin for prolonged periods or when a moist dressing is inappropriately applied, is left on too long, and/or overlaps onto intact skin. Periwound skin stripping may indicate inappropriate adhesive removal.

Venous/arterial insufficiency, infection, pressure damage, peripheral neuropathy, pyoderma gangrenosum, vasculitis, and calciphylaxis may present with distinct periwound features (Ferretti and Harkins, 2003). Table 6-6 lists some pathologies that may be revealed through a careful periwound skin inspection.

Bacterial Burden. All wounds have some degree of bioburden. The extent and significance of that bioburden is conveyed with the terms contamination, colonization, critical colonization, biofilm, and infection. The presence or absence of local signs of infection should be documented as part of the assessment. However, it's important to remember that many chronic wounds with significant bioburden may not exhibit the classic signs of infection due to factors such as immunosuppression or the presence of biofilm. Indicators of a subclinical infection or overwhelming bioburden include delayed healing despite optimal care, discolored or friable granulation tissue,

pocketing or breakdown at the wound base, and/or foul odor. A "stagnant" wound despite optimal care may indicate critical colonization or biofilm and will progress to infection without appropriate intervention (Gardner et al, 2001). Chapter 16 presents a thorough discussion of the assessment and management of bacterial burden and infection.

As the fifth vital sign, pain has gained a much-deserved focus in today's health care environment. Yet wound pain is infrequently assessed and inadequately managed. Wound pain can indicate infection or deterioration as well as inappropriate or inadequate treatment choices. Pain can be directly related to patient satisfaction and has been shown to have a negative impact on wound healing progress. Pain should be measured regularly and frequently with a validated pain assessment scale (Reddy et al, 2003). Chapters 25 and 26 provide detailed discussions related to the assessment and management of wound pain.

REASSESSMENT AND EVALUATION OF HEALING

Evaluation of healing involves wound assessment documented over time to reveal patterns and trends that indicate improvement or deterioration in the wound. In this way, assessment is linked to outcomes so that an evaluation of the plan of care can follow objective criteria.

Frequency of Reassessment

In general, the patient's overall condition, wound severity, health care setting, type of dressings used, and goals determine the appropriate frequency of wound assessment. Because frequency of reassessment is dependent on so many variables, the frequency interval commonly changes over time and across care settings. For example, a patient who is immunosuppressed and in acute care has greater risk for developing a wound infection and may warrant more frequent monitoring. Once the patient is

TABLE 6-6	Common Periwound Features by Wound Pathology
Pathology	**Periwound Feature**
Venous insufficiency	Edema, brawny discoloration, hemosiderin-staining lipodermatosclerosis, dermatitis, scaling, weeping
Arterial	Pale color, cool, dependent rubor, absent hair, xerosis
Infection	Erythema, pain, heat, swelling, induration
Pressure	Hyperemia, edema, induration, discoloration
Peripheral neuropathy	Insensate, edema, cellulitis, erythema, induration
Pyoderma gangrenosum	Ragged and boggy borders, elevated borders, dusky red or purple, halo of edema
Vasculitis	Palpable, nonblanchable purpura; may be associated with petechiae; nodules and vesicles may be present
Calciphylaxis	Dusky, purple, and palpable nodules progress to necrosis and ulceration; associated with renal disease; may include mottled, reticulated patches, plaques with focal central necrosis
Candidiasis	Pustular or macular-papular rash; erythematous satellite lesions

stable in long-term care, the "at-risk" patient's skin should be monitored daily but may require a full wound assessment only on admission and weekly. Once the patient is home, assessments are generally dependent on the frequency of home health worker or clinic visits. Family members should be instructed to make assessments between clinic visits and may be able and willing to monitor for trends.

The Wound Ostomy and Continence Nurses (WOCN) Society's "Guideline for Prevention and Management of Pressure Ulcers" makes specific recommendations on the frequency of monitoring, assessment, and evaluation of pressure ulcer healing (WOCN Society, 2003, 2010). (1) Patients at risk for skin breakdown should have a daily skin inspection (Bergstrom and Braden, 1992; WOCN Society, 2003, 2010). (2) Pressure ulcers should be assessed and monitored at each dressing change, or sooner if the wound or the patient's condition deteriorates (van Rijswijk and Braden, 1999; WOCN Society, 2003, 2010). (3) Evaluation of pressure ulcer healing should occur within 1 to 2 weeks, or sooner if the patient or wound condition deteriorates (van Rijswijk and Braden, 1999; van Rijswijk and Polansky, 1994; WOCN Society, 2003).

When topical wound therapy is being selected, the frequency with which the wound should be assessed must be considered. For example, a hydrocoloid on a stable wound should not be removed daily simply to conduct a wound assessment. Rather the assessment should be obtained at the time the dressing is scheduled to be changed (i.e., every 4 days). Chapter 18 discusses the principles of wound management and the various features of local wound care options.

Predicting Wound Healing

It is generally agreed that percent reduction in wound surface area during the initial weeks of treatment is the most reliable indicator for complete healing. van Rijswijk and the Multicenter Leg Ulcer Study Group (2003) monitored the healing of 61 patients with 72 full-thickness venous leg ulcers. They found that a greater than 30% reduction in ulcer area after 2 weeks of treatment was a significant ($p = .004$) predictor of the time required for healing. Kantor and Margolis (2000) conducted a cohort multicenter study of 104 patients and found that the percentage change in ulcer area during the first 4 weeks of treatment was the best prognostic indicator that the ulcers would eventually heal within 24 weeks. Similarly, Phillips et al. (2000) found baseline ulcer area and duration of leg ulcer were important predictors of healing in a multicenter retrospective review of 165 patients with venous ulcers. Falanga and Sabolinski (2000) reported data based on randomized, controlled, clinical trials and presented reliable and specific findings for predicting complete healing. Initial healing time of 0.1 cm/wk or greater predicts healing, whereas rates of 0.6 cm/wk or less predict nonhealing.

Studies of neuropathic and ischemic ulcers suggest a linear relationship between initial wound radius or size and healing time (Robson et al, 2000; Zimny et al, 2002). Additional studies conclude that wounds that maintain a linear relationship between wound margin size and wound surface size have faster healing rates. During a controlled prospective trial examining 338 serial tracings of venous ulcers, Cardinal et al (2009) noted faster healing rates with wounds that maintained a linear relationship between margin size and wound surface size ($p = .001$). A prospective multicenter study of 203 patients with diabetic foot ulcers found that 4-week healing rates correlated significantly with healing at 12 weeks ($p = .01$) (Sheehan et al, 2003).

Jones et al. (2007) conducted a multisite retrospective review of medical records of patients from a variety of care settings to determine factors that influence wound healing within 3 months and nonhealing after 5 months. Researchers evaluated at least 3 months of data from 400 patients with pressure, venous, and diabetic wounds who received routine wound care by typical staff. Results showed a difference in wound healing by size, location, and socioeconomic status. Large and deep wounds were less likely to heal than small and shallow wounds. Lower extremity wounds were more likely to heal than wounds located on the iliac crest or trochanter. Patients who were not Caucasian and patients on Medicare had poor healing outcomes. Not surprisingly, nonhealing wounds were also associated with infection, heavy exudate, necrosis, and inappropriate use of wound care dressings.

Tools for Documentation and Evaluation of Healing

Several tools that enable the clinician to predict and assess wounds are available; they are presented throughout the text and in Appendix B. Clinicians should be familiar with the strengths and limitations of the several methods currently available for assessing wound status. Staging and assessment tools are not designed to replace a comprehensive ongoing assessment. Ideally, tools should be reliable, valid, clinically useful, and theoretically based.

The ASEPSIS (Additional treatment, presence of Serous discharge, Erythema, Purulent exudate, Separation of deep tissues, Isolation of bacteria, and duration of inpatient Stay) Incision Assessment Tool for evaluating wound healing is discussed in Chapter 34. International Guidelines for pressure ulcers recommend evaluation of healing every 2 weeks with a validated tool such as the Pressure Ulcer Scale for Healing (PUSH) or the Bates-Jensen Wound Assessment Tool (BWAT) (NPUAP and EPUAP, 2009). The BWAT is also used to evaluate healing of non–pressure-related wounds. As with most assessment tools, they should be used in conjunction with clinical judgment.

Bates-Jensen Wound Assessment Tool. The BWAT, originally known as the PSST, takes approximately 10 to 15 minutes to complete and addresses 15 macroscopic wound characteristics (Woodbury et al, 1999). Specific definitions are provided for each characteristic. Individual items are scored on a modified Likert scale (ranging from 1 for best for that characteristic to 5 for worst). Individual items are summed, and the total provides a measure of overall wound status. Total scores range from 13, which indicates tissue health, to 65, which indicates wound degeneration.

Although the tool is now intended for use with a variety of wound types, validity and reliability has been mostly tested with pressure ulcers utilizing the original PSST. Content validity of the PSST with a nine-member expert judge panel was 0.91. Interrater reliability coefficient was 0.915; intrarater reliability was 0.975 when used with wound specialists in an acute care hospital. The interrater reliability of the PSST in long-term care with licensed practical nurses, registered nurses, and physical therapists who had no experience in wound care yielded a mean of 0.78; intrarater reliability for this group was 0.89, and agreement with an expert was 0.82. A benefit of the PSST is that it allows tracking of total score and each item or wound characteristic over time. Thus each item can be monitored for improvement or deterioration. In this way, the PSST can be used to evaluate the effectiveness of specific interventions or achievement of short-term outcomes, such as to manage wound infection or to debride the wound (Bates-Jensen, 1994, 1997). More than a decade later, researchers adapted the tool by adding a patient-reported pain scale and a "none" option for assessing undermining, peripheral tissue induration, or edema for *any* chronic wound. Content validity then was established with 33 multidisciplinary international wound care experts (Bolton et al, 2004).

Pressure Ulcer Scale for Healing. The PUSH was developed by the National Pressure Ulcer Advisory Panel (NPUAP) to monitor pressure ulcer healing over time and takes approximately 5 minutes to complete (Woodbury et al, 1999). The PUSH tool is designed to monitor three parameters that are considered the most indicative of healing: size (length and width), exudate amount, and tissue type. Each parameter has at least four sublevels. The subscore for each parameter is totaled, and the overall total score is calculated ranging from 0 to 17 (0 = healed). A comparison of total scores measured over time provides an indication of wound improvement or deterioration (Günes, 2009; WOCN Society, 2003).

Numerous validation studies have been conducted using the PUSH tool. Initial validity was established with pressure ulcers ($p<0.01$). Subsequent studies found the PUSH tool to be valid and responsive for assessing healing for pressure, venous, and diabetic lower extremity ulcers (Hon et al, 2010).

Outcome and Assessment Information Set (OASIS). Medicare's payment to home health care agencies is based on the OASIS comprehensive patient assessment which includes several wound-related questions and some diagnoses. The OASIS is completed by the registered nurse or physical therapist on admission, at recertification, and at discharge. The most extensive OASIS assessment is done on admission and contains questions that cover the patient's clinical condition and functional status and includes several questions on services received. Because payment is directly affected by how several wound-related questions are answered, the Wound, Ostomy and Continence Nurses (WOCN) Society developed an OASIS Guidance Document for clarification of how these questions could best be answered. This document is available in Appendix B.

Photography

Conventional, Polaroid, or digital photographs are commonly used in practice today to facilitate wound measurement, assessment, and evaluation of healing. Accurate photography may provide a template against which changes in wound status can be observed and compared. However, if photography is to be used, it should only be used as an *adjunct* to support written wound documentation. The WOCN Society and the NPUAP neither recommend nor discourage the use of photography for pressure ulcer documentation. However each organization provides documents to guide the use of photography in the clinical setting (WOCN Society, 2005; NPUAP, 2009). When photography is used, the facility should have specific protocols or policies in place. Checklist 6-4 provides issues to be addressed in a wound photography protocol or policy.

Health Insurance Portability and Accountability Act (HIPAA) guidelines for privacy must be followed when using wound photography; they include patient authorization for use of images beyond the purpose of treatment, payment, or health care operations (Hjort et al, 2001). Informed consent should be obtained prior to photographing, filming, or videotaping. In the situation where informed consent cannot be obtained prior to photographing, The Joint Commission recommends that images be sequestered or not finalized as part of the documentation until appropriate consent is obtained. The American Health Information Management Association (AHIMA) suggests that consent for photographs be included in the consent for treatment (Hjort et al, 2001). AHIMA's suggestions for how to phrase the consent statement can be found in the WOCN position statement (WOCN, 2005).

The debate over wound photography often leads to a discussion of litigation. A blurred photograph or photography that does not follow facility policy can give the impression of poor work quality, supporting negative outcomes in a court room rather than the intended purpose of conveying progression of healing. If a photograph of the wound is not available, the jury could be shown a

CHECKLIST 6-4

Issues to Address in Policy or Protocol for Wound Photography

✓ Informed consent (who can obtain the consent and what is included)
✓ Timing of photographs (when or under what circumstances photographs are to be taken and repeated)
✓ Criteria about who can take the photographs
✓ Method of validating competency to photograph wounds (include frequency of competency revalidations)
✓ Type of camera being used
✓ Techniques used to ensure consistency in photographing and methods used to ensure photographs are not enhanced or altered (e.g., image size, distance from the wound, sample measure in frame, such as measuring guide)
✓ Appropriate patient identification (initials, medical record number, date and time markings)
✓ Maintenance and storage of photographs effectively (where they will be stored and who will have access to them)
✓ Method for releasing copies to patients upon request (authorization form)

Data from Wound, Ostomy and Continence Nurses Society (WOCN Society): *Photography in Wound Documentation*. In: Wound, Ostomy and Continence Nurses Society Professional Practice series, 2005, available at http://www.wocn.org/pdfs/WOCN_Library/Position_Statements/photoposition.pdf, accessed August 13, 2010.

photograph of a different wound as an example of how bad it could be. Controversies related to wound photography include film type: use of Polaroid film, which cannot be altered but may soon be unavailable, versus digital film, which can be altered (Sullivan, 2008). The NPUAP (2009) recommends digital photography with a density of at least 1.5 megapixels. However, 3 megapixels or greater is preferable and offers the best ratio of picture clarity versus equipment cost. States differ regarding their stance on the admissibility of photographs in court cases (WOCN, 2005).

SUMMARY

Few pathologic conditions are evaluated with a single instrument or parameter. The more intricate the process (e.g., congestive heart failure), the more clinicians rely on several measures (e.g., radiologic examination, physical examination, pulse characteristics, treadmill tests, hematocrit) to accurately capture a full description of the extent of the condition. Similarly, several parameters are required to best capture the condition of the wound.

Recognizing the difference between simply measuring the dimensions of a wound and the more complex process of assessing the status of the wound's multiple components and healing status is essential to successful wound management and holistic patient care. It is clear that evaluating wounds as if they exist separately from the patient not only is inadequate but also is inconsistent with evidence-based practice.

REFERENCES

Bates-Jensen BM: The pressure sore status tool: an outcome measure for pressure sores, *Top Geriatr Rehabil* 9(4):17, 1994.

Bates-Jensen BM: The pressure sore status tool a few thousand assessments later, *Adv Wound Care* 10(5):65, 1997.

Bates-Jensen BM et al: Subepidermal moisture is associated with early pressure ulcer damage in nursing home residents with dark skin tones: pilot findings, *J Wound Ostomy Continence Nurs* 36(3):277-284, 2009.

Baumgarten M et al: Black/white differences in pressure ulcer incidence in nursing home residents, *J Am Geriatr Soc* 52(8):1293-1298, 2004.

Bennett AM: Report of the task force on the implications for darkly pigmented intact skin in the prediction and prevention of pressure ulcers, *Adv Wound Care* 8(6):34-35, 1995.

Bergstrom N, Braden B: A prospective study of pressure sore risk among institutionalized elderly, *J Am Geriatr Soc* 40(8):747, 1992.

Bolton L et al: Wound-healing outcomes using standardized assessment and care in clinical practice, *J Wound Ostomy Continence Nurs* 31(2):65-71, 2004.

Bryant J et al: Reliability of wound measuring techniques in an outpatient wound center, *Ostomy Wound Manage* 47:44-51, 2001.

Cardinal M et al: Wound shape geometry measurements correlate to eventual wound healing, *Wound Repair Regen* 17(2):173-178, 2009.

Crawford PE, Fields-Varnado M: Guideline for management of wounds in patients with lower-extremity neuropathic disease. In *WOCN clinical practice guideline series no. 3*, Glenview, Ill, 2004, Wound, Ostomy and Continence Nurses Society.

Doughty DB: Wound assessment: tips and techniques, *Adv Skin Wound Care* 17:369, 2004.

Falanga V, Sabolinski ML: Prognostic factors for healing of venous ulcers, *Wounds* 12(5 Suppl A):42A-46A, 2000.

Ferretti DE, Harkins SM: Assessment of periwound skin. In Miline C, Corbett L, Dubuc D, editors: *Wound, ostomy, and continence nursing secrets*, Philadelphia, 2003, Hanley & Belfus.

Gardner SE et al: A tool to assess clinical signs and symptoms of localized infection in chronic wounds: development and reliability, *Ostomy Wound Manage* 47(1):40, 2001.

Günes UY: A prospective study evaluating the Pressure Ulcer Scale for Healing (PUSH Tool) to assess Stage II, Stage III, and Stage IV pressure ulcers, *Ostomy Wound Manage* 55(5):48-52, 2009.

Hjort B et al: Practice brief. Patient photography, videotaping, and other imaging (updated), *J AHIMA* 72(6), 64M-64Q, 2001.

Hon J, et al: Prospective, multicenter study to validate use of the pressure ulcer scale for healing (PUSH(c)) in patients with diabetic, venous, and pressure ulcers, *Ostomy Wound Manage*, 56(2):26-36, 2010.

Jones KR et al: Chronic wounds: factors influencing healing within 3 months and nonhealing after 5-6 months of care, *Wounds* 19(3):51-63, 2007.

Kantor J, Margolis DJ: A multicentre study of percentage change in venous leg ulcer area as a prognostic index of healing at 24 weeks, *Br J Dermatol* 142(5):960-964, 2000.

Keast DH et al: Measure: a proposed assessment framework for developing best practice recommendations for wound assessment, *Wound Rep Regen* 5:S1, 2004.

Langemo DK et al: Measuring wound length, width, and area: which technique? *Adv Skin Wound Care* 21:42-45, 2008.

Murphy RM: Legal and practical impact of clinical practice guidelines on nursing and medical practice, *Adv Wound Care* 9(5):31, 1996.

National Pressure Ulcer Advisory Panel (NPUAP): *FAQ: Photography for pressure ulcer documentation*, available at http://www.npuap.org/faq.htm, accessed August 18, 2009.

National Pressure Ulcer Advisory Panel (NPUAP) and European Pressure Ulcer Advisory Panel (EPUAP): Treatment of pressure ulcers, Washington, DC, 2009, National Pressure Ulcer Advisory Panel.

Office for National Statistics (ONS): *Final results on 2001 census for England and Wales*, London, 2002, Author.

Phillips TJ et al: Prognostic indicators in venous ulcers, *J Am Acad Dermatol* 43(4):627-630, 2000.

Reddy M et al: Practical treatment of wound pain and trauma: a patient centered approach, *Ostomy Wound Manage* 49(4A Suppl):2-15, 2003.

Robson MC et al: Wound healing trajectories as predictors of effectiveness of therapeutic agents, *Arch Surg* 135(7):773-777, 2000.

Rosen J et al: Pressure ulcer prevention in black and white nursing home residents: a QI initiative of enhanced ability, incentives, and management feedback, *Adv Skin Wound Care* 19(5):262-268, 2006.

Salcido RS: Finding a window into the skin, *Adv Skin Wound Care* 15(3):100, 2002.

Sheehan P et al: Percent change in wound area of diabetic foot ulcers over a 4 week period is a robust predictor of complete healing in a 12 week prospective trial, *Diabetes Care* 26:1879, 2003.

Sullivan V: In focus: the photography forecast, *Today's Wound Clinic* April 15, 2008, available at http://www.todayswoundclinic.com/in-focus-the-photography-forecast, accessed October 16, 2009.

van Rijswijk L, Braden BJ: Pressure ulcer patient and wound assessment: an AHCPR clinical practice guideline update, *Ostomy Wound Manage* 45(Suppl 1A):56S, 1999.

van Rijswijk L, Lyder C: Pressure ulcer prevention and care: implementing the revised guidance to surveyors for long-term care facilities, *Ostomy Wound Manage* 51(Suppl 4):7, 2005.

van Rijswijk L, Multicenter Leg Ulcer Study Group: Full-thickness leg ulcers: patient demographics and predictors of healing, *J Fam Pract* 36(6):625-632, 2003.

van Rijswijk L, Polansky M: Predictors of time to healing deep pressure ulcers, *Ostomy Wound Manage* 40(8):40, 1994.

Woodbury MG et al: Pressure ulcer assessment instruments: a critical appraisal, *Ostomy Wound Manage* 45(5):42, 1999.

Wound, Ostomy and Continence Nurses Society (WOCN Society): Guideline for management of patients with lower extremity arterial disease, In *WOCN clinical practice guideline series no. 1*, Glenview IL, 2002, Author.

Wound, Ostomy and Continence Nurses Society (WOCN Society): Guideline for prevention and management of pressure ulcers, In *WOCN clinical practice guideline series no. 2*, Glenview IL, 2003, Author.

Wound, Ostomy and Continence Nurses Society (WOCN Society): Photography in Wound Documentation. In *Wound, Ostomy and Continence Nurses Society Professional Practice series*, 2005, available at http://www.wocn.org/pdfs/WOCN_Library/Position_Statements/photoposition.pdf, accessed August 18, 2009.

Wound, Ostomy and Continence Nurses Society (WOCN): *Guideline for management of pressure ulcers*, WOCN *clinical practice guideline series* #2, Glenview, IL, 2010, Author.

Zimny S et al: Determinants and estimation of healing times in diabetic foot ulcers, *J Diabetes Complications* 16:327-332, 2002.

Pressure Ulcers

7

Pressure Ulcers: Impact, Etiology, and Classification

Barbara Pieper

OBJECTIVES

1. Describe the incidence and prevalence of pressure ulcers in various clinical settings and vulnerable patient populations.
2. Define pressure ulcer.
3. Identify the three most common locations at which pressure ulcers develop.
4. Describe the role of subcutaneous tissue and muscle in preventing pressure ulcers.
5. Describe the role of the causative factors for pressure ulcer formation.
6. Differentiate between capillary pressure and capillary closing pressure.
7. Describe the phenomena of reactive hyperemia, blanching erythema, and nonblanching erythema.
8. Describe the pathophysiologic consequences of pressure damage, including the changes that occur at the cellular level and the cone-shaped pressure gradient.
9. List five variables that influence the extent of tissue damage as a consequence of pressure.

Pressure ulcers present a significant health care threat to patients with restricted mobility or chronic disease and to older patients. Because of this threat, more documents about pressure ulcers are being published, such as the *International Pressure Ulcer Guidelines for Prevention and Treatment* (NPUAP and EPUAP, 2009), the Wound, Ostomy and Continence Nurses (WOCN) Society *Guideline for Prevention and Management of Pressure Ulcers* (WOCN Society, 2003, 2010), the Registered Nurses Association of Ontario (RNAO) *Risk Assessment and Prevention of Pressure Ulcers Guideline* (RNAO, 2005), "Guidelines for the prevention of pressure ulcers" by the Wound Healing Society (Stechmiller et al, 2008), the Canadian Association of Wound Care "Best practice recommendations for the prevention and treatment of pressure ulcers: update 2006" (Keast et al, 2007), and *Healthy People 2010* (U.S. Department of Health and Human Services, 2000). The Institute for Healthcare Improvement identified pressure ulcers as one of its primary goals in the "Save 5 Million Lives" campaign (Padula et al, 2008). The Cochrane Wounds Group also covers the prevention and treatment of pressure ulcers (Bell-Syer et al, 2007).

SCOPE OF THE PROBLEM

The scope of the pressure ulcer problem in the United States is examined in terms of the patient's age and diagnosis and the setting. Statistics about pressure ulcers vary because of how data were collected, variations in terminology about prevalence and incidence, concern about litigation, and political and social events that changed American health care. The concepts of prevalence and incidence and methods for calculation are discussed in Chapter 1.

Prevalence

The WOCN Society (2004) defines *pressure ulcer prevalence* as the number of patients with at least one pressure ulcer who exist in a given patient population at a given point in time. In the United States, the 6-year sequential analysis of pressure ulcer prevalence ranges from 14% to 17% (Whittington and Briones, 2004). The prevalence of pressure ulcers in long-term care has been reported as 27.3%, with 8.5% being nosocomial (VanGilder et al, 2008; Whitney et al, 2008). The prevalence of pressure ulcers in home care ranges from 3% to 10% (Bolton et al, 2008). The 2003 National Pediatric Pressure Ulcer and Skin Breakdown Prevalence Survey found a pressure ulcer prevalence of 4%; 92% of pressure ulcers were partial-thickness ulcers and 66% were facility acquired (McLane et al, 2004). The discrepancies in prevalence can be attributed to the fact that some studies include intact pressure-damaged skin (suspected deep tissue injury, or Stage I), whereas other studies exclude such lesions. Prevalence is lower when intact pressure-damaged skin is excluded from the sample. Pressure ulcers in dark-skinned persons may also be difficult to detect (Black et al, 2007). Some skin conditions, such as candidiasis and herpetic lesions, may be misclassified as pressure ulcers. In infants and children, the diagnosis of a pressure ulcer is carefully considered because the most common types of skin breakdown in this group include diaper dermatitis, skin tears, and intravenous extravasation (McLane et al, 2004). Data collectors must accurately distinguish between pressure ulcers and other causes of erythema and skin ulcerations.

Incidence

The WOCN Society (2004) defines *incidence* as the number of patients who initially were ulcer-free who develop a pressure ulcer within a particular time period in a defined population. Incidence measures new conditions (e.g., pressure ulcers) and therefore is considered more reflective of the quality of care within that setting. It is a measure used to evaluate the effects of preventive and therapeutic interventions. Determining the incidence of pressure ulcers is inherently difficult because such studies require longitudinal observations. As with prevalence, incidence will vary by setting. The incidence of pressure ulcers in acute care ranges from 7% to 9% (Whittington and Briones, 2004). The incidence in long-term care ranges from 3% to 31% (Shukla et al, 2008) and in home care ranges from 0% to 17% (NPUAP, 2001).

Considerable methodologic issues surround the calculation of incidence. For example, defining who is at risk (the number used in the denominator of the incidence formula) can have a significant influence on the resulting value, which actually may overestimate or underestimate the true frequency of the condition. Consequently, variation in reports of incidence may reflect a real difference in the frequency of the condition or simply different data collection techniques, definitions, and methods. Although differences in methodology make comparisons difficult, incidence remains an important measure. Consistency in data collection technique within the health care setting is essential to generate data that can be compared over time. National standards for the definition of terms and the process for conducting prevalence and incidence studies will also increase the comparability of these kind of data (WOCN Society, 2004). The National Database of Nursing Quality Indicators (NDNQI) includes pressure ulcer prevention and hospital-acquired pressure ulcer reports from more than 1,100 facilities in the United States designed for comparisons between hospitals of similar sizes and practice levels (Montalvo, 2007).

Economic Effects

In fiscal year 2007, a preventable pressure ulcer was listed as a secondary diagnosis for 257,412 Medicare patients. The average payment for admission in which a pressure ulcer was present was $43,180 (Armstrong et al, 2008). In 2008, the Centers for Medicare and Medicaid Services (CMS) ceased payment for hospital complications considered reasonably preventable, including Stage III or IV pressure ulcers (see Chapter 8). CMS with the Centers for Disease Control and Prevention (CDC) released new codes for pressure ulcers capturing wound severity (Krapfl, 2008).

Research on the costs incurred while a pressure ulcer is being managed must be viewed cautiously; the studies are not all comparable. Some studies account for all costs: room, nursing care, supplies, medications, physician fees, and so forth. Other studies examine only direct costs, such as the supplies or medications specifically indicated for that particular problem.

Facility-associated pressure ulcers add to the patient's length of stay, delay the patient's recuperation, and increase the patient's risk for developing complications. In addition, pressure ulcers often necessitate hospitalization (in certain patient populations such as the elderly and patients with a spinal cord injury) because of sepsis or the need for debridement or surgical repair. At a time of increasingly scarce health care dollars, pressure ulcers consume intense resources in the form of dressing changes, nursing care, physical therapy, medications, nutritional support, and clinician services.

Literature reports a range of costs for pressure ulcer management. Approximately, 2.5 million patients are treated each year in U.S. acute care facilities for pressure ulcers, and the cost of treating pressure ulcers is estimated at $11 to $17.2 billion annually (Ayello and Lyder, 2008; Bolton et al, 2008). Pressure ulcers lead to loss of function, infection, and extended hospital stays, all of which can increase cost. Hospital length of stay for a principal pressure ulcer diagnosis was 14.1 days compared to 12.7 days for a secondary pressure ulcer diagnosis. The average cost per hospital day for a principal pressure ulcer diagnosis was $1,200 compared to $1,600 for a secondary pressure ulcer diagnosis. Three of four hospitalizations with a pressure ulcer diagnosis were billed to Medicare; Medicaid patients accounted for additional 12.5% of hospitalizations with a principal pressure ulcer. More than half of patients with pressure ulcer stays were discharged to long-term care, which is more than three times the rate of hospitalizations for all other causes (Russo et al, 2008).

Impact on Quality and Duration of Life

Pressure ulcers may affect psychosocial needs and quality of life in terms of occurrence, recurrence, ulcer characteristics, and ulcer demands. Pressure ulcers may cause social isolation and add burden and frustration for the patient, the family, and care providers. Aspects of quality of life include change in body image, pain, odor and drainage, and financial impact (Langemo, 2005). Quality-of-life research studies about persons with pressure ulcers tend to have small sample sizes, so additional research is needed. Important factors to assess are the patient's social networks, the patient's living space and environment, and the patient's mental status, learning needs, and personal goals. Pain is an ever-present problem with pressure ulcers and must be assessed (Pieper et al, 2009). Pain assessment and management is discussed in detail in Chapters 25 and 26.

Pressure ulcers have been examined in terms of their effects on mortality rates. In 2006, hospital mortality among persons with a secondary diagnosis of a pressure ulcer was 11.6% and was 4.2% among those with a pressure ulcer as a principal diagnosis (Russo et al, 2008). Approximately 60,000 patients die each year from pressure ulcer complications (Ayello and Lyder, 2008). Pressure ulcers were reported as a cause of death among 114,380 persons (1990–2001), and the age-adjusted mortality rate was 3.79 per 100,000 population. Pressure ulcers deaths occurred mostly in persons at least 75 years old, and septicemia was reported in 39.7%. Mortality rates were higher in African Americans than in persons of other racial/ethnic groups (Redelings et al, 2005). In a home care project in Italy, residents with a pressure ulcer had a relative risk of dying of 1.92 after adjusting for age, gender, and all significant variables between the two groups of patients (Landi et al, 2007).

VULNERABLE PATIENT POPULATIONS

A variety of specific patient populations have been discussed in the literature as being at increased risk for pressure ulcer formation: older adults, persons with spinal cord injury, surgical patients, obese patients, underweight patients, children, and patients at end of life. These particular patient populations are introduced here and discussed in greater detail throughout the text.

Historically, older adults admitted to acute and long-term care facilities have been a vulnerable population. Nearly 3 (72%) of 4 older adult patients hospitalized with a secondary pressure ulcer diagnosis and 56.5% of adults with a principal diagnosis of a pressure ulcer were 65 years of age or older (Russo et al, 2008). Among persons admitted to long-term care, 10.3% to 18.4% had one or more pressure ulcers on admission (Baumgarten et al, 2003; Siem et al, 2003). The presence of an existing pressure ulcer at the time of admission to acute care was 26.2% among persons admitted from a nursing home and 4.8% among those admitted from another living situation (Keelaghan et al, 2008). For older adults with a pressure ulcer, coexisting conditions were fluid and electrolyte disorders, nutritional disorders, diabetes mellitus without complications, and dementia (Russo et al, 2008).

Pressure ulcer prevalence for persons with spinal cord injuries ranges from 20% to 66% (Schubart et al, 2008). Paralysis and spinal cord injury were common coexisting conditions among younger adults hospitalized principally

for pressure ulcers (Russo et al, 2008). Those with the greatest level of disability and mobility impairment have the highest pressure ulcer risk. Other risk factors are history of pressure ulcers, coexisting medical conditions, rehospitalizations, nursing home stays, less than high school education, older adult, male, African American, and single (Schubart et al, 2008).

In a study involving 37 facilities, the incidence of pressure ulcers related to the surgical event was 3.5% (Aronovitch, 2007). Associated factors were at least one comorbidity, managed with a warming device, receipt of three or more anesthetic agents, and median operative time of 4.48 hours (Aronovitch, 2007). Tissue damage may become apparent within hours or may be delayed for up to 3 days. Initial manifestations may be skin discoloration (e.g., bruising) that evolves into blister formation or necrosis. Because this process transpires over several days (i.e., 2–6 days), isolating the time of the original injury is complicated (Price et al, 2005). Because the length of surgery and other variables for the surgical patient cannot be changed, the surgical team must aim to decrease pressure and shear not only during the procedure but also when transferring the patient into position before and after the procedure (Schoonhoven et al, 2002).

Both the obese and the underweight patient populations are vulnerable to pressure ulcer development. The morbidly obese are at risk for pressure ulcers due to their inability to turn themselves, underlying diseases, improper equipment, lack of adequate pressure redistribution, inadequate staff numbers, or staff not trained in how to turn and move such patients (Knudsen and Gallagher, 2003; Mathison, 2003). In a study of elderly patients admitted to acute care, the odds of developing a pressure ulcer in patients who were obese and those who were severely obese were very low (odds ratio 0.7 and 0.1, respectively). In contrast, the odds of the underweight patient developing a pressure ulcer was almost doubled (odds ratio 1.8) (Compher et al, 2007).

Two additional vulnerable patient populations are children and patients at end of life. Pressure ulcer prevalence, incidence and risk factors for these two patient populations are presented in Chapters 36 and 37 respectively.

TERMINOLOGY

Over the years, several terms have been used to describe pressure ulcers: bedsore, decubitus ulcer, decubiti, and pressure sore. *Pressure ulcer* is the accepted term because it is more accurate and descriptive. The origin of the term *bedsore* is not known, but it predates the term *decubitus*. *Decubitus*, a Latin word referring to the reclining position (Fox and Bradley, 1803), dates from 1747 when the French used it to mean bedsore. However, this term is inaccurate because it does not convey the tissue destruction associated with these lesions and because these lesions result from positions other than the lying position (such as sitting) (Arnold, 1983).

A *pressure ulcer* is defined as localized injury to the skin and/or underlying tissue usually over a bony prominence as a result of pressure or of pressure in combination with shear and/or friction. A number of contributing or confounding factors are associated with pressure ulcers, but the significance of these factors has not yet been elucidated (NPUAP, 2007).

Pressure ulcers occur most commonly over a bony prominence, such as the sacrum, ischial tuberosity, trochanter, and calcaneus; however, they may develop anywhere on the body (e.g., underneath a cast, splint, or cervical collar). Figure 7-1 shows common sites for pressure ulcers and frequency of ulceration per site. The majority of pressure ulcers occur in the pelvis, but other more common locations are the sacrum and the heels (VanGilder et al, 2008).

Bony locations are most prone to pressure ulcer formation because a person's body weight is concentrated on these areas when resting on an unyielding surface. Those who have atrophy of the subcutaneous and muscle tissue layers are at even greater risk for the "mechanical load" of pressure and thus increased soft tissue and capillary compression. The coccyx, sacrum, and heel are particularly vulnerable because less soft tissue is present between the bone and skin.

CAUSATIVE FACTORS

Pressure is the major causative factor in pressure ulcer formation. However, several factors play a role in determining whether pressure is sufficient to create tissue ischemia proceeding to tissue death. The pathologic effect of excessive pressure on soft tissue can be attributed to (1) intensity of pressure, (2) duration of pressure, and (3) tissue tolerance (ability of skin and its supporting structures to endure pressure without adverse sequelae). Braden and Bergstrom (1987) presented a model of the factors that contribute to the intensity and duration of pressure ulcers (Figure 7-2), in combination with intrinsic and extrinsic factors that affect tissue tolerance.

Intensity of Pressure

To understand the importance of intensity of pressure, it is important to review the terms *capillary pressure* and *capillary closing pressure*. *Capillary pressure* tends to move fluid outward through the capillary membrane. Exact capillary pressure is not known because of the difficulty of obtaining the measurement. Various methods have been used to estimate capillary pressure. A normal hydrostatic pressure is approximately 32 mm Hg at the arterial end of a capillary bed and 12 mm Hg at the venous end (Figure 7-3) (Kumar et al, 2005a). The mean colloidal osmotic pressure in tissue is approximately 25 mm Hg.

The term *capillary closing pressure*, or *critical closing pressure*, describes the minimal amount of pressure

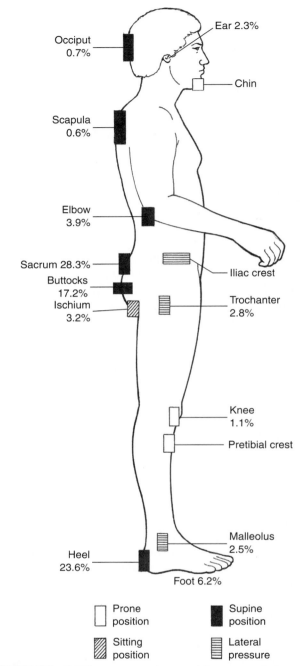

FIGURE 7-1 Sites for pressure ulcers and frequency of ulceration per site (N = 85,838). *Note:* Sites for device-related pressure ulcers, which may not involve bony prominences, are not included.

required to collapse a capillary (Burton and Yamada, 1951). Tissue anoxia develops when externally applied pressure causes vessels to collapse. It is believed that the amount of pressure required to collapse capillaries must exceed capillary pressure, which is considered to be 12 to 32 mm Hg, the numerical "standard" for capillary closing pressure.

To quantify the intensity of pressure being applied externally to the skin, interface pressures are measured. Numerous studies measuring interface pressures have

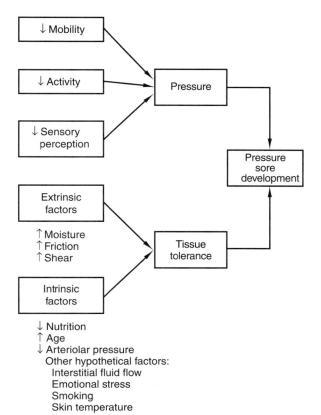

FIGURE 7-2 Factors contributing to the development of pressure ulcers. *(From Braden B, Bergstrom N: A conceptual schema for the study of the etiology of pressure sores, Rehabil Nurs 12(1):9, 1987.)*

been conducted (Kosiak, 1961; Kosiak et al, 1958; Lindan, 1961). These studies showed that interface pressures attained while a person is in the sitting or supine position commonly exceed capillary pressures (Bennett et al, 1984). In 1961, Lindan used an experimental "bed" to calculate the pressure distribution over the skin

of a healthy adult male in the supine, prone, side-lying, and sitting positions. Interface pressures ranged from 10 to 100 mm Hg. Interface readings as high as 300 mm Hg have been obtained over the ischial tuberosity of healthy, able-bodied male subjects when sitting in an unpadded chair (Kosiak, 1961).

Because head of bed elevation is important for mechanically ventilated patients in critical care and head of bed elevation greater than 30 degrees exposes the patient to increased shear injury and unrelieved pressure, Peterson et al. (2008) examined sacral interface pressures at elevations of 0, 10, 20, 30, 45, 60, and 75 degrees in 15 healthy subjects. The elevations 30 degrees or greater had peak interface pressures significantly higher than supine. In addition, elevations 45 degrees or higher had bed interface pressures greater than 32 mm Hg (Peterson et al, 2008).

Interface pressures in excess of capillary pressure will not routinely result in ischemia. Healthy people with normal sensation regularly shift their weight in response to the discomfort associated with capillary closure and tissue hypoxia. Unfortunately, pathologic processes such as spinal cord injury or sedation impair a person's ability to recognize or respond to this discomfort. Tissue hypoxia then can develop and progress to tissue anoxia and cellular death.

Duration of Pressure

Duration of pressure is an important factor that influences the detrimental effects of pressure and must be considered in tandem with intensity of pressure. An inverse relationship exists between duration and intensity of pressure in creating tissue ischemia. Specifically, low-intensity pressures over a long period can create tissue damage just as high-intensity pressure can over a

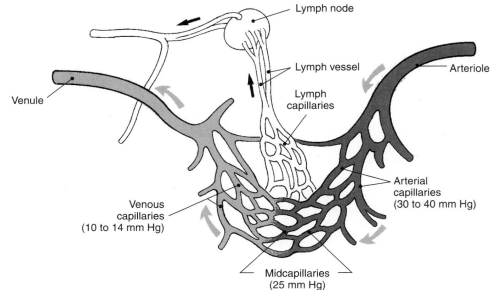

FIGURE 7-3 Capillary pressure within the capillary bed.

short period (Figure 7-4). Husain (1953) underscored the significance of the relationship between duration and intensity of pressure. Husain found that a pressure of 100 mm Hg applied to rat muscle for 2 hours was sufficient to produce only microscopic changes in the muscle. However, the same pressure applied for 6 hours was sufficient to produce complete muscle degeneration.

Tissue Tolerance

Tissue tolerance is the third factor that determines the pathologic effect of prolonged pressure. It describes the condition or integrity of the skin and supporting structures that influence the skin's ability to redistribute the applied pressure. Compression of tissue against skeletal structures and the resulting tissue ischemia can be prevented by effective redistribution of pressure.

The concept of tissue tolerance was first discussed with the need to identify how much pressure skin could "tolerate." Later, Husain (1953) introduced the concept of sensitizing the tissue to pressure and consequently to ischemia. Rat muscle was sensitized with a pressure of 100 mm Hg applied for 2 hours. Seventy-two hours later, a mere 50 mm Hg pressure applied to the same tissue caused muscle degeneration in only 1 hour. This muscle destruction resulted during the second application of pressure, even though the intensity and duration of pressure were lower than the initial intensity and duration. This finding has significant implications for the patient population at risk for pressure ulcers. It indicates that episodes of deep tissue ischemia can occur without cutaneous manifestations and that such episodes can sensitize the patient's skin. In vitro findings show that relatively small loads cause structural changes to the

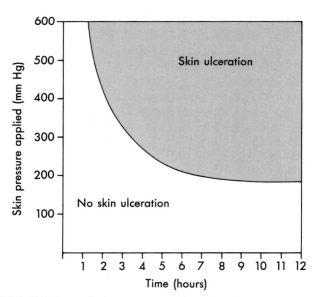

FIGURE 7-4 Graph demonstrating relationship between intensity and duration of pressure. (From Kosiak M: Etiology of decubitus ulcers, *Arch Phys Med Rehabil* 42:191, 1961.)

dermal component of tissue. Human tissue exhibits changes visible at the surface that often are minor compared to damage seen in deeper tissue layers (Edsberg, 2007). Small increments of pressure, even if only slightly above normal capillary pressure ranges, may then result in breakdown.

Tissue tolerance is influenced by the ability of the skin and underlying structures (e.g., blood vessels, interstitial fluid, collagen) to work together as a set of parallel springs that transmit load from the surface of the tissue to the skeleton inside (Krouskop, 1983). Several intrinsic and extrinsic factors can alter the ability of the soft tissue to perform this task.

Extrinsic Factors that Affect Tissue Tolerance.

Shear. Shear is caused by the interplay of gravity and friction. It exerts a force parallel to the skin and is the result of both gravity pushing down on the body and resistance (friction) between the patient and a surface, such as the bed or chair. For example, when the head of the bed is elevated, the effect of gravity on the body is to pull the body down toward the foot of the bed. In contrast, the resistance generated by the bed surface tends to hold the body in place. However, what is actually held in place is the skin, while the weight of the skeleton continues to pull the body downward.

Because the skin does not move freely, the primary effect of shear occurs at the deeper fascial level of the tissues overlying the bony prominence. Blood vessels, which are anchored at the point of exit through the fascia, are stretched and angulated when exposed to shear. This force also dissects the tissues, resulting in undermining.

Shear causes much of the damage often observed with pressure ulcers. In fact, some lesions that may result solely from shear are misinterpreted as pressure ulcers. Conversely, pressure ulcers may also be misinterpreted. Vascular occlusion is enhanced if shear and pressure occur together. For example, when the head of the bed is elevated more than 30 degrees, shear force occurs in the sacrococcygeal region. The sliding of the body transmits pressure to the sacrum and the deep fascia; the outer skin is fixed because of friction with the bed. The vessels in the deep superficial fascia angulate, leading to thrombosis and undermining of the dermis (see Figure 5-1). Dressings with a low-friction external surface have been reported to reduce shear force but do not significantly reduce interface pressures (Nakagami et al, 2006).

Friction. Friction is a significant factor in pressure ulcer development because it acts in concert with gravity to cause shear. Alone, its ability to cause skin damage is confined to the epidermal and upper dermal layers. In its mildest form, friction abrades the epidermis and dermis similar to a mild burn, and sometimes is referred to as "sheet burn." This type of damage most frequently develops in patients who are restless. To prevent friction when moving up in bed, a patient who can lift independently should do so with a lift device or with use of the hands and arms. A patient who is dependent in care may need multiple caregivers to assist with moving up in bed while using a lift sheet or lift device to prevent the body from dragging.

When friction acts with gravity, the effect of the two factors is synergistic, and the outcome is shear. It is not possible to have shear without friction. However, it is possible to have friction without significant shear (such as from moving the heels repeatedly against the bed sheets).

Moisture. Moisture, specifically incontinence, is frequently cited in the literature as a predisposing factor to pressure ulcer development (Braden and Bergstrom, 1987). Persistent moisture alters the resiliency of the epidermis to external forces by weakening the lipid layer of the stratum corneum and collagen. Both shear and friction are increased in the presence of mild to moderate moisture but may be decreased in the presence of profuse moisture. The high-moisture environment created by urinary incontinence can impact the skin by alkalinizing the skin's pH, thereby altering normal skin flora. Persons with fecal incontinence are 22 times more likely to develop pressure ulcers than are persons without this condition (Thompson et al, 2005). The negative impact of prolonged moisture on the skin is discussed in greater detail in Chapter 5.

Intrinsic Factors that Affect Tissue Tolerance.

Nutritional Debilitation. Although good nutrition is necessary for wound healing, the role of significant nutritional debilitation in producing pressure ulcers is often less appreciated. Severe protein deficiency renders soft tissue more susceptible to breakdown when exposed to local pressure because hypoproteinemia alters oncotic pressure and causes edema formation. Oxygen diffusion and transport of nutrients in ischemic and edematous tissue are compromised. In addition, resistance to infection is decreased at low protein levels because of the effect on the immune system. Malnutrition has also been associated with altered tissue regeneration and inflammatory reaction, increased postoperative complications, increased risk of infection, sepsis, increased length of hospital stay, and death.

Certain vitamin deficiencies, particularly of vitamins A, C, and E, are a concern when assessing pressure ulcer risk. Vitamin A has a role in epithelial integrity, protein synthesis, and immune function; therefore a deficiency of vitamin A delays reepithelialization, collagen synthesis, and cellular cohesion. Vitamin C plays a role in collagen synthesis, enhanced activation of leukocytes and macrophages at a wound site, and immune function. Specific to wound healing, vitamin E aids in collagen synthesis, metabolism of fat, and stabilization of cell membranes (Posthauer, 2006).

All nutrients have an important role in maintaining skin integrity and in wound repair. Still, questions remain regarding how much supplementation of nutrients will positively affect outcomes. Meta-analyses of the clinical benefits of nutritional support in patients with or at risk for pressure ulcers showed an oral nutritional supplement was associated with a significantly lower incidence of pressure ulcer development in at-risk patients of 25% compared to routine care (Stratton et al, 2005). A Cochrane evaluation of enteral and parenteral nutrition on pressure ulcer prevention and treatment was not able to draw conclusions about the effect of such nutrition because of the small number of studies and methodologic issues with the studies (Langer et al, 2004). Researchers conclude that more research is needed about the impact of oral nutritional supplements and enteral tube feeding on prevention and treatment of pressure ulcers.

Advanced Age. Several changes occur in the skin and its supporting structures with aging. The dermoepidermal junction flattens, less nutrient exchange occurs, and less resistance to shear force is present (Pittman, 2007; Reddy, 2008). With aging, gradual atrophy and greater heterogeneity of blood and lymph vessels of human skin occur (Fore, 2006; Reddy, 2008). Changes in the cutaneous nerves lead to impaired early pain warning (Fore, 2006). Skin tears occur more commonly. Loss of dermal thickness occurs; the skin appears paper-thin and nearly transparent. Aging skin experiences decreased epidermal turnover, decreased surface barrier function, decreased sensory perception, decreased delayed and immediate hypersensitivity reaction, increased vascular fragility, loss of subcutaneous fat, and clustering of melanocytes (Fore, 2006; Pittman, 2007). With these changes, the ability of the soft tissue to distribute the mechanical load without compromising blood flow is impaired.

These changes combine with many other age-related changes that occur in other body systems to make the skin more vulnerable to pressure, shear, and friction (Pittman, 2007). For example, studies have shown that blood flow in the area of the ischial tuberosity while sitting on an unpadded surface is lower in paraplegic and geriatric populations than in normal patients.

Low Blood Pressure. Mayrovitz et al (2003) noted in a study about heels that persons with lower blood pressure need lower levels of pressure to cause breakdown to the heels. When interface pressures are near diastolic pressure, little if any functional pressure redistribution is realized. When perfusion is decreased by hypotension, shock, or dehydration, blood flow to the skin is likely to be compromised, thus increasing ischemia; deep tissues may be particularly vulnerable because of their extensive vascular supply (Berlowitz and Brienza, 2007). Hypotension may shunt blood flow away from the skin to more vital organs, thus decreasing the skin's tolerance for pressure by allowing capillaries to close at lower levels of interface pressure.

Stress. Early research identified psychosocial issues, such as emotional stress, as having an association with pressure ulcers. Cortisol may alter the mechanical properties of the skin by disproportionately increasing the rate of collagen degradation over collagen synthesis.

Glucocorticoids may trigger structural changes in connective tissue and may affect cellular metabolism by interfering with the diffusion of water, salt, and nutrients between the capillary bed and the cells. Hospitalization in acute or long-term care is stressful. In examining the relationship between stress and wound healing, stress has been negatively associated with healing. Cortisol may be the trigger for lowered tissue tolerance when a person is under stress. Cortisol is the primary glucocorticoid secreted when a person is exposed to a stressor and lacks appropriate coping mechanisms to mediate the stress-related hormonal response. Higher cortisol levels were related to longer time to heal (Ebrecht et al, 2004; Gouin et al, 2008). Many factors affect cortisol; they include advanced age, immobility, body fat, recent surgery, stroke, and malnutrition.

Smoking. Smoking is associated with tissue hypoxia, nicotine-induced stimulation of the sympathetic nervous system resulting in epinephrine that causes peripheral vasoconstriction and decreased circulation, carbon monoxide shift of the oxygen dissociation curve, and hydrogen cyanide interference with cellular oxygen metabolism (Ahn et al, 2008). Smoking must be considered in patients at risk for pressure ulcers. For patients with spinal cord injury, cigarette smoking was associated with a 1.16 incidence rate ratio for one or more pressure ulcers during the previous year (Smith et al, 2008).

Elevated Body Temperature. The body experiences a 10% increase in tissue metabolism with each 1°C rise in skin temperature (Aronovitch, 2007). Elevated body temperatures increase metabolic rates and subsequently increase oxygen consumption rates. Elevated skin temperature exacerbate the effects of ischemia by increasing the need for oxygen (Berlowitz and Brienza, 2007).

Miscellaneous Factors. Other conditions, such as those that create sluggish blood flow, anemia, blood dyscrasias, or poor oxygen perfusion, may be significant intrinsic factors jeopardizing tissue tolerance. For example, greater tissue damage has been associated with increased blood viscosity and high hematocrit level. This may explain why dehydration is sometimes mentioned as a contributing factor in pressure ulcer development.

PATHOPHYSIOLOGIC CHANGES

Two primary theories explain the mechanism of pressure ulcer formation and progression (Niezgoda and Mendez-Eastman, 2006). The deep tissue injury theory holds that pressure ulcers begin from the bone and move outward. Deep tissue injury occurs first near the bone, with ischemic injury and tissue destruction continuing in an outward manner. Deep muscle tissue appears to be more susceptible to pressure damage than are skin and fat (Berlowitz and Brienza, 2007). Although it is the less favored model of pressure ulcer development, the top-to-bottom model states pressure ulcer formation results from skin destruction

that occurs at the epidermis and proceeds to deeper tissue (Niezgoda and Mendez-Eastman, 2006).

If pressure is not relieved, ischemic changes occur as a consequence of decreased perfusion; however, the occlusion also triggers a cascade of events that intensifies the extent of tissue ischemia. Hence the tissue damage typically seen with pressure is precipitated by pressure but then worsened by a series of events, such as venous thrombus formation, endothelial cell damage, redistribution of blood supply in ischemic tissue, alteration in lymphatic flow, and alterations in interstitial fluid composition.

Berlowitz and Brienza (2007) listed the four commonly hypothesized pathophysiologic explanations for pressure ulcers: (1) ischemia caused by capillary occlusion; (2) reperfusion injury; (3) impaired lymphatic function that results in accumulation of metabolic waste products, proteins, and enzymes; and (4) prolonged mechanical deformation of tissue cells. Prolonged mechanical deformation of tissue cells refers to unrelieved pressure. The remaining three hypothesized pathophysiologic explanations for pressure ulcers are described here.

Ischemia Caused by Capillary Occlusion

Obstruction of capillary blood flow by externally applied pressure creates tissue ischemia (hypoxia). If the pressure is removed in a short period, blood flow returns and the skin can be seen to flush. This phenomenon, known as *reactive hyperemia,* is a compensatory mechanism whereby blood vessels in the pressure area dilate in an attempt to overcome the ischemic episode. Reactive hyperemia by definition is transient and may also be described as blanching erythema. Blanching erythema is an area of erythema that becomes white (blanches) when compressed with a finger. The erythema promptly returns when the compression is removed. The site may be painful for the patient with intact sensation. Blanching erythema is an early indication of pressure and usually will resolve without tissue loss if pressure is reduced or eliminated.

When hyperemia persists, deeper tissue damage should be suspected. Nonblanching erythema is a more serious sign of impaired blood supply and suggests that tissue destruction is imminent or has already occurred; it results from damage to blood vessels and extravasation of blood into the tissues. The color of the skin can be an intense bright red to dark red or purple. Many providers misdiagnose pressure-induced nonblanching erythema as hematoma or ecchymosis. When deep tissue damage is also present, the area is often either indurated or boggy when palpated.

When pressure occludes capillaries, a complex series of events is set into motion. Surrounding tissues become deprived of oxygen, and nutrients and metabolic wastes begin to accumulate in the tissue. Damaged capillaries become more permeable and leak fluid into the interstitial space, causing edema. Because perfusion through edematous tissue is slowed, tissue hypoxia worsens. Cellular death ensues, and more metabolic wastes are released into the surrounding tissue. Tissue inflammation is exacerbated, and more cellular death occurs (Figure 7-5). Considering data from surgical patients, animal models and in-vitro cell culture models, pressure ulcers in subdermal tissue under bony prominences very likely occur approximately between the first hour and 4 to 6 hours after sustained loading (Gefen, 2008).

Muscle damage may occur with pressure ulcers and is more significant than cutaneous damage. Pressure is highest at the point of contact between the soft tissue (e.g., muscle or fascia) and the bony prominence. This cone-shaped pressure gradient indicates that deep pressure ulcers initially form at the bone–soft tissue interface, not the skin surface, and extend outward to the skin (Figure 7-6). Thus deep tissue damage may occur with relatively little initial superficial evidence of damage to alert caregivers of its extensiveness. The skin damage seen in pressure ulcers is often referred to as the "tip of the iceberg" because a larger area of necrosis and ischemia is assumed to be present at the tissue–bone interface. Muscle and fat tissue loading over a bony prominence is substantially higher during sitting than lying down, so pressure ulcer and deep tissue injury development are likely to occur sooner while sitting versus lying down (Gefen, 2008).

Muscle tissue is the most vascularized tissue layer between bone and skin. It is the tissue with the highest metabolic demand and the lowest tolerance to mechanical compression (Gefen, 2008). In addition, atrophied,

scarred, or secondarily infected tissue has an increased susceptibility to pressure because of injured cells (Kumar et al, 2005b). An understanding of the structure of the vascular system allows formation of a rationale for this enhanced muscle damage.

The vascular circulation can be divided into three sections: segmental, perforator, and cutaneous. The segmental system is composed of the main arterial vessels arising from the aorta. The perforator system supplies the muscles but also serves as an interchange supply to the skin. The cutaneous system consists of arteries, capillary beds, and veins draining at different levels of the skin; it serves to provide thermoregulation and limited nutritional support. This indicates that occlusion of the perforator system may initiate muscle damage and may also create some of the cutaneous ischemia. The significance of perforator blood flow to skin damage has been demonstrated when musculocutaneous flaps have been elevated surgically.

Reperfusion Injury

As blood returns to tissue where it was occluded, an accumulation of damaged cellular byproducts and white blood cells obstructs the capillaries, and free radicals are released. The free radicals damage cellular proteins, DNA, and cell membranes and contribute to cell death (Fowler et al, 2008). Tissue injury increases with each ischemia–reperfusion cycle, the duration of ischemia, and the frequency of ischemia–reperfusion cycles (Farid, 2007).

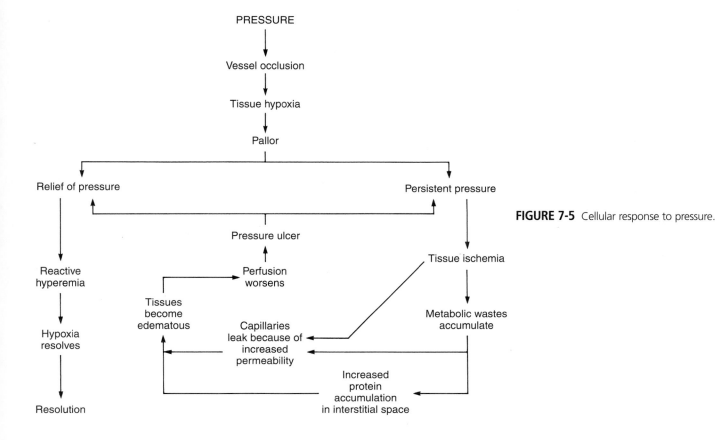

FIGURE 7-5 Cellular response to pressure.

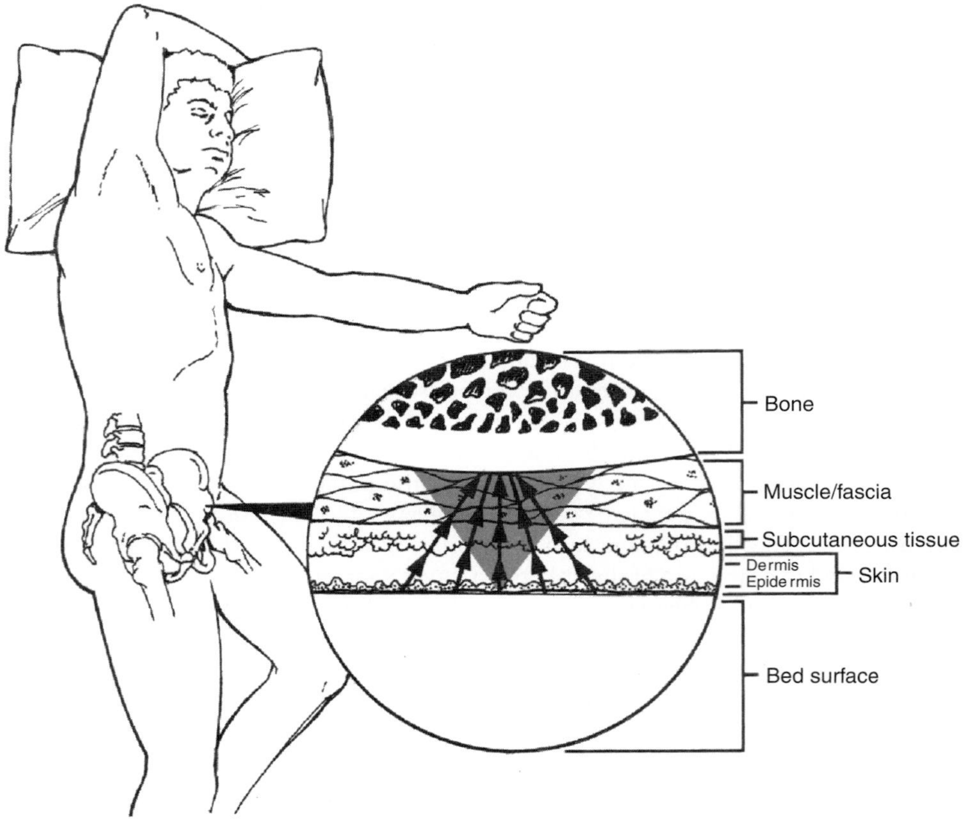

FIGURE 7-6 Amount of pressure exerted at skin level is dispersed over a large area and tapers to a point at the bone level (as indicated by the arrows), while the amount of tissue damage at the skin level is pinpoint and broadens to a larger amount of tissue damage at the bone interface (indicated by the shaded area).

Externally applied high pressures, even when applied for a short duration, damage the blood vessels directly, which in turn causes tissue ischemia. The changes in larger vessels and the formation of venous thrombi impair the normal reactive hyperemia that should occur once pressure is removed. Tissue remains ischemic even after the pressure has been alleviated.

Compression of the capillary wall also damages the endothelium. Complex pathologic changes in diverse cellular systems occur with ischemia. Up to a certain point and varying among different cell types, injury is amenable to repair, but with extension of ischemic duration, cell structures continue to deteriorate (Kumar et al, 2005b). Once pressure is removed and reperfusion begins, injury can be paradoxically exacerbated and proceed at an accelerated pace, and loss of additional cells occurs. As the endothelium is shed, platelets are activated by the underlying collagen, and clot formation is triggered. Furthermore, damaged endothelial cells lose their usual anticoagulant characteristics and release thrombogenic substances that exacerbate vessel occlusion and ultimately cause increased tissue ischemia.

The redistribution of the blood supply that occurs in ischemic skin further aggravates pressure-induced tissue hypoxia. Because of the externally applied pressure, blood flow to surface capillaries is reduced, and the reduction renders these vessels more vulnerable and more permeable than before.

Impaired Lymphatic Function

The lymphatic system has a critical role in body fluid and many other functions. It must act as a conduit that directs and regulates lymph flow and as a pump that generates lymph flow (Muthuchamy and Zawieja, 2008). Thus, the lymphatics are affected by pressure-induced ischemia. Lymphatic flow in pressure-damaged skin ceases. Likewise, the normal movement of interstitial fluid is inhibited by both pressure and ischemia. Consequently, protein is retained in the interstitial tissues, causing increased interstitial oncotic pressure, edema formation, dehydration of cells, and tissue irritation.

In summary, extensive or extended pressure occludes blood flow, lymphatic flow, and interstitial fluid movement. Tissues are deprived of oxygen and nutrients, and toxic metabolic products accumulate. Interstitial fluids retain proteins that dehydrate cells and irritate tissues. The ensuing tissue acidosis, capillary permeability, and edema contribute to cellular death.

CLASSIFICATION OF PRESSURE ULCERS

History and Purpose

During the 1980s the International Association for Enterostomal Therapy, now known as the WOCN Society, modified the Shea staging system, which originally was developed in 1975 (WOCN Society, 2003). In 2007, the

National Pressure Ulcer Advisory Panel (NPUAP) released an updated staging system (Box 7-1). The new system improved clarity and accuracy by adding more descriptors and creating definitions for suspected deep tissue injury and unstageable pressure ulcers (NPUAP, 2007). In 2009, international pressure ulcer guidelines were released. These guidelines use the same definitions but have added the term *category* and specify that the suspected deep tissue injury and unstageable are categories used in the United States (NPUAP and EPUAP, 2009).

Staging of tissue layers provides increased uniformity of language and a beginning basis for evaluation of protocols. Accurate staging requires knowledge of the anatomy of skin and deeper tissue layers, the ability to recognize these tissues, and the ability to differentiate among them. Careful evaluation of the wound bed facilitates accurate staging. Staging wounds is a complex skill that can take time to develop. The staging system, which is designed for use with pressure-induced ulcers only, is based on the ability to assess the type of tissue in the wound bed. Therefore a wound bed in which the base is covered with necrotic tissue cannot be accurately staged because of the inability to visualize the normal architecture of the wound bed. In such situations, "unstageable" should be documented. Examples of Stage I to IV pressure ulcers, suspected deep tissue injury, and unstageable pressure ulcers are provided in Plates 27 through 33. Box 7-2 gives the differential diagnosis of suspected deep tissue injury due to pressure (Ankrom et al, 2005).

Darker Skin Tones

Identifying deep tissue injury (suspected) and Stage I pressure ulcers in darker skin tones is difficult. Redness and other color changes are not as detectable with darker skin tones. Therefore other observable, pressure-related alterations of intact skin compared with the adjacent or opposite area on the body should be documented. Such

---

BOX 7-1	National Pressure Ulcer Advisory Panel (NPUAP) Pressure Ulcer Stages

Suspected Deep Tissue Injury
Purple or maroon localized area of discolored intact skin or blood-filled blister due to damage of underlying soft tissue from pressure and/or shear. The area may be preceded by tissue that is painful, firm, mushy, boggy, warmer or cooler compared to adjacent tissue.

Further Description
Deep tissue injury may be difficult to detect in individuals with dark skin tones. Evolution may include a thin blister over a dark wound bed. The wound may further evolve and become covered by thin eschar. Evolution may be rapid, exposing additional layers of tissue even with optimal treatment.

Stage I
Intact skin with nonblanchable redness of a localized area usually over a bony prominence. Darkly pigmented skin may not have visible blanching; its color may differ from the surrounding area.

Further Description
The area may be painful, firm, soft, warmer or cooler compared to adjacent tissue. Stage I may be difficult to detect in individuals with dark skin tones. May indicate "at risk" persons (a heralding sign of risk)

Stage II
Partial thickness loss of dermis presenting as a shallow open ulcer with a red–pink wound bed, without slough. May also present as intact or open/ruptured serum-filled blister.

Further Description
Presents as shiny or dry shallow ulcer without slough or bruising.* This stage should not be used to describe skin tears, tape burns, perineal dermatitis, maceration, or excoriation.

Stage III
Full-thickness tissue loss. Subcutaneous fat may be visible, but bone, tendon, or muscle is not exposed. Slough may be present but does not obscure the depth of tissue loss. May include undermining and tunneling.

Further Description
The depth of a Stage III pressure ulcer varies by anatomic location. The bridge of the nose, ear, occiput, and malleolus do not have subcutaneous tissue, and Stage III ulcers can be shallow. In contrast, areas of significant adiposity can develop in extremely deep Stage III pressure ulcers. Bone/tendon is not visible or directly palpable.

Stage IV
Full-thickness tissue loss with exposed bone, tendon, or muscle. Slough or eschar may be present on some parts of the wound bed. Often include undermining and tunneling.

Further Description
The depth of a Stage IV pressure ulcer varies by anatomic location. The bridge of the nose, ear, occiput, and malleolus do not have subcutaneous tissue, and these ulcers can be shallow. Stage IV ulcers can extend into muscle and/or supporting structures (e.g., fascia, tendon, joint capsule), making osteomyelitis possible. Exposed bone/tendon is visible or directly palpable.

Unstageable
Full-thickness tissue loss in which the base of the ulcer is covered by slough (yellow, tan, gray, green, or brown) and/or eschar (tan, brown, or black) in the wound bed.

Further Description
Until enough slough and/or eschar is removed to expose the base of the wound, the true depth, and therefore the stage, cannot be determined. Stable (dry, adherent, intact without erythema or fluctuance) eschar on the heels serves as the "body's natural (biologic) cover" and should not be removed.

From National Pressure Ulcer Advisory Panel (NPUAP) and European Pressure Ulcer Advisory Panel (EPUAP): Treatment of pressure ulcers, Washington DC, 2009, National Pressure Ulcer Advisory Panel.
*Bruising indicates suspected deep tissue injury.

BOX 7-2 | **Differential Diagnosis of Suspected Deep Tissue Injury Due to Pressure**

Bruise: Extravasation of blood in the tissues as a result of blunt force impact to the body. Usually about 2 weeks is required for a bruise to heal under normal conditions. History of trauma is common.

Calciphylaxis: Vascular calcification and skin necrosis most common in patients with long-standing history of chronic renal failure and renal replacement therapy. Lesions may have a violaceous hue and be excruciatingly tender and extremely firm. Lesions are most commonly seen on the lower extremities, not over bony prominences. The incidence of these lesions is very low in general patient populations.

Fournier's gangrene: Intensely painful necrotizing fasciitis of the perineum. May manifest initially as cellulitis.

Hematoma: Deep-seated purple nodule from clotted blood, usually associated with trauma.

Perirectal abscess: First sign commonly is a dull, aching, or throbbing pain in the perianal area. The pain worsens when sitting and immediately before defecation; the pain abates after defecation. A tender, fluctuant mass may be palpated at the anal verge. These abscesses can open to reveal large cavities, which can be confused with deep pressure ulcers.

---

indicators include changes in skin tissue consistency (firm versus boggy when palpated), sensation (pain), and warmer or cooler temperature (Black et al, 2007). Box 3-1 lists unique characteristics of darker versus lighter pigmented skin, and Checklist 6-1 gives points to consider when assessing darkly pigmented skin.

Mucosal Pressure Ulcers

Mucous tissues (i.e., lining of the gastrointestinal [GI] tract, oral cavity, nares, etc.) are also vulnerable to pressure ulcers from the presence of medical devices such as oxygen tubing, endotracheal tubes, bite blocks, nasogastric tubes, urinary catheters and fecal containment devices. These ulcers cannot be staged using the pressure ulcer staging system nor classified as partial or full thickness because the histology of mucous membrane tissue is different than skin. Therefore, pressure ulcers on mucous membranes should be documented simply as mucosal pressure ulcers (NPUAP, 2009).

Reverse Staging

The practice of reverse staging, in which the wound is described as progressing from a Stage III to a Stage II to a Stage I pressure ulcer, is incorrect. Once layers of tissue and supporting structures are gone (such as with full-thickness wounds), they are not replaced. Instead, the wound is filled with granulation tissue. This staging system is to be used for describing wounds in their most

severe state and once the wounds are accurately described, these descriptor levels endure, even in the presence of healing (Black et al, 2007). Negative outcomes of reverse staging can lead to (1) denial of acute or skilled care after Stage IV ulcers have been restaged as Stage II ulcers; (2) withdrawal of pressure-reducing support surfaces when ulcers have "healed" from Stage III or Stage IV to Stage II; and (3) lower fees paid to extended-care facilities for care of patients with healing Stage III and Stage IV ulcers that have been reclassified as Stage II or Stage I pressure ulcers. Therefore a Stage III pressure ulcer that appears to be granulating and resurfacing is described as a healing Stage III pressure ulcer.

SUMMARY

Pressure ulcers present a significant economic, quality-of-life, and overall health care threat worldwide. Standards for assessment and care initially presented by the WOCN Society have now been published by a number of dedicated disciplines and groups around the world. Once a problem considered a side effect of aging, pressure ulcers have captured the attention of payers and regulators. Pressure ulcers now are more commonly considered preventable and unacceptable (in most cases) and are considered an indicator of quality care.

REFERENCES

Ahn C et al: Smoking—the bane of wound healing: biomedical interventions and social influences, *Adv Skin Wound Care* 21:227, 2008.

Ankrom M et al; for the National Pressure Ulcer Advisory Panel (NPUAP): Pressure-related deep tissue injury under intact skin and the current pressure ulcer staging systems, *Adv Skin Wound Care* 18:35-42, 2005.

Armstrong DG et al: New opportunities to improve pressure ulcer prevention and treatment: implications of the CMS inpatient hospital care present on admission (POA) indicators/hospital-acquired conditions (HAC) policy. A consensus paper from the international expert wound care advisory panel, *J Wound Ostomy Continence Nurs* 35:485, 2008.

Arnold HL: Decubitus: the word. In Parish LC et al, editors: *The decubitus ulcer,* New York, 1983, Masson.

Aronovitch SA: Intraoperatively acquired pressure ulcers: are there common risk factors? *Ostomy Wound Manage* 53:57, 2007.

Ayello EA, Lyder CH: A new era of pressure ulcer accountability in acute care, *Adv Skin Wound Care* 21:134, 2008.

Baumgarten M et al: Pressure ulcers and the transition to long-term care, *Adv Skin Wound Care* 16:299, 2003.

Bell-Syer SE et al: The Cochrane Wounds Group: systematically reviewing the wound care literature, *Adv Skin Wound Care* 20:283, 2007.

Bennett LM et al: Skin stress and blood flow in sitting paraplegic patients, *Arch Phys Med Rehabil* 65:1861, 1984.

Berlowitz DR, Brienza DM: Are all pressure ulcers the result of deep tissue injury? A review of the literature, *Ostomy Wound Manage* 53:34, 2007.

Black J et al: National Pressure Ulcer Advisory Panel's updated pressure ulcer staging system, *Adv Skin Wound Care* 20:269, 2007.

Bolton L et al: Assessing the need for developing a comprehensive content-validated pressure ulcer guideline, *Ostomy Wound Manage* 54:22, 2008.

Braden BJ, Bergstrom N: A conceptual schema for the study of the etiology of pressure sores, *Rehabil Nurs* 12(1):81, 1987.

Burton AC, Yamada S: Relation between blood pressure and flow in the human forearm, *J Appl Physiol* 4:3291, 1951.

Compher C et al: Obesity reduces the risk of pressure ulcers in elderly hospitalized patients, *J Gerontol A Biol Sci Med Sci* 62:1310, 2007.

Ebrecht M et al: Perceived stress and cortisol levels predict speed of wound healing in healthy male adults, *Psychoneuroendocrinology* 29:798, 2004.

Edsberg LE: Pressure ulcer tissue histology: an appraisal of current knowledge, *Ostomy Wound Manage* 53:40, 2007.

Farid KJ: Applying observations from forensic science to understanding the development of pressure ulcers, *Ostomy Wound Manage* 53:26, 2007.

Fore J: A review of skin and the effects of aging on skin structure and function, *Ostomy Wound Manage* 52:24, 2006.

Fowler E et al: Practice recommendations for preventing heel pressure ulcers, *Ostomy Wound Manage* 54:42, 2008.

Fox J, Bradley R: *A new medical dictionary*, London, 1803. Darton & Harvey.

Gefen A: Bioengineering models of deep tissue injury, *Adv Skin Wound Care* 21:30, 2008.

Gouin JP et al: The influence of anger expression on wound healing, *Brain Behav Immun* 22:699, 2008.

Husain T: An experimental study of some pressure effects on tissues, with reference to the bedsore problem, *J Pathol Bacteriol* 66:3471, 1953.

Keast DH et al: Best practice recommendations for the prevention and treatment of pressure ulcers: update 2006, *Adv Skin Wound Care* 20:337, 2007.

Keelaghan E, Margolis D, et al: Prevalence of pressure ulcers on hospital admission among nursing home residents transferred to the hospital, *Wound Repair Regen.* 16(3):331-336, 2008.

Knudsen A, Gallagher S: Care of the obese patient with pressure ulcers, *J Wound, Ostomy and Continence Nursing* 30(2):111-118, 2003.

Kosiak M, et al: Evaluation of pressure as a factor in the production of ischial ulcers, *Arch Phys Med Rehabil* 39:623-629, 1958.

Kosiak M: Etiology of decubitus ulcers, *Arch Phys Med Rehabil* 42:191, 1961.

Krapfl LA: Inpatient prospective payment changes: a guide for the WOC nurse, *WOCNews* 3:16, 2008.

Krouskop TA: A synthesis of the factors that contribute to pressure sore formation, *Med Hypotheses* 11(2):2551, 1983.

Kumar V et al: Acute and chronic inflammation, in *Robbins and Cotran pathologic basis of disease*, Philadelphia, 2005a, Elsevier Saunders.

Kumar V et al: Cellular adaptations, cell injury, and cell death, in *Robbins and Cotran pathologic basis of disease*, Philadelphia, 2005b, Elsevier Saunders.

Landi F et al: Pressure ulcer and mortality in frail elderly people living in community, *Arch Gerontol Geriatr* 44(Suppl 1):217, 2007.

Langemo DK: Quality of life and pressure ulcers: what is the impact? *Wounds* 17:3, 2005.

Langer G et al: Nutritional interventions for preventing and treating pressure ulcers, *Cochrane Database Syst Rev* 2, 2004.

Lindan O: Etiology of decubitus ulcers: an experimental study, *Arch Phys Med Rehabil* 42:774, 1961.

Mathison CJ: Skin and wound care challenges in the hospitalized morbidly obese patient, *J WOCN* 30:78, 2003.

Mayrovitz HN et al: Effects of support surface relief pressures on heel skin blood perfusion, *Adv Skin Wound Care* 16:141, 2003.

McLane KM et al: The 2003 National Pediatric Pressure Ulcer and Skin Breakdown Prevalence Survey: a multisite study, *J Wound Ostomy Continence Nurs* 31:168, 2004.

Montalvo I: The National Database of Nursing Quality Indicators™ (NDNQI®), *OJIN: The Online Journal of Issues in Nursing*, 12(3), 2007. Available at www.nursingworld.org/MainMenuCategories/ANAMarketplace/ANAPeriodicals/OJIN/TableofContents/Volume122007/No3Sept07/NursingQualityIndicators.aspx. Accessed 10/11/2009

Muthuchamy M, Zawieja D: Molecular regulation of lymphatic contractility, *Ann N Y Acad Sci* 1131:89, 2008.

Nakagami G et al: Comparison of two pressure ulcer preventive dressings for reducing shear force on the heel, *J Wound Ostomy Continence Nurs* 33:267, 2006.

National Pressure Ulcer Advisory Panel (NPUAP): *Pressure ulcers in America: prevalence, incidence, and implications for the future*, Cuddigan J et al, editors, Reston, Va, 2001, Author.

National Pressure Ulcer Advisory Panel (NPUAP): *Pressure ulcer stages revised by NPUAP 2007*, available at http://www.npuap.org/pr2.htm, accessed January 27, 2009.

National Pressure Ulcer Advisory Panel (NPUAP): *Mucosal pressure ulcers an NPUAP position statement, 2009*. Available at http://www.npuap.org/Mucosal_Pressure_Ulcer_Position_Statement_final.pdf, accessed April 27, 2010.

National Pressure Ulcer Advisory Panel (NPUAP) and European Pressure Ulcer Advisory Panel (EPUAP): Pressure ulcer prevention & treatment: clinical practice guideline, In Cuddigan J, Langemo D, editors: *International pressure ulcer guidelines for prevention and treatment*, Washington DC, 2009, Author.

Niezgoda JA, Mendez-Eastman S: The effective management of pressure ulcers, *Adv Skin Wound Care* 19(Suppl 1):3, 2006.

Padula CA et al: Prevention and early detection of pressure ulcers in hospitalized patients, *J Wound Ostomy Continence Nurs* 35:65, 2008.

Peterson M et al: Effects of elevating the head of bed on interface pressure in volunteers, *Crit Care Med* 36:3038, 2008.

Pieper B et al: Pressure ulcer pain: a systematic literature review and National Pressure Ulcer Advisory Panel white paper, *Ostomy Wound Manage* 55:14, 2009.

Pittman J: Effect of aging on wound healing, *J Wound Ostomy Continence Nurs* 34:412, 2007.

Posthauer ME: The role of nutrition in wound care, *Adv Skin Wound Care* 19:43, 2006

Price MC et al: Development of a risk assessment tool for intraoperative pressure ulcers, *J WOCN* 32:19, 2005.

Reddy M: Skin and wound care: important considerations in the older adult, *Adv Skin Wound Care* 21:424, 2008.

Redelings MD et al: Pressure ulcers: more lethal than we thought? *Adv Skin Wound Care* 18:367, 2005.

Registered Nurses Association of Ontario (RNAO): *Risk assessment and prevention of pressure ulcers*, Toronto, 2005, Author.

Russo CA et al: *Hospitalizations related to pressure ulcers among adults 18 years and older, 2006*, HCUP Statistical Brief #64, 2008. Available at http://www.hcup-us.ahrq.gov/reports/statbriefs/sb64.pdf. Accessed 10/11/2009

Schoonhoven L et al: Risk indicators for pressure ulcers during surgery, *Appl Nurs Res* 15(3):163, 2002.

Schubart JR et al: Pressure ulcer prevention and management in spinal cord-injured adults: analysis of educational needs, *Adv Skin Wound Care* 21:322, 2008.

Shukla VK et al: Risk assessment for pressure ulcer: a hospital-based study, *J Wound Ostomy Continence Nurs* 35:407, 2008.

Siem CA et al: Skin assessment and pressure ulcer care in hospital-based skilled nursing facilities, *Ostomy Wound Manage* 49(6):42, 2003.

Smith BM et al: Factors predicting pressure ulcers in veterans with spinal cord injuries, *Am J Phys Med Rehabil* 87:750, 2008.

Stechmiller JK et al: Guidelines for the prevention of pressure ulcers. *Wound Repair Regen* 16(2): 151-168, 2008.

Stratton RJ et al: Enteral nutritional support in prevention and treatment of pressure ulcers: a systematic review and meta-analysis, *Ageing Res Rev* 4:422, 2005.

Thompson P et al: Skin care protocols for pressure ulcers and incontinence in long-term care: a quasi-experimental study, *Adv Skin Wound Care* 18:422, 2005.

U.S. Department of Health and Human Services: *Healthy people 2010*, Washington, DC, 2000, Author.

VanGilder C et al: Results of nine international pressure ulcer prevalence surveys: 1989 to 2005, *Ostomy Wound Manage* 54:40, 2008.

Whitney J et al: Guidelines for the treatment of pressure ulcer, *Wound Repair Regen* 14(6):663-679, 2008.

Whittington KT, Briones R: National prevalence and incidence study: 6-year sequential acute care data, *Adv Skin Wound Care* 17:490, 2004.

Wound, Ostomy and Continence Nurses (WOCN) Society: *Guideline for prevention and management of pressure ulcers*, Glenview, IL, 2003, Author.

Wound, Ostomy and Continence Nurses (WOCN) Society: *Prevalence and incidence: a toolkit for clinicians*, Glenview, IL, 2004, Author.

Wound, Ostomy and Continence Nurses (WOCN) Society: *Guideline for prevention and management of pressure ulcers*, Glenview, IL, 2010, Author.

8

Developing and Maintaining a Pressure Ulcer Prevention Program

Ruth A. Bryant and Denise P. Nix

OBJECTIVES

1. Explain three justifications for a pressure ulcer prevention program.
2. Distinguish between an avoidable and an unavoidable pressure ulcer.
3. List components of a best practice bundle of a pressure ulcer prevention program.
4. Distinguish between a pressure ulcer risk assessment and a skin assessment.
5. Identify the risk factor subscales in the Braden Scale for Predicting Pressure Sore Risk.
6. Distinguish between turning and repositioning.
7. Describe five repositioning techniques.
8. Describe why infrastructure is important to the maintenance of a successful pressure ulcer prevention program.
9. Provide examples of how an organization demonstrates skin safety as an organizational priority.

Every health care facility and health care unit needs a pressure ulcer prevention program (PUPP). When creating a PUPP, both the structure of the program (best practice bundle) and the operations of the program (infrastructure) must be addressed. From a structural perspective, the best practice bundle of the PUPP has six basic components: skin inspection, risk assessment, pressure redistribution and offloading, maintaining skin health, nutrition and hydration, and patient and family education. For a successful PUPP, the bundle must then be integrated into the culture and infrastructure of the health care system, and all caregivers and administration must share the belief that pressure ulcers are a negative outcome and that all health care providers play a role in prevention. In this chapter, we define and discuss the structure of a PUPP and steps for integration into the care delivery system to ensure ongoing viability and growth of the program.

PUPP JUSTIFICATION

There are numerous reasons to justify a PUPP. Certainly economics has heightened the interest of some, but the most important reasons stem from a concern for patient safety and quality care.

Effectiveness

The most compelling argument for implementing a PUPP is that such programs have been shown to be effective in reducing the incidence of nosocomial pressure ulcers which has become a national priority. After implementing a statewide safe skin initiative, the Minnesota Department of Health (2009) reported a 25% decrease in Stage III and IV pressure ulcers over the course of 2 years. The website for the Institute for Healthcare Improvement (IHI) (2008) reports a number of PUPPs (e.g., Children's Healthcare of Atlanta at Eggleston, Nebraska Medical Center, Yuma Regional Medical Center) that have successfully decreased the incidence of pressure ulcers to a range from 1% to 3.5%.

National Priority

As early as 2000, the U.S. Department of Health and Human Services (2000) document, *Healthy People 2010: Understanding and Improving Health*, listed reducing pressure ulcer incidence as an objective for all health care providers. According to the National Priorities Partnership (2008), medical errors kill 98,000 Americans each year and are a leading cause of mortality and morbidity in the United States, with an estimated cost of $17 to $29 billion per year. It is estimated that the United States spends approximately $11 billion on pressure ulcers alone each year (Redelings et al, 2005). These statistics are startling when we consider the fact that people come to the hospital when they are ill, trusting that they will be taken care of and protected from adversities. Medical errors that are clearly identifiable, preventable, and associated with serious consequences have been termed *never events* by the National Quality Forum. In its mission to "fundamentally transform health care," the National Priorities Partnership, which consists of members from 26 different national organizations and is convened by the National Quality Forum, announced six national priorities to direct health care reform to eliminate waste, harm and inequities. Safety (the elimination of errors whenever and wherever possible) is one such priority and incorporates severe pressure ulcers, defined as Stage III or IV (Robert Wood Johnson Foundation, 2008). The IHI also identified the prevention of pressure ulcers as one of the 12 interventions in its 5 Million Lives campaign (Duncan, 2007).

These positions represent a dramatic shift in public policy. Pressure ulcer prevention has been in the mission of the Wound, Ostomy and Continence Nurses (WOCN) Society (previously known as the International Association for Enterostomal Therapy [IAET]) and is included in the curriculum for WOC nursing education programs since 1982 (Alterescu, 1991; Goode, 1991; IAET, 1987; Wright, 1991). As new technology evolved, risk assessment refined, and pressure ulcer prevention interventions better understood, it was generally accepted by wound care experts that all pressure ulcers could be prevented and that their presence was a reflection on quality of care. In fact, the 5 Million Lives campaign by the IHI launched in 2007 specifically states "the goal for pressure ulcer incidence should be zero" (Duncan, 2007). Most recently, the concept of attaining a zero incidence of facility-acquired pressure ulcers is increasingly being challenged.

Reimbursement for Present on Admission Only

In addition to the effectiveness of a PUPP in reducing injury to patients, implementation of these programs can affect facility reimbursement. Noting that hospital-acquired conditions could be *reasonably prevented* with evidence-based guidelines, the Centers for Medicare & Medicaid Services (CMS) discontinued additional payment to hospitals for pressure ulcers that were not present on admission (POA). Because patients with hospital-acquired pressure ulcers tend to have a longer length of stay (12–14 days), reimbursement for hospital care may be further compromised. Checklist 8-1 provides the indicators for Stage III or IV pressure ulcers POA. The WOCN Society (2008) has published a useful guidance document to assist with interpreting the POA

CHECKLIST 8-1
Indicators for Stage III to IV Pressure Ulcers POA

✓ Present at time the order for inpatient admission occurs. Pressure ulcer that developed during an outpatient encounter, including the emergency department, observation, or outpatient surgery, is considered POA.
✓ Pressure ulcer diagnosis documented by "provider." A provider is a physician or any qualified health care practitioner who is legally accountable for establishing the patient's diagnosis.
✓ Determination of whether the pressure ulcer was POA is based on the provider's best clinical judgment anytime during the hospital stay.
✓ Inconsistent, missing, or conflicting documentation issues are resolved by the physician.
✓ Pressure ulcer is POA when the patient is discharged with a facility-acquired pressure ulcer and later readmitted with a different diagnosis.

Adapted from Wound, Ostomy and Continence Nurses (WOCN) Society: *Inpatient prospective payment changes: a guide for the WOC nurse*, 2008, available at http://www.wocn.org/About_Us/News/30/, accessed August 17, 2010. *POA*, Present on admission.

---

rule. The document clarifies the role of the WOC nurse, coder, and physician in determining whether the pressure ulcer is POA and what code to assign. For example, a suspected deep tissue injury (sDTI) is coded as an unstageable pressure ulcer. The POA rule emphasizes the importance of the PUPP component of skin inspection upon admission to any health care facility to establish a baseline for the patient so that subsequent pressure-related abnormalities in the skin can be identified.

Ability to Identify the Unavoidable Pressure Ulcer

By stating "hospital-acquired conditions (such as pressure ulcers) could be *reasonably prevented* with evidence-based guidelines," the CMS introduces the possibility that some pressure ulcers cannot be avoided. The paucity of evidence of the ability to bring the incidence of pressure ulcers to zero despite extensive prevention interventions further challenges the long-held belief that all pressure ulcers are preventable (Thomas, 2003). When Hagisawa and Barbenel (1999) reported 4.4% as the lowest incidence of pressure ulcers in severely ill patients despite receiving comprehensive and extensive pressure ulcer prevention care, they suggested the concept of a "limit of prevention." This idea supports the argument that not all pressure ulcers are avoidable even with risk assessment and appropriate preventive interventions.

Prior to the introduction of POA for hospitals, CMS defined the term *unavoidable pressure ulcer* (for the long-term care setting) as a pressure ulcer that develops in spite of the facility's best efforts at prevention (Checklist 8-2). However, a similar definition by the CMS for the hospital or home care setting does not exist. The WOCN Society recognized the absence of a definition for acute care as a

CHECKLIST 8-2

Avoidable and Unavoidable Pressure Ulcers

Avoidable

The resident developed a pressure ulcer and the facility did *not* do one or more of the following:

✓ Evaluate the resident's clinical condition and pressure ulcer risk factors

✓ Define and implement interventions that are consistent with the resident's needs and goals and with recognized standards of practice

✓ Monitor and evaluate the impact of interventions

✓ Revise the interventions as appropriate

Unavoidable

The resident developed a pressure ulcer even though the facility *did* the following:

✓ Evaluated the resident's clinical condition and pressure ulcer risk factors

✓ Defined and implemented interventions that were consistent with the resident's needs and goals and with recognized standards of practice

✓ Monitored and evaluated the impact of interventions

✓ Revised the interventions as appropriate

CHECKLIST 8-3

Pressure Ulcer Prevention Best Practice Audit

✓ Pressure ulcer risk assessment was documented on admission and daily.

✓ Skin inspection was documented on admission and daily.

✓ Removal of devices, such as stockings and splints, at least twice a day was documented.

✓ Devices that cannot be removed, such as indwelling tubes and drains, are stabilized and repositioned for daily skin inspection.

✓ Documented care plan linked risk assessment findings to specific preventive interventions.

✓ Patients with impaired sensory perception, mobility, and activity as defined by the risk assessment scale had the following applicable interventions documented:

• Repositioning every 2 hours

• Heels off bed

• Appropriate support surfaces (mattresses, chair cushions) for pressure redistribution

✓ Patients with friction/shear risk as defined by the Braden scale had head of bed elevated ≤30 degrees documented (if medically contraindicated, physician's order and alternative plan to prevent shear injury were documented).

✓ Patients with nutritional deficits as defined by the Braden scale were followed by dietary services once the deficit was identified.

✓ Patients with incontinence have documentation that perineal cleanser and barrier were used and the underlying cause addressed.

✓ Patient/family skin safety education and patient response were documented.

✓ Standard skin safety interventions that were determined to be medically contraindicated or inconsistent with the patient's overall goals were documented or ordered by a physician and reevaluated routinely.

✓ Inability to adhere to standard skin safety interventions (i.e., noncompliance) was documented with evidence of patient/family education and ongoing efforts to reeducate or modify care plan.

potential problem. To fill this gap, the WOCN Society released a position statement *(Avoidable versus Unavoidable Pressure Ulcers)* using the CMS definition of an unavoidable pressure ulcer and refuting the assumption that all pressure ulcers are preventable (WOCN Society, 2009).

A PUPP is based on evidence-based guidelines or best practice and therefore provides a structure in which unavoidable pressure ulcers may be identified. Identifying a potentially unavoidable pressure ulcer may not assist with reimbursement in hospitals. However, it will help to identify whether best practice was delivered and therefore may be useful in protecting against litigation. In addition, this definition of avoidable and unavoidable is useful in the population of patients at end of life who may develop a pressure ulcer. While there is support for the concept of skin failure (NPUAP, 2010) as end of life is near, there is no definitive confirmation that this concept is real. For now, the current definition of avoidable and unavoidable pressure ulcers allows for the possibility that a patient at the end of life could develop a pressure ulcer despite appropriate care. However, this definition also protects the patient from the assumption that all pressure ulcers at the end of life are unavoidable. Under the current definition, documentation is the only way to determine if a pressure ulcer was or was not avoidable. See Checklist 8-3 for examples of relevant audit questions for the patient's medical record.

Protect Facility's Reputation

Patient trust and facility reputation are another justification for PUPP implementation as patient safety becomes transparent through published reports on the Internet

and the ability of consumers to compare facility outcomes. Beyond the financial, physical, and psychological impact, errors in patient care are costly in terms of loss of trust in the system by patients, diminished satisfaction by both patients and health professionals, and loss of morale by health care professionals who are not able to provide the best care possible.

COMPONENTS OF A PUPP

A PUPP consists of a *best practice bundle* and *infrastructure* (operations). The components of a PUPP have been widely adopted by WOC nurses for years (Bryant et al, 1992) and were included in the 1992 AHCPR Pressure Ulcers Prevention Guideline. Historically, PUPPs have been demonstrated to be effective at reducing the incidence of pressure ulcers. However, the implementation, maintenance, and survival of the PUPP was often dependent on WOC nurse involvement. While the successful PUPP may be coordinated by the wound specialist, it should not be owned or dependent on one individual or group. Rather, it must be adopted into the facility's overall patient safety culture of the facility, supported and protected by administration, and therefore integrated into the facility's infrastructure.

ESTABLISHING A BEST PRACTICE BUNDLE

From a structural perspective, the best practice bundle of the PUPP has six components: skin inspection, risk assessment, maintain skin health, pressure redistribution, nutrition and hydration, and patient education. The best practice bundle includes research-based evidence and, when a higher level of evidence is not available, expert opinion.

Skin Inspection and Assessment

A skin inspection should be obtained for all patients upon admission. Because the admission inspection serves as a baseline for comparisons and pressure ulcers can develop quickly, this skin inspection should be obtained as soon as possible. Although the exact time frame for obtaining a skin inspection is not specified in the literature, physiologically a pressure can develop as soon as one hour (Gefen, 2008). Therefore, it may be reasonable to inspect the skin within the first few hours of admission given the need for patient repositioning and other cares that are conducive for skin inspection (see Table 6-1). Subsequent inspection and monitoring by trained staff is recommended at least daily for patients at risk for pressure ulcers or who have impaired skin integrity (NPUAP and EPUAP, 2009). Deviations from normal should be compared with the adjacent skin or contralateral body part and documented. Optimal visualization and palpation of skin changes require adequate lighting, removal of garments, repositioning of medical devices, and the spreading of skin folds, buttocks, and toes. Unlike inspection, skin *assessment* involves interpretation and synthesis of additional data gathered from the comprehensive holistic patient assessment such as nutrition, perfusion, medications, and other comorbidities. Chapter 6 presents a detailed discussion related to skin assessment, inspection, and monitoring, including considerations for darkly pigmented skin (see Checklist 6-1).

Risk Assessment and Screening

Chapter 7 presents a theoretical framework of pressure ulcer development and a description of intrinsic and extrinsic factors that place a patient at risk for pressure ulcer development (Figure 7-2). As with other assessments, pressure ulcer risk assessment includes identification of subjective, objective, and psychosocial factors to determine and assess the risk and care needs of the patient (Stechmiller et al, 2008). Many of these risk factors at first glance seem intuitive. However, due to highly variable experiences and knowledge among caregivers, the accuracy of clinical judgment and intuitive sense in identifying those at risk is not reliable (Bolton, 2007; Pancorbo-Hidalgo et al, 2006). Furthermore, the assumption that all patients are at risk and that preventive measures should be universally applied is difficult to defend due to the inefficient use of resources. Therefore, to enhance the accuracy of pressure ulcer risk assessment a validated risk screening scale must be inluded (NPUAP and EPUAP, 2009; WOCN Society 2003, 2010; Stechmiller et al, 2008).

A risk scale is a noninvasive, cost-effective method for distinguishing between patients who are at risk for developing a pressure ulcer from those who are not. Scales identify the extent to which a person exhibits a specific risk factor, thus directing the selection of interventions needed (Braden, 2010). In selecting a scale for predicting a condition such as a pressure ulcer, the scale must have demonstrated reliability and validity. *Reliability* refers to the degree to which the results obtained by the measurement procedure can be replicated. For example, if two nurses administered a pressure ulcer risk scale on the same patient at the same time and their scores were the same, the reliability of the scale would be a perfect 1.0, or 100% agreement. *Validity* refers to accuracy. A screening test such as a pressure ulcer risk scale should provide a good preliminary test of which individuals actually are at risk and which are not. Validity has two components: *sensitivity,* which correctly identifies patients at risk, and *specificity,* which correctly identifies patients not at risk. An ideal risk scale would be 100% sensitive and 100% specific, so it does not overpredict (therefore no false-positive scores) or underpredict (no false-negative scores). However, 100% is rarely achieved due to an inverse relationship between sensitivity and specificity; as the scale becomes more sensitive, specificity declines. Nevertheless, these measures of predictability are invaluable when comparing tools that attempt to predict a condition such as pressure ulcer.

The validity and reliability of several pressure ulcer risk assessment scales have been reported in the literature and summarized in a synthesis and systematic review (Bolton, 2007; Pancorbo-Hidalgo, 2006). Recommendations related to pressure ulcer risk assessment, such as frequency, who should administer, and which patients should be assessed, are summarized in Box 8-1 (see Appendix B for examples of risk assessment scales).

Using the Braden Scale. One of the most widely used and researched pressure ulcer risk tools is the Braden Scale for the Prediction of Pressure Ulcer Risk (Stechmiller et al, 2008). Translated into many languages, numerous reports attest to the reliability (0.83–0.95) of the scale with adequately trained registered nurses and licensed practical nurses (Magnan and Maklebust, 2008, 2009). Following meta-analysis, specificity and sensitivity of the Braden scale are reported to be 68% and 57%, respectively. In the same analysis, the percent correctly classified was reported

- Pressure ulcer risk assessment scales should be administered to all patients with one or more risk factors for pressure ulcer development when admitted to a hospital's medical, surgical, intensive care, orthopedic, cardiovascular, or step-down unit, home care, hospice, or extended care facility (Bolton, 2007).
- Reassessment should occur
  - Regularly and frequently as required by the patient's condition (NPUAP and EPUAP, 2009, WOCN Society, 2010)
  - When the patient's condition changes (NPUAP and EPUAP, 2009)
  - Acute care: At least every 48 hours or whenever the patient's condition changes (WOCN Society, 2003, 2010)
  - Long-term care: Weekly for the first 4 weeks, monthly, then quarterly after that or when the patient's condition changes (WOCN Society, 2003).
  - Home care: Every Nurse Visit (WOCN Society, 2010)
- The Braden scale (Table 8-1) then the Norton and Waterloo scales (Appendix B) have strongest body of evidence supporting validity and reliability (Bolton, 2007).
- Pressure ulcer risk assessment scales should be administered by professional nurse (Bolton, 2007).
- Braden and Norton scales have demonstrated interrater reliability when administered by both registered nurses and licensed practical nurses (Bolton, 2007).
- Risk assessment is not valid and reliable unless those administering the assessment have access to the complete scale and subscale descriptors (Bolton, 2007).

as 67%, the positive predictive value was 23%, and the negative predictive value was 91% (Bolton, 2007).

The Braden scale is composed of six risk factor subscales that conceptually reflect degrees of sensory perception, skin moisture, physical activity, nutritional intake, friction and shear, and ability to change and control body position. All subscales are rated from 1 (most risk) to 4 (least risk), except for the friction and shear subscale, which is rated from 1 to 3. Each rating is accompanied by a brief description of criteria for assigning the rating. Therefore the subscales identify which risk factors are present so that interventions can be targeted to reduce specific risk factors (Table 8-2) (WOCN Society, 2010).

Potential total scores range from 4 to 23. Based on research in three types of settings, the critical cutoff score has been set at 18. A score of 18 results in higher overprediction but decreases the number of false-negative results (Bergstrom et al, 1998). Braden scale scores can be grouped according to level of risk: not at risk (>18), mild risk (15–18), moderate risk (13–14), high risk (10–12), and very high risk (≤9) (Ayello and Braden, 2002). When a patient has a pressure ulcer or a history of a pressure ulcer but is rated "not at risk" according to the Braden scale, it is recommended to automatically place the patient in the "at-risk" category (Maklebust et al, 2005). Likewise, the level of risk should be increased for any patient whose Braden score indicates he or she is

"at risk" and who also has a fever, diastolic blood pressure less than 60, or low albumin/prealbumin (WOCN Society, 2010). For example, a patient with a Braden score of 12 would be considered at moderate risk but should be "upgraded" to the high-risk category if he or she also has a fever.

Accurate use of the Braden scale requires user training and retraining, even when nurses use the tool regularly and for a long period of time. A study involving more than 2,500 nurses in Detroit Medical Center showed that only 75.5% of nurses correctly rated Braden scale levels (Maklebust et al, 2005). Although the two extremes of risk levels, "not at risk" and "severe risk," were most often rated correctly, the subscales "moisture" and "sensory perception" were most often misunderstood. Therefore annual competencies for risk assessment are justified (Magnan and Maklebust, 2008; Maklebust et al, 2005). Similarly, the definitions for risk factors and subscales for each risk factor are essential in both paper or electronic documentation systems. The following section discusses the Braden subscales and measurement of risk factors.

Sensory Perception. With respect to pressure ulcers, *sensory perception* refers to the patient's ability to respond meaningfully to pressure-related discomfort. The extent of the deficit is dependent upon the degree to which a patient is able to feel or communicate pressure-related discomfort. Patients without a sensory impairment move or ask to be moved if they are lying on intravenous tubing or feel pain on their tail bone. They remove or request removal of shoes, stockings, or medical devices that feel uncomfortable or too tight. Examples of patients with sensory deficits who cannot adequately communicate discomfort include those with confusion, disorientation, oversedation, or unresponsiveness. Patients who are alert and oriented may be unable to communicate discomfort if they are on a ventilator, speak a different language than their caregivers, or cannot feel pain due to paralysis or neuropathy.

Moisture. The more the skin is exposed to moisture, especially near a bony prominence, the more vulnerable the skin becomes to the mechanical forces of pressure, friction, and shear. Clinical examples include the patient with incontinence who is exposed to pressure, the critically ill patient with fever and diaphoresis, or the bedbound patient with poorly contained wound exudate from a perirectal abscess.

Activity. *Degree of activity* refers to how much a patient is in the bed or chair or is ambulating. Again, reading the subscale definitions is important. For example, "walks occasionally" means the patient spends most of the time in the chair. Therefore a few steps to the bedside commode should be scored as "walks occasionally."

Mobility. One of the problems encountered with this subscale is the tendency to confuse activity (e.g., getting up in the chair) with mobility. *Mobility* refers to the patient's ability to change or control body position. The score assigned is based on what the patient demonstrates, such as the degree to which he or she is able to

TABLE 8-1　Braden Scale for Predicting Pressure Sore Risk

Patient's Name _____　Evaluator's Name _____　Date of Assessment _____

	1	2	3	4
SENSORY PERCEPTION ability to respond appropriately to pressure-related discomfort	**1. Completely limited** Unresponsive (does not moan, flinch, or grasp) to painful stimuli, due to diminished level of consciousness or sedation. OR limited ability to feel pain over most of body.	**2. Very limited** Responds only to painful stimuli. Cannot communicate discomfort except by moaning or restlessness OR has a sensory impairment which limits the ability to feel pain or discomfort over ½ of body.	**3. Slightly limited** Responds to verbal commands, but cannot always communicate discomfort or the need to be turned. OR has some sensory impairment which limits ability to feel pain or discomfort in 1 or 2 extremities.	**4. No impairment** Responds to verbal commands. Has no sensory deficit which would limit ability to feel or voice pain or discomfort.
MOISTURE degree to which skin is exposed to moisture	**1. Constantly moist** Skin is kept moist almost constantly by perspiration, urine, etc. Dampness is detected every time patient is moved or turned.	**2. Very Moist** Skin is often, but not always, moist. Linen must be changed at least once a shift.	**3. Occasionally moist** Skin is occasionally moist, requiring an extra linen change approximately once a day.	**4. Rarely moist** Skin is usually dry, linen only requires changing at routine intervals.
ACTIVITY degree of physical activity	**1. Bedfast** Confined to bed.	**2. Chairfast** Ability to walk severely limited or nonexistent. Cannot bear own weight and/or must be assisted into chair or wheelchair.	**3. Walks Occasionally** Walks occasionally during day, but for very short distances, with or without assistance. Spends majority of each shift in bed or chair.	**4. Walks Frequently** Walks outside room at least twice a day and inside room at least once every two hours during waking hours.
MOBILITY ability to change and control body position	**1. Completely immobile** Does not make even slight changes in body or extremity position without assistance	**2. Very Limited** Makes occasional slight changes in body or extremity position but unable to make frequent or significant changes independently.	**3. Slightly Limited** Makes frequent though slight changes in body or extremity position independently.	**4. No Limitations** Makes major and frequent changes in position without assistance.
NUTRITION usual food intake pattern	**1. Very poor** Never eats a complete meal. Rarely eats more than ⅓ of any food offered. Eats 2 servings or less of protein (meat or dairy products) per day. Takes fluids poorly. Does not take a liquid supplement. OR is NPO and/or maintained on clear liquids or IV's for more than 5 days.	**2. Probably Inadequate** Rarely eats a complete meal and generally eats only about ½ of any food offered. Protein intake includes only 3 servings of meat or dairy products per day. Occasionally will take a dietary supplement. OR receives less than optimum amount of liquid diet or tube feeding	**3. Adequate** Eats over half of most meals. Eats a total of 4 servings of protein (meat, dairy products) per day. Occasionally will refuse a meal, but will usually take a supplement when offered OR is on a tube feeding or TPN regimen which probably meets most of nutritional needs	**4. Excellent** Eats most of every meal. Never refuses a meal. Usually eats a total of 4 or more servings of meat and dairy products. Occasionally eats between meals. Does not require supplementation.
FRICTION & SHEAR	**1. Problem** Requires moderate to maximum assistance in moving. Complete lifting without sliding against sheets is impossible. Frequently slides down in bed or chair, requiring frequent repositioning with maximum assistance. Spasticity, contractures or agitation leads to almost constant friction	**2. Potential Problem** Moves feebly or requires minimum assistance. During a move, skin probably slides to some extent against sheets, chair, restraints, or other devices. Maintains relatively good position in chair or bed most of the time but occasionally slides down.	**3. No Apparent Problem** Moves in bed and in chair independently and has sufficient muscle strength to lift up completely during move. Maintains good position in bed or chair.	

Total Score _____

TABLE 8-2	Skin Safety Interventions by Risk Factor
Risk Factor	**Interventions (Skin Safety Precautions)**
Impaired sensory perception, mobility, activity	1. Preventive (group 1) pressure-redistribution support surface for patients with multiple intact turning surfaces and Braden Score ≤18 2. Obtain therapeutic (group 2) pressure redistribution support surface (i.e., low air loss) for patients with: • Full-thickness or suspected deep tissue injury on the trunk • Wounds on multiple turning surfaces 3. Reposition every 2 hours in bed *regardless* of bed/mattress type • Avoid positioning directly on trochanter • Collaborate with physician for pain control as needed to promote appropriate repositioning • Use pillows to keep bony prominences from direct contact with surfaces (including keeping heels off bed) • Stabilize and position tubes to prevent them from creating pressure 4. Reposition once every hour in chair • Use pressure-redistribution chair cushion • Return to bed after 1 hour if unable to reposition in chair 5. Moisturize dry skin; do *not* massage reddened bony prominences 6. Remove or reposition devices (stockings, masks, tubes) every shift for skin inspection
Moisture	1. Address cause and offer bedpan/urinal/toileting every 2 hours 2. Notify physician and registered dietitian if patient has loose stools 3. Use absorbent pads that wick moisture away from the body (avoid diapers/briefs with plastic backing) 4. Skin care twice per day and after each incontinent episode to include • Perineal cleanser and barrier in one • Moisture barrier paste if stools are loose or perineal skin is red or open 5. Consider containment devices for frequent loose stools (rectal pouches, Food and Drug Administration–approved indwelling fecal containment device)
Nutritional deficit	1. Consult nutritional services 2. Maintain adequate hydration
Friction and shear	1. Limit head of bed elevation to ≤30 degrees (unless contraindicated) 2. Use knee gatch as needed to keep patient from sliding down in bed 3. Use trapeze when indicated 4. Use lift sheet or air transfer device (HoverMatt) to move patient and prevent lateral shear 5. Protect elbows and heels with skin barriers or dressings if exposed to friction

change or control body position (i.e., shifting weight in the chair or turning or repositioning in bed). A patient may be able to sit in a chair (activity) but may not be able to shift their weight (mobility). In contrast, a patient who is agitated and moving frequently may still have a mobility deficient because the movements are not purposeful or controlled.

Nutrition. One mistake made with the Braden nutrition subscale is failure of the rater to consider "usual food intake pattern." For example the patient who is NPO (nil per os [nothing by mouth]) after midnight does not constitute a low nutrition score if his or her usual food intake pattern is adequate. Conversely, the patient's nutritional status may be rated "adequate" when the patient is receiving total parenteral nutrition or a tube feeding documented to "meet nutritional needs" even though the patient is malnourished as evidenced by abnormally low laboratory test results, such as prealbumin. This occurs because the regimen "that meets nutritional needs" requires time to reverse the malnutrition that existed before supplementation was initiated. Therefore, patients at risk for pressure ulcers with an adequate nutrition score should be placed at a higher risk level if laboratory test results are abnormally low.

Friction and Shear. *Friction* occurs when the skin rubs against another surface. Patients who are restless or agitated commonly create friction on their elbows and heels from constant movement and rubbing against the bed surface. Friction also can occur with a brace or shoe as it slides back and forth during ambulation. *Shear* occurs when friction acts with gravity. Classic examples of actions that cause shear injury include a patient sliding down in bed after the head of the bed has been elevated for lunch or allowing the patient's buttocks to drag across the bed, stretcher, or procedure table during transfer.

Maintain Skin Health

The third component of the PUPP's best practice bundle is preserving the protective function of the skin. Threats to the protective function of the skin include xerosis, incontinence, chemicals, friction, and shear. Interventions that minimize threats to skin integrity, including xerosis, need to be part of routine baseline standard of care for all patients (Box 8-2).

BOX 8-2	Interventions to Maintain Skin Health

- Avoid alkaline soaps so that pH and normal flora of skin remain intact.
- Do not use friction when washing skin to avoid traumatizing epidermis.
- Apply moisturizer or emollient frequently to prevent xerosis.
- Encourage adequate fluid intake to prevent dehydration, which contributes to xerosis.
- Use moisture barrier ointments as needed to protect skin from chemical irritants such as fecal incontinence.
- Do *not* massage reddened areas.
- Move and transfer with lift sheet, Hoyer lift, or HoverMatt to avoid shear on buttocks due to dragging.

A commonly overlooked threat to skin integrity is xerosis (pruritic, erythematous, dry, scaly, cracked, or fissured skin). Xerosis is a problem for 59% to 85% of people 64 years and older. It results from loss of natural moisturizing factors, barrier abilities, and epidermal water. Linked to infection, skin tears, and pressure ulcers, xerosis should be prevented or minimized by frequent application of moisturizers and emollients in addition to adequate water intake.

Optimize Nutrition and Hydration

The fourth component of a PUPP's best practice bundle is maintenance of adequate nutrition and hydration compatible with the individual's wishes and conditions (Whitney et al, 2006; WOCN Society, 2010). With weight loss and dehydration from sustained nutritional deficiencies, muscle mass is decreased so that less padding is available to distribute the patient's weight over a bony prominence (Reddy et al, 2006). In addition, malnourished patients may be twice as likely to develop skin breakdown (Thomas et al, 1996). Routinely, patients at risk should be assisted with meals, snacks, and hydration. If the pressure ulcer risk assessment indicates the patient is nutritionally compromised, a registered dietician should be consulted for a more comprehensive nutritional assessment and specific recommendations (WOCN Society, 2010). Depending upon the patient's comorbidities, the registered dietician's recommendations may include offering fluids every 2 hours, high-protein supplements, swallowing studies, and enteral or parenteral nutrition. Chapter 27 discusses the details of nutritional assessment and management.

Pressure Redistribution and Offloading the Patient At Risk

Pressure redistribution is accomplished with the use of support surfaces (see Chapter 9). Offloading is accomplished by turning and repositioning. Pressure redistribution and offloading are required for the at-risk patient whether he or she is in a chair, on a transport or procedure cart, in the operating room, or in a bed.

Repositioning Frequency. Repositioning is used to reduce the duration and intensity of pressure exerted over a bony prominence. In 1961, Kosiak recommended the frequency of repositioning to be hourly to every two hours, based on the interface pressure readings from healthy, able-bodied subjects (Kosiak, 1961). Today, international guidelines for pressure ulcer prevention and treatment recommend a reposition frequency that is determined by tissue tolerance, level of activity and mobility, general medical condition, overall treatment objectives, skin condition, and support surface (NPUAP and EPUAP, 2009). Although some of these factors are easily determined and remain constant (support surface), others cannot be measured with current technology (e.g., tissue tolerance) or may be unpredictable and labile (e.g., mobility, activity, and medical condition). Therefore guideline recommendations for frequency are given as a range of every 2 to 4 hours while in bed and every 15 minutes to 1 hour while in the chair (WOCN Society, 2003).

Much like determining frequency for pain medications, the effectiveness of repositioning should be assessed, adjusting frequency as needed to achieve the desired outcome (e.g., no erythema). Specifically, positioning frequency might be determined by beginning with a schedule of every 2 hours. Persistent redness from a previous episode of pressure loading, seen when the patient is repositioned, indicates that pressure is not adequately relieved. Therefore, a different support surface may be indicated or the repositioning frequency may need to be increased. Ultimately, a 4-hour repositioning schedule may be most appropriate when the patient is on a support surface, the patient's skin has remained intact and without erythema, and the patient does not have an acute illness that would precipitate a sudden change in medical condition (e.g., hemodynamic instability). Although an every-4-hour positioning schedule may be adequate in some situations for keeping the skin intact, it may be insufficient to prevent other complications associated with immobility (e.g., thromboembolism, atelectasis, aspiration).

Repositioning Techniques. Although repositioning does not reduce intensity of pressure, it does reduce the duration, which is the more critical element of pressure ulcer formation. Repositioning contributes to the patient's comfort, dignity, and functional ability (NPUAP and EPUAP, 2009). Repositioning techniques differ according to the patient's activity (chairbound, bedbound), location (operating room [OR], transport, emergency room, special procedures), comfort, and hemodynamic stability.

Turning. Turning the patient in bed is a universally accepted staple in preventing the complications associated with immobility and pressure ulcers. The proper technique for turning is placing the patient in a 30-degree side-lying position with a pillow between the knees (Figure 8-1). The patient should be turned alternately from right side, to back, to left side, to back. The proper technique avoids bony prominences, nonblanchable erythema, existing wounds, and medical devices such as tubes and catheters. For example, a 90-degree side-lying position is generally undesirable because it places the patient directly on a bony prominence (trochanter) (NPUAP and EPUAP, 2009). When an ulcer is present on a turning surface, the turning schedule may be customized so that that time spent on that turning surface is minimized.

If turning is medically contraindicated, minor shifts of the shoulders and hips should be used to allow some reperfusion (WOCN Society, 2010). For example, pillows that have been propped under the patient can be incrementally removed. Ideally the patient should also be placed on an active support surface (see Chapter 9).

Limiting Head of Bed Elevation. Chapter 5 discusses the effects of shear injury on the skin. Shear injury is seen after the skin is dragged over a surface either laterally (during transfers) or vertically (sliding up or down in bed). Keeping the head of the bed at an angle of 30 degrees or less prevents shear (Figure 5-1). To minimize the pull of gravity, the knee gatch should be used. When the head of bed must be temporarily elevated over 30 degrees, such as when eating or drinking or during procedures, the caregiver needs to monitor the patient closely so that the head of bed is not left in the elevated position longer than needed (e.g., 1 hour) (WOCN Society, 2010). When having the head of bed at 30 degrees or less is medically contraindicated, the sacral region must be frequently monitored for shear injury (WOCN Society, 2010), and a different type of support surface may be indicated (see Chapter 9). When the patient does slide down in bed, a draw sheet (or alternative transfer assist device) should be used to move the patient back to a desirable position without allowing the skin to drag across the bed surface.

Transferring without Lateral Shear. Lateral shear results from dragging the patient across a surface or onto another surface such as an operating room surface, procedure table, or cardiac chair. Traditionally, patients have been dragged with a sliding board onto another surface, or they are requested to slide (if possible) onto the new surface. Transfer assist devices are available that can safely facilitate patient movement without dragging while decreasing risk of back injury for the staff. If patients must move themselves onto the next surface, they should be asked to do so without sliding. After transfer is complete, patients should move or be moved to release any tangential forces that may have been created by the move.

Floating Heels. Heels are the second most common anatomic location for pressure ulcers (Fowler et al, 2008). The plantar aspect of the heel is well constructed to resist the forces of standing and walking. However, the posterior heel has only a thin layer of fat that is bound tightly to the underlying fascia and Achilles tendon fibers and has limited ability to (1) redistribute pressure over the small area of skin overlying the posterior tubercle of the calcaneus and (2) absorb the compressive forces of shear generated during movement or transfers. Additionally, the small branches from the calcaneal and peroneal arteries and prolonged pressure on these relatively small vessels can lead to ischemia (Wong and Stotts, 2003). Patients with diabetes and vascular disease are at increased risk for pressure ulcers on the heel, as evidenced by their diminished hyperemic response to pressure offloading (Mayrovitz and Sims, 2004). As a result, patients with vascular disease and diabetes are always at risk for pressure ulcers on the heel despite having an adequate Braden score.

Offloading products are used to "float" the heels or redistribute pressure. Options include pillows, support surfaces, and heel protectors. Offloading devices and pillows should distribute the weight of the leg *without* putting pressure on the Achilles tendon. Water-filled gloves, cut-out devices, and donuts are contraindicated (NPUAP and EPUAP, 2009; WOCN Society, 2010).

The advantage to using pillows is that they are inexpensive, readily available, and, in some studies, shown to be more effective than commercial products (Wong and

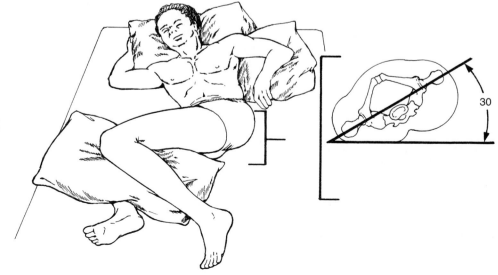

FIGURE 8-1 Thirty-degree lateral position.

30

Stotts, 2003). The disadvantage of pillows is that they do not prevent footdrop, and they can be difficult to keep in place for patients with contractures, agitation, and spasms. When pillows are used, they should be positioned under the calf muscle so that the heels do not come into contact with the mattress. Patients must be closely monitored to ensure the pillow remains properly positioned to keep the heels off the surface sufficiently.

A variety of pressure redistribution devices for the heel are commercially available in numerous shapes and sizes. The pressure redistribution medium used may be air, foam, or gel. In addition to pressure ulcer prevention, some devices provide additional functions, such as safe weight bearing, insulation (beneficial to the patient with vascular conditions), and prevention and treatment of footdrop.

Product selection should address the needs of the patient. Depending on the setting, collaboration with an occupational therapist or a physical therapist may be wise to select a device that not only will float the heels but will be compatible with ambulation or address footdrop. Use of any device, especially with patients who have a sensory perception deficit, can actually cause skin damage (see Plate 33); therefore, routine repositioning, device removal, and skin inspection are critical to prevent unintended harm. Routine repositioning varies by the device and manufacturer's instructions. For example, a splint could be repositioned four times per day to be consistent with a footdrop schedule, an endotracheal tube repositioned every 2 hours to be consistent with the every-2-hour standard of care for oral care of intubated patients, and antiembolism stockings removed twice daily in keeping with manufacturer's instructions.

Seating. Moving from the bed to the chair is a position change that may decrease the patient's overall risk for pressure ulcers by making the patient more active. However, the patient in a seated position remains at risk for pressure ulcers on the coccyx and develops a new pressure point on the ischial tuberosities. Patients at risk require a pressure-redistribution chair cushion (further discussed in Chapter 9). Foam or rubber rings (i.e., donuts) are never indicated to relieve pressure because they concentrate the intensity of the pressure on the surrounding tissue (NPUAP and EPUAP, 2009; WOCN Society, 2010). Patients expected to be chairbound for the long term should be evaluated and routinely reassessed by a seating specialist or team.

The type of chair the patient will be seated in impacts the patient's position and posture. The posture and position prescribed should minimize pressure and shear while maximizing safety, stability, and a full range of activities (NPUAP and EPUAP, 2009). For example, a reclining chair will offload the ischial tuberosities but will place more pressure on the coccyx. In contrast, a commonly used straight-back chair facilitates an upright position, with most of the pressure on the ischial tuberosities, but the coccyx again becomes vulnerable for pressure damage if the patient slouches or slides.

If the patient's feet do not touch the floor while seated, the feet should be positioned on a foot rest. The foot rest should be at a height that does not raise the knees above the patient's lap, which would create more pressure under the coccyx and ischial tuberosities.

Pressure *relief* in the chair can be attained by standing up, performing pressure relief push ups, having the wheelchair tilted back 65% or more, leaning forward, or by the patient shifting his or her weight from side to side every 15 minutes to 1 hour sufficiently enough to offload the ischial tuberosities and coccyx (WOCN Society, 2010). If pressure relief cannot be achieved, the patient should be put back to bed within an hour. If seating is necessary for the patient with an existing coccyx or ischial tuberosity wound, sitting should be limited to 1 hour or less, three times per day with a cushion and in a posture that minimizes pressure to the wound (NPUAP and EPUAP, 2009). Acutely ill patients at risk for pressure ulcers should not sit longer than two hours at a time and not return to sitting for at least one hour (WOCN Society, 2010).

Special Settings

Emergency Center and Special Procedures. Little is known about the risk of pressure injury to the patient undergoing procedures in ancillary service, such as radiology, dialysis, and special procedures. One prospective study using data from 80 patients found a 53.8% incidence of pressure ulcer development in patients undergoing lengthy radiology procedures (Brown, 2002). Hand-off communication when a patient moves from an inpatient unit to an ancillary service may be limited to pressure ulcer location and preferred positions for optimal offloading and comfort. This information, although limited, is vital for the prevention of pressure ulcers by promoting communication and troubleshooting to determine creative position strategies on surfaces and challenging environments. Facilities are now investing in larger carts with support surface pads to accommodate a population of patients with a higher acuity and greater body mass index. Simple interventions such as placing a pillow under the legs can rescue the heels from a long wait or procedure.

Operating Room. Beckrich and Aronovitch (1999) calculated the cost of treating pressure ulcers using data from the Universal Healthcare Almanac (Cherner, 1998) and from the American Hospital Association (1998). Their analysis estimated that up to 42% of all hospital-acquired pressure ulcers occur in surgical patients and cost from $750 million to $1.5 billion annually. Intraoperatively acquired pressure ulcers are not always recognized in the immediate postoperative period. Visual skin changes can appear immediately, in a few hours, or up to 72 hours following surgery. The affected area may become ecchymotic or bruised, and it may blister. Necrosis can occur within 2 to 7 days. Patients with vascular compromise and subsequent altered skin integrity may present with an area of skin that has a mottled irregular pattern that may resolve, or they reveal full-thickness skin breakdown (Aronovitch, 2007; Walton-Geer, 2009).

To date, a validated pressure ulcer risk screening tool for the intraoperative patient population has not been published. Patients assessed as low risk using a risk assessment scale commonly used outside of the OR have been known to develop pressure ulcers in the OR (Aronovitch, 2007; Grous et al, 1997). Therefore pressure ulcer risk assessment should be refined for individuals undergoing surgery (NPUAP and EPUAP, 2009). Checklist 8-4 lists pressure ulcer risk factors for intraoperative patients described in the Association of periOperative Registered Nurse's Standards, Recommended Practices, and Guidelines, which also include a 23-page guideline for positioning patients in the perioperative setting (AORN, 2008). Minimally, staff should float the heels and use a pressure-redistribution mattress on the OR table for individuals at risk for pressure ulcers (NPUAP and EPUAP, 2009). Studies have demonstrated that the standard OR mattress, defined as a 2-inch foam mattress, increases pressure ulcer risk (Armstrong and Bortz, 2001; Aronovitch, 2007; Defloor and de Schuijmer, 2000). Appendix C contains a perioperative guidance document for pressure ulcer prevention used in the state of Minnesota. Box 9-1 presents factors to consider when purchasing a support surface for the OR.

Medical Devices. The incidence of device-related pressure ulcers nationwide is unknown. Recently, 25% of full-thickness hospital-acquired pressure ulcers reported to the state of Minnesota developed secondary to pressure from medical devices (Minnesota Department of Health, 2009). Baharestani and Ratliff (2007) report that more than 50% of pediatric pressure ulcers are related to medical equipment and devices. With the exception of cervical collars, little is written about the growing problem (Jacobson et al, 2008; Powers et al, 2006; Tescher et al, 2007).

Patients with impaired sensory perception tend to be at risk for device-related pressure ulcers. Patients with sensory impairment may not remove or request removal of shoes, stockings (Plate 33), or medical devices that feel uncomfortable or too tight because paralysis, neuropathy, confusion, disorientation, or oversedation may prevent them from being able to adequately communicate discomfort. In the presence of nasal, oral, or gastric secretions or oxygen humidity, moisture also can contribute to skin breakdown caused by some devices.

Device-related pressure ulcers are generally located under or near a medical device, may not be associated with a bony prominence, and often present in the shape of the device. Because many devices are near anatomic locations without fatty tissue (e.g., nares, behind ears, occiput, bridge of nose), rapid deterioration to suspected deep tissue injury or Stage III, IV, or unstageable pressure ulcers is often seen. Table 8-3 lists common devices associated with pressure ulcers as well as suggested preventive interventions.

Provide Patient and Family Education

Formal programs for patient and family education in pressure ulcer prevention are critical to reduce the incidence of pressure ulcers in any care setting. Such education assists the patient and caregivers to better understand why repositioning should not be delayed even when the patient "just got comfortable" or "just got to sleep." Patients and family can be empowered as advocates by reminding staff of the repositioning schedule. Formal programs for patients with a spinal cord injury are common in rehabilitation centers and could serve as a model for similar educational programs for patients with any chronic disease that limits mobility as the disease progresses (e.g., multiple sclerosis, terminal cancer).

Educational materials for patients must be at an appropriate reading level and be evaluated for design features such as organization, writing style, appeal, and appearance (Wilson and Williams, 2003; WOCN Society, 2003). It may be helpful to request that caregivers come to the hospital to work with a nurse to learn techniques of care before the patient's discharge.

The importance of preventive interventions *that are consistent with the patient's needs and goals* is articulated by both the WOCN Society position statement and the CMS definitions so that caregivers can respect the informed choices of individuals who decline interventions. For example, a patient facing end of life may decline an intervention such as tube feeding to optimize nutrition. In this case, if a pressure ulcer developed, documentation of patient education could be sufficient to demonstrate *informed* refusal of care and thereby the pressure ulcer deemed to be unavoidable.

CREATING INFRASTRUCTURE TO SUSTAIN THE PUPP

Creating the best practice bundle for pressure ulcer prevention is only the first step of a PUPP. For a successful PUPP, the bundle must be integrated into the culture and infrastructure of the health care system. However, many hurdles have been identified that threaten the implementation and utilization of a PUPP: difficulty identifying

---

CHECKLIST 8-4

Pressure Ulcer Risk Factors for Intraoperative Patients

✓ Vascular, cardiac, thoracic, orthopedic surgery
✓ Impaired blood flow and hypotensive episodes
✓ Long surgeries (>4 hours)
✓ Thin stature
✓ Poor nutritional status
✓ Diabetes or vascular disease
✓ Specific positions (e.g., lithotomy, lateral supine)
✓ General anesthesia
✓ Thermoregulatory devices
✓ Age >70 years
✓ Preoperative Braden score <20
✓ Use of standard operating room mattresses during surgery

TABLE 8-3	Prevention of Devices—Related Pressure Ulcers
Device	**Preventive Interventions**
Nasogastric tube	Daily site care Move tube to different area of nose (slight changes make a difference) Consider commercial stabilizers to facilitate easier repositioning and inspection than possible with tape Proper application of stabilizers to keep clamp from touching skin Use skin sealants and commercial feeding tube stabilizer to prevent accidental dislodgment; change every other day Document skin condition with site care
Oxygen mask	Consult with respiratory therapist for proper sizing and fitting Refitting may be indicated as edema changes Consider alternative masks such as full face masks or masks with gel borders for select patients Apply minimal tension to mask strap required to create adequate seal Add skin checks under respiratory equipment to respiratory therapist worklists or documentation
Nasal oxygen	Use commercially available foam ear protectors that can be attached to tubing Make ear protectors easily accessible (i.e., place near oxygen tubing) Purchase oxygen tubing with protectors already attached to tubing Use foam tracheostomy straps to hold oxygen cannula in place and away from the ears
Endotracheal tube	Combine endotracheal tube site care with oral care Reposition tube to different locations in mouth Consider commercial stabilizers instead of tape to facilitate easier repositioning and inspection Proper application of stabilizers to keep clamp from touching mouth
Removable splint/protector/brace	Consult physical therapist/occupational therapist for proper selection, sizing, fitting Keep manufacturer's application instructions accessible Keep schedule accessible; if not available, ask for one Add device removal twice per day for skin inspection to documentation
Collar	Consult with orthotics for proper sizing and fitting Palpate for skin changes within hairline Use collars that cause lower levels of mandibular and occipital pressure
Tracheostomy straps	Use commercially available foam/collar type adjustable straps instead of ties or twill tape for comfort, pressure redistribution, easy adjustment, and to prevent inadvertent extubation

appropriate interventions based on level of risk, knowledge, and skill deficiencies; absence of adequate and straightforward documentation tools; no clear champion for the program; lack of accountability; time management; lack of administrative support; and absence of process or outcomes measures (Cranney et al, 2001; Krishnagopalan et al, 2002). Even when a PUPP is implemented, time has shown that a PUPP is difficult to sustain. Because pressure ulcers are a complex, multifactorial problem, a holistic view of the hospital system and a change in culture are required to reduce incidence. All caregivers and administration must share the belief that pressure ulcers are a negative outcome and that all health care providers play a role in protecting the patient from this adverse event. Implementation of a vital and enduring PUPP requires participation and oversight by management and critical scrutiny of the system's operations. The PUPP must become integrated into the day-to-day operations at the unit and systems level so that it is embedded into the infrastructure of education, documentation, decision making, and communication and handoffs (Bryant and Rolstad, 2001; IHI, 2008). Further evidence of the importance of infrastructure to the success of a PUPP is given in the international guidelines for pressure ulcer

prevention, which include specific recommendations that address facility policies (NPUAP and EPUAP, 2009).

PUPP Team

Pressure ulcer prevention is not exclusively under the control of nurses (Jacobson et al, 2008; Padula et al, 2008). A multidisciplinary team (described in Chapter 1) is necessary to accommodate the increasing complexity of patients at risk for pressure ulcers as well as the ever-changing amount of literature and guidelines that precipitate needed changes in policy, materials and equipment distribution, and staff education. In addition, making a sustainable change in the incidence of pressure ulcers requires a change in the culture of the organization such that the top administrators are monitoring process and outcomes data and allocating resources (e.g., staffing and time) to maintain the PUPP (Reinertsen et al, 2008). One measure of the extent of administrative support of the PUPP is the appointment of a system-wide leader or coordinator of the PUPP who has designated accountability and time for program implementation and maintenance. The PUPP coordinator should meet certain requirements for the position, primarily expertise in wound care.

Documentation

A key part of maintaining program infrastructure is providing a specific location in the medical record to document assessments and interventions relative to skin care, pressure prevention, and pressure ulcer management. To facilitate accurate documentation, a flow sheet with descriptor choices should be used rather than a narrative or progress note so that staff is prompted for documentation parameters and the form is completed in its entirety. This will also provide uniformity in the use of terms so that data collection for monitoring, auditing, and trending will be expedited. The documentation forms should include risk assessment terms and definitions with subscale and total scores, skin inspection terms (intact, within defined limits, and terms to describe deviations), wound assessment parameters, offloading and positioning options, continence care, nutrition, and device removal. See Appendix B for sample documentation forms.

Documentation should record when interventions are performed or omitted (with rationale) and when instructions are given to patients and their response. Documentation of repositioning should specify the body position in which the patient was left (back, left, or right) and the patient's tolerance (e.g., condition of offloaded bony prominence) (NPUAP and EPUAP, 2009). With such clarity and consistency in documentation, the risk of litigation is decreased should an adverse event occur (Brown, 2006). Frequency of documentation will vary by type of facility and the patient's overall condition. Checklist 8-5 includes items that must be documented, including those for which a designated space would facilitate ease, accuracy, and compliance.

Patient Handoffs

The frequency with which patients are harmed as a result of problematic "handoffs" is unknown, yet care plan communication lapses at the time of patient handoffs are common (Kitch et al, 2008). The Joint Commission states that an organization must define, communicate to staff, and implement a process in which information about patient care is communicated in a consistent manner. Therefore, any hand off communications should include relevant information about the patient's risk of developing a pressure ulcer, or the treatment and status of any existing pressure ulcers (The Joint Commission, 2008).

A standardized process for handoffs reinforces to staff the importance of pressure ulcer prevention and facilitates consistency throughout the organization. For example, a posted turning schedule can serve as a reminder to the nurse or caregiver as well as any other health care provider who enters the patient's room of the time to turn a patient and the position to use (Figure 8-2).

Handoff communications between similar units for patients at high risk or with actual or potential pressure ulcers should include the following:

- Time and results of recent pressure ulcer risk assessment
- Time and results of recent skin inspection
- Location and stages of pressure ulcers
- Time of last wound assessment and dressing change
- Current offloading device(s)
- Time and position last placed
- Toleration of repositioning frequency

Handoffs from the patient care unit to another department (e.g., radiology department, operating room) also necessitate communications concerning the patient's skin status and pressure ulcer risk. In particular, the staff of the receiving department should be made aware of the location and severity of any existing pressure ulcer, any positions that should be avoided, and the need for

---

CHECKLIST 8-5

Pressure Ulcer Prevention Documentation

✓ Pressure ulcer risk: Baseline and reassessments
✓ Skin inspection: Baseline and reassessments
✓ Routine device removal
✓ Plan of care and patient response
✓ Ongoing patient/family teaching
✓ Floating heels
✓ Repositioning frequency and position (ride side, left side, etc.)
✓ Head of bed position
✓ Type of support surface
✓ Application of incontinent devices and barriers
✓ Nutritional supplements
✓ Tube site care
✓ Relevant consultations

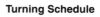

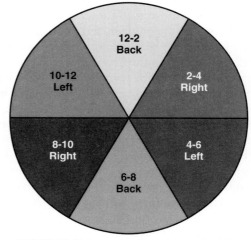

FIGURE 8-2 Example of a turning schedule.

offloading (especially heels and sacrum). Appendix C provides an example of an interdepartmental handoff communication tool.

The concept of handoffs is also applicable to the transferring of the patient out of the facility at discharge. Accurate and thorough documentation is critical for continuity of care. In addition to the items listed earlier, the handoff communication should include pressure ulcer risk score, current plan of care for pressure ulcer prevention, the patient's individual response to the plan of care, and pain.

Formularies and Decision-Making Tools

A significant and valuable contribution the wound specialist can bring to any facility and any PUPP is to standardize and organize products available within their health care system. To bring order to the utilization of these products and enhance the quality of care provided, decision-making tools are used to facilitate the accuracy and efficiency of decision making, guide treatment selection, and educate the clinician concerning a particular disease entity. Annual review of these tools is recommended because changes in the pathophysiology of pressure ulcers and product research and development are ongoing and quickly paced. Decision-making tools must use language that is consistent with policies, procedures, documentation, supply order menus, and current contracts for products. If any of these factors change, revisions are necessary to keep the tools accurate and user friendly. Examples of decision-making tools include interventions based on risk factors (see Table 8-2), support surface selection (see Table 9-1), and formularies for skin care products (see Table 5-4 and throughout textbook) and wound care dressings (see Chapters 5, 16, 18, 31, and 37).

Investing in Technology

Access to, and utilization of, appropriate technology involves not only patient care items (e.g., support surfaces or devices) but also medical record documentation so that information is complete and readily available at all times. In creating the documentation system, skin care, risk assessment, nutritional assessment, and the other critical elements of a best practice bundle must be incorporated, which requires direct input of the wound specialist. As technological advances in existing PUPP tools, such as support surfaces, transferring devices, and heel protectors, occur, the advantages of these products should be methodically reviewed by the wound specialist and presented to the PUPP team members for discussion. Similarly, the team should have a mechanism for keeping abreast of new developments in technology that may improve efficiency and reliability of interventions and the PUPP and ultimately reduce the patient's risk of pressure ulcers.

Staff Education and Competencies

All health care personnel providing care to the patient must appreciate the role they have in pressure ulcer prevention. In addition, it should not be assumed that the formal curriculum of the registered nurse, nurse practitioner, physician, physician assistant, physical therapist, and occupational therapist adequately incorporated pressure ulcer prevention and management (Odierna and Zeleznik, 2003). To keep the PUPP infrastructure strong, pressure ulcer education (including how to document) should be included in new employee orientation and annual competencies for nurses and nursing assistants. The content of the education is based on the scope of practice for the position. For example, the registered nurse should minimally demonstrate competency related to pressure ulcer etiology, skin inspection, risk assessment, wound assessment, and implementation of a full range of appropriate interventions to minimize or eliminate risk factors (WOCN Society, 2003). Nursing assistants may require education and competency related to monitoring the skin, reporting changes to the nurse, continence skin care, importance of nutrition, and appropriate positioning. To keep pace with the rapid changes in the science of pressure ulcer prevention and treatment, the health professional's knowledge and skills require routine and frequent updating through annual programs, at a minimum.

Staff Accountability

Corporate culture must convey that facility-acquired pressure ulcers are no longer tolerable or "acceptable" unless documentation indicates the pressure ulcer was unavoidable. Although it is important to encourage employees to "self-report," they still must be held accountable for any errors. Just as it is unhealthy to create a punitive environment where employees are fearful of admitting errors, so too it is unhealthy to create an environment of toleration of less than best practice, which can lead to errors and complications such as pressure ulcers. Expectations for employees to meet this standard need to be communicated during orientation and annual education and through activities that encourage transparency and sharing of experiences and learnings (both successful and unsuccessful). Examples of methods for improving accountability for pressure ulcers are given in Box 8-3.

Quality Tracking and Evaluation

Once a program as extensive and system-wide as the PUPP is implemented, feedback is needed that comes from routine measurements and quality tracking. Such feedback provides the affirmation participants need to reinforce the value of their efforts and investment in the program. Routine measurements and quality tracking

BOX 8-3	Improving Staff Accountability for Pressure Ulcer Prevention

1. Create newsletters, blogs, and emails that share experiences and learnings.
2. Post commitment statements on units or in patients' rooms informing patients and families that they can expect to be repositioned and that it is OK to ask.
3. Arrange time for involved staff members to participate in relevant root cause analysis (RCA).
4. Audit compliance with pressure ulcer preventive interventions (similar to handwashing audits).
5. Post dashboards on units sharing nosocomial rates with staff and visitors.
6. Have celebrations (with treats) when nosocomial rates drop.
7. Provide performance reviews that evaluate individual performance with pressure ulcer prevention audits, attendance and participation with relevant RCAs, unit-specific skin care initiatives, and prevalence incident studies.

will also identify areas for improvement. Once a plan for reducing or eliminating pressure is developed and the plan is implemented, the effectiveness of the intervention (turning, support surface) should be evaluated at regular intervals. Daily skin inspection should provide the information needed to determine if the pressure ulcer prevention plan is sufficient or requires modification. As a general rule, resolution of the intensity of erythema, if present, should become apparent within 24 hours of placement upon a support surface. A patient's risk for pressure ulcer formation will vary as his or her overall condition changes; therefore routine and regular reassessment and modification of the plan of care are warranted.

Quality tracking of the PUPP should include (1) concurrent 24/7 self-reporting of nosocomial pressure ulcers, (2) process measures, and (3) outcome measures. Concurrent daily reporting of nosocomial pressure ulcers for all patients is perhaps a more important measure than are quarterly or annual incidence studies. A simple 24/7 mechanism for staff to report nosocomial pressure ulcers through quality tracking (event reports, incident reports, root cause analysis) leads to more accurate reporting of nosocomial pressure ulcers, more timely root cause analysis and action plans, as well as early identification of weakening infrastructure. For example, a rise in the number of pressure ulcers secondary to oxygen masks may have resulted from a contract change to an inferior mask. Concurrent reporting of nosocomial pressure ulcers can uncover the problem quickly so that disciplines can unite, identify the root cause, and correct the problem quickly before more patients are injured. Conversely, a facility-wide incidence study that is not performed daily cannot lead to problem resolution and pressure ulcer reduction as quickly. With an average length of stay in acute care of just a few days, countless patients are missed with such infrequent incident studies.

Process measures capture compliance with designated components of the PUPP, for example, pressure ulcer risk assessment within 8 hours of admission, skin inspection upon admission, or daily risk assessments of "at-risk" patients. The value of process measures is heightened when correlated with concurrent self-reports. This will also be beneficial when targeting staff education.

The key outcome measure of a PUPP is the incidence of pressure ulcers and can be tabulated to reflect unit-based incidence or system-wide incidence. Pressure ulcer incidence can be obtained once yearly and compared to concurrent daily self-reporting data to essentially validate the accuracy of self-reported numbers. However, these kinds of incidence calculations cannot be considered reliable data collection for mandated public reporting. Pressure ulcer incidence can be calculated and reported in many ways, which contributes to the confusion and the wide range of data when comparisons to other facilities are attempted. To be most relevant, incidence should be reported as pressure ulcers per 100 admits or pressure ulcers per 1,000 patient-days (IHI, 2008).

SUMMARY

Pressure ulcers are a global health concern because, for the most part, they are a costly *preventable* complication. As a consequence of unrelieved pressure, capillaries are occluded and tissue damage ensues, and the extent of tissue damage is influenced by numerous variables. Pressure ulcer prevention requires a comprehensive multidisciplinary plan that includes risk assessment; regular and routine skin assessment; reducing risk factors; patient, family, and staff education; and evaluation. Ongoing maintenance of program infrastructure is critical to sustain a low incidence of pressure ulcers. This is accomplished through (1) embedding education into patient education tools, staff orientation, and annual competencies, (2) ensuring thorough and user-friendly documentation methods and decision-making tools, (3) concurrent and reliable quality tracking, and (4) a team approach with safe handoffs and communication across settings.

REFERENCES

Alterescu V: Reflections upon the history and future of the IAET, *J ET Nurs* 18(4):126-131, 1991.

American Hospital Association: *Hospital statistics*, Chicago, Ill, 1998, Healthcare Infosource.

AORN: *AORN recommended practices for positioning the patient in the perioperative practice setting. AORN standards, recommended practices, and guidelines*, Denver, 2008, Author.

Armstrong D, Bortz P: An integrative review of pressure relief in surgical patients, *AORN J* 73(3): 645-648, 650-653, 2001.

Aronovitch SA: Intraoperatively acquired pressure ulcers: are there common risk factors? *Ostomy Wound Manage* 53(2):57-69, 2007.

Ayello EA, Braden B: How and why to do pressure ulcer risk assessment, *Adv Skin Wound Care* 15:125, 2002.

Baharestani MM, Ratliff CR: Pressure ulcers in neonates and children: an NPUAP white paper, *Adv Skin Wound Care* 20:208, 2007.

Beckrich K, Aronovitch SA: Hospital-acquired pressure ulcers: a comparison of costs in medical versus surgical patients, *Nurs Econ* 17(5):263-271, 1999.

Bergstrom NI et al: Predicting pressure ulcer risk: a multisite study of the predictive validity of the Braden scale, *Nurs Res* 47(5):261, 1998.

Bolton L: Which pressure ulcer risk assessment scales are valid for use in the clinical setting? *J Wound Ostomy Continence Nurs* 34:368-381, 2007.

Braden BJ: *Protocols by level of risk*, 2001, available at http://bradenscale.com/images/protocols_by_level_of_risk.pdf accessed April 27, 2010.

Brown A: *Pressure ulcer prevention in x-ray departments*, Sixth European Pressure Ulcer Advisory Panel meeting, September 20, 2002, available at http://www.epuap.org/review5_1/page5c.html, accessed June, 15, 2009.

Brown G: Wound documentation: managing risk, *Adv Skin Wound Care* 19(3):155-165, 2006.

Bryant RA, Rolstad BS: Utilizing a systems approach to implement pressure ulcer prediction and prevention, *Ostomy Wound Manage* 47(9):26, 2001.

Bryant R et al: Pressure ulcer prevention and management, In Bryant R, editor: *Acute and chronic wounds: nursing management*, St. Louis, 1992, Mosby.

Cherner LL, editor: *The universal healthcare almanac*, Phoenix, Ariz, 1998, Silver & Chernes.

Cranney M et al: Why do GPs not implement evidence-based guidelines? A descriptive study, *Fam Pract* 18:359-363, 2001.

Defloor T, de Schuijmer JD: Preventing pressure ulcers: an evaluation of four operating-table mattresses, *Appl Nurs Res* 13: 134-141, 2000.

Duncan KD: Preventing pressure ulcers: the goal is zero, *Jt Comm J Qual Patient Saf* 33(10):605-610, 2007.

Fowler E. et al: Heels Practice recommendations for preventing heel pressure ulcers, *Ostomy Wound Manage* 54(10), 2008.

Gefen A: How much time does it take to get a pressure ulcer? Integrated evidence from human, animal, and in vitro studies, *Ostomy Wound Manage* 54(10), 2008.

Goode PS: Pressure ulcer prevention and early treatment, *J ET Nurs* 18(5):149-150, 1991.

Grous CA et al: Skin integrity in patients undergoing prolonged operations, *J Wound Ostomy Continence Nurs* 24(2):86-91, 1997.

Hagisawa S, Barbenel J: The limits of pressure sore prevention, *J R Soc Med* 92(11):576-578, 1999.

Institute for Healthcare Improvement (IHI): *5 million lives campaign. Getting started kit: prevent pressure ulcers how-to guide*, Cambridge, Mass, 2008, Author.

International Association for Enterostomal Therapy (IAET): *Standards of care. Dermal wounds: pressure ulcers*, Santa Ana, Calif, 1987, Author.

Jacobson TM et al: Improving practice. Efforts to reduce occipital pressure ulcers, *J Nurse Care Qual* 23(3):283-288, 2008.

Kitch BT et al: Handoffs causing patient harm: a survey of medical and surgical house staff, *Jt Comm J Qual Patient Saf* 34(10): 563-570, 2008.

Kosiak M: Etiology of decubitus ulcers, *Arch Phys Med Rehabil*, 42:191, 1961.

Krishnagopalan S et al: Body positioning of intensive care patients: clinical practice versus standards, *Crit Care Med* 30(11):2588-2592, 2002.

Magnan MA, Maklebust J: The effect of Web-based Braden Scale training on the reliability and precision of Braden Scale pressure ulcer risk assessments, *J Wound Ostomy Continence Nurs* 35(2):199-208, 2008.

Magnan MA, Maklebust J: The effect of Web-based Braden Scale training on the reliability of Braden subscale scores, *J Wound Ostomy Continence Nurs* 36(1):51-59, 2009.

Maklebust J, Sieggreen MY, Sidor D, et al: Computer-based testing of the Braden Scale for predicting pressure sore risk, *Ostomy Wound Manage* 51(4):40-52, 2005.

Mayrovitz HN, Sims N: Effects of support surface relief pressures on heel skin blood flow in persons with and without diabetes mellitus, *Adv Skin Wound Care* 17:197, 2004.

Minnesota Department of Health: *Adverse health events in Minnesota 2009*, Fifth annual public report, 2009, available at http://www.health.state.mn.us/patientsafety/ae/09ahereport.pdf, accessed November 10, 2009.

National Pressure Ulcer Advisory Panel (NPUAP) and European Pressure Ulcer Advisory Panel (EPUAP): *Prevention and treatment of pressure ulcers: quick reference guide*, Washington DC, 2009, NPUAP.

National Pressure Ulcer Advisory Panel (NPUAP): *Not all pressure ulcers are avoidable*. March 3, 2010 available at http://www.npuap.org/A_UA%20Press%20Release.pdf accessed April 27, 2010

National Priorities Partnership: *National priorities and goals for healthcare reform*, executive summary, 2008, available at http://www.nationalprioritiespartnership.org/PriorityDetails.aspx?id=612, accessed October 15, 2009.

Odierna E, Zeleznik J: Pressure ulcer education: a pilot study of the knowledge and clinical confidence of geriatric fellows, *Adv Skin Wound Care* 16(1):26, 2003.

Padula CA et al: Prevention and early detection of pressure ulcers in hospitalized patients, *J Wound Ostomy Continence Nurs* 35(1):65-75, 2008.

Pancorbo-Hidalgo PL et al: Risk assessment scales for pressure ulcer prevention: a systematic review, *J Adv Nurs* 54(1):94-110, 2006.

Powers J et al: The incidence of skin breakdown associated with use of cervical collars, *J Trauma Nurs* 13(4):198-200, 2006.

Reddy M, Gill SS, Rochon PA: Preventing pressure ulcers: A systematic review, *JAMA*. 296:974-984, 2006.

Redelings MD et al: Pressure ulcers: more lethal than we thought? *Adv Skin Wound Care* 18(7):367-372, 2005.

Reinertsen JL et al: *Seven leadership leverage points for organization-level improvement in health care*, ed 2, IHI Innovation Series white paper, Cambridge, Mass, 2008, Institute for Healthcare Improvement, available at http://www.ihi.org/IHI/Results/WhitePapers/SevenLeadershipLeveragePointsWhitePaper.htm.

Robert Wood Johnson Foundation: *National priorities partnership sets action agenda to improve health care*, 2008, available at http://www.rwjf.org/pr/product.jsp?id=33971, accessed October 260, 2009.

Stechmiller JK, Cowan L, Whitney JD, Phillips L, et al: Guidelines for the prevention of pressure ulcers, *Wound Rep Reg* 16:151-168, 2008.

Tescher AN et al: Range-of-motion restriction and craniofacial tissue-interface pressure from four cervical collars, *J Trauma* 63(5):1120-1126, 2007.

The Joint Commission: Hand-off communications, December 09, 2008, available at http://www.jointcommission.org/AccreditationPrograms/LongTermCare/Standards/09_FAQs/NPSG/Pressure_ulcers/NPSG.14.01.01/Pressure+ulcers.htm accessed April 15, 2010.

Thomas DR et al: Hospital acquired pressure ulcers and risk of death, *J Am Geriatr Soc* 44:1435-1440, 1996.

Thomas DR: Are all pressure ulcers avoidable? *J Am Med Dir Assoc* 4: 43-48, 2003.

U.S. Department of Health and Human Services: *Healthy people 2010: understanding and improving health*, ed 2, Washington DC, 2000, U.S. Government Printing Office.

Walton-Geer PS: Prevention of pressure ulcers in the surgical patient, *AORN J* 89(3):538-548, 2009.

Wilson FL, Williams BN: Assessing the readability of skin care and pressure ulcer patient education materials, *J Wound Ostomy Continence Nurs* 30:224, 2003.

Wong VK, Stotts NA: Physiology and prevention of heel ulcers: the state of science, *J WOCN* 30:191, 2003.

Wound, Ostomy and Continence Nurses (WOCN) Society: *Guideline for prevention and management of pressure ulcers*, Glenview, IL, 2003, Author.

Wound, Ostomy and Continence Nurses (WOCN) Society: *Inpatient prospective payment changes: a guide for the WOC nurse*, 2008, available at http://www.wocn.org/About_Us/News/30/, accessed October 10, 2009.

Wound, Ostomy and Continence Nurses (WOCN) Society: *Position statement: avoidable versus unavoidable pressure ulcers*, 2009, available at http://www.wocn.org/WOCN_Library/Position_Statements/, accessed October 26, 2009.

Wound, Ostomy and Continence Nurses (WOCN) Society: *Guideline for prevention and management of pressure ulcers*, Glenview, IL, 2010, Author.

Wright K: President's message: pressure ulcer prediction, prevention, and early treatment, *J ET Nurs* 18(4):115-116, 1991.

9

Support Surfaces

Denise P. Nix and Dianne M. Mackey

OBJECTIVES

1. List three limitations to the reliance of capillary closing values for support surface evaluation.
2. List four factors to consider when interpreting the significance of interface tissue pressure readings.
3. Define pressure redistribution, immersion, and envelopment.
4. Explain the difference between a reactive and an active support surfaces.
5. Compare the advantages and disadvantages of support surface categories and features.
6. List factors to consider for appropriate selection of a support surface.

A support surface is a specialized device for pressure redistribution designed for the management of tissue loads (NPUAP, 2007). Depending on the composition of the support surface and its mechanism of action, additional therapeutic functions may include reduction of shear, friction, and moisture. Support surfaces are available in different sizes and shapes and are made for chairs as well as for horizontal surfaces, such as mattresses, examination and procedure tables, operating room (OR) surfaces, and, more recently, emergency and transport stretchers or gurneys.

Although there is insufficient evidence to specify a particular brand of support surface (NPUAP and EPUAP, 2009; Whitney et al, 2006; WOCN Society, 2003, 2010), a variety of pressure-redistribution devices can help lower the incidence of pressure ulcers up to 60% (Cullum et al, 2004; Whitney et al 2006). This chapter reviews factors to consider for the (1) evaluation of support surfaces, (2) selection/evaluation of support surfaces based on individual patient assessment, and (3) creation/evaluation of a facility- or agency-wide support surface formulary. General guidance for the care of the patient requiring a support surface is given in Box 9-1.

INTERFACE TISSUE PRESSURES: PAST AND PRESENT

Interface tissue pressure is the force per unit area that acts perpendicularly between the body and the support surface and is measured by a sensor placed between the skin and support surface. This process is also known as *pressure mapping* (Figure 9-1). A review of 29 randomized controlled trials concluded that these measurements do not reliably predict support surface performance (Cullum et al, 2004). However, pressure mapping continues to be used to (1) produce images for product literature that appears to show pressure redistribution, (2) compare measurements from the same patient on two different surfaces, (3) assist with adjusting inflation of a chair cushion, or (4) teach a chairbound patient what type of position change will decrease pressure over an ischial tuberosity. Box 9-2 summarizes factors to consider when reviewing literature that includes interface tissue pressures (Reger et al, 1988; WOCN Society, 2003).

Historically, support surfaces have been categorized by comparing interface tissue pressure measurements obtained on a support surface to a standard capillary closing value. Surfaces were then placed into categories called *pressure reduction* and *pressure relief* based on how close the interface tissue pressures were to the standard capillary closing value; these terms are now considered invalid (NPUAP, 2007). However, because the concept of a standardized capillary closing pressure is affected by many variables (Box 9-2) and is unlikely to exist (Le et al, 1984), attempting to employ such a simplistic scheme to guide a process as complex as support surface selection is flawed. It is more useful to formulate a framework for support surface selection that is based on such traits as physical concepts, therapeutic functions, medium, forms and features.

PHYSICAL CONCEPTS AND THERAPEUTIC FUNCTIONS

Physical concepts are performance-related terms used to provide standard discussions about how support surfaces perform (Christian and Lachenbruch, 2007). *Life expectancy* refers to the period of time during which

BOX 9-1	General Guidance for Care of Patient Requiring a Support Surface

- Support surfaces alone neither prevent nor heal pressure ulcers and should be incorporated into a comprehensive individualized care plan.*
- Patient with or at-risk* for pressure ulcers should be placed on a support surface rather than a standard hospital mattress.
- Patient with or at risk* for pressure ulcers who sits should have a chair cushion and a sitting plan* that specifies frequency, duration, posture, and positioning needs.
- Support surfaces must be compatible with the care setting while meeting the individual needs of the patient.
- Support surfaces function best with minimal linens and pads under the patient.
- Patient must be able to assume a variety of positions on the selected surface (bed or chair) without bottoming out.
- Patient should be turned and repositioned regardless of support surface features.
- Multiple factors determine the frequency of repositioning* and must not be based solely on the features of the support surface.
- Use positioning devices and continence pads compatible with the support surface.
- A support surface that dissipates moisture (low air loss) may be indicated when skin barriers and dressings do not adequately protect the skin from moisture/incontinence.
- A reactive support surface with features and components such as low air loss, alternating pressure, viscous or air fluids should be considered for patients who:
  - can NOT be effectively positioned off their wound
  - have pressure ulcers involving multiple turning surfaces
  - have pressure ulcers that fail to improve despite optimal comprehensive management
- An active support surface (alternating pressure) should be considered when effective repositioning is determined by an MD to be medically contraindicated (frequent re-evaluation should be documented).

*See Chapter 8 for details.

BOX 9-2	Capillary Closing and Interface Tissue Pressures

A *capillary closing* pressure value should not be used to compare support surfaces for the following reasons:
- Capillary closing values are based on measurements obtained from the fingertips of young healthy males.
- Pressure is three to five times greater at the bone than at the surface of the skin.
- Lower capillary closing pressures have been reported in older patients.
- Tissue interface pressures do not ensure that blood flow through the capillaries is unimpeded.

Interface tissue pressure measurements (pressure mapping) should be reported with the following disclosures:
- Population tested (healthy subject will demonstrate lower pressure readings than debilitated subjects because normal muscle mass supports and distributes weight more effectively)
- How often equipment was recalibrated (sensors are fragile and may malfunction)
- Number of readings conducted per site (range based on multiple readings is more reliable than one single reading per site)
- Factors known to affect results:
  - Stiffness of support surface
  - Composition of body tissue
  - Transducer size and shape
  - Method of equilibrium detection
  - Uniformity of measurement technique
  - Load shape and its interaction with support material
  - Skill of person taking measurements (uniformity of technique for measuring interface tissue pressure is necessary for accuracy)

a product is able to effectively fulfill its purpose. It may be impacted by *fatigue* or a reduced capacity to perform due to intended or unintended use and/or prolonged exposure to chemical, thermal, or physical forces (NPUAP, 2007). Both of these factors will impact the ability of the support surface to redistribute pressure and control friction and shear.

Pressure Redistribution (Immersion and Envelopment)

Support surfaces are designed to prevent pressure ulcers and, through pressure redistribution, provide an environment more conducive to pressure ulcer healing. Support surfaces redistribute interface pressure by conforming to the contours of the body so that pressure is redistributed over a larger surface area rather than concentrated on a more circumscribed location. The therapeutic function of pressure redistribution is accomplished through immersion and envelopment. *Immersion* refers to the depth of penetration or sinking into the surface allowing the pressure to be spread out over the surrounding area rather than directly over a bony prominence. Immersion is dependent on factors such as the stiffness and thickness of the support

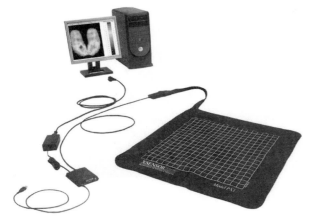

FIGURE 9-1 Pressure mapping device (XSensor pressure mapping system). (Courtesy the ROHO Group, Belleville, IL.)

surface and the flexibility of the cover. *Envelopment* refers to the ability of the support surface to conform to irregularities (e.g., clothing, bedding, bony prominences) without causing a substantial increase in pressure (Brienza and Geyer, 2005; Christian and Lachenbruch, 2007; NPUAP, 2007). In contrast to the therapeutic functions of immersion and envelopment, *"bottoming out"* occurs when the depth of penetration or sinking is excessive, allowing increased pressure to concentrate over one area or bony prominence. Whitney et al (2006) define bottoming out as less than 1 inch of material between the surface and the skin when feeling under a support surface with the palm of a hand. Factors that may lead to bottoming out include (1) weight exceeds manufacturer's recommendations; (2) disproportionate weights and sizes, such as with bilateral lower extremity amputation; (3) tendency to keep the head of the bed greater than 30 degrees; and (4) inappropriate support surface settings, such as over or underinflation. All support surfaces function best with less linen between the patient and the surface.

Friction and Shear Reduction

Friction and shear are physical concepts associated with pressure ulcer formation. *Shear stress* refers to force on the tissue; *shear strain* refers to the resulting deformation (Christian and Lachenbruch, 2007). A support surface reduces shear and friction by strategic placement of mediums and covers that allow for low-friction positioning without excessive sliding. However, the best support surface cover will not eliminate the need for additional interventions to minimize friction and shear as described in Chapters 5 and 8.

Microclimate (Temperature and Moisture) Control

Microclimate control is a therapeutic function some support surfaces may provide. Excess moisture of the skin is a well-known factor associated with pressure ulcer development. Control of temperature at the interface surface (patient–bed boundary) helps to maintain normal skin temperature, which in turn inhibits sweating and lowers skin hydration (Mackey, 2005). A support surface should be designed to help maintain normal skin hydration and temperature (Brienza and Geyer, 2005). Porous covers help reduce moisture by allowing air to transfer between the skin and surface so that moisture and body heat can dissipate. Some mediums may be nonpermeable and prevent liquid or air to escape, whereas others interact with the body to effect microclimate, such as with continuous pumped air flowing across the skin.

COMPONENTS

Components of a support surface are manufactured from various mediums as a means of creating pressure redistribution. Mediums are solid, fluid, and air used alone or in combination. The means of encapsulating the medium is considered another component of the support surface and is called cell or bladder (NPUAP, 2007). Multiple cells can be individual or interconnected, configured in a longitudinal or latitudinal pattern (Figures 9-2 and 9-3).

Foam

Foam is available in chair cushions, overlays, mattresses for beds, transport gurneys, and stretchers, and OR and procedure tables. Most foam overlays and cushions are indicated for single-patient use, whereas mattresses are intended for multiple-patient use. Both are designed for a specific weight limit and lifespan. Foam can be the sole medium or consist of hybrids that include composites of gel, air, or other more fluid materials to enhance envelopment in key areas. Benefits associated with foam support surfaces include their relatively low cost, light weight, and minimal maintenance. A disadvantage is the limited lifespan due to fatigue caused by flexion and compression over time.

Foam can be closed cell or open cell. *Closed-cell* foam is a nonpermeable formulation in which a barrier between cells prevents gases or liquids from passing through the

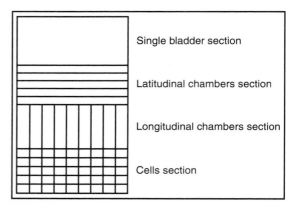

FIGURE 9-2 Interconnected, single bladder, longitudinal, or latitudinal cells.

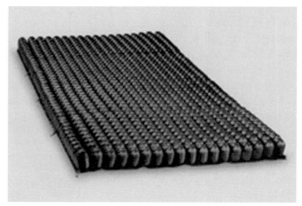

FIGURE 9-3 Nonpowered static air support surface consists of hundreds of individual air cells. (Courtesy the ROHO Group, Belleville, IL.)

foam (NPUAP, 2007), potentially increasing skin temperature by preventing dissipation of body heat (Nicholson et al, 1999). *Open-cell* foam is higher-specification foam that is more effective in preventing pressure ulcers than is closed-cell foam. Examples of higher-specification foams are elastic and viscoelastic. There is no evidence that one type of high-specification foam is better than another (NPUAP and EPUAP, 2009).

Elastic Foam.   Elastic is high-specification foam made of porous polymer material that conforms in proportion to the applied weight. Air enters and exits the open-cell foam rapidly due to its greater density (NPUAP, 2007). The surface continues to conform until the resistance to compression exceeds the weight being applied (Christian and Lachenbruch, 2007). The combination of density and hardness determines compressibility and conformity, ultimately establishing the ability of the support surface to mechanically redistribute loading force. Density describes foam weight, reported as either pounds per cubic foot or kilograms per cubic meter. Greater density provides more durability.

Indentation force deflection (IFD) also known previously as indentation load deflection (ILD), is a measure of firmness or resistance to compression. In the United States, IFD is reported as the force in pounds required to compress a prescribed size of foam by 25%. The more global foam industry tends to report the amount of force in "Newtons" necessary to compress a prescribed size of foam by 40% after a process of preconditioning. Surfaces can be made with a combination of foams strategically placed to optimize pressure redistribution in targeted locations (PFA, 2010). For example, a relatively lower-density IFD foam located closer to the patient to enhance conformation and a higher-density IFD foam located more deeply in the mattress to prevent compression or bottoming out.

A foam overlay is a single-user form of support surface placed on a mattress. If used for pressure redistribution, an overlay should have a base height of at least 3 inches measured from the base (or bottom) to the lower level of convolution (Figure 9-4), suitable density to ensure durability (1.3–1.6 lb/ft^3), IFD of 30, and ideally a ratio of 25% to 40% for compression of 2.5 or greater (Whittemore, 1998).

Viscoelastic (Memory) Foam.   *A viscoelastic* is another high-specification open-cell foam made of porous polymer material that conforms in proportion to the applied weight. Air enters and exits the foam cells slowly, which allows the material to respond slower than elastic foam. Viscoelastic foams are a subset of urethane polymer foams that exhibit a slow recovery

(memory) property. A viscoelastic foam product generally has a higher density and a lower IFD. Because of their fluid nature, when an object is placed on a viscoelastic support surface, the viscoelastic tends to displace quickly and conform to the shape of the object, with low resistance. Viscoelastic foam is available in many grades and qualities, each having properties that affect pressure redistribution and microclimate performance in unique ways. Some viscoelastic foams are engineered to change hardness within a specific temperature range. These materials tend to get softer as the material warms to body temperature, resulting in conformation similar to that of a gel. Viscoelastic support surfaces are often used in the OR (AORN, 2008) and have been shown to effectively decrease the incidence of pressure ulcers in high-risk elderly patients with fractures of the neck and femur (Cullum et al, 2001). One study of 838 patients at risk for pressure ulcers found a significantly lower pressure ulcer incidence when patients were turned every 4 hours on a viscoelastic surface compared to patients who were turned every 2 hours on a standard mattress (Defloor et al, 2005).

Gel

Gel contains a network of solid aggregates, colloidal dispersions, or polymers that may exhibit elastic properties (NPUAP, 2007). Some gel products are called *viscoelastic gel* because they respond similarly to viscoelastic foam. Gel support surfaces are intended for multiple-patient use. Because of the consistency of the medium, gels have been found to be especially effective in preventing shear. Other advantages include easy cleaning and no electricity. Disadvantages of gel support surfaces are that they tend to be heavy and are difficult to repair. Skin humidity can increase due to the nonporous nature of the gel and the lack of air flow. Although the gel is cool upon initial contact, skin temperature may increase after hours of constant contact. Gel must be carefully monitored, and the material must be manually moved back to the areas under bony prominences if it has migrated (Brienza and Geyer, 2005).

Fluids (Viscous Fluid, Water, Air)

Fluids are considered substances whose molecules flow freely past one another. Fluids have no fixed shape, so they take on the shape of the load with less resistance than a gel or solid component, creating a high degree of immersion. Fluid mediums include viscous fluid, water, and air. Moisture control characteristics are dependent on the ability of the medium to conduct heat and the composition of the product's cover.

Viscous Fluid.   Viscous fluid contains materials such as silicon elastomer, silicon, or polyvinyl (Brienza and Geyer, 2005). At first glance, viscous fluid can be mistaken for gel. Although many of its advantages and disadvantages

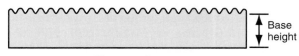

Foam overlay

FIGURE 9-4   Measuring the depth of foam overlay.

are similar to those of gels, viscous fluid is free flowing and has a similar pressure-redistribution response as air or water. Compared to air and water, viscous fluid is thicker, with a relatively higher resistance to flow (NPUAP, 2007).

Water. Water is a moderate-density fluid with moderate resistance to flow (NPUAP, 2007). Studies have demonstrated that water-filled support surfaces provide lower interface pressure than a standard mattress (Cullum et al, 2001). Although popular at home, water mattresses are undesirable in the hospital or long-term care setting due to multiple management concerns including the following:

- Need for a heater to control the temperature
- Time and labor needed to drain and move bed
- Potential for leaking
- Difficulty with repositioning and transferring and with performing cardiopulmonary resuscitation (CPR)

Air. Air is a low-density fluid with minimal resistance to flow (NPUAP, 2007). Air may be the sole redistribution medium, or it may be combined with other mediums (NPUAP, 2007). Support surfaces that incorporate air are available as chair cushions, overlays, mattresses, and bed systems. Most air support surfaces are easy to clean and can be reused. Air products have the potential to leak if damaged and require adequate inflation so that the body can immerse into the product. Air mattresses and overlays have the advantage of being lightweight and easy to clean.

CATEGORIES AND FEATURES

Categories of pressure redistribution support surfaces include overlays, mattress replacements, integrated bed systems. Pressure redistribution may be purchased in the form of a chair cushion, transport, procedure, emergency room, or perioperative surface. All of these surfaces may be powered or nonpowered, active or reactive. Features or functional components such as low air loss, air fluidization, lateral rotation, and alternating pressure may be used alone or in combination. A variety of pressure-redistribution capabilities can exist in single or multi-zoned surfaces. A zone, is a segment with a single pressure redistribution capability. Therefore, a multi-zoned surface has different segments with different pressure redistribution capabilities (NPUAP, 2007).

Mattress Overlays

The mattress overlay is a support surface that is placed on top of an existing mattress (Christian and Lachenbruch, 2007; NPUAP, 2007). Gel, water, and some air-filled overlays are intended for multiple-patient use and have the advantage of requiring much less storage space than mattresses and bed systems. Other overlays, such as foam and some air products, are for

single-patient use and present environmental concerns relative to disposal of the product. Overlays are thinner than mattress replacements, so there is potential for the patient to bottom out onto the mattress below. Because they are applied over an existing mattress, mattress overlays increase the height of the bed and may complicate patient transfers, alter the fit of linens, or increase the risk for patient entrapment and falls (U.S. FDA, 2006).

Mattresses

A mattress is composed of any medium or combination of mediums that is placed on an existing compatible frame. Mattresses reduce some of the high-profile–related disadvantages experienced with overlays and appear to have fewer issues with bottoming out. When first introduced, the majority of support surfaces were rented integrated support surfaces or overlays that were rented or purchased. When support surfaces called "replacement mattresses" entered the marketplace, many facilities realized improved skin and wound outcomes by replacing their standard mattresses with replacement mattresses (Cullum et al, 2004; Gray et al, 2001). This investment reduced lead time and labor by eliminating the need to wait for delivery of bed systems or for staff to help move the patient once risk or pressure ulcers were identified. Today, some companies no longer make mattresses that do not redistribute pressure, so their standard mattress *is* a support surface. Mattresses may include a variety of therapeutic functions such as shear and friction reduction.

Transport, Procedure, Emergency Room, and OR Mattresses. It stands to reason that patients who require a support surface in bed would benefit from a support surface during special procedures, surgeries, and long waits on emergency room and transport gurneys. In fact, patients on these surfaces may be more at risk for pressure ulcer development due to limited space for moving and repositioning in addition to their potential need for sedation or anesthesia. Although not yet presented in peer-reviewed publications, manufacturers now are creating support surface mattresses (sometimes called *pads*) with a pressure-redistribution option for emergency room, transport, and procedure tables. Some companies will custom-fit their pressure-redistribution products to fit surfaces other than beds.

Chapter 8 provides information related to unique risk factors specific to patients in the OR. A perioperative guidance document for pressure ulcer prevention can be found in Appendix C. The international guidelines recommend that the at-risk individual in the OR should have a mattress with pressure-redistributing properties greater than those of the standard OR mattress (AORN, 2008; NPUAP and EPUAP, 2009). However, a review of the literature suggests that, due to uncontrolled variables (e.g., reaction to anesthesia, discoveries leading to longer surgery), all surgical patients should be considered at risk and placed on a mattress with pressure-redistributing properties greater than those of the standard OR mattress (Walton-Geer, 2009). A standard OR mattress is defined as a 2-inch foam surface covered with a vinyl or nylon fabric (AORN, 2008).

A number of support surface options are available for the OR, including air, gel, and high-specification foam mattresses. The best OR surface for preventing pressure ulcers has not been determined. Therefore, selection of a support surface in the OR requires careful analysis of a number of factors to ensure the product provides pressure redistribution while demonstrating compatibility with the facility's most common surgical positions, safety procedures, transfer equipment, and budget (Box 9-3).

Of note, the number of pads and blankets, including warming blankets placed beneath the patient and the OR mattress, interferes with the pressure-redistribution properties of the mattress. If a cooling blanket is placed between the patient and the OR table mattress, a higher-grade surface should be considered to account for the change in pressure redistribution (AORN, 2008).

Integrated Bed Systems

An integrated bed system is a bed frame and support surface combined into a single unit. It is a rented or purchased unit whose components do not function separately (Christian and Lachenbruch, 2007; NPUAP, 2007); therefore, it is used in place of an existing bed. With the integrated bed system, the features of both the frame and the support surface must be evaluated. Frames come in different widths and lengths and support a specified amount of weight. Some frames have the ability to adjust or fold for storage or transport through narrow doors and elevators. Most frames today are electric, but alternatives are available. When selecting a frame, the population to be served and the setting in which it will be used should be considered. For example, frames with built-in bed exit alarms may be needed for patients who are confused and at risk for falls. Frames with built-in bed scales may be needed for the intensive care unit, where daily weights are a necessity, although many frames today include scales as standard operating equipment. Advantages and disadvantages mostly depend on whether or not the surface is rented (discussed later in this chapter).

Chair Cushions

Pressure redistribution in the chair often goes overlooked. Wounds that develop from sitting are located on the ischia during upright sitting and on the coccyx when slouching, sliding, or reclining. ressure-redistribution chair cushions should be used with seated individuals who are at risk for pressure ulcers and have reduced mobility (NPUAP and EPUAP, 2009). Selecting a cushion of appropriate size for the seated patient is extremely important given the potential for the patient to

BOX 9-3	AORN Selection Recommendations for Operating Room Support Surfaces

- Facilitates ability to hold patient in desired position
- Available in variety of shapes and sizes
- Ability to support maximum weight requirements
- Durable material and design
- Evidence that it can disperse skin interface pressure
- Resistance to moisture
- Smooth and intact surfaces
- Low risk for moisture retention
- Radiolucent as needed
- Fire retardant
- Nonallergenic
- Promote air circulation
- Low risk of harboring bacteria
- Easy to use and store
- Cost-effective

"bottom out" as most of the weight is applied to a relatively small body surface.

They are available in foam, air, and gel, and they come in bariatric sizes. Ring cushion (doughnut) devices increase venous congestion and edema and should not be used for pressure ulcer prevention and management (NPUAP and EPUAP, 2009; Whitney et al 2006; WOCN Society, 2003; 2010). Once implemented, chair cushions must be inspected regularly for wear and tear. Improper inflation, overcompression, or displaced gel can impair adequate pressure redistribution and lead to bottoming out.

Active (Alternating-Pressure)

An *active* support surface is a powered mattress or overlay that changes its load-distribution properties with or without an applied load (NPUAP, 2007). An active support surface moves even if nobody is in the bed (Christian and Lachenbruch, 2007). Active mattresses or overlays should be selected for high-risk patients when frequent repositioning is not possible (NPUAP and EPUAP, 2009). As of 2010, the only active support surfaces on the market are those that include the feature of alternating pressure therapy. An example of an alternating pressure therapy surface is shown in Table 9-1.

Alternating-pressure is a feature found in overlays and mattress. Alternating pressure products have cells arranged in various patterns that are inflated and deflated with air. Rather than pressure being distributed by increasing the surface area through immersion and envelopment, pressure is periodically redistributed across the body by inflating and deflating the cells of alternating zones. *Pulsating pressure* refers to shorter-duration inflation and higher-frequency cycling for which there is less direct evidence (Gunther and Clark, 2000). The individual cell that composes the

TABLE 9-1	Example of Support Surface Decision-Making Tool and Formulary
Criteria	**Support Surface**
Weight < _____ lbs AND Braden Score 13-18 (at risk to mod risk) AND one of the following: ✓ Intact skin ✓ CAN be effectively positioned off wound	REACTIVE SUPPORT SURFACE 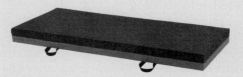 Example: Viscoelastic foam mattress (Visco 1) *(Image courtesy of EncompassTSS)*
Weight < _____ lbs AND one of the following: ✓ Intact skin with Braden Score less than 13 ✓ Patient can NOT be effectively positioned off wound ✓ Patient has less than 2 intact turning surfaces	REACTIVE SUPPORT SURFACE with features and components such as low air loss, viscous fluid or air fluids, OR active support surface (alternating pressure) 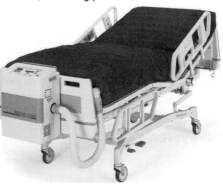 Example: low air loss mattress (Flexicair Eclipse Low Airloss Therapy Unit) *(Image courtesy of Hill-Rom Services, Inc., © 2005)*
Weight > _____ lbs or BMI > _____ **AND** Braden Score 13-18 (at risk to mod risk) AND one of the following: ✓ Intact skin ✓ CAN be effectively positioned off wound	BARIATRIC REACTIVE SURFACE 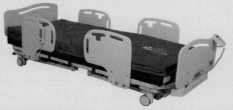 Example: Bariatric with viscoelastic foam mattress *(Image courtesy of Sizewise)*
Weight > _____ lbs or BMI > _____ **AND** one of the following: ✓ Intact skin with Braden Score less than 13 ✓ Patient can NOT be effectively positioned off wound ✓ Patient has less than two intact turning surfaces	BARIATRIC REACTIVE SUPPORT SURFACE with features and components such as low air loss, viscous fluid or air fluids. OR Active support surface (alternating pressure) 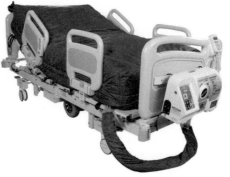 Example: Bariatric with low air loss mattress *(Image courtesy of Sizewise)*

Continued

TABLE 9-1	Example of Support Surface Decision-Making Tool and Formulary—cont'd

Criteria	Support Surface
Effective repositioning is determined by an MD to be medically contraindicated (frequent re-evaluation should be documented) *Specify bariatric option for weight > _____ lbs or BMI >_____*	CONSIDER ACTIVE SUPPORT SURFACE* 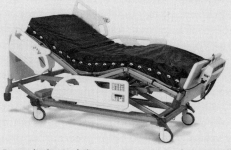 Example: 'Active' Therapy Mattress Replacement (Alternating) *(Image courtesy of ArjoHuntleigh)*
Extensive debridement or flap surgery OR Patient is on bedrest and wound(s) have deteriorated on a low air loss surface despite optimal wound management	AIR FLUIDIZED 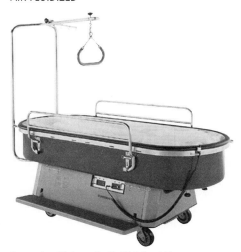 Example: Clinitron® Air Fluidized Therapy *(Image courtesy of Hill-Rom Services, Inc., © 2005)*
Patient meets three of the following criteria: Artificial airway, PaO2/FiO2<250 with FiO2>0.40, requires >10 PEEP (regardless of FiO2), desaturates with manual turning, immobile/exhibits ineffective mobility, receiving neuromuscular blockade therapy or continuous IV sedation, difficulty mobilizing secretions, ventilated with sepsis/ARDS	LATERAL ROTATION 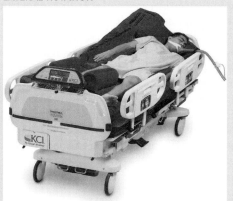 Example: TriaDyne Proventa™ Kinetic Therapy System *(Image courtesy of KCI Licensing, Inc.)*

*Refer to Active support surface (alternating pressure) section of chapter for explanation.

alternating-pressure mattress and/or overlay must be 10 cm or greater to effectively redistribute pressure (NPUAP and EPUAP, 2009). Alternating pressure and pulsating pressure can be found in combination with foam and low air loss products.

International pressure ulcer guidelines suggest the use of an active support surface (mattress or overlay) for patients at higher risk for pressure ulcer development where frequent manual repositioning is not possible. This recommendation was derived indirectly from two studies; one of which was recognized as a poor quality study.

Iglesias and colleagues (2006) noted that pressure ulcers occurred almost 11 days sooner on an alternating pressure overlay when compared to an alternating pressure mattress. However, in a study cited by International Pressure Ulcer Guidelines, no significant difference between alternating pressure mattresses and overlays were found, which lead to the guidelines statement that alternating-pressure mattresses and overlays have similar efficacy in terms of pressure ulcer incidence (Nixon et al, 2006; NPUAP and EPUAP, 2009).

Reactive

A *reactive* support surface will move or change load-distribution properties only in response to an applied load, such as the patient's body (Christian and Lachenbruch, 2007). Unlike active support surfaces that must be powered, reactive support surfaces are powered or nonpowered with the potential to avoid the noise of a motor. Examples of reactive support surfaces include mattresses and overlays filled with foam, air, or a combination of foam and air. Gel surfaces, which may be in the form of chair cushions, overlays, mattresses, and pads for stretchers, OR tables, and procedure tables, are nonpowered. Nonpowered air-filled support surfaces range from low-end prevention products that encapsulate air into a single bladder or cell to therapeutic products containing hundreds of individual interconnected cells (Figure 9-3). All reactive support surfaces are appropriate for pressure ulcer prevention in the patient who is frequently repositioned. Some are appropriate for patients with pressure ulcers. With few exceptions, reactive support surfaces are compatible with long-term care facilities, hospitals, and home settings.

Continuous Lateral Rotation. Continuous lateral rotation is a feature that has been used for the past 30 years for the prevention and treatment of selected cardiopulmonary conditions. Continuous lateral rotation therapy bed rotates the patient in a regular pattern around a longitudinal (i.e., head to foot) axis of 40 degrees *or less* to each side. In contrast, kinetic therapy is defined as the side-to-side rotation of 40 degrees *or more* to each side. Drawing firm conclusions regarding effectiveness in the patient with cardiopulmonary disease is difficult, as these surfaces are primarily intended to facilitate pulmonary hygiene in the patient with acute respiratory conditions. Use of adult specialty beds in the rotation mode is ineffective for small children because their small bodies are confined to one section or pillow of the surface (McCord et al, 2004).

Lateral rotation has been incorporated into some low air loss and air/foam mattresses, overlays and integrated bed systems as shown in Table 9-1. One descriptive study of 30 patients on continuous lateral rotation therapy incorporated into a foam mattress replacement noted no new pressure ulcer development, with improvement of trunk and pelvis wounds (Anderson and Rappl, 2004). However, knowledge of the effects of continuous lateral rotation therapy on pressure redistribution is limited.

Therefore, it is important to emphasize that continuous lateral rotation therapy does not eliminate the need for routine manual repositioning. Staff will need to take extra precautions to prevent shear, including aligning and securing the patient with bolster pads that are provided by the manufacturer and frequent turning to inspect the skin for signs of shear. Optimally, if shear injury develops, the patient would be positioned off the injured area and an alternative support surface method used. However, if the patient is still in respiratory distress, the risks and benefits of continuous lateral rotation therapy should be carefully considered prior to making a change (NPUAP and EPUAP, 2009).

Low Air Loss. One commonly misunderstood feature related to support surfaces is low air loss. The NPUAP (2007) defines low air loss as a feature that provides a flow of air to assist in managing the head and humidity (microclimate) of the skin. Low air loss consists of a series of connected pillows. A pump provides slow continuous air flow allowing for even distribution into the porous mattress and continuous air flow across the skin (Table 9-1). The amount of pressure in each pillow is controlled and can be calibrated according to height and weight distribution to meet the individual needs of the patient. As the patient settles down into the mattress, weight is distributed more evenly for pressure redistribution. There may be an additional component placed at the base of the product, such as foam or air pillows, when "bottoming out" is problematic. Low air loss can be found alone or in combination with alternating pressure, lateral rotation, and air-fluidized technology that is incorporated into overlays, mattresses, bed systems, and even a chair cushion.

The construction of a low air-loss surface in addressing the microclimate of the skin can be achieved in two ways; with air-flow under the cover or with an air-permeable cover. Most familiar to clinicians is the air-permeable cover which allows for the slow, evenly distributed release of air *through* the cover and directly to the skin. Low air-loss surfaces with airflow *under* the cover addresses skin microclimate by receiving heat, gas, and water molecules through a moisture vapor permeable cover (conducted downward from the skin), into the air stream inside mattress which eventually exits along the sides or ends of the mattress.

The smooth covers for low air-loss surfaces are generally made of nylon or polytetrafluoroethylene fabric and have a low coefficient of friction. The covers are waterproof, impermeable to bacteria, and easy to clean. In order to receive the full benefits of low air-loss, minimal linen and special underpads with a high level of moisture vapor permeability (rather than plastic back pads) should be used.

Low air-loss support surfaces have been reported as an effective treatment surface and may improve healing rates of pressure ulcers. Because of the two aforementioned constructions (air-permeable cover verses air-flow under the cover), low air loss is associated with decreasing moisture, which may lead to skin damage such as incontinence-associated dermatitis or maceration (Cullum et al, 2004; WOCN Society, 2003). Wound desiccation however is also possible and may be prevented by using a moisture donating rather than absorptive dressing if the wound begins to dry.

Low air-loss surfaces come with important safety features, such as controls that instantly inflate the cushions, thus facilitating patient positioning. Fowler boost controls help prevent bottoming out by adding more air under the buttocks when the patient's head is elevated. Controls that instantly flatten the air cushions are activated prior to administration of CPR so that effective chest compressions are possible.

Due to the lack of stability compared to a firmer mattress, low air loss is contraindicated for patients with an unstable spine. Some patients lose their ability to effectively self-position on a low air loss surface again due to the lack of firmness in the surface. Additional disadvantages of low air-loss surfaces include increased risk of bed entrapment, especially if the device is not properly adjusted. It is imperative that clinicians and involved staff are familiar with the manufacturer's recommended instructions for use. Once the proper weight setting is established, it is prudent to record the setting to assure consistency of product use. Low air-loss surfaces can be costly, require electricity and special underpads that cost more than the standard underpad.

Air-Fluidized. The feature of air-fluidization, can only be found in an integrated bed system (Table 9-1) and was initially developed to treat patients with burns. Also known as high air loss, the surface contains silicone-coated beads that become incorporated into both air and fluid support; by pumping air through the beads, the beads behave like a liquid. The person "floats" on a sheet, with one third of the body above the surface and the rest of the body immersed in the warm, dry, fluidized beads. Body fluids flow freely through the sheet and cover, but contamination is prevented through continuous pressurization (Holzapfel, 1993). When the air-fluidized bed is turned off, it quickly becomes firm enough for repositioning or CPR.

Air-fluidized beds are most commonly used for patients with burns, myocutaneous skin flaps, and multiple Stage III or IV pressure ulcers. Using a subset of retrospectively collected National Pressure Ulcer Long-Term Care Study data, Ochs et al (2005) compared pressure ulcer outcomes of 664 residents placed on several types of support surfaces, including air-fluidized, low air loss, powered and nonpowered overlays, and hospital mattresses. Results indicated that residents placed on air-fluidized support surfaces had larger and deeper pressure ulcers and higher illness severity scores than did residents placed on the other support surfaces. However, residents who used air-fluidized surfaces had better healing rates, fewer emergency visits, and fewer hospital admissions. These findings, although significant, warrant more research on variables such as initial wound size, use of dressing, debridement, nutritional status, and presence of infection and incontinence.

In the institutional environment, these products are not ideally suited to facility ownership because of the complexity and the high costs of maintenance. An air-fluidized bed system is one of the most expensive support surfaces. Air-fluidized products have a warming feature for the pressurized air, which can be comforting or harmful depending on the overall condition of the patient. Hydration issues may be more pronounced than that experienced with low air-loss surfaces. Because air-fluidized beds are heavy, they may not be safe for use in older homes. Traditional air-fluidized beds are not recommended for the patient with pulmonary disease or an unstable spine. However, air-fluidized therapy in the lower half of the bed has been combined with low air loss in the upper portion of the surface to create an adjustable bed for the patient who needs to be more upright. This bed is similar in size to a hospital bed, the head of the bed is readily adjustable, and the bed is lighter than a total air-fluidized system.

SUPPORT SURFACE SELECTION CRITERIA

Despite the lack of evidence specifying any particular brand of support surfaces, guidelines for selecting a support surface for specific patients are necessary to facilitate appropriate staff decision making and proper product use. Because multiple forms of support surfaces with a full range of features are available, it is possible to create setting-specific formularies with options compatible with the individual needs of the typical patient population for that setting.

Individual Patient Needs

Individuals with pressure ulcers or those at risk for pressure ulcers should be placed on a support surface rather than a standard hospital mattress (Cullum et al, 2004; NPUAP and EPUAP, 2009; Whitney et al, 2006; WOCN Society, 2010). As described throughout this chapter, each support surface has disadvantages and contraindications. Therefore, support surfaces must not be selected based *solely* on the patient's wound assessment but rather the patient's individual needs (NPUAP and EPUAP, 2009). Individual needs of the patient with pressure ulcers or who is at risk for pressure ulcers are dependent on the condition and location of wounds (if applicable), activity and positioning, risk for falls and entrapment, size, weight, and patient response. Critical analysis of these needs weighted with support surface indications, advantages, and disadvantages will lead to appropriate selection.

Condition and Location of Wounds. For the individual with large Stage III or IV pressure ulcers or pressure ulcers involving multiple turning surfaces, a support surface should be considered that includes features and components such as low air loss, alternating pressure, viscous fluid, or air fluids. A support surface that dissipates moisture (low air loss) may be indicated when skin barriers and dressings do not adequately protect the skin from moisture/incontinence (Cullum et al, 2004; Whitney et al, 2006; WOCN Society, 2003). As discussed in the chair cushion section of this chapter, patients with sitting surface pressure ulcers require a support surface for the chair.

Activity and Positioning. If frequent repositioning is not possible, an active support surface is indicated (NPUAP and EPUAP, 2009). Low air loss overlays may need to be changed to mattresses to prevent bottoming out if an elevated head of bed for prolonged periods of time cannot be avoided. The patient who self-repositions, gets in and out of bed, or is attempting to increase and restore mobility and independence should use a support surface that facilitates rather than impairs his or her activity and mobility.

Risk for Falls or Entrapment. A surface that raises the patient higher in the bed or creates more distance between the mattress and frame or side rails increases the risk for entrapment and falls. When possible, a pressure-redistribution support surface that minimizes height and gaps should be selected for patients at risk for falls (U.S. FDA, 2006). Some facilities are adding fall risk assessment scores to support surface selection criteria. If the patient becomes at risk for falls or entrapment on a selected support surface, additional monitoring will be necessary or an alternative support surface should be selected.

Size and Weight. Bed frame and mattress specifications for weight capacity must be considered. Low air-loss products designed for adults do not provide options to accommodate the height and weight of small children (WOCN Society, 2010). Children and infants can sink into and between cushions, leading to risk for entrapment and falls (McLane et al, 2004).

Many adult hospital bed frames manufactured today hold up to 500 lb. However, older frames may not be designed to hold more than 350 lb and have a width

that precludes the ability of obese patients to effectively reposition for any period of time. Bariatric support surfaces are available in foam, air, gel, and water with or without microclimate and moisture control features. Care of the obese patient and bariatric support surface considerations are discussed in Chapter 35.

Patient Response. Once a product is selected, its effectiveness for any given patient must be reevaluated at regular intervals with the plan of care (Checklist 9-1, *A*). If expected outcomes are not achieved, an alternative support surface should be selected. Expected outcomes may include prevention of pressure ulcers, patient comfort, or moisture control. Wound healing may not be an expected outcome if it is not realistic or consistent with the patient's overall goals. If wound healing is an expected outcome after support surface implementation, it must be used in conjunction with documented and comprehensive pressure ulcer management.

CHECKLIST 9-1
Evaluating Support Surface Effectiveness

A. Individual Needs
✓ Has there been an increase in factors that place a patient at risk for pressure ulcers?
- Hemodynamic instability
- Frequent repositioning not possible
- Moisture management problems
- Increased need to keep head of the bed elevated

✓ Has the support surface caused any problems for the patient?
- Mobility impairment
- Pain or discomfort
- Sleeplessness
- Bottoming out
- Excessive dryness
- Skin breakdown

✓ Is the wound deteriorating despite appropriate care?
- Patient and caregiver education for pressure ulcer prevention and management
- Regular skin and risk assessment
- Appropriate turning and repositioning
- Appropriate wound care, including ongoing assessments and evaluation of healing
- Management of moisture and incontinence
- Nutritional support

B. Care-Setting Compatibility
✓ Does the formulary include enough options to meet the needs of the patient population?
✓ Does the formulary and selection criteria meet the fiscal needs of the setting?
✓ Is the staff competent with product procedures, such as setup, maintenance, and cleaning?
✓ Does the staff express overall satisfaction with the products?
✓ Is there an increase in entrapment, back injuries, or falls?
✓ Do the products conform with essential regulations?
✓ Are environmental concerns addressed?
✓ Does the company live up to promises for support and value-added services? (see Table 9-2)

The same factors that guided initial support surface selection should be reevaluated. Changes in patient status may guide the decision to discontinue or change a support surface. For example, the patient who once was comatose and hemodynamically unstable may require a different support surface to facilitate independence with self-positioning. Likewise, the patient on an overlay who was achieving expected outcomes may suddenly start bottoming out due to prolonged head of bed elevation because of respiratory distress. A patient on an overlay that previously was acceptable may be at increased risk for falling due to the onset of delirium.

Care Setting–Specific Formulary

A formulary of standardized products not only controls costs but is necessary to minimize confusion and mistakes related to appropriate selection and safe use (Whittemore, 1998). Considerations for compatibility with care setting include reimbursement, renting versus owning, product maintenance, safety, and facility response. Once these considerations are analyzed, a formulary can be created with a range of products intended to meet the individual needs of the patient population. Attention must then turn to creating decision-making tools and educating staff for effective product selection and safe use. Table 9-1 and Appendix C provide examples of decision-making tools to guide support surface selection.

Reimbursement. When patients covered by Medicare Part A need a support surface, hospitals and skilled nursing facilities are financially responsible for acquiring and supplying the appropriate product. Hospitals receive a diagnosis-related group (DRG) payment based on patient diagnosis. Likewise, skilled nursing facilities receive a per diem payment based on the resource utilization group. Therefore, facilities must select the support surface that will provide the most cost-effective clinical outcome during a patient's stay.

When a patient is discharged to the home setting or converts from Medicare Part A to Medicare Part B, local coverage determination (LCD) fee schedules for support surfaces take effect. According to a report from the Office of Inspector General (Levinson, 2009), inappropriate Medicare payments for group 2 support surfaces amounted to approximately $33 million during the first half of 2007. Of the 362 claims reviewed, 86% did not meet group 2 coverage criteria, 38% were undocumented, 22% were medically unnecessary, and 17% had insufficient documentation.

When possible, selecting a support surface that matches the needs of the patient *and* meets Medicare reimbursement criteria would be ideal for patients making the challenging transition from the hospital or long-term care to home. Centers for Medicare & Medicaid Services (CMS) reimbursement criteria and product examples are listed in Appendix C. Reimbursement criteria change as technology and knowledge about support surfaces and wounds evolve. It is important to contact insurance companies, health maintenance organizations (HMOs), Medicaid, and Medicare for the most up-to-date information. Payer sources change as the patient moves through the continuum of care, and it is critical that the clinician work with the appropriate liaisons and provide documentation stating the rationale for product selections.

Renting (Leasing). For many facilities, renting support surfaces is the best option. Renting enables access to the most current technology free of any concerns about the need to update equipment. Renting support surfaces places the responsibility of maintenance and much of the liability for malfunctioning equipment with the rental company. Companies that rent equipment must provide or facilitate in-services to educate the staff on safety issues and proper use of the equipment. Rental costs may be as variable as the technology and customer service, ranging from as little as a few dollars to roughly $150 per day. Some health care agencies negotiate individual contracts with manufacturers, based on the volume of product used. However, it is important to choose a rental company that is compatible with more than just the financial needs of the facility. Table 9-2 provides a list of customer service-related items to consider during contract negotiation.

Purchasing (Owning). Advantages of owning support surface equipment include improved accessibility, decreased lead time for implementation, and potential decrease in rental expenses, particularly for critical care and bariatric surfaces. Prior to purchasing a product, the warranty information, guidelines for weight limit, setup, maintenance, and cleaning should be analyzed. Some frames of complete bed systems are not designed to accommodate certain mattresses. This will clearly restrict options for the facility's support surface formulary and usually more than once because frames tend to last longer than mattresses. However, many bed frame manufacturers have an "open architecture" design in which any mattress will fit the frame, allowing the clinician to choose the frame and the mattress that will best meet the needs of the patient population while opening up the possibility of mattress replacements as technology and patient needs evolve. Once the facility owns the equipment, it is responsible for storage, setup, and maintenance, which can be resource intensive for certain products or a safety/liability issue when the product is inadequately executed. Any cost analysis prior to purchase should consider these potential and actual financial consequences.

Product Maintenance and Safety. Keeping patients safe on a support surface is accomplished by making appropriate equipment selections; establishing proper setup, monitoring, and maintenance; facilitating optimal pressure-redistribution capacity; and maintaining the barrier to environmental hazards such as fire and infectious body fluids. Maintenance requirements of support

TABLE 9-2	Negotiating Rental Contracts/Service Expectations
Company Service Provided	**Examples**
Product standardization	All low air-loss mattresses have the CPR lever in one standard place (e.g., left side of foot of bed)
Standardized delivery and pickup times	2–4 hours
Safety and quality check on all units prior to product delivery	Flammability Product integrity (infection control/hygiene) Entrapment Labeling Biocompatibility Weight/weight capacity (maximum weight limits, safe working loads) Product expiration/lifespan
Conservation of the environment	Recycling of packaging materials Disposal and recycling of product Product is free from known harmful chemicals (PVC, DEHP, mercury, latex, etc) Disclose all materials that compose product content/mattress core
Troubleshooting information accessible to all	Troubleshooting guides affixed to product 24-hour phone number for questions affixed to product
Daily rounds on beds by consistent and knowledgeable staff	Check whether product is in working order, appropriate labels/instructions are present and legible, patient is comfortable and is not bottoming out, timely staff education (review CPR procedures, appropriate linens and pads, etc.), interaction of surface to other products/supplies (frame, underpads, etc.)
Education	Timely in-services during daily rounds as previously described, education per 24/7 hotline calls, group in-services (orientation, yearly reviews)

AORN, Association of periOperative Registered Nurses; *CPR,* cardiopulmonary resuscitation; *DEHP,* diethylhexyl phthalate; *PVC,* polyvinyl chloride.

surfaces vary by design, composition, and technology. For example, support surfaces with heel zones or head zones must be placed on the bed frame in a specific orientation. Others must be turned (or flipped) regularly to maintain efficacy and checked for wear, proper inflation, and resilience. Top covers that are water repellent, antimicrobial, or flame retardant need to be routinely inspected and replaced if damaged. Repairing or replacing loose or broken side rails, bed controls, and CPR levers (where applicable) will help to prevent some occurrences of entrapment and falls.

Fatigue is the reduced capacity of a surface or its components to perform as specified. This change may result from intended or unintended use and/or prolonged exposure to chemical, thermal, or physical forces (NPUAP, 2007). A designated process is needed to identify fatigue and verify the functional life of the support surface as indicated by the manufacturer's or industry recommended test method *before* the product is placed under a new patient (NPUAP and EPUAP, 2009). Unfortunately, this is an area that has been greatly ignored, with many facilities unaware of the age and condition of their surfaces. Some facilities have incorporated this process into housekeeping policies for terminal cleaning and bedmaking. Purchased items are marked with the month and year of delivery, preferably with indelible ink and in a consistent location. After the patient is discharged, the designated department (e.g., housekeeping) inspects the surface for proper placement and inflation (if applicable) as well as excess wear, damage, and expiration date. Torn covers or

mattresses can be replaced prior to making the bed for the newly admitted patient. This process not only protects the patient from ineffective, damaged, or contaminated products; it may save money when a warranty for non-expired products applies. Some warranties allow for full mattress replacement as indicated over a specified time frame. Others are prorated according to the age of the product. Some of the more complicated support surfaces may require a different process that includes accessible personnel with bioengineering expertise to maintain, repair, and troubleshoot the product.

Evaluation of Outcomes. Factors to consider when evaluating a care setting–specific formulary are listed in Checklist 9-1, *B*. Successful implementation and ongoing use of any product will be dependent on compliance with standardization, manufacturer's customer service, effectiveness of staff education on selection criteria, and staff competency with product use, especially safety features such as CPR levers, max inflate mode, and other bed controls.

SUMMARY

Well-designed clinical research on the effectiveness of various support surface devices is needed. NPUAP's Support Surface Initiative (S3I) has focused efforts on the testing and reporting of terms such as immersion, envelopment, and microclimate as they relate to support surfaces. Additional evidence-based data are still years away as the next steps bring these standardized tests into the clinical setting for evaluation of efficacy. Ideally, clinical trials should measure the effects of particular support surfaces on outcomes such as incidence, comfort, cost, and satisfaction. Small sample sizes may increase the risk of false-positive results (i.e., lead to the conclusion that a product makes a significant difference when it does not). In addition, sample sizes should be appropriate to allow for the most relevant and meaningful type of statistical analysis.

It is the responsibility of health care providers involved in product selection to maintain up-to-date knowledge regarding factors relevant to support surface selection. The prudent wound specialist must be familiar with the operation, indications, and contraindications of the specialty support surface products in the facility, the agency, or the patient's home.

REFERENCES

Anderson C, Rappl L: Lateral rotation mattresses for wound healing, *Ostomy Wound Manage* 50(4):50-62, 2004.

Association of periOperative Registered Nurses (AORN): AORN standards of perioperative professional practice. In: *Perioperative standards and recommended practices,* Denver, Co, 2008.

Brienza DM, Geyer MJ: Using support surfaces to manage tissue integrity, *Adv Skin Wound Care* 18(3):151-157, 2005.

Christian W, Lachenbruch C: Standardizing the language of support surfaces, *Remington Rep* 15(3):11-14, 2007.

Cullum N et al: Systematic reviews of wound care management: (5) beds; (6) compression; (7) laser therapy, therapeutic ultrasound, electrotherapy and electromagnetic therapy, *Health Technol Assess* 5(9):1-221, 2001.

Cullum N et al: Support surfaces for pressure ulcer prevention, *Cochrane Database Syst Rev* (3):CD001735, 2004.

Defloor T, De Bacquer D, Grypdonck MH. The effect of various combinations of turning and pressure reducing devices on the incidence of pressure ulcers, *Int J Nurs Stud* Jan;42(1):37-46, 2005.

Gray D, Cooper PJ, Stringfellow S: Evaluating pressure-reducing foam mattresses and electric bed frames, *Br J Nurs* 10(Suppl 22):s23, 2001.

Gunther RA, Clark M: The effect of dynamic pressure-redistributing bed support surface upon systemic lymph flow and composition, *J Tissue Viability* 10(3):10-15, 2000.

Holzapfel SK: Support surfaces and their use in the prevention and treatment of pressure ulcers, *J ET Nurs* 20(6):251, 1993.

Iglesias C et al: Pressure relieving support surfaces (PRESSURE) trial: cost effectiveness analysis, *BMJ* Jun 17;332(7555): 1416, 2006.

Le KM et al: An in-depth look at pressure sores using monolithic silicon pressure sensors, *Plast Reconstr Surg* 74(6):745, 1984.

Levinson D: *Inappropriate Medicare payments for pressure reducing support surfaces,* Department of Health and Human Ser-

vices, Office of Inspector General (OIG), August 2009, available at http://www.oig.hhs.gov/oei/reports/oei-02-07-00420.pdf, accessed November 6, 2009.

Mackey D: Support surfaces: beds, mattresses, overlays-oh my! *Nurs Clin North Am* 40(2):251-265, 2005.

McCord S et al: Risk factors associated with pressure ulcers in the pediatric intensive care unit, *J Wound Ostomy Continence Nurs* 31(4):179-183, 2004.

McLane KM et al: The 2003 national pediatric pressure ulcer and skin breakdown prevalence survey: a multisite study, *J Wound Ostomy Continence Nurs* 31(4):168-178, 2004.

National Pressure Ulcer Advisory Panel (NPUAP) and European Pressure Ulcer Advisory Panel (EPUAP): *Prevention and treatment of pressure ulcers,* Washington DC, 2009, NPUAP.

National Pressure Ulcer Advisory Panel (NPUAP): *NPUAP support surface standards initiative: terms and definitions related to support surfaces,* 2007, available at http://www.npuap.org/NPUAP_S3I_TD.pdf, accessed May 11, 2009.

Nicholson GP et al: A method for determining the heat transfer and water vapour permeability of patient support systems, *Med Eng Phys* 21(10):701, 1999.

Nixon J et al: Randomised, controlled trial of alternating pressure mattresses compared with alternating pressure overlays for the prevention of pressure ulcers: PRESSURE (pressure relieving support surfaces) trial. *BMJ* 2006 Jun 17;332(7555):1413.

Ochs RF et al: Comparison of air-fluidized therapy with other support surfaces used to treat pressure ulcers in nursing home residents, *Ostomy Wound Manage* 51(2):38, 2005.

Polyurethane Foam Association (PFA): Joint industry foam standards and guidelines. Indentation force deflection (IFD) standards and guidelines available at http://www.pfa.org/jifsg/jifsgs4.html. accessed 5-10-2010.

Reger SI et al: Correlation of transducer systems for monitoring tissue interface pressures, *J Clin Eng* 13(5):365-371, 1988.

U.S. Food and Drug Administration (U.S. FDA), Center for Devices and Radiological Health: *Hospital bed system dimensional and assessment guidance to reduce entrapment,* March 10, 2006, available at http://www.fda.gov/MedicalDevices/DeviceRegulationandGuidance/GuidanceDocuments/ucm072662.htm, accessed on May 11, 2009.

Walton-Geer P: Prevention of pressure ulcers in the surgical patient, *AORN J* 89(3):538-552, 2009.

Whitney J et al: Guidelines for the treatment of pressure ulcers, *Wound Repair Regen* 14(6):663-679, 2006.

Whittemore R: Pressure-reduction support surfaces: a review of the literature, *J Wound Ostomy Continence Nurs* 25:6, 1998.

WOCN Society: *Guideline for management of pressure ulcers,* WOCN Clinical Practice Guideline Series #2, Glenview, IL, 2003.

WOCN Society: *Guideline for management of pressure ulcers,* WOCN Clinical Practice Guideline Series #2, Glenview, IL, 2010.

SECTION III

Lower Extremity Wounds

Lower Extremity Assessment

JoAnn Ermer-Seltun

OBJECTIVES

1. Identify critical assessment parameters of the lower extremity physical assessment.
2. For each indicator used to assess perfusion, describe the techniques and results.
3. Identify two methods for describing lower extremity edema.

4. Compare and contrast assessment parameters indicative of lower extremity venous disease (LEVD) and lower extremity arterial disease (LEAD).

Chronic lower extremity ulcers are thought to affect from 0.5 to 1 million people in the United States at any given time (Bonham, 2003). Most of these wounds are chronic in nature, impact the individual's quality of life, drain monetary and health care resources, and may even progress to possible limb loss if not managed appropriately. The key to successful management of any wound is an insightful assessment to determine the underlying cause so that treatment modalities address the pathologic factors. The etiologic factors of a lower extremity wound can be a myriad of diseases, infection, trauma, drugs, insect bites, pressure, or a combination thereof. Therefore, the wound specialist must be knowledgeable regarding clinical presentation and skilled in differential assessment. Critical assessment parameters are listed in Checklists 10-1 and 10-2 and described in this chapter.

GENERAL APPEARANCE OF THE LIMB

The wound specialist must become familiar with, and proficient in, using proper descriptive dermatologic terms to describe primary or secondary lesions, the pattern of distribution, and the arrangement of lesions or other abnormalities. Careful description often leads the examiner to a specific disease state. Limb appearance should be compared with that of the contralateral limb to identify or rule out trophic changes. With the patient's shoes and socks off, the wound specialist should visually assess both extremities for varicosities, color, pigmentation, turgor, texture, dryness, fissures, hair distribution, calluses, abnormal nails, fungus, bunions, corns, bony deformities, and skin integrity. The web between the toes should be assessed for hygiene issues (Bonham and Kelechi, 2008).

Trophic Changes

Trophic changes can occur when diminished blood flow can no longer support normal growth and development of the skin, hair, and nails. For example, thin and shiny epidermis, loss of hair growth, and thickened nails are often associated with, but are not diagnostic of, lower extremity arterial disease (LEAD). Conversely, edema, hyperpigmentation, scaly, eczematous skin, and varicosities (dilated, swollen, torturous) may be indicative of lower extremity venous disease (LEVD).

Trophic changes, however, are not definitive indicators of disease. Patterns of hair growth are affected by age and ethnicity as well as perfusion status, as hair growth may be diminished or absent in the elderly and certain ethnic groups. Nail growth is also affected by factors other than perfusion, including age and fungal infections.

Appearance of Veins

The leg should be visually inspected or palpated for dilated veins, especially along the saphenous vein, beginning at the medial marginal vein on the dorsum of the foot and terminating at the femoral vein (about 3 cm below the inguinal ligament). Normally, healthy distended veins can only be visualized at the foot and ankle; the presence of dilated veins anywhere else on the leg may imply venous pathology and often is the first sign of venous insufficiency. *Dilated veins,* or *varicose veins,* are bluish, enlarged, and palpable. Often described as tortuous or rope-like, varicose veins are most often present on the back of the calf or on the inner aspect of the leg.

Small vessel changes can be detected with visual inspection. Small reddish or bluish "broken" vessels that cluster near the medial malleolus of the ankle are called *spider* or *reticular veins*; these can also be visualized anywhere on the leg. *Ankle flare,* a larger cluster of small vessels or sunburst, occurs around the ankle. *Telangiectasias* is the presence of fine, dilated capillaries.

Skin Color, Shape, and Integrity

The presence of any discoloration in the skin should be noted. For example, reddish-gray-brown hyperpigmentation in the gaiter region, more specifically hemosiderin staining (see Plate 34), is another skin color change that should be noted. Hemosiderin staining is hailed as the "classic" sign of LEVD, but it also can be found if significant trauma has occurred to the lower extremity. This type of discoloration develops after extravasated red blood cells break down and release the pigment hemosiderin.

Atrophie blanche, also seen with LEVD, is an atrophic, thin, smooth, white plaque with a hyperpigmented border, often "speckled" with tortuous vessels, occurring near the ankle or foot. Due to its scar-like appearance, atrophie blanche is easily and often mistaken for a previously healed ulcer (see Plate 35). Its presence is considered high risk for impending ulceration.

Tiny individual reddish-purple, nonblanching discolorations on the lower extremity may be observed. When the individual discolorations are larger than 0.5 cm, they are called *purpura;* when they are smaller than 0.5 cm they are called *petechiae.* Small blood vessels may leak under the skin and cause a blood or hemorrhagic patch that is a sign of some type of intravascular defect in individuals with normal or abnormal platelet counts. Purpura and petechiae (see Plates 36 and 37) are most often associated with LEAD (secondary to blood thinners) or vasculitis disorders such as systemic lupus erythematosus and polyarteritis nodosa (PAN). Purpura associated with vasculitis disorders is referred to as *palpable* purpura. Purpura that occurs in the elderly due to fragility of the vessels is known as *senile* purpura.

The presence of a condition known as *lipodermatosclerosis* should be noted as present or not present. Lipodermatosclerosis, a condition of the skin and soft tissues that develops in the presence of chronic swelling, is a progressive hardening or fibrosis of the soft tissues. Usually confined to the gaiter or "sock" area, lipodermatosclerosis may cause an inverted "champagne bottle" or "apple core" deformity of the lower extremity in sharp contrast to the unaffected leg.

Dermatitis (see Plate 38) manifested by scaling, crusting, weeping, excoriations (linear erosions due to scratching) from intense pruritus, erythema, or inflammation should be noted. Often these symptoms of dermatitis are misdiagnosed as cellulitis (see Table 12-3). Ulcers on the lower extremity should be noted in terms of their appearance, location, size, pain, and duration.

Edema (Extent, Pattern, Distribution)

Edema is a localized or generalized abnormal accumulation of fluid in the tissues (WOCN Society, 2005). Numerous conditions can cause swelling of the lower extremity; examples include chronic venous disease, post phlebitis syndrome, iliac compression syndrome, lymphedema or lipedema, and systemic disease such as chronic heart failure, pulmonary hypertension and renal failure (Buczkowski et al, 2009). Edema causes swelling that may obscure the appearance of normal anatomy. To determine the presence of edema in the lower extremities, the appearance of one extremity should be compared with the other, noting the relative size and the prominence of veins, tendons, and bones. Edema is a significant finding in the examination of the lower extremity and should be investigated.

Extent. Evaluating edema is challenging due to lack of objective measurement methods. One method is to have the patient sit or stand and, using a flexible tape, obtain measurements of the lower extremity at the calf and the ankle. For valid comparisons, subsequent measurements must be obtained with the patient in the same position and exact location. Calf circumference is obtained by first marking the largest part of the inner calf with a marker and then taking a measurement from the floor up to this mark (in centimeters). This is the floor-to-calf length, and all future measurements should occur at this level. Second, the calf circumference (in centimeters) at the largest portion of the calf that was previously marked is measured. The ankle circumference is measured 5 cm above the ankle. Likewise, the floor-to-ankle length is determined by placing the tape measure at 0 cm on the floor and making a dot on the skin 5 cm above the medial malleolus and then determining the circumference of the ankle (in centimeters).

The extent of edema can also be assessed by pressing firmly but gently with the index finger for several seconds on the dorsum of each foot, behind each medial malleolus, and over the shins. Edema is "pitting" when there is a visible depression that does not rapidly refill and resume its original contour (Figure 10-1 and Box 10-1). Severity of edema can be categorized by either estimating the depth of the indentation (Figure 10-1) or the length of time for the indentation to resolve (Box 10-1). For clarity, the type of scale used should be recorded (e.g., 3+ pitting edema on a 4 point scale (Seidel et al, 2003).

The perometer, which is a computerized digital scanner, can be used to measure limb volume and is particularly useful with lymphedema and fitting compression garments. The perometer uses digital infrared technology to measure the girth and volume of an extremity (Stanton et al, 1997).

Pattern and Distribution. The pattern and distribution of edema should be noted. For example, dependent edema is the accumulation of fluid in the lowest body parts, such as the feet and legs (WOCN Society, 2005).

BOX 10-1	Grading Scale for Severity of Edema
1+	Slight pitting, no visible distortion Disappears rapidly
2+	Somewhat deeper pit than in grade 1, but no readily detectable distortion Disappears in 10–15 seconds
3+	Pit is noticeably deep and may last more than 1 minute Dependent extremity looks fuller and swollen
4+	Pit is very deep and lasts as long as 2–5 minutes Dependent extremity is grossly distorted

From Seidel HM et al, editors: Blood vessels. In: *Mosby's guide to physical examination*, ed 6, St. Louis, 2006, Mosby, Elsevier Science.

With LEAD, dependent edema generally develops gradually, worsens with prolonged standing, and diminishes when the patient rests in a recumbent position with the legs elevated. However, the pattern of edema associated with lymphedema does not resolve with leg elevation and usually encompasses the entire leg. Another distinguishing feature of lymphedema is the presence of a positive Stemmer sign, in which a skin fold at the base of the second toe is too thick to lift. Types of edema are listed in Table 10-1. Chapter 13 provides an in-depth discussion of lymphedema.

FUNCTIONAL–SENSORY STATUS

Functional assessment includes observation for impairments in ambulation, gait, balance, use of walking aids (walker, cane), and ability to remove shoes and socks. Because loss of function may be neuropathic in origin, a focused sensory examination is an essential component of any lower extremity assessment. Sensory assessment (the ability to feel pain, pressure, temperature changes, and friction in the lower extremities and feet) is particularly relevant to the patient with a lower extremity wound. Failure to detect touch indicates loss of protective sensation and warrants caution if compression wraps will be applied because the patient may not sense ischemic changes in a timely manner (Bonham, 2003). Likewise, in patients with diabetes who also have neuropathy, motor neuropathy leads to flexion in the toes (hammer toes, claw toes), flattening of the arch, and

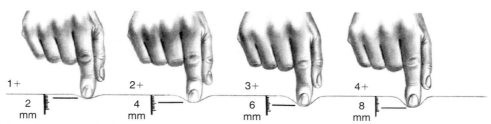

FIGURE 10-1 Pitting edema may also be categorized by depth of depression. (From Cannobio MM: *Cardiovascular disorders,* St. Louis, 1990, Mosby.)

TABLE 10-1	Types of Edema		
	Venous Edema	**Lymphedema**	**Lipedema**
Distribution	Ankle to knee May have limited foot involvement Usually unilateral	Toes to groin Usually unilateral	Ankle to groin Bilateral and symmetrical
Characteristics	Pitting edema of variable severity In long-standing disease, nonpitting edema may result from tissue fibrosis	Brawny nonpitting edema Skin and soft tissue changes common (e.g., papilloma formation, hyperkeratosis) Positive Stemmer sign (not possible to pinch fold of skin over dorsum of second toe) is early indicator Advanced disease: elephantiasis (loss of normal architecture/massive enlargement of limb)	Soft, rubbery tissue Pain on palpation common Painful bruising common Negative Stemmer sign Abnormal fat distribution extends to involve hips
Management	Elevation and compression (toes to knees) are primary approaches Intermittent pneumatic compression typically beneficial Surgery sometimes beneficial	Elevation and standard compression beneficial only in early stages Manual lymphatic drainage and inelastic compression are key elements of management Intermittent pneumatic compression frequently contraindicated	No effective treatment available Management focus is treatment of any comorbidities, patient education, support
Risk factors	Deep vein thrombosis or thrombophlebitis Thrombophilia Obesity or multiple pregnancies Sedentary lifestyle Calf muscle pump failure	Filariasis (third-world countries) Radical cancer surgery plus radiation Long-standing venous disease Vein harvesting/reconstruction	Heredity

bones shifting that deteriorates into prominent plantar metatarsals. When combined with sensory (loss of sensation) and autonomic neuropathy (diminished capillary perfusion and sweat and oil gland production), a neuropathic ulcer may easily develop. In the case of LEAD, several studies confirmed peroneal nerve injury resulting in reduced nerve conduction velocity, poor functional outcomes, and loss of muscle strength in the lower extremities (WOCN Society, 2008). These findings suggest that poor arterial flow has a direct harmful effect on peroneal nerve function (McDermott et al, 2006). Signs of neuropathy include reduced sensation (detected by Semmes-Weinstein 5.07 monofilament), gait abnormalities caused by foot drop/drag, weakness of the ankles or feet, and loss of vibration and deep tendon reflexes (Bonham and Kelechi, 2008; Steed et al, 2006). Sensorimotor assessment is discussed in greater detail in Chapter 14.

Range of Motion of the Ankle Joint

The calf muscle pump is a critical contributor to normal venous return. Normal function of the calf muscle pump is dependent on a normally moving ankle joint. A "normal" walking motion requires flexion of the ankle joint past the 90-degree position. Therefore, routine assessment of ankle range of motion should be incorporated into the physical assessment of a patient with known or suspected

LEAD because elevated ankle stiffness has been associated with calf muscle pump impairment (Padberg et al, 2004). Ankle stiffness due to edema and fibrosis should be quantified according to severity: 0 = none, 1 = reduced stiffness, and 2 = nonreducible or ankylosis (Carpentier et al, 2003). A goniometer device, often used by physical therapists to measure ankle flexion/stiffness, is an objective measurement of range of motion (Bonham and Kelechi, 2008). Ankle joint equinus (the inability to dorsiflex the ankle joint less than 90 degrees) may occur with peripheral neuropathy. This loss of dorsiflexion can place extraordinary pressure on the sole of the foot, which in turn elevates the incidence of diabetic neuropathic ulceration (Caselli et al, 2002).

Pain

Effective pain management is a critical aspect of care for any patient with an ulcer; thus the assessment must always include determination of the type and severity of pain (both baseline and procedural), exacerbating and relieving factors, and past and present attempts to manage the pain. For the patient with a lower extremity ulcer, the pain history provides additional important etiologic clues (Table 10-2). Chapter 11 describes ischemic pain that is relieved by placing the leg in a dependent position (Box 11-3). In contrast, leg pain that is relieved by elevation is more consistent with a venous etiology. The

TABLE 10-2	Pain Assessment of Patient with Leg Ulcer		
Factors to be Assessed	**Typical Findings**		
	Venous	*Arterial*	*Neuropathic*
Characteristics	Dull Aching	Intermittent claudication Nocturnal pain Rest pain (see Box 11-3)	Burning/tingling "Shooting" "Pins and needles"
Severity	Variable Typically moderate to severe	Variable Frequently severe	Variable Commonly severe
Exacerbating factors	Dependency Increased edema Infection	Elevation Activity Infection	Variable Inactivity sometimes a precipitating factor
Relieving factors	Elevation Edema control Reduction of bacterial burden	Dependency Rest Reduction of bacterial burden	Activity such as walking

patient with diabetes who is complaining of leg pain described as "pins and needles," a shooting "electrical shock," or burning sensation that is relieved by walking probably is experiencing neuropathic pain (WOCN Society, 2004, 2005). Because patients with lower extremity disease may limit walking and other activities because of discomfort and comorbidities, "classic" signs of pain may not be appreciated. Extreme pain that seems out of proportion to the type of ulcer present (hyperalgesia) or pain associated with nonpainful stimuli (allodynia) should alert the clinician to further investigate for other conditions that may lead to atypical leg wounds. Further discussion related to the assessment and management of pain is presented in Chapters 25 and 26.

PERFUSION

Extent of perfusion can be derived though inspection of leg temperature, position-related color changes, quality of pulses, and blood flow. Diagnostic tests used to assess perfusion include venous filling time, ankle-brachial index, and transcutaneous oxygen pressure measurements (Seidel et al, 2003).

Elevational Pallor and Dependent Rubor

Presence of permanent discoloration (cyanosis, dark brown to black, pallor) of the digit and increased pain with or without ulceration may be evidence of critical digital ischemia and merits prompt investigation of the peripheral vascular system. Position-related color changes in one or both legs provide important information concerning adequacy of arterial perfusion.

Elevational pallor. With the patient supine on the examination surface, the leg is raised to a 60-degree angle for 15 to 60 seconds. The color of the soles of the feet is observed. Normally, color should not

change. When perfusion is impaired, pallor is observed in fair-skinned individuals and gray (ashen) hues in dark-skinned individuals. Box 10-2 correlates the severity of arterial occlusion with the amount of time needed for elevation pallor to occur (Lesho et al, 2004).

Dependent Rubor. As for the examination for elevational pallor, the leg is raised 60 degrees while the patient is supine on the examination surface for 15 to 60 seconds. The normal leg will remain a healthy color when dependent. Initially the ischemic limb will slowly turn from white to pink and progress to a purple-red discoloration, referred to as *dependent rubor*. Color change occurs as a result of retention of deoxygenated blood in the dilated skin capillaries (Lesho et al, 2004).

Skin Temperature

Skin temperature of the leg is assessed by palpating lightly with the palmar surface of the fingers and hands, moving from proximal to distal, and comparing each limb to the opposite limb (e.g., right leg with left leg). Findings of unilateral coolness and a sudden marked change from proximal to distal are possible indicators of LEAD (Hopf et al, 2006). In contrast, patients with LEVD have been shown to have higher

BOX 10-2	Assessment of Elevational Pallor

1. Raise leg to 60-degree angle for 15–60 seconds
2. Observe amount of time needed for pallor to appear:
   - Pallor within 25 seconds indicates severe occlusive disease
   - Pallor within 25–40 seconds indicates moderate occlusive disease
   - Pallor within 40–60 seconds indicates mild occlusive disease

From Seidel HM et al, editors: Blood vessels. In: *Mosby's guide to physical examination*, ed 6, St. Louis, 2006, Mosby, Elsevier Science.

skin temperatures at the ankle (Kelechi et al, 2003; WOCN Society, 2005).

When localized inflammation occurs, a slight elevation in skin temperature (2.2°C [4°F]) at that location can be detected, referred to as *dermal thermometry*. Such an elevation in skin temperature was reported to be highly predictive of impending ulceration (within 7–10 days) in patients with lower extremity neuropathic disease (LEND) (Armstrong et al, 2007). Several studies have suggested that self-monitoring of skin temperature for patients with high-risk diabetes may reduce the incidence of ulceration by modifying activity to reduce the local inflammation (Armstrong et al, 2007; Lavery et al, 2007). Although some evidence suggests dermal thermometry may also be useful to screen for pending ulceration in patients with LEVD (Kelechi et al, 2003; Sayre et al, 2007), more studies are needed to support use of home thermometry for patients with LEVD (Kelechi and Bonham, 2008).

Blood Flow (Bruit/Thrill)

Blood flow through the artery should move in a laminar flow pattern. Turbulence in the flow of arterial blood occurs when some pathology, such as a clot, compression, or fatty deposit, develops within the vessel. Velocity of blood flow will slow around the source of the turbulence and cause blood cells to adhere to vessel lining, thus forming a clot. Turbulent blood flow through an artery may be auscultated with the bell of a stethoscope and is heard as a blowing or rushing sound, which is called a *bruit* (Hirsch et al, 2006; Rumwell and McPharlin, 2004). Presence of a bruit is indicative of arterial narrowing, but because of the low-frequency sound the bruit may not always be heard. Turbulent blood flow may also be palpated, which is referred to as a *thrill*.

Capillary Refill

The capillary bed consists of small-diameter vessels that lie between the arterial and the venous systems. The time needed for the capillary bed to fill after it is occluded by pressure (capillary refill time) gives some indication of the health of the system. Delayed capillary refill (greater than 3 seconds) may indicate LEAD (WOCN Society, 2008). However, the patient with LEAD may have normal capillary refill because the emptied vessels may refill in a retrograde manner from surrounding veins even if arterial inflow is markedly impaired or absent. Environmental factors such as temperature also may influence the speed of capillary refill; therefore this assessment is vulnerable to considerable subjective interpretation and should be used only to confirm a clinical judgment. Box 10-3 explains how and why capillary refill time is assessed (Seidel et al, 2003).

BOX 10-3	Assessment of Capillary Refill Time

- Blanch toenail bed with sustained pressure for several seconds
- Release pressure
- Observe time elapsed before nail regains full color
- In presence of arterial occlusion, refill time will be longer than 2–3 seconds

Caution: Decreased temperature can prolong capillary refill time.

Data from Seidel HM et al, editors: Blood vessels. In: *Mosby's guide to physical examination*, ed 6, St. Louis, 2006, Mosby, Elsevier Science.

Assessment of Pulses

Pulses should be compared with the contralateral pulses and assessed in a proximal-to-distal direction. Normally pedal pulses can be palpated at both the dorsalis pedis and the posterior tibialis locations (Figure 10-2). Presence or absence of palpable pulses is not diagnostic of LEAD (Collins et al, 2006). If pulses are palpable, the patient may still have LEAD. If pulses are not palpable, a Doppler probe must be used to determine the presence or absence of pulses.

The absence of Doppler pulse usually should lead to referral. However, in healthy individuals, dorsalis pedis (DP) pulse is absent in 8.1% and posterior tibialis (PT) pulse in 2.9% and both are absent in less than 2%. Therefore, it is important to assess all dorsalis pedis and posterior tibialis pulses (Hopf et al, 2006).

The best way to document pulses is to use descriptive terms such as *present* or *absent,* followed by clarifying terms such as *weak* or *bounding.* Box 10-4 presents a 4-point scale that describes the amplitude of the pulse (WOCN Society, 2008). Because a variety of 3- and 4-point scales are used in clinical practice, it is important to specify the type of scale used (e.g., 3+ pedal pulse on a 4-point scale).

DIAGNOSTIC TESTING

When the diagnosis is unclear or wound healing fails, diagnostic studies are indicated. Vascular referral and studies are indicated to identify the components of the vascular system involved in the disease process, the specific pathologic process, the anatomic level of the lesions or dysfunction, and the severity of dysfunction. With the exception of the ankle-brachial index, these tests involve

BOX 10-4	Assessment of Amplitude of the Pulse
4	Bounding
3	Full, increased
2	Expected
1	Diminished, barely palpable
0	Absent, not palpable

Data from Seidel HM et al, editors: Blood vessels. In: *Mosby's guide to physical examination*, ed 6, St. Louis, 2006, Mosby, Elsevier Science.

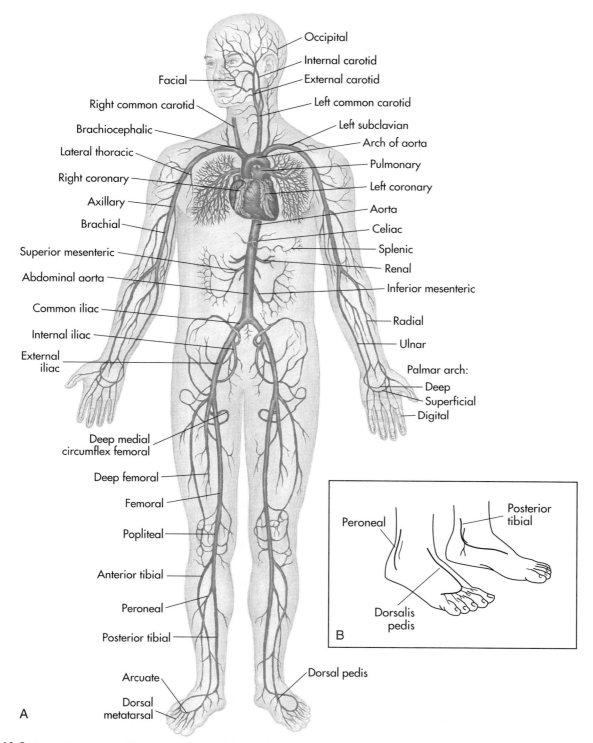

Occipital

Internal carotid

Facial

External carotid

Right common carotid

Left common carotid

Brachiocephalic

Left subclavian

Lateral thoracic

Arch of aorta

Right coronary

Pulmonary

Axillary

Left coronary

Brachial

Aorta

Superior mesenteric

Celiac

Abdominal aorta

Splenic

Common iliac

Renal

Internal iliac

Inferior mesenteric

External
iliac

Radial

Ulnar

Palmar arch:

Deep

Superficial

Digital

Deep medial
circumflex femoral

Deep femoral

Femoral

Popliteal

Peroneal

Posterior
tibial

Anterior tibial

Peroneal

Posterior tibial

Dorsalis
pedis

B

Arcuate

Dorsal pedis

Dorsal
metatarsal

A

FIGURE 10-2 Arterial structure of lower extremity. **B** delineates approximate location of peroneal artery, posterior tibialis, and dorsalis pedis pulses. (**A,** From Seidel HM et al, editors: Blood vessels. In: *Mosby's guide to physical examination,* ed 6, St. Louis, 2006, Mosby.)

equipment that is reserved for use in a vascular laboratory by a trained technician and reviewed by a vascular radiologist or surgeon. Checklist 10-2 lists diagnostic tests used for the patient with a wound resulting from lower extremity disease. Diagnostic tests are described in detail in Chapters 11 through 15.

SUMMARY

Lower extremity ulcers are an increasingly common problem and may be caused by compromised function in any component of the circulatory system (e.g., arterial, venous, lymphatic). Table 10-3 provides a brief

TABLE 10-3	Characteristics of Arterial, Venous, and Neuropathic Ulcers		
	Arterial	**Venous**	**Neuropathic**
Location	Tips of toes (spontaneous necrosis) Pressure points (e.g., heel, lateral foot) Areas of trauma (nonhealing wounds)	Between ankles and knees; "classic" location is medial malleolus	Plantar surface over metatarsal heads Areas of foot exposed to repetitive trauma (toes, sides of feet)
Wound bed	Pale or necrotic	Dark red, "ruddy" May be covered with fibrinous slough	Typically red (if no coexisting ischemia)
Exudate	Minimal	Moderate to large amounts	Moderate to large amounts
Wound edges	Well defined	Poorly defined, irregular	Well defined Frequently associated with callous formation
Other	Infection common, but signs and symptoms muted Typically painful Typically associated with other indicators (ischemia, diminished/absent pulses, elevational pallor, dependent rubor, thin fragile skin) See Plate 39	Edema common Hyperpigmentation surrounding skin common Feet typically warm with good pulses (if no coexisting arterial disease) See Plates 34,35,38	Infection common, but signs and symptoms may be muted May have coexisting ischemia See Plate 40

summary of key assessment distinctions among arterial, venous, and neuropathic ulcers. However, multiple other causes of lower extremity ulcers, including vasculitis, autoimmune disorders, neuropathy, and metabolic derangements, can precipitate ulcerations on the leg, with unique manifestations. To further complicate the picture, many patients have ulcers of mixed etiology or comorbidities that affect management and the potential for healing. The wound specialist must utilize astute physical assessment skills and clearly and accurately document findings to facilitate an accurate differential assessment that leads to the correct diagnosis in a timely manner.

REFERENCES

Armstrong DG et al: Skin temperature monitoring reduces the risk for diabetic foot ulceration in high-risk patients, *Am J Med* 120(12):1042-1046, 2007.

Bonham P: Assessment and management of patients with venous, arterial, and diabetic/neuropathic lower extremity wounds, *AACN Clin Issues Adv Pract Acute Crit Care* 14(4):442-456, 2003.

Bonham P, Kelechi T: Evaluation of lower extremity arterial circulation and implications for nursing practice, *J Cardiovasc Nurs* 23(2);144-152, 2008.

Buczkowski G et al: Chronic venous insufficiency, *Clin Rev* 19(3):19, 2009.

Carpentier PH et al: Appraisal of the information content of the C classes of CEAP clinical classification of chronic venous disorders: a multicenter evaluation of 872 patients, *J Vasc Surg* 37(4):827-833, 2003.

Caselli A et al: The forefoot-to-rearfoot plantar pressure ratio is increased in severe diabetic neuropathy and can predict foot ulceration, *Diabetes Care* 25(6):1006, 2002.

Collins T et al: An absent pulse is not sensitive for the early detection of peripheral arterial disease, *Fam Med* 38(1):38-42, 2006.

Hirsch A et al: ACC/AHA 2005 Practice Guidelines for the management of patients with peripheral arterial disease (lower extremity, renal, mesenteric, and abdominal aortic): a collaborative report from the American Association for Vascular Surgery/Society for Vascular Surgery, Society for Cardiovascular Angiography and Interventions, Society for Vascular Medicine and Biology, Society of Interventional Radiology, and the ACC/AHA Task Force on Practice Guidelines (Writing Committee to Develop Guidelines for the Management of Patients With Peripheral Arterial Disease): endorsed by the American Association of Cardiovascular and Pulmonary Rehabilitation; National Heart, Lung, and Blood Institute; Society for Vascular Nursing; TransAtlantic Inter-Society Consensus; and Vascular Disease Foundation, *Circulation*, 113(11):e463-e654, 2006.

Hopf HW et al: Guidelines for the treatment of arterial insufficiency ulcers, *Wound Repair Regen* 14(6):693-710, 2006.

Kelechi TJ et al: Skin temperature and chronic venous insufficiency, *J Wound Ostomy Continence Nurs* 30(1):17, 2003.

Kelechi TJ, Bonham PA: Lower extremity venous disorders: Implications for nursing practice, *J Cardiovasc Nurs* 23(2):132-143, 2008.

Lavery LA et al: Preventing diabetic foot ulcer recurrence in high-risk patients: the use of temperature monitoring as a self-assessment tool, *Diabetes Care* 30(1):14-20, 2007.

Lesho E et al: Management of peripheral arterial disease, *Am Fam Physician* 69(3):525, 2004.

McDermott M et al: Lower extremity nerve function in patients with lower extremity ischemia, *Arch Intern Med* 166(18): 1986-1992, 2006.

Padberg FT et al: Structured exercise improves calf muscle pump function in chronic venous insufficiency: a randomized trial, *J Vasc Surg* 39(1):79-87, 2004.

Rumwell C, McPharlin M: *Vascular technology*, ed 3, Pasadena, Calif, 2004, Davies Publishing.

Sayre EK et al: Sudden increase in skin temperature predicts venous ulcers: a case study, *J Vasc Nurs* 25(3):46-50, 2007.

Seidel HM et al, editors: Blood vessels. In: *Mosby's guide to physical examination*, ed 5, St. Louis, 2003, Mosby, Elsevier Science.

Stanton AWB et al: Validation of an optoelectronic limb volumeter (perometer), *Lymphology* 30(2):77-97, 1997.

Steed DL et al: Guidelines for the treatment of diabetic ulcers, *Wound Repair Regen* 14(6):680-692, 2006.

Wound, Ostomy, and Continence Nurses (WOCN) Society: *Guideline for management of patients with lower extremity neuropathic disease,* WOCN clinical practice guideline series #3, Glenview Ill, 2004, Author.

Wound, Ostomy, and Continence Nurses (WOCN) Society: *Guideline for management of patients with lower extremity venous disease,* WOCN clinical practice guideline series #2, Glenview Ill, 2005, Author.

Wound, Ostomy, and Continence Nurses (WOCN) Society: *Guideline for management of patients with lower extremity arterial disease,* WOCN clinical practice guideline series #1, Mount Laurel, NJ, 2008, Author.

11

Arterial Ulcers

Dorothy B. Doughty

OBJECTIVES

1. Describe etiologic factors, risk factors, pathophysiology, typical presentation, and principles of management for arterial ulcers.
2. Describe essential assessment for the patient with a suspected arterial ulcer, including history, pain assessment, physical assessment, and laboratory studies.
3. Outline a patient teaching plan for the individual with ischemic disease of the lower extremity, including lifestyle changes to maximize perfusion and measures to prevent trauma.
4. Distinguish between *critical* limb ischemia and *acute* limb ischemia, including assessment parameters and implications for management.
5. Identify indications and options for surgical revascularization and for amputation.
6. Describe pharmacologic options for management of arterial ulcers.
7. Recommend appropriate topical therapy for each of the following: ischemic ulcer covered with dry eschar and no signs of infection; ischemic ulcer covered with dry eschar and mild erythema and fluctuance of surrounding skin; open ischemic ulcer with and without signs of infection.

Arterial ulcers (also known as *ischemic ulcers*) occur as a result of severe tissue ischemia and are extremely painful. In addition, ischemic ulcers represent potential limb loss. These lesions are generally refractory to healing unless tissue perfusion can be improved, and they are prone to progress to invasive infection and/or gangrene, which may necessitate amputation (Bonham et al, 2008). Of further concern is the likelihood of coexisting, and possibly unrecognized, cardiovascular or cerebrovascular disease. Thus any patient with an ulcer caused or complicated by arterial insufficiency requires thorough physical assessment and aggressive management. The treatment plan for these patients must be multifaceted, including measures to maximize perfusion and minimize risk of infection, evidence-based wound care, and ongoing assessment and management of ischemic pain. Effective management of ischemic disease frequently requires significant lifestyle modifications; thus patient education and counseling are essential elements of the management plan.

EPIDEMIOLOGY

Many terms are used to describe the anomalies that can affect the peripheral vascular system. *Peripheral vascular disease* describes noncardiac disease that includes a myriad of conditions affecting the arterial, venous, and lymphatic circulation. *Peripheral arterial disease* (PAD) specifically refers to a range of noncoronary arterial syndromes caused by an alteration in the structure and function of the arteries that supply the brain, visceral organs, and limbs; it is the preferred term for stenotic, occlusive, and aneurysmal diseases (Hirsch et al, 2006). *Peripheral arterial occlusive disease* describes arterial disease that is specifically occlusive in nature. Finally, *lower extremity arterial disease* (LEAD) includes only arterial disease that affects the leg arteries and excludes arterial diseases of the aorta, carotid, upper extremity, or visceral arteries (Hirsch et al, 2006). Most ischemic ulcers develop as a result of LEAD.

Although ischemic ulcers are much less common than those resulting from venous insufficiency or neuropathy, the underlying disease process (LEAD) is quite prevalent, especially among the elderly. Current data suggest prevalence rates ranging from 18% to 29% among those 60 years of age or older; similar prevalence rates have been reported for individuals older than 50 years of age who are high risk due to diabetes or tobacco use. Altogether an estimated 5 to 10 million people in the United States have LEAD, many of whom are undiagnosed; recent data suggest that "silent" disease accounts for almost half of cases (Aronow, 2008; Bonham et al, 2008; Sigvant et al, 2009).

The high prevalence of undiagnosed disease is explained by the fact that vascular disease frequently is asymptomatic until the disease process is advanced; this is true of coronary artery disease and cerebrovascular disease as well as PAD. Unfortunately, the failure to diagnose vascular disease at an earlier time results in failure to treat until the disease is advanced and the patient becomes symptomatic. Advanced (symptomatic) disease is associated with much greater risk of morbidity and mortality (e.g., myocardial infarction, cerebrovascular accident, limb loss), and is much less amenable to effective treatment; thus the focus in management of patients with any form of vascular disease (coronary artery disease, cerebrovascular disease, PAD) must shift to routine screening to detect asymptomatic disease. Because atherosclerotic disease is the most common disease process affecting the arterial system and is a systemic phenomenon, the patient with disease in one vascular bed (e.g., coronary artery bed) is at greater risk for disease in another vascular bed (Hirsch et al, 2006). Studies indicate that patients with PAD are very likely to have coexisting coronary artery disease or cerebrovascular disease and are at significantly greater risk for early death due to a cardiac event (Aronow, 2008; Bonham et al, 2008; Sigvant et al, 2009). Ankle-brachial index (ABI) testing with a handheld Doppler is an effective bedside screening procedure. Because ABI less than 0.9 is an independent predictor for increased risk of cardiovascular death, individuals with ABI less than 0.9 should be referred for further assessment to rule out "silent but treatable" cardiac disease (Bonham et al, 2008; Hopf et al, 2006).

As noted, a significant proportion of individuals with PAD are asymptomatic. Patients who are symptomatic most commonly present with intermittent claudication (pain with walking that is relieved by rest). Others present with vague complaints of impaired mobility and leg weakness; the diagnosis is frequently "missed" in these individuals, whose symptoms may be attributed to aging or sedentary lifestyle.

Critical and Acute Limb Ischemia

Critical limb ischemia refers to patients with chronic (more than 2 weeks) ischemic rest pain, ulcers, or gangrene attributable to objectively proven arterial occlusive disease. *Acute limb ischemia* refers to a quickly developing or sudden decrease in limb perfusion that threatens limb viability (Hirsch et al, 2006; Norgren et al, 2007). Signs of acute limb ischemia include the six *P*s: pain, paralysis, paresthesias, pulselessness, pallor, and polar (cold extremity). Arterial embolism, however, can occur without symptoms (Hirsch et al, 2006). Because irreversible nerve and muscle damage may occur within hours, all patients with suspected acute limb ischemia should be evaluated immediately by a vascular specialist (Norgren et al, 2007).

ETIOLOGY

Arterial insufficiency and arterial ulcers are most common among older adults and middle-aged adults who have additional risk factors, such as diabetes or tobacco use. The most common causative factor in these cases is atherosclerotic disease. Arterial ulcers also occur with thromboangiitis obliterans (Buerger disease), sickle cell disease, and vasculitis but are less common and can occur among younger individuals. Least common are arterial ulcers that develop as a result of entrapment syndromes, acute embolic syndromes, and arterial trauma (Hirsch et al, 2006).

Atherosclerosis

The most common cause of LEAD and arterial ulceration among older adults is atherosclerosis involving the peripheral circulation. Atherosclerotic disease can occur in any vessel in the body. In the peripheral circulation the aortic, iliac, femoral, and popliteal arteries (see Figure 10-2) are the vessels most commonly affected (Dillavou and Kahn, 2003).

Although the pathology of atherosclerotic disease is not completely understood, it is known to involve two primary processes: plaque formation and enlargement, which cause narrowing of the vessel lumen, and endothelial injury subsequently triggering an inflammatory process that ultimately results in fibrosis and hardening of the vessel wall (Hirsch et al, 2006).

Plaque formation begins with the lesion known as a "fatty streak," which is a gray or pearly white lesion that adheres to the intima (inner layer of the arterial wall). This lesion consists of a lipid core and a connective tissue covering. As further lipid accumulation occurs, the plaque enlarges, which results in progressive narrowing of the vessel lumen. Over time the plaques harden as a result of deposition of calcium salts and cholesterol crystals, causing loss of vessel elasticity, which further compromises blood flow (Hirsch et al, 2006).

The second process contributing to vessel narrowing and hardening is triggered by damage to the vessel lining. Endothelial damage results in areas where the intimal lining is denuded. Platelets aggregate over these denuded areas, causing clot formation and the subsequent release of growth factors that stimulate mitosis of the vascular smooth muscle cells and promote synthesis of connective tissue proteins such as collagen. The end result is thickening and fibrosis of the vessel wall, which further contributes to narrowing and hardening of the involved arteries. Clinically these changes result in a chronic reduction in blood flow to the tissues and a loss of the ability to respond with increased blood flow when metabolic demands are increased. In addition, acute vessel occlusion may occur as a result of sudden plaque enlargement or plaque rupture (Hirsch et al, 2006).

Thromboangiitis Obliterans (Buerger's Disease)

Thromboangiitis obliterans, also known as Buerger's disease and arteriosclerosis obliterans, is a rare condition almost exclusively limited to adults younger than 50 years who are heavy smokers (Hirsch et al, 2006). The disease typically involves the small- and mid-sized arteries in both the upper and lower extremities. The process is always bilateral and frequently involves all four limbs. The cause of the disease is not known but does not involve plaque formation or hypercoagulability. Instead the lesions appear to be inflammatory in origin, which suggests an autoimmune process (Hanly et al, 2009). Patients may complain of cold sensitivity, rest pain, pedal claudication, digital ulceration, or gangrene. Ulceration may occur spontaneously but more commonly is precipitated by minor trauma. The most effective management is elimination of tobacco, which provides consistent interruption of the disease process. Among individuals who continue to use tobacco, digit or limb amputations are common; however, mortality is not increased (Hanly et al, 2009).

Sickle Cell Disease

Lower extremity arterial ulcers occur in 25% to 75% of patients with sickle cell disease, a hereditary disease primarily affecting those of African American descent. During physiologic stress in a person with sickle cell disease, the red blood cells become deformed into a crescent moon or sickle shape. These abnormal blood cells clump together and cause vascular occlusion and tissue necrosis. In addition, injury to the red blood cells causes increased expression of adhesion molecules on the endothelial surface to which the sickled cells attach, resulting in further occlusion and necrosis. Fortunately, once the sickle crisis is resolved, blood flow typically is restored, and the ulcer slowly heals. Unfortunately, many individuals develop chronic ulcers that are very slow to heal. Many individuals with sickle cell disease also have chronic venous insufficiency, which further delays healing. Because a sickle cell crisis is frequently precipitated by minor trauma, preventive care is a key element of management for these patients (Trent and Kirsner, 2004).

Vasculitis

Another potential cause of ischemic ulceration is vasculitis, which is a general term for inflammation of vessel walls. The inflammation may produce defects in the vessel wall, allowing leakage of blood into the surrounding tissues, or it may produce vessel occlusion and tissue necrosis. The vasculitis "umbrella" comprises a large number of specific conditions that vary significantly in clinical presentation and prognosis, depending on the size and location of the inflamed vessels. The causative factors for vasculitis are not well defined, but the condition is frequently associated with either an acute allergic reaction or an autoimmune process. When the condition is associated with an autoimmune process, the patient commonly presents with systemic symptoms such as malaise, joint pain, and low-grade fever in addition to the specific symptoms produced by the inflamed vessels. Vasculitic conditions producing lower extremity ulcers typically involve mid-sized and small arteries and are characterized by a petechial rash, purpura, tissue necrosis, and extreme pain. Diagnosis is suggested by patient history, clinical presentation, and high serum levels of inflammatory markers and is confirmed by biopsy demonstrating vessel inflammation. Management primarily involves systemic antiinflammatory agents and pain management. Topical therapy is based on the principles of wound bed preparation (elimination of necrotic tissue and control of bacterial burden) and moist wound healing (Xu et al, 2009).

RISK FACTORS FOR LEAD

Risk factors for LEAD (Box 11-1) are the same as those for coronary artery disease and include both modifiable factors and predisposing factors. Studies have identified a number of "emerging" risk factors that appear to be associated with the development of atherosclerotic disease, but their impact is not yet well defined (Liapis et al, 2009). While some of these risk factors, such as age, gender, and family history, are irreversible, the majority are very responsive to lifestyle modifications and pharmacologic therapy. A clear understanding of current recommendations for management of risk factors is critical because effective management of the underlying disease process is essential for wound healing, limb salvage, and longterm survival (Aronow, 2008; Bonham et al, 2008; Hopf et al, 2006; Liapis et al, 2009).

BOX 11-1   Risk Factors for Lower Extremity Arterial Disease (LEAD)

Causal Modifiable (see Table 11-1)
1. Smoking
2. Diabetes
3. Dyslipidemia
4. Hypertension

Predisposing
5. Modifiable factors (obesity, inactivity, social isolation, stress)
6. Nonmodifiable factors (advanced age, male gender, postmenopausal status, family history, African American ethnicity)

Emerging
7. Elevated homocysteine levels
8. Inflammation
9. Infection
10. Renal failure

Causal Modifiable Risk Factors

The "big four" risk factors are those that appear to play a direct causal role in the development of atherosclerosis: smoking, diabetes mellitus, dyslipidemia, and hypertension. All of these risk factors are modifiable; thus management of these factors should be the clinician's primary focus. Table 11-1 and Box 11-2 summarize goals and guidelines for the management of modifiable risk factors (Liapis et al, 2009).

Smoking. Smoking is a highly significant risk factor for atherosclerotic disease in general and for PAD in particular; smokers have a fourfold increased risk for PAD. Most studies suggest a connection between pack-year history and the number and severity of vascular complications; however, the number of pack-years that constitutes a significant increased risk for vascular disease is unknown (Bonham et al, 2008; Liapis et al, 2009; Sigvant et al, 2009). Smoking may be particularly harmful to women, who reportedly have a significant increase in risk with a 10-year pack history compared to men with a 30-year pack history (Sigvant et al, 2009). The negative effects of tobacco on the vascular system are due to its byproducts: nicotine, carbon monoxide, and hydrogen cyanide. The most significant of these is nicotine, which is a potent vasoconstrictor and also promotes platelet aggregation and clot formation. Smoking cessation can significantly reduce the progression of LEAD as well as mortality rates from other vascular complications; thus smoking cessation (see Box 11-2) should be a primary target of therapy (Aronow, 2008; Bonham et al, 2008; Hopf et al, 2008; Liapis et al, 2009).

Diabetes Mellitus. Diabetes, especially type 2, is one of the strongest predictors of PAD, representing a twofold to fourfold increase in risk. Even more significantly, patients with diabetes are at increased risk for death and limb loss caused by vascular disease; for each 1% increase in hemoglobin A_{1c} (HbA_{1c}) there is a 28% increase in risk of death. Patients with diabetes are 10 times more likely to progress to critical limb ischemia and amputation (Bonham et al, 2008; Hirsch et al, 2006; Liapis et al, 2009). Specific pathologic features associated with diabetes that contribute to LEAD include increased plaque formation, increased red blood cell (RBC) rigidity, increased blood viscosity and coagulability, hypertrophy of vascular smooth muscle, and increased vascular resistance (Gibbons, 2003). Insulin resistance and hyperinsulinemia may be one causative factor for hypertrophy of vascular smooth muscle, even in the early stages of the disease, because insulin is known to be a vascular growth factor. Fortunately, tight glycemic control (HbA_{1c} <7.0) can significantly reduce the risk of microvascular complications and amputation; thus effective diabetes management (through diet, exercise, and pharmacologic therapy) is another key element of effective therapy for the patient with LEAD (Hopf et al, 2008). However, the

TABLE 11-1	Management of Modifiable Risk Factors
Risk Factor	**Management Goals/Guidelines**
Tobacco use	*Goal:* Cessation of tobacco use *Guidelines:* See Box 11-2
Diabetes mellitus	*Goal:* HbA$_{1c}$ <7.0% (<6% if possible for high-risk patient) *Guidelines:* • Patient education and counseling regarding diet and exercise • Oral hypoglycemics and/or insulin
Dyslipidemia	*Goals:* • LDL-C <100 mg/dl (<70 mg/dl for very-high-risk patient) • HDL-C >40 mg/dl for men, >45 mg/dl for women • Triglycerides <150 mg/dl *Guidelines:* • Patient education and counseling regarding diet and exercise • Statins
Hypertension	*Goals:* <140/90 mm Hg (nondiabetic), <130/80 mm Hg (diabetic) *Guidelines:* • Patient education and counseling regarding diet and exercise • Antihypertensive medications • Thiazide diuretics as initial drug • Angiotension-converting enzyme inhibitor or angiotension receptor blocker for patient with diabetic renal disease (except patient with renal artery stenosis) or congestive heart failure • β-Adrenergic blocker for patient who also has coronary artery disease • Calcium channel blocker as needed for uncontrolled hypertension *Note:* Multiple agents should be used as needed to maintain blood pressure within accepted range.

HDL-C, High-density lipoprotein cholesterol; *LDL-C,* low-density lipoprotein cholesterol.

BOX 11-2 | **Interventions to Promote Cessation of Tobacco Use**

1. General education concerning the negative effects of tobacco use on health status.
2. Specific and consistent advice from health care team to eliminate tobacco use.
3. Establishment of patient–provider contracts in which the patient commits to a date on which he or she will eliminate tobacco use.
4. Anticipatory guidance (e.g., counseling to help the patient identify triggers of tobacco use and specific strategies for managing triggering events and situations).
5. General stress management and support.
6. Appropriate use of adequate doses of nicotine replacement agents (nicotine replacement therapy) and/or medications for nicotine addiction.
7. Frequent follow-up during the critical weeks after initial termination of tobacco use (by phone or office visit).
8. Appropriate counseling after any relapse on recognition that most individuals who successfully stop smoking have one to four relapses.

---

goals for glycemic control must be individualized based on the patient's overall clinical profile. Early results from the Action to Control Cardiovascular Risk in Diabetes (ACCORD) study suggest that aggressive glycemic control (see Table 11-1) could increase mortality among patients with type 2 diabetes (Aronow, 2008).

Dyslipidemia. Elevated levels of cholesterol, low-density lipoprotein cholesterol (LDL-C), triglycerides, and lipoprotein(a) are independent risk factors for LEAD. Each 10 mg/dl rise in total cholesterol is associated with a 10% increase in risk (Bonham et al, 2008; Hirsch et al, 2006; Liapis et al, 2009). In contrast, elevated levels of high-density lipoprotein cholesterol (HDL-C) appear to play a protective role. Recommended target levels for lipid management and strategies for maintaining normal lipid levels are provided in Table 11-1.

Hypertension. Elevated blood pressure (BP) is associated with up to a threefold increase in risk for LEAD in addition to a significant increase in risk for cardiovascular disease. Although treatment with antihypertensive medication has not been shown to improve LEAD outcomes, it is an essential element of care because of its impact on morbidity from cardiovascular and cerebrovascular disease (Lesho et al, 2004). Current goals and guidelines for maintaining BP are listed in Table 11-1 (Aronow, 2008; Bonham et al, 2008; Liapis et al, 2009).

Predisposing Risk Factors

Although predisposing risk factors *may* increase risk independently, they primarily act to increase the impact of primary (causative) risk factors. Predisposing risk factors include both modifiable factors (e.g., obesity, inactivity, social isolation, stress) and nonmodifiable

factors (e.g., advanced age, male gender, postmenopausal status, family history, African American ethnicity). Clinicians should work with patients and other providers to eliminate or minimize modifiable factors through diet, exercise, and strategies that reduce stress and isolation. Clinicians should educate patients about the impact of nonmodifiable risk factors and the critical importance of attention to smoking cessation, glycemic control, BP control, and correction of dyslipidemia (Bonham et al, 2008; Hopf et al, 2008; Liapis et al, 2009).

Emerging Risk Factors

Emerging risk factors include conditions such as elevated homocysteine levels, inflammation, infection, and indicators of renal failure.

Homocystinemia. Homocystinemia is a rare autosomal dominant disease found in 30% to 40% of individuals with LEAD. Studies suggest that elevated homocysteine levels may cause a mild increase in risk for LEAD; however, whether homocystinemia plays an etiologic role in LEAD is unclear. The abnormal metabolism of homocysteine (a thiol-containing amino acid) can be easily normalized through administration of vitamin B_6, vitamin B_{12}, and/or folic acid. Although there are no proven benefits in terms of reduced cardiovascular risk, current recommendations suggest treatment for those at risk for LEAD, with a treatment goal <10 μmol/L (Bonham et al, 2008; Liapis et al, 2009).

Inflammation. Inflammation is known to play a role in the development of atherosclerotic lesions in that endothelial injury triggers an inflammatory response that ultimately results in fibrosis. Some investigators suggest that repeated episodes of tissue ischemia (as evidenced by claudication) may trigger a low-grade inflammatory response that contributes to disease progression. Others have hypothesized that rapid progression of the disease process in a subset of patients may be the result of an underlying inflammatory disorder. The role of inflammation in the progression of the disease seems to be supported by studies demonstrating elevated levels of inflammatory markers such as C-reactive protein, fibrinogen, and interleukin-6 among patients with advanced PAD. The link between inflammation and the progression of PAD is unclear, and at present there are no recommendations for routine assessment of inflammatory markers such as C-reactive protein levels or for intervention (Bonham et al, 2008; Chaparaia et al, 2009; Liapis et al, 2009).

Infection. Inflammation, specifically both periodontal disease and *Chlamydia pneumoniae* (CPN), has been associated with increased risk and severity of LEAD. Acute CPN infections have been associated with increased lipid abnormalities and endothelial dysfunction. Antibiotic treatment of LEAD resulted in better clinical outcomes in patients who were seropositive for CPN than in seropositive controls who did not receive antibiotic therapy.

Although more research is needed, prompt treatment of any infectious process is recommended for all patients (Bonham et al, 2008; Liapis et al, 2009).

Renal Failure. Data suggest that there is a parallel between advancement of vascular disease and renal disease, and that renal failure increases the risk of death in patients with advanced LEAD. Although more study is needed, it appears clear that early intervention to preserve both vascular function and renal function is warranted (Liapis et al, 2009).

PATHOLOGY OF ARTERIAL ULCERATION

The exact pathologic mechanisms producing ulceration in the ischemic limb have not been clearly defined. Spontaneous ulceration typically involves the toes or distal foot and most likely is the result of progressive occlusion leading to cellular ischemia and tissue necrosis. Arterial ulcers may also be precipitated by minor trauma, which results in nonhealing wounds because the damaged vessels are unable to meet the increased demands for oxygen associated with tissue injury and the healing process (Hirsch et al, 2006). Patients with LEAD and compromised mobility are at greater risk for pressure ulcer development because they have an existing baseline of diminished blood flow. Therefore heel ulcers may occur rapidly in a bedbound patient with preexisting vascular impairment. It should be emphasized that pressure ulcers in these patients are *not* unavoidable; they can be prevented with standard interventions such as heel elevation.

ASSESSMENT

A comprehensive assessment provides the essential data for appropriate management of any patient with a lower extremity ulcer (see Checklist 11-1). Although "pure" arterial ulcers are relatively uncommon, other disease processes such as venous insufficiency and neuropathy frequently coexist with arterial disease, and the management plan may require modification depending on the severity of the coexisting arterial disease. In addition, a comprehensive assessment assists the clinician to identify patients with asymptomatic (early) arterial insufficiency; these patients should be referred for cardiac workup even if the level of LEAD is mild and does not interfere with wound healing.

Palpable pulses alone do *not* rule out arterial disease. Dependence on such unreliable assessment methods is a major contributing factor to the high incidence of unrecognized and untreated LEAD.

A comprehensive assessment for any patient with a lower extremity ulcer should include the patient's medical/surgical history, history of ulcer onset, previous management, lower extremity assessment, ulcer characteristics, and simple noninvasive vascular studies. Select patients may require laboratory studies or more complex or invasive vascular studies.

Patient History

The patient interview should include queries regarding any past illnesses or surgical procedures. Specific questions should be posed regarding history of angina, myocardial infarction, cardiovascular procedures, or "problems with circulation." The patient should be specifically queried regarding the major risk factors for LEAD: history of smoking/tobacco use, including any past attempts to stop smoking and willingness to consider smoking cessation; history of diabetes, including onset, type, management, usual fasting glucose level, and last HbA_{1c}; history of hypertension, including onset, duration, management, and usual BP; and lipid levels (if known) as well as any measures in place to manage dyslipidemia (Hopf et al, 2008). The history must include a review of all medications, including herbal agents, over-the-counter medications, and prescription drugs (see Appendix B for a sample assessment form). The patient should be asked about ulcers, any associated events (e.g., trauma), past treatments, and ulcer response.

Pain History

As described in Chapter 10, the patient should be questioned about the location, duration, and intensity of pain to assist with differential diagnosis (see Table 10-2). Pain in the lower extremity is often the first indication of LEAD. Location may suggest the level of the occlusion. In general, the patient will report pain in one joint distal to the stenosis or occlusion (Table 11-2) (Cimminiello, 2002). Aggravating and relieving factors help determine categories of pain that indicate severity of ischemia (Box 11-3).

Unfortunately, the patient with LEAD does not always experience or report "classic" ischemic pain symptoms. Intermittent claudication, for example, is normally described as reproducible cramping, aching, fatigue, or weakness as well as a distinct discomfort in the buttock, thigh, or calf muscle precipitated by exercise and rapidly disappearing after 10 minutes of rest (Hirsch et al, 2006). However, because the patient with LEAD may limit walking or activities to avoid pain, signs of claudication may be absent or reported as "leg weakness." Patients with sensory neuropathy (e.g., mixed neuropathic and

TABLE 11-2	Correlation between Site of Occlusion and Location of Pain
Site of Occlusion	**Location of Pain**
Iliofemoral arteries	Thighs, buttocks, calves
Superficial femoral artery	Calf artery
Infrapopliteal artery	Foot

From Cimminiello C: PAD: epidemiology and pathophysiology, *Thromb Res* 106(6):V295, 2002.

BOX 11-3	**Categories of Ischemic Pain**
Intermittent claudication pain	Occurs with moderate to heavy activity; relieved by approximately 10 minutes of rest. Typically occurs when involved vessel is approximately 50% occluded.
Nocturnal pain	Develops as occlusion worsens. Occurs when patient is in bed. Caused by combination of leg elevation (to horizontal position) and reduced cardiac output. Relieved by placing limb in a dependent position.
Rest pain	Occurs in absence of activity and with legs in a dependent position. Rest pain signals advanced occlusive disease (typically >90% occlusion).

arterial disease) may also have absent or blunted awareness of ischemic pain (Hopf et al, 2008).

Rest pain is perceived as a "constant deep aching pain." However, the patient with advanced LEAD may shift from nociceptive pain, typically described as "aching" or "throbbing," to neuropathic pain, which usually is described as "tingling, burning, electric-shock" type pain (Ruger et al, 2008). Further discussion related to the assessment and management of pain is given in Chapters 25 and 26.

Lower Extremity Assessment

With LEAD, legs generally appear cool, pale, thin, and shiny, with loss of hair. Pulses often are diminished or absent. Absence of pedal pulses mandates referral to a vascular surgeon. However, diminished or absent pulses cannot be used as a sole measure of arterial insufficiency, because some individuals with normal perfusion lack one or both pedal pulses (Hopf et al, 2006). Functional and sensory deficits are often observed, especially when combined with LEND. Positional color changes, such as elevational pallor (with fair skin) or ashen tones (with dark skin), and dependent rubor may be noted. Permanent ischemic changes (mottled or blue) require an immediate vascular referral.

The classic arterial ulcer (see Plate 39) is frequently described as having a "punched out" appearance that is well defined and located on tips of toes, areas of trauma, or pressure points on the heel or foot. Arterial ulcers are very frequently infected because hypoxia compromises bacterial control; however, the infection may be missed because the signs of inflammation are very subtle in ischemic tissue (faint halo of erythema, moderate amounts of exudate). Table 10-3 gives a comparison of arterial, venous, and neuropathic ulcer characteristics.

Checklist 11-1 provides a simple list of possible findings specific to lower extremity assessment of the patient with LEAD. However, few lower extremity ulcers are "pure" arterial without mixed disease (venous/arterial or neuropathic/arterial). Therefore Chapter 10 should be

CHECKLIST 11-1
Lower Extremity Arterial Disease (LEAD) Assessment

✓ General appearance
  • Trophic changes: thin, shiny epidermis
  • Hair and nail patterns: loss of hair growth, thickened nails
  • Edema: variable based on need to keep leg dependent and coexisting disease
  • Skin color: pale or ischemic colors (possibly purpura and petechiae secondary to blood thinners)
✓ Functional sensory status: may be diminished with deformities
✓ Range of motion of ankle joint: stiffness
✓ Pain: ischemic (see Box 11-3)
✓ Perfusion
  • Dependent rubor and elevational pallor: present (see Box 10-2)
  • Skin temperature: cool
  • Capillary refill time: delayed
  • Blood flow: abnormal turbulence (bruit)
  • Pulses: diminished or absent
  • ABI: diminished
  • TBI: diminished
✓ Diagnostic tests
  • ABI and TBI (see Table 11-3)
  • Transcutaneous partial pressure of oxygen
  • Skin perfusion pressure
  • Pulse volume recording and Doppler waveform study
  • Segmental limb pressure measurements
  • Magnetic resonance angiography
  • Duplex angiography
  • Computed tomographic angiography
  • Arteriography

ABI, Ankle-brachial index; *TBI,* toe-brachial index.

carefully reviewed for a detailed description of lower extremity assessment regardless of etiology, including simple perfusion assessments such as assessment of pulses, capillary refill, dependent rubor, and elevational pallor (see Boxes 10-2, 10-3 and 10-4).

NONINVASIVE TESTING FOR LEAD

When the diagnosis is unclear or the wound fails to improve, diagnostic studies are indicated. The most common diagnostic tests for LEAD are listed in Checklist 11-1. With the exception of the ABI, these tests involve equipment that is reserved for use in vascular laboratories by trained technicians and reviewed by vascular radiologists or surgeons.

Ankle-Brachial Index (ABI)

ABI, also known as *ankle-arm index,* is a simple bedside comparison of perfusion pressures in the lower leg with those in the upper arm using a blood pressure cuff and a portable handheld battery-operated continuous-wave Doppler ultrasound device with a Doppler probe (Figure 11-1). The Doppler probe generates the correct

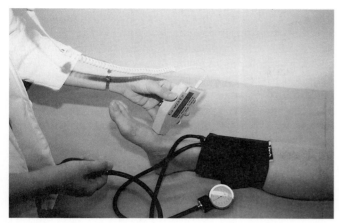

FIGURE 11-1 Handheld Doppler probe being used to obtain an ankle-brachial index.

TABLE 11-3	Interpretation of Noninvasive Tests for LEAD
Value	**Interpretation/Clinical Significance**
ABI	
>1.3	Abnormally high range, typically because of calcification of the vessel wall in patient with diabetes
	Renders ABI test invalid as a measure of peripheral perfusion
	TBI indicated
1.0–1.3	"Normal" range
≤0.9	LEAD
0.6–0.8	Borderline perfusion
≤0.5	Severe ischemia; wound healing unlikely unless revascularization can be accomplished
TBI	
<0.7	LEAD
TcPO$_2$ (Obtain if ABI or TP cannot be performed due to calcification or amputations of ankle or toes)	
≥40 mm Hg	Normal
<40 mm Hg	Hypoxia with impaired wound healing
AP	
AP <40 mm Hg	Limb threatened
TP	
<30 mm Hg	Critical limb ischemia (<50 mm Hg in patient with diabetes)
SPP	
>30 mm Hg	Required for healing to occur

ABI, Ankle-brachial index; *AP*, ankle pressure; *LEAD*, lower extremity arterial disease; *SPP*, skin partial pressure; *TBI*, toe-brachial index; *TP*, toe pressure; *TcPO$_2$*, transcutaneous partial pressure of oxygen.

frequency (8–9 MHz) for assessment of skin-level vessels (Bonham et al, 2007). This noninvasive test is used to screen patients for evidence of significant arterial insufficiency and to identify patients who require further workup. An ABI of 0.90 or less is approximately 95% sensitive for detecting LEAD compared to angiography-proven ischemic disease (Norgren et al, 2007). The ABI is also an excellent diagnostic tool for monitoring LEAD progression and is useful for detecting restenosis after revascularization. A 15% change from the baseline ABI is indicative of disease progression (Hirsch et al, 2006). Finally, the Wound, Ostomy and Continence Nurses Society Society (2002) recommends conducting an ABI test every 3 months in patients suffering from LEAD and nonhealing wounds to identify severe or critical limb ischemia that warrants referral or a change in the plan of care (Table 11-3).

The procedure for conducting an ABI test is outlined in Box 11-4. Guidelines for interpretation of ABI and toe–brachial index are provided in Table 11-3. A research-based protocol should be used to measure ABIs with a pocket Doppler to enhance achieving valid and reliable results compared to results obtained from a vascular laboratory (Bonham et al, 2007).

ABI provides only an indirect measure of peripheral perfusion and cannot be considered accurate in patients with noncompressible vessels (e.g., patient with diabetes, renal failure, and vessel calcification) (Bonham et al, 2007). Patients with diabetes who have clinical evidence of ischemia but normal or elevated ABI measurements should be referred for more definitive testing, such as toe-brachial index (TBI). A normal resting ABI in the presence of claudication suggests severe arterial stenosis (Bonham et al, 2007). Therefore referral to a vascular laboratory for ABI testing at rest and treadmill exercise testing or segmental pulse volume recording (PVR) tests is recommended (Hirsch et al, 2006).

Toe-Brachial Index (TBI)

TBI, also known as the *toe-arm index,* is indicated when ABI is greater than 1.3, which is suggestive of noncompressible arteries (Steed et al, 2006). This procedure can be performed by a trained clinician and conducted in the same manner as the ABI test, although a small digit cuff is placed around the great toe or the second toe and a transducer in the toe pad is used to detect pulsatile cutaneous blood flow (photoplethysmography). Cold toes and vasospastic disease produce constricted arteries, so continuous-wave Doppler devices are neither reliable nor recommended for measuring toe pressures (Bonham et al, 2007). Guidelines for interpretation of toe pressure measurements are provided in Table 11-3.

Exercise Stress Testing

Exercise stress testing is an effective diagnostic study for symptomatic patients with normal ABI readings and is sometimes used to assess the functional impact of

---

BOX 11-4   Procedure for Obtaining an ABI

1. Place patient in supine position in warm, tranquil environment for at least 10 minutes before the test (prevents vasoconstriction of arteries). Provide blankets if necessary.
2. Obtain brachial pressure in each arm using Doppler probe and 12- to 14-cm cuff placed 3 cm above cubital fossa. Inflate cuff 20–30 mm Hg above the last sound; slowly deflate cuff until initial sound is heard. Record highest brachial pressure.
3. Place appropriately sized cuff (10–12 cm) around lower leg 3 cm above malleolus.
4. Apply acoustic gel over dorsalis pedis pulse location.
5. Hold Doppler probe over pedal pulse according to manufacturer's guidelines (e.g., pen-style Doppler devices should be held at 45-degree angle). Be careful not to occlude the artery with excessive pressure; hold the probe lightly!
6. Inflate cuff to level 20–30 mm Hg above point where pulse is no longer audible.
7. Slowly deflate cuff while monitoring for return of pulse signal. The point at which the arterial signal returns is recorded as the dorsalis pedis pressure.
8. Apply acoustic gel over posterior tibial pulse location and repeat procedure. The higher of the two values is used to determine the ABI.
9. Calculate ABI by dividing the higher of the two ankle pressures by the higher of the two brachial pressures.

ABI, Ankle-brachial index.

LEAD. A baseline ABI is performed, then the patient walks on a treadmill set at a constant speed and grade. A patient who is unable to walk on a treadmill can be asked to stand with knees fully extended and to repeatedly raise the heels off the floor. The stress activity (treadmill walking or repetitive heel raises) is continued until the patient becomes symptomatic or until a set limit is reached (e.g., 5 minutes on the treadmill or 50 heel raises). A repeat ABI is obtained 1 minute after completion of the stress activity. Individuals with normal perfusion exhibit no change or a slight increase in ABI, whereas individuals with LEAD exhibit a clear drop in ABI. Contrast-enhanced ultrasound has also been used to assess perfusion of skeletal muscle at rest and following exercise and was found to accurately reflect severity of vascular impairment (Begelman and Jaff, 2006; Lindner et al, 2008).

Transcutaneous Oxygen Pressure (TcPO₂)

Transcutaneous partial pressure of oxygen ($TcPO_2$) measurements provide information about the adequacy of oxygen delivery to the skin and underlying tissues. This test is valuable for determining skin perfusion when a wound fails to improve or when ABI and TBI are not valid or are not possible due to incompressible arteries or amputation of feet or toes. $TcPO_2$ is a simple test that usually is performed in a vascular laboratory, specialty clinic, or hyperbaric oxygen therapy (HBOT) center. To obtain a $TcPO_2$ measurement, an oxygen sensor and a particular electrode are attached to the skin to quantify oxygen diffusion through the skin. Values less than 40 mm Hg reflect tissue hypoxia and are associated with delays in wound healing (Norgren et al, 2007).

Skin Perfusion Pressure (SPP)

Laser Doppler skin perfusion pressure (SPP) is another noninvasive measurement used for predicting successful wound healing in critical limb ischemia or for planning the lowest possible level of amputation for maximal preservation of functionality and mobility (Tsuji et al, 2008). SPP has been identified as an alternative when TBI and ABI measurements cannot be accurately obtained due to incompressible arteries or are impossible due to amputation of feet and toes (Okamoto et al, 2006). Unlike $TcPO_2$, SPP results are not influenced by factors such as local edema and anemia, and the procedure is less time consuming. An SPP value is obtained by using a laser Doppler probe and placing a cuff around the forefoot (including the five metatarsal and 14 phalange bones and surrounding soft tissues) of a patient lying supine in a thermoregulated room. SPP greater than 30 mm Hg is requisite for wound healing (Tsuji et al, 2008).

Pulse Volume Recordings (PVR) and Doppler Waveform Studies

PVR provides a reflection of actual perfusion volume during the cardiac cycle and is recommended when ABI is greater than 1.3. PVRs are obtained with cuffs that incorporate pneumoplethysmograph capability (i.e., the ability to detect changes in blood volume in the underlying arteries). The cuffs are inflated to a preset level, and the machine provides tracings that reflect blood volume within the underlying arteries throughout the cardiac cycle. A similar tracing of flow within a single vessel may be obtained using a Doppler probe; this tracing is commonly referred to as a *Doppler waveform study*. Normal tracings for both PVRs and Doppler waveform studies are triphasic, showing a clearly defined systolic peak, followed by a dicrotic notch that represents reversal of blood flow during early diastole, and finally a diastolic wave (Figure 11-2, *A*). With mild LEAD, the waveform changes to a biphasic pattern, whereas with advanced LEAD the waveform becomes monophasic or severely blunted (Figure 11-2, *B* and *C)*. Waveforms can also be obtained for the digital vessels by wrapping a cuff around the arch of the foot or the

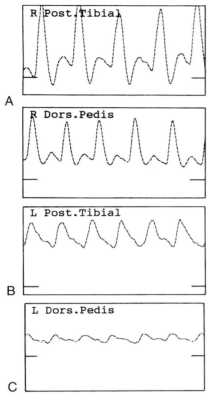

FIGURE 11-2 A, Normal Doppler waveforms from normal vessels (right posterior tibialis and right dorsalis pedis). Signal is triphasic, showing systolic peak, dicrotic notch representing blood flow reversal during early diastole, and a diastolic wave. **B,** Doppler waveform of vessel with moderately severe occlusive disease as evidenced by a monophasic waveform. **C,** Doppler waveform of vessel with advanced occlusive disease. Note that waveform is severely blunted.

the same leg is indicative of a possible occlusive lesion between the cuffs. A 20 to 30 mm Hg pressure difference between the contralateral positions may indicate stenosis or an occlusive lesion in the extremity with the lower pressure. The pressures are then compared, and a difference of 20 mm Hg or more between two adjacent cuff positions localizes the occlusion to the intervening vessels (Begelman and Jaff, 2006).

SLP and PVR measurements are often obtained in combination. SLP and PVR measurements alone are 85% accurate compared with angiography in detecting and localizing significant occlusive lesions (see Figure 11-2, *A*). When SLP and PVR are used together, however, the accuracy is closer to 95%. Additionally, the patient with diabetes and calcified arteries who produces a falsely elevated SLP will be accurately assessed by PVR when the two tests are done in combination (Norgren et al, 2007).

Magnetic Resonance Angiography

Magnetic resonance angiography (MRA), with or without gadolinium enhancement, can be helpful in determining the location and severity of stenosis and is one option for obtaining the detailed anatomic information required for accurate decision-making regarding surgical intervention. Benefits of MRA include its noninvasive nature, its minimal risk, and its ability to provide impressive images of the pedal arteries; fewer followup diagnostic tests are required with the contrast enhanced MRA when compared with the duplex ultrasound (de Vries et al, 2006). MRA is not an option for patients with implanted defibrillators, permanent pacemakers, intracranial aneurysm clips, or claustrophobia, and gadolinium enhancement may be contraindicated in patients with chronic renal insufficiency. In addition, MRA does not reliably detect calcification and is not currently able to image endovascular stents constructed of metal alloys (Begelman and Jaff, 2006; Hirsch et al, 2006; Rybicki et al, 2008).

Duplex Angiography (Ultrasound Imaging)

Ultrasonography uses sound waves to reveal characteristics of tissue or organs. By combining ultrasonography with Doppler technology, duplex angiography provides imaging of arteries and visualization of blood flow in order to identify the location and severity of stenosis, thrombi, or occlusive lesions (Ajijola and Jaff, 2008; Hirsch et al, 2006). Duplex angiography has a sensitivity of 99% and 80% and specificity of 94% and 91% for the femoropopliteal and tibial segments, respectively, compared with arteriography (Hopf et al, 2006). Results are comparable to contrast enhanced MRA and costs less however necessitates more follow-up diagnostic tests (de Vries et al, 2006).

great toe; waveforms that are dampened or flat suggest small vessel disease (Aronow, 2008; Begelman and Jaff, 2006; Rybicki et al, 2008). Results, however, can be influenced by factors such as local edema and anemia (Tsuji et al, 2008).

Segmental Limb Pressure (SLP)

Segmental limb pressure (SLP) measurements are used to determine the location of an occlusion when a surgical intervention is contemplated for critical limb ischemia (Hirsch et al, 2006). Cuffs are placed at high and low thigh level, below the knee, and just above the ankle. A Doppler probe is used to localize the most distal pulses (dorsalis pedis and posterior tibialis), and the ankle cuff is inflated until the arterial signal is obliterated. The cuff then is deflated until the arterial signal again is audible. The pressure at which the signal is heard is recorded as the ankle systolic pressure. The procedure is repeated with inflation of the "below-the-knee" cuff and then with the thigh cuff. A 30 mm Hg decrease in pressure between two adjacent levels on

INVASIVE TESTING FOR LEAD

Prior to revascularization, an anatomic roadmap is needed. This can be obtained with duplex angiography, MRA, angiography, or computed tomographic angiography (CTA).

Arteriography

Contrast angiography was once considered the "gold standard" for diagnosing LEAD and planning surgical intervention. However, it is an invasive procedure that now is used only in planning surgical intervention, primarily for patients in whom MRA and multidetector CTA are contraindicated or would provide insufficient anatomic data. When performed, angiography utilizing digital subtraction technology is the usual choice. A plain film of the involved area is taken prior to injection of contrast material, and the computer then "subtracts" the plain film image from the postcontrast images. As a result, the final films show only the arteries, allowing for clear identification of the site and severity of stenotic lesions (Hopf et al, 2006; Norgren et al, 2007).

Computed Tomographic Angiography

CTA utilizes iodinated contrast agent and X-rays to visualize arterial anatomy and to localize stenosis in patients who are candidates for surgical revascularization or endovascular procedures. The use of CTA is increasing, due in part to improvements in image detail provided by new 64-channel "multidetector" channels. Multidetector CTA can be used to image the arterial system all the way down to the pedal arteries and to evaluate the patency of bypass grafts (Begelman and Jaff, 2006; Rybicki et al, 2008; Schernthaner et al, 2009). CTA is faster than MRA and is safer than digital subtraction. CTA is an alternative for the patient with a pacemaker or implanted defibrillator who cannot undergo MRA. CTA has reduced accuracy in extensive vessel calcification and cannot be used with the patient who cannot tolerate iodine-based contrast and exposure to ionizing radiation (Hirsch et al, 2006).

MANAGEMENT OF THE PATIENT WITH ARTERIAL ULCERATION

The primary focus in management of the patient with an arterial ulcer is improving perfusion because the ability to heal is directly correlated with the ability to provide sufficient oxygen and nutrients to support the repair process. Secondary concerns include systemic support for wound healing, prevention and management of infection, appropriate topical therapy, and patient education and counseling regarding lifestyle changes and limb preservation. The patient must be monitored carefully for indicators of advancing necrosis, which may mandate amputation.

Measures to Improve Perfusion

Strategies for improving blood flow include surgical revascularization, aggressive management of modifiable risk factors to prevent disease progression, pharmacologic therapy, HBOT, intermittent pneumatic compression devices, and lifestyle modifications.

Surgical Options

Revascularization is the intervention most likely to provide healing, and data indicate that approximately 10% to 20% of individuals with LEAD will require revascularization (Hirsch et al, 2006). Patients who should be referred for surgical evaluation include those with critical limb ischemia and those with ulcers that are not healing with appropriate therapy. According to the AHA/ACC guidelines for the management of patients with peripheral arterial disease, patients with incapacitating claudication should be evaluated for revascularization if there is a reasonable likelihood that symptoms will improve and there is an absence of another diagnosis that would limit exercise, such as angina or heart failure (Hirsch et al, 2006). Appropriate evaluation is needed to ensure the patency of distal vessels and may involve MRA, multidetector CTA, or contrast angiography using digital subtraction techniques. Options for revascularization include open bypass grafting and endovascular procedures (angioplasty and placement of endovascular stents) (Hopf et al, 2006).

Bypass Grafts. Bypass grafts have been considered the "gold standard" for revascularization and are most commonly done using the patient's own saphenous vein (autologous saphenous vein bypass) (Figure 11-3). If the saphenous vein is damaged or unavailable, a synthetic graft (e.g., heparin-bonded expanded polytetrafluoroethylene) may be used. Long-term results are generally good, with 5-year patency rates of approximately 70%. Distal bypass procedures involving smaller vessels have slightly lower long-term patency rates. Smoking cessation can improve patency rates and is a key element of a comprehensive management program (Bonham et al, 2008; Daenens et al, 2009; Hopf et al, 2006).

Endovascular Procedures. Endovascular procedures are advantageous because they are less invasive and therefore are associated with lower risk. Although these procedures may provide less durable results, their increased use is associated with reduced numbers of amputations (Cao and DeRango, 2009; Hopf et al, 2006; Rowe et al, 2009). Patient selection is critical for achieving optimal outcomes with endovascular procedures. Angioplasty is generally not a good option for patients with extensive occlusive disease or for lesions longer than 10 cm, and it may not be feasible for use in smaller vessels. Approximately one third of patients with severe ischemic disease of the lower leg are candidates for angioplasty, and initial results are generally

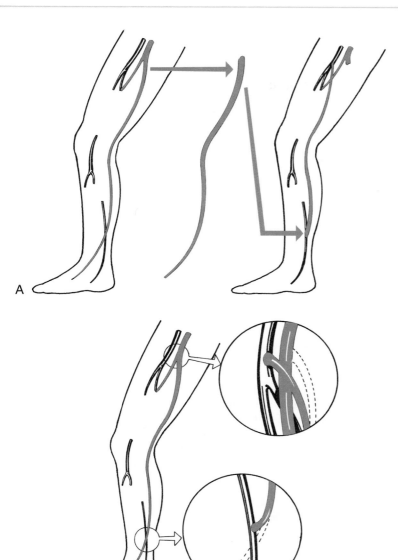

FIGURE 11-3 Illustration of bypass grafts using an autologous saphenous vein in a reversed saphenous vein procedure **(A)** and an in situ procedure **(B).**

good. Long-term patency rates have been enhanced by placement of endovascular stents into the stenotic area immediately after angioplasty (Ellozy and Carroccio, 2003; Wipke-Tevis and Sae-Sia, 2004). Cilostazol may also be of benefit in reducing recurrent stenosis caused by intimal hyperplasia (Dindyal and Kyriakides, 2009).

Management of Modifiable Risk Factors

In addition to managing the primary (causative) contributing risk factors and the emerging risk factors for LEAD (as summarized in Table 11-1), the patient must be counseled regarding simple strategies that improve perfusion, such as maintenance of adequate hydration and avoidance of cold and constriction (Hopf et al, 2006; Zeymer et al, 2009). Strategies for patients with mild to moderate LEAD and patients who have been

effectively revascularized include a supervised graduated walking program (Bonham et al, 2008; Hopf et al, 2008).

Supervised Walking Program. Supervised walking programs have been shown to improve walking distance, reduce claudication pain, and reduce cardiovascular morbidity and mortality by reducing plasma viscosity. Patients who are candidates for a walking program should be counseled regarding the benefits and should be strongly encouraged to enroll in a supervised program that provides three exercise sessions per week. Each session should involve 30 to 60 minutes of treadmill or track walking to the point of pain, followed by rest. Self-directed walking programs are an alternative to supervised programs for patients who are medically cleared for such programs (Bonham et al, 2008; Hafner et al, 2009; Hopf et al, 2008; Sakamoto et al, 2009).

Pharmacologic Therapy

The mainstays of pharmacologic therapy for LEAD include antiplatelet drugs, cilostazol, statins, and analgesics.

Antiplatelet agents work primarily by reducing platelet aggregation. The most commonly used antiplatelet agent is low- to medium-dose aspirin (75–325 mg/day), which may delay the rate at which LEAD progresses and may improve long-term patency of bypass grafts. However, the primary benefit of aspirin is the reduction in morbidity and mortality related to cerebrovascular and cardiovascular disease (stroke and myocardial infarction). Clopidogrel (75 mg/day) is currently recommended as an effective alternative to aspirin (Aronow, 2008; Berger et al, 2009; Bonham et al, 2008; Hopf et al, 2008).

Cilostazol has both antiplatelet and vasodilatory effects and is currently the most commonly recommended drug for symptomatic LEAD. Benefits include increased walking distance, reduced intermittent claudication, improved ABI, and favorable modification of plasma lipoprotein levels. The recommended dose is 100 mg twice per day, and the drug is generally well-tolerated. Approximately one third of patients report mild side effects, which subside in about 6 weeks. New onset of congestive heart failure is a contraindication (Aronow, 2008; Hopf et al, 2006; O'Donnell et al, 2009).

Statins are lipid-lowering drugs used to treat systemic atherosclerosis. They slow disease progression, improve the ABI, improve walking distance, and reduce the risk of adverse cardiovascular events. Statins are currently considered to be standard therapy for patients with LEAD (Bonham et al, 2008; Hopf et al, 2008; Liapis et al, 2009). Niacin or vitamin B_6 also may be helpful in reducing triglyceride levels and increasing HDL-C levels. The recommended dose of niacin is up to 3 g/day for as long as 60 weeks, as tolerated (Bonham et al, 2008).

Analgesics, specifically opioid analgesics, may be required for patients with advanced ischemia to relieve chronic pain and thus improve quality of life. Effective pain management also contributes to improved perfusion by preventing the vasoconstriction caused by sympathetic stimulation (Wipke-Tevis and Sae-Sia, 2004).

Investigational agents, such as the angiogenic growth factor vascular endothelial growth factor, are being used in patients with advanced ischemic disease and ulceration to improve perfusion by inducing new vessel growth (Hopf et al, 2006).

Hyperbaric Oxygen Therapy

HBOT increases the amount of oxygen dissolved in the plasma, which results in the delivery of "oxygen-enriched" blood to the tissues. HBOT has been shown to increase tissue oxygen levels in ischemic tissues where positive plasma flow exists; it has also been shown to support angiogenesis and wound healing. Candidates for HBOT include patients with significant ischemic disease who are not candidates for revascularization and patients who have undergone revascularization but who still demonstrate significant tissue hypoxia and impaired healing. Patients should be evaluated carefully to ensure responsiveness to HBOT (i.e., reversal of tissue-level hypoxia). Responsiveness can be evaluated by obtaining $TcPO_2$ measurements while the patient is breathing room air and then repeating $TcPO_2$ measurements while the patient is breathing 100% oxygen. Normally the $TcPO_2$ level will rise to greater than 100 mm Hg when the patient is breathing 100% oxygen, which signifies a good potential for enhanced healing with HBOT. In contrast, a patient who demonstrates minimal response (<10 mm Hg increase) is not likely to benefit from HBOT (Fife et al, 2009; Hopf et al, 2006). HBOT is discussed in greater detail in Chapter 22.

Intermittent Pneumatic Compression

Intermittent pneumatic compression devices (see Figure 12-8) promote venous return without impairing arterial inflow and may actually improve distal perfusion. Further studies are needed before intermittent pneumatic compression can be considered primary therapy for arterial disease (Bonham et al, 2008; Hopf et al, 2006; Hopf et al, 2008).

Modified Compression for Patients with Mixed Arterial-Venous Disease

Because edema further compromises perfusion, strategies for edema control should be considered when managing the patient with arterial disease complicated by lower limb edema. However, the use of sustained compression devices must be modified based on the severity of the arterial disease. Current evidence supports reduced or modified compression (23–30 mm Hg at the ankle) for patients with ABI greater than 0.5 and less than 0.8 (Bonham et al, 2008).

Patients with ABI of 0.5 or less should be managed with intermittent pneumatic compression or low-level elevation; they should not receive sustained compression (Bonham et al, 2008). Intermittent compression devices are discussed further in Chapter 12.

Systemic Support for Wound Healing

Nutritional support, tight glucose control, and control of other comorbidities are critical elements of care for the patient with an arterial ulcer (Bonham et al, 2008; Hopf et al, 2006). These issues are discussed in greater depth in Section 6 (Critical Cofactors) and Chapters 14 and 27.

Prevention and Management of Infection. Ischemia increases the risk for infection, and both ischemia and infection are significant impediments to the repair process. Thus prompt recognition and aggressive treatment of infectious complications are critical to positive outcomes. However, this can be a challenge because signs of infection are frequently muted (and therefore easy to miss) in ischemic conditions. Clinicians must routinely assess for subtle indicators of infection, such as a faint halo of erythema extending circumferentially around the wound edge. In wounds that present with signs of infection, systemic antibiotic therapy should be promptly initiated. When viable tissue is present in the wound bed, a culture should be obtained to ensure appropriate antibiotic selection. Some evidence indicates that "neuroischemic" wounds (wounds caused by a combination of neuropathy and ischemia) may be critically colonized even without obvious indicators; therefore a short course of antibiotic therapy may be appropriate for nonhealing mixed neuroischemic wounds. Effective management of infected ischemic wounds involves revascularization when indicated and possible, aggressive debridement of all necrotic tissue (including any necrotic bone), and appropriate antibiotic therapy. Topical antimicrobial dressings can be used in conjunction with systemic antibiotic therapy and may be helpful in controlling bacterial loads as well as *preventing* infection in clean open wounds. However, antimicrobial dressings should not be used as sole therapy for infected ischemic wounds (Bonham et al, 2008; Hopf et al, 2006).

Topical Therapy. The principles of topical therapy for ischemic ulcers are generally the same as for all other wounds. They involve wound bed preparation (removal of necrotic tissue and control of bacterial burden) followed by moisture retentive dressings to keep the wound surface clean, moist, and protected. However, specific wound characteristics should be considered when selecting dressings, and distinctly different guidelines for the management of closed necrotic wounds should be followed.

Guidelines for Dressing Selection. Ischemic ulcers typically have minimal exudate and are at very high risk for infection; therefore hydrating dressings with sustained release antimicrobial properties and a nonocclusive outer layer are likely to be of particular benefit. In addition, the periwound skin typically is very fragile; thus nonadherent dressings or those with silicone adhesive are frequently indicated, as is protection of the periwound skin with a skin sealant or moisture barrier ointment.

Management of Closed Necrotic Wounds. Although necrotic tissue is clearly a potential medium for bacterial growth, a dry intact eschar also can serve as a bacterial barrier. A closed wound surface is advantageous when managing a very poorly perfused wound in which any bacterial invasion is likely to result in clinical infection and

limb loss. A closed wound should be maintained when (1) the involved limb is clearly ischemic with limited or no potential for healing, (2) no indications of infection are present, and (3) the wound surface is dry and necrotic. A sample topical therapy protocol for this type of ulcer is outlined in Box 11-5. Note that this protocol applies only to *uninfected* wounds covered with dry intact eschar. If the wound develops clinically significant infection, the patient should be promptly referred for surgical evaluation (for debridement and hopefully revascularization) (Bonham et al, 2008; Hopf et al, 2006).

PATIENT EDUCATION

Lifestyle changes may be more difficult for the patient than either a surgical procedure or drug therapy; therefore effective introduction of such changes requires in-depth education and supportive, goal-directed patient counseling. In addition to receiving education regarding the specific plan of care and rationale, the patient should be taught the importance (and specifics) of protective lower limb care (Box 11-6) (Aronow, 2008; Bonham et al, 2008; Lesho et al, 2004).

Amputation

Amputation is reserved as the "treatment of last resort" and is indicated primarily for patients with irreversible ischemia (i.e., tissue necrosis) and invasive infection. $TcPO_2$ measurements may be used to accurately predict the level of amputation at which healing is most likely (Aronow, 2008; Bonham et al, 2008; Fife et al, 2009; Hopf et al, 2006; Palmer-Kazen and Wahlberg, 2003).

SUMMARY

Arterial ulcers are most commonly caused by peripheral arterial occlusive disease and may progress to critical limb ischemia and limb loss. Risk factors for peripheral arterial occlusive disease and arterial ulcers are the same as those for coronary artery disease and cerebrovascular disease. They include tobacco use, diabetes mellitus, dyslipidemia, and hypertension, as well as family history and age. Arterial ulcers typically present as spontaneous ulceration of the toes and distal foot or as a nonhealing

BOX 11-5	Topical Therapy for Dry, Necrotic, Uninfected Ischemic Wound

1. Inspect for subtle indicators of infection. If any signs or symptoms of infection develop, immediate referral for debridement and initiation of antibiotic therapy are critical.
2. Paint with antiseptic solution (e.g., povidone-iodine 10% solution); allow to dry.
3. Apply dry gauze dressing and secure with wrap gauze.

traumatic injury. Ulcers usually are painful, with a pale or necrotic wound bed, well-demarcated edges, and minimal exudate. Arterial ulcers are commonly infected; however, the signs of infection are muted due to the underlying ischemia. Successful management of an arterial ulcer is dependent upon measures to improve perfusion and oxygenation (revascularization, HBOT, and lifestyle measures such as smoking cessation). Positive long-term outcomes are dependent on lifestyle modifications to correct reversible risk factors and a progressive walking program to improve lower limb perfusion, as well as measures to prevent injury.

REFERENCES

Ajijola OA, Jaff MR: Noninvasive evaluation of peripheral arterial disease. In Kandarpa K, editor: *Peripheral vascular interventions,* Philadelphia, 2008, Lippincott Williams & Wilkins.

Aronow H: Peripheral arterial disease in the elderly: recognition and management, *Am J Cardiovasc Drugs* 8(6):353-364, 2008.

Begelman S, Jaff M: Noninvasive diagnostic strategies for peripheral arterial disease, *Cleve Clin J Med* 73(Suppl4):S22-S29, 2006.

Berger J et al: Aspirin for the prevention of cardiovascular events in patients with peripheral artery disease: a meta-analysis of randomized trials, *JAMA* 301(18):1909-1919, 2009.

Bonham P et al: Are ankle and toe brachial indices (ABI-TBI) obtained by a pocket Doppler interchangeable with those obtained by standard laboratory equipment? *J Wound Ostomy Continence Nurs* 34(1):35-44, 2007.

Bonham P et al: *Guidelines for management of wounds in patients with lower-extremity arterial disease,* Mt. Laurel, NJ, 2008, Wound Ostomy Continence Nurses Society.

Cao P, DeRango P: Endovascular treatment of peripheral artery disease (PAD): so old yet so far from evidence! *Eur J Vasc Endovasc Surg* 37(5):501-503, 2009.

Chaparaia R et al. Inflammatory profiling of peripheral arterial disease, *Ann Vasc Surg* 23(2):172-178, 2009.

Cimminiello C: PAD: epidemiology and pathophysiology, *Thromb Res* 106(6):V295, 2002.

Daenens K et al: Heparin-bonded ePTFE grafts compared with vein grafts in femoropopliteal and femorocrural bypasses: 1 and 2 year results, *J Vasc Surg* 49(5):1210-1216, 2009.

de Vries M et al: Peripheral arterial disease: clinical and cost comparisons between duplex US and contrast-enhanced MR angiography—a multicenter randomized trial, *Radiology* 240(2):401-410, 2006.

Dillavou E, Kahn M: Diagnosing and treating the 3 most common peripheral vasculopathies, *Geriatrics* 58(2):37-42, 2003.

Dindyal S, Kyriakides C: A review of cilostazol, a phosphodiesterase inhibitor, and its role in preventing both coronary and peripheral arterial restenosis following endovascular therapy, *Recent Pat Cardiovasc Drug Discov* 4(1):6-14, 2009.

Ellozy S, Carroccio A: Drug-eluting stents in peripheral vascular disease: eliminating restenosis, *Mount Sinai J Med* 70(6):417, 2003.

Fife C et al: Transcutaneous oximetry in clinical practice: consensus statement from an expert panel based on evidence, *Undersea Hyperb Med* 36(1):43-53, 2009.

Gibbons G: Lower extremity bypass in patients with diabetic foot ulcers, *Surg Clin North Am* 83(3):659, 2003.

Hafner H et al: Influence of controlled vascular training on the pain free walking distance and plasma viscosity in patients suffering from peripheral arterial occlusive disease, *Clin Hemorheol Microcirc* 41(1):73-80, 2009.

Hanly E et al: *Buerger's disease (thromboangiitis obliterans): differential diagnosis and workup,* E-Medicine from Web MD, Updated May 2009. http://emedicine.medscape.com/article/460027-overview. Accessed April 27, 2010

Hirsch A et al: ACC/AHA 2005 practice guidelines for the management of patients with peripheral arterial disease (lower extremity, renal, mesenteric, and abdominal aortic): a collaborative report from the American Association for Vascular Surgery/Society for Vascular Surgery, Society for Cardiovascular Angiography and Interventions, Society for Vascular Medicine and Biology, Society of Interventional Radiology, and the ACC/AHA Task Force on Practice Guidelines, *Circulation* 113(11):1474-1547, 2006.

Hopf H et al: Guidelines for the prevention of lower extremity arterial ulcers. *Wound Repair Regen* 16(2):175-188, 2008.

Hopf H et al: Guidelines for the treatment of arterial insufficiency ulcers, *Wound Repair Regen* 14(6):693-710, 2006.

Lesho E et al: Management of peripheral arterial disease, *Am Fam Phys* 69(3):525, 2004.

Liapis C et al: What a vascular surgeon should know and do about atherosclerotic risk factors, *J Vasc Surg* 49(5):1348-1354, 2009.

Lindner J et al: Limb stress-rest perfusion imaging with contrast ultrasound in the assessment of peripheral arterial disease severity, *JACC Cardiovasc Imaging* 1(3):343-350, 2008.

Norgren L et al: Inter-society consensus for the management of peripheral arterial disease (TASC II), *J Vasc Surg* 45(Suppl S): S5-S67, 2007.

O'Donnell M et al: The vascular and biochemical effects of cilostazol in patients with peripheral arterial disease, *J Vasc Surg* 49(5):1226-1234, 2009. Cited in Text

Okamoto K et al: Peripheral arterial occlusive disease is more prevalent in patients with hemodialysis: Comparison with the findings from multidetector-row computed tomography, *Am J Kidney Dis* 48(2):269-76, 2006.

Palmer-Kazen U, Wahlberg E: Arteriogenesis in peripheral arterial disease, *Endothelium* 10(4):225, 2003.

Rowe V et al: Patterns of treatment for peripheral arterial disease in the United States: 1996–2005, *J Vasc Surg* 49(4):910-917, 2009.

Ruger L et al: Characteristics of chronic ischemic pain in patients with peripheral arterial disease, *Pain* 139(1):201-208, 2008.

Rybicki F et al: ACR appropriateness criteria on recurrent symptoms following lower-extremity angioplasty, *J Am Coll Radiol* 5(12):1176-1180, 2008.

Sakamoto S et al: Patients with peripheral artery disease who complete 12-week supervised exercise training program show reduced cardiovascular mortality and morbidity, *Circ J* 73(1):167-173, 2009.

Schernthaner R et al: Value of MDCT angiography in developing treatment strategies for critical limb ischemia, *AJR Am J Roentgenol* 192(5):1416-1424, 2009.

Sigvant B et al: Risk factor profiles and use of cardiovascular drug prevention in women and men with peripheral arterial disease, *Eur J Cardiovasc Prev Rehabil* 16(1):39-46, 2009.

Steed DL, et al: Guidelines for the treatment of diabetic ulcers, *Wound Repair Regen* 14(6):680-692, 2006.

Tsuji Y et al: Importance of skin perfusion pressure in treatment of critical limb ischemia, *Wounds* 20(4):95-100, 2008.

Trent J, Kirsner R: Leg ulcers in sickle cell disease, *Adv Skin Wound Care* 17(8):410-416, 2004.

Wipke-Tevis D, Sae-Sia W: Caring for vascular leg ulcers, *Home Healthcare Nurse* 22(4):237, 2004.

Wound, Ostomy Continence Nurses Society (WOCN Society): Guideline for management of patients with lower extremity arterial disease, WOCN clinical practice guideline series #1, Glenview IL, 2002, Author.

Xu L et al: Cutaneous manifestations of vasculitis, *Semin Arthritis Rheum* 38(5):348-360, 2009.

Zeymer U et al: Risk factor profile, management and prognosis of patients with peripheral arterial disease with or without coronary artery disease: results of the prospective German REACH registry study, *Clin Res Cardiol* 98(4):249-256, 2009.

12

Venous Ulcers

Jane E. Carmel[1]

OBJECTIVES

1. Discuss venous ulcers in terms of etiologic factors, risk factors, assessment, diagnostic criteria, pathophysiology, typical presentation, and principles of management.
2. Describe Laplace's law in predicting sub-bandage pressure and the level of compression applied to the lower leg.
3. Explain the mechanism of action underlying effective compression therapy for the individual with chronic venous insufficiency.
4. Discuss considerations for use of inelastic compression, short-stretch bandages, long-stretch bandages, compression stockings, and intermittent pneumatic compression.
5. Identify adjunctive therapies that may be of benefit to the patient with a venous ulcer.
6. List three key points to teach a patient being treated with a multilayer compression wrap.

Chronic venous disorders include a wide range of morphologic and functional abnormalities of the venous system, that includes mild conditions (e.g., uncomplicated telangiectasias and varicose veins) to complex conditions (e.g., deep vein thrombosis, and venous ulcers). The majority of chronic venous disorders exist in the healthy patient population. The term chronic venous disease is used when referring to the subset of chronic venous disorders that are more complicated; those that are associated with signs and symptoms significant enough to require medical care, such as deep vein thrombosis, chronic venous insufficiency, and venous ulcers. Lower extremity venous disease (LEVD) is synonymous with chronic venous disease. Chronic venous insufficiency (CVI) refers to leg-related manifestations of venous hypertension and functional abnormalities of the venous system (edema, skin changes, ulceration) (Meissner, 2009). Venous ulcers are the most common lower extremity ulcers, accounting for 70% to 90% of all leg ulcers (WOCN Society, 2005). These lesions develop as a result of skin and tissue changes caused by CVI and the associated ambulatory venous hypertension.

Management of patients with venous ulcers must include measures to optimize wound healing through reduction of edema, prevention of complications, and appropriate topical therapy to promote healing (de Araujo et al, 2003; Moffat et al, 2007; Robson et al, 2006). Once the ulcer is healed, the emphasis shifts to long-term disease management and prevention of recurrence.

EPIDEMIOLOGY

The exact prevalence of venous ulcers is not known, although prevalence estimates in developed countries range from less than 1% to greater than 3% of the population (Bolton, 2008; Kerstein, 2003). Venous disease and venous ulcers occur in individuals as young as 20 years. "Peak" incidence occurs between the ages of 60 and 80 years (de Araujo et al, 2003). Although no racial predilection is apparent, most studies report female gender is a risk factor (de Araujo et al, 2003; Kalra and Gloviczki, 2003). In addition, an increased incidence of obesity is seen in 25% of patients with venous ulcers (Benigni et al, 2006).

LEVD affects approximately six to seven million individuals in the United States, and approximately one million of these persons will develop ulcerations (WOCN Society, 2005). The impact of venous disease is tremendous as it relates to the individual and costs to the health care system and society. Individuals with venous disease report pain, itching, anxiety, social isolation, and reduced ability to perform usual activities as their areas of greatest concern (de Araujo et al, 2003). In contrast, nurses caring for these patients rated pain control as a less important aspect of care than wound healing and limb preservation, which indicates the need for increased awareness and focus on quality-of-life issues on the part of health care providers (Ryan et al, 2003).

[1]The author and editors acknowledge Rhonda Holbrook and Dorothy Doughty for their work on developing content of this chapter in the third edition of *Acute & Chronic Wounds: Nursing Management*. Many of the concepts and comments they developed in the previous edition are reflected in this chapter. Their significant contribution is well appreciated.

Approximately $2.5 to $3.5 billion is spent annually on management of venous ulcers (Bolton, 2008). The average lifetime cost of care for an individual with LEVD can exceed $40,000 (Weingarten, 2001). Cost per occurrence in the home care or wound clinic setting is estimated at $1,621 to $3,279 without calculating lost wage time (Bolton et al 2006; Korn et al, 2002; McGucklin et al, 2002).

The negative impact of venous ulcers is compounded by recurrence rates of 26% to 28% in the first year and is as high as 76% within 3 to 5 years, which reflects the chronicity of the underlying condition (Bolton et al, 2006; Castonguay, 2008) Frequent recurrence is attributed to a failure to adequately address the primary problems of venous insufficiency and venous hypertension (WOCN Society, 2005).

VENOUS STRUCTURE AND FUNCTION

The veins of the lower extremity venous system include deep veins, superficial veins, and perforator veins. The deep veins include the posterior and anterior tibial and the peroneal veins; these veins are located in the deep tissue adjacent to the calf muscle. The superficial venous system is also known as the *saphenous system* because the two major vessels are the greater saphenous vein and lesser saphenous vein. These two vessels are located just below the superficial fascia and have multiple tributaries located in the superficial tissues (Figure 12-1) (Kalra and Gloviczki, 2003). The perforator veins "connect" the two systems, transporting blood from the superficial system into the deep system, from which point the blood is propelled back to the heart. The number of perforator veins per leg can vary greatly; the typical patient can have 200 perforator veins below the knee and 20 above the knee (Hussein, 2008).

Veins fill normally via slow capillary inflow, which takes more than approximately 20 seconds. All veins are equipped with one-way valves that support a unidirectional flow of blood toward the heart. Because these valves prevent reflux of blood from the high-pressure deep venous system to the low-pressure superficial venous system, they play an essential role in normal venous function. Further protection is provided by the fact that the perforator veins follow an oblique course through the fascia and muscle layers, which provides additional support for the connecting veins and their valves. The closed valves in the perforator veins prevent transmission of the high resting pressures back into the superficial system, so long as the valves remain competent (Kalra and Gloviczki, 2003). Approximately 50% to 60% of patients with venous ulcers have incompetent superficial and perforator vein valves (Agren and Gottrup, 2007).

Returning blood from the feet and legs to the heart is a major physiologic challenge because the blood must flow "uphill" against the forces of gravity. When an individual is standing upright, the gravitational force creates a column of hydrostatic pressure of approximately 90 mm Hg at the ankle. The primary mechanisms by which venous blood is returned to the heart are the smooth muscle tone within the venous walls, the contraction of the calf muscles (gastrocnemius and soleus), and the negative intrathoracic pressure created during inspiration. Of these three mechanisms, contraction of the calf muscle pump is by far the most essential (Meissner, 2009).

The calf muscle pump and one-way valves normally work together to propel venous blood back toward the heart. Calf muscle contraction forces the blood out of the deep veins and into the central circulation. While blood is being pumped from the deep veins, the one-way valves in the perforator system are closed to prevent backflow of the venous blood into the superficial veins. As the calf muscle relaxes, the valves in the perforator veins open to permit the blood in the superficial system to flow into the deep veins. At the onset of calf muscle contraction, the pressures within the deep venous system peak at 120 to 300 mm Hg. These pressures then fall rapidly as the veins empty and the calf muscle relaxes (Figure 12-2). Thus high resting (filling) pressures, but low walking (emptying) pressures, characterize normal venous function (Figure 12-3).

CHRONIC VENOUS INSUFFICIENCY

The three elements most essential to normal venous function are competent valves, the physical properties of the venous wall, and the normally functioning calf muscle pump. With the loss of valvular competence, veins no longer fill normally via slow capillary inflow alone. Retrograde flow (reflux or back flow) of venous blood occurs during calf muscle pump relaxation preventing a reduction in the venous pressure and a rapid (<20 second) venous refill time. This sustained high pressure or failure to lower venous pressure in the deep veins via the action of the calf pump muscle can be transmitted into the perforator veins and into the normally low-pressure superficial venous system. Incompetent valves subsequently contribute to venous hypertension and the condition known as CVI. Conditions that cause or contribute to valvular incompetence include those that cause direct damage to the valve leaflets and those that cause venous distention. Distention contributes to valve dysfunction by causing mechanical stretch that results in loss of coaptation of the valve leaflets.

Valve failure changes the normal unidirectional flow of blood into a "bidirectional" flow. As a result, blood refluxes back into the superficial system, causing distention and congestion of the superficial veins and capillaries, which manifest clinically as edema. The deep veins are incompletely emptied, causing increased pressures within the deep system, which create resistance to blood draining from the superficial veins. Resistance to flow creates congestion and distention of the superficial

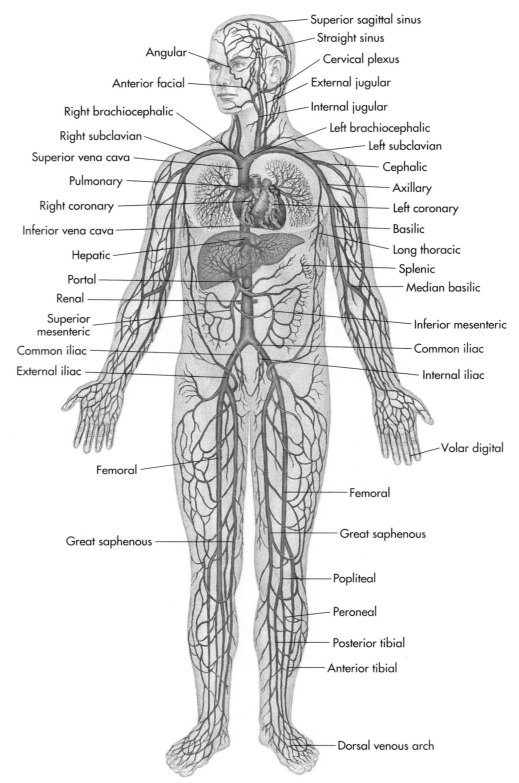

FIGURE 12-1 Systemic circulation: veins. (From Seidel HM et al: *Mosby's guide to physical examination,* ed 6, St. Louis, 2006, Mosby.)

and perforator veins, which cause loss of valve coaptation. The incompetent valves then permit backward transmission of the high pressures in the deep system (Meissner, 2009). The failure to adequately lower venous pressure with the pumping of the calf muscle or by the incompetence of the valves creates ambulatory venous hypertension. Venous ulceration is a direct result of ambulatory venous hypertension from CVI. A clear understanding of the anatomy and physiology of the lower extremity venous system provides the framework for determining the pathology of LEVD, ambulatory venous hypertension, and venous ulceration.

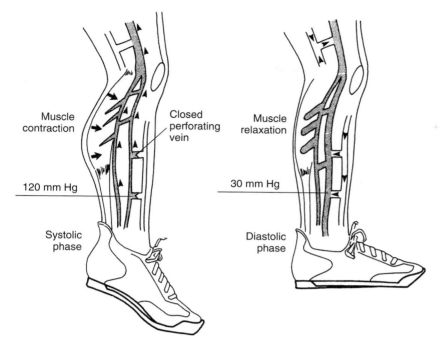

FIGURE 12-2 Anatomy of the perforating (communicating) veins. During the systolic phase of calf muscle contraction, the one-way valves of the perforating veins are closed, which prevents deep-to-superficial blood flow. During the diastolic phase the valves of the perforating veins are open, allowing superficial-to-deep blood flow to refill the deep veins. (From O'Donnell TF Jr, Shepard AD: Chronic venous insufficiency. In Jarrett F, Hirsch SA, editors: *Vascular surgery of the lower extremities,* St. Louis, 1996, Mosby.)

The majority of patients have multisystem valvular incompetence (i.e., incompetent valves in at least two of the three venous systems) (Meissner, 2009). Perforator valve incompetence is particularly common and clinically significant. At least two thirds of patients with venous hypertension and venous ulcers have incompetent perforator valves, which can result in supramalleolar pressures well above 100 mm Hg and a "reflux rate" greater than 60 ml/min. When multiple valves become incompetent, the effect is magnified and clinically evident disease becomes much more likely (Kalra and Gloviczki, 2003; Meissner, 2009).

Of the three leg muscle pumps responsible for venous return in lower extremities (foot, calf, and thigh), the calf muscle pump is of greatest importance and generates the highest pressure. Among the venous pumps, the ejection fraction of the calf muscle pump is 65% compared to only 15% from the thigh muscle. In the limb with active ulceration, the ejection fraction can decrease to 35% (Meissner, 2009).

Ultimately, the end result of prolonged ambulatory venous hypertension is damage to the skin and soft tissues that renders these structures vulnerable to minor trauma and susceptible to spontaneous ulceration. Venous ulcers are caused primarily by chronic valvular disease of the deep venous system and perforators (Hussein, 2008). In the past, the cutaneous inflammation observed with venous insufficiency was believed to the result of blood pooling (thus the term *stasis*) with low oxygen tension in the superficial veins, which precipitated hypoxic damage to the overlying skin. Today, no evidence supports the theories of stasis or hypoxia, prompting discontinuation of the terms *stasis dermatitis* and *stasis ulcers* (Flugman and Clark, 2009).

Classification

CVI is classified according to: Clinical indicators, Etiologic factors, Anatomic location of the dysfunctional venous structures, and specific Pathophysiologic processes (CEAP). This system is presented in Table 12-1 (Agren and Gottrup, 2007; WOCN Society, 2005).

Risk Factors

Risk factors for CVI include a history of major leg trauma, hip or knee surgery, and vein stripping. However, factors that lead to valvular or calf muscle dysfunction are the most common risk factors; they are listed in Table 12-2 along with other key elements of the medical history that must be obtained for the patient with a venous ulcer.

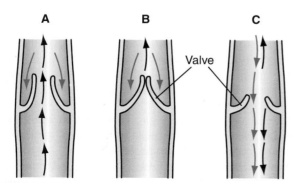

FIGURE 12-3 Venous valves. **A,** Open valves allow forward blood flow. **B,** Closed valves prevent back flow. **C,** Incompetent valves unable to fully close, causing blood to flow backward and producing venous insufficiency.

TABLE 12-1	CEAP Classification for Lower Extremity Venous Disease		
Clinical Classification	Etiologic Classification	Anatomical Classification	Pathophysiologic Classification
C_0: No visible or palpable indicators of venous disease C_1: Telangiectases C_2: Varicosities C_3: Edema C_4: Venous skin changes (hemosiderosis, dermatitis, lipodermatosclerosis) C_5: Venous skin changes *plus* healed ulceration C_6: Venous skin changes *plus* active ulceration	E_c: Congenital E_p: Primary E_s: Secondary (post-thrombosis) E_n: No venous cause identified	A_s: Superficial veins A_d: Deep system A_p: Perforator system A_n: No venous identified	P_r: Reflux P_o: Obstruction P_{ro}: Combination of reflux and obstruction
	S: Symptomatic (aches, pain tightness, skin irritation) A: Asymptomatic		

An example of using CEAP classification is C_{6s}; E_p; A_{pd}; P_r.

TABLE 12-2	Key Elements of History for Patients with Venous Ulcers
Element	Description
Risk factors for valvular dysfunction	Obesity, pregnancy, thrombophlebitis, leg trauma (e.g., fracture), thrombophilic conditions
Risk factors for muscle dysfunction	Sedentary lifestyle, prolonged standing, advanced age, altered or "shuffling" gait, musculoskeletal conditions and surgeries that compromise calf muscle function (e.g., paralysis, arthritis)
Factors that impede healing	Diabetes, tobacco, malnutrition, unplanned weight loss, medications
Factors that impede treatment	Limited activity and mobility, cardiac disease, heart failure (clinically significant heart failure is contraindication to compression)
Ulcer history	Previous ulcers, onset, duration, precipitating event (duration >6 months is negative predictor for wound healing)
History of prior treatment	Surgical, pharmacologic, compression (venous ulcers that consistently fail to respond to treatment should be evaluated for misdiagnosis, malignant or mixed disease)
Patient concerns and anticipated barriers	Pain, itching, anxiety, anticipated barriers, transportation, ability to apply compression, job/financial limitations, impact on activities of daily living, treatment goals and priorities

Valvular Dysfunction. Numerous risk factors for valvular dysfunction have been identified and include the following (Burrows et al, 2007; WOCN Society, 2005):

- Obesity, which creates resistance to venous return due to pressure on pelvic veins
- Pregnancy, especially multiple pregnancies or pregnancies that are close together, because of increased pressure against pelvic veins and compromised venous return
- Thrombophlebitis (e.g., deep vein thrombosis, pulmonary embolism), which triggers an inflammatory response that can cause direct damage to the valve leaflets, or chronic partial deep vein obstruction due to incomplete recanalization of the vein, which in turn causes venous distention and valvular compromise
- Leg trauma (e.g., fracture), which suggests undiagnosed damage to the vessel walls and valves
- Thrombophilic conditions (e.g., protein S deficiency, protein C deficiency, factor V [Leiden mutation]), which increase the coagulability of venous blood, thus increasing the risk of deep vein thrombosis and microvascular thrombosis; thrombophilic conditions have been identified in as many as 50% of patients with venous ulcers

Calf Muscle Dysfunction. The dynamics of the calf muscle pump can be adversely affected by changes that accompany major injuries, neurologic disease, and bone or joint pain. The calf muscle becomes weak with disuse; gait changes can exacerbate venous hypertension and calf muscle atrophy (Burrows et al, 2007). Risk factors for compromised calf muscle function include the following:

- Sedentary lifestyle
- Occupations that require prolonged standing
- Musculoskeletal conditions that compromise calf muscle function (e.g., paralysis, arthritis)
- Advanced age, which is associated with decreased elasticity of the calf muscle tendon
- Reduced mobility
- Altered or "shuffling" gait that fails to induce calf muscle contraction; reduced mobility and gait do not relate to calf muscle dysfunction
- Arthroscopic surgery, which could cause fixation of the hip, knee, or ankle, leading to loss of calf muscle pump
- Injection drug use due to progressive deterioration of the venous function of the legs (Pieper et al, 2008)

Pathology of Venous Ulceration

Whereas CVI is clearly precipitated by ambulatory venous hypertension, the reason for venous ulceration as a consequence of venous hypertension is not well understood. This mystery is compounded by the fact that only a minority of patients with chronic venous disease actually progress to ulceration.

Fibrin Cuff Theory. Browse and Burnand (1982) initially postulated that capillary bed distention permitted leakage of large molecules such as fibrinogen into the dermal tissue, and that the fibrinogen then polymerized to form a thick perivascular cuff composed of fibrin, fibronectin, laminin, tenascin, and collagen. These cuffs do not pose any barrier to the diffusion of oxygen and nutrients into the tissues; therefore skin hypoxia cannot be the ultimate factor in the pathogenesis of venous ulcerations (Meissner, 2009).

White Blood Cell Activation and Trapping Theory. The trap hypothesis suggests that venous hypertension reduces the velocity of blood flow in the postcapillary bed. When blood flow becomes sluggish, leukocytes begin to adhere to each other (leukocyte aggregation) and/or to the capillary walls (leukocyte margination). This triggers the release of toxic oxygen metabolites, proteolytic enzymes, and cytokines causing tissue inflammation and dermal fibrosis (Meissner, 2009). Dermal capillary loops also become plugged with leukocytes so that fibrin and other macromolecules leak out of the permeable capillary beds into the dermis, further aggravating inflammatory and fibrotic changes in the subcutaneous tissues and rendering them very susceptible to ulceration, which can occur spontaneously or as a result of minor trauma. Leukocyte migration and activation and the interaction of leukocytes with the endothelium in the presence of venous hypertension play considerable roles in the pathophysiology of venous ulcerations (Agren and Gottrup, 2007; Kalra and Gloviczki, 2003; WOCN Society, 2005).

ASSESSMENT

Key assessment parameters for patients with a leg ulcer include medical history, ulcer history, previous treatments, clinical examination, inspection of the ulcer, and Doppler assessment of pulses (Nelzen, 2007). Assessment of Doppler pulses are discussed in Chapters 10 and 11 and illustrated in Figure 11-1.

Patient History

Risk factors for CVI are identified through the patient history. Of particular importance are risk factors that differentiate venous insufficiency from arterial disease and other pathologies that may cause ulceration in the lower extremity (see Table 12-2). Because of the contraindications to sustained compression, pretreatment

evaluation must include a cardiac history and any indicators of uncompensated heart failure.

Lower Extremity Assessment

Both legs need to be examined by the clinician to ascertain if the manifestations are bilateral or more severe on one extremity. Findings unique to LEVD include edema, hemosiderosis, dermatitis, lipodermatosclerosis, atrophie blanche, varicose veins, ankle flaring, and scarring from previous ulcers (WOCN Society, 2005). Checklist 12-1 gives a list of assessment findings unique to the leg of a patient with CVI.

Arterial Perfusion. Concomitant arterial disease occurs in as many as 25% of patients with venous ulcers (de Araujo et al, 2003; Ryan et al, 2003). Therefore an ankle-brachial index (ABI) should be obtained to determine if some degree of arterial insufficiency is present. An ABI of 1.0 indicates a "pure" venous ulcer (no coexisting arterial insufficiency). An ABI of 0.9 or less indicates arterial insufficiency is present; these ulcers are referred to as *mixed arterial/venous ulcers*. This is an important initial assessment because compression (critical for treatment of venous ulcers) must be modified or, in some cases, omitted. Wounds that begin specifically as a venous ulcer can develop an arterial component, so monitoring for signs of arterial disease at regular intervals is necessary (WOCN Society, 2008).

Edema. Edema is a classic indicator of venous insufficiency because of the combination of capillary bed distention and elevated intracapillary pressures. As described in Chapter 10, the severity of edema varies among patients and from time to time throughout the day. The classic pattern is pitting edema (see Figure 10-1) that worsens with dependency and improves with elevation. Box 10-1 describes the assessment of pitting edema. With prolonged disease and gradual fibrosis of the soft tissues, edema may become "brawny," that is, nonpitting. Thus

---

CHECKLIST 12-1

Lower Extremity Assessment for Chronic Venous Insufficiency

✓ General Appearance
- Trophic changes: lipodermatosclerosis
- Edema: present from ankle to knee, often pitting
- Color: hemosiderin staining, atrophie blanche
- Dermatitis or varicosities may be present

✓ Pain
- Dull aching (see Table 10-2)
- Exacerbates with dependency, improves with compression

✓ Wound Characteristics
- Gaiter area (see Table 10-3)
- Exudative and shallow

✓ Perfusion
- Diminished only with coexisting arterial disease
- Diagnostic evaluation: duplex ultrasound

the characteristics of the edema are a clue to the duration of the underlying disease process.

The distribution of edema is also indicative of the underlying process. Venous edema primarily involves the lower leg between the ankle and the knee. In contrast, lymphedema and lipedema involve the entire extremity. Table 10-1 gives a comparison of the edema associated with these three conditions. Measuring the circumference of the calf and gaiter area is another method for assessing edema, especially if it is unilateral. Thus changes in these circumferential measurements provide an indication of the effectiveness of compression therapy (Nelzen, 2007). Circumferential measurements usually are taken weekly when the compression bandage is changed.

Hemosiderin Staining (Hemosiderosis). Another "classic" indicator of venous insufficiency is hemosiderosis, the discoloration of the soft tissue located in the gaiter area that results when extravasated red blood cells break down and release the pigment hemosiderin. The result is a gray-brown pigmentation of the skin known also as *hyperpigmentation* or *tissue staining* (de Araujo, et al, 2003) (see Plate 34). Hemosiderin plays a role in the evolution of skin changes toward lipodermatosclerosis and ulceration (Caggiati et al, 2008).

Lipodermatosclerosis. Lipodermatosclerosis (see Plate 38), a term used to denote fibrosis, or "hardening," of the soft tissue in the lower leg, is indicative of long-standing venous insufficiency. The fibrotic changes typically are confined to the gaiter, or "sock," area of the leg, which results in an inverted "champagne bottle" or "apple core" appearance of the affected lower leg. The fibrosis causes abnormal narrowing of the affected area, which contrasts sharply with the normal tissue in the proximal limb, and a "woody," hard texture when the area is palpated. These fibrotic changes are thought to result from a combination of fibrin deposits, compromised fibrinolysis, and deposition of collagen in response to growth factors produced by activated white blood cells (de Araujo et al, 2003). A body mass index greater than 34 has been found to predispose to lipodermatosclerosis (Bruce et al, 2002).

Varicosities. Varicose veins are swollen and twisted veins that appear blue, are close to the skin's surface, may bulge or throb, cause the legs to swell, and precipitate a feeling of heaviness. They are most often seen in the back of the calf or the medial aspect of the leg. Varicosities precede valvular incompetence and appear to develop as a consequence of intrinsic structural and biochemical abnormalities of the vein wall (Meissner, 2009). Patients with varicosities should manage their weight and exercise and avoid crossing their legs and wearing constrictive garments (WOCN Society, 2005).

Skin Changes Near the Ankle. *Ankle blowout* has been described as uncommon painful clusters of tiny venous ulcers located near the medial malleolus originating from dilated ruptured vessels (Kunimoto, 2001), but no further discussion related to ankle blowout has been noted in recent literature or evidence-based guidelines. *Malleolar flare* has been described in recent guidelines as visible capillaries from distention of small veins around the medial malleolus (WOCN Society, 2005).

Atrophie Blanche Lesions. Atrophie blanche lesions (see Plate 35) can be found in as many as one third of patients with LEVD. These lesions are smooth white plaques of thin, "speckled" atrophic tissue with tortuous vessels on the ankle or foot with hemosiderin-pigmented borders. Sometimes mistaken for scars of healed ulcers, this clinical finding actually represents spontaneously developing lesions. Prompt recognition is important so that a plan can be established to protect these high-risk areas from ulceration due to the thin, atrophic epidermis (de Araujo et al, 2003; Ryan et al, 2003; WOCN Society, 2005). Ulcers occurring in this area usually are small, very painful, and hard to heal. Topical steroids should be avoided because they can cause further damage to the very fragile skin.

Venous Dermatitis. Venous dermatitis is a common but distressing inflammation of the epidermis and dermis on the lower extremity of the patient with LEVD (see Plate 38). Often the earliest cutaneous sequelae of venous insufficiency, they most commonly affect middle-aged to elderly patients (Flugman and Clark, 2009). Venous dermatitis is characterized by scaling, crusting, weeping, erythema, erosions, and intense itching; symptoms may be acute or chronic. The cutaneous inflammation of venous dermatitis is often confused with cellulitis. Factors that distinguish between dermatitis and cellulitis are listed in Table 12-3 (WOCN Society, 2005).

Venous dermatitis results from the release of inflammatory mediators from activated leukocytes that are trapped within the fibrin cuffs and surrounding perivascular space (Flugman and Clark, 2009). Dermal fibrosis, a hallmark of venous dermatitis, develops as a result of fibrin cuff formation, decreased fibrinolysis, and release of transforming growth factor-β_1 (a mediator of dermal fibrosis) by the leukocytes. Potent chemoattractants (intercellular adhesion molecule-1 and vascular cell adhesion molecule-1) keep leukocytes active in the perivascular environment and perpetuate cutaneous inflammation with fibrosis. Why venous dermatitis is common among some patients but is rare among others is unclear (Ryan et al, 2003; WOCN Society, 2005).

Venous dermatitis increases the risk of developing contact sensitivity due to the presence of chronic inflammation of the skin (Flugman and Clark, 2009). Exposure to usually benign topical substances (e.g., wound exudate, skin sealants, adhesives, silver sulfadiazine) easily exacerbates venous dermatitis. Frequent contact allergens include lanolin, balsam of Peru, and fragrances (Romanelli and Romanelli, 2007). Patients also can become sensitized to rubber products contained in some compression wraps and stockings. More than 30% of patients with contact dermatitis developed sensitivity to the topical antibiotics

TABLE 12-3	Distinguishing Between Dermatitis and Cellulitis	
	Dermatitis	**Cellulitis**
Symptoms	Afebrile Itching Varicose veins/deep vein thrombosis	May have fever Painful No relevant history
Signs	Normal temperature Erythema, inflammation May be tender Vesicles and crusting Lesions on other parts of the body (e.g., other leg, arms) May be unilateral or bilateral	Elevated temperature Erythema, inflammation Tenderness One or a few bullae No crusting No lesions elsewhere Unilateral
Portals of entry	N/A	Usually unknown; breaks in skin, ulcers, trauma, tinea pedis, intertrigo implicated
Laboratory	Normal white blood cell count Negative blood cultures Skin swabs (*Staphylococcus aureus* common)	Leukocytosis Blood cultures usually negative Skin swabs usually negative except for necrotic tissue

DVT, Deep vein thrombosis; *WBC*, white blood cell.
From Wound, Ostomy and Continence Nurses Society (WOCN Society): *Guideline for management of patients with lower extremity venous disease*, WOCN clinical practice guideline series #1, Glenview Ill, 2005. Data from Quartey-Papafio CM: Lesson of the week: importance of distinguishing between cellulitis and varicose eczema of the leg, *BMJ* 318(7199):1672-1673, 1999.

neomycin and bacitracin (Alguire and Mathes, 2007). Although less common, sensitization of the skin to topical corticosteroids can develop, triggering an allergic contact dermatitis. When the clinical manifestations of the limb affected with venous dermatitis worsen despite appropriate topical therapy, contact dermatitis should be considered.

To prevent venous dermatitis, product ingredients should be carefully scrutinized before topical therapy is selected, and products containing sensitizers should be avoided (de Araujo et al, 2003). Skin moisturizers such as bland, perfume-free topical emollients and white petrolatum, can be used to maximize epidermal integrity. An essential component of prevention and treatment of venous dermatitis is graduated compression (discussed later in this chapter), which may require considerable patient education and encouragement due to the discomfort associated with an inflamed, edematous limb. Patients need reassurance that the discomfort should decrease as the edema resolves. Exudate absorbers such as alginates and hydrofibers are commonly indicated, often in combination with a secondary foam dressing to adequately absorb and contain exudate.

To reduce inflammation and itching, mild-potency topical corticosteroids (e.g., triamcinolone 0.1% ointment) can be used short term (i.e., 2 weeks) but sparingly because of the risk for skin atrophy. High-potency topical corticosteroids are rarely used because of the risk for skin atrophy as well as systemic absorption through open denuded skin. Systemic corticosteroids are seldom warranted for treatment of venous dermatitis (Flugman and Clark, 2009). Cool compresses with Burow's solution (aluminum acetate) followed by an application of plain petrolatum also can be used to relieve itching. Additional remedies for venous dermatitis include Condy

solution (potassium permanganate), dilute vinegar compresses, and cool tar ointment. Patients with severe or nonresponsive dermatitis should be referred to dermatology for management (Bonham, 2003; Ryan et al, 2003).

Ulcer Characteristics. The classic venous ulcer is located in the gaiter area and around the medial malleolus, due to the greatest hydrostatic pressure at these sites. Typically, the ulcers are shallow, with moderate to high exudate and a dark red "ruddy" wound base or a thin layer of yellow slough. Islands of eschar may be present. Ulcers that are deep and may have exposed tendon are likely not to be of pure venous origin (Nelzen, 2007). Venous ulcers usually have irregular edges and periwound maceration, crusting, scaling, and/or hemosiderin staining (Wipke-Tevis and Sae-Sia, 2004) (see Plates 34 and 38). See Table 10-3 for a comparison of features that distinguish venous, arterial, and neuropathic ulcers.

Diagnostic Evaluation

In order to effectively diagnose and safely manage the patient with a CVI wound, the patient must first be evaluated for the presence of arterial insufficiency because standard therapy for venous ulcers (compression) may be contraindicated or may require modification of therapy in the presence of arterial disease (Robson et al, 2006). Arterial insufficiency is diagnosed with an ABI of 0.9 or less or a toe-brachial index of 0.6 or less (see Table 11-3). Chapter 11 describes diagnostic tests for arterial disease.

CVI is the result of either venous reflux or venous obstruction. Noninvasive vascular tests are used to distinguish between these two conditions. Traditionally, tourniquet test, photoplethysmography, and venography were used. However, poor reliability and inability to provide visualization of the venous system compromised the utility of the tests. Therefore these tests have been largely replaced by duplex ultrasound imaging (Meissner, 2009; Min et al, 2003). However, Kelechi and Bonham (2008) propose further clinical studies to examine the utility of a hand-held noninvasive photoplethysmography instrument that measures venous filling time to facilitate early diagnosis of chronic venous insufficiency that might otherwise go unrecognized.

Duplex Ultrasound. Duplex ultrasound scanning is now recognized as the gold standard for accurate evaluation of the highest point of valve failure and the extent of reflux (Whiddon, 2007).

Duplex ultrasound imaging is noninvasive and has a high degree of sensitivity. Duplex imaging technology uses two-dimensional ultrasound and Doppler shift to produce images of blood flow through the superficial, deep, and perforating veins, pinpointing the anatomic site of reflux, obstruction such as deep vein thrombus, and abnormal vein walls as well as reflux through delicate venous valves (Kelechi and Bonham, 2008; WOCN Society, 2005). Color duplex ultrasound scanning performed with proximal compression or a Valsalva maneuver helps to confirm a venous etiology and assists the clinician to determine if radiologic (laser ablation) or surgical intervention is warranted, especially in patients with nonhealing or recurrent venous ulceration (Robson et al, 2006).

MANAGEMENT

As outlined in the LEVD guideline (WOCN Society, 2005) and the Wound Healing Society's guidelines for the treatment of venous ulcers (Robson et al, 2006), primary interventions for correcting the underlying cause of venous insufficiency and venous hypertension include lifestyle adaptations and compression therapy; pharmacologic agents and surgical procedures do not play a large role in the management of LEVD.

Limb Elevation

Limb elevation is a simple but effective strategy for improving venous return by making use of gravitational forces. This is an important component of management for any patient with venous insufficiency, but it is an essential element of therapy for patients who are unable to adhere to a compression therapy regimen. Patients should be taught to lie down and elevate the affected leg above the level of the heart for at least 1 to 2 hours twice daily as well as during sleep. This position may be difficult for the obese person to manage comfortably. In addition, patients should be taught to strictly avoid prolonged standing or prolonged sitting with the legs dependent. Periods of standing or sitting must be interspersed with

walking. Having the patient keep a "legs-up" chart can reinforce the importance of leg elevation. This chart should be reviewed with the patient at each visit (Wipke-Tevis and Sae-Sia, 2004).

Exercise

Normal function of the calf muscle pump is essential to venous return, and effective contraction of the calf muscle requires a mobile ankle and routine dorsiflexion beyond 90 degrees. The patient with limited mobility is a challenge for clinicians. A patient with reduced ankle mobility or a "shuffling" gait should undergo a physical therapy evaluation to determine if he or she can benefit from gait retraining and routine exercises to increase ankle strength and range of motion (Burrows et al, 2007). A home-based exercise program that includes isotonic exercise can improve poor calf muscle and calf muscle pump function (WOCN Society, 2005). The Wound Healing Society's Prevention of Venous Ulcers Guidelines recommends calf muscle pump exercises as helpful in long-term maintenance and venous ulcer prevention (Robson, et al, 2006). All patients with venous insufficiency should be encouraged to perform ankle pumps routinely while standing or sitting and to intersperse standing and sitting with walking (Wipke-Tevis and Sae-Sia, 2004). Primarily used to assess the elderly for fall risk, the Tinetti Balance and Gait Scale was found to be reliable and valid in evaluating the walking mobility of patients with venous ulcers using injectable drugs. The wound specialist may find it beneficial to incorporate this scale (available in Appendix B) into the workup of the patient with venous ulcers.

Weight Control

Obesity interferes with venous return, thus increasing the risk for LEVD. Morbid obesity can cause insufficiency in the deep venous system. In addition, significant obesity makes it very difficult for the patient to adhere to compression therapy and to avoid prolonged sitting. With the increase in obesity in younger people, the incidence of venous insufficiency and ulcers will continue to rise. Therefore it is important to educate patients regarding the relationship between weight and venous disease and to strongly encourage patients to reduce their weight to a healthy level. Patients who are morbidly obese should be referred to a bariatric treatment center for evaluation and management (Wipke-Tevis and Sae-Sia, 2004).

Pharmacologic Therapy

Treating venous ulcers with pharmacologic means is based on the hypothesis of venous insufficiency pathogenesis. Inappropriate leukocyte activation, which has been shown to be present in chronic venous disease, can lead to the development of a venous ulcer (Coleridge-Smith et al, 2005). Diuretics and topical corticosteroids reduce edema and pain in the short term but offer no long-term treatment. Herbal supplements decrease the inflammatory response to venous hypertension but are not licensed by the U.S. Food and Drug Administration (FDA) and can vary in efficacy and safety.

Several pharmacologic agents have demonstrated benefit in the management of venous disease. The three agents with documented efficacy in the management of venous disease are pentoxifylline (Trental), micronized purified flavonoid fraction (Daflon), and horse chestnut seed extract (HCSE).

Pentoxifylline (Trental). In the United States, pentoxifylline (Trental) is the drug most commonly prescribed for venous disease and appears to be an effective adjunct to compression therapy. Its mechanism of action appears to be reduced aggregation of platelets and white blood cells, which reduces capillary plugging, and enhanced blood flow in the microcirculation, which reduces tissue ischemia (Jull et al, 2004, 2007). Dosages of 400 mg orally three times daily can accelerate healing of venous ulcers and should be considered for slow-healing venous ulcers (Jull, 2007; WOCN Society, 2005).

Pentoxifylline may also promote healing even in the absence of compression. However, the beneficial effects of pentoxifylline must be balanced against its potential adverse effects (e.g., diarrhea, nausea) and its cost. Therefore pentoxifylline is generally reserved for patients who do not respond to standard therapy and is not used for routine care (Jull, 2007).

Micronized Purified Flavonoid Fraction (MPFF). Although not available in the United States, the phlebotropic drug known as micronized purified flavonoid fraction (MPFF; Daflon) has been approved by Europe and other countries to improve outcomes for patients with LEVD. The specific mechanisms of its action include the following: (1) enhances venous tone, which promotes venous return; (2) reduces capillary permeability, which reduces edema formation; and (3) reduces expression of endothelial adhesion molecules, which reduces margination, activation, and migration of leukocytes (Robson et al, 2006). These mechanisms reduce the release of inflammatory mediators, which is thought to be the primary pathologic event resulting in dermatitis, lipodermatosclerosis, and ulceration (Coleridge-Smith et al, 2005; Lyseng-Williamson and Perry, 2003; Simka and Majewski, 2003).

The combination of MPFF with standard therapy (compression plus topical therapy) resulted in a statistically significant improvement in healing rates compared to standard therapy alone or to placebo in a double-blind trial, with a side effect profile comparable to that of placebo (Coleridge-Smith et al, 2005). A meta-analysis of MPFF as adjunct therapy for venous ulcers concluded that venous ulcer healing was accelerated and recommended MPFF use for large and long-standing ulcers (Coleridge-Smith et al, 2005). In addition, cost analysis studies have demonstrated a significant reduction in cost of healing compared to conventional therapy. Finally, studies indicate significant improvement in quality-of-life scores for patients with LEVD treated with MMPF (Coleridge-Smith, 2003; Simka and Majewski, 2003).

Horse Chestnut Seed Extract. The herbal agent HCSE containing aescin is commonly used in Europe as a method for managing CVI (Jull, 2007; Leach et al, 2006). The mechanism of action appears to be an inhibitory effect on the catalytic breakdown of capillary wall proteoglycans (Suter et al, 2006). Several placebo-controlled trials have demonstrated decrease in leg size, pain, pruritus, and tenseness. Preliminary evidence suggests comparable outcomes between HCSE and compression therapy. Available as an oral tincture, topical gel, and tablets (20 mg, 50 mg), the recommended oral dosage is 300 mg every 12 hours for 12 weeks (Pittler, 2006). Severe allergic reactions have been reported when HCSE was given intravenously, and hepatitis has been associated with intramuscular injections. More studies are needed to clearly verify the efficacy of HCSE in treatment, especially in long-term use and as an adjunct to compression therapy.

COMPRESSION THERAPY

Venous insufficiency is associated with increased hydrostatic pressure in veins in the legs. Compression therapy is used to reduce hydrostatic pressure and aid venous return (Vowden & Vowden, 2006). Compression is provided by wraps, bandages, garments or devices. Compression wraps are products that specifically wrap around the extremity. Bandage is the more common term used in European literature in place of wrap or compression dressing, however. Garment refers to compression products that are a clothing item such as compression stockings. The intermittent pneumatic compression device is the only product that is powered. Compression products apply pressure externally from the base of the toes to the knee to support the calf muscle pump during ambulation and dorsiflexion. The increased interstitial tissue pressure serves to oppose leakage of fluid into the tissues and to return interstitial fluid to the blood and lymph vessels, thus eliminating edema. Compression of the superficial veins promotes coaptation and normal function of the valves; it also increases the velocity of blood flow, which reduces the aggregation and extravasation of white blood cells (Weingarten, 2001).

Features

Compression products share many different features and these features guide the selection of the most appropriate compression option for each individual. Compression therapy can be either sustained (i.e., continuous) pressure or intermittent pressure. Products that remain in place and are removed after several days or only at night provide continuous pressure; the majority of products on the market provide continuous compression (Table 12-4). Products that provide intermittent compression are applied 2-3 times per day for 1- to 2-hour intervals; intermittent compression is particularly beneficial to the patient who cannot tolerate continuous compression or is unable to apply the continuous compression wraps or stockings.

Another feature of compression products is based on the type of material used to deliver the pressure: elastic or inelastic. *Elastic compression* adapts to changes in limb volume. The product exerts external pressure while the leg is at rest as well as when the calf muscle expands during ambulation, thus continuing to provide external pressure. Elastic compression products are appropriate choices for patients who are relatively sedentary or who have a "shuffling" gait that fails to engage the calf muscle (de Araujo et al, 2003). *Inelastic (or nonelastic) compression* will not expand during ambulation. As the calf muscle expands while walking, pressure is created by the muscle pressing against the "semi-rigid" bandage/dressing. At rest, when there is no calf pump muscle activity, only limited compression occurs. Therefore inelastic compression products are most appropriate for patients who are actively ambulating.

Compression products can be disposable or reusable. Many compression products are disposable and are used early in treatment when significant edema or an ulcer is present. Reusable compression products can be removed,

TABLE 12-4	Formulary of Compression Therapy Products							
			Features					
Category	**Type**	**Examples***	**Elastic**	**In-elastic**	**Disposable**	**Reusable**	**Therapeutic pressure**	**Modified pressure**
Wraps	Multilayer	Profore/ProGuide (Smith & Nephew) Dyna-Flex (Systagenix Wound Management) Coban™ 2 Layer (3M™) ThreePress (Hartmann-USA Inc.)	X		X		X	X
	Long stretch	SurePress (ConVaTec) Setopress (Mölnlycke Health Care)	X			X	X	X
	Short stretch	Comprilan (BSN Medical) Farrow wrap (Farrow Medical Innovation)		X		X		X
	Paste	Viscopaste (Smith & Nephew) Unna-Flex (ConvaTec) Gelocast (BSN Medical) Unna Press (Derma Sciences)		X	X			X
Garments	Reusable inelastic device	CircAid (CircAid Medical Products)		X	X	X		X
	Tubular sleeve	Tubigrip (Mölnlycke Health Care) Medigrip (Medline)	X			X		X
	Stockings	Jobst Juzo Sigvaris Medi-Strumpf TheraPress DUO	X			X	X	X
Intermittent pneumatic Pumps		Mobility (Derma Science Inc.)		X		X	X	X

*=Not inclusive.

cleaned, and then reused. The reusable products are non-adhesive wraps or garments. The nonadhesive reusable wraps can be used while edema and/or ulcer are present. The reusable garments are primarily used for "maintenance compression" once the edema has resolved and the ulcer is significantly healed or at least no longer exudative.

A key feature of compression wraps/garments is that they can provide a range of pressures. The amount of compression considered "therapeutic" for venous insufficiency (effective in controlling venous hypertension and preventing edema formation) is 30 to 40 mm Hg at the ankle (de Araujo et al, 2003; O'Meara et al, 2009; Paquette and Falanga, 2002; Vowden & Vowden, 2006). Some clinicians recommend even higher levels of compression (40 to 50 mm Hg) for patients with severe venous insufficiency (Robson et al, 2006). While the evidence is clear that 30 mm Hg or more is considered high compression and is the preferred level of pressure, many patients experience discomfort with high levels of pressure or are unable to physically apply the garment. In these situations, lower levels of pressure are more appropriate (Table 12-4). A general guide to categories of pressure is as follows: high pressure (30-40 mm Hg), medium pressure (20-30 mm Hg), and low pressure (15 mm Hg) (Nelson et al, 2000). Many compression wraps have "indicators" to guide the amount of tension or stretch to use when applying the wraps so that the desired amount of pressure can be attained. Similarly, compression stockings are manufactured to provide a specific range of pressure.

Clues for Compressing Correctly

1. Follow manufacturer's instructions for application technique to assure attaining the appropriate level of compression.
2. Measure the extremity accurately when using compression garments.
3. Assess patient mobility and activity carefully when selecting elastic versus inelastic compression products. Inelastic compression products will not be effective if the patient is unable to perform very frequent calf muscle pumps, such as with ambulation.
4. Compression should be used with caution if the patient has decreased leg sensation, infection in the leg, or allergies to ingredients in the compression materials.
5. All patients with a leg ulcer should be screened for arterial disease using a Doppler measurement of the ABI. Use modified or lower levels of compression (23-30 mm Hg at the ankle) when coexisting arterial disease is present. An ABI greater than 0.5 and less than 0.8 precludes high levels of sustained compression (Kelechi and Bonham, 2008; Cullum et al, 2003; Robson et al, 2006). Patients with venous insufficiency and ABI ≤0.5 who require compression

should be managed with IPC (Kelechi and Bonham, 2008).

6. Monitor the skin around and under the compression wrap or device closely and particularly during dressing changes to prevent pressure ulcers. External compression at high pressures will reduce blood supply to the skin and may lead to pressure damage. Similarly, impaired arterial blood supply to the legs may also result in pressure damage. If the patient expresses complaints about the extremity that is suggestive of device-related pressure damage, the compression may need to be removed so that the extremity can be assessed.
7. Patients with venous hypertension need to understand that "compression is for life!" It is not a treatment that can be discontinued once the ulcer heals or the edema resolves. This ongoing compression is often referred to as "maintenance" compression. When the patient fails to adhere to maintenance compression, a 70% recurrence rate of venous ulcers has been reported (Nelson et al, 2000). Furthermore, a normal ABI can potentially deteriorate over time, thus requiring a modification in the recommended level of compression. Diligent monitoring by the wound specialist is essential for continued follow-through with the plan of care (Robson et al, 2006; Wipke-Tevis and Sae-Sia, 2004; WOCN Society, 2005). The wound specialist is challenged to recommend the most clinically effective and "patient-friendly" system for each patient based on individual assessment, indications, contraindications, advantages and disadvantages, and special considerations of the many available compression products.

Contraindications

All compression is contraindicated in the patient with a coexisting venous thrombosis in the extremity with the ulcer and uncompensated heart failure. When compression of any kind is used with uncompensated (unstable) heart failure, edema fluid can mobilize into the circulatory system, potentially increasing preload volume and precipitating pulmonary edema (de Araujo et al, 2003; Weingarten, 2001). In most cases, sustained compression is contraindicated in the presence of severe peripheral vascular disease (i.e., ABI ≤ 0.6) because sustained tissue pressure could further compromise tissue perfusion and potentially cause ischemic tissue death (Hopf et al, 2006). In these situations, *intermittent* pneumatic compression is a safe and viable option.

COMPRESSION WRAPS

Wraps are one of the most commonly used compression products, especially during the initial phase of treatment when limb volumes are changing rapidly as a result of edema reduction. Compression wraps are identified by the number of components in the wrap. Single-layer wraps contain a single component while a multi-layer wrap may have 2, 3, or 4 components that are applied to the extremity. All wraps have a bandage layer; this bandage determines whether the wrap is elastic or inelastic. In addition to the bandage layer, the two-layer wrap also has either an orthopedic wool layer placed against the skin under the bandage wrap or a tubular sleeve over the bandage wrap. The components of a three-layer wrap include the orthopedic wool, a bandage wrap, and a tubular sleeve. The four-layer wrap contains the orthopedic wool, a crepe support bandage, a bandage wrap, and a self-adherent bandage (O'Meara et al, 2010).

Generally, compression wraps are applied by professionals and left in place for 3 to 7 days. Most wraps are capable of providing modified compression. The most commonly used wraps are inelastic paste wraps, multilayer elastic wraps, and single-layer inelastic (short-stretch) bandages (see Table 12-4). Although individual clinical trials have reported multilayer and single-layer compression systems to be equally effective (Burrows et al, 2007; Castonguay, 2008), a recent systematic review of literature conducted by the Cochran Collaboration reported that multi-component systems achieve better healing outcomes than single-component compression (O'Meara et al, 2009).

Application Technique

All compression wraps are designed based on *Laplace's law of physics,* which states that sub-bandage pressure is directly proportional to the tension and number of bandage layers and inversely proportional to leg circumference and bandage width (Figure 12-4). Laplace's law explains why application of a wrap with constant tension will create graduated pressure. Bandage tension is held constant while the circumference of the leg increases steadily from ankle to knee, and sub-bandage pressure will be highest at the ankle and lowest at the knee (Burrows et al, 2007; Ghosh et al, 2008; Moffat et al, 2007).

Some wraps are designed to be applied with a spiral technique, whereas others require a figure-of-eight

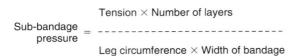

$$\text{Sub-bandage pressure} = \frac{\text{Tension} \times \text{Number of layers}}{\text{Leg circumference} \times \text{Width of bandage}}$$

FIGURE 12-4 Laplace's law of physics as it applies to compression bandaging. Laplace's law demonstrates how compression therapy is a function of tension, number of layers, leg circumference, and bandage width. Increases in tension and/or layering increase sub-bandage pressure, whereas increases in leg circumference and/or bandage width decrease sub-bandage pressure.

application to achieve optimal results. Application techniques must follow the manufacturer's instructions. Some layers require 100% stretch and others 50% stretch; some may incorporate a visual indicator to achieve the correct level of pressure (Wipke-Tevis and Sae-Sia, 2004).

The skill of the clinician applying the wrap will impact tension (Moore, 2002; O'Meara et al, 2009). Studies indicate that even when nurses are experienced with application, they frequently wrap with insufficient tension to produce therapeutic pressure levels. Training has been shown to significantly improve accuracy, but further studies are needed to quantify the interval at which this training should be repeated (Feben, 2003). An accurate and precise sub-bandage pressure monitor may be an option for assessing the clinician's ability to apply safe, graduated pressure.

The patient with a large calf or uneven contours can experience difficulty in keeping the bandage in place. Slippage of the bandage can lead to a tourniquet effect, which can cause edema above the wrap and injury to the skin. Compression wraps must be replaced when slippage occurs. One technique for preventing slippage is the use of extra padding to recontour the leg to a normal shape (Moffat et al, 2007). It has been found that bandages applied in a figure-of-eight configuration tend to stay in place better, especially for the person with a large leg. However, the manufacturer's instructions for wrapping must be followed to accommodate differences in product materials and layers, all of which impact the level of compression achieved. The best time of day to apply compression is when the least amount of edema is present: first thing in the morning before getting out of bed and before hanging the legs over the side of the bed. Patients who are unable to lift their leg(s) should be wrapped by two clinicians to ensure an even application (Moffatt et al, 2007).

Multi-layer Wraps/Bandages

Multi-layer wraps are disposable, elastic, provide sustained compression, and can be applied to provide either a modified or therapeutic level of pressure. These wraps therefore provide compression when the patient is active as well as when they are at rest (Figure 12-5). Multilayer wraps cannot be reused and should be changed when they begin to loosen, slip, or become saturated (typically in 3–7 days). A key feature of multi-layer wraps is absorption of exudate. In many settings, these devices have become the product of choice for early intervention because of their ability to absorb exudate, adapt to changes in limb size, and provide sustained compression at rest and with activity.

Paste Wraps. Paste wraps are inelastic wraps that cannot be reused and provide sustained compression at a modified level of pressure. Dr. Paul Unna was the first to introduce

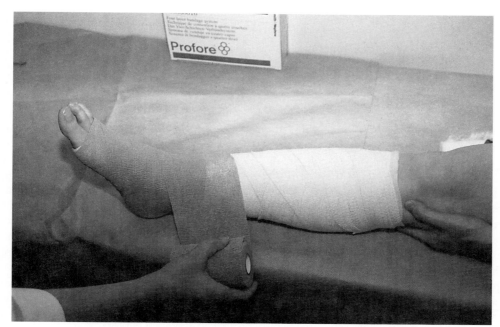

FIGURE 12-5 Compression wraps: layered bandage system.

use of a zinc paste bandage to create a conformable but inelastic "boot" around the leg; thus a paste-type compression wrap is commonly referred to as an Unna's boot (Weingarten, 2001). Today various inelastic paste wraps exist and are impregnated with any of the following products: zinc, glycerin, gelatin, or calamine (Wipke-Tevis and Sae-Sia, 2004). Thus the paste wraps are not identical and an adverse reaction to one does not predict a reaction to another.

Inelastic paste wraps should be applied without tension, beginning at the base of the toes and extending to the tibial tuberosity below the knee. The patient must be reminded to maintain the foot in a dorsiflexed position while the paste wrap is applied (Box 12-1). Common and appropriate techniques used to ensure a smooth conformable fit include open or closed heel, pleating, reverse folding, and cutting and restarting (Davis and Gray, 2005; Wipke-Tevis and Sae-Sia, 2004). If the paste layer is left open to air, it dries to a "semi-cast" consistency. Often the paste layer is covered with a self-adherent wrap to protect clothing from the paste. Paste bandages should be changed when they begin to loosen, slip, or become saturated (typically in 3–7 days). Problems associated with paste bandages include skin reaction to certain paste ingredients (e.g., calamine), maceration due to lack of an absorptive layer, slippage, poor fit, and inability to bathe (Davis and Gray, 2005). As with all inelastic compression devices, paste bandages are most appropriate for actively ambulating patients.

Short-Stretch (Single-Layer) Reusable Wraps. Short-stretch reusable wraps are inelastic, single-layer wraps that provide sustained compression at a modified or

BOX 12-1	Procedure for Paste Bandage Application

1. Apply gloves after assembling supplies and washing hands.
2. Gently wash and dry extremity. Replace gloves.
3. Place patient in supine position with affected leg elevated and not in dependent position.
4. Foot should be dorsiflexed so foot and leg are at 90-degree angle while applying initial bandage layers around the foot and ankle.
5. Open all paste bandage wrappers and cover wrap. Estimate amount of material based on size of leg(s).
6. Hold paste bandage roll in nondominant hand. Begin to apply bandage at base of toes.
7. If an ulcer is present, apply appropriate topical dressing to ulcer and secondary dressing (if indicated) before applying paste bandage.
8. Treat periwound (if indicated) and moisturize rest of leg.
9. Wrap twice around base of toes without using tension.
10. Continue wrapping bandage around foot, ankle, and heel, using a circular technique, with each strip overlapping previous strip by approximately 50% to 80%. Do not apply tension to the wrap.
11. Smooth paste bandage while applying and remove any wrinkles and folds (may pleat, reverse fold, or cut to ensure smooth bandage).
12. Wrap up to knee and finish smoothing.
13. Remove gloves.
14. Apply cover wrap using recommended amount of tension (e.g., 50% stretch) and 50% overlap.
15. Remove twice weekly or weekly as indicated by leakage, slippage, hygiene, wound care, complaint of numbness, or anticipated decrease in edema.

therapeutic level. Because they are inelastic they are most appropriate for the actively ambulating patient. These short-stretch wraps or single-layer wraps must not be confused with *Ace-type bandages,* which provide low levels of compression and are not considered therapeutic for patients with venous hypertension or insufficiency. Ace-type bandages tend to stretch when the calf expands and thus fail to provide calf muscle support during ambulation. In addition, they are very user dependent and are frequently applied incorrectly.

A major advantage of short-stretch reusable wraps is their "wash and reuse" feature. This feature permits more frequent removal of wraps for bathing and dressing changes and contributes to cost-effective care. Many of these wraps incorporate a visual indicator of correct tension, which is advantageous when teaching caregivers how to apply the wrap correctly to achieve the prescribed level of pressure (Wipke-Tevis and Sae-Sia, 2004).

Long-Stretch Reusable Wrap. The long-stretch wrap is also a reusable, single-layer product that provides sustained compression at either a therapeutic or modified level of pressure. However, the distinctive feature of the long-stretch reusable wrap is that it is elastic so it can be used for both the sedentary and the actively ambulating patient. Much like the short-stretch wrap, the long-stretch wrap also can be washed and reused and should not be confused with Ace-type bandages.

COMPRESSION GARMENTS

Compression garments are essentially cloth products that can be reused: reusable inelastic device, tubular sleeve, and compression stockings.

Stockings

Compression stockings are reusable, elastic garments that are most commonly used for patients with stable venous insufficiency to prevent ulceration (either initial or recurrent). These garments are appropriate for sedentary as well as actively ambulating patients. Compression stockings must not be confused with *antiembolism* stockings, which provide 15 to 17 mm Hg of pressure and are therefore not appropriate for therapeutic compression (WOCN Society, 2005).

Stockings are generally not a good choice for compression during the initiation of therapy because of the rapid changes in limb circumference associated with edema reduction. They should be used once the edema has been controlled and limb circumference has stabilized. Another relative contraindication for stocking use is severe lipodermatosclerosis because the "inverted champagne bottle" configuration of the leg typical of this condition makes obtaining a good fit difficult. If necessary, however, customized stockings can be made after a referral to a trained "stocking fitter."

Stockings are available in a variety of colors, styles and sizes. Accurate measurement for safe sizing must be done according to careful review of the manufacturer's instructions. Stockings may be knee high or thigh high; most patients with venous insufficiency are effectively managed with knee-high stockings. Compression stockings are classified according to the pressure produced at the ankle (Kline et al, 2008): class I (light support), class II (medium support), class III (strong support), and class IV (very strong support). The actual amount of pressure (in mm Hg) appointed to each classification varies by country and manufacturer. Compression stockings are produced as either a circular knit or a flat knit garment. The circular knit stocking is a thin, lightweight material without a seam; it is not available in high levels of compression (Moffatt et al, 2007).

Stockings are the "mainstay" of maintenance compression but are effective only if the patient wears them. Therefore it is critical for the wound specialist to educate and ensure that the patient understands the importance of life-long compression and is able to correctly don the stocking (Moffatt et al, 2007). If barriers are identified, resources and devices to assist with application or other options for compression must be explored. Tips for applying compression stockings (including assist devices) and other key points for patient education are outlined in Box 12-2. One example of a device that facilitates stocking application is shown in Figure 12-6.

Tubular Sleeve

The tubular sleeve is reusable, elastic and, when measured and applied correctly as a double layer, provides sustained compression at a modified level of pressure (O'Meara et al, 2009). A tubular sleeve may be selected when the patient cannot tolerate other types of compression. It also may be used as a temporary intervention while a more permanent solution is pending. Application and removal are easy and require minimal, if any, education; therefore the tubular sleeve is an excellent option when simplicity is the top priority.

Reusable Inelastic Device

Many of the compression garments and devices used for managing lymphedema can be used to manage the edema associated with venous hypertension. For example, the CircAid (CircAid Medical Products, San Diego, CA, USA) is an inelastic reusable compression device that is secured with overlapping bands. By securing the bands according to the pressure indicators, the device can provide therapeutic or modified levels of pressure (Figure 12-7). The ability to easily reapply and readjust the straps helps prevent slippage as edema fluctuates and permits frequent bathing and wound care. Ease of

BOX 12-2 | Patient Education: Compression Stockings

Tips for Putting On Stockings

- Don stockings immediately upon awakening, before getting out of bed.
- For easier application of stockings, wear rubber gloves; apply talcum powder (light dusting) first to foot and leg.
- Apply heavy stockings over light silk stocking or silky stocking "liner."
- Use commercial device designed to facilitate stocking application:
  - Stocking butler or donning gloves (Jobst)
  - Easy-slide toe sleeves for open-toe stockings (Jobst, Juzo, Sigvaris)
  - Stocking donner (Beiersdorf-Jobst)
  - Slippie Gator (Juzo)
- Wash new stockings before wearing (follow manufacturer's directions) to reduce stiffness and difficulty in application.
- Use a "layered" approach: either two-piece stockings (TheraPress DUO) or two layers of lower-compression stockings (e.g., two layers of stocking, each of which provides 15 mm Hg compression).
- Turn leg portion of stocking inside-out down to heel. With stocking stretched, slip foot in while pulling stocking by its folded edge over heel. Gently work stocking up leg, gradually turning stocking right-side out.
- Conduct foot exercises with stockings on: move toes in circular motion (make big circles) both clockwise and counterclockwise. Repeat exercise at least 10 times per day.

Care and Management

- Purchase two pairs of stockings to permit laundering.
- Launder with mild detergent and line dry (follow manufacturer's guidelines).
- Replace stockings every 3–4 months to maintain therapeutic efficacy.
- If stockings become too tight or too loose, contact wound care nurse, wound program, or physician for refitting.
- For person having problems with stocking sliding down, use roll-on adhesive applicator (It Stays by Jobst).

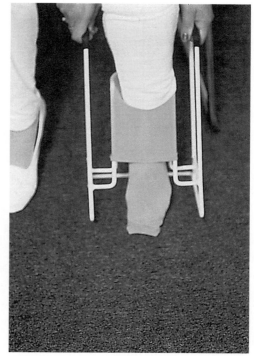

FIGURE 12-6 Application of a therapeutic support stocking with a "stocking donner."

removal and application may improve compliance among individuals who are unable to tolerate other forms of compression therapy. The product is washable and reusable, and it comes with a warranty for 3-6 months.

INTERMITTENT PNEUMATIC COMPRESSION (IPC)

IPC (also known as *dynamic compression therapy*) is a reusable compression device that involves the use of an air pump to intermittently inflate a sleeve applied to the lower extremity (Figure 12-8). IPC may be used for patients with LEVD who are mobile or for those who are immobile and need higher levels of compression than can be provided with stockings or wraps. IPC may be used as adjunct therapy to sustained compression, or an alternative for patients unable to tolerate sustained compression or who are too compromised for sustained

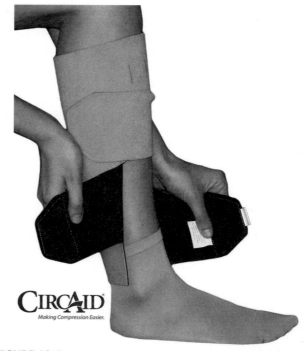

FIGURE 12-7 An example of an inelastic reusable device. *(Courtesy CircAid® Medical Products, San Diego, CA).*

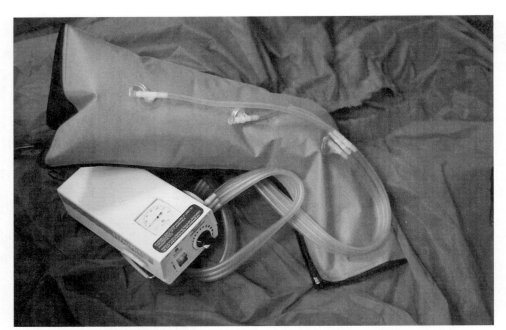

FIGURE 12-8 Dynamic compression device: sequential compression therapy.

compression (Robson et al, 2006). The basic effects of IPC are increase venous velocity, reduce edema, increase popliteal artery blood flow and increase nitric oxide synthase (Comerota, 2009).

Intermittent compression devices vary in terms of the inflation–deflation cycle, amount of pressure exerted against the leg, and number of compartments in the sleeve. Single-compartment sleeves simply inflate and deflate on a cyclic basis, whereas multicompartment sleeves provide sequential compression (i.e., distal to proximal "milking" compression wave). Computer-simulated models suggest that sequential compression devices have the greatest impact on venous return (Chen et al, 2001). Typically, patients are instructed to apply the therapy once or twice daily for 1 to 2 hours each time.

Benefits of IPC include mobilization of interstitial (edema) fluid back into the circulation and enhanced venous return without impairing arterial flow. In fact, IPC may actually improve distal perfusion, making the therapy safe for patients with coexisting arterial disease (Kelechi and Bonham, 2008; Hopf et al, 2006). IPC is thought to exert antithrombotic and vasodilatory effects, possibly as a result of the marked increase in velocity of blood flow and the resultant "shear stress" at the level of the endothelial cells (Chen et al, 2001). IPC therapy may contribute to healing of long-standing venous ulcers that have "failed" standard compression therapy. Studies also report higher levels of patient satisfaction and adherence to IPC therapy (Berliner et al, 2003; Mani et al, 2001).

A disadvantage to most IPC devices is the need for the patient to stay immobile during the therapy.

However, a newer dynamic device (MOBILITY1 Derma Sciences) comes with a small compressor that allows mobility of patients while they are receiving optimal therapy. Medicare and Medicaid reimbursement only covers patients with venous ulcers that have "failed" to heal after a 6-month trial of conservative therapy directed by a physician. The trial of conservative therapy would be expected to include a compression bandage system or garment, an appropriate dressing for the ulcer, exercise, and elevation of the limb(s) (Medicare Determination Manual, 2010).

LOCAL WOUND CARE

As with all wounds, topical therapy for the venous wound is selected based upon wound characteristics (see Chapter 18). Initially, the venous ulcer may present with copious amounts of exudate. Black necrotic tissue is seldom seen in venous ulcers except when infection or trauma is present. Therefore an appropriate rule of thumb is to select dressings that minimize potential allergens while effectively managing the exudate to prevent periwound maceration and control bioburden. Interventions to prevent and manage venous dermatitis were described earlier in the chapter. As edema decreases, the volume of exudate from the venous ulcer also will diminish, and the types of dressings will need to be modified.

When a wound fails to progress, the entire treatment plan must be reevaluated; if the plan remains appropriate and implemented, the diagnosis should be reevaluated. Many other causes of lower extremity ulcers can present as venous ulcers, such as mixed venous/arterial, lymphedema, vasculitis, autoimmune disease, and malignancy.

If a biopsy and differential diagnosis again confirm a venous etiology, failure to heal may be due to the negative cellular environment of a chronic wound. In this case, a product or therapy designed to convert the chronic wound environment into an environment that supports repair should be considered. Skin grafts, bioengineered human skin equivalents, negative pressure wound therapy, electrical stimulation, and selected growth have shown varying degrees of success in the management of refractory venous ulcers if the underlying cause is appropriately addressed. However, laser therapy, phototherapy, and ultrasound therapy have not been shown to statistically improve venous healing (Robson et al, 2006). Biophysical and biological agents are described in detail in Chapters 19 through 24.

SURGICAL INTERVENTIONS

Appropriate topical therapy and compression are not sufficient to heal all venous ulcers (Robson et al, 2006). Factors associated with failure to heal include increased ulcer size (>5 cm^2), longer duration (>6 months), and failure to show significant progress toward healing during the first 3 to 4 weeks of compression therapy. Coexisting arterial disease, persistence of fibrin throughout the wound bed, reduced mobility, and history of vein ligation or knee or hip replacement have been reported as negative prognostic indicators (Paquette and Falanga, 2002).

The procedure of choice for patients with significant perforator and/or deep vein incompetence is ligation of the incompetent perforator veins, which acts to prevent transmission of the elevated pressures within the deep system to the vulnerable superficial veins and tissues. This procedure may be combined with superficial vein stripping for patients who also have significant saphenous vein incompetence. In the past, ligation of perforator veins was performed as an open (Linton) procedure, but the classic Linton procedure has fallen out of favor. In its place is an endoscopic procedure—subfascial endoscopic perforator surgery (SEPS). Wide excision of diseased tissue and free flap transfer of healthy tissue with its own microvasculature and uninjured venous valves can benefit the patient with severe lipodermatosclerosis and persistent, recurrent ulcers (Robson et al, 2006). The Wound Healing Society Guidelines recommend the SEPS procedure of choice to address underlining venous etiology of the venous ulcer by preventing backflow from deep to the superficial venous system. The procedure is not effective if the patient has severe deep venous disease with either reflux or obstruction (Robson et al, 2008).

Less extensive procedures are available for the patient who has not responded to conservative treatments. Duplex Doppler studies can demonstrate an intact deep venous system with abnormal perforators or superficial valves (Tenbrook et al, 2004). Procedures such as superficial (saphenous) venous ablation, endovenous laser ablation, and valvuloplasty can help to decrease venous hypertension and prevent the recurrence of venous ulcers when combined with compression therapy (Robson et al, 2006; Vowden and Vowden, 2006). A new approach of injecting ultrasound-guided foam into refluxing superficial and perforator veins has been reported to be safe and effective (Whiddon, 2007).

FOLLOW-UP AND LIFELONG MAINTENANCE

With recurrence rates ranging between 26% and 69% during the first 12 months following ulcer healing, the emphasis of management must shift to prevention of recurrence once the ulcer is healed (Nelson et al, 2000). Lifelong exercise, weight control, and compression therapy are ongoing challenges. Many patients fail to utilize compression consistently for a variety of reasons (Jull et al, 2004; Nelson et al, 2000). In one study, the two factors that were most predictive of patients' continued use of compression therapy were their perception of the value of compression and their level of comfort/discomfort with the stockings (Jull et al, 2004).

These findings clearly speak to the importance of effectively communication with the patient, stressing the importance of lifelong compression and identifying barriers and solutions to the issues that impair intervention adaptation (Wipke-Tevis and Sae-Sia, 2004). Solutions may involve placing the patient in a lower level of compression so that he or she is able to apply the garment. Although some evidence suggests that high-level compression stockings are more effective in preventing recurrence, other evidence indicates that medium-level compression stockings are associated with significantly higher compliance rates (Jull et al, 2004; Nelson et al, 2000). The Wound Healing Society's Guidelines recommend the use of compression stockings constantly and forever and attempts must be made to aid the patient's compliance (Robson, 2008). Education that includes the families and caregivers as well as the patient is critical to achieving optimal outcomes (Burrows et al, 2007). Chapter 29 provides more strategies for facilitating the patient's adaptation to therapy rather than simply labeling the patient as "noncompliant."

REFERENCES

Agren M, Gottrup, F: Causation of venous ulcers. In Morison M et al, editors: *Leg ulcers: a problem-based learning approach,* Edinburgh, 2007, Elsevier.

Alguire P, Mathes P: *Treatment of chronic venous insufficiency,* Retrieved March 8, 2009 from 2007 Up To Date: http:www.uptodate.com.

Benigni JP, Cazoubon M, Mathieu M, Achammer I. Chronic venous disease in the obese male: an epidemiological survey. *Phlebolymphology* 14:47-49, 2006.

Berliner E et al: A systematic review of pneumatic compression for treatment of chronic venous insufficiency and venous ulcers, *J Vasc Surg* 37(3):539, 2003.

Bolton L: Compression in venous ulcer management, *J Wound Ostomy Continence Nurs* 35(1):40-49, 2008.

Bolton L et al: Development of a content-validated venous ulcer guideline, *Ostomy Wound Manage* 52(11):32-48, 2006.

Bonham P: Assessment and management of patients with venous, arterial, and diabetic/neuropathic lower extremity wounds, *AACN Clin Issues Adv Pract Acute Crit Care* 14(4):442, 2003.

Browse NL and Burnand KG: The cause of venous ulceration *The Lancet*, Vol. 320 No. 8292, pp 243-245, 1982.

Bruce A et al: Lipodermatosclerosis: a review of cases evaluated at Mayo Clinic, *J Am Acad Dermatol* 46:187-192, 2002.

Burrows C et al: Best practice recommendations for the prevention and treatment of venous ulcers: update 2006, *Adv Skin Wound Care* 20(11):611-621, 2007.

Caggiati A et al: The nature of skin pigmentations in chronic venous insufficiency, *Eur J Vasc Endovasc Surg* 35(1):111-118, 2008.

Castonguay G: Short-stretch or four-layer compression bandages: an overview of the literature, *Ostomy Wound Manage* 54(3):50-55, 2008.

Chen A et al: Intermittent pneumatic compression devices-physiological mechanisms of action, *Eur J Vasc Endovasc Surg* 21:383, 2001.

Coleridge-Smith P: From skin disorders to venous leg ulcers: pathophysiology and efficacy of Daflon 500 mg in ulcer healing, *Angiology* 54(Suppl 1):S45, 2003.

Coleridge-Smith P et al: Venous leg ulcer: a meta-analysis of adjunctive therapy with micronized purified flavonoid fraction, *Eur J Vas Endovasc Surg* 30(2):198-208, 2005.

Comerota A: Treatment of chronic venous disease of the lower extremities: what's new in guidelines? *Phlebolymphology* 16(4): 313-320, 2009.

Davis J, Gray, M: Is Unna's boot bandage as effective as a four-layer wrap for managing venous leg ulcers? *J Wound Ostomy Continence Nurs* 32(3):152-156, 2005.

de Araujo T et al: Managing the patient with venous ulcers, *Ann Intern Med* 138(4):326, 2003.

Eklof B et al: Revision of the CEAP classification for chronic venous disorders: consensus statement, *J Vasc Surg* 1248:40-52, 2004.

Feben K: How effective is training in compression bandaging techniques? *Br J Community Nurs* 8(2):80, 2003.

Flugman SL, Clark RA: Stasis dermatitis, updated March 23, 2009. Available at http://emedicine.medscape.com, accessed April 13, 2009.

Ghosh S et al: Pressure mapping and performance of compression bandage/garment for venous leg ulcer treatment, *J Tissue Viability* 17(3):82-94, 2008.

Hopf HW, Ueno C, Aslam R, Burnand K, Fife C et al: Guidelines for the treatment of arterial insufficiency ulcers, *Wound Repair Regen* Nov-Dec;14(6):693-710 2006.

Hussein R: Chronic venous ulcer an end of long term suffering, *Internet J Plast Surg* 5(1): 2008.

Jull A: An overview of pharmacological treatment options for venous leg ulcers. In Morison M et al, editors: *Leg ulcers: a problem-based learning approach*, Edinburgh, 2007, Elsevier.

Jull A et al: Pentoxifylline for treating venous leg ulcers, *Lancet* 359(9317):1550-1554, 2004.

Jull A et al: Pentoxifylline for treating venous leg ulcers, *Cochrane Database Syst Rev* 3:CD001733, 2007.

Kalra M, Gloviczki P: Surgical treatment of venous ulcers: role of subfascial endoscopic perforator vein ligation, *Surg Clin North Am* 83:671, 2003.

Kelechi T, Bonham P: Measuring venous insufficiency objectively in the clinical setting, *J Vasc Nurs* 26(3):67-73, 2008.

Kerstein M: Economics of quality ulcer care, *Dermatol Nurs* 15(1):59, 2003.

Kline C et al: Inelastic compression legging produces gradient compression and significantly higher skin surface pressures compared with an elastic compression stocking. *Vascular* 16(1):25-30, 2008.

Korn P et al: Why insurance should reimburse for compression stockings in patients with chronic venous stasis, *J Vasc Surg* 35(5):950-957, 2002.

Kunimoto B: Assessment of venous leg ulcers: an in depth discussion of a literature-guided approach, *Ostomy Wound Manage* 47(5):38, 2001.

Leach M et al: Using horsechestnut seed extract in the treatment of venous leg ulcers: a cost-benefit analysis, *Ostomy Wound Manage* 52(4):68-70, 72-74, 76-78, 2006.

Lyseng-Williamson K, Perry C: Micronised purified flavonoid fraction, *Drugs* 64(1):71, 2003.

Mani R et al: Intermittent pneumatic compression for treating venous leg ulcers, *Cochrane Database Syst Rev* 2001.

McGucklin M et al: Validation of venous leg ulcer guidelines in the United States and United Kingdom, *Am J Surg* 183(2):132-137, 2002.

Medicare National Coverage Determination Manual, Part 4: Section 280.6: Pneumatic Compression Devices Retrieved May 2, 2010 from http://www.4.cms.hhs.gov/manuals.

Meissner MH: Pathophysiology of varicose veins and chronic venous insufficiency. In Hallett JW Jr et al, editors: *Comprehensive vascular and endovascular surgery,* Philadelphia, 2009, Mosby.

Min RJ et al: Duplex ultrasound evaluation of lower extremity venous insufficiency, *J Vasc Interv Radiol* 14(10):1233-1241, 2003.

Moffat C et al: Compression therapy in leg ulcer management. In Morison M et al, editors: *Leg ulcers: a problem-based learning approach,* Edinburgh, 2007, Elsevier.

Moore Z: Compression bandaging: are practitioners achieving the ideal sub-bandage pressures? *J Wound Care* 11(7):265-268, 2002.

Nelson E et al: Compression for preventing recurrence of venous ulcers, *Cochrane Database Syst Rev* 1, 2000.

Nelzen O: Venous ulcers: patient assessment. In Morison M et al, editors: *Leg ulcers: a problem-based learning approach,* Edinburgh, 2007, Elsevier.

O'Donnell TF Jr, Shepard AD: Chronic venous insufficiency. In Jarrett F, Hirsch SA, editors: *Vascular surgery of the lower extremities,* St. Louis, 1996, Mosby.

O'Meara S et al: Compression for venous leg ulcers (review). *Cochrane Database of Syst Rev* 1, 2009. Art. No.:CD000265. DOI:10.1002/14651858. CD000265.pub2.

Paquette D, Falanga V: Leg ulcers, *Geriatr Dermatol* 18(1):77, 2002.

Pieper B et al: Chronic venous disorders and injection drug use, *J Wound Ostomy Continence Nurs* 35(3):301-310, 2008.

Pittler M: Horse chestnut seed extract is effective for symptoms of chronic venous insufficiency, *ACP J Club* 145(1):20, 2006.

Robson M et al: Guidelines for the treatment of venous ulcers, *Wound Repair Regen* 14:649-662, 2006.

Romanelli M, Romanelli P: Dermatological aspects of leg ulcers. In Morison M et al, editors: *Leg ulcers: a problem-based learning approach,* Edinburgh, 2007, Elsevier.

Ryan S et al: Venous leg ulcer pain, *Ostomy Wound Manage* 49(4A Suppl):16, 2003.

Seidel HM et al: *Mosby's guide to physical examination,* ed 6, St. Louis, 2006, Mosby.

Simka M, Majewski E: The social and economic burden of venous leg ulcers: focus on the role of micronized purified flavonoid fraction adjuvant therapy, *Am J Clin Dermatol* 4(8):573, 2003.

Suter A et al: Treatment of patients with venous insufficiency with fresh plant horse chestnut seed extract. A review of 5 clinical studies, *Adv Ther* 23(1):179-190, 2006.

Tenbrook J et al: Systematic review of outcomes after surgical management of venous disease incorporating subfascial endoscopic perforator surgery, *J Vasc Surg* 39(3):583, 2004.

Vowden KR, Vowden P: Preventing venous ulcer recurrence: a review, *Int Wound J* 3:11-21, 2006.

Weingarten M: State-of-the-art treatment of chronic venous disease, *Clin Infect Dis* 32:949, 2001.

Whiddon L: The treatment of venous ulcers of the lower extremities, *Proc Baylor Univ Med Center* 20(4):363-366, 2007.

Wipke-Tevis D, Sae-Sia W: Caring for vascular leg ulcers, *Home Healthc Nurse* 22(4):237, 2004.

Wound, Ostomy and Continence Nurses Society (WOCN Society): *Guideline for management of patients with lower extremity venous disease,* WOCN clinical practice guideline series #1, Glenview IL, 2005.

Wound, Ostomy and Continence Nurses Society (WOCN Society): *Guideline for management of patients with lower extremity arterial disease,* WOCN clinical practice guideline series #1, Glenview, IL, 2008.

13

Lymphedema

Catherine R. Ratliff

Lymphedema is a chronic disease characterized by swelling of the affected body part, usually the limb, because of impaired flow of lymph fluid. Accumulation of lymph fluid results in swelling in the affected limb. The swelling may be mild or it may be severe, such that the individual is unable to use the affected limb. Lymphedema primarily occurs in the subcutaneous fatty tissues of the arms or legs (Lawenda et al, 2009; Sieggreen and Kline, 2004).

The clinical presentation of lymphedema results from the subcutaneous accumulation of fluid. With interstitial fluid accumulation comes an inflammatory response, slowed lymphatic flow, which causes lipogenesis, and fat deposition. Patients develop firmer subcutaneous tissue in the limb as fibrosis as well as hypertrophy of the adipose tissue occur. These physical changes present clinically as soft and pitting edema but later progress to induration and fibrosis with nonpitting edema (Warren et al, 2007b).

EPIDEMIOLOGY

As the third component of the vascular system, the lymphatic system receives the least attention. Similarly, lymphedema and related pathologies have received much less attention than the pathologies associated with venous and arterial ulcers. Chronic lymphedema has no cure, and long-term management with patient involvement is critical to control the lymphedema. Lymphedema is frequently undertreated, and an insufficient number of lymphedema centers and specialists are addressing the problem. Among breast cancer patients undergoing surgery and radiation in the United States, the incidence of lymphedema ranges from 10% to 40%. Globally, 140 to 250 million cases of lymphedema are estimated to exist (Revis, 2008). The incidence of lymphedema is expected to rise as a result of the increasing numbers of obese persons and elderly persons who often have many medical comorbidities but have limited ability to care for themselves as well as limited social and financial resources (Cheville, 2007).

Lymphedema in cancer patients (e.g., breast, gynecologic, colon, bladder cancer; sarcoma) is seen today at more advanced stages of the cancer than in the past because cancer patients are living longer as a result of more effective cancer treatments. With the increased survival of these patients, the numbers of cancer patients with lymphedema is also expected to increase. However, these patients may be sicker and less able to care for themselves, including managing their lymphedema (Cheville, 2007).

PATHOPHYSIOLOGY

The lymphatic system is composed of lymphatic vessels and lymphatic tissue, which function as a drainage and transport system. When fluid from the interstitial space enters the lymphatic system, it is considered lymph fluid. Lymph fluid consists of protein, water, fatty acids, salts, white blood cells, microorganisms, and debris. It is absorbed from the interstitial spaces into the lymphatic vessels, where it is transported to the venous system (Holcomb, 2006; Lawenda et al, 2009).

The major function of the lymphatic system is to return fluid and protein from interstitial spaces to the vascular system. Because lymphatic vessels often lack a basement membrane and have thinner vessel walls, they can reabsorb molecules too large for the venous system (Holcomb, 2006; Sieggreen and Kline, 2004). Usually tissue fluid and protein macromolecules filtrated by the arterial capillaries are reabsorbed and returned to the circulation through the lymphatic system. From 50% to 100% of the intravascular proteins are filtered this way in the interstitial space. The lymphatic vessels absorb 2 to 4 L of protein-rich fluid retained in the interstitial space per day. This fluid is picked up by the lymphatic capillaries and returned to the circulation, thus maintaining normal plasma volume and preventing interstitial edema. If the system is overloaded, fluid and protein accumulate in the interstitial space, forming a high-protein edema that triggers an inflammatory response with deposition of collagen (Holcomb, 2006; Macdonald et al, 2003).

Two systems of lymphatic drainage work similarly to the venous system. The superficial system drains the skin and subcutaneous tissues, and the deep system drains the tissues to the fascia and below. The lymphatic vessels in the superficial system are located in the subcutaneous tissues, whereas those of the deep system are aligned with the blood vessels, especially the veins. These two systems of lymphatic drainage are connected by perforating vessels just like the veins (Lawenda et al, 2009; Macdonald et al, 2003).

The lymphatic system is composed of lymphatic capillaries, precollectors, lymph collectors, and lymphatic trunks. Capillaries absorb lymph fluid and transport it to lymph nodes, lymphatic trunks, and lymphatic ducts. The lymphatic capillaries are larger than the blood capillaries, are more permeable with thinner walls, and have no basement membranes allowing them to absorb fluids. The lymphatic capillaries do not have valves, so lymph flows in the direction of the lower pressure. The precollectors connect the lymphatic capillaries with the lymph collectors. The lymph collectors are similar to veins; they have valves and transport lymph fluid to the lymph nodes and lymphatic trunks. The precollectors and collectors are the principal vessels of the lymphatic system and eventually filter through to the lymph nodes (Lawenda et al, 2009; Macdonald et al, 2003).

Lymph drains from the legs into the lumbar lymphatic trunk to the intestinal lymphatic trunk and cisterna chyli to the thoracic duct, which drains into the left subclavian vein (Figure 13-1). The thoracic duct empties approximately 3 L of lymph fluid per day into the venous circulation (Lawenda et al, 2009). From the left side of upper body, the lymphatic vessels of the left arm drain into the left subclavian lymphatic trunk, which then drains into the left subclavian vein. Lymph is drained from the right side of the head, neck, thorax, and right arm into the right subclavian vein by way of the right thoracic duct (Sieggreen and Kline, 2004).

Lymphedema is caused by dysfunction of the lymphatic system, where accumulation or pooling of lymph fluid into the interstitial space occurs. The dysfunction is most commonly caused by external forces such as surgery, radiation, or infection, which can damage the lymphatic system. With an impaired lymphatic system, the amount of lymphatic fluid in the interstitial space becomes more than the body's lymph system can handle. Plasma oncotic pressure decreases, oncotic pressure of tissue fluid increases, and lymphatic blockage or obstruction occurs (Sieggreen and Kline, 2004). With retention of fluid and large protein molecules within this interstitial space, the space swells (Lawenda et al, 2009). With swelling, the large protein molecules leak into the tissues, causing fibrosis. Over time progressive obstruction to lymphatic flow occurs by distortion or obliteration of the lymphatic channels from the fibrotic changes in the tissues (Macdonald et al, 2003; Sarvis, 2003; Tiwari et al, 2003).

TYPES OF LYMPHEDEMA

Lymphedema may be *acute* or *chronic*. Acute lymphedema is a condition that lasts less than 6 months and is associated with pitting edema with pressure and lack of brawny skin changes. Risk factors for acute lymphedema include surgical drains with extravasation into the surgical site, acute injury to the limb, radiation therapy, infection, and phlebitis (Sieggreen and Kline, 2004). Chronic lymphedema, unlike acute lymphedema, is not reversible and requires lifetime management. Lymphedema may be classified as *primary* (idiopathic) or *secondary* (acquired) (Holcomb, 2006).

Primary (Idiopathic) Lymphedema

Primary lymphedema is caused by congenital absence or abnormalities of lymphatic tissue. It affects between one and two million individuals in the United States and usually involves the leg (Holcomb, 2006; Revis, 2008). Primary lymphedema may be classified by time of onset: *congenital lymphedema* is detected at less than 1 year of age, *lymphedema praecox* is detected from ages 1 to 35 years, and *lymphedema tarda* is detected after age 35 years (Holcomb, 2006; Kerchner et al, 2008). The congenital type may be sporadic or familial. The familial form is called Milroy disease and is thought to be linked to autosomal inheritance of a mutated gene. Congenital lymphedema affects both lower extremities but can involve the upper extremities as well as the face. The most common type of primary lymphedema is lymphedema praecox (Meige disease). It usually affects adolescent women. Meige disease occurs when some lymphatics that are present at birth become damaged by infection or when the number of lymphatics is inadequate as the individual grows and matures. The condition usually is unilateral, involving the foot and calf. Lymphedema tarda is seen in individuals after age 35 years who have congenitally weakened lymphatics so that a precipitating event such as injury can result in lymphedema (Kerchner et al, 2008).

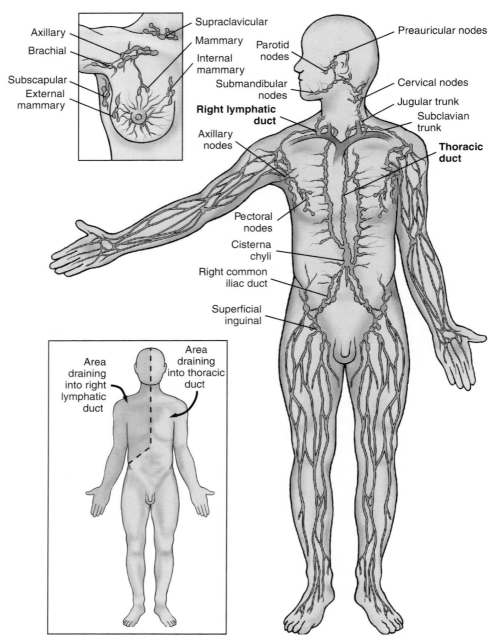

FIGURE 13-1 Anatomy of the lymphatic system. (From Monahan FD, Neighbors M: *Medical surgical nursing: foundations for clinical practice*, ed 2, Philadelphia, 1998, WB Saunders.)

Secondary (Acquired) Lymphedema

Secondary lymphedema affects between two and three million individuals in the United States (Holcomb, 2006). The most common cause of secondary lymphedema in the United States is related to malignancy and its subsequent treatment. The types of cancers associated with secondary lymphedema include breast cancer, gynecologic cancer, lymphoma, melanoma, and urologic cancers. Secondary lymphedema is caused by dysfunction or obstruction of the lymphatic system that usually occurs at proximal limb segments (i.e., lymph nodes) due to surgery, radiation, trauma, infection, malignancy, or scar tissue. Surgery may include the removal of one or more lymph nodes. If the remaining lymph nodes and vessels cannot compensate for those that have been removed, then lymphedema can result. The current use of sentinel node biopsy (e.g., with cancer surgery) has helped reduce the risk of patients developing lymphedema because fewer lymph nodes are removed. Radiation can cause scarring and inflammation of the lymph system, which can restrict the flow of lymph fluid, thus increasing the risk for lymphedema. Cancer can block the lymphatic vessels, which also increases the risk for lymphedema.

Infection from parasites can infiltrate the lymph vessels and block the flow. The cause of the most common form of infection, called *filariasis,* is the nematode *Wuchereria bancrofti,* which is transmitted to humans by mosquitoes. When the filarial larvae mature into adult worms in the lymphatic channels, they block the lymph channels, causing severe lymphedema in the arms, legs, and genitalia, a condition also known as *elephantiasis.* It infects more than 90 million people globally, occurs mainly in southeast Asia, India, and Africa, and is the most common cause of lymphedema worldwide (Macdonald et al, 2003; Tiwari et al, 2003).

Once damage has occurred to the lymphatic system, transport capacity is permanently decreased predisposing to lymphedema. The pelvic and inguinal nodes in the lower limbs and the axillary nodes of the upper limbs are the primary sites of obstruction (Sieggreen and Kline, 2004). Lymphedema has been reported 20 to 30 years after the precipitating event (e.g., surgery).

With the rise in obesity rates comes an increase in the number of cases of secondary lymphedema in the morbidly obese. In a review of wound clinic data of approximately 15,000 patients from 17 wound centers in the United States, Fife and Carter (2008) found 74% prevalence of secondary lymphedema in morbidly obese patients. Morbidly obese patients also have been observed to have lymphedema in conjunction with venous ulcer disease. Obesity impedes lymphatic flow, leading to accumulation of lymphatic fluid in the subcutaneous tissue (Kerchner et al, 2008). The risk for lymphedema increases as body mass index increases (Dell and Doll, 2006). Sizable weight gain has been shown to increase a woman's risk for lymphedema following breast cancer (Warren et al, 2007b). With the increase of lymphatic fluid in the setting of decreased oxygen tensions, fibrosis with chronic inflammation and increased risk for infection result. In addition to occurring in the extremities, lymphedema can be seen in the overhanging abdominal pannus of the morbidly obese (Kerchner et al, 2008).

STAGES OF LYMPHEDEMA

The International Society of Lymphology recognizes four categories or classifications for staging (Table 13-1). Stage 0 is a subclinical lymphedema in which swelling is not evident despite impaired lymphatic function. Stage 0 (reversible) may exist for months or years before edema occurs. Stage I (reversible) is defined as lymph fluid with a high protein content (in contrast to venous ulcer disease edema) that dissipates after limb elevation. Pitting may occur. Pitting edema is considered present when, 5 seconds after a finger is pressed into the edematous tissue, an indentation remains. In stage II (irreversible), pitting edema is present but limb elevation alone does not reduce edema. As stage II progresses, tissue fibrosis develops, and pitting may or may not be present. Stage III (irreversible) is elephantiasis in which pitting is not

TABLE 13-1 Stages of Lymphedema

Stage	Manifestations
0	Subclinical lymphedema with edema that is not evident despite impaired lymphatic function
I	Reversible pitting edema that begins distally (at foot) Negative or borderline Stemmer sign No palpable fibrosis
II	Minimally pitting or nonpitting (brawny) edema that is not reduced by conservative measures such as elevation Positive Stemmer sign Pronounced fibrosis Hyperkeratosis (thickening of skin) Papillomatosis (skin has rough cobblestone appearance and texture)
III	Lymphostatic elephantiasis (massive enlargement and distortion of limb caused by breakdown of skin's elastic components) Progressive fibrosis, acanthosis, hyperkeratosis, papillomatosis Ulceration

Data from the International Society of Lymphology, The diagnosis and treatment of peripheral lymphoma: 2009 Consensus Document, *Lymphology* 42(2):51-60, 2009, available at http://www.lymphnotes.com, accessed April 14, 2009.

present but skin changes in the limb, such as acanthosis (increase in thickness of the epidermis), fatty deposits, and warty growths, may be present. Within each stage, limb volume differences can be categorized as minimal (<20% increase in size), moderate (20%–40% increase in size), and severe (>40% increase in size) (Holcomb, 2006; Macdonald et al, 2003).

LIPEDEMA

Lipedema, often confused with lymphedema, is a syndrome of bilateral adipose deposition that almost always occurs in overweight women. Lipedema usually presents around puberty with a familial tendency of enlarged or fatty legs and buttocks (hips and thighs). Features distinguishing lymphedema from lipedema are listed in Table 13-2 (Fonder et al, 2007; Warren et al, 2007a). Table 10-1 compares characteristics of venous edema to lipedema and lymphedema.

The diagnosis of lipedema usually is based on history and physical examination. Diagnostic tests, such as those done with lymphedema, may be conducted and usually only show subcutaneous fat hypertrophy. Treatment options for lipedema are mainly dietary and lifestyle modifications. However, research now is assessing the role of liposuction in treating lipedema patients. Schmeller and Meier-Vollrath (2006) treated 28 female patients with liposuction. Twenty-one patients were reevaluated after an average of 12 months. All patients showed an improvement in body proportions. Eighteen patients suffered from pain before the procedure;

TABLE 13-2	Comparison of Lymphedema and Lipedema	
	Lymphedema	Lipedema
Gender	Male and female	Female
Age	Any age	After or during puberty
Edema	Pitting progresses to firm fibrotic	Nonpitting
Epidermal skin changes	Common	Uncommon
Cellulitis	Common	Uncommon
Stemmer sign	Positive	Negative
Distribution	Unilateral or bilateral, toes to groin	Always bilateral, ends at ankles
Tenderness	None	Tender to palpation Bruising common
Magnetic resonance imaging	Honeycomb pattern	Normal

10 patients had improvement in pain levels after liposuction. All patients complained of sensitivity to pressure. After the liposuction, this symptom disappeared in 8 patients and improved in 13 patients. Generally lipedema responds poorly to compression therapy and leg elevation, although low-level compression therapy usually is recommended to prevent the disease from progressing to lipolymphedema, which is a combination of lipedema and lymphedema (Fonder et al, 2007; Kerchner et al, 2008; Schmeller and Meier-Vollrath, 2006).

DIAGNOSTIC TESTS

Diagnosis of lymphedema typically is made through clinical presentation and history. Diagnostic confirmation can be made with isotopic lymphoscintigraphy, in which a radionuclide is injected into the lymphatic tissue between the first and second digits of the affected limb to identify abnormalities of the lymphatic pathways, including enlarged vessels and backflow problems due to obstruction. Lymphoscintigraphy is considered the gold standard for imaging studies for lymphedema (Holcomb, 2006; Kerchner et al, 2008; Lohrmann et al, 2006; Warren et al, 2007b). However, lymphoscintigraphy is expensive and invasive. Because radioactive dye must be injected into an already compromised limb, lymphoscintigraphy generally is indicated only if the patient is a surgical candidate and a definitive diagnosis is needed. Computed tomography scans or magnetic resonance imaging (MRI) can be performed to evaluate for the presence of lymphedema, but these procedures also are expensive and so are not routinely recommended. However, because MRI can detect a honeycomb pattern of the subcutaneous tissue from fibrosis and lymph fluid, a finding that is not seen with other forms of edema, it can be helpful for diagnosis (Kerchner et al, 2008; Warren et al,

2007b). Lymph fluid analysis with protein content between 1 and 5.5 g/dL usually indicates lymphedema (Holcomb, 2006). Other laboratory studies, such as serum albumin and urinalysis, should be performed to rule out other causes of edema, such as renal or hepatic impairment. Edema can be classified by its protein content. Low-protein edema is composed of less than 1 g of protein per 100 mL of fluid; high-protein edema is composed of greater than 1 g of protein per 100 mL of fluid (Lawenda et al, 2009). Lymphedema is a high-protein edema. Ultrasound can provide an analysis of soft tissue changes but does not provide any information about the lymphatics. Duplex doppler studies may be required if venous ulcer disease is also suspected. Genetic testing may be recommended for patients with primary lymphedema.

Bioimpedance spectroscopy (BIS) is a procedure in which an electrical current is passed through the limb and impedance flow is measured. This technique, also known as bioelectrical impedance analysis, measures the composition of tissues, especially the presence of fluids such as lymph. Reduced impedance values are indicative of lymphedema. In lymphedema management, BIS can be used for early detection and ongoing measurements of fluid buildup in the affected limb to determine the effectiveness of therapy. Warren et al. (2007c) studied 15 patients with either upper or lower limb lymphedema who underwent BIS analysis. Participants underwent BIS of both limbs so that they could serve as their own control. The average ratio of impedance to current flow of the affected extremity to the unaffected extremity was 0.9. The authors concluded that BIS can be used as a tool for documenting the presence of lymphedema in patients with lymphedema and may be useful in long-term monitoring of patients (Warren et al, 2007b).

ASSESSMENT

Assessment of the patient with limb enlargement should begin with a history of risk factors for lymphedema, such as surgeries (especially nodal dissections), radiation therapy, trauma, infection, malignancy, obesity, familial history, and travel to areas with endemic filariasis. To determine if lymphedema is the cause of swelling, knowing the onset of limb enlargement and associated symptoms is important. Symptoms of lymphedema include feelings of heaviness, aching, and fatigue in the affected limb. A history of recurrent infections (e.g., cellulitis) is an important clue to lymphedema. Individuals may report less flexibility in the extremities and difficulty fitting into clothing, hardening of the skin, and paresthesias (Neese, 2000).

Knowing if the patient has a history of comorbid conditions that can cause swelling of the extremities, such as cardiac disease, venous ulcer disease, renal disease, hepatic disease, trauma, and infection, also is important. Patients with rheumatoid arthritis, obesity, lipedema, and venous ulcer disease are at greater risk for lymphedema because these conditions further stress the already impaired lymphatics. Lymph nodes are located around most joints, so patients undergoing surgical procedures such as total knee replacements may be at greater risk for developing lymphedema because these lymph nodes may become damaged during the surgery. Some relatively minor conditions, such as vein stripping, can exacerbate mild lymphedema (Tiwari et al, 2003). Yellow nail syndrome is an uncommon disorder that may be seen with lymphedema. The pathophysiology of the syndrome remains unclear, but lymphatic abnormalities as well as chronic pulmonary disease and genetic predisposition may play a role (Maldonada et al, 2009).

Physical Assessment

Physical assessment parameters for lymphedema include skin texture (soft vs hard), papillomatosis (cobblestone skin appearance), skin color (erythema, unusually dark), lymphangiomas (blisters containing lymph fluid), presence of skin fissures, presence of skin folds, presence of pedal pulses, edema, range of motion of the limb, neurologic deficits, and signs of venous ulcer disease. Mushroom-like papules may be present. In normal persons, leg circumference varies as the leg is measured from ankle to knee. However, in lymphedema patients the circumference from ankle to knee is almost the same. The Stemmer sign (or Kaposi-Stemmer sign) is another clinical indication of lymphedema. In this test, the examiner is unable to pinch a fold of skin at the base of the second toe on the dorsal aspect of the foot or between the second and third finger. Skin that does not fold up into a pinch is considered a positive sign of lymphedema (Kerchner et al, 2008; Sarvis, 2003).

Physical examination and history usually are sufficient to make a diagnosis of lymphedema. Lymphedema is evaluated by visual inspection and palpation. Initially there will be soft, painless pitting edema, but over time fibrosis, nonpitting edema, and induration may be present in the affected limb. The characteristic lymphatic swelling in the lower extremity is edema from the ankle up toward the knee. Occasionally swelling includes the feet. Depending on the extent of the disease, the edema may extend into the groin. The skin has a roughened leathery appearance resembling an elephant's skin. Because of this appearance, the name *elephantiasis* was coined for the lymphedema caused by the filarial infection. The skin over the lymphedema does not usually have the darkened brown pigment skin changes seen with venous ulcer disease unless the patient has venous ulcer disease. Patients with lymphedema and venous ulcer disease may have a leathery appearance of the skin with dark-brown hemosiderin-pigmented skin changes.

Measuring Limb Size. Two methods for measuring the size of the limb affected by lymphedema are girth and volume. Girth measurements should include 3 cm above the lateral malleolus, 12 cm above the lateral malleolus, and 18 cm above the lateral malleolus. Using a flexible tape to measure circumference around these areas, the clinician should then compare those measurements with the contralateral limb (Fowler and Carson, 2007) and measurements for each assessment recorded. The clinician should measure the limb in the same position each time and try to measure the limb at the same time of day because girth may increase during the day because of swelling. An increase in limb size by 1.5 cm or more, is suspicious for lymphedema (Dell and Doll, 2006; Fowler and Carson, 2007). Other methods of measurement, such as water displacement of the limb, can be used to determine limb volume. For this method, a container is filled with tepid water and the limb is immersed in the water. The amount of overflow is measured to determine the volume of fluid displaced. Both limbs are assessed and results are compared. A volume difference of 20% or more is considered significant. Even though this method may be more precise than tape measurements and is often considered the gold standard for measuring girth it is not user friendly for the clinician (Dell and Doll, 2006; Fowler and Carson, 2007). To clinically define the presence of lymphedema, Spillane et al (2008) assessed 66 patients who had undergone inguinal or ilio-inguinal lymph node dissection for metastatic melanoma. They found that a change in limb volume of 15% or more and an increase of 7% or more in the sum of limb circumferences of the defined points on the limb provided a more standardized definition of lymphedema in those patients (Spillane et al, 2008).

PREVENTION

Prevention of lymphedema in high-risk individuals, especially those undergoing surgery and radiation for cancer, is paramount. The importance of skin integrity in preventing injury and infection cannot be overemphasized (Box 13-1).

Skin Care

Skin care is important in the prevention of infection, dermatitis, and hyperkeratosis. Lanolin or fragrances can cause sensitization in this population and so should be avoided. However, routine use of fragrance-free, lanolin-free emollients to prevent cracking and promote suppleness of the skin is encouraged. Any break in the skin can be an entry site for bacteria, and the protein-rich lymphedema fluid is a great medium for bacterial proliferation. Foot care with daily cleansing and drying of the toe web spaces will help to prevent fungal infections of the edematous feet. A common symptom of lymphedema is pruritus. Scratching from pruritus can cause breaks in the skin, which contribute to infection and cellulitis. Pruritus is thought to be caused by factors in the lymphedematous skin that lower the threshold for

BOX 13-1	Teaching Points for the Patient with Lymphedema

- Avoid sauna, hot tub, tanning booths.
- Do not use heating pad on affected limb.
- Do not use chemical hair remover, wax, hair laser on affected limb.
- Use electric razor to avoid cuts or nicks in skin.
- Blood pressure, blood draws, vaccinations should be administered on unaffected limb.
- Wear gloves to protect limb from hot water and potential trauma when washing dishes, cleaning, gardening.
- Protect lymphedema extremity from sun exposure at all times.
- Protect lymphedema extremity and foot from all types of trauma.
- Apply sunscreen and insect repellent on lymphedema extremity prior to going outside.
- Avoid heavy lifting with affected limb (arm); do not carry handbag or other bags on shoulder of affected side.
- Do not restrict fluid or protein intake in attempt to prevent fluid buildup.
- Maintain or lose weight.
- Exercise in moderation wearing compression garment in place.
- Carry lymphedema alert card and wear lymphedema alert bracelet or necklace.

degranulation of dermal mast cells. With the degranulation of mast cells comes a subsequent release of histamine, which potentiates the itch. McCord and Fore (2007) evaluated nine patients with mild to severe pruritus associated with lymphedema over a 6-month period who were treated with olivamine-based products. The average pruritus evaluation score before treatment with the products was 2, which corresponds to mild to moderate pruritus; after treatment the average score was 0.11, which corresponds to absent pruritus. Additional research is needed to determine which products work best for the management of pruritus associated with lymphedema (McCord and Fore, 2007).

Protect from Injury

Protecting the limb from injury is important to prevent infection. For example, using an electric razor and wearing gloves when gardening or washing dishes are advisable. Many of the interventions for protection are based on common sense to prevent injury to an already compromised limb. Greene (2005) suggests that avoidance of blood pressure measurements and venipuncture in patients at risk for lymphedema does not appear to be evidence based. According to Greene, the treatment of lymphedema is compression therapy, including compression pumps, so pumping the cuff for blood pressure readings should not cause injury. He reports no cases of cellulitis from venipuncture were published in the literature between 1966 and 2004. In addition, no cases of cellulitis resulting from the use of lymphoscintigraphy (i.e., injection of dye into the compromised limb) in the

diagnosis of lymphedema have been reported in the literature (Greene, 2005). As we continue to search for evidence that determines best practice, additional common sense approaches may be challenged.

Promote Lymphatic Flow

Placing limbs in gravity-dependent positions for long periods promotes swelling and should be avoided. The patient should avoid constricting garments, weight gain, heavy lifting, extreme heat (e.g., from heating pad or sauna), and rapid altitude changes seen with flying for 2 hours. Exercises that do not make the patient feel fatigued can increase movement of lymph fluid out of the limb and decrease the risk for lymphedema. Wrapping the limb with bandages can promote lymphatic flow and drainage.

MANAGEMENT

Chronic lymphedema has no known cure. Positive clinical outcomes depend on prompt recognition of lymphedema and initiation of treatment to interrupt the cycle of fluid retention, lymphatic obstruction, and soft tissue fibrosis. Effective management of the patient with lymphedema requires a comprehensive lifelong program of exercise, massage, skin care, and compression garments and is most effectively carried out in a lymphedema center. Patients and care providers need to understand that conservative therapies are aimed at reducing symptoms and will not cure the underlying lymphatic dysfunction.

The goals of lymphedema management include (1) moving the "trapped" lymph from the interstitial space, (2) eliminating edema, (3) restoring normal limb contours, (4) maintaining the "restored" limb state, and (5) preventing infection. The components of treatment are highlighted in Table 13-3, with key points discussed by Macdonald et al (2003), Sarvis et al (2003), and Tiwari et al (2003).

Complete Decongestive Physiotherapy

Complete decongestive physiotherapy is the gold standard for management of moderate to severe lymphedema. Patients should be referred to a lymphedema therapist, who might be an occupational therapist, physical therapist, or nurse practitioner who is specially trained in complete decongestive physiotherapy. Unlike Europe where patients can undergo a 4-week intensive inpatient stay, in the United States the focus is on short outpatient programs that focus on self-care (Neese, 2000).

Complete decongestive physiotherapy is a specialized massage technique designed to stimulate the lymph vessels, break up subcutaneous fibrous tissue, and redirect lymph fluid to areas where lymph flow is normal. The therapy involves four steps: manual lymph drainage, compression bandaging, exercises, and skin/nail care.

TABLE 13-3	Lymphedema: Treatment Components		
Intervention	**Desired Effect**	**Action**	**Cautions**
Complex decongestive physiotherapy Therapeutic massage Compression bandages applied immediately after treatment	Mobilization of retained lymph	Mobilize lymphatic fluid in channels adjacent and proximal to involved site	Performed only by therapist trained in the technique Usually requires treatments daily for 1–3 weeks
Sequential compression therapy	Mobilization of retained lymph	Dynamic compression pumps with limb sleeves compress lymphatic and mobilize lymph	Risk of displacing fluid to proximal leg or genitalia Risk of further damage to lymphatics
Limb elevation	Edema reduction	Counter effect of gravity on lymph flow	Effective only in early phase of disease
Compression bandaging	Critical component of maintenance therapy Nonelastic or short-stretch bandages and custom-fitted sleeves or stockings most effective	Apply pressure to tissues to facilitate compression of lymph channels and movement of lymph from interstitial space into circulation	Should provide 40–60 mm Hg sub-bandage pressure Replace regularly to prevent loss of therapeutic effectiveness
Exercise (light movement exercise with compression bandage or garment in place)	Maintenance of lymph reduction	Stimulate intact lymphatics to increase rate of lymph transport	Should not be strenuous or cause fatigue
Skin and nail care (avoid trauma, apply moisturizer, regular nail care)	Infection control during restorative and maintenance phases	Keep skin supple and prevent breaks in skin to reduce risk of infection	Recommend having standing prescription for antibiotic should signs of infection appear Do not cut cuticles

Complete decongestive physiotherapy is administered in two phases. In the first restorative phase, manual lymph drainage involves daily to weekly sessions for up to 8 to 12 weeks. The lymphedema therapist uses specialized massage techniques to (1) activate the lymphatic channels proximal to the affected limb, (2) mobilize lymph in the proximal tissues, and (3) mobilize lymph in the distal tissues. Manual lymph drainage is accompanied by range-of-motion exercises, short-stretch compression bandages (worn between treatments), and meticulous skin/nail care to prevent skin infections. When the extremity has been reduced in size, a compression garment is ordered and the maintenance phase begins.

Compression wraps and stockings are an important component of therapy for all patients with lymphedema to continue to prevent the reaccumulation of lymph fluid in the limb. Compression garments must be worn between manual lymph drainage treatment sessions during the restorative phase and throughout the day and night thereafter. During the first phase of manual lymph drainage, short-stretch bandages are used in multilayers. These bandages may be difficult to apply for some patients with physical impairments. Devices such as the Reid Sleeve and the CircAid (see Figure 12-4) might be recommended because they are easier to apply (Neese, 2000).

Intermittent pneumatic compression pumps (see Figure 12-8) are another method for decreasing the volume of the affected limb. The pump, which can be used in the home, consists of a sleeve with several compartments that are serially inflated by a pump to push the fluid out of the extremity from the distal to the proximal portion. After the daily or twice-daily treatments, which lasts for several hours, the patient should continue with compression through either a garment or bandaging. Reassessment determines frequency and duration of treatments. For example, if the treatments are not effective after two weeks of therapy, they should be discontinued. These pumps are very expensive and currently are covered by Medicare only if other therapies initially attempted were unsuccessful (Kerchner et al, 2008).

Badger et al (2004) examined randomized controlled clinical trials that tested physical therapy modalities with a follow-up of at least 6 months. Only three studies with 150 patients were included. Because none of the studies examined the same intervention, combining the data was not possible. One crossover study of manual lymph drainage followed by self-administered massage versus no treatment concluded that improvements seen in both groups were attributed to compression sleeves and that manual lymph drainage provided no extra benefit. Another trial of hosiery versus no treatment had a high dropout rate, with only 3 of 14 in the treatment group and 1 of 11 in the control group finishing the trial. Clearly more well-controlled clinical trials on the physical therapy modalities used to treat lymphedema are needed (Badger et al, 2004).

Adjunctive Therapy

Selenium therapy for lymphedema is currently being studied. The hypothesis is that lymphedema is caused by excessive generation of oxygen free radicals and that selenium, an antioxidant, consumes oxygen radicals, which might decrease the damage to the lymph system (Holcomb, 2006). The use of hyperbaric oxygen is also being studied. Hyperbaric oxygen may stimulate growth of new lymphatic channels in breast cancer patients (Holcomb, 2006). The role of thermal therapy and pulsed radiofrequency energy in the treatment of lymphedema remains unclear (Holcomb, 2006).

Kinesio taping is a type of compression therapy that is being tested in trials of lymphedema patients. Kinesio taping is a thin elastic tape invented by Kenzo Kase in 1996. The tape can be stretched up to 140% of its original length, making it very elastic (Fu et al, 2008). The wrapping technique with the Kinesio tape is thought to reduce swelling by improving blood and lymphatic fluid flow and is beginning to be used with lymphedema patients. However, research regarding its effectiveness in lymphedema patients currently is lacking (Fu et al, 2008).

Barclay et al (2006) described a randomized trial determining the effect of self-massage and skin care using a cream with aromatherapy oils versus a cream without aromatherapy oils on limb volume measurements and symptom relief in 81 people with lymphedema. Results showed that self-massage and skin care significantly improved patient-identified symptom relief and well-being but did not significantly reduce limb volume. Aromatherapy oils did not appear to improve limb volume measurements (Barclay et al, 2006).

Surgery

Surgery is reserved for individuals with a positive lymphoscintigram who do not respond to more conservative methods such as complete decongestive physiotherapy. Surgery for lymphedema can be restorative and debulking. Reconstructive or restorative procedures create lymph-venous shunts or autologous vessel transplantations. Debulking procedures remove excess tissue to reduce the size and weight of the limb (Kerchner et al, 2008). However, with debulking procedures the superficial lymphatics and collaterals are removed, which can further compromise the lymphatics.

Surgical treatment can be divided into three types: resection procedures, microsurgical procedures, and suction-assisted lipectomy (liposuction) procedures. *Resection or debulking procedures* remove redundant skin folds and subcutaneous tissues but do not address the lymphatic vessel dysfunction and usually are performed to promote comfort. Subcutaneous excisions may require multiple surgeries and are associated with infection, thromboembolism, dehiscence, and scarring complications. *Microsurgical procedures* are performed in an attempt to correct the underlying lymphatic pathology, usually lymphaticovenous anastomoses. Microsurgery uses a lymphatic collector or vein segment to restore the continuity of the lymphatics. *Suction-assisted lipectomy,* which is the removal of subcutaneous fatty tissue through circumferential liposuction of the affected limb, is less invasive and has fewer complications. However, patients undergoing all of these procedures are placed immediately postoperatively in compression garments, so complete assessment of the effectiveness of the procedure is difficult (Warren et al, 2007b).

Salgado et al (2007) reviewed 15 patients with lymphedema who had not responded to conventional therapy and were treated by surgical reduction of lymphedema tissue with preservation of perforating skin vessels from posterior tibial and peroneal arteries. This procedure allowed for reduction of lymphedema tissue in a single procedure while preserving blood supply to the skin. In these 15 patients, the average lymphedema reduction was 52%. At follow-up of 13 months, no cases of skin flap necrosis or incisional wound breakdown were seen. Three patients had cellulitis, and one patient had a seroma and hematoma (Salgado et al, 2007).

Campisi and Boccardo (2004) reviewed 676 patients with lymphedema treated with microsurgical lymphatic-venous anastomoses. They found that of the 447 patients who were available for follow-up, 380 (85%) had been able to discontinue conservative methods for managing the disease, with an average reduction in limb volume of 69%. An 87% reduction in cellulitis after the microsurgery also was noted (Campisi and Boccardo, 2004). Koshima et al. (2004) studied the effectiveness of lymphaticovenular anastomoses for lower leg lymphedema in patients under local anesthesia and reported that 17 patients had a greater than 4-cm reduction in leg circumference.

Pharmacology

Diuretics are not beneficial for lymphedema because they may promote volume depletion. Diuretics draw off excess water but not protein from the interstitial spaces. As soon as the diuretic is stopped, the concentrated proteins pull more water back into the interstitial space, increasing the edema (Holcomb, 2006). Diuretics act to remove water from the cells. Lymphedema is a high-protein edema, and the high osmotic pressure from the increased protein in the interstitial space causes rapid reaccumulation of edema. In addition, the higher concentration of protein in the edema fluid causes increased fibrosis and induration of the skin. Diuretics are not contraindicated for treatment of other conditions in lymphedema patients, but they should not be used as primary treatment of lymphedema (Neese, 2000).

BOX 13-2	Lymphedema Resources
Circle of Hope Lymphedema Foundation	http://www.lymphedemacircleofhope.org
Lymphatic Research Foundation	http://www.lymphaticresearch.org
Lymphology Association of North America	http://www.clt-lana.org
National Lymphedema Network	http://www.lymphnet.org

Benzopyrones (e.g., coumarin) are thought to hydrolyze tissue proteins and facilitate absorption while stimulating lymphatic collectors. However, because of their hepatic toxicity and dose regimens, benzopyrones are not approved for use in the United States and consequently are not manufactured in the United States (Macdonald et al, 2003). Treatment with benzopyrones is thought to decrease fluid formation in the subcutaneous tissues and to reduce pain and discomfort of the affected area. However, in a systematic review published in the *Cochrane Library*, Badger et al (2004) could not draw any conclusions from the current trials about the effectiveness of benzopyrones in the management of lymphedema.

COMPLICATIONS

Common skin complications seen with lymphedema include lymphangitis and cellulitis. Lymphangitis has a distinctive erythematous linear pattern (red streak) that travels along the lymphatics. Fever, chills, headache, muscle aches, and loss of appetite are common presenting symptoms. Lymphangitis often results from a streptococcal or staphylococcal infection of the skin, which causes the lymph vessels to become swollen and tender. Antibiotics, analgesics, and antiinflammatory drugs may be prescribed and elevation of the extremity recommended.

Cellulitis involves the subcutaneous tissue. It usually has an indistinct border and is characterized by pain, warmth, and edema, with red appearance of the skin. Fever, chills, headache, muscle aches, and fatigue may be presenting symptoms. Cellulitis occurs in approximately 50% of patients with lymphedema and usually occurs when a crack or fissure in the skin serves as the portal entry for bacteria. The most common pathogen is β-hemolytic streptococcus. According to Badger et al (2004), penicillin V is the antibiotic of choice because streptococcus is believed to be the most common infecting organism. Antibiotics should be used at the first sign of cellulitis. Penicillin 250 mg orally four times per day for 7 to 10 days usually is effective. Patients who are prone to cellulitis should have medication on hand at home (Badger et al, 2004; Neese, 2000).

Macdonald et al (2003) reported that compression bandaging is indicated for treatment of cellulitis. However, other sources do not recommend compression bandaging until the patient is afebrile and erythema is resolving (Feldman, 2005). Fungal infections with itching and burning between the toes increase the risk for cellulitis in the lower extremity (Feldman, 2005). Meticulous skin care, including washing with soap and water and applying emollients to dry skin areas, decreases the risk of cellulitis.

SUMMARY

Lymphedema is a chronic disease. Treatment focuses on managing the symptoms of the disease, mainly the high-protein edema and its effects on the limb. Lymphedema management crosses all care settings. The numbers of lymphedema patients, especially among the obese and the elderly, are increasing. Management of the disease relies on patients and caregivers assuming lymphedema care practices in the home setting. Most care providers are not familiar with the specialized care required for lymphedema patients, and local resources may be unavailable (Box 13-2). Health care providers need to become more knowledgeable about lymphedema practices because many lymphedema patients have comorbid conditions that necessitate their admission to acute and long-term care.

REFERENCES

Badger C et al: Physical therapies for reducing and controlling lymphoedema of the limbs, *Cochrane Database Syst Re*, 4:CD003141, 2004.

Barclay J et al: Reducing the symptoms of lympheoedema: is there a role for aromatherapy? *Eur J Oncol Nurs* 10(2):140-149, 2006.

Campisi C, Boccardo F: Microsurgical techniques for lymphedema treatment: lymphatic-venous microsurgery, *World J Surg* 28(6):609-613, 2004.

Cheville AL: Current and future trends in lymphedema management: implications for women's health *Phys Med Rehabil Clin N Am* 18(3):539-553, 2007.

Dell DD, Doll C: Caring for a patient with lymphedema, *Nursing* 36(6):49, 2006.

Feldman JL: The challenge of infection in lymphedema, *Lymph Link Article* 17(4):1, 2005.

Fife CE, Carter MJ: Lymphedema in the morbidly obese patient: unique challenges in a unique population, *Ostomy Wound Manage* 54(1):44-56, 2008.

Fonder MA et al: Lipedema, a frequently unrecognized problem, *J Am Acad Dermatol* 57(2):51-53, 2007.

Fowler E, Carson S: Management of edema. In Sussman C & Bates-Jensen B editors: *Wound care: a collaborative practice manual for health professionals*, Baltimore, Md., 2007, Lippincott Williams & Wilkins.

Fu TC et al: Effect of kinesio taping on muscle strength in athletes- a pilot study, *J Sci Med Sport* 11(2):198-201, 2008.

Greene AK: Blood pressure monitoring and venipuncture in the lymphedematous extremity, *Plast Reconstr Surg* 116(7): 2058-2059, 2005.

Holcomb SS: Identification and treatment of different types of lymphedema, *Adv Skin Wound Care* 19(2):103-108, 2006.

International Society of Lymphology: The diagnosis and treatment of peripheral lymphoma: 2009 Consensus Document, *Lymphology* 42: 51-60, 2009, available at http://www.lymphnotes.com, accessed April 14, 2009.

Kerchner K et al: Lower extremity lymphedema update: pathophysiology, diagnosis, and treatment guidelines, *J Am Acad Dermatol*, 59(2):324-331, 2008.

Koshima I et al: Minimal invasive lymphaticovenular anastomosis under local anesthesia for leg lymphedema: is it effective for stage III or IV? *Ann Plast Surg* 53(3):261-266, 2004.

Lawenda BD et al: Lymphedema: a primer on the identification and management of a chronic condition in oncologic treatment, *CA Cancer J Clin* 59(1):8-24, 2009.

Lohrmann C et al: Chronic lymphedema: detected with high-resolution magnetic resonance lymphangiography, *J Comput Assist Tomogr* 30(4):688, 2006.

Macdonald JM et al: Lymphedema, lipedema, and the open wound the role of compression therapy, *Surg Clin North Am* 83(3):639-658, 2003.

Maldonada F et al: *Yellow nail syndrome: analysis of 41 consecutive patients*, 2009, available at http://www.chestjournal.org/cgi/content/abstract/134/2/375, accessed January 2, 2009.

McCord D, Fore J: Using olivamine-containing products to reduce pruritic symptoms associated with localized lymphedema, *Adv Skin Wound Care* 20(8):441-442, 444, 2007.

Monahan FD, Neighbors M: *Medical surgical nursing: foundations for clinical practice*, ed 2, Philadelphia, 1998, WB Saunders.

Neese PY: Management of lymphedema, *Lippincott's Prim Care Pract* 4(4):390-399, 2000.

Revis D: *Lymphedema*, 2008, available at http://emedicine.medscape.com, accessed April 11, 2009.

Salgado CJ et al: Radical reduction of lymphedema with preservation of perforators, *Ann Plast Surg* 59(2):173-179, 2007.

Sarvis C: When lymphedema takes hold, *RN* 66(9):32-36, 2003.

Schmeller W, Meier-Vollrath I: Tumescent liposuction: a new and successful therapy for lipedema, *J Cutan Med Surg* 10(1):7-10, 2006.

Sieggreen MY, Kline RA: Current concepts in lymphedema management, *Adv Skin Wound Care* 17(4):174-178, 2004.

Spillane AJ et al: Defining lower limb lymphedema after inguinal or ilio-inguinal dissection in patients with melanoma using classification and regression tree analysis, *Ann Surg* 248(2):286-293, 2008.

Tiwari A et al: Differential diagnosis, investigation, and current treatment of lower limb lymphedema, *Arch Surg* 138(2):152-161, 2003.

Warren AG et al: Evaluation and management of the fat leg syndrome, *Plast Reconstr Surg* 119(1):9e-15e, 2007a.

Warren AG et al: Lymphedema a comprehensive review, *Ann Plast Surg* 59(4):464-472, 2007b.

Warren AG et al: The use of bioimpedance analysis to evaluate lymphedema, *Ann Plast Surg* 58(5):541-543, 2007c.

14

Neuropathic Wounds: The Diabetic Wound

Vickie R. Driver, Jonathan M. LeBretton, Mary Anne Landowski, and J. L. Madsen

OBJECTIVES

1. Describe three types of neuropathy that may occur in the patient with diabetes.
2. Identify critical factors to be included in the history and physical examination of the patient with lower-extremity neuropathic disease.
3. Describe the correlation of protective sensation with risk for diabetic foot ulcer.
4. Distinguish from among the musculoskeletal foot deformities that lead to focal areas of high pressure in the patient with peripheral neuropathy.
5. Identify key components of a patient education program for the patient with lower extremity neuropathic disease.
6. Identify key concepts in effective and appropriate offloading.

Lower extremity neuropathic disease (LEND) develops as a result of damage to nerve structures. In the case of diabetic foot ulcers, lower extremity metabolic changes and peripheral arterial disease (PAD) exacerbate neuropathy. Diabetic foot ulcers are sometimes referred to as *neurotrophic, trophic, perforating,* or *mal perforans* ulcers (see Plate 40). The presence of possible coexisting factors, such as impaired perfusion, susceptibility to infection, neuropathy, biochemical abnormalities, repeated or continuous trauma, or a combination of these factors, in the patient with LEND who has diabetes creates a particularly challenging situation for ulcer healing (Frykberg, 2003). This chapter presents the assessment, prevention, and management of the diabetic foot ulcer.

EPIDEMIOLOGY

The prevalence of diabetes in the United States is 7.8% of the population or 23.6 million people (2007 estimate) and is increasing. Of these cases, 5.7 million are undiagnosed (Centers for Disease Control and Prevention [CDC], 2007). Cases of type 2 diabetes in the United States are steadily increasing. In the 12 years from 1990 to 2002, the prevalence of diagnosed diabetes doubled (CDC, 2004b). Data from 2007 indicate that 57 million adults age 20 years and older qualify as prediabetic, that is, they have fasting glucose levels that are elevated but still below the threshold for a diagnosis of diabetes (CDC, 2007). The increasing prevalence of diabetes is

due to a wide variety of causes, with the obesity epidemic and an aging population heading the list. Although population-based prevalence data are lacking, statistics indicate that type 2 diabetes is on the rise among Americans 10 to 19 years old (American Academy of Pediatrics, 2009). An increase in type 2 diabetes is expected, with an estimated 7% of adolescents in the United States meeting criteria of prediabetes (CDC, 2007). These data lay the foundation for future research into the causative factors and lifetime risk of diabetes.

Using the Behavioral Risk Factor Surveillance System (BRFSS), a national survey database, the CDC (2003) estimated a 12.7% prevalence of patients with diabetes who had a history of foot ulcers. In the BRFSS, foot ulcers are defined as "any sores or irritations on the feet that took greater than 4 weeks to heal." Reiber et al (1995) estimated a slightly higher 15% to 20% prevalence of diabetic foot ulcers during the lifetime of a patient with diabetes. Within a given year, the incidence of patients with diabetes who develop foot ulcers ranges from 1.0% to 4.1%, with a potential lifetime risk of 25% (Abbott et al, 2002; Muller et al, 2002; Singh et al, 2005).

Foot ulcers precede lower extremity amputations in 85% of cases (Larsson et al, 1998; Pecoraro et al, 1990). The leading nontraumatic cause of lower extremity amputations in the United States is attributed to diabetes. Of all the nontraumatic amputations in the United States, 50% to 75% are caused by diabetic foot ulcers (CDC, 2001). The national average annual incidence of

Copyright © 2011, Elsevier Inc.

patients with diabetes having a lower extremity amputation was approximately 4.8 per 1,000 (age-adjusted) for the year 2005 (CDC, 2008a).

After decades of steady increase, the percentage of amputations in the diabetic population compared to total amputations appears to be decreasing. Department of Veterans Affairs data show that in 1986, 59% of all amputations were because of diabetes. In 1998, 66% of all amputations were because of diabetes (Mayfield et al, 2000). In 1997 the total number of lower extremity amputations for patients with diabetes in the United States peaked at 84,000 (excluding military health care facilities), and the total figure remained above 80,000 annually until 2001 and then dropped to 71,000 in 2005 (CDC, 2004a, 2008b). Presumably, advancements in therapeutic modalities and diagnostics, implementation of multidisciplinary teams, and advanced wound care have supported this downtrend. Although overall lower extremity amputation rates are declining, they continue to rise with patient age (CDC, 2008c). The rate of lower extremity amputation for patients with diabetes is 28 times greater than for individuals without diabetes. Furthermore, amputation of the contralateral limb within 2 to 3 years is 50% to 84%, although implementation of a multidisciplinary foot care service has been shown to lower contralateral amputation rates to as low as 7% and to lower the odds ratio for lower extremity amputation in diabetics compared to nondiabetics (Van Gils et al, 1999). Driver et al (2005) reported an 82% reduction in amputations using a multidisciplinary approach, despite a 48% increase in diagnosed diabetics receiving treatment. Three years after a patient with diabetes has a lower extremity amputation, the mortality rate is 20% to 50% (Reiber et al, 1995). Five-year survival rates among patients with diabetes who undergo above-knee and below-knee amputations were as low as 28% (Aulivola et al, 2004).

Economic Burden

The economic burden of diabetes in the United States is enormous and is growing. Direct medical and indirect expenditures due to diabetes in 2007 were estimated to be $174 billion (CDC, 2007). Lower extremity amputations in patients with diabetes and their consequences represent a significant portion of these costs (not to mention the cost in quality of life). Using 1992 to 1995 data from a private health maintenance organization, Ramsey et al (1999) estimated the 2-year medical costs for a middle-aged man with a diabetic foot ulcer to be $27,900. Using Medicare data from 1995 to 1996, Harrington et al (2000), found a 20-week healing rate for diabetic foot ulcers to be only 31% and estimated the annual cost for lower extremity ulcer treatment in patients with diabetes to be $15,300, with 74% of the costs from inpatient charges.

The cost of care increases significantly when a diabetic foot ulcer proceeds to amputation. Using 2001 costs, the total event cost ranges from $23,700 for a toe amputation to $51,300 for an above-the-knee amputation (Gordois et al, 2003). An earlier, comprehensive study of amputation costs from Sweden that includes all inpatient, outpatient, and home care costs over a 3-year period estimated a cost of $43,100 for a minor amputation and $63,100 for a major amputation (Apelqvist et al, 1995). Shearer et al (2003) reported that the cost to treat an uninfected foot ulcer was $775.00 per month, increasing to $2,049.00 per month for an ulcer with cellulitis and $3,798.00 for an ulcer with osteomyelitis. Driver et al (2005) found that hospitalizations involving osteomyelitis were 2.5 times more expensive as those with no infection. Economic data support early identification and intervention of diabetic foot ulcers to prevent not only amputations but also the vast increases in costs associated with recurring infections, comorbid disease progression, and hard-to-close wounds (ADA, 2003a).

PATHOGENESIS

The origin and development of a diabetic foot ulcer have several components. An in-depth causal pathway study with two patient cohorts from different parts of the world identified 32 unique causal pathways for developing foot ulcers. The study found three components present in the majority (63%) of the identified pathways: peripheral neuropathy, structural foot problems, and minor trauma (Reiber et al, 1999). In another study, peripheral neuropathy was the major contributing factor leading to the development of 90% of all foot ulcers (Boulton, 1994). The risk of developing a diabetic foot ulcer is seven times more likely in diabetic patients with neuropathy than in their nonneuropathic counterparts (Rathur and Boulton, 2007). Other less prevalent causes were edema, callus, and peripheral ischemia resulting from PAD. Diabetics with PAD have been shown to have more distal disease coupled with poorer mortality and amputation outcomes than nondiabetic patients (Jude et al, 2001; Rathur and Boulton, 2007). Although infection is a common factor (59%) associated with lower extremity amputation in the patient with diabetes, it is not a common cause leading to diabetic foot ulcers (Pecoraro et al, 1990).

Neuropathy

Peripheral neuropathy is involved in 78% of diabetic foot ulcers (Reiber et al, 1999). The incidence of neuropathy in patients with diabetes appears to be linked to the duration of diabetes and, to some extent, to glycemic control. Prospective studies comparing patients with standard versus those with tighter control of blood glucose have shown that patients with better glucose control have better nerve conduction velocity as well as less retinopathy and nephropathy (Diabetes Control and Complications Research Group, 1993). Lowering hemoglobin A_{1c} values have been shown to decrease the neuropathic and micro-vascular complications of diabetes (American Diabetes Association [ADA], 2007). The exact etiology of peripheral neuropathy is unknown but likely is the result of metabolic events, including accrual of glucose, sorbitol, and fructose, reduction in myoinositol (needed for nerve conduction), and nerve ischemia due to reduction in the number and diameter of vessels in the vasa nervosum (Levin, 2002). The predominant structural mechanism affected by the various metabolic components may be the microvascular component. Under normal conditions the arteriole-venule (AV) shunts in the sole of the foot are closed, and blood flows through the nutrient capillaries (capillary dermal papillae loops). With diabetic neuropathy a decrease in the sympathetic innervation of the highly innervated AV shunts results in a greater dilation in the arterioles, which leads to a shunting away of blood from the capillary dermal papillae loops. This results in lower skin temperature and a decrease in transcutaneous oxygen tension at the skin. Theoretically the metabolic components may be reversible, but structural component changes (shunting) apparently cannot be undone once changed (Tanneberg and Donofrio, 2008). However, recent advances and several randomized clinical trials in various areas of gene therapy and angiogenesis show promise in changing this long-standing convention and expanding our insight into the disease process (Driver and LeBretton, 2008). A more detailed explanation of the many etiologic pathways that lead to diabetic neuropathy is beyond the scope of this chapter.

Neuropathy can be either focal or diffuse. *Focal neuropathies* can be divided into ischemic and entrapment types. *Focal ischemic neuropathies* are caused by an acute event to the nerves. Examples include cranial and femoral neuropathies. These types of neuropathy are characterized by sudden onset and are asymmetric in distribution. *Focal entrapment neuropathies* occur when a nerve is compressed in a specific area of the body. These neuropathies tend to be more progressive in development and are also often asymmetrically located. Examples include carpal tunnel syndrome and tarsal tunnel syndrome.

Diffuse neuropathies can be divided into *distal symmetric polyneuropathy,* which includes motor and sensory neuropathies, and *autonomic neuropathy* (Tanneberg and Donofrio, 2008). Diffuse neuropathies are caused by abnormal structural, vascular, and metabolic conditions. They have a symmetric distribution and are progressive in nature. Diffuse neuropathies are the type encountered frequently in patients with diabetes.

Neuropathy is a frequent risk factor for diabetic foot ulcers and can include (1) sensory nerves (controlling sensation), (2) motor nerves (controlling musculature), and (3) autonomic nerves (controlling functions, e.g., sweating and oil production, vascular flow, and heart rate) (Sumpio, 2000; Tanneberg and Donofrio, 2008). Sensory, motor, and autonomic neuropathies represent the most common complications affecting the lower extremities of patients with diabetes (Mulder et al, 2003). Although diabetes is the most common cause of lower extremity neuropathy, other well-defined causes include uremia, acquired immunodeficiency syndrome (AIDS), nutritional deficiencies, nerve compression, trauma, fractures, prolonged use of crutches, tumors, radiation and cold exposure, certain medicines, systemic lupus erythematosus, and rheumatoid arthritis (National Institute of Neurological Disorders and Stroke [NINDS], 2003).

Sensory and Motor Neuropathy. Sensory and motor neuropathies are grouped under the frequently cited category of "peripheral neuropathy" rather than distal symmetric polyneuropathy. The vast peripheral nervous system connects the nerves running from the brain and spinal cord (the central nervous system) and transmits information to the rest of the body (arms, legs, hands, feet). This distal and dying-back progression of neuropathy is often referred to as a "stocking and glove" pattern.

In *sensory neuropathy* the loss of protective sensation leads to a lack of awareness of pain and temperature change, resulting in increased susceptibility to injury. However, the eventual lack of pain awareness is generally preceded by 8 to 10 years of painful neuropathy. Persons with this condition will have worse pain at night, and relief will come from movement rather than rest (Tanneberg and Donofrio, 2008). Once the painful phase ends, minor trauma caused by poor-fitting shoes or an acute injury can precipitate a chronic ulcer. Patients may not realize they have a foot wound for some time because of lack of sensation in their feet. The loss of pain sensation can reach to the knees.

Motor neuropathy affects the muscles required for normal foot movement and can result in muscle atrophy. The distal motor nerves are the most commonly affected and cause atrophy of the small intrinsic muscles of the foot. Often the wasting of the lumbrical and interosseous muscles of the foot will result in collapse of the arch (Sumpio, 2000). Cocked-up or claw toes, hammer toes (Figure 14-1), and weight redistribution from the toes to the metatarsal heads lead to increased pressures and subsequent ulceration (Levin, 2002). Generally, patients with diabetes develop both kinds of distal symmetric polyneuropathy (Sumpio, 2000).

Autonomic Neuropathy. Autonomic neuropathy—a disease of the involuntary nervous system—can affect a wide range of organ systems throughout the body. Diabetic autonomic neuropathy frequently coexists with other peripheral neuropathies and other diabetic complications (Vinik et al, 2003). Autonomic neuropathy results in decreased sweating and oil production, loss of skin temperature regulation, and abnormal blood flow in the soles of the feet. The resulting xerosis can precipitate fissures, cracks, callus, and finally ulceration (Mulder et al, 2003; Tanneberg and Donofrio, 2008).

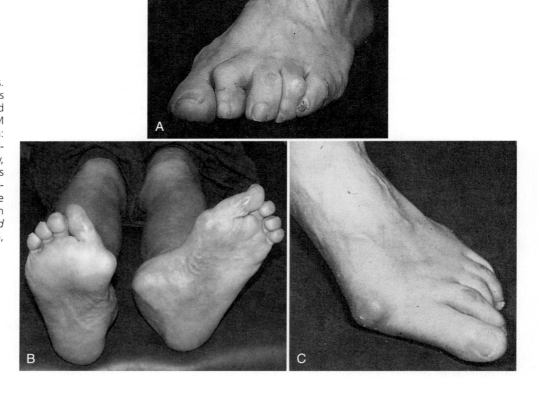

FIGURE 14-1 A, Hammer toes. **B,** Charcot foot. **C,** Hallux valgus (lateral deviation of hallux) and bunions. (**A, C** From Seidel HM et al, editors: Blood vessels. In: *Mosby's guide to physical examination,* ed 6, St. Louis, 2006, Mosby, Elsevier Science. Courtesy Charles W. Bradley, DPM, MPA, and Caroline Harvey, DPM, California College of Podiatric Medicine. **B** From Bowker JH, Pfeifer MA: *Levin and O'Neal's the diabetic foot,* ed 6, St. Louis, 2001, Mosby.)

Musculoskeletal Abnormalities

Foot deformities (Table 14-1) are very common in patients with diabetes and peripheral neuropathy and lead to focal areas of high pressure. These deformities are also associated with thinning of the fat pad under the metatarsal heads. Diabetic foot ulcers generally result from repetitive stress on "hot spots" that develop from bone deformities and/or callus buildup (Levin, 2002). The areas at the top of the toes, the tips of the toes, under the metatarsal heads, and the heels are vulnerable to ulceration and infection. Atrophied or dislocated fat pads beneath the metatarsal heads increase the pressure under them. This situation can lead to skin loss or callus development and increases the risk of ulceration (Sumpio, 2000). A 28% incidence of ulcers among neuropathic patients with elevated plantar pressures has been observed compared to patients with normal plantar pressures. Notably, no ulcers were observed in the normal pressure group (Boulton, 2004).

Associated callus can increase foot pressure by as much as 30% (Young et al, 1992). Callus presence has been associated with a 77-fold increase in ulceration in one cross-sectional study. Further follow-up data showed that plantar ulcers in neuropathic patients formed only at callus sites, suggesting an infinite risk for ulcer development (Murray et al, 1996). In the absence of neuropathy, the patient can feel the presence of a fissure, blister, or bony prominence and will take corrective action. However, with neuropathy the protective response is diminished or

TABLE 14-1	Brief Descriptions for Selected Foot Malformations
Malformation	**Characteristics**
Plantar fasciitis	Heel pain caused by inflammation of long band of connective tissue running from calcaneus to ball of foot
Heel spurs	Bony growths on underside, forepart of calcaneus bone; may lead to plantar fasciitis
Bunions (hallux valgus)	First joint of large metatarsal slants outward, with tip angling toward other toes; may lead to edema, tenderness
Hammer (claw) toes	Toes appear bent into claw-like position, often seen in second metatarsal when bunion slants large metatarsal toward and under it
Neuromas	Enlarged, benign growths of nerves, most commonly between third and fourth toes; caused by bones or other tissue rubbing against and irritating the nerves
Charcot arthropathy	Disruption or disintegration of some foot and ankle joints; frequently associated with diabetes, resulting in erythema, edema, deformity
Pes cavus	High arch or instep
Pes covus	Flat foot

even nonexistent. Thus foot ulcers can get progressively worse before any action is taken. Individuals with diabetic neuropathy have been known to walk around for days in shoes containing shoehorns. Abnormalities in foot biomechanics from the previously described deformities and possible ulceration often cause a dysfunctional gait, which leads to further damage to the structure of the foot.

Ankle Joint Equinus. Ankle joint equinus, defined as less than 0 degrees of ankle joint dorsiflexion, occurs in some patients with peripheral neuropathy. With ankle joint equinus the range of motion of the foot joint becomes limited, which increases pressure on the sole of the foot (Caselli et al, 2002). Of all patients with diabetes, 10.3% develop ankle joint equinus; this risk increases with duration of disease (Lavery et al, 2002). High plantar pressures from ankle equinus can increase the incidence of ulceration in patients with diabetes (Caselli et al, 2002).

Charcot Foot. Charcot foot or Charcot neuroarthropathy (or arthropathy) is a classic and increasingly common diabetic foot deformity affecting nearly 10% of diabetics with neuropathy and greater than 16% of those with a history of neuropathic ulcer (Reiber et al, 1995). Lavery et al (2003) found the incidence of Charcot arthropathy for non-Hispanic whites with diabetes to be 11.7 per 1,000 per year. A long duration of diabetes is an important factor in the development of Charcot neuroarthropathy; greater than 80% of patients with Charcot foot had diabetes for more than 10 years (Cofield et al, 1983).

The precise neural mechanism causing Charcot foot is unknown, and a number of different theories have been proposed to explain the underlying etiology (Yu and Hudson, 2002). Despite conventional thinking that many diabetic lower extremities are ischemic, overwhelming evidence indicates that many patients with diabetic neuropathy have increased blood and pooling in their feet. This condition has been directly correlated with decreased bone density in Charcot foot, possibly as a result of autonomic neuropathy. Charcot foot may well be due to a combination of neurotraumatic and neurovascular mechanisms (Yu and Hudson, 2002).

Progression of Charcot disease is divided into three radiographically different stages: development, coalescence, and reconstruction. *Development* represents the acute, destructive phase characterized by joint effusions, edema, subluxation, formation of bone and cartilage debris, intraarticular fractures, and bone fragmentation. This period is often initiated by minor trauma and is aggravated by persistent ambulation. The second stage, *coalescence,* is marked by a reduction in edema, absorption of fine debris, and healing of fractures. The final phase of bone healing is *reconstruction,* in which further repair and remodeling of bones takes place along with fusion and rounding of large bone fragments and decreased joint mobility. Early diagnosis and treatment (i.e., offloading) in the development stage are critical in the treatment of this disease (Sanders and Frykberg, 2008).

The Charcot foot is prone to increased pressures because of its deformity and possible bone or joint collapse. The patient with Charcot neuroarthropathy is four times more likely to develop a foot ulcer (Jeffcoate and Harding, 2003; Yu and Hudson, 2002).

Peripheral Arterial Disease

PAD is a major risk factor for lower extremity amputation, particularly in patients who have diabetes, because the accompanying inadequate oxygenation and perfusion of tissues significantly impair wound healing (see discussion of PAD in Chapter 11) (Mulder et al, 2003). In a comparison between patients with diabetes and patients without diabetes and PAD, patients with diabetes were five times more likely to have an amputation (Jude et al, 2001).

The incidence of ischemic diabetic foot ulcers is relatively low. However, because more than half of people with PAD are asymptomatic, determining the true prevalence in patients with diabetes is difficult. Peripheral ischemia was present in 35% of ulcerations in a two-center causal pathway study (Reiber et al, 1999). Oyibo et al (2002) found that 11% of diabetic foot ulcers were ischemic (52.3% neuroischemic, 36% neuropathic). In contrast, a study from England found that only 16% of new diabetic foot ulcers were ischemic (24% neuroischemic). Incongruence in ulcer classification rates could indicate greater awareness spawned by the advent of multidisciplinary teams (Rathur and Boulton, 2007) as well as improvements in classification and stratification of ulcer presentation as diagnostic technology, research, and our understanding of causative factors continue to advance. Although ischemic foot ulcers are relatively less common than neuropathic or neuroischemic diabetic foot ulcers, they are more serious and lead to higher rates of amputation in patients with diabetes who do not have peripheral neuropathy (Moulik et al, 2003). Amputations of lower extremities in patients with diabetes are almost always due to multiple causes, including ischemia, infection, and neuropathy. Van Gils et al. (1999) found that 55% of amputations required within a high-risk foot clinic were due to the combination of ischemia and infection. Their study supported the findings of Prompers et al (2008), who showed a negative healing impact of infection among patients with PAD and infection compared to patients with infections and no PAD. Additionally, infection was the only predictor of healing in patients with PAD.

Relatively little is known about the biology of PAD in patients with diabetes; however, it is thought to be similar to other manifestations of atherosclerotic disease, such as coronary artery disease and carotid artery disease (ADA, 2003b). Seventy percent of deaths among type 2 diabetics can be attributed to vascular disease (National Diabetes Advisory Board, 1983). PAD typically results from gradual diameter reduction of the lower extremity arteries and from the progression of atherosclerotic changes in arterial circulation in the lower extremities. Endothelial injury and resulting endothelial dysfunction occur in the earliest stages of the disease. The endothelial surface can be injured by various means, including hyperlipidemia and diabetes (Levy, 2002). The atherosclerotic plaque that develops in the patient with diabetes and PAD is no different than the plaque that develops in the patient without diabetes (Levin, 2002). The pattern of PAD in patients with diabetes is such that medium-size arteries, mainly at the popliteal trifurcation, are affected. However, distal pedal vessels are spared (Steed et al, 2006).

Microvascular tissue perfusion, in contrast to macrocirculation, may present problems for patients with diabetes. Whereas PAD in persons with diabetes normally spares the small pedal arteries, microcirculation abnormalities in the foot as a result of neuropathy are common. Diabetic neuropathy impairs the nerve axon reflex and causes local vasodilation in response to a painful stimulus. The impaired vasodilation in diabetic neuropathic lower extremities can create a functional ischemia.

ASSESSMENT

The components of assessment for any patient with signs or symptoms of LEND include the patient history and risk factors, physical examination, and simple noninvasive tests. Select patients may require more complex studies. Appendix B contains an example of an assessment form for patients with lower extremity ulcers.

Patient History

The patient history includes general state of health, a record of diabetic complications and treatments, walking difficulties, shoe problems, pain in the extremity, medications (prescribed and over-the-counter), glycosylated hemoglobin level, and risk factors for LEND and diabetic foot ulcers. Because diabetic foot ulcers can occur as a consequence of neuropathy and lower extremity arterial disease (LEAD), specific questions regarding any LEAD risk factors should be posed (see Box 11-1).

Risk Factors. A number of studies have quantified the relative significance of various risk factors associated with the presence of foot ulceration. Lavery et al (1998) found that the risk of ulceration increases dramatically based on the number and type of risk factor associated with a patient with diabetes. They found the following increases in relative risk:

- 1.7 in persons with peripheral neuropathy
- 12.1 in persons with peripheral neuropathy *and* foot deformity
- 36.4 in persons with peripheral neuropathy, foot deformity, *and* a history of previous amputation

In a large multicenter study that lasted 30 months, Pham et al (2000) analyzed the incidence of new foot ulceration in patients with diabetes and various measurable risk factors. Of the patients enrolled in their study, 29% developed one or more foot ulcers over the 30-month period (a very high incidence). Nearly all (99%) of these patients had a high neuropathy disability score and/or a poor score on the Semmes-Weinstein monofilament examination for sensation. Additional factors that yielded a statistically significant odds ratio for foot ulceration during the study include the following:

- Gender (male)
- Ethnic background (Native American)
- Duration of diabetes (long)
- Palpable pulses
- History of foot ulceration
- High vibration threshold score
- High foot pressures

Foot ulcers often have a multifactorial etiology. Although the earlier studies list the most commonly associated risk factors, the clinician must recognize many other risk factors in order to comprehensively assess a patient. Box 14-1 contains a list of the most commonly recognized risk factors for ulceration (Abbott et al, 2002; Lavery et al, 1998). As with the presence of infection, vascular insufficiency has a much more important role in delaying wound healing and subsequent amputation than as a risk factor contributing to ulceration (Lavery et al, 1998).

Classification of Risk. Many specialized foot treatment clinics use a foot risk classification system for patients with diabetes to allocate resources such as therapeutic shoes, education, and frequency of clinic visits (Peters and Lavery, 2001). The International Working Group on the Diabetic Foot (Apelqvist et al, 1999) recommends the "international" system as listed in Box 14-2. Risk classification systems have been

---

BOX 14-1 | Diabetic Foot Ulcer Risk Factors

- Absence of protective sensation due to peripheral neuropathy
- Vascular insufficiency
- Structural deformities and callus formation
- Autonomic neuropathy causing decreased sweating and dry feet
- Limited joint mobility
- Long duration of diabetes
- Long history of smoking
- Poor glucose control
- Obesity
- Impaired vision
- Past history of ulcer or amputation
- Male gender
- Increased age
- Ethnic background with high incidence of diabetes (e.g., Native American)
- Poor footwear inadequately protecting skin from high pressures

BOX 14-2	Foot Risk Classification by the International Working Group on the Diabetic Foot

Group 0: Patients have diabetes but no other risk factors
Group 1: Patients have both diabetes and neuropathy
Group 2: Patients have diabetes, neuropathy, vascular disease, and/ or foot deformities
Group 3: Patients have a history of foot ulcers or previous amputation and further specified as:
    Group 3A: Patients with history of foot ulcers
    Group 3B: Patients with previous amputation

shown to be very effective in predicting future diabetic foot ulcers (Lavery et al, 1998; Peters and Lavery, 2001). Additional risk classification systems are provided in Tables 14-2 and 14-3.

Lower Extremity and Foot Physical Examination

Chapter 10 describes how to conduct a comprehensive lower extremity assessment and should be carefully reviewed. The following section discusses the aspects of the lower extremity examination that are unique to the patient with LEND.

Protective Sensation. Screening for neuropathy can be done rapidly and reliably using a Semmes-Weinstein 5.07 (10-g) monofilament test or a vibration tuning fork test with the on–off method (ADA, 2007; Perkins et al, 2001). Biothesiometry expands on the traditional tuning fork, allowing for quantification of the vibration thresh-

old (Figure 14-2, *A*). An electric oscillator is applied to the traditional assessment landmarks (Figure 14-2, *B*) and "dialed in" until the patient is able to perceive the vibration (Figure 14-2, *C*). The value obtained can be used to follow the progression of neuropathy and qualify future assessment findings. As shown in Figure 14-3, the monofilament line used for the Semmes-Weinstein test is normally mounted on a rigid paper holder. The line has been standardized to deliver a 10-g force when pushed against an area of the foot. Regardless of which method is used, the patient should be placed in a room that is quiet and relaxed. Boxes 14-3 and 14-4 provide procedures for conducting these examinations.

Pain. A description of neuropathic pain is an important assessment parameter and may be specific to the disease state. In general, neuropathic pain varies in severity and is described as "burning," "tingling," "shooting," or "pins and needles." Activity can alleviate or exacerbate neuropathic pain. Because of the potential for LEAD, the patient should be assessed for ischemic pain (see Box 11-3). A comparison of pain characteristics of venous, arterial, and neuropathic wounds is given in Table 10-2. Chapters 25 and 26 provide a detailed discussion on the assessment and management of wound-related pain.

Musculoskeletal Abnormalities. Loss of motor nerve function affects the intrinsic foot muscles. When imbalances due to weakening of the intrinsic muscles occur, it can cause changes in foot structure and gait and muscle wasting. Plantar fat pads also become displaced, and the metatarsal heads become prominent. These changes may predispose the patient to ulceration. Each foot has 26 bones, 29 joints, and 42 muscles; thus there are

TABLE 14-2	Foot Risk Classification System and Management Considerations	
Low-Risk Diabetes	**Moderate-Risk Diabetes**	**High-Risk Diabetes**
Classification		
Intact sensation (neurologic)	Intact sensation (neurologic)	Absence of sensation (neurologic)
and/or	*and/or*	*and/or*
Intact pulses (vascular)	Intact pulses (vascular)	Absence of pulses (vascular)
Absence of foot deformities	Presence of foot deformities	Presence or absence of foot deformities
Management		
Education emphasizing disease control, proper shoe fit/design, daily self-inspection, early reporting of foot injuries or breaks in skin	Education emphasizing disease control, proper shoe fit/design, daily self-inspection, early reporting of foot injuries or breaks in skin	Education emphasizing disease control, proper shoe fit/design, daily self-inspection, early reporting of foot injuries or breaks in skin
Proper fitting/design footwear with orthotics as needed	Proper fitting/design footwear with orthotics as needed; depth-inlay footwear, molded/ modified orthosis may be required	May require modified or custom footwear
Annual follow-up for foot screening	Routine follow-up every 6 months for foot examination	Routine follow-up every 1–12 weeks for foot ulcer evaluation and callus/nail care
Follow as needed for skin/callus/nail care or orthosis	Referral to foot and ankle care specialist if deformity is causing pressure point and conservative measures fail	Referral to foot and ankle care specialist

Data from Driver VR, Madsen J, Goodman RA: Reducing amputation rates in patients with diabetes at a military medical center: the limb preservation service model, *Diabetes Care* 28(2):248-253, 2005.

TABLE 14-3	Lower Extremity Amputation Prevention Program (LEAP) and Management Categories for the Foot	
Risk Categories	**Definition**	**Management Categories**
0	No loss of protective sensation of the feet	Education emphasizing disease control, proper shoe fit/design Follow-up yearly for foot screen Follow as needed for skin, callus, nail care, or orthosis
1	Loss of protective sensation of the feet	Education emphasizing disease control, fit/design, daily inspection, skin/nail care, early reporting of foot injuries Proper fitting/design footwear with soft inserts/soles Routine follow-up every 3–6 months for foot/shoe examination and nail care
2	Loss of protective sensation of the feet with either high-pressure deformity or poor circulation	Education emphasizing disease control, proper shoe fit/design, daily inspection, skin/nail care, early reporting of foot injuries Depth-inlay footwear, molded/modified orthoses Modify shoes as needed; footwear with soft inserts/soles Routine follow-up every 1–3 months for foot/activity/footwear evaluation and callus/nail care
3	History of plantar ulcer or neuropathic fracture	Education emphasizing disease control, proper fitting footwear, daily inspection, skin/nail/callus care, early reporting of foot injuries Depth-inlay footwear, molded/modified orthoses; modified/custom footwear, ankle footwear orthoses as needed Routine follow-up every 1–12 weeks for foot/activity/footwear evaluation and callus/nail care

Note: "Loss of protective sensation" is assessed with a Semmes-Weinstein monofilament examination using a 5.07 monofilament at nine locations on each foot. Foot clinic visit frequency may vary based on individual patient needs.
From WOCN Society: *Guideline for management of wounds in patients with lower-extremity neuropathic disease,* WOCN Clinical Practice Guideline Series #3, Glenview, Ill, 2004.

numerous potential locations for problems. A few structural foot deformities are briefly described in Table 14-1. Figure 14-1 provides illustrations of selected structural foot deformities.

Claw, hammer, and mallet toes are signs of distal muscle atrophy and foot neuropathy. When muscles weaken, other muscles can overpower them, leading to contractures. *Hammer toe* is a contracture of the proximal joint, which is further from the front (or top) of the toe. *Mallet toe* refers to the distal joint, closer to the end of the toe, and is almost identical to hammer toe. When both joints are contracted, the condition is called *claw toe.* Prominent metatarsal heads occur if one of the metatarsal bones is longer or lower than its neighboring bones. This may lead to uneven weight distribution between the heads and subsequent pain, callus, and ulceration. Bunions are caused by an enlarged head of the first metatarsal bone just below the first toe joint (ADA, 2004a).

When changes in the gait or foot structure are observed, the patient should be referred for more testing. Patients with Charcot foot normally have a rocker-bottom foot that is hot, erythematous, and edematous with bounding pedal pulses and prominent veins (see Figure 14-1). Pain is normally, but not always, minimal in the early stages. The foot may be 10°F to 12°F warmer than the rest of the skin (Yu and Hudson, 2002). A history including an absence of trauma, a portal of entry for infection, or other signs of infection is suggestive of an acute Charcot foot (Levin, 2002).

Vascular Status. The coexisting calcification of arteries that occurs with diabetes and PAD leaves the blood vessels difficult to compress and therefore difficult to assess (Levin, 2002; Sumpio, 2000). When pulses cannot be palpated, use of a Doppler probe will allow the skilled examiner to determine whether pulses are triphasic, biphasic, or monophasic. The absence of pedal pulses despite the presence of popliteal pulses is a classic finding for patients with diabetes who also have PAD. If pedal pulses are not detectable with a Doppler device, a referral to a vascular specialist is warranted (Hopf et al, 2006).

In the absence of pedal pulses, additional noninvasive vascular tests may be conducted to obtain a better indication of the condition: (1) segmental pressures (i.e., taken at the thigh, calf, and ankle); (2) toe pressures; or (3) transcutaneous oxygen readings (Steed et al, 2006). Transcutaneous oximetry ($TcPO_2$) is an assessment of the microcirculatory system, which can be impaired in persons with diabetes and peripheral neuropathy. Zimny et al (2001a) found that patients with diabetes and neuropathy had significantly higher sitting to supine $TcPO_2$ differences than patients with diabetes only, indicating microcirculatory impairment.

Vasodilation in diabetic, neuropathic lower extremities can create a functional ischemia. Symptoms of impaired microcirculation are discussed in Chapters 10 and 11. Armstrong et al (2003a) showed that skin temperature is a poor indicator of vascular status, neuropathy, or future foot complications in patients with diabetes. The only

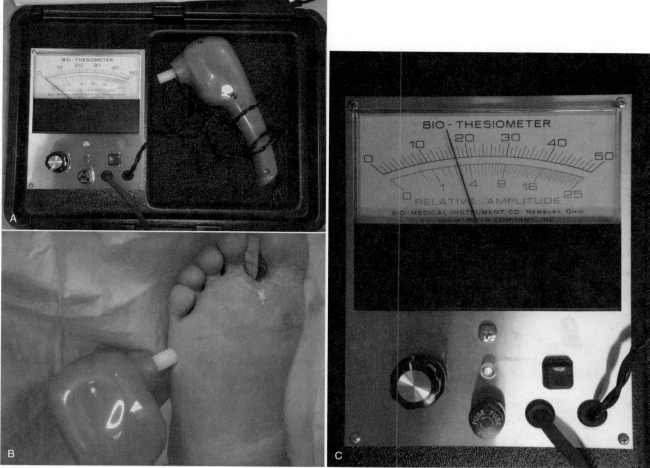

FIGURE 14-2 A, Biothesiometer. **B,** Application of biothesiometer oscillator head to patient's foot during peripheral neuropathy assessment. **C,** Oscillator amplitude knob to determine level of sensation. (Courtesy J. LeBretton and V. Driver.)

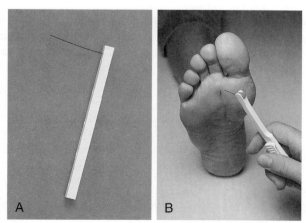

FIGURE 14-3 A, Monofilament. **B,** Press the monofilament against the skin hard enough so that it bends. (From Seidel HM et al, editors: Blood vessels. In: *Mosby's guide to physical examination,* ed 5, St. Louis, 2003, Mosby.)

BOX 14-3	**Procedure for Semmes-Weinstein 5.07 (10-g) Monofilament Examination (SWME)**

1. Explain procedure to patient.
2. Position patient in sitting position, resting patient's lower leg on examiner's lap.
3. Demonstrate monofilament on patient's hand so that he or she knows what to expect.
4. Explain to patient to that he or she should respond with a "yes" when he or she feels the filament touching the skin.
5. Have patient close his or her eyes. Sites to be tested should be shown on examination form.
6. Apply monofilament perpendicular to skin's surface. Apply sufficient force to cause the filament to buckle or bend. Use a smooth, not jabbing, motion.
7. Total duration of the approach, skin contact, and departure of filament from each site should be approximately 1–2 seconds.
8. Apply filament along margin of callus, ulcer, scar, and/or necrotic tissue; do *not* apply filament over these lesions.
9. Record and, if appropriate, map the results on examination form.

BOX 14-4	Procedure for Biothesiometry Examination (Amplitude of Vibration)

1. Explain procedure to patient.
2. Position patient in sitting position, resting patient's lower leg on examiner's lap.
3. Demonstrate oscillator on patient's hand so that he or she knows what to expect.
4. Explain to patient that he or she should respond with a "yes" when he or she feels the oscillator vibrating.
5. Have patient close his or her eyes. Sites to be tested should be shown on examination form.
6. Apply oscillator perpendicular to (flat against) skin's surface. Apply just enough force for the oscillator head to make total contact with skin. Use a smooth, not jabbing, motion.
7. The amplitude of the vibration should be slowly increased until the patient perceives the vibration and the value on the meter noted.
8. Apply oscillator along margin of callus, ulcer, scar, and/or necrotic tissue; do *not* apply oscillator over these lesions.
9. Record and, if appropriate, map the results on examination form.

significant association found in their study was higher skin temperatures in patients with Charcot arthropathy. However, a difference in skin temperature may be an indication of trauma, fracture, and/or infection. Skin temperature should be assessed in both feet using the back of the examiner's hand or an infrared temperature scanner.

Skin and Nail Condition. Skin and nail condition is an important component of the assessment for the patient with LEND. Descriptions of foot lesions and nail disorders are given in Chapter 15. Loss of sweating and oil production may cause cracking of the skin and fissures that can become infected. The presence of eczema, dermatitis, and/or psoriasis should be noted. The web spaces between the toes should be examined for moisture and/or fungal problems. The patient's skin condition should be documented and any corns, calluses, preulcerative lesions (e.g., blisters, hematomas), or open ulcers measured and drawn on the documentation form. If the patient has coexisting vascular disease, additional skin changes may be apparent. Table 10-3 lists characteristics of lower extremities and wounds in patients with LEAD, LEND, and LEVD.

Callus formation is a natural protective response to repetitive stress. It is characterized by thickened hyperkeratotic skin. The problem with this buildup is that accumulation of callus can increase pressure 25% to 30%, resulting in an ulcer below the callused area that is not visible to the examiner and/or is not palpable. Hemorrhage into a callus is a principal indicator of ulceration (Wound, Ostomy and Continence Nurse [WOCN] Society, 2004). A callus usually is painless but in some cases can cause pain because nerve endings close to the surface layers are irritated. Callus buildup is a

result of a biomechanical problem. Unless the underlying cause is eliminated, callus will continue to occur. Based on the duration and amount of pressure applied, the skin may eventually break down and an ulcer will develop.

Thickened nails are common. In addition, any abnormalities under the nail and any sign of nail infections should be noted. Nails bear the brunt of daily activities: running, walking, participating in sports, and just wearing shoes. When feet are abused and/or injured, a portion or all of the nail plate can be damaged. Repeated trauma, improper trimming, and minor injuries can result in nail problems. If the toe box is pressing down on the nails, bleeding may occur under the nail. Some nail disorders are hereditary. Ingrown toenails (onychocryptosis) may have a convex deformity. As pressure is exerted on the tissues, callus builds up. Nails that are red, brown, or black may indicate trauma (acute or chronic). Any discharge from around the nail or under the nail may indicate an infection process. Fungal infections are common. A nail that curves inward in the corners is called a *paronychia*. If present, remove nail polish to better view the nails.

Footwear

Evaluation of the patient's shoes is as important as taking a good history and/or examining the patient's feet. The majority of injuries to the foot are not recognized by the person with diabetes because of neuropathy. Most skin injuries on the foot of the person with diabetes are located on either the dorsal or the plantar surface. Many ulcers on the dorsum are located at sites of high pressure where the patient's footwear creates a lesion, implying a biomechanical etiology. Due to the lack of clinical outcome studies guiding practice, assessment of footwear should follow a logical progression, observing for pressure points, wear, and areas of friction. Checklist 14-1 outlines the items that should be investigated when evaluating the patient's shoes. Boxes 14-5 and 15-5 provide tips for appropriate footwear selection.

Foot Imprints (Harris Mat). Although a number of commercial devices exist for barefoot or in-shoe plantar pressure measurement, an inexpensive method that can be used to identify areas of increased pressure and

---

CHECKLIST 14-1

Items to Investigate When Evaluating Shoes in a Patient with Diabetes

- ✓ Bulges on outside of shoes
- ✓ Wear patterns on soles of shoes
- ✓ Wearing down on heels
- ✓ Worn lining inside shoes
- ✓ Shoe cushioning
- ✓ Foreign objects in shoes

BOX 14-5   Instructions for Care of Diabetic Feet

Inspection
- Inspect feet and toes daily for blisters, cuts, swelling, redness, and any other discolored areas. If you are unable to see the bottom of your feet, use a mirror.
- Look for dry areas and cracks in the skin.
- Apply a thin coat of lubricating oil after bathing.
- If your vision is impaired, have a family member inspect your feet daily and trim nails and buff calluses when required.

Bathing
- Wash your feet daily. Dry them carefully, including between the toes. Test the water with hands or elbow to ensure it will not burn your feet.
- Do not soak your feet. Soaking actually dries the skin by removing natural oil and can cause maceration (wrinkled appearance).
- Apply moisturizing cream to feet (but not between toes) after bathing.

Toenail Care
- Cut toenails after bathing, when they are soft and easier to trim.
- Never cut nails too short. Leave $\frac{1}{16}$ to $\frac{1}{8}$ inch of the nail. Nails should be cut straight across the top or shaped to follow the contour of the toe. Sharp edges should be filed smooth with an emery board to avoid cutting adjacent toes.
- Ingrown nails or other problematic nails should be cared for by a foot care provider.
- Avoid using sharp objects to clean under the toenail.

Corns and Calluses
- Do not use chemical corn or callus removers or corn pads. They can damage or burn the skin.
- When feet are dry, file away calluses with a pumice stone.
- Corns and calluses are a response to pressure from poorly fitting shoes. Change footwear to reduce these pressure "hotspots."
- Never use a razor blade yourself to reduce corns or calluses.

Shoes and Socks
- Wear clean socks every day. Avoid nylon socks as much as possible.
- Socks need to fit well, with no tight elastic at the top or seams.
- Do not walk barefoot, even in your home. Wear slippers with a rubber sole. Wear shoes and socks outside at all times.
- In winter, take special precautions to prevent foot damage from the cold.
- Inspect shoes for objects inside before you put them on.
- Buy shoes later in the day when feet are their largest. Do not depend on breaking in shoes.
- Shoes should be sufficiently wide for your feet and should have thick, flexible rubber soles, closed toes, and closed heels, as in running or walking shoes.
- Avoid pointed-toe shoes or boots. Do not wear sandals with strap between your toes.
- Wear new shoes for short periods each day, from 1–2 hours. Watch for signs of poor fit.

Circulation
- Do not smoke. If you do, stop!
- Exercise regularly.
- If your feet are cold, wear socks to keep your feet warm.
- Do not use a heating pad or hot water bottle.

---

unequal weight distribution of the patients' feet is the Harris mat (Tanneberg and Donofrio, 2008). The mat (foot imprint system) has two compartments. One side of the mat is inked. Paper is placed facing the inked surface. Two sheets are required; one for each foot. The inked side is closed, and the mat is reversed. The patient is asked to remove his or her shoes, leaving socks and/or hose on. The patient is asked to take a normal step down on the side that does not have ink. Stepping on the mat leaves an impression of the foot on the paper that indicates areas of high pressure and uneven weight distribution (Figure 14-4, *A*). Use of the mat identifies high-risk areas and is a good motivator for getting patients to wear their orthotics because they can see where problem areas exist.

Forefoot Test. The forefoot test shows patients how well their shoes fit their feet. First, have the patient remove his or her socks and/or hose. Instruct the patient to stand on a piece of paper with both feet. Trace the outline of both feet on the paper. Next, take the patient's shoes and just place the edge of the shoe over the traced outline. If any of the lines are visible, the shoes are too tight (see Figure 14-4, *B).* Again, this is a highly visual cue that helps the patient realize the importance of wearing shoes that fit his or her feet.

Diabetic Foot Ulcer Evaluation

The initial description of the foot ulcer is critical for mapping of its development during treatment. Detailed wound assessment and evaluation of healing are described in Chapter 6.

Characteristics. Common locations and causes of diabetic foot ulcers are listed in Table 14-4. Ulcers with a LEND etiology may resemble a laceration, puncture, or blister with a rounded or oblong shape. The wound base may be necrotic, pink, or pale, with well-defined, smooth edges and small-to-moderate amounts of serous or clear exudate. The periwound skin often presents with callus.

Diabetic Foot Ulcer with LEAD. Although ischemic foot ulcers are relatively less common than neuropathic or neuro-ischemic diabetic foot ulcers, they are more serious and lead to higher rates of amputation in patients with diabetes (Moulik et al, 2003). A comparison of the characteristics of neuropathic, arterial, and venous wounds is given in Table 10-3. Trophic changes for arterial disease alone are not diagnostic of arterial insufficiency and should be interpreted with caution. Characteristics of ischemic foot ulcers include pain, absence of bleeding, presence of an underlying deformity, or history

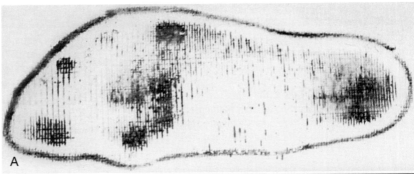

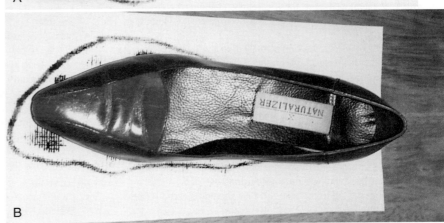

FIGURE 14-4 A, Example of Harris ink mat impression. **B,** Patient's shoe laid over traced image of foot. (Courtesy David M. Osterman.)

of a trauma (Sumpio, 2000). Ischemic ulcers on the dorsum are uncommon because perfusion usually is better and pressures are reduced at that location (Sumpio, 2000). Additional indicators of ischemia are discussed in detail in Chapter 11.

Diabetic Foot Ulcer Classification. Numerous diabetic ulcer classification systems have been reported in the literature (Lavery et al, 1996; Sims et al, 1988; Van Acker

TABLE 14-4	Common Lower Extremity Neuropathic Disease (LEND) Wound Sites and Causative Factors
Wound Site	**Causative Factor**
Toe interphalangeal joints	Limited interphalangeal joint flexibility
Metatarsal head	High pressure, limited joint flexibility
Interdigital	Increased moisture, footwear too narrow, toe crowding, deformity
Bunion sites	Footwear too narrow, foot deformity
Dorsal toes	Hammer or claw toe deformity, footwear too shallow in toe box
Distal toes	Poor arterial perfusion, external force, footwear too short
Midfoot (dorsal or plantar surface)	Charcot fracture, external trauma
Heels	Unrelieved pressure

From WOCN Society: *Guideline for management of wounds in patients with lower-extremity neuropathic disease,* WOCN Clinical Practice Guideline Series #3, Glenview, Ill, 2004.

et al; 2002; Wagner, 1981). These systems are useful for guiding treatment regimens, facilitating communication among care providers, predicting future outcomes, and conducting clinical trials. The various systems often include location, depth, necrotic characteristics, and presence of infection, ischemia, and/or neuropathy.

The widely used Wagner foot wound classification system divides foot ulcers into six grades based on the depth of the lesion and the presence of osteomyelitis or gangrene (Wagner, 1981). The Wagner system does not include presence of infection, ischemia, or neuropathy. The WOCN Society (2004) modified the Wagner system to address ischemia and infection (Table 14-5).

Another popular diabetic foot ulcer classification system, the University of Texas (UT) system (Table 14-6), utilizes a matrix structure with four grades of wound depth and four associated stages to specify ischemia, infection, both ischemia and infection, or neither (Lavery et al, 1996). The University of Texas system has been judged superior to the original Wagner system as a predictor of patient outcomes (Oyibo et al, 2001). Another system is the Size (Area and Depth) (SAD) classification system, which grades the wound according to area, depth, sepsis, quality of pulses, and accuracy of sensation (Table 14-7) (Macfarlane and Jeffcoate, 1999).

Infection. Infection rarely causes diabetic foot ulcers. Rather, ulcers provide a portal for the entry of pathogens, which often thrive because of the impaired host response of the person with diabetes (Steed et al, 2006). Infection is a causal component in 59% of

TABLE 14-5	Wagner Ulcer Classification System (Modified)*
Grade	**Description**
0	At-risk foot Preulcer No open lesions; skin intact May have deformities, erythematous areas of pressure or callus formation
1	Superficial ulcer Disruption of skin without extending into subcutaneous fat layer* Superficial infection with or without cellulitis may be present*
2	Full-thickness ulcer Penetrates through fat to tendon or joint capsule, without abscess or osteomyelitis
3	Deep ulcer that may probe to the bone, with abscess, osteomyelitis, or joint sepsis Includes deep plantar space infections or abscesses, necrotizing fasciitis, or tendon sheath infections*
4	Gangrene of geographic portion of foot (e.g., toes, forefoot, heel) Remainder of foot is salvageable but may be infected*
5	Gangrene of whole foot beyond salvage Required limb- or life-sparing amputation*

*Modification was added to the Wagner scale to identify ischemia and infection.
From WOCN Society: *Guideline for management of wounds in patients with lower-extremity neuropathic disease,* WOCN Clinical Practice Guideline Series #3, Glenview, Ill, 2004.

diabetic limb amputations (Pecoraro et al, 1990). In a Swedish study, Eneroth et al (1997) found that 42% of patients with diabetes who had deep foot infections required lower extremity amputations and 86% required surgery.

The person with diabetes is more prone to infection than is the person without diabetes (Shah and Hux, 2003), most likely due to impaired leukocyte function in patients with chronic hyperglycemia. However, infected diabetic foot wounds often are less symptomatic than nondiabetic wounds, exhibiting only subtle or even a complete absence of signs (Frykberg, 2003). Recalcitrant hyperglycemia may be the only clinical finding indicating a severe infection of a diabetic foot ulcer (Frykberg, 2002). The presence of probable infection needs to be noted during the initial examination, although culturing is best done after surgical debridement.

Wound culture technique is important to ensure surface colonies are not included and therefore confused with infection (see Chapter 16). Wound cultures should be taken by obtaining tissue from the debrided wound base or by aspirating pus. If swabs are the only option, ensure they are taken from the wound base after cleansing. The gold standard for infection assessment is the quantitative biopsy (Frykberg, 2003). Evaluation does not end after initial culturing. Wounds must be continually monitored for bacterial colonization.

Like the classification of diabetic foot ulcers in general, the classification of diabetic foot infections can be useful for determining appropriate treatment. Diabetic foot infections are subdivided into either non–limb-threatening or limb-threatening categories (Table 14-8), with the understanding that the latter classification can become life-threatening (ADA, 1999). Research indicates that stratification is warranted to distinguish wounds with vascular insufficiency from those without. Prompers et al (2008) suggest that diabetic foot ulcers with and without PAD be classified as different disease states due to vastly different predictors of healing between diabetic wounds with and those without concomitant PAD.

One of the most important assessments at this stage is wound depth and, more importantly, presence of osteomyelitis, which is surprisingly common. It is found in approximately 60% of moderate to severe diabetic foot ulcers (Eneroth et al, 1997). Bone biopsy gives a

TABLE 14-6	University of Texas at San Antonio Diabetic Wound Classification System			
	Grade			
Stage	**0**	**I**	**II**	**III**
A	Preulcerative or postulcerative lesion completely healed	Superficial wound not involving tendon, capsule, or bone	Wound penetrating to tendon or capsule	Wound penetrating to bone or joint
B	Preulcerative or postulcerative lesion completely epithelialized with infection	Superficial wound not involving tendon, capsule, or bone with infection	Wound penetrating to tendon or capsule with infection	Wound penetrating to bone or joint with infection
C	Preulcerative or postulcerative lesion completely epithelialized with ischemia	Superficial wound not involving tendon, capsule, or bone with ischemia	Wound penetrating to tendon or capsule with ischemia	Wound penetrating to bone or joint with ischemia
D	Preulcerative or postulcerative lesion completely epithelialized with infection and ischemia	Superficial wound not involving tendon, capsule, or bone with infection and ischemia	Wound penetrating to tendon or capsule with infection and ischemia	Wound penetrating to bone or joint with infection and ischemia

From Lavery LA, Armstrong DG, Harkless, LB: Classification of diabetic foot wounds, *J Foot Ankle Surg* 35:528, 1996.

TABLE 14-7	Size (Area and Depth) (SAD) Classification				
Grade	Area	Depth	Sepsis	Arteriopathy	Denervation
0	Skin intact	Skin intact	No infection	Pedal pulses palpable	SWMT (Semmes Weinstein monofilament test) Normal (see Box 14-3 for procedure) VPT normal
1	<10 mm²	Skin and subcutaneous tissue	Superficial slough or exudate	Diminution of both pulses or absence of one	Reduced or absent pinprick sensation VPT raised
2	10–30 mm²	Tendon, joint, capsule, periosteum	Cellulitis	Absence of both pedal pulses	Neuropathy dominant, palpable pedal pulses
3	>30 mm²	Bone and/or joint spaces	Osteomyelitis	Gangrene	Charcot foot

VPT, Vibration perception threshold.
From Macfarlane R, Jeffcoate W: Classification of diabetic foot ulcers: the size (area and depth) (SAD) system, *Diabetic Foot* 2(4):123, 1999.

TABLE 14-8	Signs of Limb-Threatening and Non–Limb-Threatening Diabetic Foot Infections
Non–Limb-Threatening	**Limb-Threatening**
Less than 2 cm of surrounding cellulitis	Greater than 2 cm of surrounding cellulitis
No systemic toxicity signs	Deep abscess or osteomyelitis, gangrene
No deep abscess, osteomyelitis, gangrene	

definitive diagnosis, but less invasive techniques are useful in establishing a diagnosis with a high degree of sensitivity and specificity. Appropriate diagnostic measures include probing the wound, serial X-ray films, magnetic resonance imaging, computed tomography, and radionuclide imaging (Steed et al, 2006). The ulcer normally is examined with a blunt sterile probe. Either direct exposure of bone or a positive "probe to bone" test is used to determine the presence of osteomyelitis (Steed et al, 2006). Probing can also detect sinus tract formations and undermining along the ulcer margins (Frykberg, 2002). X-ray studies are inexpensive, readily available, and useful for *excluding* an inflammatory process such as osteomyelitis. However, evidence of changes on X-ray films generally take about 2 weeks after bone infection, giving X-ray films a sensitivity of approximately 55% (Sinacore and Mueller, 2008). Magnetic resonance imaging offers high-resolution views not only of bone but also of soft tissue, has a sensitivity and specificity of greater than 90% and 80%, respectively, and, therefore, tends to be the diagnostic procedure of choice.

MANAGEMENT

The level of expertise and knowledge required to manage LEND and diabetic foot ulcers is constantly increasing. Because of the complex nature of diabetic foot ulcers and the numerous comorbidities that can occur in patients with diabetes, a multidisciplinary team approach to management is recommended (ADA 2007; Driver et al, 2005; Frykberg, 2002). An ideal foot care team should include the following: (1) podiatric/orthopedic surgeon; (2) vascular surgeon; (3) infectious disease specialist; (4) endocrinologist or family practice or internal medicine physician; (5) orthopedic/podiatric technician; (6) certified wound care nurse; (7) orthotist; and (8) certified diabetes educator. Numerous references from the U.S. and European literature document improvements in patient outcomes, including reduction of lower extremity amputation rates, as a result of implementing a multidisciplinary approach to diabetic foot care (Driver et al, 2005; Meltzer et al, 2002; Muller et al, 2002). Rates of avoidance of lower extremity amputation after implementation of a multidisciplinary team have been shown to be as high as 86.5% after 3 years and 83% after 5 years (Van Gils et al, 1999). However, health care providers frequently work in situations without this level and variety of expertise; thus patients with diabetes who develop a foot problem will often require referral to consultants. In fact, the standards of medical care in diabetes recommend the referral of high-risk patients to foot specialists for surveillance and preventative care (ADA, 2004b).

Diabetic neuropathy is associated with a reduced blood supply to the nerves, a microcirculatory network called the *vasa nervosum*. Currently, no prescription therapy in the United States is approved for treatment of the underlying process of microvascular damage that leads to diabetic peripheral neuropathy, although lowering of hemoglobin A_{1c} levels has been shown to decrease the microvascular complications of diabetes (ADA, 2007). Research has demonstrated that capillary vascular perfusion is inversely correlated with the degree of peripheral neuropathy (Nabuurs-Franssen et al, 2002). Nerve ischemia leads to poor nerve function. Based on earlier research in which certain prostacyclins (vasodilators) or their analogues gained approval for treatment of critical limb ischemia in Europe, Remodulin (United Therapeutics Corp.) is being tested in patients with diabetes and neuropathic ulcers. Preliminary results demonstrated that treatment significantly increased lower limb blood flow in these patients (Mohler et al, 2000).

Another new area of investigation for neuropathy treatment of the patient with diabetes involves the enzyme protein kinase C-beta (PKC-β). Current hypotheses concerning the pathogenesis of diabetic neuropathy suggest that PKC-β (which is stimulated by hyperglycemia) may be involved in the process that leads to microvascular dysfunction, impairment of endoneural blood flow, and damage of nerves (Vinik et al, 2003). The PKC-β inhibitor LY333531 (Eli Lilly) is currently being tested and has shown encouraging results in improving diabetic peripheral neuropathy (Litchy et al, 2002). Advancements in gene therapy have shown promise as potential treatments of diabetic complications such as neuropathy and neuropathic wounds, and research continues to broaden our understanding of the biochemical and molecular bases of diabetes and associated complications (Driver and LeBretton, 2008).

Early Intervention (Prevention)

Careful and frequent inspection of the diabetic foot is the most effective and least expensive method for preventing diabetic foot ulcers and possibly lower extremity amputations. Abnormalities, whether age related, structural, or pathologic, can be assessed and documented. The ADA (2007) recommends patients with diabetes undergo a comprehensive annual foot examination.

At least 50% of all amputations due to diabetic neuropathy are preventable with early intervention (Reiber et al, 1995). Given the life-altering and life-threatening risks associated with the development of a diabetic foot ulcer, it is incumbent upon the health care professional to identify patients with lower extremity peripheral neuropathy as early as possible so that preventive interventions can be implemented. Preventive interventions for the patient with LEND must become a routine that the patient incorporates into everyday life. Specific instructions concerning inspection of the foot, bathing, nail care, care of corns and calluses, shoes, socks, and circulation should be enforced in writing and verbally as outlined in Box 14-5. Clearly, one of the most important components of the clinician's role is providing patient education.

Using the patient's foot risk classification, a management plan (i.e., education, diagnostic studies, footwear recommendations, referrals, and follow-up visits) can be developed in order to minimize the odds of developing a foot ulcer (Driver, 2004). Tables 14-2 and 14-3 lists programs that correlate specific preventive interventions with each level of risk. Implementing these early interventions and adhering to preventive interventions (e.g., moisturizing the foot and inspecting the shoe before putting it on) address the first two principles of wound management (i.e., control or eliminate causative factors,

and provide systemic support to reduce existing and potential cofactors).

Glycemic Control

The prevalence of undiagnosed diabetes is approximately 24% of the total number of people in the United States with diabetes (CDC, 2007). A similar percentage of people admitted to the hospital for treatment also have undiagnosed diabetes. A study by Umpierrez et al (2002) documented that 31% of persons—with diabetes—admitted to an urban hospital had no known history of diabetes and were diagnosed during their stay.

Inadequate glycemic control is key in the development of neuropathy in the extremity of the person with diabetes (Steed et al, 2006). Hyperglycemia results in leukocyte dysfunction and suppression of lymphocytes, high blood pressure, and impaired endothelial function, among other dangers. Because of their impaired immune response, persons with hyperglycemia will respond poorly to a severe foot infection. Armstrong et al (1996) found that 56% of persons being admitted for diabetic foot infections had normal white blood cell counts. Improved blood glucose levels will increase the immune defenses of patients and thus should be a component of clinical care of infected diabetic foot ulcers. Elevated hemoglobin A_{1c} levels in a patient with diabetes who is infected may be the only sign alerting the provider to the problem (Frykberg, 2003). Thus patients with diabetes must be managed with a high index of suspicion for soft tissue infection, deep space infection, and osteomyelitis.

Offloading

Offloading and redistributing pressure is a basic principle involved in the prevention of foot ulcers and lower extremity amputations as well as the healing of existing diabetic foot ulcers. Numerous books, references, and websites discuss the various offloading modalities used for patients with diabetic foot ulcers or at risk for developing foot ulcers. Orthotists and pedorthists are frequently consulted for assistance in managing foot problems. Orthotists and pedorthists are trained specifically to make and fit orthopedic footwear (and other appliances) that can accommodate the patient with diabetes. Table 15-5 lists various methods and considerations for offloading the foot. Options for offloading include bed rest, wheelchairs, crutches, surgical shoes, custom sandals, healing shoes, cast shoes, and foam dressings (Steed et al, 2006). The following section discusses total contact casts, removable cast walkers, felted foam dressings, orthotics and orthopedic footwear, and surgical offloading procedures.

The total contact cast (TCC) has been shown to be very effective at relieving pressure and healing diabetic foot ulcers. The cast is designed to equalize pressure loading of the plantar surface by equal "total contact" of the plantar skin with the cast material (Figure 14-5). Repetitive injury to the wound site is reduced while the patient ambulates. Epidemiologic studies have shown that TCC healing rates are between 73% and 100%, with healing times between 30 and 63 days (Bus et al, 2008). A study of the histologic features of patients undergoing ulcerectomy after 20 days in a TCC versus patients undergoing ulcerectomy at presentation showed marked increases in granulation and angiogenesis in the TCC group (Piagessi et al, 2003). TCCs are absolutely contraindicated for patients with acute deep infection, sepsis, or gangrene. Relative contraindications include patients with ulcers with depth greater than width, fragile skin, or excessive edema; noncompliant patients; and those who would be unstable with a cast (Sinacore and Mueller, 2008).

A test of the effectiveness of TCCs, removable cast walkers (RCWs), and half-shoes in healing neuropathic diabetic foot ulcers demonstrated that patients with a TCC had significantly better healing rates at 12 weeks than did patients treated with the other two offloading modalities. Interestingly, patients with a TCC were significantly less active than were patients with half-shoes. No activity difference was noted between patients with the TCC and those with the RCW (Armstrong et al, 2001). Armstrong et al. (2003b) devised an activity test for patients with diabetic foot ulcers wearing RCWs. Total daily activity was recorded per patient. In addition, unbeknownst to patients, the daily activity of the RCW also was recorded. Results showed that patients wore the RCW only 28% of the time.

A study of 50 patients with neuropathic foot ulcerations compared healing rates of wounds offloaded with RCW to wounds offloaded with RCW wrapped with a cohesive bandage. Results showed that the wounds offloaded with the RCW wrapped with a cohesive bandage healed significantly sooner *(p = .02)* than did those with only the RCW, which could be removed more easily (Armstrong et al, 2005b). These studies suggest that pro-

tective footwear that is less easily removed may increase the odds of healing diabetic foot ulcers by increasing patient compliance. Interestingly, a 2008 study showed that only 1.7% of the 895 clinical respondents used a TCC as a treatment modality for diabetic foot ulcer, and 45.5% reported no use of a TCC. Patient tolerance and application requirements were the predominant reasons indicated for lack of TCC use (Wu et al, 2008).

Often described as a "poor man's TCC," the felted foam dressing (FFD) has been shown to provide the offloading benefits of a TCC while allowing appropriate management of patients with typical contraindications (Figure 14-6). A 2001 report from German researchers indicates that FFD reduces plantar loading at the ulcer site while allowing for daily dressing changes (Zimny et al, 2001b). Whether used as an adjunct to a surgical shoe, a healing shoe, or a walking splint, FFD has been found to be equally as effective as a TCC in time to healing and healing proportion (Birke et al, 2002). FFD requires less skill to apply and reduces or eliminates some of the inherent challenges and risks of TCC, such as limited assessment ability (Wu et al, 2008) and edema-related compromise. FFD helps to foster compliance levels while eliminating the bulk and relative immobility of TCCs. It also allows for direct offloading of a diabetic foot ulcer while permitting the use of orthotics to meet concurrent offloading needs. When felted foam is being applied, all edges must be beveled to prevent improper redistribution of forces (edge effect).

Customized orthotics include extra-depth shoes, PPT and Plastazote (foam) inserts, custom-molded foot beds, and molded orthotics such as the Charcot restraint orthotic walker (CROW) (Figure 14-7). Shoe modifications are the predominant method of pressure management in the patients with diabetes (Figure 14-8) (Wu et al, 2008). Patients who used a Plastazote arch filler in conjunction with an RCW showed healing of recalcitrant plantar ulcers within 4 months (Ritz et al, 1996). Patients who

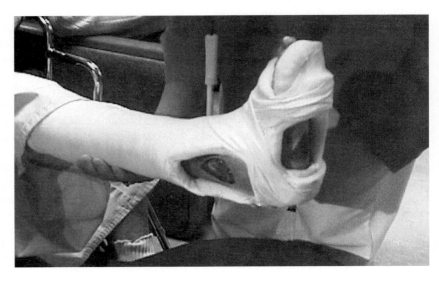

FIGURE 14-5 Modified total contact cast applied to offload pressure from neuropathic plantar ulcer that developed after prolonged use of a multipodus boot. A window around the wounds allows dressing changes without cast removal. The cutout portion of the cast is secured with self-adhering wrap. (Courtesy Ted Tomter, RN, CWOCN, St. Joseph's Candler Health System, Savannah, Ga.)

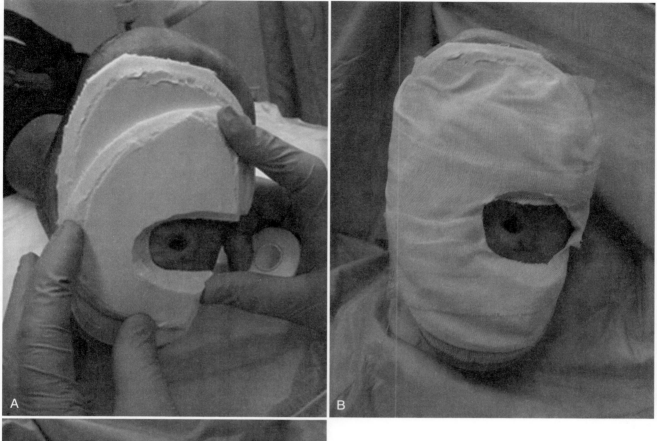

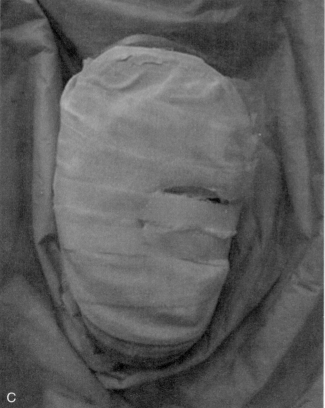

FIGURE 14-6 A, Felted foam applied to plantar aspect of foot to decrease loading forces directly over an ulcer. **B,** Foam secured in place using cloth mesh tape and rubber cement. A cutout is made in the tape to allow for dressing changes between office visits. **C,** Felted foam dressing with concurrent dressing applied. Gauze roll is used to further secure the dressing in place and then is covered in a sock or stockinette. (Courtesy J. LeBretton and V. Driver.)

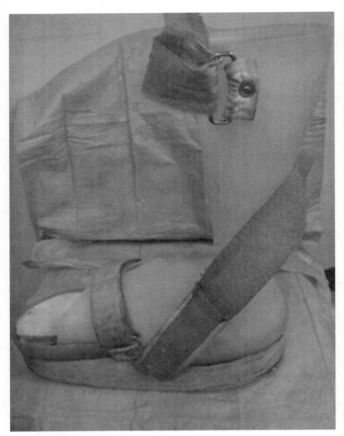

FIGURE 14-7 Customized removable offloading walker (Charcot Restraint Orthotic Walker) boot. (Courtesy J. LeBretton and V. Driver.)

used various foam inlays applied to their shoes and rocker-bottom outsoles demonstrated a reduction in peak plantar pressures (Praet and Louwerens, 2003).

Offloading can also be achieved with prophylactic and corrective surgical procedures such as Achilles tendon lengthening, sometimes referred to as tendo-Achilles

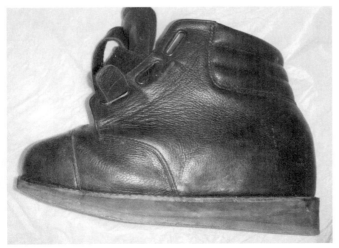

FIGURE 14-8 Custom-molded shoe for a transmetatarsal amputation. (Courtesy J. LeBretton and V. Driver.)

lengthening (TAL), joint arthroplasty, and excision or resection of bony prominences. Patients who may be considered for TAL include those with peripheral neuropathy and equinus contracture. Equinus causes high forefoot pressure that contributes to plantar surface ulceration (LaBorde, 2003). A randomized clinical trial of patients with plantar diabetic foot ulcers compared TCC with and TCC without TAL. The study showed that all ulcers in the TAL plus TCC group healed with a risk of recurrence that was 75% less at 7 months and 52% less at 2 years than in the TCC-only treatment group (Mueller et al, 2003). However, a follow-up to this study found that patients who had undergone the TAL plus TCC procedure had decreased physical functioning compared to the TCC-only patients after 8 months (Mueller et al, 2004). Although joint arthroplasty in combination with TCC showed no difference in healing proportions compared to TCC alone, significantly shorter healing time was observed in the arthroplasty group (Armstrong et al, 2003c; Lin et al, 2003). Metatarsal head resection has also been demonstrated to shorten healing time compared to a control group (Armstrong et al, 2005a). Increases in pressure in other areas of the foot have been observed with metatarsal head resection, necessitating a multidisciplinary approach and accommodative orthotics or other offloading to compensate for changes in pressure and to support prevention of new, recurrent, or recalcitrant ulceration.

Structural Foot Deformities. The traditional treatment for Charcot arthropathy (without ulceration) is cast immobilization. Few patients require surgery for this condition; however, exostectomy has been shown to be an appropriate method of treatment of Charcot prominences (Catanzariti et al, 2000) should nonsurgical interventions fail. Before immobilization, compression bandages are applied at weekly intervals until all edema has subsided. This period can last 2 to 3 weeks. A short non–weight-bearing cast is generally required for 12 to 16 weeks. The cast can be changed once or more times during this period. Gradual weight-bearing is started when the surface of the skin has returned to near-normal temperature (Yu and Hudson, 2002). Noninvasive bone stimulation such as electrostimulation can be a valuable adjunctive treatment of Charcot arthropathy (Grady et al, 2000). If edema and inflammation persist, administration of pamidronate is recommended to prevent further deterioration (Guis et al, 1999). Table 14-9 lists the healing phases of Charcot foot.

Wound Management

The principles of wound management and goals of topical therapy are described in Chapter 18. Jeffcoate and Harding (2003) listed the following priorities specifically for treating diabetic foot wounds: (1) aggressively treat infections; (2) establish whether ischemia is present and revascularization is required; (3) relieve pressure to the

TABLE 14-9	Healing Phases of Charcot Foot		
Clinical Presentation	Dissolution Phase	Coalescence Phase	Remodeling Phase
Edema	May be profound	Decreased	Decreased
Erythema	May be severe	Generally absent	Generally absent
Temperature compared to contralateral foot	May be increased 3°C to 7°C	Generally more than compared to 2°C increased	Generally less than compared to 2°C increased
X-ray image	May demonstrate fractures, dislocations, subluxations May not show abnormality during earliest acute phase of injury	May demonstrate early consolidation, formation of bone callus	Demonstrates consolidation stability

From WOCN Society: *Guideline for management of wounds in patients with lower-extremity neuropathic disease,* WOCN Clinical Practice Guideline Series #3, Glenview, Ill, 2004.

wound; and (4) improve the wound condition by debridement, dressings, and advanced care treatments where appropriate. Ultimately, the principal goal in the treatment of diabetic foot ulcers is wound closure.

Debridement and Callus Management. Wound and callus debridement is integral in the management of diabetic foot wounds. Key benefits of debridement in the diabetic wound include removal of free-living bacteria and biofilms, stimulation of growth factors, removal of senescent cells, and removal of hyperproliferative nonmigratory tissue (i.e., callus) (Steed et al, 2006). Serial debridement of wounds for the first 4 weeks of treatment has been shown to reduce median wound area by as much as 54% compared to wounds not undergoing serial debridement. Notably, this was the first study to evaluate healing rates and debridement across multiple chronic wound etiologies (Cardinal et al, 2009). Methods of debridement may change over time or may be performed in combination as conditions change. Debridement is repeated as often as needed, depending on the formation of new necrotic tissue. Weekly debridement is common and is generally referred to as *maintenance debridement* (Steed et al, 2006).

Hyperkeratotic callus buildup is frequently seen in the patient with diabetes due to the drying effects of autonomic dysfunction secondary to neuropathy and the natural response to repetitive minor trauma over pressure points. The callus development increases peak plantar pressures, fostering hematoma development and ulceration. A vicious circle is created in which high pressure causes callus buildup, which in turn leads to higher pressures and further callus development. Callus management is integral in the prevention and treatment of diabetic foot ulcer. Callus removal (see Plate 41) should be performed regularly and combined with effective orthotics or shoe modifications to better distribute pressures and prevent callus buildup. Supportive therapy, such as daily application of moisturizer, will assist in counteracting decreases in skin oil production seen in the patient with diabetes who has neuropathy.

Traditionally, callus has been removed by means of a scalpel or tissue nipper, but difficulty in smoothing the edges of the callus where tissue has been removed can result in areas of micropressure. Rotary files use a small drum covered with sandpaper or various burrs spun at rates of 1,000 to 3,000 rpm. Due to the high revolution, rotary files allow the skilled clinician to "shape" the callus (McLaughlin, 2008) rather than excise hyperkeratotic tissue, which can create minute pressure points and a potential portal of entry for infection. Removal of dry hyperkeratotic tissue decreases pressure and can reveal ulcerations and undermining of tissue under the callus that otherwise would not be visible.

When selecting a specific method of debridement of diabetic foot ulcers, many factors must be considered: pain, arterial insufficiency, antiembolic medications, patient setting, resources, characteristics of the wound, as well as the type of debridement. Methods of debridement and factors to consider for selection are discussed in detail in Chapter 17.

Considerations specific to patients with LEND and diabetic foot ulcers are highlighted by the ADA and the WOCN Society:

- Revascularization and surgical removal of necrotic tissue from an infected wound on an ischemic leg or foot is the treatment of choice for limb salvage.
- All ulcers with extensive cellulitis and/or osteomyelitis should be debrided and referred for pharmacologic (intravenous) intervention.
- Evidence supporting the use of whirlpool or pulsatile jet irrigation in neuropathic ulcers is insufficient.
- Caution must be exercised to prevent immersion burns from whirlpools because of reduced sensitivity in the neuropathic leg.
- Maintain dry, stable eschar on noninfected, ischemic, neuropathic wounds.

Infection. The assessment and treatment of infection is discussed in detail in Chapter 16. The classification of the infection, allergies, medical condition of the patient, and culture results (often not available initially) usually guide antibiotic therapy (Frykberg et al, 2000). The ADA (1999) cites categories of infection for the patient with diabetes as limb-threatening infections, non–limb-threatening infections, and osteomyelitis.

No antibiotics are recommended for the patient with an ulcer that is not clinically infected. However, remember that the patient with diabetes often does not show common symptoms of infection and thus must be monitored closely. Limb-threatening infections (see Table 14-9) require immediate hospitalization. Additional conditions of limb-threatening infections may include necrotizing fasciitis, ischemia, hyperglycemia, and leukocytosis (ADA, 1999; Eneroth et al, 1997; Frykberg, 2003).

Patients with non–limb-threatening infections require immediate antibiotic therapy, generally beginning the same day as the diagnosis is made. For mild and most moderate infections, therapy can be an oral agent, although certain patients may require parenteral therapy. Commonly used oral agents include cephalexin, clindamycin, levofloxacin, and amoxicillin/clavulanate. Trovafloxacin is appropriate for polymicrobial infections. Patients may be treated on an outpatient basis but only if certain criteria are met. Those who require surgical procedures, multiple diagnostic tests, or consultations or who are immunocompromised may be better treated and evaluated in a brief hospitalization.

Patients with limb-threatening infections need to be hospitalized and treated parenterally with antibiotics. Empirical therapy for these infections should be broad in spectrum, including aerobic, gram-positive, and gram-negative organisms as well as resistant organisms. Examples of antibiotic therapies include imipenem/cilastatin or vancomycin plus aztreonam plus metronidazole. Antibiotics should be reassessed when culture results are available.

Healing osteomyelitis with antibiotics alone is difficult but possible. Treatment usually lasts 6 weeks or more, often with 1 to 2 weeks of parenteral therapy. Infected bones that can be easily resected should be removed to speed recovery and reduce the need for antibiotic therapy (Steed et al, 2006). Additional regimens for treating diabetic foot infections can be found in the new international consensus guidelines for diagnosing and treating infected diabetic feet (Frykberg, 2003; Lipsky, 2004).

Methicillin-resistant *Staphylococcus aureus* (MRSA) and other resistant bacteria are a major new challenge in the treatment of diabetic foot ulcer infections (Frykberg, 2003). Using data from a multihospital study in the United States, Pfaller et al. (2001) reported that the percentage of MRSA of all *S. aureus* isolates increased from 22% to 34% from 1997 to 2000. Vancomycin (Vancocin HCl, Eli Lilly) or linezolid (Zyvox, Pfizer) is frequently prescribed for control of MRSA. Vancomycin-resistant *S. aureus* (VRSA), the evolution of MRSA in response to current practices in antibiotic therapy, has been reported (Tenover et al, 2004).

Topical Wound Care. Evidence does not support the use of one dressing over the other for the treatment of diabetic foot ulcers (WOCN Society, 2004). Topical therapy for diabetic foot ulcers is based on the principles outlined in Chapter 18, and a formulary of multiple dressing options will be necessary to meet the needs of the wound as its characteristics (e.g., size, depth, exudate) change.

The increase in bacterial resistance to antibiotics has changed how some clinicians view the use of topical antimicrobials. There is a lack of consensus on the use of topical antimicrobial therapy for infected or ischemic neuropathic ulcers (WOCN Society, 2004). A short course of a topical antimicrobial may be considered if the ulcer has a high level of bacteria (Steed et al, 2006; WOCN Society, 2004). However, wounds treated with topical antimicrobials can develop resistant organisms over time. Topical creams, ointments, and gels containing antimicrobials may also cause sensitivity reactions.

Advanced care has been described as "the use of drugs, devices, or treatment regimens that may be experimental, newly approved, or above and beyond treatment modalities routinely used in the general community for a specific medical problem." Advanced care may sometimes be the only means of rapidly and effectively attaining wound closure (Mulder et al, 2003). Diabetic foot ulcers that are limb threatening (based on ADA criteria) and require hospitalization, antibiotics, and debridement may not progress to this level (or any further) if early advanced care interventions are made. Early, advanced, or "appropriate" care practices may be more cost-effective than standard care practices in decreasing the incidence of lower extremity amputations (Apelqvist et al, 1995; Warriner and Driver, 2006).

When confronted with a wound that fails to progress, the clinician must carefully reevaluate the entire treatment plan to ensure appropriateness and should consider biopsy to rule out malignancy. If the biopsy result is negative and the management plan is appropriate, the most likely reason for failure to heal is the negative cellular environment of a chronic wound. In this case, the clinician should consider implementing an interactive wound therapy, that is, a product or therapy designed to convert the chronic wound environment into an environment that supports repair (Driver, 2004). Specific therapies that have shown varying degrees of success in the management of diabetic foot ulcers include contact and noncontact ultrasound technologies, regenerative tissue matrix, electrical stimulation, negative pressure wound therapy, hyperbaric oxygen therapy, angiogenic stimulators, and protease inhibitors (Cullen et al, 2002; Driver and Fabbi, 2009; Driver and LeBretton, 2008; Steed et al, 2006). These therapies are discussed in Chapters 18 through 24.

Pain Control

A variety of interventions can be used for the treatment of neuropathic pain; management of pain is presented in Chapter 26. In some cases, referral of the patient to a pain clinic and to neurologists for pain management may be necessary (WOCN Society, 2004).

Education

Basic knowledge assessment of patients with diabetes, regardless of the length of time since their diagnosis, often reveals a lack of understanding about the principles of diabetes self-management. Education must be relevant, simple, complete, and ongoing in order to assist the patient to achieve and maintain the highest possible level of functioning. However, education does not equal knowledge. Achieving understanding often requires presentation of material multiple times in different formats and by different health care team members.

Key components of the patient's education plan require behavioral change on the part of the patient, which can leave the patient feeling overwhelmed. The inability of the patient to follow through with a treatment plan should be carefully scrutinized and explored. The patient's behavior should not be assumed to be intentional, nor should the patient be erroneously labeled as "noncompliant," as many factors can contribute to an individual's ability to succeed or fail in the treatment plan. Key among these factors is expecting the patient to implement a therapy that he or she is physically unable to perform or that conflicts with another activity in his or her life. Probably the best advice to health care professionals was provided by Heisler et al. (2002), who stated that to facilitate patients' self-management, there is a need for a paradigm shift in the relations between provider and patients from directive to a more collaborative interactive style in which problems, treatment goals, and management stratagems are defined together. Strategies for achieving a sustainable plan are discussed further in Chapter 29.

Studies have documented the success of diabetes and foot care education in reducing the incidence of diabetic foot ulcers (Dargis et al, 1999; Ollendorf et al, 1998). However, many of the studies documenting success of educational efforts at reducing diabetic foot problems compared comprehensive programs that may not exist in more operational settings. In real-world situations, both patients and providers face significant challenges in the areas of diabetes and diabetic foot care education. A study in south Texas showed contextual factors such as time constraints, practice economics, and low reimbursement rather than physician knowledge and attitude affected caregivers' performance in delivering diabetes care education. The study also found that patients with a lower income had a decreased awareness of diabetic care principles (Larme and Pugh, 2001).

Appropriate measures should be implemented for patients who have limited mobility, cognitive problems, and visual difficulties. Other family members and/or friends can assist with visual assessments. Many patients diagnosed with diabetes participate in general diabetes self-management education programs through their primary health care provider (ADA, 2004a). Some clinics include a preexamination and a postexamination test on diabetes and foot care knowledge, providing an opportunity to build on the patient's knowledge base. The test is scored at the time of the visit, and the patient is told that the test will be repeated at the end of the visit.

It is imperative that patients understand the importance of daily foot examinations, the implications of losing protective sensation, their risk for ulceration and amputation, and the methods for minimizing or eliminating factors that place them at risk for ulceration and amputation. Box 14-5 provides an example of general foot care instructions that can be given to patients (Steed et al, 2006).

Teaching appropriate footwear selection is essential. All patients need to pay special attention to the fit and style of their shoes. Shoes need to fit the foot, so patients should avoid tight-fitting shoes, pointed-toe or open-toe shoes, flip-flops, and high heels. The shoes should be able to breathe; plastic shoes are inelastic and do not breathe. Finally, shoes should be adjustable with hook and loop closures, laces, and/or buckles. Shoes with soft insoles that cushion the feet may do well at reducing plantar pressure, but injury to the dorsum may result if the upper part of the shoes does not fit when the insole is inserted (Cavanagh and Ulbrecht, 2008).

SUMMARY

Peripheral neuropathy, structural foot problems, and minor trauma are the primary causative factors for a diabetic foot ulcer in the patient with LEND, and 25% of patients with a diabetic foot ulcer require lower extremity amputation. The ultimate goals of the care of the patient with LEND and a diabetic foot ulcer are to reduce the incidence of lower extremity amputations and to increase the frequency of minor or partial foot amputations as a percentage of all lower extremity amputations. A team approach is required for comprehensive management of the patient with LEND to adequately address the complex needs of this patient population: prevention of injury or trauma, frequent inspection, diligent daily foot care, education and support, and appropriate offloading (i.e., use of shoes and orthotics).

REFERENCES

Abbott CA et al: The North-West Diabetes Foot Care Study: incidence of, and risk factors for, new diabetic-foot ulceration in a community-based patient cohort, *Diabetes Med* 19(5):377-384, 2002.

American Academy of Pediatrics: *An update on type 2 diabetes in youth from the National Diabetes Education Program,* available at http://www.pediatrics.org/cgi/content/full/114/1/259, accessed February 23, 2009.

American Diabetes Association (ADA): Consensus Development Conference on Diabetic Foot Wound Care, 7-8 April 1999, Boston, Mass, *Diabetes Care* 22(8):1354-1360, 1999.

American Diabetes Association (ADA): Economic costs of diabetes in the U.S. in 2002, *Diabetes Care* 26(3):917-932, 2003a.

American Diabetes Association (ADA): Peripheral arterial disease in people with diabetes, *Diabetes Care* 26(12):3333-3341, 2003b.

American Diabetes Association (ADA): Preventative foot care in diabetes, *Diabetes Care* 27(Suppl 1):S63-S64, 2004a.

American Diabetes Association (ADA): Standards of medical care in diabetes, *Diabetes Care* 27(Suppl 1):S15-S35, 2004b.

American Diabetes Association (ADA): Standards of medical care in diabetes—2007, *Diabetes Care* 30(Suppl 1):S4-S41, 2007.

Apelqvist J et al: Long-term costs for foot ulcers in diabetic patients in a multidisciplinary setting, *Foot Ankle Int* 16:388-394, 1995.

Apelqvist J et al: International consensus on the diabetic foot. In: *The International Working Group on the Diabetic Foot*, Amsterdam, The Netherlands, 1999, John Wiley & Sons.

Armstrong DG et al: Value of white blood cell count with differential in the acute diabetic foot infection, *J Am Podiatr Med Assoc* 86(5):224-227, 1996.

Armstrong DG et al: Off-loading the diabetic foot wound: a randomized clinical trial, *Diabetes Care* 24(6):1019-1022, 2001.

Armstrong DG et al: Skin temperatures as a one-time screening tool do not predict future diabetic foot complications, *J Am Podiatr Med Assoc* 93(6):443-447, 2003a.

Armstrong DG et al: Activity patterns with diabetic foot ulceration: patients with active ulceration may not adhere to a standard pressure off-loading regimen, *Diabetes Care* 26(9):2595-2597, 2003b.

Armstrong DG et al: Clinical efficacy of the first metatarsophalangeal joint arthroplasty as a curative procedure for hallux interphalangeal joint wounds in patients with diabetes, *Diabetes Care* 26(12):3284-3287, 2003c.

Armstrong DG et al: Efficacy of fifth metatarsal head resection for treatment of chronic diabetic foot ulceration. *J Am Podiatr Med Assoc* 95(4):353-356, 2005a.

Armstrong DG et al: Evaluation of removable and irremovable cast walkers in the healing of diabetic foot wounds: a randomized controlled trial, *Diabetes Care* 28(3):551-554, 2005b.

Aulivola B et al: Major lower extremity amputation: outcome of a modern series, *Arch Surg* 139(4):395-399, 2004.

Birke JA et al: Comparison of forefoot ulcer healing using alternative off-loading methods in patients with diabetes mellitus, *Adv Skin Wound Care* 15(5):210-215, 2002.

Boulton AJM: The diabetic foot: of neuropathic aetiology? *Diabetes Care* 7:852-858, 1994.

Boulton AJM: Pressure and the diabetic foot: clinical science and offloading techniques, *Am J Surg* 187(5A):17S-24S, 2004.

Bus SA et al: The effectiveness of footwear and offloading interventions to prevent and heal foot ulcers and reduce plantar pressure in diabetes: a systematic review, *Diabetes Metab Res Rev* 24(Suppl 1):S162-S180, 2008.

Cardinal M et al: Serial surgical debridement: A retrospective study on clinical outcomes in chronic lower extremity wounds, *Wound Repair Regen*, 17(3):306-311, 2009.

Caselli A et al: The forefoot-to-rearfoot plantar pressure ratio is increased in severe diabetic neuropathy and can predict foot ulceration, *Diabetes Care* 25(6):1066-1071, 2002.

Catanzariti AR et al: Ostectomy for diabetic neuroarthropathy involving the midfoot, *J Foot Ankle Surg* 39(5):291-300, 2000.

Cavanagh PR, Ulbrecht JS: The biomechanics of the foot in diabetes mellitus. In: Bowker JH, Pfeiffer MA, editors: *Levin and O'Neal's the diabetic foot*, ed 7, St. Louis, 2008, Mosby.

Centers for Disease Control and Prevention (CDC): *National health interview survey*, Washington, DC, 2001, National Center for Health Statistics.

Centers for Disease Control and Prevention (CDC): History of foot ulcer among persons with diabetes—United States, 2000–2002, *MMWR Morb Mortal Wkly Rep* 52(45):1098-1102, 2003.

Centers for Disease Control and Prevention (CDC): *Data and trends, diabetes surveillance system. Nontraumatic lower extremity amputation with diabetes*, 2004a, available at http://www.cdc.gov/diabetes/statistics/lea/fig1.htm, accessed April 23, 2004.

Centers for Disease Control and Prevention (CDC), National Center for Chronic Disease Prevention and Health Promotion: *Data and trends, diabetes surveillance system, prevalence of diabetes*, 2004b, available at http://www.cdc.gov/diabetes/statistics/prev/national/figpersons.htm, accessed May 16, 2004.

Centers for Disease Control and Prevention (CDC): *National diabetes fact sheet*, 2007, available at http://www.cdc.gov/diabetes/pubs/pdf/ndfs_2007.pdf, accessed February 10, 2009.

Centers for Disease Control and Prevention (CDC): *Data and trends, national data. Age-adjusted hospital discharges per 1,000 diabetic population, by level of amputation, United States, 1993–2005*, 2008a, available at http://www.cdc.gov/diabetes/statistics/lealevel/fig8.htm, accessed February 10, 2009.

Centers for Disease Control and Prevention (CDC): *Data and trends, national data. Number (in thousands) of hospital discharges for nontraumatic lower extremity amputation with diabetes as a listed diagnosis, United States, 1980-2005*, 2008b, available at http://www.cdc.gov/diabetes/statistics/lea/fig1.htm, accessed February 10, 2009.

Centers for Disease Control and Prevention (CDC): *Data and trends, national data. Hospital discharge rates for non-traumatic lower extremity amputation per 1,000 diabetic population, by level of amputation and age, United States, 2005*, 2008c, available at http://www.cdc.gov/diabetes/statistics/lealevel/fig9.htm, accessed February 10, 2009.

Cofield RH et al: Diabetic neuroarthropathy in the foot: patient characteristics and patterns of radiographic change, *Foot Ankle* 4(1):15-22, 1983.

Cullen B et al: Mechanism of action of PROMOGRAN, a protease modulating matrix, for the treatment of diabetic foot ulcers, *Wound Repair Regen* 10(1):16-25, 2002.

Dargis V et al: Benefits of a multidisciplinary approach in the management of recurrent diabetic foot ulceration in Lithuania: a prospective study, *Diabetes Care* 22(9):1428-1431, 1999.

Diabetes Control and Complications Research Group: The effect of intensive treatment of diabetes on the development and progression of long-term complications in insulin-dependent diabetes mellitus, *N Engl J Med* 329(4):977-986, 1993.

Driver VR: Treating the macro and micro wound environment of the diabetic patient: managing the whole patient, not the hole in the patient, *Foot Ankle Q* 16(2):47-56, 2004.

Driver VR, Fabbi M: Recent advances in the use of ultrasound in wound care. In Sen CK, editor: *Wound Healing Society, advances in wound care: volume 1*, New Rochelle, NY, 2009, Mary Ann Liebert.

Driver VR, LeBretton JM: "Gene therapy"-therapeutic angiogenesis-does it have an impact for wound healing and limb preservation, *Podiatr Today* August, 2008, pp 74-78.

Driver VR et al: Reducing amputation rates in patients with diabetes at a military medical center: the limb preservation service model, *Diabetes Care* 28(2):248-253, 2005.

Eneroth M et al: Clinical characteristics and outcome in 223 diabetic patients with deep foot infections, *Foot Ankle Int* 18(11):716-722, 1997.

Frykberg RG: Diabetic foot ulcers: pathogenesis and management, *Am Fam Physician* 66:1655-1662, 2002.

Frykberg RG: An evidence-based approach to diabetic foot infections, *Am J Surg* 186/5A:44S, 2003.

Frykberg RG et al: *Diabetic foot disorders—a clinical practice guideline*, Brooklandville, Md, 2000, Data Trace Publishing.

Gordois A et al: The health care costs of diabetic peripheral neuropathy in the U.S., *Diabetes Care* 26(6):1790-1795, 2003.

Grady JF et al: Use of electrostimulation in the treatment of diabetic neuropathy, *J Am Podiatr Med Assoc* 90(6):287-294, 2000.

Guis S et al: Healing of Charcot's joint by pamidronate infusion, *J Rheumatol* 26(8):1843-1845, 1999.

Harrington C et al: A cost analysis of diabetic lower-extremity ulcers, *Diabetes Care* 23(9):1333-1338, 2000.

Heisler M et al: The relative importance of physician communication, participatory decision-making, and patient understanding in diabetes self-management, *J Gen Intern Med* 17(4):243-252, 2002.

Hopf HW et al: Guidelines for the treatment of arterial insufficiency ulcers, *Wound Repair Regen* 14(6):693-710, 2006.

Jeffcoate WJ, Harding KG: Diabetic foot ulcers, *Lancet* 361(9368):1545-1551, 2003.

Jude EB et al: Peripheral arterial disease in diabetic and nondiabetic patients: a comparison of severity and outcome, *Diabetes Care* 24(8):1433-1437, 2001.

Laborde JM: Treatment of forefoot ulcers with tendon lengthenings, *J South Orthop Assoc* 12(2):60-65, 2003.

Larme AC, Pugh JA: Evidence-based guidelines meet the real world, *Diabetes Care* 24(10):1728-1733, 2001.

Larsson J et al: Long term prognosis after healed amputations in patients with diabetes, *Clin Orthop* 350:149-158, 1998.

Lavery LA et al: Classification of diabetic foot wounds, *J Foot Ankle Surg* 35(6):528-531, 1996.

Lavery LA et al: Practical criteria for screening patients at high risk for diabetic foot ulceration, *Arch Intern Med* 158(2):157-162, 1998.

Lavery LA et al: Ankle equinus deformity and its relationship to high plantar pressure in a large population with diabetes mellitus, *J Am Podiatr Med Assoc* 92(9):479-482, 2002.

Lavery LA et al: Diabetic foot syndrome: evaluating the prevalence and incidence of foot pathology in Mexican Americans and non-Hispanic whites from a diabetes disease management cohort, *Diabetes Care*, 26(5):1435-1438, 2003.

Levin ME: Management of the diabetic foot: preventing amputation, *South Med J* 95(1):10-20, 2002.

Levy PJ: Epidemiology and pathophysiology of peripheral arterial disease, *Clin Cornerstone* 4(5):1-15, 2002.

Lin SS et al: Total contact casting and Keller arthroplasty for diabetic great toe ulceration under the interphalangeal joint, *Foot Ankle Int* 24:680-684, 2003.

Lipsky BA: A report from the international consensus on diagnosing and treating the infected diabetic foot, *Diabetes Metab Res Rev* 20(Suppl 1):S68, 2004.

Litchy W et al: *Diabetic peripheral neuropathy (DPN) assessed by neurological examination (NE) and composite scores (CS) is improved with LY 333531 treatment*, 2002, program and abstracts of the 62nd Scientific Sessions of the American Diabetes Association, June 14–18, 2002, San Francisco, California, Abstract 321-OR.

Macfarlane R, Jeffcoate W: Classification of diabetic foot ulcers: the size (area and depth) (SAD) system, *Diabetic Foot* 2(4):123, 1999.

Mayfield JA et al: Trends in lower limb amputation in the Veterans Health Administration, 1989–1998, *J Rehabil Res Dev* 37(1):23-30, 2000.

McLaughlin C. *Healing from the toes up. Nurse's foot care system helps prevent amputations in diabetic patients*, 2008, available at http://nursing.advanceweb.com/Editorial/Content/Editorial.aspx?CC=119624, accessed March 20, 2009.

Meltzer DD et al: Decreasing amputation rates in patients with diabetes mellitus. An outcome study, *J Am Podiatr Med Assoc* 92(8):425-428, 2002.

Mohler ER 3rd et al: Trial of a novel prostacyclin analog, UT-15, in patients with severe intermittent claudication, *Vasc Med* 5(4):231-237, 2000.

Moulik PK et al: Amputation and mortality in new-onset foot ulcers stratified by etiology, *Diabetes Care* 26(2):491-494, 2003.

Mueller MJ et al: Effect of Achilles tendon lengthening on neuropathic plantar ulcers. A randomized clinical trial, *J Bone Joint Surg Am* 85(8):1436-1445, 2003.

Mueller MJ et al: Impact of Achilles tendon lengthening on functional limitations and perceived disability in people with a neuropathic plantar ulcer, *Diabetes Care* 27(7):1559-1564, 2004.

Mulder G et al: Standard, appropriate, and advanced care and medical-legal considerations. Part one—diabetic foot ulcerations, *Wounds* 15(4):92, 2003.

Muller IS et al: Foot ulceration and lower limb amputation in type 2 diabetic patients in Dutch primary health care, *Diabetes Care* 25(3):570-574, 2002.

Murray HJ et al: The relationship between callus formation, high pressures and neuropathy in diabetic foot ulceration. *Diabet Med* 13:979-982, 1996.

Nabuurs-Franssen MH et al: The effect of polyneuropathy on foot microcirculation in Type II diabetes, *Diabetologia* 45(8):1164, 2002.

National Diabetes Advisory Board: *The prevention and treatment of five complications of diabetes: a guide for primary care practitioners*, HHS Pub. No. 83-8392, Atlanta, Ga, 1983, Centers for Disease Control.

National Institute of Neurological Disorders and Stroke (NINDS), National Institutes of Health: *NINDS peripheral neuropathy information page*, 2003, available at http://www.ninds.nih.gov/health_and_medical/disorders/peripheralneuropathy_doc.htm, accessed December 1, 2003.

Ollendorf DA et al: Potential economic benefits of lower-extremity amputation prevention strategies in diabetes, *Diabetes Care* 21(8):1240-1245, 1998.

Oyibo SO et al: A comparison of two diabetic foot ulcer classification systems: the Wagner and the University of Texas wound classification systems, *Diabetes Care* 24(1):84-88, 2001.

Oyibo SO et al: Clinical characteristics of patients with diabetic foot problems: changing patterns of foot ulcer presentation, *Pract Diabetes Int* 19:10-12, 2002.

Pecoraro RE et al: Pathways to diabetic limb amputation. Basis for prevention, *Diabetes Care* 13(5):513-521, 1990.

Perkins BA et al: Simple screening tests for peripheral neuropathy in the diabetes clinic, *Diabetes Care* 24(2):250-256, 2001.

Peters EJG, Lavery L: Effectiveness of the diabetic foot risk classification system of the International Working Group on the Diabetic Foot, *Diabetes Care* 24(8):1442-1447, 2001.

Pfaller MA et al: *Trends in antimicrobial susceptibility of bacterial pathogens isolated from patients with bloodstream infections (BSI) in North America (NA): SENTRY Program*, 1997–2000, 2001. Program and abstracts of the 41st Interscience Conference on Antimicrobial Agents and Chemotherapy, Chicago, Illinois, December 16–19, 2001.

Pham H et al: Screening techniques to identify people at high risk for diabetic foot ulceration: a prospective multicenter trial, *Diabetes Care* 23(5):606-611, 2000.

Piagessi A et al: Semiquantitative analysis of the histopathological features of the neuropathic foot ulcer: effects of pressure relief, *Diabetes Care* 26(11):3123-3128, 2003.

Praet SF, Louwerens JW: The influence of shoe design on plantar pressures in neuropathic feet, *Diabetes Care* 26(2):441-445, 2003.

Prompers L et al: Prediction of outcome in individuals with diabetic foot ulcers: focus on the differences between individuals with and without peripheral arterial disease. The EURODIALE Study, *Diabetologia* 51(5):747-755, 2008.

Ramsey SD et al: Incidence, outcomes, and cost of foot ulcers in patients with diabetes, *Diabetes Care* 22(3):382-387, 1999.

Rathur HM, Boulton AJM: The diabetic foot, *Clin Dermatol* 25:109-120, 2007.

Reiber GE et al: Lower extremity foot ulcers and amputations in diabetes. In: *Diabetes in America*, ed 2, Bethesda, Md, 1995, National Institutes of Health.

Reiber GE et al: Causal pathways for incident lower-extremity ulcers in patients with diabetes from two settings, *Diabetes Care* 22(1):157-162, 1999.

Ritz G et al: Use of the Cam walker in treating diabetic ulcers. A case report. *J Am Podiatr Med Assoc* 86(6):253-256, 1996.

Sanders LJ, Frykberg RG: The Charcots foot (pied de Charcot). In Bowker JH, Pfeiffer MA, editors: *Levin and O'Neal's the diabetic foot*, ed 7, St. Louis, 2008, Mosby.

Seidel HM et al, editors: Blood vessels. In: *Mosby's guide to physical examination*, ed 5, St. Louis, 2003, Mosby.

Seidel HM et al, editors: Blood vessels. In: *Mosby's guide to physical examination*, ed 6, St. Louis, 2006, Mosby, Elsevier Science.

Shah BR, Hux JE: Quantifying the risk of infectious diseases for people with diabetes, *Diabetes Care* 26(2):510-513, 2003.

Shearer A et al: Predicted costs and outcomes from reduced vibration detection in people with diabetes in the U.S., *Diabetes Care* 26(8):2305-2310, 2003.

Sims DS et al: Risk factors in the diabetic foot: recognition and management, *Phys Ther* 68(12):1887-1902, 1988.

Sinacore DR, Mueller MJ: Off loading for diabetic foot disease. In: Bowker JH, Pfeiffer MA, editors: *Levin and O'Neal's the diabetic foot*, ed 7, St. Louis, 2008, Mosby.

Sinacore DR, Mueller MJ: Infectious problems of the foot in diabetic patients. In Bowker JH, Pfeiffer MA, editors: *Levin and O'Neal's the diabetic foot*, ed 7, St. Louis, 2008, Mosby.

Singh N et al: Preventing foot ulcers in patient with diabetes, *JAMA* 293(2):217-228, 2005.

Steed DL et al: Guidelines for the treatment of diabetic ulcers, *Wound Repair Regen* 14(6):680-692, 2006.

Sumpio B: Primary care: foot ulcers, *N Engl J Med* 343(1):787-793, 2000.

Tanneberg RJ, Donofrio PD: Neuropathic problems of the lower limbs in diabetic patients. In Bowker JH, Pfeiffer MA, editors: *Levin and O'Neal's the diabetic foot*, ed 7, St. Louis, 2008, Mosby.

Tenover FC et al: Vancomycin-resistant *Staphylococcus aureus* isolate from a patient in Pennsylvania, *Antimicrob Agents Chemother* 48(1):275-280, 2004.

Umpierrez GE et al: Hyperglycemia: an independent marker of in-hospital mortality in patients with undiagnosed diabetes, *J Clin Endocrinol Metab* 87(3):978-982, 2002.

Van Acker K et al: The choice of diabetic foot ulcer classification in relation to the final outcome, *Wounds* 14(1):16, 2002.

Van Gils et al: Amputation prevention by vascular surgery and podiatry collaboration in high-risk diabetic and nondiabetic patients, *Diabetes Care* 22(5):678-683, 1999.

Vinik AI et al: Diabetic autonomic neuropathy, *Diabetes Care* 26(5):1553-1579, 2003.

Wagner FW: The dysvascular foot: a system for diagnosis and treatment, *Foot Ankle* 2(2):64-122, 1981.

Warriner RA, Driver VR: The true cost of growth factor therapy in diabetic foot ulcer care, *Wounds* 2006, Supplement to July 2006.

WOCN Society: *Guideline for management of wounds in patients with lower-extremity neuropathic disease*, WOCN Clinical Practice Guideline Series #3, Glenview, IL, 2004.

Wu SC et al: Use of pressure offloading devices in diabetic foot ulcers, *Diabetes Care* 31(11):2118-2119, 2008.

Young MJ et al: The effect of callus removal on dynamic plantar foot pressures in diabetic patients, *Diabetic Med* 9(1):55-57, 1992.

Yu GV, Hudson JR: Evaluation and treatment of stage 0 Charcot's neuroarthropathy of the foot and ankle, *J Am Podiatr Med Assoc* 92(4):210-220, 2002.

Zimny S et al: Early detection of microcirculatory impairment in diabetic patients with foot at risk, *Diabetes Care* 24(10):1810-1814, 2001a.

Zimny S et al: Effects of felted foam on plantar pressures in the treatment of neuropathic diabetic foot ulcers, *Diabetes Care* 24(12):2153-2154, 2001b.

15

Foot and Nail Care

Sheila Howes-Trammel, Ruth A. Bryant, and Denise P. Nix

OBJECTIVES

1. Correlate medical conditions with potential foot problems.
2. Describe the structure and function of the foot and nails.
3. Compare and contrast foot malformations addressing key features, prevention, and management.
4. Describe common foot lesions, including their etiology, manifestations, treatment, and prevention.
5. Distinguish between two toenail disorders and their treatments.
6. Develop an appropriate plan for routine care of the foot.

Foot problems occur in at least 75% of Americans (Menz et al, 2001). The five most common problems in the elderly population are *toenail disorders* (75%), *toe deformities* (60%), *corns and calluses* (58%), *bunions* (37%), and *dry skin, fungal infections,* or *maceration between the toes* (36%). Most of these foot problems can be prevented by proper foot care performed on a regular basis (Badlissi et al, 2005).

Age-related changes (e.g., impaired vision, inability to reach feet, thinning of epidermis and dermis), vascular-related skin changes (e.g., trophic, edema), and deformed hardened toenails impact on foot hygiene. An age-related change of the foot and lower extremity is loss of hair, which leads to increased dry skin. Trophic changes in the skin are related to loss of vasculature (e.g., pigmentation changes; shiny, red skin; hair loss).

Chronic foot problems (i.e., those lasting more than 2 weeks) are associated with diabetes, peripheral vascular disease, neuropathy, atherosclerosis, arthritis, and obesity. In fact, the signs and symptoms of many of these systemic disorders manifest initially in the feet. Improper shoe wear, overuse, or systemic disease can trigger chronic foot pain. These issues magnify the importance of a good foot assessment (Popoola and Jenkins, 2004).

QUALITY OF LIFE

Foot diseases and their treatments have a tremendous impact on quality of life (Katsambas et al, 2005). In fact, patients with diabetes who have foot ulcers report a poorer quality of life than patients with diabetes who have amputations (Price and Harding, 2000). In a large-scale, quality-of-life survey of 45,593 patients with various foot diseases representing 17 countries (the Achilles Project), the researchers found that 40.3% of the respondents experienced discomfort in walking, 30.7% had pain, 27.3% had embarrassment, and 19.6% experienced limitations in their activities of daily living (Katsambas et al, 2005).

Overall, foot disease has a significantly greater effect on the quality of life of women than of men with regard to their experience of pain, discomfort in walking, and embarrassment (Katsambas et al, 2005; Leveille et al, 1998). One explanation is that the many types of shoes typically worn by women are tighter-fitting, which increases their risk of developing toenail onychomycosis, which is associated with pain and discomfort in walking.

STRUCTURE AND FUNCTION

The foot has two key functions: weight bearing and propulsion. To perform properly, the foot requires a high degree of stability and must be flexible to adapt to uneven surfaces. Flexibility is provided by the numerous bones and joints in the foot; these bones also form the arch to support weight (Quinn, 2009). Each foot contains 26 bones, 33 joints, and a network of more than 100 tendons, muscles, ligaments, blood vessels, nerves, and nails. Together, the feet comprise a quarter of the 206 bones in the body. An average day of walking brings a force equal to several hundred tons to bear on the feet. As such, feet are more subject to injury than is any other part of the body (Cavanagh and Ulbrecht, 2008; Mix, 1999).

Skeletal Components

The three functional units of the foot are the hindfoot (2 bones), midfoot (5 bones), and forefoot (19 bones). All units must work together to provide both flexibility and stability (Figure 15-1).

Within the forefoot are the phalanges (toes) and the five metatarsal bones. Each toe (phalanx) is made up of several bones. The great toe (also called the hallux) consists of two phalanx bones: proximal and distal; these phalanges are larger than all the other phalanges. Phalanges two through five have three phalanx bones each: proximal, distal, and intermediate (an additional middle bone). Each phalanx is connected to a metatarsal at the metatarsophalangeal (MTP) joint; together the MTP joints form the ball of the foot. The proximal portion of a metatarsal is called the *base,* the middle is the *shaft,* and the distal is the *head* (Figure 15-2). Each of the five metatarsals is unique in size. The first metatarsal is the shortest in length, the largest in diameter, bears the most weight and plays the most important role in propulsion (Quinn, 2009). At the head of the first metatarsal bone on the plantar surface of the foot are two sesamoid bones that serve to attach small muscles and aid in stabilizing the first MTP joint. (A sesamoid bone is a bone imbedded within a tendon and functions to protect the tendon where it passes over a bony prominence.) The second, third, and fourth metatarsal bones are the most stable metatarsal bones. At the fifth metatarsal base is an eminence on the lateral aspect called the

tuberosity of fifth metatarsal or *styloid process.* This area is easily palpated on the lateral aspect of the foot.

In the midfoot, five of the seven tarsal bones are located (Figure 15-2). These irregularly shaped tarsals (the navicular, cuboid, and three cuneiform) form the arch and contain multiple joints. The three cuneiform bones articulate with the navicular bone in the proximal midfoot. The midfoot connects with the forefoot at the five tarsometatarsal (TMT) joints and connects to the hindfoot by muscles and ligaments.

The hindfoot links the midfoot to the ankle and consists of two of the seven tarsal bones, the talus and the calcaneus. The talus sits on top of the calcaneus and articulates with the tibia and fibula at the calcaneus and navicular bones, allowing the foot to move up and down. The calcaneus forms the heel and is the largest tarsal and the largest bone in the foot. It allows the foot to become rigid or loose to accommodate the process of walking. It is also the cause of numerous heel-related pains (Jolly et al, 2005).

Ligaments hold the bones together at the joints. The Achilles tendon stretches from calf muscle to heel and is the largest, strongest tendon in the foot. The planter fascia is the longest ligament and forms an arch on the sole of the foot from the heel to the toes. These long fibrous strands are vulnerable to injury (e.g., a strain or sprain in the foot or ankle) because the ligaments can overstretch, break, and curl back on themselves. Over time the strain heals with scar tissue; however, the scar is never as strong as the original fibers of the ligament.

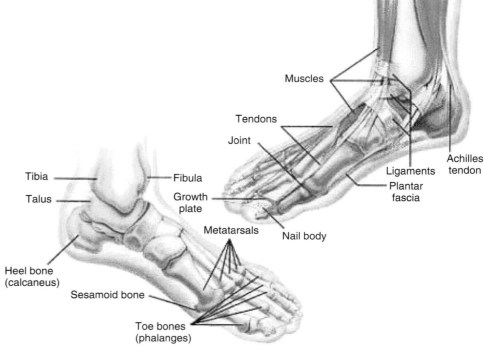

FIGURE 15-1 Anatomic structures of the foot. (Courtesy Fort Worth Orthopaedics.)

Tibia
Talus
Heel bone (calcaneus)
Sesamoid bone
Toe bones (phalanges)
Fibula
Growth plate
Metatarsals
Nail body
Joint
Tendons
Muscles
Ligaments
Plantar fascia
Achilles tendon

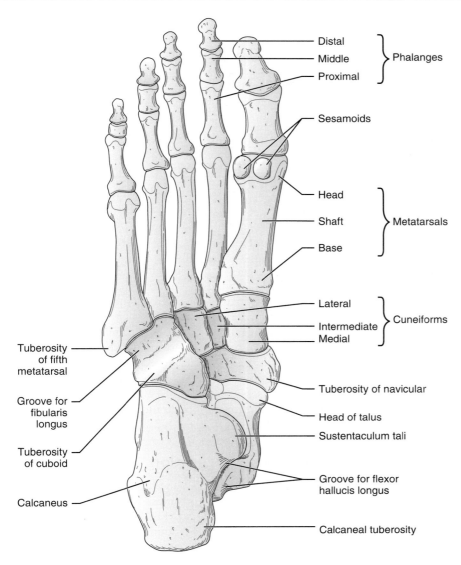

Distal
Middle } Phalanges
Proximal

Sesamoids

Head
Shaft } Metatarsals
Base

Lateral
Intermediate } Cuneiforms
Medial

Tuberosity of fifth metatarsal
Groove for fibularis longus
Tuberosity of cuboid
Calcaneus

Tuberosity of navicular
Head of talus
Sustentaculum tali
Groove for flexor hallucis longus
Calcaneal tuberosity

FIGURE 15-2 Dorsal view of anatomic structures of foot. (From Jenkins DB: *Hollinshead's functional anatomy of the limbs and back,* ed 9, St. Louis, 2009, Saunders/Elsevier, p 333.)

Muscular Components

The foot is constructed of 20 muscles. These muscles hold the bones in place, providing the foot with its shape and contracting and relaxing to allow for movement. Key muscles are the anterior tibial (moves foot upward), posterior tibial (supports arch), peroneal tibial (controls lateral ankle movements), extensors (help ankle raise toes to begin walking), and flexors (stabilizes to the ground).

Neurovascular

The feet are innervated by the sciatic nerve, which branches off the spinal cord at the sacral level. As it descends, the sciatic nerve divides into the tibial and common peroneal nerves and further subdivides into numerous branches.

Branching off the popliteal artery in the lower leg are the anterior tibial artery and the posterior tibial artery.

The anterior tibial artery becomes the dorsalis pedis (dorsum of the foot). The posterior tibial artery passes posterior to the medial malleolus, divides into the peroneal and plantar arteries, and then feeds into the lateral plantar and medial plantar arteries. The two most dominant arteries in the foot are the dorsalis pedis and the posterior tibial artery. Two sets of veins drain the leg and foot: deep veins and superficial veins.

As shown in Figure 10-2, the dorsalis pedis pulse is palpated or auscultated over the navicular and middle cuneiform bones. The posterior tibial pulse is palpated over the medial malleolus of the tibia.

Cutaneous and Subcutaneous Components

The skin on the plantar surface of the foot is thick and hairless and contains numerous sweat glands. *Eccrine* sweat glands are densely populated on the soles of the feet, palms, and axillae. Their primary function is thermoregulation through evaporation of sweat. The sebaceous and apocrine sweat glands empty into the upper portions of the hair follicles. Sebaceous glands produce lipid-rich sebum that prevents the skin and hair from drying out. Because the foot has little hair growth and therefore very few *sebaceous* glands, the foot is extremely vulnerable to dryness and xerosis.

Three anatomic areas on the plantar surface of the foot have increased fat in the form of fat pads: the calcaneus, the metatarsals, and the lateral longitudinal arch. Contained by the subcutaneous tissue, the fat pad absorbs impact and tolerates weight-bearing as a means of protecting the underlying bones. With age, these fat pads thin and provide less shock absorbency. More pressure is then exerted over the calcaneus and metatarsal. Thinning of the fat pad is accelerated by obesity, diabetes, and constant high impact. The thinning process begins as early as 30 years of age. An orthotic or insole cushioning can be used to provide additional shock absorption (Ozdemir et al, 2004).

Nail Structure

Nails are made of epidermal cells converted to hard plates of keratin. The highly vascular nail bed lies beneath the plate, giving the nail its pink color. The stratum corneum layer of the skin covering the nail root is the eponychium (cuticle), which forms a seal between the nail and the digit to prevent foreign matter from entering. The paronychia is the soft tissue surrounding the nail border. The normal nail is composed of six parts: nail root, nail bed, nail plate, eponychium (cuticle), perionychium, and hyponychium as illustrated in Figure 15-3 and described in Box 15-1.

Nails grow all the time, but their rate of growth slows with age and poor circulation. Fingernails grow faster than toenails. They grow at a rate of 3 mm per month and take 6 months to grow from root to free edge. Toenails grow approximately 1 mm per month and require 12 to 18 months to be completely replaced. Actual growth rate is dependent upon age, gender, season, exercise level, diet, and hereditary factors (Sinni-McKeehen, 2007).

PHYSICAL ASSESSMENT

Components of an initial evaluation of the patient with an actual or potential foot disorder are listed in Checklist 15-1. Because so many patients with foot disorders have concomitant lower extremity disease, perfusion and sensation must be assessed (see Chapters 10, 11, 12, and 14), and a baseline health history is essential. The following discussion presents the unique assessment parameters for the foot and nail.

Specific information should be elicited about routine care of the foot, any history of foot and nail problems, and how these problems were treated either personally or by a health care provider. Effects of prior treatments, including prescription and over-the-counter medications, should be assessed (Piraccini, 2004; Sprecher, 2005). Quality-of life-information should be solicited (Garrow et al, 2004; Vileikyte et al, 2003).

Musculoskeletal Function

Musculoskeletal function of the foot involves assessment of range of motion, deformities, and strength. Passive range of motion of the first MTP joint and the subtalar joint should be assessed. Maximal range of motion is

FIGURE 15-3 Anatomic structures of the nail. (From Thompson JM et al: *Mosby's clinical nursing*, ed 5, St. Louis, 2002, Mosby.)

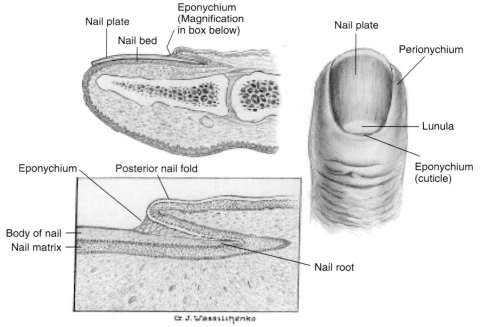
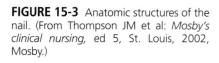

BOX 15-1 | Nail Anatomy

Nail Root (Matrix): Root of fingernail is also known as the *matrix.* The matrix begins 7 to 8 mm under proximal nail fold to lunula (white crescent at distal nail). Fingernail root produces most of volume of nail plate and nail bed.

Nail Bed: Part of nail matrix, under the nail plate. Extends from lunula (white crescent at distal nail) to hyponychium. Nail bed contains blood vessels, nerves, and melanocytes or melanin-producing cells. As nail is produced by root, it streams down along the nail bed, which adds material to the undersurface of the nail, making it thicker.

Nail Plate: The actual fingernail, made of translucent keratin. Pink appearance of nail comes from blood vessels underneath nail. Underneath surface of nail plate has grooves along length of nail that help anchor it to the nail bed.

Eponychium (Cuticle): Fold at proximal end of nail plate. Nail plate has very firm adhesion to the cuticle. Both epidermal structures are directly continuous with one another, overlapping the lunula. Fusing of these structures provides a waterproof barrier.

Perionychium: Skin that overlies nail plate on its sides. Also known as the *paronychial edge.* Site of hangnails, ingrown nails, and infection of skin called *paronychia.*

Hyponychium: Area between free edge of nail plate and epidermis of toe. Continuous fusing of these areas to epidermal structures provides waterproof barrier.

Periungual: Tissue around nail plate.

Subungual: Tissue under nail plate.

Ungual: Pertaining to the nail.

From Mix G: *The salon professional's guide to foot care,* Albany, NY, 1998, Milady Salon Ovations.

CHECKLIST 15-1

Components of Initial Evaluation of Patient with Foot Disorder

History

✓ Presenting complaint including detailed description of pain
✓ General: vision, strength, dexterity, mobility
✓ Blood glucose readings for past month
✓ Personal or family history: skin, hair, or nail disease (especially rashes), lichen planus, psoriasis, diabetes, heart or vascular disease, obesity
✓ Specific history of foot problems: foot malformations, lesions, skin alterations, nail disorders, changes in sensation, foot/ankle strength
✓ Current and prior treatments and medications (including over-the-counter) used to treat nail and foot problems
✓ Health habits: smoking, exercise, hygiene, nutrition, weight management

Physical Assessment

✓ Overall skin condition
✓ Lesions on foot
✓ Foot malformations
✓ Condition of nails
✓ Perfusion and sensation, pulses, blanching, capillary refill, microvascular function (laser Doppler flowmetry), ankle-brachial index or toe-brachial index, temperature, hair growth
✓ Musculoskeletal function: gait, mobility, balance, hand strength and dexterity, visual cognition

Risk Assessment

✓ Ulceration risk
✓ Amputation risk

Equipment

✓ Footwear (including socks)
✓ Mobility aids (canes, walkers)

---

determined from maximal inversion to maximal eversion of the subtalar joint of the foot (Figure 15-4). If available, a goniometer can be used to quantify the arc or range of motion (Badlissi et al, 2005) (Figure 15-5). Range of motion can also be tested by supporting the heel with the hand and grasping the foot with the other hand, then moving the foot in dorsiflexion, plantar flexion, eversion, and inversion. The dorsiflexion position tests for shortening of the Achilles tendon. Inversion will be limited by a spasm of the peronei. Eversion will be limited with a rigid flat foot. Restrictions in range of motion of the ankle might limit the ability to correct a loss of balance (Duthie, 2007).

The strength of the anterior leg muscles can be tested by having the patient stand on the heels. Muscle strength can also be assessed by comparing both feet as the patient walks a few steps on the toes and then the heels. If the patient has difficulty with balance, cannot walk, or both, strength can be assessed with the patient sitting. With the clinician's hand under the patient's foot, the patient is asked to flex and extend the foot against resistance by "pressing down on the gas pedal." Next, with the clinician's hand positioned on the top of the patient's foot and the clinician's thumbs underneath, the patient is instructed to pull the "toes toward the nose" while

the clinician applies gentle pressure downward. Any differences in strength currently or in the past 6 months should also be recorded (Frey, 2005).

To assess toe flexibility, the patient can be instructed to pick up a marble or a small dishtowel with the toes (Table 15-1). To test ankle flexibility, the patient is instructed to stand on a stair step, hang his or her heel off a step, and let the heel drop below the level of the stair. If this motion causes pain, the exercise should be stopped. The heel should be able to drop below the level of the stair without causing strain in the calf. Some strain can be improved with flexibility exercises (Frey, 2005).

To examine the medial longitudinal arch, have the patient stand with feet parallel, separated by 4 inches. Note if the arch flattens with weight-bearing and if it resumes to normal shape without weight-bearing.

Muscle strength reflexes (deep tendon reflexes) usually show no changes in the elderly patient, although nearly half have a diminished Achilles tendon reflex. This is likely due to slow nerve conduction and

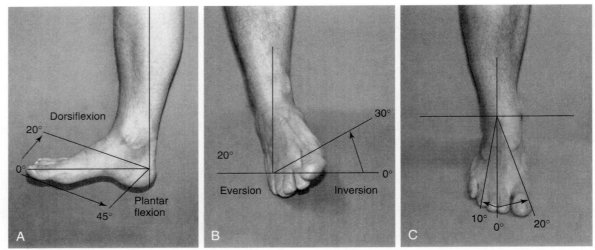

FIGURE 15-4 Range of motion of the foot and ankle. (From Seidel HM et al: *Mosby's guide to physical examination,* ed 6, St. Louis, 2006, Mosby.)

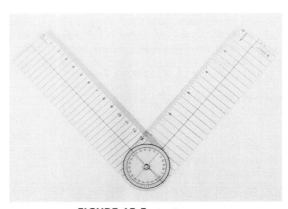

FIGURE 15-5 Goniometer.

decreased tendon elasticity. Hyperactive deep tendon reflexes suggest upper motor neuron disease; hypoactive reflexes suggest lower motor neuron dysfunction. Tone is assessed through passive motion. Increased tone is suggestive of upper motor neuron dysfunction; decreased tone is suggestive of lower motor neuron dysfunction.

Functional Ability

The patient's functional ability is a significant factor influencing his or her ability for self-care and safety. Assessments of functional ability should address cognition, vision, strength–hand dexterity, coordination, balance, proprioception, and gait. Because key interventions in the prevention and management of foot and nail disorders are patient education and self-care, the patient will need adequate cognition to conduct self-care or commu-

nicate pain. Vision and strength–hand dexterity are essential so that patients will be able to inspect their feet and remove footwear (Duthie, 2007). Many of these functional abilities can be assessed through observation and demonstration return.

Coordination can be determined with a rapid alternating movement that includes heel to shin testing. Another test in which the patient taps the feet rhythmically against the floor will assess the accuracy and reproducibility of endpoints as well as the ability to maintain motor movements over time. The coordination testing is documented qualitatively because no quantification guidelines are available (Duthie, 2007).

Proprioception is the awareness of the body's position in context with the surrounding environment. Disturbed proprioception (loss of position sense) in the feet is disabling; the patient may be clumsy, bump into things, or have an abnormal gait. In practice, the patient often comes down hard on the heels and then slaps the sole of the foot (high stepping and stamping) in an attempt to increase sensory feedback and restore proprioception. Proprioception disturbances are always worse in the dark when vision cannot be used to compensate for loss of position sense.

The Romberg test (Box 15-2) is positive in the patient with proprioception disturbances (Jarvis, 2004). In addition, the patient's gait may be slightly wide while the stride length is normal or a little reduced (Willacy, 2008). Gait should be assessed without an assistive device if possible so as not to mask deviations. Proprioception and vibration sense are carried by the same nerve pathways. Therefore, testing vibration may reveal proprioception disturbances. To test vibration sense, a 128-Hz tuning fork is applied over a bony prominence such as the medial malleolus and the

TABLE 15-1	Foot Flexibility Exercises		
	Exercise	Instructions	Recommendations
	Toe raise, toe point, toe curls	Hold each position for 5 seconds and repeat 10 times.	Individuals with hammer toes or toe cramps
	Golf ball roll	Roll a golf ball under the ball of your foot for 2 minutes—great massage for bottom of foot.	Individuals with plantar fasciitis (heel pain), arch strain, or foot cramps
	Towel curls	Place small towel on floor and curl it toward you, using only your toes. You can increase resistance by putting a weight on end of towel. Relax and repeat exercise five times.	Individuals with hammer toes, toe cramps, and pain in the ball of the foot
	Marble pickup	Place 20 marbles on floor. Pick up one marble at a time with your toes and put it in a small bowl. Do this exercise until you have picked up all 20 marbles.	Individuals with pain in the ball of the foot, hammer toes, and toe cramps
	Sand walking	Any chance you get, take off your shoes and walk in the sand at the beach. This not only massages your feet but also strengthens your toes.	Good for general foot conditioning Watch out for glass!

Modified from American Orthopaedic Foot and Ankle Society: *Keep your foot flexible*, available at http://www.aofas.org/Scripts/4Disapi.dll/4DCGI/cms/review.html?Action=CMS_Document&DocID=71, accessed September 2, 2010.

BOX 15-2	Romberg (Equilibrium) Test

- Have patient stand with arms at side and feet together.
- Have patient maintain position for 20 seconds with only minimal swaying.
- Have patient perform initially with eyes open and then with eyes closed.
- Stand close to patient to prevent falls.

patient is asked to report when the vibration stops (Jarvis, 2004).

Condition of Legs, Feet, Toes, and Nails

Lower extremity assessment should include all of the components discussed in Chapter 10. In addition to examining skin integrity, color changes, sensation, pain, and vascular conditions, the foot must be inspected for skin that is too dry or too moist, evidence of fungal or bacterial infection, lesions, foot malformations, and nail conditions (Boulton and Armstrong, 2008). All surfaces (dorsal, plantar, medial, lateral, posterior surfaces) of the heel, areas between the toes (interdigitally), and each nail should be examined. Note the character of skin changes from the proximal leg to the distal foot. Compare the skin on the lower extremity and feet to the skin on the arms and hands.

Ulceration and Amputation Risk

The data collected during the examination will assist in identifying risk for ulceration and amputation. Risk assessment tools with management strategies are given in Tables 14-2 and 14-3. Risk factors include history of plantar ulcer, presence of foot deformity, presence of protective sensations, and presence of diseases that lead to decreased sensation. Risk categories range from 0 (no risk) to 3 (greatest risk). The level of risk determines the patient's management strategy. Yetzer (2004) recommends foot examinations at each visit (at least four times per year) regardless of risk score.

PREVENTION AND ROUTINE MANAGEMENT

Maintaining healthy nails and feet requires daily attention to the skin of the foot and ankle, nails and footwear. Routine over the counter remedies can be used to correct common problems and hopefully prevent deterioration into a serious condition.

Routine Foot Hygiene

Routine foot care includes daily inspection and moisturizing. Cleansing and bathing should be based on the individual needs of the patient and should consist of mild skin cleansers and lukewarm water to minimize drying effects.

After bathing, the feet must be dried completely, especially between the toes. Patients should wear socks to provide extra padding to bony prominences and to wick away moisture from the skin. Socks may need to be changed more than once per day if feet sweat excessively.

Maceration between the toes (interdigital) and under the toes (subdigital) is a very common foot problem. Such overhydration of the skin, characterized by a white, "waterlogged" appearance, weakens collagen, promotes overgrowth of bacterial and fungal species of skin flora, and decreases the skin's ability to resist trauma (Kelechi, 2005; Stroud and Kelechi, 2006). Pseudomonads as well as gram-negative organisms are common etiologic agents (Schwartz, 2009). Overhydration of the skin can occur with excessive perspiration (hyperhidrosis) related to endocrine, neurologic, or sweat gland disorders.

Maceration is prevented by keeping the skin dry and protected. Absorbent foot powder (e.g., Zeasorb) can be used twice per day. After bathing, the patient should pay special attention to drying the interdigit spaces; using a hair dryer on a cool setting may be helpful. Skin sealants may be used to protect the skin from moisture. If maceration persists after 1 week of care, consider the presence of interdigital tinea (Table 15-2) or superimposed bacterial infection. Treatment includes drying the interdigital web spaces, topical econazole, and daily to three times a day local application of Castellani paint (a drying agent containing 1.5% phenol in a water and alcohol base) (Schwartz, 2009).

Foot odor is caused by excessive perspiration from the more than 250,000 sweat glands in the foot. Bacteria living in shoes and socks metabolize the sweat to form isovaleric acid, which is responsible for foot odor. In addition to washing the feet and changing shoes and socks even more frequently than daily, the patient can dust the feet with a nonmedicated spray, foot powder, or antiperspirants. Soaking feet in vinegar and water can help lessen odor (American Podiatric Medical Association, 2010). Severe cases of foot odor may be caused by hyperhidrosis (excessive perspiration formation related to endocrine, neurologic, or sweat gland disorders). The prescription-strength antiperspirant Drysol can be used if over-the-counter antiperspirants or sprays fail (Hill, 2010). In severe cases the nerve controlling the sweat glands in the feet may be surgically severed, but compensatory sweating in other areas of the body may occur after surgery.

Anhidrosis (inability to produce sweat) is associated with autonomic dysfunction caused by endocrine or neurologic disorders, environmental conditions, and aging. Xerosis is a consequence of the skin's loss of natural moisturizing factors and loss of moisture from the stratum corneum and intercellular matrix (Hill, 2008). Clinically, xerosis appears as excessively dry, rough, uneven, and cracked skin. Raised or uplifted skin edges (scaling), desquamation (flaking), chapping, and pruritus may be present. This condition occurs particularly on the heels and bottoms of the feet. A person who has a decrease or loss of function of the sweat glands on the plantar surface of the foot will experience xerosis or anhidrosis of the feet (Kelechi, 2005). *Xerosis* can lead to fissures (linear cracks in the skin), which may serve as a portal of entry for bacteria. Consequently, fissures are associated with increased risk of cellulitis and foot ulceration (Hill, 2008). *Fissures* are treated with humectants and exfoliant moisturizers or sealants, such as Dermabond. Prevention includes ongoing use of moisturizers and exfoliants and wearing of shoes that do not flop at the heel. Hyperkeratotic tissue is common around fissures and often necessitates debridement and exfoliation. Table 15-3 provides a formulary of products for the prevention and treatment of dry skin.

Cuticles and Nails

About half of the foot care professional's activity is nail care and specifically nail debridement. Nail debridement and trimming can be accomplished with manual nippers (Box 15-3) or with a mechanical rotary tool (Box 15-4). The use of proper and professional-quality instruments is key to providing proper foot and nail care. Five basic instruments are recommended for providing foot and nail care: toenail nippers, curette, rasp, ingrown nail shaver, and cuticle nippers.

Nippers. Podiatry toenail cutters or pedicure nail nippers are best suited for trimming thicker toenails and lateral curves of the nail. This instrument should be used like scissors. The nail should be removed incrementally to avoid injuring the hyponychium and thus breaking the seal on the nail plate, which would open a portal of entry for fungal or bacterial infections (Godfrey, 2006). There is much debate regarding the best methods for debriding or trimming toenails: straight across versus rounding, or following the shape or contouring of the top of the toe. If the patient has a problem with nail corners curving and causing pain and thickening of the skin at the distal aspect of the nail groove, it is recommended that the corners be slightly rounded. Patients who have puffy or a thick skin folds might require nails that are cut straight across so that the corners grow up out of the grooves to prevent ingrown toenails (Katoh, 2008). Box 15-3 gives a procedure for basic cuticle and nail trimming using a nipper.

Curette. The dull-edged curette is a small spoon-shaped instrument that allows for removal of debris under the nail margins. A scooping motion is used along the nail plate to remove debris from the nail groove. This process may need to be repeated until all the debris is removed.

Nail Rasp or Nail File. The medical field calls the nail file a nail rasp. It is used to smooth the distal edges of the nail in the nail groove. The file is placed gently in the nail groove against the free (distal) edges of the nail plate. The rasp is then pulled along the edges of the rough nail plate. Each nail should be smoothed with the nail rasp,

TABLE 15-2	Assessment, Prevention, and Management of Common Foot Lesions and Infections			
Name	**Description**	**Common Locations**	**Prevention**	**Treatment**
Soft corn (heloma molle)	End of phalange is too wide, causing friction between toes Aggravated by tight shoes	Between fourth and fifth toes	Properly fitting shoes	Wider shoes Surgically reshape phalange
Hard corn (heloma durum)	Toes curl inside of shoes, creating pressure between toes against the sole Aggravated by narrow-toed shoes	Sides and tops of toes		Use wider shoes or sandals Reduce corn with file, pumice, rotary tool Assess for underlying ulceration Offload and pad as needed Surgically straighten toes
Callus (keratoma or tyloma) (see Plate 41a)	Thickened areas of skin without distinct borders caused by repeated pressure Aggravated by narrow-toed shoes and high heels	Planter surface, heel, under metatarsal head	Properly fitting shoes	Reduce with file, pumice, rotary tool Assess for underlying ulceration Moisturize and exfoliate (best applied to damp skin after bathing) Offload and pad as needed Use shoes with soft soles, lower heels, arch support, extra width
Planter wart (verruca plantaris)	Caused by a contagious viral infection (human papillomavirus) Overproliferation of skin and mucosa growing downward (iceberg effect) Single lesion or clustered Yellow, brown, gray, or black Vesicular inclusion from dried capillary ends leads to black/red appearance	Pressure points on sole, heel, ball of foot	Change socks and shoes daily Do not share shoes Keep feet clean and dry Avoid direct contact with warts on other people Use water-resistant footwear in showers, locker rooms, pools	Reduce with file or pumice Salicylic acid or cryotherapy Surgical curettage or laser removal Human papillomavirus dies within 1–2 years and wart disappears
Tinea pedis (interdigital)	Dermatophyte infection White macerated, denuded, vesicles, scales, or fissures	Between fourth and fifth toes		Topical antifungal twice daily for minimum of 1 week Urea cream for scaling, itching
Tinea pedis (planter)	Dermatophyte infection Itchy, hyperkeratotic scaling, cracking, peeling, dry patches Chronic, diffuse, noninflammatory	Sole, heel, side of foot (moccasin)		Topical antifungal twice daily for minimum of 1 week Urea cream for scaling, itching
Tinea pedis (vesiculobullous)	Dermatophyte infection Acute highly inflammatory eruptions	Arch, side of foot		Topical or systemic antifungals and corticosteroids (depending on severity)

beginning with healthy nails to prevent transmission of infection.

Ingrown Nail Shaver and Cuticle Nippers. These tools are used when a little more nail needs to be removed from the lateral nail margins. The nail shaver is shaped like a small paddle and has a slot in the middle of the paddle; the end of the slot is filed to a sharp cutting edge. The paddle portion of the nail shaver is placed in the nail groove so that the end of the nail edge is in the slot to trim the spicule of nail present (Mix, 1999).

Mechanical Rotary Tool. The mechanical rotary tool (Dremel drill, cordless or plug-in) is a standard tool used

TABLE 15-3	Formulary of Moisturizing Products: Descriptions, Examples, and Indications		
Moisturizer	**Indications and Actions**	**Ingredient Examples***	**Product Examples***
Emollients	Prevent dry skin Fill in cracks between clusters of desquamating corneocytes Not occlusive unless applied heavily	Lipids Oils Dimethicone	Keri Original (Bristol Myers Squibb) Cavilon Emollient Cream (3M) Cetaphil Lotion (Galderma Laboratories)
Occlusives	Treat dry skin Reduce transepidermal water loss by creating hydrophobic barrier over skin Has most pronounced effect when applied to slightly damp skin	Petrolatum Lanolin Mineral oil Dimethicone	Cetaphil Cream (Galderma Laboratories) Remedy Skin Repair Cream (Medline) Sween 24 Cream (Coloplast)
Humectants and exfoliants	Treat dry skin, xerosis, fissures, ichthyoses Contains urea, lactic acid, or both, which are naturally present in healthy skin and markedly reduced in dry skin Enhance water absorption by drawing and absorbing water from environment and retaining moisture within skin cells Keratolytic effects soften scales to be easily released from skin surface Urea has antipruritic effects	Urea Lactic acid	Eucerin 10% Urea Lotion (Beiersdorf) Lac-Hydrin Lotion (Bristol Myers Squibb) Atrac-Tain Lotion (Coloplast)

*Concentrations and total formulation determine actions and effectiveness. List is not all inclusive.
Data from Pham HT et al: A prospective, randomized, controlled double-blind study of a moisturizer for xerosis of the feet in patients with diabetes, *Ostomy Wound Manage* 48(5):30, 2002; *Ostomy/Wound Management (OWM) 2009 Buyers' Guide,* 55(7) Malvern, PA, 2009, HMP Communications; Loden M: Role of topical emollients and moisturizers in the treatment of dry skin barrier disorders, *Am J Clin Dermatol* 4:771, 2003.

for nail debridement. Use of a rotary tool disperses nail dust into the air, which can be inhaled by the patient as well as the clinician and can settle on surfaces throughout the room. Aerosol nail dust, particularly from onychomycotic toenails, can lead to conjunctivitis, rhinitis, asthma, coughing, hypersensitivity, and impaired lung function (Ward, 2005). These hazards have resulted in a great deal of controversy within the nursing community about the appropriateness of using drill types of mechanical nail avulsion and debridement tools (Rees, 2008). Box 15-4 lists equipment options and sterilization tips that enhance safety and effectiveness. For example, a drill with an attached vacuum is available that will automatically contain large particles. However, personal protection equipment is still required to prevent exposure to small particles.

Footwear

The main purpose of the shoe is to protect and cushion the foot. Incorrectly fitting footwear is common in older people and is strongly associated with forefoot pathology (hallux valgus, lesser toe deformities, corns, calluses), foot pain, skin breakdown, abnormal foot pressures, ischemia, and inflammation from repetitive stress (Menz and Morris, 2005; Ward, 2005). Although foot size increases with age, surprisingly, many people continue to wear the same size shoe throughout their lifespan. As a result, the foot will take on the shape of the shoe regardless of the fit. A proper shoe fit requires

appropriate length and width measurements as well as an assessment of the person's style of arch. Box 15-5 provides several considerations for selecting and maintaining appropriate footwear.

Any patient with foot or ankle problems should have their shoes evaluated. Assessment parameters include wear pattern, a tracing of the weight-bearing foot, footprints, and use of heels, arch supports, and heel cushions. Normal wear patterns occur on the outsole and slightly medial at the great toe and lateral calcaneus. Different wear patterns may be indicative of underlying foot problems or problems with alignment and gait as illustrated in Figure 15-6. For example, wear on the ball of the foot may indicate that the heel tendon is tight, in which case heel-raising exercises can be recommended to release this tendon. Toe-shaped ridges on the upper toe box may indicate that the shoes are too small or that hammer toes are developing. A bulge and wear to the side of the great toe may indicate that the shoe is too narrow or that a bunion is present. Finally, unridged wear on the upper toe box generally indicates that the front of the shoe is too low (Ward, 2005).

A tracing of the weight-bearing foot is useful in assessing the fit of the shoe in terms of length and width. The foot tracing is compared to the current shoe to objectively reveal the flaw in the fitting, whether the foot is wider or longer than the shoe (see Figure 14-4). For example, toe box width plays an enormous role in the development of bunions, toe deformities, and corns. This type of foot tracing will also reveal the source of

BOX 15-3	**Basic Cuticle and Nail Trimming Using Toenail Nippers**

1. Begin cuticle and nail care after bathing when nails are softer.
2. Examine nails.
   A. Observe for presence of hyponychium that has hypertrophied, hypergranulation tissue, ingrowing corners of nail borders, hyperkeratosis, or other abnormal findings. Patients with very thick or ingrown nails require referral to foot care professional.
   B. Define the free nail border by assessing the tissue underneath the nail, using beveled edge of orangewood stick.
   C. Unhealthy nails should be trimmed last to prevent the transmission of infection.
3. Remove any loose debris from under the nail.
4. Gently trim excessively thick or loose cuticles.
   A. Avoid excess manipulation of the cuticle, which may lead to infection.
5. Decide between slightly rounded cut and straight across cut:
   A. *Straight across* (not too short) for puffy or thick skin folds prone to ingrown toenails
   B. *Slightly rounded* for problems with nail corners curving and causing pain and thickening of skin at distal aspect of nail groove
6. Remove free edge of nail.
   A. Do not trim nail off in one clip; make small cuts.
   B. Begin at one edge of nail, nip smoothly working across entire nail border no lower than $\frac{1}{16}$ to $\frac{1}{8}$ inch from end of toe (lateral plate should extend beyond nail fold).
   C. Do not cut deeply into lateral corners of nail bed.
   D. Avoid cutting skin; openings in skin are avenues of entry for bacteria and other infectious agents.
7. Use fine point of nipper to trim out sharp edge of lateral aspect of nail that curves deeply in nail margin.
8. Smooth nail with emery board.

BOX 15-4	**Nail Debridement Using Mechanical Rotary Tool**

1. Before using a Dremel drill, patients should be informed that they will feel a vibration while the nail is being debrided.
2. Don appropriate personal protective equipment.
3. Remove most of fungal nail with quality nippers before using drill to minimize dust.
4. Support toe between index finger and thumb of nondominant hand to prevent toe from moving during debridement. The other toes should be held away from the bur during the procedure.
5. Set grinder speed to 10,000–15,000 rpm.
6. Debride nail by slowly and gently applying pressure as grinder is moved from proximal to distal portion of plate.
7. Keep nail plate visible at all times. Frequently stop grinding to wipe away dust with a cloth (do not blow).
8. Stop grinding when nail is thin or when dust becomes very fine and is not visibly produced during debridement.
9. *Do not grind through nail plate!* Soft underlying layers of plate can be abraded, possibly resulting in subungual wound to nail bed.
10. Avoid surrounding tissue, which can become abraded.

Equipment Options
- Drill with attached vacuum
- Room air circulators with high-efficiency particulate air (HEPA) filters
- Tungsten carbide burs and bits are preferable because they run cold, do not abrade skin, and produce big particles rather than dust
- Ruby carvers and diamond bits are preferable to steel

Equipment Sterilization
- Proper cleansing of equipment between patients is single most important task in reducing or eliminating spread of infection.
- Sterilize in autoclave or use antifungal cold soaking solution (glutaraldehyde, phenol, sodium hypochlorite, sodium bromide, iodophors).
- Alcohol does not kill fungus and should not be used for cleansing nail equipment.

Personal Protective Equipment and Back Safety
- Gloves, mask, goggles, gown, hair covering
- Height-adjustable chair or examination table for patient
- Height-adjustable chair for clinician
- Change positions frequently; stretch back muscles

any foot pain. This tracing can be used to reinforce teaching to the patient about proper shoe fitting. Because the proper fitting of shoes is not an exact science, the patient should be encouraged to take the tracing to the shoe store when purchasing new shoes.

To evaluate the arch, a footprint can be made by placing the foot into a bucket of water and making a footprint on a piece of brown paper (Figure 15-7). A footprint that is very wide in the middle is indicative of flat feet. With flat feet, the foot rolls excessively to the inside (i.e., overpronation), which leads to arch strain and pain on the inside of the knee. Adaptations to overcome flat feet and overpronation include molded leather arch supports (available over the counter) and athletic shoe styles. These types of shoes are designed with "control" features that aid in preventing the rolling-in motion of the ankle. If arch supports or sports shoes are ineffective, a foot specialist can fabricate a custom-molded orthotic shoe insert.

If the footprint shows little or no connectedness between the heel and the forefoot, the person has a high arch (underpronation). In this case, the foot rolls too much laterally, with a lot of weight landing on the outside edge of the foot. With this type of situation, the ankle becomes more susceptible to sprains and stress fractures. Again, athletic shoes are most appropriate because (1) "stability" athletic shoes are built with extra cushioning and (2) high-top athletic shoes cover the foot and ankle snugly to reduce the risk of ankle sprains and minimize damage to the ankle from twists (American Orthopaedic Foot & Ankle Society, 2010).

High heels increase torque on the knee and increase pressure on the forefoot. In addition, women naturally pronate more than men and naturally rely heavily on heel cushioning and arch support to reduce pronation. Unfortunately, high heels and arch supports restrict the

---

BOX 15-5	Selecting and Maintaining Appropriate Footwear

Shoe Size
- Do not select shoes by size marked inside shoe; sizes vary among shoe brands and styles.

Measurement
- Measure *both* feet regularly; size of feet change with age.

Fitting
- Fit to larger foot.
- Fit at end of the day when feet are at their largest.
- Stand during fitting process.
- Hold new shoe over foot tracing to be certain entire tracing is covered by shoe.
- There should be ⅜ inch to ½ inch between longest toe and end of each shoe.
- Stand next to shoes to determine if shoes are shaped like feet or if there are areas of constriction.
- Shoe should conform as much as possible to shape of foot.
- Heel should fit comfortably in shoe with minimum amount of slippage.
- Ball of foot should fit comfortably into widest part (ball pocket) of shoe.
- Do not purchase shoes that feel too tight, expecting them to "stretch" to fit.
- Examine inside of shoe by hand to check for seams, tacks, rough places.
- Walk in shoe to make sure it fits and feels right.

Shoe Type
- A healthy shoe is one that is shaped like the foot. Shoe has deep, roomy, and rounded or square toe box (area of shoe over toes).
- Shoe should be made of very soft material similar to glove leather.

- Flat shoes (with heel height of 1 inch or less) are the healthiest shoes for feet. If high-heeled shoes are needed, keep to heel height of 2 inches or less, limit wearing of shoes to 3 hours at a time, and take shoes off coming to and from work, dinner, or church.
- Soles should be shock-absorbing and skid-resistant (rubber rather than smooth leather).
- Avoid shoes that have seams over areas of pain (e.g., bunion).
- Avoid shoes with heavy rubber soles that curl over top of toe area (e.g., some running shoes) because they can catch on carpets and cause accidental falls.
- Lace-up rather than slip-on shoes provide more secure fit and can accommodate insoles and orthotic devices.
- Select and wear shoe appropriate to activity (e.g., steel-toed boots for farm work, running shoes for running).

Additional Tips
- Wear new shoes initially for short intervals (e.g., 20 minutes twice per day) and check feet and toes upon removal.
- Indentations, skin discoloration, warmth may be signs of mechanical trauma (pressure points, friction, repetitive stress).
- Do not wear same pair of shoes every day.
- Prior to putting on shoes, shake them and feel inside them to remove any foreign objects
- Note lumpy insoles or torn linings. Replace worn-out shoes as soon as possible.
- White or light-colored socks are preferred so that any drainage (suggestive of ulceration) is readily apparent.
- Avoid walking barefoot, even at home, because feet are more susceptible to injury and infection.
- Apply sun block to feet when wearing sandals or at the beach.
- Discard socks with holes, socks that have been darned.
- Tops of socks should not restrict circulation.

Data from Orthopaedic Foot and Ankle Society, the National Shoe Retailers Association, and the Pedorthic Footwear Association (*Am Orthop Foot Ankle Soc*, 2003).

---

natural movement of the ankle. Furthermore, by reducing pronation, the natural function in ankle motion also increases torque on the knee (Godfrey, 2006).

Offloading and Padding

Offloading and padding are used to protect bony structures of the foot, such as prominent metatarsal heads, or toe deformities from mechanical trauma caused by seams in the socks or shoes. Offloading techniques such as those summarized in Table 15-4 and illustrated in Figures 14-5, 14-6, 14-7, and 14-8 include total contact casts, removable splints and casts, and customized shoes, pads, and inserts.

Over-the-counter and custom-molded padding and inserts can be used to redistribute pressure, reduce hyperkeratotic lesions, and eliminate repetitive stress and friction (Freeman, 2002; Wound, Ostomy and Continence Nurses [WOCN] Society, 2004). Pads can be used

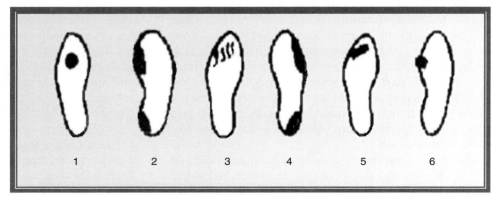

FIGURE 15-6 How to "read" your shoes. **1,** Wear on the ball of the foot. **2,** Wear on the inner sole. **3,** Toe-shaped ridges on the upper toe box. **4,** Outer sole wear. **5,** Bulge and wear to the side of the big toe. **6,** Wear on the upper and above the toes. (Modified from American Orthopaedic Foot & Ankle Society: *How to "read" your shoes,* available at http://www.aofas.org/Scripts/4Disapi.dll/4DCGI/cms/review.html? Action=CMS_Document &Doc ID=78, accessed September 2, 2010.)

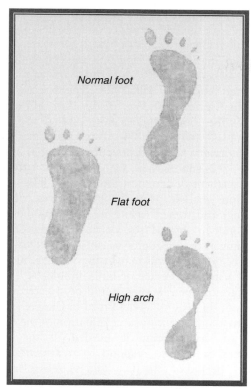

FIGURE 15-7 How to "read" your footprint. (From American Orthopaedic Foot & Ankle Society: *How to "read" your footprints,* available at http://www.aofas.org/Scripts/4Disapi.dll/4DCGI/cms/review. html?Action=CMS_Document&DocID=168, accessed September 2, 2010.)

to protect diminished fat pads on the plantar surface of the foot. However, pads with aggressive adhesives should be avoided on fragile elderly skin. Nonadherent silicone pads should be used and can be held in place with socks over prominent metatarsal heads. Tubular pads can be fit on the tips of toes to protect at-risk areas or used between toes where intradigital calluses may form. Lamb's wool can be woven between all toes or placed between at-risk toes. The wool provides inherent moisturizing from the lanolin while also absorbing perspiration and excess moisture (Kelechi and Lukacs, 1996; Ozdemir et al, 2004).

MANAGEMENT OF SPECIFIC CONDITIONS

Many conditions and circumstances can greatly affect the integrity and function of the foot, such as obesity, anemia, renal insufficiency, impaired circulation, gout, warfarin therapy, Raynaud disease, immunosuppression, and recurrent cellulitis. The 33 joints in each foot must accommodate an extraordinary weight load, making the feet particularly susceptible to arthritic inflammation and swelling of the cartilage and lining of the joints. Individuals older than 50 years are at greatest risk for arthritis. Osteoarthritis is the most common form of arthritis and is associated with

TABLE 15-4	Techniques for Offloading the Foot
Method	**Characteristics**
Bed rest	Total non–weight-bearing Patient adherence is difficult Presents quality-of-life issues Promotes hyperglycemia Promotes patient debilitation Increases risk of posterior heel pressures
Total contact cast	Forces adherence Allows for limited ambulation Requires specialized skill to make Not advisable for infected or highly exudative wounds
Walking splints/ removable casts	Allows for daily wound surveillance and care Requires strict patient adherence
Wedge-soled shoe	Commercially available Can be customized May cause balance problems
Healing shoe with large toe box and customized inserts	Provides offloading to specific wound locations Requires specialized equipment Requires specialized skill to make
Adhesive felt pad	Simple to make Inexpensive Easy to use with dressings Requires at least weekly dressing changes
Felted foam pads	Simple to make Inexpensive Easy to use with dressings Requires replacement every 3–4 days
Crest pads (adjunct for hammer or claw toes)	Simple to make Commercially available Inexpensive May be used for wound prevention Requires frequent replacement
Interdigital pads	Commercially available May be used for wound prevention Ineffective if shoes are too narrow
Lamb's wool	Commercially available Inexpensive May cause toe constriction
Padded socks	Commercially available May be cause of foot pressure and/or toe constriction if shoe fit does not allow for increased padding

From WOCN Society: *Guideline for management of wounds in patients with lower-extremity neuropathic disease,* WOCN Clinical Practice Guideline Series #3, Glenview, IL, 2004.

aging, injury, or overuse. The foot is one of the first places for osteoporosis to appear; a stress fracture of the foot is often its first sign. A variety of normal age-associated changes occur in the foot: the foot becomes wider, longer, and flatter; the fat pad on the bottom of the calcaneus thins; and the foot and ankle lose some degree of range of motion and become stiff, which contributes to some loss of balance with ambulation (Ozdemir et al, 2004; Willacy, 2008). Impaired circulation due to lower extremity arterial disease or lower extremity venous disease as well as decreased foot sensation due to lower extremity neuropathic disease, syphilis, leprosy, myelomeningocele, syringomyelia, hereditary neuropathies, or traumatic nerve injury contribute to problems with the foot (Adler et al, 1999; Younes et al, 2004). Superficial as well as deep lesions and skin alterations can potentially lead to significant infection.

Skin Conditions

A variety of skin conditions (e.g., vesicles, bullae, or ulcers) can develop on the feet due to repetitive friction and prolonged pressure from ill-fitting shoes. Infection can develop in the foot triggered by a moist environment and require treatment with appropriate medications (antifungal, antibacterial, or antiviral). Hyperkeratotic lesions (corns and calluses) are among the most common foot problems among older people (Figure 15-8). Ulcers can develop under these hyperkeratotic lesions with long-term low-level insult and become particularly problematic in the person with loss of protective sensation (Spink et al, 2009).

Warts *(Verruca papilloma)* are common dermatologic infections. Plantar warts, specifically, are caused by the human papillomavirus, affect persons of all ages, are contagious, and will spread to other people especially where the epidermal barrier is disrupted (Watkins, 2006). Plantar warts can also spread to other histologically similar sites (Lichon and Khachemoune, 2007).

Fungal infections may develop and include candida (rarely seen on the feet) and dermatophytes. More commonly called tinea, dermatophyte lesions are discussed in detail in Chapter 5. Dermatophyte symptoms may be less pronounced in elderly individuals and in individuals with altered sensation (Hill, 2008). The moccasin type of tinea pedis is often mistaken for dry skin on the plantar surface of the foot but does not respond to emollient application (Crawford, 2004). Tinea pedis may co-exist with a secondary bacterial infection (Erbagci, 2004).

Table 15-2 summarizes the assessment, prevention, and management of common foot lesions. The variety of interventions include properly fitting shoes, offloading, positioning, and topical agents such as emollients, antifungals, and, in some cases, corticosteroids. Offloading and padding as described previously is needed to interrupt the presence of the stressors causing vesicles, ulcers, and corns. In general, a vesicle or bulla should be left intact. Topical care of open lesions should be selected based on the needs of the wound as described in Chapter 18.

As with all interventions, reevaluation of the effectiveness of the intervention is needed. If the problem deteriorates or fails to respond to treatment within a reasonable period of time (i.e., 7 days), reassessment and modification of the treatment should be conducted. For example, topical antibiotics and corticosteroids may need to be delivered systemically rather than topically. However, use of these medications should be recommended only by a practitioner who is well informed of their potential complications and side affects, which can include conditions such as skin reactions, liver enzyme abnormalities, diarrhea, and visual and taste disturbances.

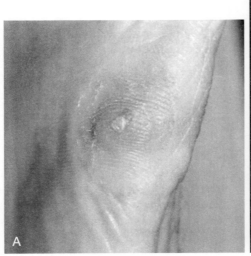
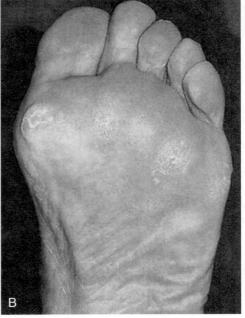

FIGURE 15-8 Selected lesions and skin alterations. A, Corn. B, Callus. (From Seidel HM et al, *Mosby's guide to physical examination* ed 5, St. Louis, MO, 2003.)

Foot Conditions (Malformations)

Foot malformations can affect all three sections of the foot: forefoot, midfoot, and hindfoot. Charcot arthropathy (see Figure 14-1, *B*) is a fairly rare but serious condition caused by the disruption or disintegration of some of the foot and ankle joints. Redness, swelling, and deformity may develop and may be misinterpreted as cellulitis. Charcot arthropathy is frequently associated with diabetes (discussed in greater detail in Chapter 14).

Forefoot. The forefoot area has the highest prevalence of foot malformations. The most common problems that arise in the forefoot are hallux valgus (bunions), bunionettes, hallux rigidus, claw toes, hammer toes and mallet toes, metatarsalgia, and interdigit neuromas (Morton neuroma). Forefoot problems are painful and are generally accompanied by ingrown toenail, calluses, and corns (Hsi et al, 2005). Forefoot problems occur nine times more often in women than in men and are most commonly associated with wearing shoes with high heels and a narrow toe box. Once forefoot problems develop, finding footwear can be difficult. Brief descriptions of forefoot malformations are provided in Table 15-5 and illustrated in Figure 14-1 (Ferrari et al, 2004; Larson et al, 2005; Thomson et al, 2004). Forefoot pain, specifically metatarsalgia, results from an abnormal metatarsal length with alteration of the weight-bearing forces. Symptoms of metatarsalgia include callus formation and localized pain in the plantar aspect of the forefoot over the metatarsal heads. Treatment of forefoot pain involves the application of a metatarsal pad and paring down of calluses (Hsi et al, 2005).

Midfoot. The primary midfoot problem is pain. Midfoot pain is commonly caused by arthritis in the midfoot joints, including the tarsometatarsal joint, subtalar joint, and talonavicular joint. The exact area of pain is easily pinpointed with palpation. The palpation of a bony prominence that is an osteophyte or dorsal bossing corresponds with the joint with the arthritis. Although less common, soft tissue pain can be present on the plantar aspect of the midfoot, which occurs with plantar fasciitis; this is discussed in more detail in the "Hindfoot" section below (Frey, 2005).

Hindfoot. Heel pain, a typical hindfoot problem, is caused by stress on the calcaneus and results from poorly made footwear and walking or jumping on hard

TABLE 15-5	Types of Forefoot Malformations	
Name	**Description**	**Common Location(s)**
Hallux valgus (bunion) (see Figure 14-1C)	Lateral deviation of great toe (hallux) Produces abnormal hypertrophic bursa over medial eminence of first metatarsal Diagnostic testing includes examination and radiograph to determine degree of deviation Symptoms include pain, redness, and swelling at or near the joint; as toe devastation progresses, bunion becomes more painful	First MTP joint
Bunionette (tailor's bunion)	Less common than bunion; see description above	Fifth MTP joint
Hallux rigidus	Degenerative arthritis of MTP joint Presents with pain in great toe with activity, especially in toe-off phase of gait Stiffness of great toe and loss of extension at MTP joint Toe in normal alignment Radiographs show narrowing of MTP joint of great toe	First MTP joint
Interdigit neuroma (Morton neuroma)	Not a true neuroma Perineural fibrosis of common digital nerve as it passes through metatarsal head; fibrosis results from repeated irritation of nerve that may be caused by bones or other tissue rubbing against and irritating the nerves Plantar pain in forefoot is most common presenting symptom Pain usually is alleviated by rubbing ball of the foot after removing shoes	Metatarsal head
Claw toe	Usually associated with neurologic disorder or inflammatory arthritis	Lesser toes
Hammer toe (see Figure 14-1A)	Fixation of proximal dorsiflexion, middle joint is fixed in plantar flexion, distal joint is moveable Usually bilateral Often accompanied by hallux valgus	Lesser toes
Mallet toe	Distal interphalangeal joint is plantarflexed on intermediate phalanx with rest of joint in normal position	Lesser toes
Charcot arthropathy (see Figure 14-1B)	Fairly rare but serious; associated with diabetes Caused by disruption or disintegration of some of the foot and ankle joints Redness, swelling, and deformity may develop and may be misinterpreted as cellulitis (Discussed in greater detail in Chapter 14)	Foot

MTP, Metatarsophalangeal.

surfaces. Common causes include plantar fasciitis, heel spur, tarsal tunnel syndrome, and Achilles tendonitis (Labib et al, 2002). Additional causative factors include arthritis, gout, ankylosing spondylitis, Reiter syndrome, radiculopathy, inferior calcaneal bursitis, calcaneal fracture, foreign bodies, circulatory problems, and obesity. Calcaneus pain can be palpated directly over the plantar medial calcaneal tuberosity. A heel spur, an osteophyte bony growth on the underside, foremost part of the calcaneus bone, is commonly associated with plantar fasciitis, as illustrated in Figure 15-9 (Frey, 2005).

Plantar fasciitis is the most common condition causing heel pain. This pain occurs with weight-bearing or faulty biomechanics that place too much stress on the calcaneus bone, ligaments, or nerves in the area (Jolly et al, 2005; La Porta and La Fata, 2005). Plantar fasciitis is essentially an inflammation of the long band of connective tissue running from the calcaneus to the ball of the foot that forms the arch of the foot (Lemont et al, 2003). Symptoms include pain on the plantar surface of the heel and pain that is worse upon arising or after sitting a long time and increases over a few months. Plantar fasciitis is most likely to develop in people with either overly flat feet or high arched feet.

Posterior heel pain causes symptoms behind the foot rather than underneath, is likely related to irritation from shoes, and presents with a prominence over the superior process of the calcaneus. A common cause of posterior heel pain is Achilles tendonitis, considered a jumping injury. The Achilles tendon connects the calf muscle to the heel bone and facilitates walking by helping raise the heel off the ground. Symptoms of Achilles tendon pathology includes pain along the tendon (aching, stiff, soreness) and pain that begins upon arising and after periods of rest, improves slightly with movement, then worsens with increased activity. Athletes are at high

risk for developing Achilles tendon pathology. Tarsal tunnel syndrome causes heel pain similar to carpal tunnel syndrome in the hand and is a repetitive motion injury (Badlissi et al, 2005).

The cause of heel pain must be determined before a plan of treatment is initiated. General treatments include rest or avoiding the precipitating activity (e.g., jogging), icing the heel, exercises and stretches, and nonsteroidal antiinflammatory medications. An orthotic device, such as a silicone heel pad insert with shock absorbing soles, is often key to successful treatment of calcaneus pain. Exercises such as "alphabet exercise," where the patient moves the ankle in multiple planes of motion by drawing both lowercase and uppercase letters of the alphabet with the foot, is particularly beneficial for heel spurs. Cortisone injections as well as over-the-counter heel cups or custom-made orthotics also may be warranted.

Nail Conditions (Onychopathy)

Onycho means "nail." Onychopathy is any disease or deformity of the nail. Abnormal nails are clues to multisystem diseases. The growth rate, discoloration, thickness, and structural changes can be equated to specific disease processes. Nails should be inspected for general appearance; nail plate for length, color, thickness, presence of subungual debris, odor, hyponychium or eponychium for separation from the nail plate; and paronychial edge for infection, ingrown nails, hangnails, and pain. The toenails should be assessed for changes in color, continuity of the nail plate, missing nails or nail malformations, and infection. Selected nail disorders, descriptions, symptoms, and causes are listed in Table 15-6. This section describes management strategies.

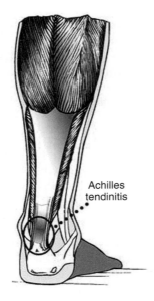

FIGURE 15-9 Locations of Achilles tendonitis and heel spur. (From American Physical Therapy Association, 1996.)

Achilles tendinitis

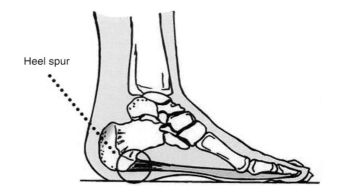

Heel spur

TABLE 15-6	Selected Nail Disorders		
Name	**Description**	**Symptoms**	**Cause**
Paronychia (see Figure 15-10A)	Painful infection of tissue around base of nail (perionychium)	Swelling and tenderness posterior or lateral to nail folds. May progress to superficial abscess	Bacteria enter break in skin caused by damage, trauma (e.g., nail biting, chemical irritants)
Onychocryptosis (ingrown nail) (see Figure 15-10B)	Penetration of segment of nail plate into nail sulcus and subcutaneous tissue	Acute inflammation, edema, exudate, pain. Can evolve into infection, (paronychia, cellulitis), ulceration, necrosis. Most commonly affects large toes	Improper nail trimming; Shoe pressure; Injury or fungal infection; Poor foot structure; Onychogryposis; Higher risk: male, increasing age, immunosuppression, diabetes, PVD, peripheral vascular disease
Onychomycosis (fungal infection)	Tinea unguium or dermatophyte infection. Occurs in three distinct forms: distal subungual, proximal subungual, white superficial	Painless, dystrophic changes (thick, brittle discoloration) of one or many toenails. Psoriasis, lichen planus, dermatitis, dyshidrosis may mimic onychomycosis	Infectious agent present on susceptible host; Chronic exposure to moisture; Hyperhidrosis; Tinea pedis; Poor hygiene
Onychogryposis (ram's horn nail)	Large, deformed, hypertrophic nail	Thick hard nails that curl like horn of ram	Nail was permitted to grow without trimming or debridement
Onychophosis	Localized or diffuse hyperkeratosis on lateral or proximal nail folds, in space between nail folds and nail plate	First and fifth toes are commonly affected	Poor-fitting shoes
Onychatrophia	Atrophy of nails	Softer, thinner, smaller nails. Nail detachment	Skin diseases, underlying diseases

Onychocryptosis (Ingrown Nail). Management of onychocryptosis includes education on proper nail trimming and proper fitting of shoes. The lateral plate should be allowed to grow well beyond the nail fold before trimming horizontally. The mild to moderate ingrown nail with minimal pain and erythema and no discharge can be treated with the application of a cotton wedge or dental floss underneath the lateral nail plate. This separates the nail plate from the lateral nail fold, which relieves the pressure. The moderate to severe ingrown toenail with substantial erythema and pustular discharge (Figure 15-10B) will require a digital block and removal of the involved nail wedge with a hemostat. Cleansing the area with 1:1 peroxide and water two to three times per day followed by the application of a topical antibiotic is recommended (Rounding and Bloomfield, 2005).

Onychomycosis (Fungal Infection of Nail). Fungal infections account for only 50% of the dystrophic nails. Nail conditions such as psoriasis, lichen planus, dermatitis, dyshidrosis, and other infections may mimic onychomycosis (Baran and Kaoukhov, 2005). Therefore culturing the nail has become a standard of practice before treatment with an antifungal. The antifungal chosen is usually driven by insurance reimbursement of the medication. The highest cure rates are associated with oral terbinafine and itraconazole. Topical nail

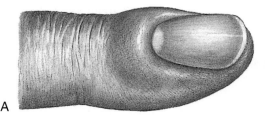

Paronychia

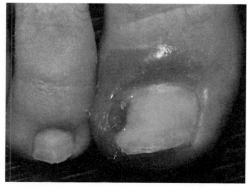

FIGURE 15-10 Selected nail disorders: **A,** Paronychia **B,** Onychocryptosis (ingrown nail). (A, From Seidel HM et al: *Mosby's guide to physical examination,* ed 6, St. Louis, 2006, Mosby. B, From White GM: *Color atlas of regional dermatology,* St. Louis, 1994, Mosby.)

lacquer containing ciclopirox is used for mild to moderate onychomycosis that does not involve the lunula (see Figure 15-3). The lacquer is applied once daily to the affected nail, 5 mm of surrounding skin, the nail bed (hyponychium), and the undersurface of the nail plate. Once per week, the nail is wiped off with alcohol. Studies have showed increased efficacy with the combination treatment (Sidou and Soto, 2004).

Paronychia. Paronychia is inflammation of the cells that grow the nail (matrix) (see Figure 15-10A) resulting in edema and erythema from many of the disorders described in Table 15-6. For chronic paronychia, treatment consists of warm soaks and topical antifungal agents. Treatment of acute paronychia includes warm compresses for 20 minutes three times per day and topical antibiotics (triple antibiotic) applied after the warm soaks. For more severe infections, oral antibiotics with gram-positive coverage may be necessary (Lee et al, 2009).

Referral

Numerous specialists (e.g., primary care provider, podiatry, orthopedics, dermatology, endocrinology, vascular surgery, general surgery, physical therapy, occupational therapy, pedorthist/orthotist, home health, pain management, diabetes education, smoking cessation, case/care manager, social worker, wound specialist) may be required to provide comprehensive foot and nail care. Results of the foot screening must be communicated to the appropriate health care provider, along with the patient's foot ulceration risk and a record of the educational materials given to the patient and family (Boulton and Armstrong, 2008; Patout et al, 2001).

Patient and Caregiver Education

Involving patients in their own care decreases foot complications therefore it is important to provide education on foot and nail care to the patient and caregiver (Howell and Thirlaway, 2004). Box 15-6 lists the components of patient and family education related to foot care (Phillip, 2005). Patients should be taught that they can protect the health of their feet by maintaining a normal weight to lessen changes due to osteoporosis (Neno, 2007; Woodrow, et al 2005). Additional foot care instructions can be found in Box 14-5. The patient should be taught to call the health care professional when problems as listed in Box 15-6 arise (American Orthopaedic Foot & Ankle Society, 2008; Gemmell et al, 2005; van Os et al, 2005).

Home Remedies

Many over-the-counter and home remedies are used for treatment of foot and nail problems. Four products are most commonly used; Vicks VapoRub, vinegar, vegetable oil, and Vaseline. Vaseline and vegetable oil (Crisco)

BOX 15-6	Components of Patient and Family Education

- Foot care (hygiene, skin care, inspection, nail care)
- Anatomy and pathophysiology affecting the foot
- Age-specific foot changes
- Ulcer and amputation risk
- Lifestyle choices that affect health (exercise, smoking, nutrition, weight management)
- Plans for preventing foot disorders
- Proper footwear (see Box 15-5)
- Plan for follow-up
- Problems that should be reported:
  - Foot or ankle pain that is intense
  - Foot or ankle pain that persists for more than 72 hours
  - Lower extremity pain that increases with exercise or ambulation, rest, or elevation
  - Swelling of one leg or foot that persists for more than 24 hours
  - Sudden progression of a foot deformity
  - Unilateral flattening of foot arch
  - Infection
  - Loss of sensation
  - Blister or ulcer on foot that developed without the patient feeling it
  - Blister or ulcer on foot that is not healing

---

are inexpensive options and can be used to moisturize the skin. Vegetable oil has a risk of bacterial growth while in the container and the risk of allergic dermatitis. Vaseline (petroleum) comes in different grades, which vary depending on composition, purity (depending on stock), production, and packaging. Petrolatum-based products have been identified as clinically effective and cost-effective. Allergic dermatitis can occur from petroleum products (Kelechi, 2005).

Vinegar and Vicks VapoRub are used to treat fungal and bacterial infections. In various dilutions, vinegar is effective in reducing or eliminating growth of bacteria. Evidence for the use of vinegar in treating fungal infection is limited. The literature has reported vinegar (one part vinegar and 2 parts water for 15 minutes per day) used as treatment of toenail fungus, athlete's foot, and foot odor and as an exfoliant. Long-term use of vinegar (regardless of concentration) is contraindicated, however, due to the drying effect and potential for skin irritation. Anecdotally, Vicks VapoRub applied topically to the nail daily has been used for treatment of toenail fungus (Kelechi, 2005).

Unsupervised home remedies for foot ailments should be avoided. Self-treatment has the potential for turning a minor problem into a major one. Persons with diabetes, poor circulation, or heart problems should not treat their own feet because they are more prone to infection. It is vital that older individuals see a foot care specialist at least once per year for a checkup (Neno, 2007; Woodrow et al 2005).

SUMMARY

Foot and nail disorders are predominantly a reflection of the patient's overall health status. By conducting a regular and routine foot and nail assessment in conjunction with a routine skin assessment, preventive interventions can be identified that will prevent the discomfort and secondary complications that arise from foot and nail disorders. Routine foot care should be integrated into everyday practice, thus keeping the skin healthy and intact and minimizing the risk of trauma or malformation (Howell and Thirlaway, 2004).

REFERENCES

American Orthopaedic Foot and Ankle Society: *How to "read" your footprints*, (copyright 2010), available at http://www.aofas.org/Scripts/4Disapi.dll/4DCGI/cms/review.html?Action=CMS_Document&DocID=168, accessed May 17, 2010.

American Orthopaedic Foot and Ankle Society: Watch out for these red flags, (copyright 2010) last updated January 2008. available at http://www.aofas.org/Scripts/4Disapi.dll/4DCGI/cms/review.html?Action=CMS_Document&DocID=75

American Podiatric Medical Association: *General foot health. A biological masterpiece, but subject to many ills,* 2010, available at http://www.apma.org/MainMenu/Foot-Health/FootHealth-Brochures/GeneralFootHealthBrochures/GeneralFootHealth.aspx, accessed May 24, 2010.

Badlissi F et al: Foot musculoskeletal disorders, pain, and foot-related functional limitation in older persons, *J Am Geriatr Soc* 53:1029-1033, 2005.

Baran R, Kaoukhov A: Topical antifungal drugs for the treatment of onychomycosis: an overview of current strategies for monotherapy and combination therapy, *J Eur Acad Dermatol Venereol* 19:21, 2005.

Boulton A, Armstrong D: Comprehensive foot examination and risk assessment, *Diabetes Care* 31:1679-1685, 2008.

Cavanagh PR, Ulbrecht JS: The biomechanics of the foot in diabetes mellitus. In Bowker JH, Pfeiffer MA, editors: *Levin and O'Neal's the diabetic foot,* ed 7, St. Louis, 2008, Mosby.

Crawford F: Athlete's foot and fungally infected toenails, *Clin Evid* June:2128-2132, 2004.

Duthie EH: History and physical exam. In Duthie EH et al, editors: *Practice of geriatrics,* ed 4, Philadelphia, 2007, Saunders Elsevier.

Erbagci Z: Topical therapy for dermatophytoses: should corticosteroids be included? *Am J Clin Dermatol* 5:375, 2004.

Ferrari J et al; Interventions for treating hallux valgus (abductovalgus) and bunions, *Cochrane Database Syst Rev* 1:CD000964, 2004.

Freeman DB: Corns and calluses resulting from mechanical hyperkeratosis, *Am Fam Physician* 65:2277, 2002.

Frey C: Plantar fasciitis. In Griffin LY, editor: *Essentials of musculoskeletal care,* ed 3, Rosemont, Ill., 2005, American Academy of Orthopaedic Surgeons.

Garrow AP et al: The Cheshire foot pain and disability survey: a population survey assessing prevalence and associations, *Pain* 110:378, 2004.

Gemmell H et al: A theoretical model for treatment of soft tissue injuries: treatment of an ankle sprain in a college tennis player, *J Manipulat Physiol Therapeut* 28:285, 2005.

Godfrey, JR: Toward the optimal health. D. Casey Kerrigan, MD., discusses the impact of footwear on the progression of osteoarthritis in women, *J Womens Health* 15:894-897, 2006.

Hill MJ: Fungal Infections, *Dermatol Nurs* 20:137-138, 2008.

Howell M, Thirlaway S: Integrating foot care into the everyday clinical practice of nurses, *Br J Nurs* 13:470, 2004.

Hsi WL et al: Optimum position of metatarsal pad in metatarsalgia for pressure relief, *Am J Phys Med Rehabil* 84:514, 2005.

Jarvis C: Neurologic system. In Jarvis C, editor: *Physical examination and health assessment,* St. Louis, 2004, Saunders.

Jolly GP et al: Neurogenic heel pain, *Clin Podiatr Med Surg* 22:101, 2005.

Katoh T: Outpatient foot care by dermatologist and specially trained nurse, *Jpn J Mycol* 49:173-174, 2008.

Katsambas A et al: The effects of foot disease on quality of life: results of the Achilles project, *J Eur Acad Dermatol Venereol* 19:191, 2005.

Kelechi T: The four V's of footcare, *Adv Nurse Pract* 12:67, 2005.

Kelechi T, Lukacs K: Intrapreneurial nursing: the comprehensive lower extremity assessment form, *Clin Nurse Spec CNS* 10:266, 1996.

La Porta GA, La Fata PC: Pathologic conditions of the plantar fascia, *Clin Podiatr Med Surg* 22:1, 2005.

Labib SA et al: Heel pain triad (HPT): the combination of plantar fasciitis, posterior tibial tendon dysfunction and tarsal tunnel syndrome, *Foot Ankle Int* 23:212, 2002.

Larson EE et al: Accurate nomenclature for forefoot nerve entrapment: a historical perspective, *J Am Podiatr Med Assoc* 95:298, 2005.

Lee S et al: *Paronychia,* updated August 11, 2009, available at http://emedicine.medscape.com/article/1106062-overview, accessed December 8, 2009.

Lemont H et al: Plantar fasciitis: a degenerative process (fasciosis) without inflammation, *J Am Podiatr Med Assoc* 93:234, 2003.

Leveille SG et al: Foot pain and disability in older women, *Am J Epidemiol* 148:657, 1998.

Lichon V, Khachemoune A: Plantar warts: a focus on treatment modalities, *Dermatol Nurs* 19(4):372-375, 2007.

Menz HB, Morris ME: Footwear characteristics and foot problems in older people, *Gerontology* 51:346-351, 2005.

Menz HB et al: The contribution of foot problems to mobility impairment and falls in community-dwelling older people, *J Am Geriatr Soc* 49:1651, 2001.

Mix G: *Salon professional's guide to foot care,* Albany, NY, 1999, Milady Salon Ovations.

Neno R: Feet for purpose? *Nurs Older People* 19(8):5-6, 2007.

Ozdemir H et al: Effects of changes in heel fat pad thickness and elasticity on heel pain, *J Am Podiatr Med Assoc* 94:47, 2004.

Patout CA Jr et al: A decision pathway for the staged management of foot problems in diabetes mellitus, *Arch Phys Med Rehabil* 82:1724, 2001.

Piraccini BM et al: Drug-induced nail abnormalities, *Expert Opin Drug Saf* 3:57, 2004.

Popoola MM, Jenkins L: Caring for the foot mobile, *Holistic Nurs Pract* 19:222-227, 2004.

Price P, Harding K: The impact of foot complications on health-related quality of life in patients with diabetes, *J Cutan Med Surg* 4:45, 2000.

Quinn E: Foot anatomy and physiology. *Sports Medicine About.com,* 2009, available at http://sportsmedicine.about.com/cs/foot_facts/a/foot1.htm, accessed May 15, 2010.

Rees HG: World at work; evidence based risk management of nail dust in chiropodists and podiatrist, *Occupat Environ Med* 65:216-217, 2008.

Rounding C, Bloomfield S: Surgical treatments for ingrowing toenails, *Cochrane Database Syst Rev,* 2:CD001541, 2005.

Schwartz R: *Gram-negative toe web infection,* 2009, available at http://emedicine.medscape.com/article/1055306-diagnosis, accessed November 15, 2009.

Sidou F, Soto P: A randomized comparison of nail surface rema-nence three nail lacquers, containing amorolfine 5%, ciclopirox 8% or tioconazole 28%, in healthy volunteers, *Int J Tissue Reactions* 26(1-2):17, 2004.

Sinni-McKeehen B: Nursing assessment. Integumentary system. In Lewis SL et al ed: *Medical-surgical nursing. Assessment and management of clinical problems*, St. Louis, 2007, Elsevier.

Spink MJ et al: Distribution and correlates of plantar hyperkera-totic lesions in older people, *J Foot Ankle Res* 30:8, 2009.

Sprecher E: Genetic hair and nail disorders, *Clin Dermatol* 23:47, 2005.

Stroud S, Kelechi T: Itching and sores between the toes. Macera-tion and fungal infection, *Adv Nurse Pract* 16(7):26, 2006.

Thomson CE et al: Interventions for the treatment of Morton's neuroma, *Cochrane Database Syst Rev* 3:CD003118, 2004.

van Os AG et al: Comparison of conventional treatment and supervised rehabilitation for treatment of acute lateral ankle sprains: a systematic review of the literature, *J Orthop Sports Phys Ther* 35:95 2005.

Vileikyte L et al: The development and validation of a neuropathy- and foot ulcer-specific quality of life instrument, *Diabetes Care* 26:2549, 2003.

Ward SA: Diabetes, exercise, and foot care, *Physician Sports Med* 33:33-38, 2005.

Watkins P: Identifying and treating plantar warts, *Nurs Stand* 20(42):50-54, 2006.

Willacy H: *Abnormal gait*, version 20, updated April 24, 2008. available at http://www.patient.co.uk/doctor/Abnormal-Gait.htm, accessed December 8, 2009.

WOCN Society: *Guideline for management of wounds in patients with lower-extremity neuropathic disease*, WOCN Clinical Practice Guideline Series #3, Glenview Ill., 2004, Author.

Woodrow P, et al: Foot care for non-diabetic older people, *Nurs Older People* 17(8):31-32, 2005.

Yetzer EA: Incorporating foot care education into diabetic foot screening, *Rehabil Nurs* 29(3):80, 2004.

Younes NA et al: Diabetic heel ulcers: a major risk factor for lower extremity amputation, *Ostomy Wound Manage* 50:50, 2004.

Wound Bed Preparation

16

Wound Infection: Diagnosis and Management

Nancy A. Stotts

OBJECTIVES

1. Compare and contrast the continuum of bacterial bio-burden, including contamination, colonization, critical colonization, biofilm, and wound infection.
2. Identify risk factors for chronic wound infection.
3. Describe the processes used in obtaining a wound culture by biopsy, aspiration, and swab.
4. Interpret laboratory data indicative of a wound infection.
5. Identify situations appropriate for debridement, topical antimicrobials, and systemic antibiotics.

The body's greatest defense against infection is intact skin. It is a mechanical barrier to microorganisms and its normal flora and acid pH control invasion of the skin by other microorganisms. When skin integrity is breached, the wound quickly becomes contaminated by body fluids and normal skin flora (Fonder et al, 2008). The effects of bacterial burden, called *bioburden*, on the wound are numerous and complex. Bacteria not only compete for the limited nutrients and oxygen present in the wound; they produce endotoxins and exotoxins that destroy or alter normal cellular activities, such as collagen deposition and cross-linking. *Endotoxins* are lipids and polysaccharides that are located in the cell wall of gram-negative organisms. When released, they activate the regulatory systems of the body (e.g., clotting, inflammation). *Exotoxins* are proteins released from bacteria that enzymatically inactivate or modify cells, causing them to die or disrupting their normal cellular functioning (Edwards and Harding, 2004). Excessive activity in these systems results in increased capillary permeability, leakage of fluid out of the vasculature, coagulopathies, and ultimately shock.

All chronic wounds contain some degree of bacterial bioburden and exhibit significantly elevated proinflammatory cytokines (interleukin-1, tumor necrosis factor-α, γ-interferon), matrix metalloproteinases (MMP-2, MMP-8, MMP-9), and neutrophils (Wolcott et al, 2009). In response to the proinflammatory proteins, neutrophils continue to arrive at the wound and release cytotoxic enzymes, free oxygen radicals, and inflammatory mediators triggering additional degradation of extracellular matrix and growth factors. Eventually protein lysis exceeds the synthesis of these proteins that are essential to wound repair so that the wound remains in the inflammatory phase and is unable to advance into the proliferative phase (Bjarnsholt et al, 2008; Woo and Sibbald, 2009).

The most common effect of this persistent chronic inflammatory state is delayed healing (Expert Working Group, 2008), which can deteriorate into infection, sepsis, multisystem organ failure, and death. Concomitantly, infection results in high cost, long hospitalization, as well as pain and suffering for patients and their families (Landis, 2008).

CONTINUUM OF BACTERIAL BIOBURDEN

All wounds have some level of bacterial burden; few wounds are infected. The presence of organisms in the wound is an expectation. Recognizing the range of wound bioburden is helpful because it provides a framework from which to assess the significance of the situation and identify appropriate interventions. The continuum of bacterial bioburden can be subdivided into five microbial states: contamination, colonization, critical colonization, biofilm, and infection (Box 16-1).

Contamination

Contamination is the presence of nonreplicating microorganisms on the wound surface (Sibbald et al, 2006). Because all open wounds are inevitably contaminated by normal skin flora, the body is continually challenged to defend itself against invasion (Basu et al, 2009).

BOX 16-1	Glossary of Terms

Antibacterial: Antiseptic that inhibits the growth of bacteria.

Antibiotic: Agent that can destroy or inhibit organisms. Has single target and therefore vulnerable to resistance.

Antimicrobial: General term for a substance that destroys or inhibits growth and replication of microorganisms.

Antiseptic/Antibacterial: Topical substance that inhibits growth and reproduction of organisms. Can be used on open wounds as well as intact skin. Strong biocidal agents and multiple pharmaceutical targets; little resistance developed to them; examples are iodine and silver. Duration of use limited to 2 weeks.

Bioburden: Presence of microorganisms on or in a wound. Continuum of bioburden ranges from contamination, colonization, critical colonization, biofilm, and infection. Bioburden includes the quantity of microorganisms present as well as their diversity, virulence, and interaction of the organisms with each other and with the body (synergism).

Biofilm: Complex community of aggregated bacteria embedded in a self-secreted extracellular polysaccharide matrix. Bacteria within biofilm respond to signals from other bacteria in the community to change their phenotype. Highly resistant to and poorly penetrated by antimicrobials. Can be removed with debridement. Reformation

is prevented with antimicrobials and maintenance debridement (including autolysis).

Colonization: Replicating microorganisms adherent to the wound surface without a host reaction. Antimicrobials are not indicated.

Contamination: **Non**replicating microorganisms **on** the wound surface without a host reaction. All open wounds are contaminated by normal skin flora. Antimicrobials are not indicated.

Critical Colonization: Replicating microorganisms present on the wound and attached to the cells and structures in the wound. Level of bacteria inhibits wound healing but host does not exhibit classic signs of infection. Topical antimicrobials are indicated.

Disinfectant: Chemical that destroys, neutralizes, or inhibits growth of microorganisms. Usually used on inanimate objects and intact skin; harmful to open tissue. Examples includes alcohol and hydrogen peroxide.

Infection: Microorganisms invade tissue and yield a local or systemic response. Cultures are obtained to direct antibiotic selection.

Osteomyelitis: Bone infection characterized by a mixture of inflammatory cells, fibrosis, bone necrosis, and new bone formation.

Planktonic Bacteria: Free-floating (not anchored) bacteria, such as occurs with contamination and colonization.

Contaminating microorganisms may be endogenous (e.g., normal skin and gastrointestinal flora) or exogenous, present in the external environment (e.g., bed linen, devices, hospital personnel) (Woo and Sibbald, 2009). Early contaminants usually are gram-positive organisms (*Staphylococcus aureus, Corynebacterium, Streptococcus,* coagulase-negative staphylococcus), followed by gram-negative organisms *(Escherichia coli, Klebsiella, Proteus.)* Later anaerobic organisms, such as *Prevotella, Bacteroides,* and *Peptostreptococcus,* and fungi are present and are difficult to isolate with routine culture techniques because they typically lodge deep in the wound (Landis, 2008). Local or systemic antibiotics are not required for the contaminated wound.

Colonization

With colonization, the microorganisms adhere to the surface of the wound and replicate. Colonization does not impair healing (Edwards and Harding, 2004). The bacteria are not pathogenic and do not require treatment with local or systemic antibiotics. Inappropriate use of antibiotics during this phase has contributed to the prevalence of antibiotic-resistant organisms (Landis, 2008).

Critical Colonization

Critical colonization describes a level of bacterial presence that affects skin cell proliferation and tissue repair; however, there is no systemic response (i.e., fever or leukocytosis) (Landis, 2008). Microorganisms are present on the surface of the wound and are attached to the wound surface but there is no invasion of the tissues by the bacteria.

The key characteristic associated with critical colonization are presented in Box 16-2 and include nonhealing (wound size fails to decrease over 2 or more weeks) (Sibbald et al, 2006). In addition to nonhealing, subtle indicators of critical colonization may include friable, unhealthy granulation tissue (dull dark red or overly bright red), exuberant granulation tissue, increased exudate, odor, and a change or increase in pain. Necrotic material or debris may be present and serve as a nutrient source for the invading organism(s) but is not an indicator of critical colonization (Sibbald et al, 2006; Woo and Sibbald, 2009). When critical colonization is suspected, topical antimicrobials should be implemented (Table 16-1) for a time-limited period (usually 2 weeks) and the situation reevaluated (EWMA, 2005).

BOX 16-2	Criteria for Colonization and Infection*

Critical Colonization (NERDS)
N = Nonhealing wound
E = Exudative wound
R = Red and bleeding wound
D = Debris
S = Smell from the wound

Deep Tissue Infection (STONEES)
S = Size is bigger
T = Temperature increased
O = Os (probes to or exposed bone)
N = New area of breakdown
E = Erythema/Edema
E = Exudate
S = Smell

*Data from Sibbald et al, 2006; Woo & Sibbald, 2009.

TABLE 16-1	Commonly Prescribed Topical Antimicrobials	
Topical Agent	**Action**	**Comments**
Acetic acid 0.25%–0.5%	Bactericidal	Effective against *Pseudomonas aeruginosa* Used as irrigant or soak Protect periwound skin, changes pH
Cadexomer iodine	Broad spectrum	Effective against Methicillin-resistant *Staphylococcus aureus* (MRSA) Slow release of iodine from beads Concentrations are nontoxic to fibroblasts Microspheres absorb bacteria and exudate while slowly releasing iodine to remove inhibitory cytokines Confirm patient is not allergic to iodine prior to use
Chlorhexidine 0.02%	Broad spectrum	Effective against *Staphylococcus aureus and Escherichia coli* Consider use in patients allergic to iodine Use as irrigant solution
Honey	Produces H_2O_2, contains antioxidants	Releases antiinflammatory products Reduces odor through bacterial metabolism that yields lactic acid instead of ammonia or sulfur Confirm patient is not allergic to honey, bee products, or bee stings prior to use
Hydrofera blue	Methylene blue and gentian violet	Effective against Methicillin-resistant *Staphylococcus epidermidis (MRSE)*, Vancomycin-resistant enterococcus (VRE), *S. aureus, S. epidermidis, Serratia, E. Coli*
Hydrogen peroxide	Oxidative debridement when necrotic tissue/debris present in wound	Not effective in reducing organisms Useful in removing debris because of its effervescent effects Use with care in closed cavities because of gas release
Mupirocin 2% ointment	Blocks activity of enzyme in bacteria responsible for making proteins	Effective against Methicillin-resistant *Staphylococcus aureus* (MRSA), β-hemolytic streptococcus, *Streptococcus pyogenes* Contraindicated for large burns Contains polyethylene glycol, which may damage kidneys if absorbed through skin
Povidone-iodine 1%–10%	Broad spectrum	No reported resistance Do not use scrub in open wound Confirm patient is not allergic to iodine prior to use
Silver dressings and creams	Broad spectrum	Concentration, rate of release, method of delivery vary by type of dressing (e.g., Acticoat provides rapid and sustained release when activated by water; Contreet hydrocolloid/foam provides sustained release as long as dressing absorbs exudate) Incorporated into cream, mesh, transparent, hydrogel, hydrocolloid, foam, alginate dressings, with selection based on wound characteristic and patient's needs (see Chapter 18) Effective against Methicillin-resistant *Staphylococcus aureus* (MRSA), Vancomycin-resistant enterococcus (VRE) Minimal allergic response Potential for tissue staining (see Plate 43)
Sodium hypochlorite (Dakin's solution)	Chlorine action kills organisms	Not usually recommended unless other alternatives are unavailable

Bacitracin zinc-neomycin, gentamycin sulfate, Polymyxin B, Garamycin for topical wound care are not commonly prescribed due to frequent development of sensitization.

Biofilms

Once microorganisms begin to adhere to the surface of the wound, they begin to develop biofilm (Pupp and Williams, 2008). A *biofilm* is a complex structure of microorganisms embedded in an extracellular matrix of hydrated polysaccharide that is permanently attached to the biologic or nonbiologic surface. Almost 70% of chronic wounds have a biofilm present, whereas only 6% of acute wounds have documented biofilm (Bjarnsholt et al, 2008). The biofilm comprises various types of organisms living together in symbiotic relationships and a harmonious community. *Proteus aeruginosa* and

S. aureus are the most common microorganisms forming chronic biofilm (Bjarnsholt et al, 2008). The number of organisms is limited by nutrient availability. Bacteria within the biofilm respond to signals from other bacteria in the community to change their phenotype, increasing the difficulty of identifying an antibiotic that is effective in eradicating the biofilm. The polysaccharide matrix protects the organism from invasion by other organisms, the phagocytic activity of polymorphonuclear neutrophils, oral or topical antibiotics, and topical antiseptics (silver, chlorhexidine, Dakin solution, povidone-iodine). Biofilms form on other moist surfaces, such as prosthetic implants and biomaterials (e.g., stainless steel pits in orthopedic surgery) (Pupp and Williams, 2008). As the biofilm progresses, the risk of difficult-to-treat infection rises.

Treatment of biofilm requires a two-pronged approach or a biofilm-based wound care plan. First the wound is surgically débrided. Sharp debridement may be adequate when it can be conducted aggressively and with minimal pain. Following debridement, topical therapy with moisture-retentive dressings and wound irrigation techniques provide continued debridement through autolysis. This approach is essential to prevent re-formation of the biofilm. Some investigators advocate weekly surgical or sharp redebridement, referred to as *continued maintenance debridement,* to keep wound biofilm in a weakened and susceptible state (Wolcott et al, 2009).

Two agents that appear promising for removing biofilm are topical doxycycline and cadexomer iodine. Doxycycline, a tetracycline, acts as a competitive inhibitor of MMPs and in studies has been applied once per day. This application of doxycycline remains under investigation and is not approved by the Food and Drug Administration. Cadexomer iodine is a topical broad-spectrum antiseptic that has been used in wound care for a number of years. The product slowly releases iodine beads into the wound and removes inhibitory cytokines while absorbing wound exudate. One study showed cadexomer iodine destroyed *Pseudomonas* biofilms after 24 hours of exposure to an in vitro biofilm model of skin wounds (Thorn et al, 2009).

Infection

Wound infection occurs when microorganisms on the wound surface penetrate into the wound tissues. A local or systemic response is indicative of an infection (Box 16-3) which may include increased exudate, erythema, odor, local warmth, edema, induration, pain, tenderness, fever, chills, and leukocytosis (Cutting and Harding, 1994; Gardner et al, 2001: Sibbald et al, 2006). Infection develops when the wound bioburden is significant enough to overwhelm the body's defenses. A quantitative bacterial count of greater than 10^5 in the wound is the gold standard for diagnosing a wound infection (Robson and Heggers, 1969). However, the concept of wound bioburden encompasses more than the number of bacteria present; it includes the diversity, virulence, and interaction of the organisms with each other and with the body (synergism). When more than one species of microorganisms exists in the wound, an infection can develop with fewer microorganisms present due to the interaction between the organisms. Greater than 90% of chronic wounds have polymicrobial flora containing up to four species, depending upon the type of wound (Woo and Sibbald, 2009). This situation also makes it extremely difficult to identify which organism is the actual pathogen.

BOX 16-3	Clinical Indications for Wound Infection*

Lack of healing after 2 weeks of topical therapy
Local signs of infection
- Increased erythema
- Increase amount and/or change in character of exudate
- Odor
- Increased local warmth
- Edema or induration
- Pain or tenderness
Systemic signs of infection
- Fever
- Chills
- Leukocytosis
Elevated glucose in patient with diabetes
Pain in neuropathic extremity

*Data from Cutting and Harding, 1994; Edwards and Harding, 2004; Gardner et al, 2001, 2007; Sibbald et al, 2006; Woo & Sibbald, 2009.

Infection depends on the adherence of the organism to the host's body. Attachment requires that the organism bond with a receptor using a ligand. Some receptors are site specific (e.g., mucous membranes), some are cell specific (e.g., T lymphocytes), and others are nonspecific (e.g., moist surface). Colonization and ultimately invasion of the tissue by microorganisms cannot occur without attachment (Bowler et al, 2001). Microorganisms have invasive factors that allow penetration of the host tissue, including enzymes (e.g., proteases) that lyse cells.

The local wound environment is important in the genesis of a wound infection. Organisms proliferate in an environment rich in necrotic tissue, foreign bodies (e.g., sutures, dirt), and hematomas. These serve as a nidus for infection, providing a medium for the growth of invading microorganisms. Inflammatory mediators and cytokines are stimulated and enzymes released that lyse proteins, such as fibrin, which is essential for fibroblast migration and maintenance of macrophage activity. The inflammatory response is augmented and prolonged. Exotoxins are released from the organisms and inhibit migration of keratinocytes and fibroblasts (Schultz et al, 2003). The organisms use oxygen and contribute to the relative hypoxia as seen in infected wounds (Falanga, 2004). In addition, if the environment is warm, moist, and slightly hypoxic, anaerobic organisms proliferate (Bowler et al, 2001; Edwards and Harding, 2004; Falanga, 2004).

Clinical Manifestations. Diagnosis of a wound infection is based primarily on the clinical assessment (see Box 16-3) and cultures are obtained to direct antibiotic selection (Expert Working Group, 2008; Gardner et al, 2006). However, the classic local signs of infection may be muted or absent when the inflammatory response is impaired, as in cases of malnutrition, steroid therapy, immunosuppression, and wound chronicity (Gardner and Frantz, 2008). Infection must be diagnosed in the context of the patient's history and risk factors (Box 16-4) as well as subtle clues such as friable granulation tissue and unexplained failure to heal (Edwards and Harding, 2004).

Research is under way to clarify and explore the reliability and validity of signs and symptoms of infection and critical colonization of the chronic wound. The Clinical Signs and Symptoms Checklist was derived from the early work by Cutting and Harding (1994) and was tested and extended by Gardner et al. (2001, 2007). Later, a review of the literature led to the acronym NERDS for identifying critical colonization (Nonhealing wound, Exudative wound, Red and bleeding wound, Debris, Smell from the wound) and the acronym STONEES (Size is bigger, Temperature increased, Os [probes to bone or exposed bone]), New area of breakdown, Erythema/Edema, Exudate, Smell) for identifying infection (see Box 16-2); subsequent research validated these categories (Woo and Sibbald, 2009). An international group led by Harding (Expert Working Group, 2008) has also proposed criteria for chronic wounds as well as acute wounds. Criteria common to each paradigm for infection in the chronic wound are erythema, edema, exudate, delayed healing, friable granulation tissue, odor, and new wound breakdown.

Each type of chronic wound may also have its own set of signs of infection (Cutting and White, 2005; EWMA, 2005; Gardner et al, 2009). For example, the criteria used to define infection in diabetic foot ulcers (anything below the malleolus) include purulence plus two cardinal signs of inflammation (Lipsky et al, 2008). Data from a Delphi study have delineated criteria for major types of wound: acute, venous, arterial, pressure ulcer, diabetic ulcer, and acute wound (Expert Working Group, 2008). Further research is needed to develop construct validity before these criteria are considered diagnostic of wound infection in various types of wounds.

Laboratory Tests and Cultures. Laboratory tests may reveal an increase in the number of white blood cells when infection is present. The differential may show an increase in bands or immature neutrophils. This "shift to the left" denotes increased immature leukocytes are released from the bone marrow into the bloodstream to fight invading organisms. Ongoing evaluation of inflammation can be monitored with erythrocyte sedimentation rate and C-reactive protein levels which are elevated with inflammation.

Cultures are indicated when clinical signs of infection are present (see Box 16-3) or when a clean wound does not show any progress in healing with 2 weeks of topical treatment (Robson et al, 2006; Steed et al, 2006; Whitney et al, 2006). A wound culture is performed primarily to identify the specific aerobic and anaerobic organisms present and their susceptibility to antibiotics. Wound culture can also be used to obtain a specimen for Gram staining, a method recognized as a rapid diagnostic technique for identifying infection (Duke et al, 1972; Levine et al, 1976). For a Gram stain, the tissue fluid is placed on a slide, treated with various stains, and viewed under a microscope. Gram stain will identify whether organisms ($>10^5$ organisms) are present and whether they are gram positive or gram negative. Results from a Gram stain can be expected in 20 minutes, a preliminary culture report in 24 hours, and a final culture and sensitivity within 48 hours. A Gram stain provides information about the type of organism present in the wound and allows the provider to prescribe a preliminary antibiotic. A wound culture must be taken from clean, healthy-appearing tissue. Because infection involves the tissue, it is important to culture the tissue rather than pus, slough, eschar, or necrotic material. Data show that culture of wound exudate, compared with tissue biopsy, has a predictive validity of 60% (Gardner et al, 2006). Although a laboratory report will be produced if pus, eschar, or necrotic tissue is cultured, the results will reflect the microflora of that site but will not provide an accurate profile of the microflora in the tissue. In fact, the results will be a false report—the only question is the type of error. It could be false positive (organisms present in the area that is cultured but not present in the tissue), false negative (organisms not present in the area that is cultured but present in the tissue), or a chance agreement (area that is cultured and tissue have the same result). A false negative is problematic in that the patient has an infection and needs to receive treatment. In this case, the patient's condition may deteriorate if the patient is not treated. A false positive is problematic if the patient is treated when there is not a need, increasing the risk of side effects and the development of organism

BOX 16-4	Risk Factors for Wound Infection Elicited Through History*

- History of prior wounds
- Family history of chronic wounds/poor healing
- Systemic conditions:
  - Human immunodeficiency virus/acquired immunodeficiency syndrome
  - Rheumatoid disease
  - Malnutrition: weight loss, obesity
  - Diabetes
  - Immune deficiency
  - Hypoxic conditions: chronic obstructive pulmonary disease, anemia
  - Ischemic disease: peripheral artery disease, congestive heart failure, shock, dehydration
  - Organ failure: heart, kidney, liver
  - Remote infection
- Health habits
  - Drug use/abuse
  - Smoking
- Drugs that impair healing
  - Corticosteroids
  - Antiinflammatory drugs
  - Chemotherapeutic agents

*Data from Fonder et al, 2008; Stojadinovic et al, 2008.

resistance. The probability is small that the number and types of organisms in the area that is cultured are the same as those in the tissue. Data indicate that even within the same wound tissue, the number and types of organisms vary (Levine et al, 1976). In general, a wound infection is present when the culture results show greater than 10^5 organisms or the presence of *any* β-hemolytic streptococcus (Robson et al, 2006; Steed et al, 2006; Whitney et al, 2006).

Three techniques can be used to obtain a wound culture: biopsy, needle aspiration culture, and swab culture.

Tissue biopsy for culture is removal of a piece of tissue with a scalpel or punch biopsy. Caution should be exercised in the use of local anesthetic because some data show that local anesthetics have antibiotic properties and may result in false-negative results (Johnson et al, 2008). The open wound is cleansed with a nonantiseptic sterile solution. A biopsy specimen is taken from clean tissue with a scalpel or punch biopsy, and bleeding is controlled. Once in the laboratory, the specimen is processed and plated (Gardner et al, 2006; Robson and Heggers, 1969).

The tissue biopsy is considered the gold standard for wound culture (Gardner et al, 2006; Robson and Heggers, 1969). A physician or wound care specialist with special training performs the biopsy. One of the limitations of the technique is that many facilities do not process tissue for culture, so the method cannot be used. In addition, obtaining a tissue culture requires disruption of the wound, which may cause the patient pain because living tissue is severed when obtaining the sample. Patients who are therapeutically anticoagulated are at risk of bleeding.

The second technique, *needle aspiration*, involves insertion of a needle in the tissue adjacent to the wound to aspirate tissue fluid. Organisms present in the tissue are detected in the aspirated tissue fluid (Lee et al, 1985). Intact skin next to the wound is disinfected and allowed to dry. Fanning the area to speed drying is not recommended because organisms in the environment are stirred up and settle on the biopsy site. Using a 10-ml disposable syringe and a 22-gauge needle, about 0.5 ml of air is drawn into the syringe, and the needle is inserted through intact skin adjacent to the wound. Suction is applied by withdrawing the plunger to the 10-ml mark. The needle is moved backward and forward at different angles for two to four explorations. After the needle is withdrawn from the tissue, excess air is removed from the syringe and the syringe is capped. The aspirated fluid is plated in the laboratory. If tissue is extracted using this technique, it is processed as described for tissue biopsy.

With the aspiration technique, the operator needs to understand the structures being penetrated by the needle. The major risk of this technique is inadvertent damage caused by the needle. Compared to tissue biopsy, needle aspiration tends to underestimate the number of organisms (Rudensky et al, 1992).

The *swab technique* is the third type of culture and is the most commonly performed. Two approaches have been used: a Z technique, in which the base of the wound is cultured by moving the swab back and forth over the surface of the wound in as criss-cross pattern, and the Levine technique. Comparison of these two swab techniques to tissue biopsy showed the Levine technique had a 91% sensitivity and 57% specificity when compared with the Z technique 63% sensitivity and 53% specificity (Gardner et al, 2006). Because of its accuracy, the method of Levine et al (1976) is recommended for swab culture. The procedure for a swab culture using the Levine technique is outlined in Box 16-5. The swab technique probably is the most frequently used because it requires the fewest clinical skills and most laboratories are accustomed to performing the analysis.

National guidelines on management of various types of chronic wounds (venous, diabetic, pressure) recommend determining the level of suspected infection by either tissue biopsy or validated quantitative swab technique (Robson et al, 2006; Steed et al, 2006; Whitney et al, 2006; WOCN, 2010). The decision of which technique to use is made by the provider considering the available equipment, the speed with which the specimen can be transported to the laboratory, and the ability of the laboratory to perform the requested culture.

A wide range of microbial flora can populate the chronic wound. The most commonly identified species in chronic wounds are *S. aureus,* coagulase-negative staphylococcus, and *Pseudomonas aeruginosa.* Additional aerobic organisms include *Klebsiella, E. coli, Proteus, Enterobacter,* and *Enterococci.* Anaerobic organisms may include *Peptostreptococcus, Prevotella,* and *Bacteroides* (Basu et al, 2009).

BOX 16-5	Procedure for Swab Wound Culture Using Levine Technique

1. Prepare to collect specimen using sterile technique (before administering antibiotics). If a Gram stain will be performed, a second swab will be obtained from the same clean tissue site
2. Identify 1 cm² of *clean wound tissue* (infection resides in viable tissue; culturing epidermis, periwound skin, or necrotic tissue will lead to false-positive results)
3. Clean wound with nonantiseptic sterile solution
4. Moisten swab or applicator with normal saline without a preservative (moist swab provides more precise data than dry swab)
5. While applying pressure, rotate applicator within 1–2 cm² of clean wound tissue (try to elicit tissue fluid)
6. When tip of swab is saturated, insert into appropriate sterile container (do not contaminate specimen when placing it in sterile container)
7. Complete the laboratory slip to provide clinical data to the microbiologist, including wound site, time collected, prior antibiotics
8. Transport culture specimen quickly (within 1 hour) to laboratory to keep the specimen stable

Treatment. As described in Chapter 18, the three principles of wound management are to eliminate or reduce causative factors, minimize cofactors, and provide an optimal physiologic wound environment. In this section, only treatment of excess bacterial burden is discussed with the understanding that appropriate interventions will be implemented to satisfy the first two principles of wound management. The goal of treatment of critical colonization and infection is to reduce the bioburden without causing tissue injury or development of drug resistance (Landis, 2008).

Local. Appropriate topical therapy focuses on removing pathogenic organisms in the wound. In conjunction with cleansing, debridement, and moist wound healing (see Chapters 17 and 18), topical antimicrobials may be necessary to control bioburden while minimizing the potential for host resistance to antibiotics. Sufficient quantities of antimicrobials are not absorbed when applied topically to effectively treat systemic infections (Landis, 2008).

The duration of topical treatment in infection is not well delineated. However, obtaining a culture can direct treatment by targeting the specific organism(s). Topical antimicrobials were out of favor for a period of time. More recently, antibiotic-resistant organisms have increased, and practitioners have realized that early control of bioburden with topical antimicrobials has the potential to reduce the need for antibiotics and prevent the development of resistant strains. Types of antimicrobials are listed in Box 16-1. Examples of commonly used topical antimicrobials are described in Table 16-1 and shown in Plate 42. The selection of antimicrobial is based on the agent's mechanism of action and its overall effectiveness (Bowler et al, 2004; Demling and DeSanti, 2002; Fumal et al, 2002; Leaper and Durani, 2008; Zhou et al, 2002).

Systemic. The primary treatment of wound infection is systemic antibiotics (Lavery et al, 2009). It is important to remember that culture and gram stain should be obtained prior to initiating antibiotic therapy. Failure to obtain the culture prior to antibiotic administration may result in false-negative culture results. Once the culture results are known, the antibiotic most specific to the identified pathogen can be used. Until then, broad-spectrum antibiotics should be prescribed. Topical antimicrobials should also be used to reach ischemic tissue or granulation tissue which systemic antibiotics cannot reach (WOCN, 2010), treat biofilm, or control odor. In order to optimize the effectiveness and safety of antibiotic therapy, consultation with an infection disease specialist and pharmacologist may be warranted.

Osteomyelitis

Osteomyelitis, infection of the bone, develops as a complication of a wound infection and is not easily diagnosed. It is characterized by a mixture of inflammatory cells, fibrosis, bone necrosis, and new bone formation (Rennert et al, 2009). Osteomyelitis is suspected when the wound is healing poorly, with or without systemic manifestations of infection (Lavery et al, 2009). The bone marrow, cortex, and periosteum and surrounding soft tissue all can be affected. Osteomyelitis can be categorized as acute (first episode resolves in less than 6 weeks) or chronic (lasts longer than 6 weeks or recurs after initial infection).

If a wound has visible signs of wound infection in combination with exposed bone, osteomyelitis should be suspected (Rennert et al, 2009). Bone biopsy that yields microorganisms with histologic findings of inflammatory cells and osteonecrosis is the gold standard for diagnosing osteomyelitis (Lipsky et al, 2008). Quite often, the less invasive technique of "probe to the bone" is used to establish the clinical diagnosis of osteomyelitis in patients with diabetes (Bonham, 2001).

Because of the invasive nature of the bone biopsy, a number of noninvasive tests for diagnosing osteomyelitis have been explored, including X-ray films, magnetic resonance imaging, bone scans (three-phase), technetium 99m-labeled antigranulocyte antibody scintillography, and leukocytes scans. Although widely accessible, flat-plate X-ray films are unreliable when observing for osteomyelitis because bony changes typical of osteomyelitis (i.e., periosteal reactive changes or erosion) can also be present in noninfected bone. In contrast, magnetic resonance imaging has demonstrated the presence of osteomyelitis with 98% sensitivity and 89% specificity (Lipsky et al, 2008; Livesley and Chow, 2002) and is the preferred technology for diagnosis of osteomyelitis (Rennert et al, 2009).

EVALUATION

As with all wounds, ongoing surveillance at regular intervals is essential; signs of critical colonization should abate within a 2-week period (Robson et al, 2006; Steed et al, 2006; Whitney et al, 2006). When the wound is infected, a response in terms of decreased erythema should be observed within 24 to 48 hours. The wound size should be decreasing, the quality of the granulation tissue improving, volume of exudate decreasing, odor resolving, and pain intensity decreasing.

The absence of a response to treatment, further deterioration, or recurrence of signs and symptoms warrant reassessment of the wound and of the interventions. When the patient has an intact immune system and the subtle signs of critical colonization are still present but no local or systemic signs of infection are seen, interventions should be modified to (1) assess adequate relief from the underlying etiology, (2) ensure adequate resolution of cofactors (e.g., tissue oxygenation, nutrition, serum glucose), and (3) alter the physiologic wound environment by using a different antiseptic dressing and increasing the frequency of dressing changes. If a quantitative tissue biopsy can be obtained, sites different from the sites that were sampled in the original biopsy should be used. Reculturing will determine whether the pathogens have changed, thereby indicating a need for a different antibiotic. Given that much of the treatment of wound infection is provided on an outpatient basis, it is critical that patients/families be given detailed instructions about what they should observe and for how long as well as how to contact the provider for continued follow-up. With a wound that is unresponsive, biopsy may be indicated to differentiate infection from atypical lesions such as cancer, calciphylaxis, or vasculitis.

SUMMARY

Creating an optimal wound environment requires diligent management of the wound bioburden. Failure to recognize the manifestations of the continuum of bioburden conditions will lead to prolonged delay of healing and eventually sepsis as well as continued growth of antibiotic resistant microorganisms. The wound care provider must be able to recognize the early, although discreet, symptoms that are indicative of biofilm formation, critical colonization, and chronic wound infection. Treatment of critical colonization and wound infection requires the appropriate use of antibiotics, antiseptics, and debridement.

REFERENCES

Basu S et al: A prospective descriptive study to identify the microbiological profile of chronic wounds in outpatients, *Ostomy Wound Manage* 55(1):14-20, 2009.

Bjarnsholt T et al: Why chronic wounds will not heal: a novel hypothesis, *Wound Repair Regen* 16(1):2-10, 2008.

Bonham P: A critical review of the literature. Part I: diagnosing osteomyelitis in patients with diabetes and foot ulcers, *J Wound Ostomy Continence Nurs* 28(2):73, 2001.

Bowler PG et al: Wound microbiology and associated approaches to wound management, *Clin Microbiol Rev* 14(2):244, 2001.

Bowler PG et al: Microbicidal properties of a silver-containing hydrofiber dressing against a variety of burn wound pathogens, *J Burn Care Rehabil* 25(2):192-196, 2004.

Cutting KF, Harding KGH: Criteria for identifying wound infection, *J Wound Care* 3:198, 1994.

Cutting KF, White RJ: Criteria for identifying wound infection-revisited, *Ostomy Wound Manage* 51(1):28, 2005.

Demling RH, DeSanti L: The rate of re-epithelialization across meshed skin grafts is increased with exposure to silver, *Burns* 28(3):264, 2002.

Duke WF et al: Civilian wounds, their bacterial flora and rate of infection, *Surg Forum* 23(0):518, 1972.

Edwards R, Harding KG: Bacteria and wound healing, *Curr Opin Infect Dis* 17(2):91, 2004.

European Wound Management Association (EWMA): *Position document: identifying criteria for wound infection*, London, 2005. MEP Ltd.

Expert Working Group: Wound infection, *Int Wound J* 5(3):1-11, 2008.

Falanga V: The chronic wound: impaired healing and solutions in the context of wound bed preparation, *Blood Cells Mol Dis* 31:88, 2004.

Fonder MA et al: Treating chronic wounds: a practical approach to the care of nonhealing wounds and wound care dressings, *J Am Acad Dermatol* 58(2):185-206, 2008.

Fumal I et al: The beneficial toxicity paradox of antimicrobials in leg ulcer healing impaired by a polymicrobial flora: a proof-of-concept study, *Dermatology* 204(Suppl 1):70, 2002.

Gardner SE, Frantz RA: Wound bioburden and infection-related complications in diabetic foot ulcers, *Biol Res Nurs* 10(1):44-53, 2008.

Gardner SE et al: The validity of the clinical signs and symptoms used to identify localized chronic wound infection, *Wound Repair Regen* 9(3):178, 2001.

Gardner SE et al: Diagnostic validity of three swab techniques for identifying chronic wound infection, *Wound Repair Regen* 14(5):548-57, 2006.

Gardner SE et al: The inter-rater reliability of the clinical signs and symptoms checklist in diabetic foot ulcers, *Ostomy Wound Manage* 53(1):46-51, 2007.

Gardner SE et al: Clinical signs of infection in diabetic foot ulcers with high microbial load, *Biol Res Nurs* 11(2):119-128, 2009.

Johnson SM et al: Local anesthetics as antimicrobial agents: a review, *Surg Infect (Larchmt)* 9(2):205-213, 2008.

Landis SJ: Chronic wound infection and antimicrobial use, *Adv Skin Wound Care* 21(11):531-540, quiz 541-542, 2008.

Lavery LA et al: Risk factors for developing osteomyelitis in patients with diabetic foot wounds, *Diabetes Res Clin Pract* 83(3):347-352, 2009.

Leaper DJ, Durani P: Topical antimicrobial therapy of chronic wounds healing by secondary intention using iodine products, *Int Wound J* 5:361-368, 2008.

Lee P et al: Fine-needle aspiration biopsy in diagnosis of soft tissue infections, *J Clin Microbiol* 22(1):80, 1985.

Levine NS et al: The quantitative swab culture and smear: a quick, simple method for determining the number of viable aerobic bacteria on open wounds, *J Trauma* 16(2):89, 1976.

Lipsky BA et al: Topical versus systemic antimicrobial therapy for treating mildly infected diabetic foot ulcers: a randomized, controlled, double-blinded, multicenter trial of pexiganan cream, *Clin Infect Dis* 47(12):1537-1545, 2008.

Livesley NJ, Chow AW: Infected pressure ulcers in elderly individuals, *Clin Infect Dis* 35(11):1390, 2002.

Pupp G, Williams C: What you should know about biofilms and chronic wounds, *Podiatr Today* 21(7):25-27, 2008.

Rennert R et al: Developing and evaluating outcomes of an evidence-based protocol for the treatment of osteomyelitis in stage IV pressure ulcers: a literature and wound electronic medical record database review, *Ostomy Wound Manage* 55(3):42-53, 2009.

Robson MC, Heggers JP: Bacterial quantification of open wounds, *Mil Med* 134(1):19, 1969.

Robson MC, et al: Guidelines for the treatment of venous ulcers, *Wound Repair Regen* 2006 Nov-Dec;14(6):649-662.

Rudensky R et al: Infected pressure sores: comparison of methods for bacterial identification, *South Med J* 85(9):901, 1992.

Schultz GS et al: Abstinence from smoking reduces incisional wound infection: a randomized controlled trial, *Ann Surg* 238(1):1, 2003.

Sibbald RG et al: Increased bacterial burden and infection: the story of NERDS and STONES, *Adv Skin Wound Care* 19(8):447-461, 2006.

Steed DL, et al: Guidelines for the treatment of diabetic ulcers, *Wound Repair Regen* 2006 Nov-Dec;14(6):680-692.

Stojadinovic A et al: Topical advances in wound care, *Gynecol Oncol* 111(2 Suppl):S70-S80, 2008.

Thorn RMS et al: In *vitro* comparison of antimicrobial activity of iodine and solver dressings against biofilms, *J Wound Care* 18(8):343-346, 2009.

Whitney J, et al: Guidelines for the treatment of pressure ulcers, *Wound Repair Regen* 14(6):663-679, 2006.

Wolcott RD et al: Regular debridement is the main tool for maintaining a healthy wound bed in most chronic wounds, *J Wound Care* 18(2):54-56, 2009.

Woo KY, Sibbald RG: A cross sectional validation study of using NERDS and STONEES to assess bacterial burden, *Ostomy Wound Manage* 55(8):40-48, 2009.

Wound, Ostomy and Continence Nurses (WOCN) Society: *Guideline for prevention and management of pressure ulcers*, Mt. Laurel, NJ, 2010.

Zhou LH et al: Slow release iodine preparation and wound healing: in vitro effects consistent with lack of in vivo toxicity in human chronic wounds, *Br J Dermatol* 146(3):365, 2002.

17

Wound Debridement

Janet M. Ramundo

OBJECTIVES

1. Describe the role of debridement in the wound healing process.
2. List contraindications to debridement.
3. Distinguish between selective and nonselective debridement.
4. Compare and contrast four methods of debridement: autolysis, chemical, mechanical, and sharp.
5. Describe the appropriate use of debridement using wet-to-dry dressings, conservative sharp debridement, and high-pressure wound irrigations.

6. List debridement options for the infected wound.
7. Describe at least five factors to consider when selecting a debridement approach.
8. For each method of debridement, list two advantages, disadvantages, and relevant special considerations.

DEFINITION AND PURPOSE

Debridement is the removal of nonviable tissue and foreign matter from a wound and is a naturally occurring event in the wound repair process. During the inflammatory phase, neutrophils and macrophages digest and remove "used" platelets, cellular debris, and avascular injured tissue from the wound area. However, with the accumulation of significant amounts of damaged tissue, this natural process becomes overwhelmed and insufficient. Buildup of necrotic tissue then places considerable phagocytic demand on the wound coupled with the continued presence of proinflammatory cells, both of which ultimately retard wound healing (Robson, 1997; Stotts and Hunt 1997). Consequently, debridement of necrotic tissue is an essential objective of topical therapy and a critical component of optimal wound management. Debridement not only is an integral component of wound bed preparation, it also facilitates bacterial balance and moisture balance (Hopf et al, 2006; Robson et al, 2006; Steed et al, 2006; Whitney et al, 2006).

Debridement is believed to achieve several objectives:

1. Reduce the bioburden of the wound. Because devitalized tissue supports the growth of bacteria, the presence of necrotic tissue places the patient at risk for wound infection and sepsis. Using external measures to remove the necrotic tissue and foreign matter reduces the volume of pathogenic microbes present in the wound.

2. Control and potentially prevent wound infections, particularly in the deteriorating wound.
3. Facilitate visualization of the wound wall and base. In the presence of necrotic tissue, accurate and thorough assessment of the viable tissue is hampered.
4. At the molecular level, debridement interrupts the cycle of the chronic wound so that protease and cytokine levels more closely approximate those of the acute wound (Schultz et al, 2003).

Necrotic tissue can appear in various forms. Eschar has the firm, dry, leathery appearance of desiccated and compressed tissue layers (see Plate 24). When the tissue is kept moist, the devitalized tissue, called *slough*, remains soft and may be brown, yellow, or gray in appearance (see Plates 14, 25, 26A, 32). Slough may be adherent to the wound bed and edges, or loosely adherent and stringy (see Plate 25). Components of slough include fibrin, bacteria, intact leukocytes, cell debris, serous exudate, and significant quantities of deoxyribonucleic acid (DNA) (Thomas, 1990). Once the eschar is removed, slough is often visible covering the wound bed. Maintaining a moist wound environment is essential because continued exposure to air dehydrates slough, causing it to return to a hard, leathery state.

Debridement is indicated for any wound, acute or chronic, when necrotic tissue (which may be slough or eschar) or foreign bodies are present. It is also indicated when the wound is infected. Once the wound bed is clean and viable tissue is present, debridement is no lon-ger indicated. Dry, stable (i.e., noninfected or nonfluctu-ant) ischemic wounds or those with dry gangrene should not be debrided until perfusion to the extremity has im-proved (Hopf et al, 2006; Robson et al, 2006; Steed et al, 2006; Whitney et al, 2006). Measurement of vascular status, including an ankle-brachial index, is an important component of the assessment process when considering debridement in a patient with lower leg ulceration. Debridement is also contraindicated for stable eschar covered heels. Treatment goals should be consistent with the goals and lifestyle of the individual (Hopf et al, 2006; Robson et al, 2006; Steed et al, 2006; Whitney et al, 2006).

METHODS OF DEBRIDEMENT

Several methods of debridement are available for removal of devitalized tissue from necrotic wounds. Debridement methods are classified as either selective (only necrotic tissue is removed) or nonselective (viable tissue is removed along with the nonviable tissue) (Table 17-1). More specifically, debridement is classified by the actual mecha-nism of action: autolysis, chemical, mechanical, biologic, or sharp (conservative or surgical). Although one method of debridement may be the primary approach selected to rid the wound of necrotic tissue, debridement typically involves a combination of methods.

Autolysis

Autolysis as a natural, highly selective painless method of debridement. Specifically, autolysis is the lysis of necrotic tissue by the body's white blood cells and natural en-zymes, which enter the wound site during the normal inflammatory process. The body's proteolytic, fibrino-lytic, and collagenolytic enzymes are released to digest the devitalized tissue present in the wound while leaving the healthy tissue intact (Rodeheaver et al, 1994). As a naturally occurring physiologic process, autolysis is stim-ulated by a moist, vascular environment with adequate leukocyte function and neutrophil count. Therefore, au-tolysis is contraindicated in patients with compromised immunity. Autolysis as a sole method of debridement is not recommended for actively infected wounds or wounds

with extensive necrotic tissue or significant tunneling and undermining (NPUAP-EPUAP, 2009).

A moist environment is facilitated by the application of a moisture-retentive dressing left undisturbed for a reasonable length of time. Maintaining a moist wound environment allows the cellular structures that are es-sential for phagocytosis (neutrophils and macrophages) to remain intact and avoid premature destruction through desiccation. An important role of macrophages is pro-duction of growth factors, so the presence of healthy macrophages in the wound fluid supports continued production of growth factors. Once autolysis is initiated, eschar will loosen from the edges, become soft, change to a brown or gray color, and eventually transform into stringy yellow slough. It is critical to monitor the wound closely during the autolysis process because as the wound is debrided, the full wound bed and walls are exposed and the true extent of the wound is revealed; consequently, the wound will increase in length, width, and depth, necessitating a change in topical therapy. Plate 26 shows the appearance of a wound before and after autolysis.

Clinicians, patients, and family members unfamiliar with the process of autolysis can misinterpret the collec-tion of wound exudate and the accompanying odor as indicative of an infection. It is important to emphasize that the wound exudate contains enzymes and growth factors that are essential to wound repair. In fact, wounds treated with moisture-retentive dressings are less likely to become infected than are wounds treated with conventional dressings because semiocclusive dressings are impermeable to exogenous bacteria. In ad-dition, viable neutrophils and other natural substances in wound fluid inhibit bacterial growth (Hutchinson, 1989; Lawrence, 1994).

The use of semiocclusive dressings to create and maintain a moist wound environment launched the use of autolysis as an alternative to surgical debridement. Semiocclusive dressings trap enzyme-rich wound exu-date at the wound site, which is very effective at detach-ing nonviable tissue from the surrounding skin and wound base. Selection of dressings that promote autoly-sis is based on the condition of the wound base, depth of the wound, presence of tunnels or undermining, volume of wound exudate, and the patient's condition. When the wound base is dry, a dressing that will add moisture, such as a hydrogel, should be used. If absorption is needed, a dressing should be selected that will absorb excess exudate without dehydrating the wound surface, such as an alginate dressing for a highly exudative wound or a hydrocolloid for the minimally exudative wound. Chapter 18 provides an in-depth discussion on dressing selection to promote autolysis while matching the needs of the wound.

Debridement by autolysis compares favorably with other methods of debridement in terms of effectiveness (Konig et al, 2005). However, the process is slower than

TABLE 17-1	Selective Versus Nonselective Debridement Methods	
Selective	**Nonselective**
Autolysis	Surgical
Enzyme	Hydrotherapy
Conservative sharp debridement	Wet-to-dry gauze
Biosurgical (maggot)	Surgical sharp
Ultrasonic mist	

alternative methods such as mechanical and sharp. A multicenter randomized trial conducted by Burgos et al (2000) showed no significant difference in healing of Stage III pressure ulcers with the use of a hydrocolloid for autolysis compared to a commercially prepared topical enzyme product. Another randomized study comparing the same products found the enzyme to be a faster when used to treat Stage IV pressure ulcers on the heel after surgical debridement (Müller et al, 2001). The time frame for the occurrence of autolysis varies depending on the size of the wound and the amount and type of necrotic tissue. Generally, the softening and separating of necrotic tissue is observed within days. If tissue autolysis is not apparent in 1 to 2 weeks, another debridement method should be used (Hopf et al, 2006; Robson et al, 2006; Steed et al, 2006; Whitney et al, 2006).

Autolysis can be used in combination with other debridement techniques. In fact, promotion of autolysis is an important adjuvant to all debridement modalities for ongoing maintenance debridement and prevention of tissue dehydration and cellular desiccation. For example, after surgical sharp debridement of a pressure ulcer, the application of a hydrogel-impregnated gauze maintains a moist wound environment, thus preventing tissue desiccation and promoting continued softening and loosening of residual necrotic tissue. It often becomes necessary to combine dressings to achieve debridement while meeting all the needs of the patient and wound. For example, a transparent dressing is inappropriate for debridement of a wound that has depth or is heavily exudative. Instead, a dressing such as an alginate is warranted because it will fill the wound depth and absorb the exudate (see Chapter 18).

Chemical

Necrotic wound tissue can be removed through a chemical process using enzymes and sodium hypochlorite (Dakin's solution). Silver nitrate is another method of chemical debridement; however, it is more commonly used on epibole (closed or rolled wound edges) as described in Chapter 4 and shown in Plate 4 and hypergranulation (see Chapter 6 and Plate 27).

Enzymes. Topical application of exogenous enzymes is a selective method of debridement. Over the years, various sources have been used to manufacture enzymes (e.g., krill, crab, papaya, bovine extract, bacteria). Today the only enzyme available in the United States is collagenase, which is derived from clostridium bacteria. Collagenase digests collagen in necrotic tissue by dissolving the collagen "anchors" that secure the avascular tissue to the underlying wound bed (NPUAP-EPUAP, 2009).

Similar to autolysis, enzymatic debridement is slower than mechanical or sharp debridement but is frequently used for initial debridement when anticoagulant therapy renders surgical debridement unfeasible (Konig et al, 2005; Ramundo and Gray, 2008). The length of time required to achieve debridement may range from several days to weeks. Unlike autolysis, enzymes may also be used to debride a wound with significant bacterial bioburden or infection (Ramundo and Gray, 2008).

Specific ions, including several commonly used antimicrobial dressings and antiseptic solutions, inhibit or inactivate collagenase. Silver dressings and cadexomer iodine have been reported to reduce collagenase activity by more than 50% and 90%, respectively. pH levels below 6.0 or above 8.0 common in antiseptic cleansers containing heavy metal ions, acetic acid, and hyperchlorite also reduce the activity of collagenase.

A secondary dressing is required when an enzyme is used and should be selected based on the needs of the wound. With the previously mentioned exceptions, manufacturer's state that most dressings can be used safely with enzymes, including gauze, hydrogels, and transparent film dressings; however, silver-impregnated dressings should be avoided. Frequency of enzyme application is at least daily and may be twice daily; therefore, the secondary dressing also should be appropriate for daily or twice-daily changes. Enzymatic debridement can be augmented by using a moisture-retentive dressing. Enzymes require a prescription, so their use has cost and reimbursement implications. In addition, daily or twice-daily dressing changes dictate considerable commitment on the part of the caregiver (patient, family, or staff) that may not always be reasonable or acceptable.

When collagenase is used on a wound with intact eschar, the eschar must be cross-hatched to allow penetration of the enzyme, and the wound surface must be kept moist. Cross-hatching the eschar is achieved by using a no. 10 blade to make several shallow slits in the eschar without damaging the viable wound base. Once the eschar begins to separate or demarcate from the surrounding skin, the enzyme can be applied to the wound edges along the line of demarcation to hasten separation. At this point, conservative sharp debridement can be used to remove softened necrotic tissue. Enzyme treatment can then be continued, or another debridement technique such as autolysis can be instituted. Because these enzymes are selective, damage to viable tissue in the wound bed should not occur if the dressing is continued once debridement is completed and viable tissue is exposed. However, enzyme application typically is discontinued when the wound bed is free of necrotic tissue. More appropriate dressings are available at a fraction of the cost and should be implemented once the wound is debrided. A transient stinging or burning sensation, particularly when the enzyme comes into contact with intact skin, has been reported (Ramundo and Gray, 2008). Barrier ointments can be used to protect the periwound skin.

Dakin's Solution. Originally used as a topical disinfectant for wounds sustained in war, Dakin's solution (diluted sodium hypochlorite solution) has a long history of being used to cleanse, debride, and control odor in wounds (Lindfors, 2004). As a debriding agent, Dakin's solution denatures protein, therefore loosening slough and rendering it more easily removed from the wound. Collagen degradation and fibroblast migration are affected by the concentration of Dakin's solution. Vick et al (2009) found that less than 0.5% concentration resulted in little or no collagen degradation, whereas 0.5% either partially or completely degraded collagen.

Dakin's solution is most appropriately used in conjunction with periwound skin protection for wounds with a large amount of slough or odor. Gauze is saturated with the diluted Dakin's solution is saturated into gauze, lightly packed into the wound, and covered with a secondary dressing. If the goal is debridement, the dressing is changed twice daily. Use of Dakin's solution should be considered a short-term treatment (fewer than 10 days). Once infection and odor are under control and viable tissue exposed, alternative dressing and debridement techniques should be implemented.

Biosurgical (Maggots)

Originating from the battlefield, maggots have been used to achieve a biologic method of debridement. Physicians noted anecdotal reports from medics who observed the rapid removal of necrotic tissue when maggots were present on the wound bed. Today, therapeutic maggot therapy involves sterilizing the eggs of *Lucilia sericata* (greenbottle fly). Once the eggs hatch (again, under sterile conditions), the sterile larvae are introduced into the wound bed.

It is theorized that larvae secrete proteolytic enzymes, including collagenase, allantoin, and other agents, which rapidly break down necrotic tissue (NPUAP-EPUAP, 2009). It is also believed that the larvae ingest microorganisms, which are then destroyed. Some researchers are investigating the effects of maggots on fibroblasts and extracellular matrix interaction and enhancement of healing beyond the debridement effects (Chambers et al, 2003; Horobin et al, 2003). Because of this reported action and the emergence of resistant organisms, there is renewed interest in maggot therapy in some centers, and more research supporting this therapy is available (Sherman 2002, 2003; Wallina et al, 2002; Wolff and Hansson, 2003).

Despite the renewed interest in clinical centers and reports in the literature, maggot therapy is still generally considered a last resort option when the patient is not a surgical candidate and the wound has not responded to conventional methods of debridement. A review of evidence concluded that maggot therapy offers no more overall effectiveness than other methods of debridement (Gray, 2008).

Care should be taken to prevent the larvae from coming in contact with healthy skin because the proteolytic enzymes can cause damage. Pain and bleeding have been reported, so the patient should be monitored for both,

particularly with the widespread use of antiplatelet therapy (Steenvorde and van Doorn, 2008; Steenvorde et al, 2005). The main disadvantage to maggot therapy is the sensation of crawling that some patients experience, but confinement of the larvae to the wound bed decreases this sensation. Various dressings have been described; most involve periwound protection with mesh or nylon net to contain the larvae and an absorbent pad to absorb exudate (Van Veen, 2008). Biosurgical therapy should not be used with wounds that are poorly perfused, require frequent inspection, or have exposed blood vessels, necrotic bone, or limb-threatening infections (NPUAP-EPUAP, 2009).

Mechanical

Mechanical modes of debridement include wet-to-dry gauze dressings, irrigation, and hydrotherapy. These techniques represent selective and nonselective modes of debridement.

Wet-to-Dry Gauze Debridement. Experts agree that wet-to-dry dressings may induce mechanical separation of eschar, but the dressings can be painful and, if dry, may damage newly formed viable tissue (Hopf et al, 2006; Robson et al, 2006; Steed et al, 2006; Whitney et al, 2006; WOCN, 2010). However, they are commonly used in clinical practice possibly due to the availability of gauze, clinician training, preference, habit, or the perception that the method is cost effective.

Wet-to-dry debridement is most appropriately used with heavily necrotic or infected wounds without visible granulation tissue. Correct technique consists of lightly packing saline-moistened (not dripping wet) gauze to the wound bed and allowing it to dry on the wound, trapping debris. Once dry, usually 4 to 6 hours after application, the dressing is pulled off the wound along with the trapped debris, the wound is cleansed, and the saline-moistened gauze reapplied. This process is continued until viable tissue is apparent. In determining debridement costs, caregiver time must be factored into the equation. If done correctly, wet-to-dry gauze debridement requires dressing changes for several days to weeks, three to six times per day.

The most effective type of dressing material for wet-to-dry gauze dressings is an open-weave cotton fabric because it adheres best to the wound bed when dry. Moistening dry gauze that is adherent to the wound bed to minimize patient discomfort prior to removal will not facilitate mechanical debridement. Nonwoven gauze is generally ineffective because the fiber composition does not allow for tissue adherence. Hypertonic saline-impregnated gauze is only indicated to absorb and contain exudate from heavily exudative wounds and should not be used for wet-to-dry debridement.

Wound Irrigation and Pulsatile Lavage. Wound irrigation and pulsatile lavage involve debridement of necrotic tissue with fluid and between 4 to 15 pounds per square inch (psi) of pressure, which is adequate to remove debris from the wound bed without damaging healthy tissue or inoculating the underlying tissue with bacteria (Hopf et al, 2006; Robson et al, 2006; Steed et al, 2006; Whitney et al, 2006). Delivering fluid under pressure to the wound bed can cause dissemination of wound bacteria over a wide area, exposing the patient and care provider to potential contamination. Consequently, the care provider should wear personal protective equipment (mask, gloves, gown, goggles) during this procedure when "splash" is expected (NPUAP-EPUAP, 2009).

Wound irrigation is accomplished using a 19-gauge angiocatheter and a 35-ml syringe (a bulb syringe does not provide enough pressure). Prepackaged canisters of pressurized saline and products that attach to saline bags for continuous acceptable pressures are available for irrigation.

A *pulsatile lavage* machine combines intermittent high-pressure lavage with suction to loosen necrotic tissue and facilitate its removal by other methods of debridement (Morgan and Hoelscher, 2000). Pulsatile lavage is an effective alternative to whirlpool for removing larger amounts of debris and should be discontinued once the wound is clean. Pulsatile lavage should be used with caution to avoid blood vessels, graft sites, and exposed muscle, tendon, and bone. Patients on anticoagulant therapy should be observed carefully for any bleeding and treatment discontinued immediately if bleeding occurs. Disadvantages of debridement with pulsatile lavage include cost and time. The hose and tip are designed for one-time use, and large necrotic wounds may require twice-daily treatments. Pulsatile lavage treatment should be delivered in an enclosed area separate from any other patients to prevent contamination with mist (Maragakis et al, 2004).

Hydrotherapy (Whirlpool). Whirlpool may be used to remove bacteria and debris from the surface of large trunk or extremity pressure ulcers. Additional benefits include softening and loosening of adherent necrotic tissue and cleansing and removal of wound exudate (NPUAP-EPUAP, 2009; Whitney et al, 2006). Prolonged use and periods of wetness may macerate the tissue or may be associated with bacterial contamination (Whitney et al, 2006).

The pathophysiology of the wound and the physical assessment of the patient must be considered before whirlpool therapy is selected. Vasodilation and increased circulation naturally occur with whirlpool therapy but are not always desirable. For example, increasing circulation in the extremity of the patient with a venous insufficiency wound contributes to venous congestion (McCulloch and Boyd, 1992). In the presence of advanced arterial disease, the vessels in the leg are likely to be maximally dilated, and the added stress locally may increase metabolic demands. Whirlpool therapy must be used cautiously in the patient with diabetes who may not be able to detect temperature changes because of sensory or autonomic neuropathy. Optimal water temperature is

37°C. Current national guidelines do not specifically address the use of whirlpool for debridement in the care of diabetic and vascular wounds (Hopf et al, 2006; Robson et al, 2006; Steed et al, 2006).

Ultrasonic Mist. Ultrasound uses acoustic energy to remove necrotic tissue from the wound bed and promote healing. Ultrasound mist therapy uses saline coupled with the acoustic wave to produce mechanical and thermal effects. When the probe delivering the mist is in contact with the wound, destruction of fibrin may occur (Stanisic et al, 2005). This debridement effect is not seen when contact with the wound is avoided, as in low-frequency, low-intensity, noncontact ultrasound. A review of the literature on the use of ultrasound noted insufficient evidence to determine the effectiveness of debridement (Ramundo and Gray, 2008). Ultrasound use for wound care is discussed in greater detail in Chapter 24.

Sharp Debridement

Sharp debridement is a rapid process that uses sterile instruments. Sharp debridement can be done sequentially in a conservative fashion (conservative sharp wound debridement), or it can be done surgically (surgical sharp debridement). Any method of sharp debridement must be performed by a specially trained, competent, qualified, and licensed health care professional consistent with local legal and regulatory statutes (NPUAP-EPUAP, 2009; Wound, Ostomy and Continence Nurses [WOCN] Society, 2005).

Conservative Sharp Wound Debridement. Conservative sharp wound debridement, also known as *conservative instrumental debridement*, is a selective debridement method for the removal of loosely adherent, nonviable tissue using sterile instruments (e.g., forceps or "pick-ups," scissors, and scalpel with no. 10 or no. 15 blades). When done correctly, the procedure is not aggressive enough to harm viable tissue and is not likely to result in blood loss.

Conservative sharp debridement has several advantages. It removes the necrotic tissue more quickly than the previously discussed methods, and it can be accomplished in a serial manner. This method of debridement can be combined with other debridement techniques (autolysis or enzymatic) to shorten this phase of wound care. Theoretically, a more rapid approach to debridement decreases the body's expenditure of energy during a time of high resource use.

Because of the low risk involved, conservative sharp debridement in many states is a delegated medical function that can be performed in a variety of settings by a non–physician clinician who is competent and credentialed in the technique. Therefore conservative sharp debridement is a viable option for patients residing in nonacute care settings without the need for transfer to a hospital. A variety of requirements may need to be satisfied, depending on the nurse practice act specific to the state and the employer's requirements. Checklist 17-1 gives factors to consider prior to performing conservative sharp debridement. Box 17-1 provides a sample policy and procedure for conservative sharp debridement.

A disadvantage of conservative sharp debridement is that, depending on the size of the ulcer and the amount of necrotic tissue involved, it could conceivably take weeks to remove all of the nonviable tissue. The procedure may be uncomfortable for the patient, so the need for analgesia should be considered. Blood loss is not expected during conservative sharp debridement but remains a possibility. As a result, the patient should be assessed for factors that place him or her at risk for clotting problems if a vessel is accidentally severed. Factors to consider include medications (e.g., heparin, warfarin, high-dose nonsteroidal antiinflammatory drugs, antibiotics) and pathologic conditions (e.g., thrombocytopenia, impaired hepatic function, vitamin K deficiency, malnutrition). When any of these factors are present, the wound specialist should confer with the physician before proceeding with conservative sharp debridement.

Infected wounds present unique considerations for conservative sharp debridement. In general, there is the potential for transient bacteremia after debridement of a wound, particularly when the wound is infected. Transient bacteremia in a patient who is nutritionally compromised, leukopenic, or otherwise immunocompromised can be devastating. Because of the lack of research on the relationship between sharp debridement and transient bacteremia, a cautious, conservative approach is warranted.

CHECKLIST 17-1

Factors to Consider Prior to Performing Conservative Sharp Debridement

✓ Is conservative sharp debridement covered under the clinician's state practice act?
✓ Are specialty education, training, and credentials in conservative sharp debridement required by the state or the employer?
✓ What formal knowledge and skill updates are required and how often?
✓ Has the individual's professional organization or employer delineated specific guidelines related to conservative sharp debridement?
✓ Are policies, procedures, and protocols in place for conservative sharp debridement?
✓ Is conservative sharp debridement considered part of the clinician's clinical privileges, or is a physician's order required for each incident of conservative sharp debridement?
✓ What level of physician supervision, if any, is required for conservative sharp debridement?
✓ Does the employer provide malpractice insurance coverage for conservative sharp debridement?
✓ Does the clinician carry malpractice insurance to cover conservative sharp debridement?

Surgical sharp debridement is the preferred method for debriding most infected wounds. However, if surgical sharp debridement is not an option because of the patient's condition or the care setting, serial conservative sharp debridement can be conducted by the non–physician wound care provider, but only in conjunction with appropriate antibiotic coverage. Although systemic antibiotics may not penetrate the necrotic tissue to reduce the bacterial load in the wound, they should reduce the potential for systemic dissemination of the pathogens. Topical antiseptic solutions may also be instrumental in reducing the bioburden of the wound. The wound specialist should be in compliance with the policies of the facility or agency on the management of infected wounds.

Surgical Sharp Wound Debridement. Surgical debridement is the fastest method for removing large amounts of necrotic tissue but is outside of the scope of practice of most nonphysician providers. This method not only removes necrotic tissue and its attached bacterial burden, but it also can result in removal of senescent cells and bleeding, thus converting a chronic wound to a pseudo-acute wound (Steed et al, 1996). In many cases, surgical debridement is performed at the bedside. However, international guidelines for the care of pressure ulcers recommend performing debridement in the operating room in the following cases (NPUAP-EPUAP, 2009):

• Presence of advancing cellulitis
• Wound-related sepsis
• Extensive necrotic tissue
• Inability to establish degree of undermining and tunneling
• Infected bone or hardware that may need to be removed

Disadvantages of surgical debridement include the potential for negative effects from anesthesia, excess bleeding, and transient bacteremia that may progress to systemic infection and patient death. The condition of the patient, aggressive nature of this procedure, and higher level of care required after debridement may require the patient to spend more time in the hospital.

Laser and Water Debridement. *Laser debridement*, a form of surgical debridement, uses focused beams of light to cauterize, vaporize, or slice through tissue. Several light sources for lasers are available: argon, CO_2, neodymium:yttrium-aluminum-garnet (Nd:YAG), and tunable (Habif, 1996). Each type of laser emits light at a specific wavelength, and different body tissues absorb different wavelengths. The part of the tissue that absorbs the light is called the *chromophore* (e.g., water is the chromophore for the CO_2 laser, and hemoglobin is the chromophore for the argon laser). When the chromophore absorbs the light, it is quickly heated and vaporized. When the beam of light is tightly focused, it is capable of cutting through human tissue like a knife (Raz, 1995).

BOX 17-1	Policy and Procedure: Conservative Sharp Wound Debridement

I. Purpose

The purpose of this policy and procedure is to outline the process by which an RN with certification in wound care may remove devitalized tissue by conservative sharp wound debridement.

II. Policy

1. Any RN performing conservative sharp wound debridement will have additional didactic education in the skill.
2. Any RN performing conservative sharp wound debridement will have additional laboratory education to develop the skill.
3. Any RN performing conservative sharp wound debridement will participate in a clinical practicum involving patients with wounds.
4. Documentation of the above will be filed with the individual's other credentialing information. (This is determined by practice setting.)

III. Authority and Responsibility

1. The individual performing conservative sharp wound debridement will provide documentation of education and competency.
2. An order from the attending physician will be obtained before the procedure, or physician practice protocols permitting the procedure will be in effect.
3. Consent will be obtained from the patient or appropriate representative. (This is determined by practice setting.)

IV. Definitions

Conservative sharp wound debridement is the removal of loose, avascular tissue using surgical instruments (e.g., scissors, scalpel, forceps) without inflicting pain or precipitating bleeding.

V. Procedure

1. Explain procedure to patient.
2. Obtain consent. (This is determined by practice setting.)
3. Assemble equipment:
   A. Sterile forceps with teeth
   B. Sterile scalpel handle with no. 15 blades
   C. Silver nitrate sticks
   D. Curved iris scissors
   E. Surgical gel foam or silver nitrate stick
   F. Gauze sponges
   G. Normal saline
   H. Clean gloves
4. Wash hands.
5. Prepare work surface.
6. Position patient for procedure.
7. Ensure adequate lighting.
8. Apply clean gloves.
9. Remove old dressing and discard.
10. Wash hands and apply clean gloves.
11. Clean wound with normal saline or appropriate surgical scrub/solution.
12. Grasp loosely adherent tissue with forceps; pull taut, exposing a clear line of dissection.
13. Cut or snip loose tissue, avoiding all vascular tissues and tissues that are not clearly identified.
14. Irrigate wound with normal saline.
15. For minor bleeding, apply silver nitrate, gel foam, or pressure.
16. Apply appropriate dressing.
17. Document procedure and patient's response to procedure and type of dressing applied.

RN, Registered nurse.
Data from Wound Ostomy and Continence (WOCN) Society: *Conservative sharp wound debridement: best practice for clinicians*, Mount Laurel, NJ, 2005.

Advantages of laser debridement are that the wound bed is sterilized and that most severed vessels are cauterized (Flemming et al, 1986). Animal studies using a laser to debride partial-thickness burns have demonstrated results similar to those of sharp debridement but with hemostasis and no disturbance of periwound skin (Graham et al, 2002; Lam et al, 2002). Disadvantages of laser debridement include risk of injury to adjacent healthy tissue and therefore delayed healing. Work with pulsed laser beams rather than continuous laser beams has decreased these negative effects (Glatter et al, 1998; Smith et al, 1997). Unfortunately, this method is not available in all settings.

The *hydrosurgical water knife* is a method of surgical debridement that dispenses normal saline at a high power, which enables debridement and cleansing of the wound base. This water jet device is regulated to precisely control the depth of debridement. The high-velocity stream runs parallel to the wound surface and creates a vacuum, which then cleanses and removes debris into a collection container. This device is designed for use only in the operating room. Limited studies have shown some promise compared with traditional surgical debridement in the treatment of burns and lower extremity ulcers (Caputo et al, 2008; Gravante et al, 2007; NPUAP-EPUAP, 2009).

SELECTION OF DEBRIDEMENT METHOD

Three general parameters guide the selection of the most appropriate debridement process: (1) overall condition and goals for the patient; (2) status of the wound and urgency of the need for debridement; and (3) skill level of the care provider. Algorithms are available to guide the clinician in selecting the appropriate debridement method. Although they are based on expert opinion and have not been validated, these algorithms can serve as a useful starting point for decision making (Figure 17-1).

Overall Condition and Goals for the Patient

Occasionally, it may be necessary to forego debridement if it is not consistent with the patient's wishes and overall goals for care (NPUAP-EPUAP, 2009). Such a decision must include input from the patient, the patient's significant others, and the primary care provider. Even if the goal is not to heal the wound, debridement of necrotic

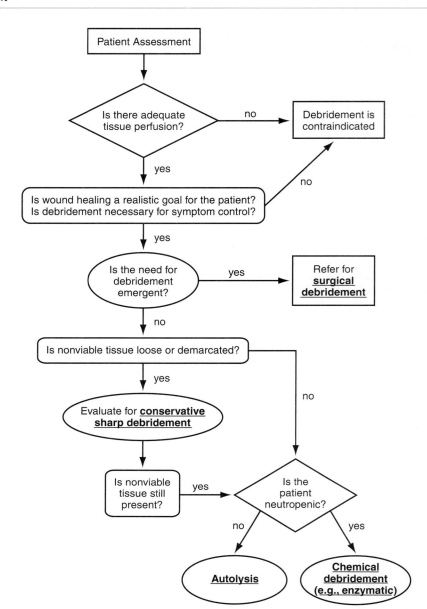

FIGURE 17-1 Debridement algorithm.

tissue will control infection and unpleasant wound odors, making the environment more comfortable for the patient, family, and caregivers.

The patient's history and coexisting morbidities affect the selection of debridement method. For example, awareness of any clotting disorders or anticoagulant medications used is critical when considering sharp debridement. When a patient has severe nutropenia (absolute count <500) and therefore at risk for severe sepsis; autolysis is not realistic or safe because of the insufficient number of neutrophils available to respond to the wound demands (Bodey et al, 1966). Generally, the wound will appear stagnant during this time. Debridement by autolysis should be postponed until the neutrophil count climbs over 1,000 mm³. Chemical debridement using enzymes is an effective option in the presence of severe neutropenia.

The risk for transient bacteremia in conjunction with any debridement technique should be considered. The release of microorganisms from the necrotic tissue of even a noninfected wound may be sufficient to overwhelm the patient's immune system, and the procedure may need to be postponed for the patient who is critically ill or neutropenic.

Wound Status

When there is no urgent clinical need for debridement, then mechanical, autolytic, enzymatic or biosurgical methods of debridement can be used. Ulcer related cellulitis, crepitus, or sepsis dictates rapid surgical debridement (NPUAP-EPUAP, 2009).

Wound pain is another critical determinant of debridement method selection. Patients who are experiencing wound pain may benefit from the less painful debridement modalities (autolysis or enzymatic). The other types of debridement (wet-to-dry, conservative sharp, and surgical sharp) may trigger or exacerbate pain. The patient's pain status during dressing changes and while resting should be assessed. Prophylactic analgesia should be administered topically or systemically.

Stable eschar (attached, noninfected, dry) on a poorly perfused limb or on a pressure ulcer on the heel should not be debrided (Hopf et al, 2006; Robson et al, 2006; Steed et al, 2006; Whitney et al, 2006; WOCN Society, 2010).

Clinician Experience and Competence

Although debridement methods such as autolysis, wound irrigation, wet-to-dry dressings, and enzymes ideally are initiated under the direction of the physician or wound care specialist, they are procedures that can be performed by nurses, physical therapists, the patient, and caregivers. However, the more aggressive methods of debridement, specifically sharp debridement, require a greater level of skill and competence. Conservative sharp debridement should be performed only by a wound specialist or physician with demonstrated and documented competence. The wound care specialist must be in compliance with his or her scope of practice, state nurse practice act, and institutional policies. Surgical sharp debridement and laser debridement are performed only by physicians.

Clinicians performing sharp debridement in the outpatient setting are cautioned to work closely with experienced coders and billing personnel. Coding errors for debridement are common. A review by the Office of Inspector General (OIG) noted an error rate of 66% in Medicare claims when the codes specific to debridement were examined. Inappropriate billing can result in underpayment or, more seriously, charges of fraud (OIG, 2007).

PROGRESSION AND MAINTENANCE OF DEBRIDEMENT

The methods of wound debridement typically used by the non–physician wound specialist do not immediately yield a completely clean wound; therefore the wound must be closely monitored for indicators of progression of the debridement process.

Deterioration of the wound requires reevaluation of the treatment selected. Assessment parameters include wound dimensions, volume of exudate, odor, type of tissue present, and condition of the periwound skin. Wound dimensions typically increase as the necrotic tissue is removed from the wound. Early in the debridement process, the wound is commonly exudative; this should decrease as the necrotic tissue is removed. As the underlying tissue is exposed, healthy viable tissue in the wound base should be present. When using autolysis, enzymes, or wet-to-dry dressings, a gradual transition in the type of necrotic tissue present in the wound

base should be observed and documented. Hydrated eschar becomes gray and soft; firmly adherent slough becomes loose and stringy. When the wound is infected, a decrease in periwound erythema and induration should be observed after debridement. If the patient was febrile or had leukocytosis before initiating debridement, a decrease should be observed as the necrotic tissue is removed and the bacterial load is reduced. However, these clinical changes may also be attributed to antibiotic therapy.

Traditionally, the clinician discontinues sharp or enzymatic debridement when the wound base is clean and free of necrotic tissue. At that point, moisture-retentive dressings are critical to the wound to maintain a clean vascular wound bed. Without this moist vascular wound environment, the wound bed will become dry, cellular desiccation will occur, and necrotic tissue will begin to re-form. Maintaining a moist wound environment with moisture-retentive dressings will prevent these negative consequences. Inevitably cellular byproducts will accumulate on the wound surface. By utilizing moisture-retentive dressings, autolysis will naturally occur and therefore essentially achieve maintenance debridement by keeping the wound bed moist.

Some clinical experts propose continuing sharp debridement even when the wound bed is visibly free of necrotic tissue, particularly in recalcitrant wound beds (Falanga et al, 2008). This theory of maintenance debridement is based on findings from clinical trials that noted improved healing rates when more frequent debridement was performed (Steed et al, 1996). This concept requires further study to determine efficacy and to guide the clinician in the decision to continue debridement, select the appropriate method of debridement, and differentiate between selection of advanced wound therapy versus maintenance debridement.

SUMMARY

Debridement is a critical component of topical therapy for necrotic wounds. The wound specialist should be knowledgeable about the various methods available for debridement and should discuss the options with the patient and with the patient's physician so that the most appropriate wound management choice can be made. Debridement methods are not used in isolation; rather, they are used in combination and are modified as the wound conditions change. For example, an eschar-covered, noninfected wound may be cross-hatched and covered with a hydrogel sheet. As the eschar softens, it may become possible to use conservative sharp debridement to facilitate removal of the bulk of the residual eschar and then continue use of the hydrogel or select another moisture-retentive dressing, depending on the wound needs. Close supervision of the patient and accurate wound assessments during the debridement phase are essential to ensure an outcome consistent with the stated wound goals.

REFERENCES

Bodey GP et al: Quantitative relationship between circulating leukocytes and infection in patients with acute leukemia, *Ann Intern Med* 64(2):328, 1966.

Burgos A et al: Cost, efficacy, efficiency and tolerability of collagenase ointment versus hydrocolloid occlusive dressing in the treatment of pressure ulcers: a comparative, randomised, multicenter study, *Clin Drug Invest* 19(5), 2000, available at http://www.medscape.com/viewarticle/406174, accessed on January 11, 2009.

Caputo WJ et al: A prospective randomised controlled clinical trial comparing hydrosurgery debridement with conventional surgical debridement in lower extremity ulcers, *Int Wound J* 5(2):288-294, 2008.

Chambers L et al: Degradation of extracellular matrix components by defined proteinases from the greenbottle larva Lucilia sericata used for the clinical debridement of non-healing wounds, *Br J Dermatol* 148:14, 2003.

Falanga V et al: Maintenance debridement in the treatment of difficult to heal wounds, recommendations of an expert panel, *Ostomy Wound Manage* June(Suppl):2-13, 2008.

Flemming A et al: Skin edge necrosis in irradiated tissue after carbon dioxide laser excision of tumor, *Lasers Med Sci* 1:263, 1986.

Glatter D et al: Carbon dioxide laser ablation with immediate auto-grafting in a full-thickness porcine burn model, *Ann Surg* 228(2):257, 1998.

Graham JS et al: Efficacy of laser debridement with autologous split-thickness skin grafting in promoting improved healing of deep cutaneous sulfur mustard burns, *Burns* 28:719, 2002.

Gravante G et al: Versajet hydrosurgery versus classic escharectomy for burn débridment: a prospective randomized trial, *J Burn Care Res* 28(5):720-724, 2007.

Gray M: Is larval (maggot) debridement effective for removal of necrotic tissue from chronic wounds? *J Wound Ostomy Continence Nurs* 35(4):378,2008.

Habif TP, editor: *Clinical dermatology: a color guide to diagnosis and therapy*, ed 3, St. Louis, 1996, Mosby.

Hopf HW et al: Guidelines for the treatment of arterial insufficiency ulcers, *Wound Repair Regen* 14(6):693-710, 2006.

Horobin AJ et al: Maggots and wound healing: an investigation of the effects of secretions from Lucilia sericata larvae upon interactions between human dermal fibroblasts and extracellular matrix components, *Br J Dermatol* 148:923, 2003.

Hutchinson JJ: Prevalence of wound infection under occlusive dressings: a collected survey of reported research, *Wounds* 1(2):123, 1989

Konig M et al: Enzymatic versus autolytic debridement of chronic leg ulcers: a prospective randomized trial, *J Wound Care* 14(7):320, 2005.

Lam DG et al: The treatment of Lewisite burns with laser debridement—lasablation, *Burns* 28(1):19, 2002.

Lawrence JC: Dressings and wound infection, *Am J Surg* 167(1A):215, 1994.

Lindfors JA: Comparison of an antimicrobial wound cleanser to normal saline in reduction of bioburden and its effect on wound healing, *Ostomy Wound Manage* 50(8):28-41, 2004.

Maragakis LL et al: An outbreak of multidrug-resistant Acinetobacter baumannii associated with pulsatile lavage wound treatment, *JAMA* 292(24):3006-3011, 2004.

McCulloch J, Boyd V: The effects of whirlpool and the dependent position on lower extremity, *J Orthop Sports Phys Ther* 16(4):169, 1992.

Morgan D, Hoelscher J: Pulsed lavage: promoting comfort and healing in home care, *Ostomy Wound Manage* 46(4):44-49, 2000.

Müller E et al: Economic evaluation of collagenase-containing ointment and hydrocolloid dressing in the treatment of pressure ulcers, *Pharmacoeconomics* 19(12):1209-1216, 2001.

National Pressure Ulcer Advisory Panal (NPUAP) and European Pressure Ulcer Advisory Panal (EPUAP): *Prevention and treatment of pressure ulcers*. Washington DC: National Pressure Ulcer Advisory Panel; 2009.

Office of Inspector General (OIG): *Medicare payments for surgical debridement services in 2004*, OEI-02-05-00390, May 2007.

Ramundo J, Gray M: Is ultrasonic mist therapy effective for debriding chronic wounds? *J Wound Ostomy Continence Nurs* 35(6):579, 2008.

Raz K: Laser physics, *Clin Dermatol* 13:11, 1995.

Robson M: Wound infection: a failure of wound healing caused by an imbalance of bacteria, *Surg Clin North Am* 77(3):637, 1997.

Robson MC et al: Guidelines for the treatment of venous ulcers, *Wound Repair Regen* 14(6):649-662, 2006.

Rodeheaver GT et al: Wound healing and wound management: focus on debridement, *Adv Wound Care* 7(1):22, 1994.

Schultz G et al: Wound bed preparation, a systemic approach to wound bed management, *Wound Rep Regen* 11(Suppl):1, 2003.

Sherman R: Maggot vs conservative debridement therapy for the treatment of pressure ulcers, *Wound Repair Regen* 10(4):208, 2002.

Sherman R: Maggot therapy for treating diabetic foot ulcers unresponsive to conventional therapy, *Diabetes Care* 26(2):446, 2003.

Smith K et al: Depth of morphologic skin damage and viability after one, two, and three passes of a high-energy, short pulse CO_2 laser (Tru-Pulse) in pig skin, *J Am Acad Dermatol* 37(2):204, 1997.

Stanisic MC et al: Wound debridement with 25 kHz ultrasound, *Adv Skin Wound Care* 18(9):484, 2005.

Steed DL et al: Effect of extensive debridement and treatment on the healing of diabetic foot ulcer, *J Am Coll Surg* 183:61, 1996.

Steed DL et al: Guidelines for the treatment of diabetic ulcers, *Wound Repair Regen* 14(6):680-692, 2006.

Steenvorde P, van Doorn LP: Maggot debridement therapy: serious bleeding can occur. Report of a case, *J Wound Ostomy Continence Nurs* 35(4):412, 2008.

Steenvorde P et al: Determining pain levels in patients treated with maggot debridement therapy, *J Wound Care* 14(10):485, 2005.

Stotts N, Hunt T: Managing bacterial colonization and infection, *Clin Geriatr Med* 13(3):65, 1997.

Thomas S: *Wound management and dressings*, London, 1990, Pharmaceutical Press.

Van Veen LJ: Maggot debridement therapy: case study, *J Wound Ostomy Continence Nurs* 35(4):432, 2008.

Vick LR et al: Effect of Dakin's solution on components of a dermal equivalent, *J Surg Res* 155(1):54-64, 2009.

Wallina U et al: Biosurgery supports granulation and debridement in chronic wounds—clinical data and remittance spectroscopy measurement, *Int J Dermatol* 41(10):635, 2002.

Whitney J, et al: Guidelines for the treatment of pressure ulcers, *Wound Repair Regen* 14(6):663-79, 2006.

Wolff H, Hansson C: Larval therapy—an effective method of ulcer debridement, *Clin Exp Dermatol* 28(2):134, 2003.

Wound, Ostomy and Continence Nursing (WOCN) Society: *Guideline for prevention and management of pressure ulcers*, Mt. Laurel, NJ, 2010, Author.

Wound, Ostomy and Continence Nurses (WOCN) Society: *Conservative sharp wound debridement: best practice for clinicians*. Mt. Laurel, NJ, 2005, Author.

18

Topical Management

Bonnie Sue Rolstad, Ruth A. Bryant, and Denise P. Nix

OBJECTIVES

1. Identify three principles of wound management.
2. Describe the characteristics of a physiologic wound environment.
3. Identify at least five objectives in creating a physiologic wound environment.
4. Define the terms occlusive, semiocclusive, moisture retentive, primary dressing, and secondary dressing.
5. List two indications and one contraindication for each dressing category.
6. Describe the factors to consider when selecting a wound dressing.

Numerous factors impact on the process of wound healing, all of which must be addressed to achieve wound closure. Topical wound management is determined based on many of these factors. Topical wound management is the manipulation of the wound to positively influence the physiologic local wound environment. Three principles of wound management provide comprehensive and holistic guidance to optimize the patient's ability to heal.

PRINCIPLES OF WOUND MANAGEMENT

Wounds do not occur as an isolated event within a patient. Consequently, the principles of effective wound management must incorporate a holistic approach that identifies and intervenes to minimize or abate the underlying etiology and any coexisting contributing factors. Box 18-1 lists the three principles of wound management and examples of how these principles can be addressed. To control or eliminate causative factors and potential cofactors, diagnostic or laboratory tests are often required. Failure to address causative factors will result in delayed healing or a nonhealing wound despite appropriate systemic and topical therapy. No dressing can compensate for an uncorrected pathologic condition. The various possible etiologies of acute or chronic wounds and the cofactors that impair wound healing are discussed throughout this textbook. This chapter focuses solely on the third principle of wound management: create a physiologic wound environment.

Characteristics of a Physiologic Wound Environment

Topical wound management is the manipulation of the wound to restore a physiologic wound environment; an environment that is "characteristic of an organism's healthy or normal functioning." Key features of a physiologic wound environment are adequate moisture level, temperature control, pH regulation, and control of bacterial burden. These various conditions create a milieu that is conducive to a successful and expedient journey from compromised skin to skin repair and restoration of function. Wound care dressings are used to mimic the skin so that a physiologic local wound environment can be created. Objectives and interventions for creating a physiologic wound environment are given in Table 18-1.

Moisture Level. The human body is more than 65% water; the primary means of maintaining this level of moisture is located within the epidermis (Spruitt, 1972). The stratum corneum layer of the epidermis prevents loss of excessive amounts of water in the form of water vapor to the external environment. Therefore, moisture levels of healthy skin are maintained by an intact stratum corneum. When the stratum corneum has been removed or compromised, tissues and cells are subject to increased loss of moisture and may desiccate and eventually die. Wound healing is slowed significantly in such a dry environment because epithelial cells must burrow below the dry surface to reach a moist surface over which they can migrate (Hinman and Maibach, 1963;

BOX 18-1   Wound Management Principles and Examples

1. Control or Eliminate Causative Factors
   - Offload pressure
   - Reduce friction and shear
   - Protect from moisture
   - Compression to improve venous return
   - Prevent trauma to insensate foot
2. Provide Systemic Support to Reduce Existing and Potential Cofactors
   - Optimize nutrition
   - Provide adequate hydration
   - Reduce edema
   - Control blood glucose levels
   - Promote blood flow (avoid cold, control pain, eliminate nicotine and caffeine)
3. Maintain Physiologic Local Wound Environment (see Table 18-1)
   - Prevent and manage infection
   - Cleanse wound
   - Remove nonviable tissue (debridement)
   - Maintain appropriate level of moisture
   - Eliminate dead space
   - Control odor
   - Eliminate or minimize pain
   - Protect periwound skin

Winter, 1962). A moist environment physiologically favors cellular migration and extracellular matrix formation which facilitates healing of wounds, reduces pain and tenderness, reduces fibrosis, decreases wound infection and produces a better cosmetic outcome (Hopf et al, 2006; Robson et al, 2006; Schultz et al, 2003; Steed et al, 2006; Whitney et al, 2006). However, the moisture level of the wound surface can range from dry (particularly nonviable tissue) to an excessively moist surface. Topical dressings are used to establish and maintain a moist—not wet—wound environment. Topical wound dressings are used to maintain adequate moisture in the wound by one of three mechanisms: containing wound fluids, absorbing excess moisture, or donating moisture. Semiocclusive dressings can keep a wound moist, even when no additional moisture is supplied, by "catching" and retaining moisture vapor that is being lost by the wound on a continual basis. Their ability to maintain tissue hydration can be characterized by a measurement known as the *moisture vapor transmission rate* (MVTR). Dressings transmit less moisture vapor than the average wound loses, thus facilitating moisture retention in the tissue as opposed to desiccation. In general, if the dressing material transmits less moisture vapor than the

TABLE 18-1   Objectives of a Physiologic Wound Environment

Objectives	Interventions
(1) Prevent and manage infection	Cover wound with dressings impermeable to bacteria to protect from outside contaminants, with the most appropriate dressing or combination of dressings based on wound assessment and overall goals for the patient Infection control precautions, no-touch dressing application Appropriate wound cleansing and debridement Antimicrobials when indicated Appropriate wound culture technique (see Chapter 16)
(2) Cleanse wound	Normal saline with 4–15 psi of pressure/force to remove debris without harming healthy tissue
(3) Remove nonviable tissue	Most appropriate debridement method or combination of debridement methods based on patient's condition and wound assessment (see Chapter 17) Method of debridement consistent with patient's overall goals
(4) Maintain appropriate level of moisture	Dressing with high moisture vapor transmission rate will allow moisture to escape and evaporate to manage minimally exudative wounds Moderate to heavily exudative wounds require absorptive dressings Select topical dressings that maintain moist wound environment to prevent tissue desiccation
(5) Eliminate dead space	Hydrating or absorbent-impregnated gauze for large, deep wounds Fluff packing material and loosely place into wound using cotton-tipped applicator Ensure packing material is in contact with wound edges and can be easily retrieved
(6) Control odor	Appropriate dressing change frequency Cleansing with each dressing change Debridement and antimicrobials as indicated Charcoal dressings
(7) Eliminate or minimize pain	Semiocclusive dressings Nonadherent dressings Dressings that require fewer changes Pain control interventions as described in Chapters 25 and 26
(8) Protect wound and periwound skin	Skin barriers (liquid, ointments, wafers) to protect the periwound skin from moisture and adhesives as described in Table 5-4 Appropriate interval for dressing changes so that exudate does not pool on surrounding skin or undermine adhesive of wound dressing

wound loses, the wound will remain moist. If the dressing material transmits more moisture vapor than the wound loses, the wound may dry out. For this reason, transparent dressings designed for intravenous sites have a higher MVTR than the transparent dressings intended for wound management.

In a wound that has excess moisture, the topical dressing must have moisture absorptive capacity to prevent the wound from becoming overly saturated and the periwound skin macerated. The process of absorption physically moves drainage away from the wound's surface and edges and into the dressing material. At the other end of the hydration spectrum, wound tissue that is dry may need to be actively rehydrated using dressing materials that donate water to the tissue (i.e., hydrogel).

Normal Temperature. Another characteristic of a physiologic wound environment is a normal body temperature. One of the functions of the skin is to provide thermoregulation. The wound dressing must restore the insulating effect formerly provided by the skin. All cellular functions are affected by temperature, including chemical reactions (e.g., metabolism, enzymatic catalysis, production of growth factors interleukin-1β and interleukin-2, protein synthesis, and oxidation) and processes (e.g., phagocytosis, mitosis, and locomotion). Local hypothermia is known to increase the risk of infection by causing vasoconstriction and increasing hemoglobin's affinity for oxygen, both of which result in a decreased availability of oxygen to phagocytes. The consequences of hypothermia on phagocytes include decreased phagocytic activity, decreased production of reactive oxygen products, and impaired ability to migrate. Topical wound dressings that reduce moisture loss from wounded tissues and do not require frequent changes will diminish local cooling (Wenisch et al, 1996).

Bacterial Balance. The importance of bacterial balance for a physiologic wound environment and interventions to control bioburden are discussed in Chapters 16 and 17. Strategies include (1) debridement, (2) appropriate wound cleansing, (3) appropriate infection control precautions, 4) use of antimicrobials, and (5) use of moisture-retentive dressings.

Semiocclusive dressings reduce wound infections by more than 50% compared with traditional gauze dressings. This finding supports the theory that semiocclusive dressings optimize the phagocytic efficiency of endogenous leukocytes by maintaining a moist wound environment and reduce airborne dispersal of bacteria during dressing changes. Semiocclusive dressings provide a mechanical barrier to the entry of exogenous bacteria. In contrast, bacteria have been reported to penetrate up to 64 layers of gauze (Ovington, 2001).

pH. A neutral pH similar to the pH of blood (7.4), is required to provide a physiologic wound environment. In a wound, the pH of the tissue becomes mildly alkaline due to the loss of moisture. The presence of urine, stool, or fistula drainage in a wound will affect the local pH as well. The consequence of an altered pH is an increased the risk of bacterial invasion and impaired function of matrix metalloproteinases (MMPs) (Armstrong and Jude, 2002; Ovington, 2002). Semiocclusive wound dressings facilitate a mildly acidic to neutral wound fluid pH (Varghese et al, 1998).

TYPES OF DRESSINGS

Wound dressings include both primary dressings and secondary dressings. The *primary dressing* is a therapeutic or protective covering applied directly to the wound bed to meet the needs of the wound. The *secondary dressing* serves a therapeutic or protective function and is used to increase the ability to adequately meet the wound needs and/or secure the primary dressing. For example, a hydrocolloid dressing is the primary dressing when it is used over a shallow minimally exudative wound but it functions as a secondary dressing when it is used over a wound filler.

Most wound dressings today are semiocclusive rather than occlusive. Semiocclusive dressings (also known as *moisture-retentive dressings*) emerged in the 1970s and currently are staples in the wound care portfolio. Wound care technologies were worth more that $2 to $3 billion in 2005 and are predicted to reach $4.6 billion in 2011 (Andrews, 2001). The wound care market is constantly changing with an extensive variety of dressings that vary by shape, size, and ingredients. They are selected based on the needs of the wound, the patient, and the care setting.

Common ingredients in wound dressings include glycerin, polymers, carboxymethylcellulose, collagen, alginate, cellulose, cotton or rayon, and polyurethane. Wound care dressings may be *single-component* dressings containing, for example, only alginate, hydrogel, or hydrocolloid, or *multicomponent* dressings in which components are mixed together, such as an alginate and a hydrocolloid to increase absorptive capacity. Multicomponent dressings are categorized and reimbursed according to the clinically predominant component (e.g., alginate, collagen, foam, gauze, hydrocolloid, hydrogel). Most of the dressing categories are available in an antimicrobial form such as silver (see Chapter 16), however reimbursement is still based upon their clinically prominent component). The effects of these products and components have been reported by a number of studies (EPUAP-NPUAP, 2009; Hopf et al, 2006; Robson et al, 2006; Steed et al, 2006; Whitney et al, 2006).

Wound care needs may change frequently throughout the various phases of wound healing. Therefore, a variety of products must be accessible. In general, dressing selection and utilization is guided by the Medicare Part B Surgical Dressing Policy. Table 18-2 is a formulary of wound care products and provides examples in addition to the Medicare Part B utilization parameters and codes.

TABLE 18-2	Wound Dressing Formulary			
Product and Examples	**Description**	**Indications for Use**	**Instructions for Use**	**Coverage Guidelines/HCPCS**
Antimicrobial: antiseptics, cadexomer iodine, honey, Hydrofera blue, mupirocin ointment, silver cream, silver dressings (Plates 42-43)	See Chapter 16 for complete descriptions	Partial- or full-thickness wound Critical colonization, infection, or biofilms Odorous wound	Cleanse wound *Avoid* saline in nanocrystalline silver products Apply to wound Apply appropriate secondary dressing as needed and secure in place	No reimbursement for antiseptics Silver dressings coded by function (i.e., silver hydrogel A6242-A6248, honey alginate A6196-A6199)
Calcium alginate: Restore CalciCare (Hollister), SeaSorb (Coloplast), Algisite (Smith & Nephew) (Plates 44-45)	Polysaccharide derived from brown seaweed Highly absorbent Converts to viscous, hydrophilic gel Provides moist environment Hemostatic properties	Partial- or full-thickness wound with or without depth Moderate to heavily exudative wound Contraindicated in third-degree burns	Cleanse wound base Place or lightly pack into wound Apply appropriate secondary dressing and secure in place Change as needed, usually every 24-48 hours	One dressing per day Fillers up to two per day Cover when used on full-thickness wound with moderate to heavy exudate Coded as alginate or other fiber gelling dressing A6196-A6199
Charcoal: CarboFlex odor control (ConvaTec), Lyofoam C (Molnlycke, ConvaTec)	Activated carbon (charcoal) Absorbs toxins and wound degradation products Absorbs volatile amines and fatty acids responsible for odor	Malodorous wound (e.g., infected, fungating) Fecal fistula Pressure ulcer	Apply as a "filter" for odor control If absorbing exudate, may need to be changed daily. Weekly if no exudate Can be reused if filter only	CarboFlex is coded as an alginate Lyofoam C is coded as a foam
Collagen: Puracol collagen (Medline), Biostep (Smith & Nephew), Cellerate gel (Hymed Group), CollaSorb (Hartmann)	May enhance deposition of organized collagen fibers Chemoattractant to granulocytes and fibroblasts Bioresorbable Hemostatic properties Most processed from bovine or porcine sources	Full-thickness wound with or without depth Noninfected wound Minimal to moderate drainage Contraindicated in bovine sensitivities and third-degree burns	Packaged as gels, alginates, sheets, powders Cleanse wound as appropriate Apply to wound base Apply appropriate secondary dressing Secure as necessary	Collagen fillers (once a day) A6010-A6011 Collagen dressings A6021-A6024 Dressing change frequency depends on product used and amount of exudate; check manufacturer's recommendations
Promogran (Systagenix Wound Management)	Some collagens also inactivate matrix metalloproteinases	Chronic wound free of necrotic tissue	Read manufacturer's instructions carefully; some may need to be moistened with saline if wound bed dry	

Category/Products	Composition/Action	Indications	Application	Frequency/Codes
Composite: Tegaderm absorbent clear acrylic dressing (3M), Alldress (Mohnlycke), Covaderm Plus (DeRoyal)	Combine physically distinct components into single dressing Functions as bacterial barrier Absorptive layer distinct from alginate, foam, hydrocolloid, hydrogel Semiadherent or nonadherent	Partial- or full-thickness wound without depth Dry to heavy exudate (depends on dressing components) Product selection varies based on wound characteristics	Cleanse wound as appropriate Dressing application dependent on product selected Can function as either primary or secondary dressing May be used with topical medications	Up to three per week A6200–A6205
Contact layer: Restore TRIACT technology (Hollister), Mepitel (Mohnlycke)	Protects wound bed from direct contact with other agents and dressings Conforms to wound shape Porous to allow exudate to pass or medication to absorb into wound	Partial- or full-thickness wounds with or without depth Infected wounds Donor sites Split-thickness skin grafts	Cleanse wound as appropriate Line wound bed Apply topical agent over contact layer or apply secondary dressing for absorption Not intended to be changed with each dressing change	One contact layer per week A6206–A6208
Fiber Gelling: Aquacel Hydrofiber (ConvaTec)	Carboxymethylcellulose Absorbs heavy exudate Converts to a gel Keeps wound base moist	Partial- or full-thickness wound with or without depth Moderate to heavily exudative wound	Cleanse wound base Place or lightly pack into wound Apply appropriate secondary dressing and secure in place Change every 24–48 hours	One dressing per day Coded as alginate or other fiber gelling dressing A6196–A6199
Foam: Biatain (Coloplast), Hydrocell (Derma Sciences), PolyMem (Ferris Mfg Corp) (Plates 46-48)	Absorptive and nonadherent Consists of hydrophilic polyurethane or film-coated layer	Partial- or full-thickness wound without depth (sheets) or with depth (fillers) Moderate to heavily exudative wound Contraindicated in ischemic wound with dry eschar and third-degree burns Frequently a secondary dressing	Cleanse wound base and dry well Apply topical agent or primary dressing to wound base Place foam dressing in wound Apply appropriate secondary dressing and secure in place Change every 24 hours or PRN	Three dressings per week Covered when used on full-thickness wound with moderate to heavy exudate Foam filler: one per day Sheets covered as primary or secondary dressing A6209–A6215
Gauze: Hypertonic saline Curasalt (Tyco Healthcare/Kendall), Mesalt (Mohnlycke Health Care)	Gauze impregnated with dry sodium chloride by the manufacturer	Full-thickness, heavily exudating wound and nonviable wound base with or without infection	Cleanse wound, apply to the wound dry, cover with secondary dressing	Coded as gauze impregnated with products *other than* water, normal saline, and hydrogel A6222-A6224

Continued

TABLE 18-2 | **Wound Dressing Formulary—cont'd**

Product and Examples	Description	Indications for Use	Instructions for Use	Coverage Guidelines/HCPCS
Hydrocolloid: DuoDERM (ConvaTec), Exuderm (Medline), Replicare (Smith & Nephew) (Plates 49-51)	Contains gel-forming agents (gelatin, pectin, carboxymethylcellulose) Forms gelatinous mass Impermeable to contaminants, reducing risk of infection Promotes autolysis Reduces pain and protects Promotes moist wound Molds to body contours Adhesive	Partial- or full-thickness wound without depth Minimal to moderately exudative wound Avoid acutely infected wound Avoid dry eschar Use with caution in persons with diabetes Contraindicated in third-degree burns	Cleanse wound and dry peri-wound area well Select dressing 1–2 inches larger than wound Apply light pressure to allow body heat to promote adhesion Change every 3–5 days as needed Use peri-wound skin preparation product	Three dressings per week per wound A6234–A6241
Hydrogel: Skintegrity (Medline), Elasto-Gel (Southwest Technologies), Vigilon (Bard) (Plates 52-54)	Maintains clean, moist wound Nonadherent Little or no absorption Various formulations: amorphous gel, sheet, impregnated gauze Cool and soothing Decreases pain Aggressive autolytic debridement by autolysis	Partial- or full-thickness wound without depth (sheet or gel) or with depth (impregnated gauze) Dry to minimally exudative wound Sterile gel for every 3-day dressing changes Nonsterile gel can be used for daily dressing changes Contraindicated in third-degree burns	Cleanse wound Apply to cover wound base Do not use as wound filler Use appropriate secondary dressing Secure as necessary Change daily	Sheets or impregnated gauze: one per day Sheets or gauze with adhesive border: three per week Hydrogel filler: 3 oz per 30 days per wound A6242—A6248
Transparent film: Tegaderm (3M) Suresite (Medline), Opsite (Smith & Nephew) (Plates 56-58)	Permeable to oxygen and water vapor Protects from environmental contaminants—good shield Maintains moist wound Creates "second skin" Reduces friction Nonabsorbent Promotes autolysis	Shallow partial-thickness wound Dry to minimally exudative wound Not recommended for acutely infected wound Contraindicated in third-degree burns	Cleanse wound and dry peri-wound area Allow for 1- to 2-inch border around wound Apply without stretching or tension Change every 4–7 days or as needed Use skin sealant around wound edges	Three dressings per week per wound A6257–A6259
Wound fillers: Flexigel strands (Smith & Nephew), Multidex maltodextrin (DeRoyal)	Pastes, granules, powders, beads, gels	Full-thickness wound with depth Minimal to moderate exudate Infected or noninfected	Cleanse wound as appropriate Apply directly to wound Use appropriate secondary to optimize moist wound environment Change every 1–2 days	A6261 (gel/paste) A6262 (dry form)

HCPCS, Healthcare Common Procedure Coding System.
Examples of product brand names within this formulary are not inclusive nor intended as a product endorsement.

Before using specific products, providers should refer to the manufacturer's product insert for the most current information on contraindications, interactions, and utilization. The policy also contains a category for pouching wounds. These products are described in Chapter 38.

Alginate and Fiber Gelling

These highly absorptive products are gelling dressings made of spun fibers of brown seaweed (alginate dressings) or carboxymethylcellulose (fiber gelling dressings). They act via an ion exchange mechanism to absorb serous fluid or exudate, forming a nonadhesive, nonocclusive hydrophilic gel that conforms to the shape of the wound. These versatile dressings are available in the form of sheets or ropes that can be cut to the size of the wound or loosely packed into wound dead space (see Plates 44–45. Because these dressings absorb and hold exudate, they create a moist environment, thus promoting autolysis, granulation, and epithelization. Alginates have hemostatic properties as well.

Alginates and fiber gelling dressings are primary dressings changed as often as daily, or they are left on for several days depending on the volume of exudate and the secondary dressing used. For example, transparent films used as secondary dressings will not add to the absorptive capacity of an alginate or fiber gelling product, whereas foams used as secondary dressings with alginates will increase overall absorptive capacity and facilitate a longer wear time. Some alginates become almost amorphous gels in the wound and will require irrigation for removal, whereas others retain their structural integrity as they "gel" and can be lifted out of the wound. Removal of the dressing need not be aggressive, as the residual fibers are biocompatible. If an alginate is used inappropriately (e.g., used with minimally exudative wounds), the wound bed may become desiccated with alginate fibers imbedded in the wound. The alginate dressing should not be moistened prior to application. If the dressing is dry at the scheduled dressing change, the dressing change frequency should be decreased or an alternative product selected (Belmin et al, 2002; NPUAP-EPUAP, 2009).

Collagen

Collagen is a body protein that is degraded in chronic wounds by proteases and elastase. Collagen dressings usually are formulated with type I bovine (cowhides or tendon) or avian collagen or with type III porcine collagen. Collagen products are nonadhesive, nonocclusive primary dressings available in a variety of formulations: particles encapsulated in nonadherent pouches or vials, gels loaded in a syringe, pads, and freeze-dried sheets. Collagen dressings chemically bind to members of the MMP family, thus reducing the levels of proteases in chronic wounds (Cullen, 2002; Nisi et al, 2005; Ovington, 2002).

A collagen dressing requires the use of a secondary cover dressing and can be safely used for a partial-thickness or full-thickness wound with granular or nonviable tissue. International pressure ulcer guidelines recommend considering the use of collagen dressings for nonhealing Stage III and IV pressure ulcers (NPUAP-EPUAP, 2009). However, they also describe a randomized controlled trial comparing collagen and hydrocolloids dressings that found no significant difference in the healing rate of Stage II and III pressure ulcers after adjusting for baseline depth (Graumlich et al, 2003). The guidelines also point out that collagen dressing are more expensive and time consuming to apply than hydrocolloid dressings.

Composite

Composite dressings are used as primary or secondary dressings. They combine physically distinct components into a single dressing that provides multiple functions. The component in the center of the composite dressing is placed over or in contact with the wound base while the attached adhesive border secures the dressing. Composite dressings should not be cut because the structure of the dressing design will be compromised. Composites should be sized to have at least 2.5 cm (1 inch) of dressing that extends onto intact surrounding skin.

Up to three composite dressing changes per week are considered medically necessary, one wound cover per dressing change, unless it is documented that more frequent changes are medically necessary. Because composite dressings, foam and hydrocolloid wound covers, and transparent film, when used as secondary dressings, are meant to be changed at frequencies less than daily, appropriate clinical judgment should be used to avoid their use with primary dressings which would require more frequent dressing changes. For these dressings, changes greater than once every other day are not considered medically necessary. While a highly exudative wound might require such a combination initially, with continued proper management the wound should progress to a point where the appropriate selection of these products should result in the less frequent dressing changes which they are designed to allow.

Contact Layers

Contact layers are nonadherent net sheets that are woven or perforated. They are intended for placement over the wound bed to protect the tissue from direct contact with other dressings. Contact layers are porous to allow wound fluid to pass through for absorption by an overlying separate or attached dressing. A single contact layer is generally applied as a liner over a granular or epithelial wound surface overlapping onto surrounding skin. The contact layer stays in place during dressing changes, protecting the wound bed from trauma while allowing for passage of exudate through its mesh or perforations. Contact layers usually are changed once per week. They are not recommended for dry wounds, those with thick viscous exudate, and wounds with tunneling and extensive undermining.

Soft silicones are polymers, are insoluble to wound exudate, are not intrinsically absorbent, and do not interact chemically with the wound. Soft silicone dressings are manufactured as single contact layers, or they are added the wound-facing layer of an absorbent dressing (e.g., foam) for management of an exuding wound (Dykes and Heggie, 2003). An international advisory group of scar management experts recommends the use of silicone gel sheeting for the prevention and treatment of hypertrophic scars and keloids in select situations (Mustoe et al, 2002). Silicone dressings are easily removed and therefore do not traumatize the wound or the surrounding skin (NPUAP-EPUAP, 2009; Mustoe, et al 2002).

Foam

Polyurethane foam dressings are sheets of foamed polymers that contain variably sized small open cells capable of holding wound exudate away from the wound bed. A moist environment is created by maintaining the exudate in the wound space. Foam dressings are adhesive or nonadhesive, primary or secondary dressings, available in widely variable formulations (see Plates 46–48). Nonadhesive foam dressings can be secured in position with a secondary dressing, such as a transparent film dressing, or a nonadhesive wrap, such as roll gauze. The foam may be of traditional thickness (4–7 mm) or thin (<1 mm). Generally, the thin foam dressing has an adhesive wound surface and an outer layer of a transparent film dressing that provides a waterproof barrier. The traditional-thickness nonadhesive foam dressings may or may not have an adhesive border or an outer transparent layer that helps prevent strikethrough exudate. Foams are available as wafers, rolls, and cavity dressings as well as shapes to fit the heel, elbow, or sacrum. *Polymeric membrane* foams combine glycerin (to soften devitalized tissue), starch (to wick away exudate), and a surfactant (to loosen necrotic tissue) (Yastrub, 2004).

The appropriately sized foam dressing extends onto the periwound skin at least 2.5 cm (1 inch). Foam other than cavity dressings can be cut or contoured to fit anatomic areas. Check the manufacturer's instructions to determine which side of the dressing is applied to the wound surface. The usual dressing change for an open-cell foam dressing is up to three times per week. Foam cavity dressings used as wound fillers may be changed as often as once per day.

Because traditional-thickness open-cell foam is one of the most absorbent materials available, foam dressings are appropriate for moderate to heavy exudative wounds with or without a clean granular wound bed (Diehm and Lawall, 2005). International pressure ulcer guidelines recommend considering foam dressings for use on exudative Stage II and shallow Stage III pressure ulcers (NPUAP-EPUAP, 2009). The traditional-thickness nonadhesive foam dressing is particularly useful for management of exudate under compression in venous ulcers and in any wound with friable or fragile periwound skin. Foam dressings can be used as secondary dressings to absorptive primary dressings (e.g., alginate, collagen, or fiber gelling) to enhance absorption of wound exudate. When applied to a dry or minimally exudative wound, the traditional-thickness foam dressing may adhere to the wound surface and require irrigation to facilitate removal. Therefore only very thin foam can be used to manage the superficial wound with minimal exudate and protect intact vulnerable skin.

When a cavity foam dressing is used to fill depth, the size of the product should be determined carefully, leaving sufficient room in the wound for the cavity dressing to expand as it absorbs wound exudate. Single small pieces of foam dressings should not be placed in cavities (NPUAP-EPUAP, 2009). Foam dressings do not redistribute pressure but have been shown to be effective in reducing shear (NPUAP-EPUAP, 2009; Ohura et al, 2005). Foam dressings are not indicated for wounds with tunneling.

Hydrocolloid

Hydrocolloid dressings are a formulation of elastomeric, adhesive, and gelling agents. The most common absorbent ingredient in the hydrocolloid is carboxymethylcellulose, which was adapted from ostomy skin barriers. Multiple meta-analyses confirm what is widely accepted in clinical practice, that hydrocolloids result in better (statistically significant) wound healing outcomes compared to gauze (Bouza et al, 2005; Bradley et al, 1999; Singh et al, 2004). Studies have also shown that hydrocolloids result in healing rates similar to those of comparable such as alginates and foams or more advanced dressings such as collagens. (Bale et al, 1997; Belmin et al, 2002; Graumlich et al, 2003).

Early versions of hydrocolloid dressings were described as being fully occlusive. Today hydrocolloids are backed with a semiocclusive film layer that renders them impermeable to fluids and bacteria and semipermeable to gas and water vapor. The wound side of this dressing is adhesive and adheres to moist surfaces as well as dry skin but does not adhere to moist wound beds. Hydrocolloid dressings provide a great degree of conformability and flexibility.

As a primary dressing, the hydrocolloid is available as a wafer in several shapes and sizes. Contoured dressings also are available that enhance adherence to anatomically challenging sites, such as the sacrum, heel, knee, and elbow (see Plates 49–51). Many hydrocolloid dressings have an adhesive border that extends beyond the actual hydrocolloid surface. This design prevents shear and friction from loosening the edges of the hydrocolloid and circumvents the need for additional tape along the borders of the dressing.

As wound fluid is absorbed, the hydrocolloid forms a viscous, colloidal gel in the wound bed, which enhances the moist wound environment needed for granulation, epithelization, and autolysis. This gel is easily irrigated out of the wound at dressing change. Hydrocolloid dressings can also be formulated to contain an alginate, which increases the dressing's absorptive capacity.

The correct size of hydrocolloid dressing should extend onto intact periwound skin at least 2.5 cm (1 inch). If the hydrocolloid is cut from a larger piece, the edges should be taped to avoid rolling or adhering to clothing or sheets. Because hydrocolloids are most effective at body temperature, the dressing should be held in place with the hand for a short period of time (30–60 seconds) after application. Dressings should be changed when the wound gel appears to have migrated beyond the margins of the wound or the seal is leaking so that periwound skin is in contact with exudates or the wound is contaminated with feces or urine.

Traditional-thickness hydrocolloid dressings are indicated as primary dressings for minimally to moderately exudate partial- and full-thickness wounds without depth. Hydrocolloids can be used as a secondary dressing over filler materials such as hydrocolloid powders, pastes, and alginates. International pressure ulcer guidelines advocate the use of hydrocolloids for clean Stage II and noninfected shallow Stage III pressure ulcers in anatomic locations where the product does not roll or melt (NPUAP-EPUAP, 2009). Due to its prescribed wear time and reimbursement, wounds that require assessment more often than twice per week should not be treated with a hydrocolloid.

As with thin foams, thin hydrocolloids absorb minimal exudate but have a lower profile and are more flexible. Therefore thin hydrocolloid dressings are indicated for the partial-thickness wound with minimal exudate or for intact skin that needs protection against friction or skin stripping.

Hydrogel

Hydrogel dressings contain hydrated (glycerin- or water-based) hydrophilic polymers that are primarily and uniquely designed to hydrate or donate moisture to the wound, thus facilitating moist wound healing and autolysis. Therefore hydrogel dressings are indicated for dry to minimally exudative wounds with or without depth, and are a good choice for painful wounds because hydrogel dressings do not adhere to the base of the wound. International pressure ulcer guidelines recommend considering the use of hydrogels for dry to minimally exudative pressure ulcers that are noninfected and granulating in anatomic locations that are not at risk for dressing migration (NPUAP-EPUAP, 2009). Hydrogel dressings are formulated as sheets or amorphous gel (see Plate 52).

Amorphous hydrogels are similar in formulation to the hydrogel sheet except that the polymer has not been cross-linked to form a sheet. Because of the absence of cross-linking, the amorphous hydrogel does not provide the same cooling effect as the sheet hydrogel. These dressings vary widely in viscosity and are available in a foil package, tube, spray bottle, impregnated gauze (see Plate 53), or ribbon gauze strips. The ability to hydrate the wound surface and resist drying out has been among the most salient selling points of hydrogel dressings, making them excellent replacements for saline-moistened gauze (Eisenbud et al, 2003). Unlike saline moistened gauze, however, amorphous hydrogel usually needs only to be changed daily. Amorphous hydrogels can be applied to shallow wounds or may be impregnated into gauze to pack wounds with depth, undermining, or tunneling (impregnated into gauze and strips). Because of the high water content of amorphous gels, care must be taken to protect the periwound skin with careful placement and/or use of periwound skin barriers.

Hydrogel sheets are three-dimensional networks of cross-linked, hydrophilic polymers intended for use on dry or minimally exudative shallow wounds. The cross-linked polymer (polyethylene oxide, polyacrylamide, or polyvinylpyrrolidone) physically traps water to form a solid sheet. Although the hydrogel sheet may contain up to 96% moisture and feel moist, water is not released when the sheet is squeezed. Hydrogel sheets have a cooling effect that can be further enhanced with refrigeration, a particularly effective intervention when a sustained "cooling sensation" is the priority (e.g., with a sunburn). Sheets may be packaged with a polymer film on one or both sides; one side is removed before the sheet is placed on the wound bed. Hydrogel sheets that are composed primarily of water should be cut to the size of the wound to avoid overlapping and maceration of intact periwound skin (see Plate 54). A skin barrier ointment or skin sealant (see Plate 55) can be applied to the immediate periwound skin to further prevent maceration. The hydrogel sheet that is predominantly glycerin can be applied to the wound and overlap onto the periwound skin with minimal risk of periwound maceration. Hydrogel sheets can be sterile or nonsterile and ar formulated with or without an adhesive border. Sheets without borders require secondary dressings. Hydrogel sheets are generally changed daily to three times per week.

Honey

The strong osmotic action of honey has demonstrated the ability to promote autolysis by pulling lymph fluid from surrounding tissues thus adding moisture to the wound. Honey's production of hydrogen peroxide may also provide broad spectrum antibacterial effect and facilitate autolysis by activating matrix metalloproteases (Pieper, 2009; WOCN, 2010). Honey for wound care can be formulated into gels that are spread onto a dressing prior to application or purchased in the form of preimpregnated pads or alginates. In 2007, the US Food and Drug Administration approved a honey-based wound dressing that uses active Manuka honey (*Leptospermum scoparium*), derived from tea plants, and *Leptospermum polygalifolium*, known as the jelly bush. The product (Medihoney, Derma Sciences) is formulated into and reimbursed as a calcium alginate dressing. Contraindications for using a honey dressings include: (1) using a honey product that is not indicated for wound care; (2) sensitivity to bee venom/stings or honey; (3) dry, necrotic wounds; (4) dressings that cannot be changed within a specific time; (5) wounds requiring surgical debridement; and (6) following an incision and drain of an abscess (Pieper, 2009).

Specialty Absorptive

Specialty absorptive dressings are unitized multilayer dressings that provide either (1) a semiadherent quality or nonadherent layer or (2) highly absorptive layers of fibers, such as absorbent cellulose, cotton, or rayon. These dressings may or may not have an adhesive border. Specialty absorptive dressings are indicated for wounds with moderate to heavy exudate. Specialty absorptive dressings without an adhesive border usually are changed daily; those with an adhesive border usually are changed every other day.

Transparent Film

Transparent film dressings are polyurethane sheets coated on one side with an acrylic, hypoallergenic adhesive. The adhesive is inactivated by moisture and will not adhere to a moist surface. Distinguishing features of film dressings are the packaging, ease of use, and application process. Film dressings are available in a variety of sizes and features (see Plates 56–57).

Film dressings have no absorbent capacity and are impermeable to fluids and bacteria. However, they are semipermeable to gas, such as oxygen and water vapor. The extent of semipermeability, measured as MVTR, is variable. Traditional film dressings have a low MVTR that ranges from 400 to 800 $g/m^2/day$. A "high-permeability" film dressing has an MVTR of 3,000 $g/m^2/day$ and higher and is specifically designed to be used over an intravenous site. High-permeability film dressings will allow an excessive amount of moisture to escape if they are used over a wound and precipitate desiccation. A collection of purulent-appearing fluid is typical when using a transparent film dressing (particularly in the presence of nonviable tissue) and should not be misinterpreted as indicative of an infection (see Plate 58).

Film dressings are commonly used as secondary dressings to other products, such as alginates and foam. Film dressings are indicated as a primary dressing for (1) prophylaxis on high-risk intact skin, (2) superficial wounds with minimal or no exudate, and (3) eschar-covered wounds when autolysis is indicated, appropriate, and safe (NPUAP-EPUAP, 2009). When a transparent dressing is being used to facilitate autolysis in an eschar-covered wound, it must be monitored closely and possibly changed more frequently. During the autolysis process, the eschar will liquefy, and the fluid that accumulates potentially can undermine the film's adhesive. As the eschar softens, liquefies, and is removed, the depth of the wound becomes apparent and alternative dressings will be indicated to fill dead space and absorb exudate.

A film dressing should be selected that allows a 2.5-cm (1-inch) perimeter of intact surrounding skin. A liquid skin barrier can be applied to the periwound skin prior to dressing application to prevent skin stripping, particularly in the presence of fragile skin. When removing the transparent film dressing, stretch the film in a direction parallel to the wound rather than pulling upward. The stretching action gently breaks the seal. Film dressings should be changed when the exudate extends beyond the edges of the wound onto periwound skin (see Plate 58). The typical dressing change frequency for the transparent dressing is every 3 days.

Transparent dressings should be avoided in the management of arterial ulcers and infected wounds that require frequent monitoring. Because transparent films do not fill dead space, they should not be used as a primary dressing on wounds with depth, undermining, or tunneling.

Gauze

Gauze is available woven or nonwoven, as cotton or synthetic blends, sterile or nonsterile, in many forms (pads, ribbon, strips, and rolls), and plain or impregnated. Nonwoven cotton-filled gauze is particularly useful for scrubbing, prepping, wiping, absorption, and protection. To increase its versatility and applicability, gauze may be impregnated by the manufacturer with substances such as iodinated agents, petrolatum, zinc paste, crystalline sodium chloride, chlorhexidine gluconate, bismuth tribromophenate, water, aqueous saline, hydrogel, or other agents. Impregnated gauze provides additional functions, such as hydrating the wound (e.g., hydrogel or aqueous saline impregnated), absorbing exudate (e.g., crystalline sodium chloride formulations), or delivering antimicrobial agents and nutrients.

Because of their low unit cost, gauze dressings are often viewed as the least expensive and most cost-effective dressing. However, when analyzing cost efficacy, it is important to take into consideration health care provider knowledge and time, frequency of dressing changes, ease of use, patient discomfort, and healing rate, as well as the unit cost of the dressing (Hopf et al, 2006; Robson et al, 2006; Steed et al, 2006; Whitney et al, 2006). Gauze does not maintain a moist wound environment unless the wound is heavily exudative, which often necessitates

TABLE 18-3	Disadvantages of Gauze Dressings	
Disadvantage	**Potential Consequences**	
Moisture evaporates quickly and dressing dries out	Painful removal Impaired cell migration Desiccation of viable tissue Impaired autolysis Removal of healthy tissue upon removal	
Requires frequent dressing changes	Dispersal of bacteria with each dressing change Increased patient discomfort and need for pain medications Increased for caregiver time and costs	
Associated with increased infection rates as compared to semiocclusive dressings	Increased cost for antimicrobials Slower healing rates Increased pain Decrease in patient satisfaction Increased caregiver time	

more frequent dressing changes. When numerous dressing changes are required each day to manage moisture, alternative dressing options are indicated to decrease pain, caregiver time, and the potential for dispersal of bacteria during dressing changes (Hopf et al, 2006; Ovington, 2001).

The many disadvantages of gauze use are summarized in Table 18-3. Unlike semiocclusive dressings, gauze lacks a mechanical barrier to the entry of exogenous bacteria. Compared to semiocclusive dressings, gauze has been associated with a 50% greater infection rate (Ovington, 2001). The Wound Healing Society states that wet-to-dry dressings are not an inappropriate wound dressing selection because they are not continuously moist (Whitney et al, 2006). Indications for use of dry gauze in wound management is also constrained by the fact that dry gauze does not maintain a moist wound environment unless the wound is heavily exudative.

Continuously Moist Saline Gauze. Continuously moist saline gauze dressings can be effective in terms of healing rate but may have other drawbacks, such as maceration of the periwound skin, practicality of use, and cost-effectiveness (Robson et al, 2006). The ability of saline-moistened gauze dressings to keep a wound from drying out depends on the amount of exudate from the wound and the frequency with which the gauze is changed or moistened. It is possible to extend the ability of saline-moistened gauze to prevent loss of moisture by incorporating petrolatum-impregnated gauze into the dressing as an upper layer. The hydrophobic nature of petrolatum will block transmission of moisture through the upper dressing. Box 18-2 contains a guide to appropriate use of gauze dressing (NPUAP-EPUAP, 2009).

Hypertonic Saline Impregnated Gauze. Hypertonic saline gauze is impregnated with dry sodium chloride. The product is applied to the wound dry, requires a secondary dressing, and is dependent upon heavy wound exudate for a moist environment. Once moistened with wound exudate, the dressing becomes isotonic and uses a wicking action to draw fluid and debris out of the wound

BOX 18-2	Guide to Appropriate Use of Gauze Dressing

- Avoid gauze dressings for clean pressure ulcers because these dressings are labor intensive and dry out easily, leading to painful removal and tissue desiccation.
- When other forms of moisture-retentive dressings are not available, use continuously moist gauze.
  - Loosely fill dead space to avoid pressure on the wound.
  - Fill dead space with single gauze piece or roll (small pieces may be left behind, creating a potential infection source).
- Use loosely woven gauze for highly exudative wounds.
- Use tightly woven gauze for minimally exudative wounds.

thereby decreasing interstitial edema; an ideal dressing for infective, exudative cavity wounds. Because they are dependent upon wound exudate for moisture, hypertonic saline dressings should not be used for dry or minimally exudative wounds. Conversely, they may not be cost effective if too many dressing changes are required. Hypertonic saline gauze should be discontinued when new growth of granulation tissue in sufficient amount is present.

Wound Filler

Wound fillers are dressing materials that are placed into open wounds to eliminate dead space, absorb exudate, or maintain a moist wound surface. Wound fillers come in hydrated forms (e.g., pastes, gels) dry forms (e.g., powder, granules, beads), and other forms (e.g., ropes spiral, pillows). Up to one dressing change per day is considered medically necessary, unless it is documented that more frequent changes are needed.

COMPONENTS OF A DRESSING CHANGE

In general, the components of a dressing change are the same: infection control, atraumatic removal, cleansing, light filling or packing, periwound skin protection, dressing application, and securement.

Infection Control

Although the wound surface is expected to be contaminated, infection control measures are needed to prevent bacteria from inoculating or escalating to an infection. This is particularly important in light of studies identifying health care workers (nurses, physicians, technicians) as the source of methicillin-resistant *Staphylococcus aureus* (MRSA). Results from studies of health care workers colonized with MRSA ranged from 15% to 50% (Bisaga et al, 2008; Johnston et al, 2007).

Standard universal precautions (gloves, eye protection when splashes are possible, etc.) and handwashing should be routinely followed during dressing changes (Stotts et al, 1997). Although handwashing is the most effective infection control practice, it is the most frequently overlooked precaution. Caregivers should wash their hands (1) before and after patient contact, (2) after contact with a source of microorganisms (e.g., body fluid and substances, mucous membranes, broken skin, soiled dressings), and (3) after removing gloves. An easily overlooked opportunity for handwashing is between care of a dirty body site and a clean body site; an analogy is the removal of a dirty wound dressing and application of a new dressing. Although the practice has not been researched specifically, two sets of gloves should be used: one set for dressing removal and wound cleansing and another set for dressing application.

Bioburden can be affected by the techniques used to apply and remove dressings and topical agents. There is no evidence that sterile technique as opposed to clean techniques for changing dressings on chronic wounds is warranted or improves outcomes. There is also a lack of agreement as to what actually constitutes sterile as opposed to nonsterile technique. *No-touch* technique is a method of changing surface dressings without directly touching the wound or any surface that might come in contact with the wound (Wound, Ostomy Continence Nurses [WOCN] Society and the Association for Professionals in Infection Control and Epidemiology [APIC], 2005). Sterile devices are used to hold and administer sterile irrigant solution. Sterile cotton-tipped applicators are used to probe the wound and insert wound fillers, gauze, or packing. Clean (rather than sterile) gloves are used to apply sterile dressings; however, the surface of the dressing that will contact the wound bed is not touched.

Atraumatic Dressing Removal

During dressing removal, the periwound skin and the wound base must be protected from trauma. Adhesives are removed in the direction of hair growth. An edge of the dressing is gently rolled or lifted to obtain a starting edge. The tissue adjacent to the dressing is supported as the dressing is gently released from the skin. Moistened gauze can be used to support the skin during dressing removal to minimize the potential for stripping. If the dressing material is attached to the wound base, saline or a wound cleanser can be used to moisten the dressing and allow gentle release of the dressing material from the tissue. Difficult or painful removal must also facilitate an alternative wound care plan (i.e., skin sealant or nonadhesive product) to decrease pain and trauma to the wound with future dressing changes. Dressing changes are performed on a scheduled basis depending on the type of dressing in use; dressings that are oversaturated or leaking should be changed promptly. Dressing materials and contaminated gloves are disposed in accordance with agency policies and procedures.

Cleansing and Irrigation

Every open wound regardless of size or depth requires cleansing with each dressing change. Wound cleansing is necessary to physically remove surface bacteria and debris from the wound bed without damaging healthy tissue or inoculating the underlying tissue with bacteria by using a force between 4 to 15 pounds per square inch (psi) (Hopf et al, 2006; Robson et al, 2006; Steed et al, 2006; Whitney et al, 2006). This is accomplished with the use of normal saline, a 19-gauge angiocatheter, and a 35-ml syringe (bulb syringes do not provide enough pressure). Commercially prepackaged canisters of pressurized saline and wound cleansers with surfactants that deliver a safe range of pressure to the wound are available. Although normal saline is generally the wound cleanser of choice in hospitals, it does not contain a preservative to prevent bacteria from growing in the container. Therefore, once opened, saline bottles must be discarded in a short period (i.e., 24 hours). Conversely, commercially prepared wound cleansers contain surfactants and therefore can be used for many dressing changes.

When the wound is suspected of having critical colonization or infection, an irrigant with a surfactant, antiseptic, or antimicrobial agent is indicated. Antiseptic solutions are generally diluted and discontinued when the condition of the wound improves (NPUAP-EPUAP, 2009). Chapter 16 provides a detailed discussion related to wound infection, diagnosis, and management including description, and indications for antimicrobials and antiseptic solutions.

Periwound Skin Protection

After dressing removal and wound cleansing, the surrounding skin is gently cleansed and dried. Wound exudate and dressing adhesives place the periwound skin at risk for maceration, skin stripping, and infection. Periwound maceration and continuous contact with wound exudate can enlarge the wound and impede healing (Robson et al, 2006; Steed et al, 2006; Whitney et al, 2006). In addition, the pathophysiologic impact of an underlying etiology such as arterial insufficiency may leave the periwound skin dry, cracked, or friable. Measures to maintain the integrity of the periwound skin include use of moisturizers when the skin is dry, use of skin sealants to

TABLE 18-4	Dressing Options Based on Wound Needs					
Dry–Minimal Exudate, Shallow	**Moderate–Heavy Exudate, Shallow**	**Dry–Minimal Exudate with Depth**	**Moderate–Heavy Exudate with Depth**	**Nonadherent**	**Conformable**	**Recalcitrant**
Foam (thin)	Specialty absorptive	Hydrogel-impregnated gauze	Alginate/Hydrofiber	Foam (nonadhesive brand)	Alginate	Antimicrobials (see Chapter 16)
Hydrocolloid	Foam (standard)	Continuously moist gauze	Foam cavity	Contact layer	Transparent	Collagen
Transparent	Hydrocolloid (moderate exudate)		Loosely woven gauze	Hydrogel	Hydrocolloid	
Hydrogel	Alginate/Hydrofiber		Hypertonic saline gauze		Thin foam	

protect the skin from moisture and adhesives (see Table 5-4), and use of nonadhesive dressings (Tables 18-2 and 18-4). Dressings should be changed or modified when the wound exudate is no longer contained by the dressing and is encroaching on the intact skin. Chapter 5 provides a detailed discussion of additional steps to prevent and manage skin stripping and candidiasis.

Dressing Application

The selected dressing is applied, according to manufacturer's instructions, without stretching the skin. In the gluteal fold, wafer dressings are folded in half before application to ensure that the adhesive seals into the anatomic contours. Applications of dressings at the heel or elbow may require cutting and shaping the dressing to customize the fit. Position the heel or elbow in the bent position during application so that the dressing does not pull the skin when the limb is extended.

Packing or Filling. The purpose of filling or packing the wound is to fill dead space and avoid the potential of abscess formation by premature closure of the wound. Packing materials should be conformable to the base and sides of the wound. In the presence of undermining, impregnated gauze, alginate rope, or fiber gelling dressings may be used to gently pack the space. When tunneling is apparent in the wound, strip gauze packing may be used to fill narrow areas so that the complete dressing can be easily removed during dressing changes. Absorbent packing dressings (e.g., alginate, fiber gelling, dry gauze) are appropriate for wounds that are exudative. Conversely, for wounds that are dry, the packing material must be hydrating so that it provides moisture to the wounds (e.g., hydrogel-impregnated gauze, continuously moist gauze). For large deep wounds, hydrating or absorbent-impregnated gauze is effective and usually requires fewer dressing changes than dry gauze. The packing material is fluffed and loosely placed into the wound with a cotton-tipped applicator so that the packing material is in contact with the wound edges and base. Gauze dressings may be necessary to act as an additional absorbent layer.

Overpacking of the wound should be avoided (WOCN Society, 2003). A secondary cover dressing is then applied and secured.

Securing the Dressing

A method of securing nonadhesive dressings is necessary to keep such dressings in place. Self-adhesive wraps, tape, Montgomery straps, gauze wraps, or tubular mesh dressings may be used. If the wound is located on the leg, a gauze wrap can be taped upon itself to avoid applying tape to the skin.

DRESSING SELECTION

Topical dressing selection is based on the wound characteristics and dressing functions. The process of dressing selection is guided by a series of questions and assessments (Checklist 18-1). Two key wound assessment parameters that most influence dressing selection are the amount of wound exudate and the depth of the wound. Not all dressing are intended nor appropriate to be used continuously until closure. Therefore, dressings should be reevaluated for appropriateness based on the wound characteristics and patient response.

CHECKLIST 18-1
Questions for Appropriate Dressing Selection

✓ Does the wound have exudate?
✓ Does the wound have depth, tunneling, or undermining?
✓ What type of tissue is present in the base of the wound?
✓ What is the condition of the periwound skin?
✓ Are there any compatibility issues to consider?
✓ What is the location of the wound?
✓ Are topical antimicrobials indicated?
✓ Is senescence suspected?
✓ Are there any special patient or caregiver considerations?

Does the Wound Have Exudate?

The volume and type of wound exudate are such sufficiently significant factors in selecting a wound dressing that the presence of exudate is the first question posed. Dry wounds require a dressing that will hydrate the tissue. Conversely, exudative wounds require absorbent dressing materials. Several dressings are available that are designed to manage the full range of exudate volume, from minimal to heavy amounts (see Tables 18-2 and 18-4). Adequate containment of exudate is critical to managing bioburden, maintaining a seal, protecting the periwound skin, controlling odor, and avoiding overuse of wound care products. In addition, the prolonged presence of excessive amounts of moisture in the wound may increase the patient's risk for developing hyperplasia or hypergranulation tissue in the base of the wound (see Plate 27). Methods of exudate management include moisture vapor transmission, as with transparent dressings, and wicking, as with alginate or foam dressings.

Does the Wound Have Depth, Tunneling, or Undermining?

Tissue that is not exposed to treatment agents cannot be expected to respond to the regimen and proceed to healing (Whitney et al, 2006). Once depth, tunneling, or undermining is identified, the dressing selected must be able to reach the extent of the wound base as well as fill the dead space to prevent abscess and premature closure of the wound. For example, a hydrocolloid paste can fill a very small amount of depth, whereas a deeper wound may require layers or strips of packing agents such as impregnated gauze to adequately fill dead space.

What Type of Tissue is Present in the Base of the Wound?

When granulation is the primary tissue in the wound, a dressing that maintains a moist wound surface usually is ideal. The presence of slough or eschar in the wound will dictate the need for some form of debridement to decrease the bioburden in the wound and remove physical obstacles to wound closure. Moisture-retentive dressings promote autolysis by maintaining a moist wound–dressing interface. The type of dressing used to achieve or assist with debridement varies depending on the form of debridement selected. All of the dressing categories in the formulary, except for dry gauze, are moisture retentive. The dressing selected is also based on the volume of exudate and the architecture of the wound. For example, when the wound is minimally exudative and eschar covered, one option for autolysis is to apply an amorphous hydrogel over the wound and cover with a transparent dressing. Within 24 hours the eschar typically is rehydrated and

loosening from the wound edges. At that time, sharp debridement may be indicated and the hydrogel may continue to be appropriate, or another dressing may be indicated if the wound depth is revealed.

What Is the Condition of the Periwound Skin?

The periwound skin can be intact, dry, cracked, macerated, erythematous, or infected (e.g., candidiasis). Dry and cracked skin may require a moisturizer before dressing application. Skin that is vulnerable to adhesives may require a nonadhesive dressing or can be protected from adhesives with the use of skin protectants, sealants, and barriers. Skin integrity is also affected by the technique used to apply and remove adhesives. When appropriate, less frequent dressing changes are preferred to prevent unnecessary exposure of the skin to adhesive removal. As previously described, less aggressive adhesives such as silicones may be indicated. Caregivers should be taught techniques for gentle removal of dressings to prevent skin stripping.

The presence of maceration indicates that wound exudate is not adequately contained or managed. Prolonged contact of wound fluid with the periwound skin predisposes the patient to development of fungal infection (most commonly candidiasis) or erythema at the periwound site. To correct this situation, either the type of dressing used should be modified to a more absorbent type (see Tables 18-2 and 18-4) or the frequency of dressing changes should be increased. A liquid skin barrier will protect the periwound skin from damp or saturated wound dressings. Occasionally the patient will require an antifungal powder or lotion to treat a fungal infection, although milder cases may resolve spontaneously when the excessive wound exudate is managed effectively. Absorbent dressings and pouching techniques are used to manage wound exudate, thus preventing or reducing periwound maceration, erythema, and candidiasis.

Are there Any Compatibility Issues to Consider?

Safety features of wound care dressings indicate that products are free from toxic chemicals and fibers and that product biocompatibility has been tested and reported by the manufacturers (Flanagan, 1997). Safety should also demonstrate that the product does not increase the patient's risk of morbidity or mortality. The wound specialist's role in safety includes correct use of the product as recommended by the manufacturer (including FDA-approved clinical indications) and proper education of the caregiver.

The wound specialist should be cautious about mixing different topical agents for use in a wound because ingredients in one agent may interact with ingredients in another. For example, the enzymatic activity of collagenase is adversely affected by certain detergents and heavy metal ions (e.g., mercury, silver), which are used in some antiseptics, and is inactivated by povidone-iodine. If the collagenase enzyme is used in combination with a secondary cover dressing that releases silver ions, the silver ions would inactivate the enzyme, resulting in no enzymatic debridement and little or no antibacterial effect of the silver. Similarly, certain foams are degraded by hydrogen peroxide, and the two should not be used sequentially. It is vitally important to thoroughly read product package inserts and instructions for use when dressings, ointments, and solutions are being used together or sequentially in the same wound.

Finally, compatibility with concurrently used therapies and procedures is an important consideration in selecting the optimal dressing. For example, some products are not compatible with electrical stimulation, hyperbaric oxygen therapy, or radiation therapy. Because various compression therapy methods have change frequencies ranging from daily to weekly, the patient with a venous insufficiency wound requires a dressing with a compatible wear time. The patient with an ostomy close to a midline incision wound will require a dressing that does not interfere with the patient's ability to empty and change the ostomy pouch.

What Is the Location of the Wound?

The dressing selected should stay in place, minimize shear and friction, and not cause additional tissue damage (Robson et al, 2006; Steed et al, 2006; Whitney et al, 2006). Wound location combined with patient activity can significantly impact the dressing's ability to stay intact. Digit dressings are useful for the toes and fingers. In some situations, flexible dressing options shaped to fit heels, elbows, and sacrum, may provide better coverage and wear time than a standard square or rectangular dressings. Wounds in locations exposed to friction and shear from sheets, clothing, or braces may require thin adhesive dressings with smooth backings and tapered edges to keep from rolling. In the presence of incontinence, wounds close to the perineal region will benefit from waterproof dressings.

Are Topical Antimicrobials Indicated?

Bacterial bioburden influences decisions on topical wound management. Therefore with each dressing change the wound should be assessed for signs and symptoms of infection. When the wound is overcolonized or infected, a complete systemic assessment and appropriate treatment must be instituted. Chapter 16 provides a detailed discussion related to wound infection, diagnosis, and management, including descriptions and indications for antimicrobial dressings and antiseptic solutions.

Generally, nonocclusive dressings are indicated as the most conservative topical wound care approach; semiocclusive dressings are not recommended for infected wounds. Semiocclusive dressings should be monitored closely and changed more frequently than generally anticipated.

Odor is also commonly associated with infected or highly colonized wounds, such as fungating lesions or pressure ulcers with necrotic debris. Improvement is generally noted as odor-causing bacteria are eliminated through the use of debridement, antimicrobials, and antiseptics. A slight odor however noted during a dressing change may not be indicative of an infection. Odor is associated with the use of certain types of dressings (e.g., hydrocolloids), strikethrough exudate and leakage, poor hygiene, and inappropriate use of dressings (e.g., extending dressing wear time beyond that which is recommended). In these situations, patient and caregiver education is indicated. Chapter 37 presents interventions (including topical dressing options) that are available when odor is an ongoing problem such as with a fungating wound.

Is Senescence Suspected?

If a wound is not progressing despite optimal care, cellular senescence (a decrease in proliferation potential of dermal fibroblasts and inability of cells to respond to growth factors) may be a factor. In the case of senescence, biophysical and biologic agents (e.g., growth factors, electrical stimulation, negative pressure wound therapy) may be considered to manipulate the repair process for successful "recruitment" of nonsenescent cells to the wound bed. These therapies are discussed in greater detail in Chapters 19 through 24.

Are There Special Patient or Caregiver Considerations?

During the initial patient interview, it is valuable to obtain a history of the patient's wound, including what dressings thus far have been used for the wound and the effect of those interventions. This information can be used to identify dressings to avoid, dressings that may require extra encouragement for the patient to use again, or dressings that will require additional periwound skin protection, such as a skin barrier ointment, cream, or sealant. Realistic goals for the wound and for the patient must be identified (WOCN, 2010). For example, the patient with a wound on a limb with an ABI of 0.6 that cannot be revascularized may not have enough blood flow to promote autolysis; thus keeping the wound dry with betadine treatments is a more appropriate plan than promoting moist wound healing.

A holistic assessment of the patient requires identifying who is (or will be) providing care and in what care setting. Box 18-1 shows the numerous variables that impact product selection and potential outcomes of care. Clearly, the caregiver has a significant impact on the ability to achieve positive wound-related outcomes. As the plan of care is being developed and dressing choices are being made, the availability, level of skill, and care-related concerns of the caregiver will be important to ascertain and explore. A primary concern of the caregiver is ease of use.

Reimbursement for supplies (and therefore access to products) is dependent on the type of health care setting and how the setting is paid for services. When the patient needs to pay out-of-pocket for wound care supplies, the risk of nonadherence with the plan of care is increased. Therefore treatment decisions should be made considering what is financially reasonable for the patient so that the patient is able to implement the plan of care. Wound care items that are not reimbursed are listed in Box 18-3. For more discussion of facilitating cooperation and establishing a sustainable plan of care, see Chapter 29.

Pain at the wound site must be adequately described and objectively quantified before the wound specialist can understand the origin of the pain and identify appropriate pain control measures. Chronic pain, as occurs with ischemia, requires maintenance pain control measures. Pain at the wound site may be relieved or minimized by the use of nonadhesive moisture-retentive dressings. Analgesics given before the dressing change also may be indicated. However, pain that occurs during dressing changes should prompt a reevaluation of dressing change technique and wound care product choices. Liquid skin sealants will protect skin from mechanical forces during dressing removal. Nonetheless, caregiver technique in the removal of tape (i.e., proper use of adhesives and supporting the tissue during dressing removal) has a dramatic effect on the patient's pain experience. Wound pain and control measures are discussed in greater detail in Chapters 25 and 26.

DOCUMENTATION AND REIMBURSEMENT

On a per-patient basis, local wound management interventions should be planned with consideration of product reimbursement for the patient. Documentation, product selection, and the care setting affect how reimbursement occurs. Some wound care items, such as skin and wound cleansers, moisturizers, and skin barriers, are not reimbursed by Medicare. If the patient is paying out of pocket for these supplies, wound care may be jeopardized. Guidelines for utilization as established by Medicare Part B require documentation of medical necessity as defined in Checklist 18-2. Guidelines for utilization and HCPCS codes are given in Table 18-2 and Box 18-3. Dressing size must be based on, and appropriate to, the size of the wound. For wound covers, the pad size usually is about 2 inches greater than the dimensions of the wound.

- No more than a 1-month supply of dressings may be provided at one time.

CHECKLIST 18-2
Documentation Requirements for Coverage and/or Medical Necessity

Wound Care Orders
- ✓ Written wound care orders every 3 months, when a new dressing is added, or if quantity increases
- ✓ Order must be signed and dated by health care provider
- ✓ Order must specify the following:
  A. Type of dressing
  B. Size of the dressing
  C. Number/amount to be used at one time
  D. Frequency of dressing changes
  E. Expected duration of need

Documentation
- ✓ Monthly documentation by nurse, physician, or other health care professional
- ✓ More frequent documentation (e.g., weekly) for patients in nursing facility or patients with heavily draining or infected wounds
- ✓ Documentation must include the following:
  A. Number of wounds being treated with a dressing
  B. Type of wound (e.g., surgical wound, debrided wound)
  C. Whether dressing is being used as primary or secondary dressing
  D. Location, size (length × width, in centimeters), depth of wound; amount of exudate
  E. Additional relevant information

Clinical Policy Bulletin: Surgical Dressings (Wound Care Supplies). Accessed May 25, 2010. Available at http://www.aetna.com/cpb/medical/data/500_599/0526.html Aetna.

BOX 18-3	Wound Care Items That are not Reimbursed

- Dressings for drainage from a cutaneous fistula which has not been caused by or treated by a surgical procedure.
- Dressings for Stage 1 pressure ulcers.
- Dressings for 1st degree burns.
- Dressings for wounds caused by trauma which do not require surgical closure or debridement (skin tears, venipuncture, arterial puncture site).
- Skin sealants or barriers, wound cleansers or irrigating solutions, solutions used to moisten gauze (e.g., saline), topical antiseptics and topical antibiotics.
- Gauze or other dressings used to debride a wound, but not left on the wound.
- Dressing kits. All dressings must be individualized for each patient.
- More than one type of wound filler or wound cover in a single wound
- Use of some combinations of a hydrating dressing and an absorptive dressing (e.g., hydrogel, alginate) on the same wound at the same time.
- More than a 1-month supply at a time

Clinical Policy Bulletin: Surgical Dressings (Wound Care Supplies). Accessed May 25, 2010. Available at http://www.aetna.com/cpb/medical/data/500_599/0526.html Aetna.

SUMMARY

Wounded skin is a complex pathophysiologic condition that necessitates a specific and intricate knowledge base, which includes assessments and interventions to achieve appropriate outcomes for the wound. Unfortunately, nonphysiologic approaches and inappropriate product use remain commonplace and are likely to delay wound closure thus increasing the overall cost of wound care.

A frequently stated axiom in wound care is "All wounds are not the same." Consequently, many aspects of local wound management differ, and numerous factors affect local wound treatment decisions. One treatment protocol is not appropriate for all wounds, and seldom does a wound progress to healing with only one type of dressing used. Most wounds require numerous modifications as wound characteristics change.

This chapter reviewed the principles of topical wound management with an emphasis on maintaining a physiologic wound environment. Even when a physiologic wound environment is maintained, realistic and appropriate goals for the patient with a wound can be obtained only when causative factors are controlled or eliminated and systemic support of the patient is provided. Furthermore, understanding the principles of wound management prepares the wound specialist to partner within interdisciplinary teams, to articulate underlying rationale, and to use a research-based approach to provide cost-effective care to the patient with a wound.

REFERENCES

Andrews L: *Market for advanced wound care technologies*, BCC research report code PHM011C, November 2001, available at http://www.bccresearch.com/report/PHM011C.html, accessed December 10, 2009.

Armstrong DG, Jude EB: The role of matrix metalloproteinases in wound healing, *J Am Podiatr Med Assoc* 92(1):12, 2002.

Bale S et al: A comparison of two dressings in pressure sore management, *J Wound Care* 6(10):463-466, 1997.

Belmin J et al; Investigators of the Sequential Treatment of the Elderly with Pressure Sores (STEPS) Trial: Sequential treatment with calcium alginate dressings and hydrocolloid dressings accelerates pressure ulcer healing in older subjects: a multicenter randomized trial of sequential versus nonsequential treatment with hydrocolloid dressings alone, *J Am Geriatr Soc* 50(2):269-274, 2002.

Bisaga A et al: Prevalence study of methicillin-resistant *Staphylococcus aureus* colonization in emergency department health care workers, *Ann Emerg Med* 52(5):525-528, 2008.

Bouza C et al: Efficacy of advanced dressings in the treatment of pressure ulcers: a systematic review, *J Wound Care* 14(5):193-199, 2005.

Bradley M et al: Systematic reviews of wound care management: (2). Dressings and topical agents used in the healing of chronic wounds, *Health Technol Assess* 3(17 Pt 2):1-35, 1999.

Cullen B: The role of oxidized regenerated cellulose/collagen in chronic wound repair. Part 2, *Ostomy Wound Manage* 48(6 Suppl):8, 2002.

Diehm C, Lawall H: Evaluation of Tielle hydropolymer dressings in the management of chronic exuding wounds in primary care, *Int Wound J* 2(1):26-35, 2005.

Dykes PJ, Heggie R: The link between the peel force of adhesive dressings and subjective discomfort in volunteer subjects, *J Wound Care* 12(7):260-262, 2003.

Eisenbud D et al: Hydrogel wound dressings: where do we stand in 2003? *Ostomy Wound Manage* 49(10):52-57, 2003.

Flanagan M: Wound cleansing. In Morison M et al, editors: *Nursing management of chronic wounds*, ed 2, London, 1997, Mosby.

Graumlich JF et al: Healing pressure ulcers with collagen or hydrocolloid: a randomized controlled trial, *J Am Geriatr Soc* 51(2):147-154, 2003.

Hinman CD, Maibach H: Effect of air exposure and occlusion on experimental human skin wounds, *Nature* 200:377-378, 1963.

Hopf HW et al: Guidelines for the treatment of arterial insufficiency ulcers, *Wound Repair Regen* 14(6):693-710, 2006.

Johnston CP et al: Staphylococcus aureus colonization among healthcare workers at a tertiary care hospital, *Infect Control Hosp Epidemiol* 28:1404-1407, 2007.

Mustoe TA et al: International clinical recommendations on scar management, *Plast Reconstr Surg* 110(2):560-571, 2002.

National Pressure Ulcer Advisory Panel (NPUAP) and European Pressure ulcer Advisory Panel (EPUAP): *Prevention and treatment of pressure ulcers*, Washington, DC, 2009, National Pressure Ulcer Advisory Panel.

Nisi G et al: Use of a protease-modulating matrix in the treatment of pressure sores, *Chir Ital* 57(4):465-468, 2005.

Ohura N et al: Evaluating dressing materials for the prevention of shear force in the treatment of pressure ulcers, *J Wound Care* 14(9):401-404, 2005.

Ovington LG: Hanging wet-to-dry dressings out to dry, *Home Healthcare Nurse* 19:477-484, 2001.

Ovington LG: Overview of matrix metalloproteinase modulation and growth factor protection in wound healing. Part 1, *Ostomy Wound Manage* 48(6 Suppl):3, 2002.

Pieper, B: Honey-based dressings and wound care journal of wound ostomy & continence nursing, 36(6):589, November/December 2009.

Robson MC et al: Guidelines for the treatment of venous ulcers, *Wound Repair Regen* 14(6):649-662, 2006.

Schultz GS et al: Wound bed preparation: a systematic approach to wound management, *Wound Repair Regen* 11(s1):s1-s28, 2003.

Singh A et al: Meta-analysis of randomized controlled trials on hydrocolloid occlusive dressing versus conventional gauze dressing in the healing of chronic wounds, *Asian J Surg* 27(4):326-332, 2004.

Spruitt D: The water barrier and its repair. In Maebashi H, Rovee D, editors: *Epidermal wound healing*, Chicago, 1972, Yearbook Medical.

Steed DL et al: Guidelines for the treatment of diabetic ulcers, *Wound Repair Regen* 14(6):680-692, 2006.

Stotts NA et al: Sterile versus clean technique in postoperative wound care of patients with open surgical wounds: a pilot study, *J Wound Ostomy Continence Nurs* 24:10, 1997.

Varghese M et al: Local environment of chronic wounds under synthetic dressings, *Arch Dermatol* 122:52,1998.

Wenisch C et al: Mild intraoperative hypothermia reduces production of oxygen intermediates by polymorphonuclear leukocytes, *Anesth Analg* 82(4):810, 1996.

Whitney J et al: Guidelines for the treatment of pressure ulcers, *Wound Repair Regen* 14(6):663-679, 2006.

Winter GD: Formation of the scab and the rate of epithelization of superficial wounds in the skin of the young domestic pig, *Nature* 193(4812):293-294, 1962.

Wound, Ostomy and Continence Nurses (WOCN) Society: *Guideline for management of pressure ulcers*, WOCN clinical practice guideline series #2, Glenview, Ill., 2010, Author.

Wound, Ostomy Continence Nurses (WOCN) Society and the Association for Professionals in Infection Control and Epidemiology (APIC): *WOCN position statement. Clean versus sterile: management of chronic wounds*, 2010 available at http://www.wocn.org/pdfs/WOCN_Library/Position_Statements/clvst.pdf, accessed December 28, 2009.

Yastrub D: Relationship between type of treatment and degree of wound healing among institutionalized geriatric patients with Stage II pressure ulcers, *Care Manage J* 5(4):213-218, 2004.

SECTION V

Biophysical and Biologic Agents

19

Skin Substitutes and Extracellular Matrix Scaffolds

Susie Seaman

OBJECTIVES

1. Differentiate between cellular and acellular products for chronic wound care.
2. Define autologous, allogeneic, xenographic, biosynthetic, and synthetic with regard to skin substitutes and extracellular matrix (ECM) scaffolds.
3. Define cell therapy.
4. Compare and contrast three types of skin substitutes and the ECM scaffolds in terms of formulation, availability, and role in wound care.
5. Summarize future directions for cell-based therapies.
6. Describe the keys to success when using these products.
7. Describe two best-practice algorithms for the use of skin substitutes in the care of patients with venous leg ulcers and diabetic foot ulcers.

When the patient with a chronic wound has not responded to optimal care, including both systemic support and local wound management, use of advanced products, such as skin substitutes and extracellular matrix (ECM) scaffolds, may be indicated to promote wound healing and closure. The field of tissue engineering has advanced significantly in the last 2 decades to the point where wound care providers have multiple products from which to choose. These products are derived from human, various animal, and synthetic sources, and they may be cellular or acellular. Depending on the material used and how it is processed, wound healing may result in a traditionally expected scar, or it may actually lead to regenerated tissue, in which the original structure and function of the skin and underlying tissue are partially or completely restored (Badylak, 2007; van Winterswijk and Nout, 2007).

Products vary in the level of evidence supporting their ability to enhance wound healing beyond what can be achieved with standard care alone. Some products are considered to be devices equivalent to collagen-based dressings, which have a long history of safety in wound care but may lack efficacy data. This chapter reviews the various skin substitutes and ECM products, and summarizes those currently available for chronic wound care.

Skin substitutes and ECM scaffolds are adjuncts to excellent wound and patient care. The ultimate success in healing a challenging wound with these products depends on meticulous wound bed and patient preparation, including aggressive correction of the underlying wound etiology and comorbidities that affect healing. Checklist 19-1 lists key points to successful use of skin substitutes and ECM scaffolds.

CLASSIFICATION OF PRODUCTS

Skin substitutes and ECM products can be classified as *cellular* (i.e., containing living cells) or *acellular* (Clark et al, 2007; Shores et al, 2007). Cellular products are frequently referred to as *skin substitutes* and acellular products as *extracellular matrix (ECM) scaffolds*. These products may be autologous (derived from the patient's own body), allogeneic (derived from other humans, also called *homografts*), xenographic (derived from nonhuman sources, e.g., porcine, bovine, equine, avian, also called *heterografts*), biosynthetic (biological and manmade materials), or synthetic (man-made materials) (Ågren and Werthén, 2007; Shores et al, 2007). These products are available as sheets (which may have to be rehydrated), gels, or granules. Some products may retain native growth factors and other polypeptides, such as fibronectin, which promote cell migration and healing in normal wound repair. Processing of skin substitutes and ECM scaffolds will affect their function. For example, products that are engineered to resist degradation will more likely evoke a chronic inflammatory response and, while enhancing wound closure, will result in a scar. In contrast, products that provide controlled degradation while allowing infiltration of and replacement by host tissue have the potential to alter the body's natural default mechanism to form scar and instead may result in regeneration of tissue layers (Badylak, 2007). Tables 19-1, 19-2, and 19-3 provide examples, descriptions, and indications for known cellular and acellular products, including those that are not available in the United States. In the following sections, products that are available in the U.S. market are presented.

CELLULAR PRODUCTS

Cellular products used in chronic wound care consist of autologous or allogeneic keratinocytes and/or fibroblasts and the ECM proteins and growth factors produced by these cells. Most products consist of confluent cells cultured on various bioabsorbable matrices. They provide cell therapy, defined as "the administration of cells to the body to the benefit of the recipient" (Harris, 2008). Autologous cellular products are expected to "take" or survive. Allogeneic cell-based products, however, rapidly die and slough off (Griffiths et al, 2004; Metcalfe and Ferguson, 2007). The primary purpose of allogeneic products is to deliver healthy living cells to the wound,

where they secrete multiple growth factors and other ECM proteins that stimulate the host to proceed with wound repair. The majority of cellular products used in chronic wound care today are produced with allogeneic cells.

Cellular skin substitutes, most of which are living when applied to wounds, can be epidermal, dermal, or bilayered. Epidermal skin substitutes consist of keratinocytes; dermal skin substitutes contain fibroblasts that are embedded in a matrix; and bilayered skin substitutes have both keratinocytes and the matrix-embedded fibroblasts to form epidermal and dermal layers. Cellular skin substitutes do not contain various skin structures (e.g., blood vessels, hair follicles, sweat glands) or cells (e.g., melanocytes, Langerhans cells, macrophages, lymphocytes). Human neonatal foreskin is the common source for allogeneic cellular products. Both the donating neonate and its mother are thoroughly screened for infectious diseases prior to use in the manufacture of these products.

Epidermal Skin Substitutes

Epidermal skin substitutes are cultured keratinocytes taken as a biopsy either from the patient (autograft) or from another human (allograft) and then expanded and enlarged in a laboratory setting. They are manufactured as sheets, gels, sprays, and suspensions, although only cultured epidermal autograft sheets are currently available in the U.S.

One of the first skin substitutes on the market is *Epicel* (Genzyme, Cambridge, Mass., USA), a cultured epidermal autograft which is indicated for patients with deep dermal to full-thickness burns affecting 30% or greater total body surface area. Epicel is not used in chronic wound care. The main advantage of Epicel in burn care is the ability to cover large wounds with permanent skin that will not be rejected because the graft is autologous (Kamolz, 2008). Enough skin to cover the patient's entire body can be ready within 4 weeks. Disadvantages to Epicel include the 2-3 week wait for product availability and its fragility. It is only 2-8 cells thick so can be difficult to handle and apply. It also lacks long-term strength which can lead to spontaneous blistering months after grafting (Woodley et al, 1998). Table 19-1 lists other epidermal skin substitutes that are not yet available in the United States.

Dermal Skin Substitutes

Dermal substitutes contain fibroblasts seeded and cultured on a bioabsorbable matrix, along with the ECM proteins and growth factors that they produce. They may be delivered fresh or cryopreserved, although only the latter is available in the U.S.

Dermagraft (Advanced Biohealing, Westport, Conn., USA) is a cryopreserved allogeneic dermal substitute

TABLE 19-1	Epidermal Skin Substitutes	
Product	**Manufacturer**	**Description**
Epicel	Genzyme (Cambridge, MA, USA)	Cultured from autologous keratinocytes obtained from skin biopsy of patient. Delivered as 30-cm² sheets, attached to a petrolatum gauze backing.
Laserskin*	Fidia Advanced Polymers (Abano Terme, Italy)	Sheet of esterified hyaluronic acid with laser-created perforations seeded with autologous keratinocytes.
Keragraf*	Healthpoint (Fort Worth, Tex., USA)	Cultured from autologous adult stem and precursor cells derived from hair plucked from the patient.
Myskin*	Altrika (Sheffield, United Kingdom)	Autologous keratinocytes cultured on silicone sheet with specially formulated surface coating that allows for growth of applied cells. Silicone removed from wound after 1week. New Myskin is applied weekly if needed.
CellSpray*	Avita Medical (Cambridge, United Kingdom)	Autologous preconfluent keratinocytes in suspension, sprayed on wound. Requires small biopsy. Suspension ready in 5 days.
CellSpray XP*	Avita Medical	Autologous preconfluent keratinocytes in suspension, sprayed on wound. Requires larger biopsy. Suspension ready in 2 days.
Bioseed-S*	BioTissue, (Freiberg, Germany)	Autologous keratinocytes suspended in thrombin solution with fibrin sealant. Packaged in syringe. Has shown efficacy in study of 225 patients with venous ulcers (Vanscheidt et al, 2007).
Cultured epidermal allografts*	Various; not all commercially available yet	Allogeneic keratinocytes cryopreserved sheets, lyophilized (freeze-dried) sheets, gels, sprays, and suspensions. Studied in leg ulcer care. (Beele et al, 2005; Horch et al, 2005; Navrátilová et al, 2004.)

*Currently not available in the United States.

with fibroblasts seeded on a bioabsorbable polyglactin mesh (Roberts and Mansbridge, 2002). Once thawed at the bedside in an easy step-by-step process, a 5- × 7.5-cm living dermal substitute can be applied onto clean, debrided wounds that are free of infection.

Dermagraft has demonstrated efficacy in the treatment of patients with diabetic foot ulcers (Gentzkow et al, 1999; Pollak et al, 1997). In a randomized controlled trial of 314 patients with diabetic foot ulcers of over 6 week's duration, 30% of Dermagraft-treated patients were healed at 12 weeks versus 18.3% in the control group *(p* = .023) (Marston et al, 2003). Dermagraft is approved by the U.S. Food and Drug Administration (FDA) for the treatment of full-thickness diabetic foot ulcers of greater than 6 weeks duration which extend through the dermis, and are without tendon, muscle, joint capsule or bone exposure. It is also recommended for use in the treatment of nonhealing diabetic foot ulcers by the Wound Healing Society (Steed et al, 2006).

Dermagraft must be used only as an adjunct to standard care, which includes off-weighting the ulcer, debridement, treatment of infection, glucose control, and assurance of adequate blood flow for healing. Optimal healing rates are associated with aggressive offloading, not only with footwear but also with crutches or wheelchairs. Dermagraft is applied with either side toward the wound bed and is covered with a nonadherent contact layer. To ensure good contact of Dermagraft with the wound bed, the wound should be lightly filled with saline-moistened gauze or a soft foam dressing. Although Dermagraft was applied weekly for up to 8 weeks in clinical trials, this frequent application should not be

necessary with most patients. The best-practice algorithms published for Apligraf (Figures 19-1 and 19-2) provide excellent guidelines for the use of any skin substitute in the clinical setting (Cavorsi et al, 2006).

Bilayered Skin Substitutes

Apligraf (Organogenesis, Canton, Mass., USA) is a living allogeneic bilayered skin substitute consisting of keratinocytes and fibroblasts. Fibroblasts are cultured in a type 1 bovine collagen gel. Keratinocytes are then seeded on this gel, cultured, and air exposed to stimulate differentiation into the layers of the epidermis, including the stratum corneum. This process results in a 44-cm², 0.75-mm-thick skin substitute delivered fresh on a Petri dish containing nutrient medium, and sealed in an airtight bag.

Apligraf, when used in conjunction with compression therapy, has been demonstrated to achieve closure of hard-to-heal venous ulcers at a significantly higher rate than seen with compression alone (Falanga and Sabolinski, 1999; Falanga et al, 1998). Apligraf is FDA-approved for the treatment of venous ulcers of greater than 1 month duration that have not adequately responded to standard care, including debridement, infection control, assurance of adequate arterial flow, and compression therapy. National guidelines support the use of bi-layered skin substitutes in conjunction with compression bandaging to improve healing rates of venous ulcers (Robson et al, 2006).

Apligraf has also demonstrated efficacy in the treatment of diabetic foot ulcers. In a trial of 208 patients with diabetic neuropathic foot ulcers, Veves et al (2001)

Text continues on page 316

TABLE 19-2	Dermal and Bilayered Skin Substitutes				
Category	**Trade Name**	**Description**	**Indications**	**References**	**Available in United States?**
Allogeneic Dermal	Dermagraft (Advanced Biohealing, Westport, CT, USA)	Fibroblasts seeded and cultured on bioabsorbable mesh, then cryopreserved; delivered on dry ice. 5 x 7.5 cm. Apply to either side of wound.	Nonhealing full-thickness diabetic foot ulcers >6 weeks duration, extending through dermis, but without tendon, muscle, joint, or bone exposure.	Multiple RCTs. Roberts and Mansbridge, 2002; Pollak et al, 1997; Gentzkow et al, 1999; Marston et al, 2003.	Yes
Allogeneic Dermal	CDS (Cultured Dermal Substitute) (Kitasato University, Japan)	Fibroblasts seeded onto two-layered sponge of lyophilized hyaluronic acid and bovine collagen, then cryopreserved.	Arterial and venous ulcers and various other chronic wounds.	Case studies and case series. No RCTs in chronic wounds. Hasegawa et al, 2007; Yonezawa et al, 2007.	No
Allogeneic Bilayered	Apligraf (Organogenesis, Canton, MA, USA)	Fibroblasts mixed with bovine collagen gel and cultured. Keratinocytes seeded and cultured on gel. 44 cm². Delivered fresh. Apply dermal side toward wound.	Venous ulcers over 1-month duration. Full-thickness diabetic neuropathic foot ulcers >3 weeks duration but without tendon, muscle, capsule, or bone exposure.	Multiple RCTs. Falanga et al, 1998; Falanga and Sabolinski, 1999; Veves et al, 2001.	Yes
Allogeneic Bilayered	OrCel (Forticell Bioscience, New York, NY, USA)	Fibroblasts seeded on porous side of bovine collagen sponge; keratinocytes seeded on nonporous side. Has been used fresh or cryopreserved.	Donor sites in burn patients, surgical wounds and donor sites in patients with epidermolysis bullosa.	Case series. RCTs in diabetic foot ulcer and venous ulcer (latter not published). Eisenberg and Llewelyn, 1998; Still et al, 2003; Lipkin et al, 2003.	No Cryopreserved version for venous ulcers under review at FDA (unpublished data, M. Silberklang, personal communication, March 2009).
Autologous Dermal	Hyalograft 3D (Fidia Advanced Biopolymers, Abano Terme, Italy)	Fibroblasts obtained from skin biopsy of patient seeded and cultured on matrix of esterified hyaluronic acid. Ready 8 days after seeding. Epidermal product, Laserskin (see Table 19-1), can be applied 7-10 days after Hyalograff 3D.	Used in Europe for many years on various chronic wounds.	Cases series and one small RCT in diabetic foot ulcers. Uccioli, 2003; Caravaggi et al, 2003; Lobmann et al, 2003.	No
Cadaver skin	GammaGraft (Promethean LifeSciences, Pittsburgh, PA, USA)	Gamma-irradiated human cadaver skin. Stored at room temperature up to 2 years. May stay in place until wound heals if it remains adherent to wound bed. Left in place while new host skin grows in under dressing. Gradually dries out and edges peel away.	Chronic wounds and burns.	Case reports only. No RCTs on use with chronic wounds. Kagan et al, 2005; Britton-Byrd et al, 2008; Humphries and Mansavage, 2006; Rosales et al, 2003.	Yes
Cadaver skin	TheraSkin (Soluble Systems, Newport News, VA, USA)	Cryopreserved human cadaver skin. Delivered on dry ice. Available in 2 sizes and meshed.	Chronic wounds and burns.	No published studies.	To be launched in 2010.

RCT, Randomized controlled trial.

TABLE 19-3	Acellular ECM Scaffolds			
Category	Trade Name	Description	Indications	References	Available in United States?
Allogeneic	AlloDerm (LifeCell, Branchburg, NJ, USA)	Derived from cadaveric human skin from tissue banks. Epidermis and all cellular components removed, leaving dermal matrix. Freeze-dried; rehydrate to use. Contains intact collagen fibers to support ingrowth of new tissue, elastin filaments to provide strength, and hyaluronan and proteoglycans for cell attachment and migration.	Burns, traumatic or oncologic wounds with deep structure exposure, hernia repair, breast and other tissue reconstruction.	Small RCTs, case series or reports in variety of wounds, but no RCTs in chronic wound care. Wainwright et al, 1996; Munster et al, 2001; Bastidas et al, 2009; Misra et al, 2008; Candage et al, 2008; Patton et al, 2007; Bindingnavele et al, 2007; Topol et al, 2008.	Yes
Allogeneic	Cymetra (LifeCell)	Injectable micronized particulate form of AlloDerm. Dry form, packaged in syringe, rehydrated prior to use with either normal saline or lidocaine for injection.	Cosmetic soft tissue augmentation and treatment of vocal cord paralysis by injection laryngoplasty.	Case reports and case series in chronic wound care. No RCTs. Levy et al, 2004; Banta et al, 2003; Allam, 2007.	Yes
Allogeneic	GraftJacket Regenerative Tissue Matrix (Wright Medical Technology, Arlington, TN, USA)	Same as Alloderm, but meshed 1:1 to allow wound exudate to pass through. Available in two sizes (4 × 4 cm and 4 × 8 cm) and one thickness (0.4–0.8 mm) for chronic wound care. Available nonmeshed and thicker for tendon and ligament repair.	Diabetic foot ulcers and other chronic wounds, ligament and tendon repair.	Small to medium sized RCTs and case series in diabetic foot ulcers. Brigido et al, 2004; Brigido, 2006; Martin et al, 2005; Winters et al, 2008; Reyzelman et al, 2009.	Yes
Allogeneic	GraftJacket Xpress (Wright Medical Technology)	Same as Cymetra. Available in a pre-filled 5-cc syringe. Once rehydrated, is injected to fill the entire dead space of a sinus tract or deep wound.	Deep wounds, tunnels or sinus tracts.	No RCTs for chronic wounds.	Yes
Allogeneic	DermaMatrix (Synthes CMF, West Chester, PA, USA)	Cadaver human skin from tissue banks. Donor skin is processed to remove all cellular components, including epidermis, and then is freeze-dried. Rehydrate to use.	Similar to indications for AlloDerm: soft tissue repair, breast reconstruction, abdominal hernia repair, head and neck reconstruction.	No RCT's in chronic wound care. No differences when compared to Alloderm in small study of breast reconstruction (Becker et al, 2009).	Yes
Allogeneic	Amniotic membrane in many forms used Biovance (Celgene Cellular Therapeutics, Summit, NJ, USA) is decellularized and lyophilized	From human placenta. Has been used fresh, frozen, lyophilized (freeze-dried) and gamma irradiated. May be decellularized. Fresh sample may have cells present.	Reported uses in burn care, skin graft donor sites, pressure ulcers, venous ulcers, diabetic foot ulcers.	Case series and case studies, no RCTs. Kesting et al, 2008; Mermet et al, 2007; Gajiwala et al, 2004; Letendre et al, 2009.	No

Xenographic Porcine	Oasis Wound Matrix (Healthpoint, Fort Worth, TX, USA)	Porcine small intestinal submucosa (SIS) with complex matrix of collagen, glycosaminoglycans, proteoglycans, cell adhesive glycoproteins, and growth factors. Freeze-dried. Available multiple sizes, fenestrated, or meshed.	Partial- and full-thickness wounds, chronic ulcers, traumatic wounds, superficial and second-degree burns, surgical wounds.	Numerous animal studies and case series in many applications. Two RCTs in chronic wounds. Hodde et al, 2005; Badylak, 2007; Mostow et al, 2005; Niezgoda et al, 2005.	Yes
Xenographic Porcine	MatriStem (Medline Industries, Mundelein, IL, USA)	Derived from porcine urinary bladder matrix (UBM) with intact basement membrane. Composed of collagen matrix, glycosaminoglycans, glycoproteins, and proteoglycans. Available as fenestrated sheets of variable sizes or as powder. Must be rehydrated prior to use and cut to size of wound.	Partial- and full-thickness wounds, traumatic wounds, surgical wounds, chronic wounds.	Animal studies, but no RCTs. Nieponice et al, 2006; Gilbert et al, 2008	Yes
Xenographic Equine	Unite Biomatrix (Synovis Orthopedic and Woundcare, Irvine, CA, USA)	Derived from decellularized equine pericardium. Available fenestrated, in three sizes. Must be rehydrated. Apply 2-4 mm larger than wound and staple in place.	Partial- and full thickness wounds, chronic wounds, traumatic wounds, surgical wounds.	Case studies and case series. No RCTs. Nataraj et al, 2007; Mulder et al, 2009a, 2009b, 2009c.	Yes
Xenographic Bovine	PriMatrix (TEI Biosciences, Boston, MA, USA)	Derived from fetal bovine dermis, which has been decellularized, freeze-dried, and sterilized. Must be rehydrated. Available nonfenestrated in various sizes and thicknesses. Must fenestrate for high exudating wounds.	Skin ulcers, second-degree burns, surgical wounds.	No published studies.	Yes
Xenographic Porcine	Mediskin and E-Z Derm (Brennan Medical, St. Paul, MN, USA)	Porcine skin with epidermis and dermis. Mediskin is frozen and irradiated, with shelf life of 24 months; stored in a standard freezer. E-Z Derm is chemically cross-linked for durability; stored at room temperature up to 18 months. Both are available in multiple sizes, perforated or nonperforated.	Temporary coverage of burns, surgical wounds, partial- and full-thickness wounds of variable etiologies.	Many small studies and case reports, mainly in burn care. No large RCTs in chronic wound care. Davis and Arpey, 2000.	Yes
Xenographic Porcine	Xelma (Mölnlycke, Göteborg, Sweden)	Consists of amelogenin proteins derived from the enamel matrix of developing porcine teeth, mixed with propylene glycol alginate and water. Administered as a gel. Promotes cell migration via ECM and cell adhesion properties.	Used in Europe for the treatment of venous ulcers, diabetic foot ulcers and pressure ulcers.	RCTs in venous ulcers. Vowden et al, 2006, 2007; Romanelli et al, 2008a, 2008b; Hoang et al 2002; Esposito et al, 2005.	No

Continued

TABLE 19-3	Acellular ECM Scaffolds—cont'd			
Category	Trade Name	Description	Indications	References	Available in United States?
Xenographic Bovine	MatriDerm (Dr. Suwelack Skin & Health Care, Billerbeck, Germany)	Engineered three-dimensional matrix consisting of native structured collagen from bovine dermis, and elastin from bovine nuchal ligament. Available in three sizes with 1 or 2 mm thickness, based on grafting needs of wound.	Burns, surgical reconstruction of soft tissue defects.	Case series in burn care and reconstruction. No RCTs. Ryssel et al, 2008; Haslik et al, 2010; Ryssel et al 2010.	No
Xenographic Porcine	E-Matrix (Pioneer Surgical, Marquette, MI, USA)	Injectable mixture of gelatin derived from porcine collagen and high-molecular-weight dextran. Injected around wound edges and under wound base at dermal–subdermal junction. Up-regulates gene expression in host cells which may result in increased growth factor production and tissue regeneration similar to fetal healing.	Studied in diabetic foot ulcers.	One case series published. Young, 2007; Marston et al, 2005.	No
Biosynthetic	*Biobrane* (UDL Laboratories, Sugar Land, TX, USA)	Very thin sheet of semipermeable silicone bonded to a knitted trifilament nylon fabric. Nylon coated with type 1 porcine collagen, which creates hydrophilic coating that facilitates adherence to wound. Silicone membrane has water vapor loss rate similar to that of intact skin; once Biobrane has adhered to a wound, it provides moist, protected environment that minimizes water loss.	Partial-thickness burns, skin graft donor sites, superficial wounds after surgery, laser resurfacing, dermabrasion. Lesions secondary to toxic epidermal necrolysis and pemphigus, as coverage for chronic wounds.	Strong data for burn care. Case reports for other uses. No RCTs in chronic wound care. Whitaker et al, 2008; Mandal, 2007.	Yes
Biosynthetic	Biobrane-L (UDL Laboratories)	Same as Biobrane, except monofilament nylon is used instead of knitted trifilament nylon, which renders it less adherent to wound bed.	Indicated where less adherence is desired (e.g., over meshed autografts).	Same as above.	Yes
Biosynthetic	TransCyte (previously named Dermagraft-TC; Advanced Biohealing, Westport, CT, USA)	Nylon mesh coated with porcine dermal collagen, bonded to semipermeable silicone membrane, and seeded with human fibroblasts, which secrete ECM proteins and growth factors. Product is frozen, killing fibroblasts; matrix and growth factors are preserved. Silicone layer functions as synthetic epidermis. Procedure for use similar to Biobrane.	Debrided full-thickness and deep partial-thickness burns that require temporary coverage prior to autografting. Primary treatment of superficial burns (remains in place until host reepithelialization occurs).	RCTs in burn care. No RCTs in chronic wound care. Purdue et al, 1997; Noordenbos et al, 1999; Kumar et al, 2004.	No

Biosynthetic	Integra Dermal Regeneration Template (IDRT) (Integra Life Sciences, Plainsboro, NJ, USA)	Bilayered product composed of outer semipermeable silicone sheet (functions as epidermal substitute) and inner ECM scaffold containing bovine cross-linked collagen and chondroitin-6-sulfate. Inner layer facilitates cell migration and tissue ingrowth, which leads to formation of neodermis, usually within 2–3 weeks of application. As neodermis is formed, ECM matrix degrades. Silicone covering is then removed.	Deep partial- or full-thickness burns, contracture release procedures, reconstructive surgery of complex wounds and surgical defects.	Multiple case reports and case studies in many acute wounds. Small RCT in burns. No RCTs in chronic wound care. Branski et al, 2007; Lee et al, 2008; Heimbach et al, 2003; Frame et al, 2004; Groos et al, 2005; Muangman et al, 2006; Tufaro et al, 2007; Helgeson et al, 2007; Silverstein, 2006.	Yes
Biosynthetic	Integra Bilayer Matrix Wound Dressing (BMWD) (Integra Life Sciences)	Same product as IDRT but repackaged for chronic wound care. Available meshed or unmeshed in multiple sizes.	Chronic wounds of various etiologies, surgical wounds, traumatic wound, can be placed over deep structures.	Same as above. No RCTs in chronic wound care.	Yes
Biosynthetic	Integra Matrix Wound Dressing (Integra Life Sciences)	The ECM scaffold of the BMWD without silicone membrane. Can be used alone or with BMWD for deeper wounds (Matrix Wound Dressing first, then covered with BMWD).	Same indications as BMWD.	Same as above	Yes
Biosynthetic	Integra Flowable Wound Matrix (Integra Life Sciences)	Same ingredients (minus silicone layer) as other Integra products. ECM matrix is provided in syringe as dry granules that are rehydrated with saline prior to one-time use. Injected directly into wound until filled.	Same indications as BMWD but use focuses on application to wounds with deep tunnels or undermining.	No published studies on Integra Flowable Wound Matrix in chronic wound care.	Yes
Synthetic	Hyalomatrix PA (Fidia Advanced Biopolymers, Abano Terme, Italy)	Bilayered with thin moisture vapor permeable silicone sheet adhered to nonwoven pad composed of the benzyl ester of hyaluronic acid (Hyaff 11). Provides matrix for cell migration while silicone maintains protected moist environment.	Most chronic wounds, partial- and full-thickness burns, surgical wounds, traumatic wounds. Widely used in Europe.	Large case series, but no RCTs. Price et al, 2006; Gravante et al, 2007; Caravaggi et al, 2009.	Received 510K clearance by FDA in 2007 but not yet marketed in United States.
Synthetic	Suprathel (PolyMedics Innovations, Denkendorf, Germany)	Synthetic epidermal substitute composed of copolymer of polylactide, trimethylene carbonate and e-caprolactone. Completely dissolves within 4 weeks.	Used in Germany since 2004 for deep partial-thickness burns, superficial full-thickness burns, skin graft donor sites, abrasions, scar revision.	RCTs in burns and donor sites; no RCTs in chronic wound care. Schwarze et al, 2007, 2008.	Has received FDA approval, but not available yet.

ECM, Extracellular matrix; *RCT*, randomized controlled trial.

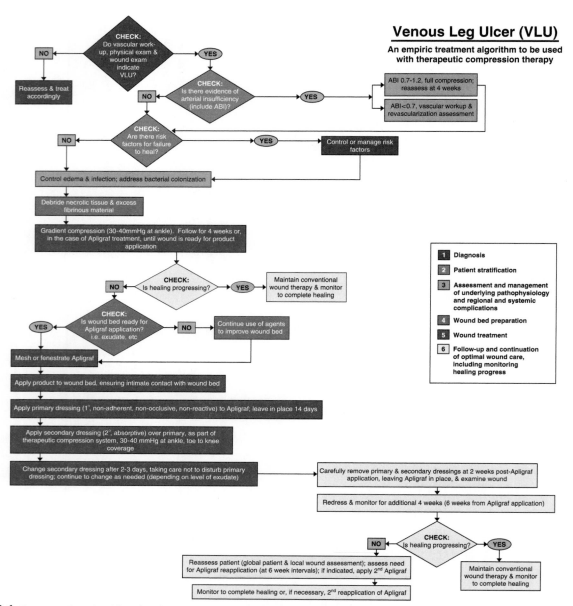

FIGURE 19-1 Best practice algorithm for the use of Apligraf® in the treatment of venous leg ulcers. (From Cavorsi J et al: Best-practice algorithms for the use of a bilayered living cell therapy (Apligraf®) in the treatment of lower-extremity ulcers, *Wound Rep Regen* 14:102-109, 2006.)

found that 56% of patients treated with Apligraf were healed at 12 weeks versus 38% in the control group *(p = .0042)*. Apligraf is FDA-approved for the treatment of diabetic neuropathic foot ulcers of at least 3 weeks duration that extend through the dermis without tendon, muscle, joint capsule, or bone exposure and which have not adequately responded to standard care, including debridement, infection control, glucose control, offweighting, and assurance of adequate arterial flow.

Like Dermagraft, Apligraf is an adjunct to standard wound care. Apligraf is applied to the wound with the dermal side contacting the wound bed. Many clinicians fenestrate Apligraf with a scalpel prior to application to allow exudate to pass through it onto bandages because pooled exudate under the product

may decrease its efficacy. Once applied, it should be anchored with Steri-strips, staples, or skin adhesive. Apligraf should be covered with a nonadherent contact layer and a secondary bandage of choice. Foam dressings work well over venous ulcers because they absorb exudate and apply local pressure under the compression wrap to keep the Apligraf in good contact with the wound bed. Secondary dressings are changed as needed based on the amount of exudate, but the contact layer over the Apligraf should not be disturbed for at least 2 weeks. Any wound cleansing over the ensuing few weeks should be very gentle so as not to disturb any lingering allogeneic cells. Figures 19-1 and 19-2 give algorithms for the use of Apligraf in the clinical setting.

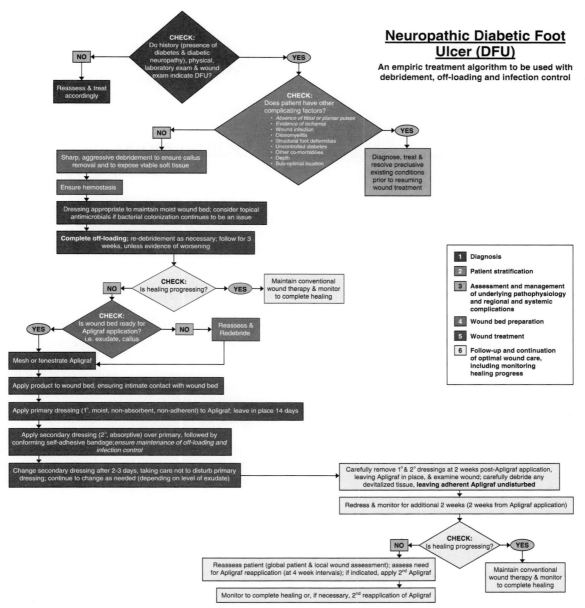

FIGURE 19-2 Best practice algorithm for the use of Apligraf® in the treatment of diabetic foot ulcers. *ABI*, Ankle-brachial index. (From Cavorsi J et al: Best-practice algorithms for the use of a bilayered living cell therapy (Apligraf®) in the treatment of lower-extremity ulcers, *Wound Rep Regen* 14:102-109, 2006.)

OrCel (Forticell Bioscience, New York, NY, USA) is a bilayered allogeneic product first developed by an Australian physician in the 1980s to treat his son, who suffered from epidermolysis bullosa. Outcomes were improved when OrCel was used in combination with split-thickness autografts in the surgical reconstruction of children with epidermolysis bullosa–related hand contractures and syndactyly (Eisenberg and Llewelyn, 1998). In 2001, the FDA approved the fresh version of OrCel under a humanitarian device exemption (HDE) for the treatment of surgical wounds and donor sites in patients with epidermolysis bullosa undergoing reconstructive hand surgery. Cryopreserved OrCel was later approved with an HDE for the same indication. In a

study of split-thickness autograft donor site treatment in burn patients, donor sites treated with Orcel healed an average of 7 days faster versus treatment with Biobrane-L *(p* < .0006) and were ready for recropping for more autografts an average of 5 days faster (Still et al, 2003). The fresh version of OrCel was FDA approved for the treatment of donor sites in burn patients in 2001. Cryopreserved OrCel has been studied in venous ulcer treatment (unpublished) and FDA approval for this indication is pending. Neither version of Orcel is currently available.

Cadaveric human skin has been used for years as temporary wound coverage in burn care (Britton-Byrd et al, 2008; Kagan et al, 2005). This nonliving product facilitates the short-term coverage of large tissue defects when autografts are not yet available, leading to reduced loss of fluid, electrolytes, and protein, decreased risk of infection, decreased wound desiccation and pain, and improved success of later autografting. One disadvantage of using cadaveric skin is the possibility of disease transmission, despite donor screening regulations by the FDA and quality control standards developed by the American Association of Tissue Banks (AATB) (Humphries and Mansavage, 2006). Another disadvantage is the fact that cadaveric skin is rejected by the host within 2 to 4 weeks. Cadaveric human skin is available fresh (used within 14 days of harvesting), cryopreserved (stored in a freezer for 3–6 months or in liquid nitrogen for up to 10 years), or irradiated (stored at room temperature).

GammaGraft (Promethean LifeSciences, Pittsburgh, Penn., USA) is gamma-irradiated human cadaver skin that provides wound coverage for chronic wounds or burns. It can remain in place until the wound is healed, depending on wound size and depth of tissue damage. GammaGraft is placed on a clean, debrided wound that is free of infection and is covered with a nonadherent dressing for 1 to 2 days. At that time, the graft should be adhered to the wound base. If the graft is not adherent, the wound may be infected, and the graft should be removed. If GammaGraft is adherent, it should be left uncovered; it will dry out and appear much like a scab. It is left in place while new host skin covers the wound underneath. As the wound heals, the edges of the GammaGraft will peel away and can be cut off. Treatment of the underlying problem, such as compression for edema or off-weighting for pressure redistribution, must be continued throughout the treatment period. Gamma-Graft may be used on any chronic wound. However, although there are case reports of GammaGraft use in chronic wounds (Rosales et al, 2003), no randomized controlled trials have demonstrated the efficacy of this product in wound healing compared to standard care.

Additional products for providing cell therapy in the treatment of chronic wounds are in development (Ehrenreich and Ruszczak, 2006; Hrabchak et al, 2006). Next-generation products may extend beyond the relative simplicity of providing keratinocytes and/or fibroblasts with their secreted growth factors and ECM proteins to a chronic wound. Melanocytes for repigmentation, endothelial cells for neovascularization, stem cells for regeneration of tissue all may be included in future products. Genetically engineered cells may be used that express specific growth factors to stimulate a particular aspect of wound healing (e.g., neovascularization) identified to be deficient in an individual patient. "Smart" skin substitutes may be developed in which genetically engineered cells respond to the wound environment by secreting or restricting secretion of certain cytokines, depending on what the wound requires to progress through repair, or better yet, regeneration (Metcalfe and

Ferguson, 2007). Cells can be engineered to secrete increased levels of natural bactericidal chemicals to decrease risk of infection (Schurr et al, 2009). As these products become available, clinicians must critically analyze data to ensure that the use of these products enhances healing while reducing complications compared with standard care.

ACELLULAR PRODUCTS

Whereas cellular products are derived from either autologous or allogeneic sources, acellular products, which are nonliving, are produced from allogeneic, xenographic, biosynthetic, or synthetic materials. Most acellular products are commonly referred to as *ECM scaffolds*. However, some products, especially those with synthetic epidermal components, are considered to be *skin substitutes* or combinations of an ECM scaffold with a synthetic epidermal layer (see Table 19-3). The goal in using ECM scaffolds in chronic wound care is to promote rapid healing while minimizing scar tissue formation. The ideal ECM scaffold provides for host cell attachment and migration of keratinocytes, fibroblasts, endothelial cells, and other cells involved in wound healing. Depending on the signaling that occurs in response to the type of ECM scaffold used, marrow-derived stem cells may be recruited to the area, differentiating into various cell types that manufacture original host tissue instead of scar (Clark et al, 2007). Angiogenesis and neovascularization occur, and, as the implanted scaffold is infiltrated by new host tissue, the scaffold undergoes controlled degradation. Products such as collagen-based dressings, which degrade almost immediately, do not last long enough to function as a scaffold for cell ingrowth. Products that have been altered to withstand degradation to the point that they persist for many months may elicit a chronic inflammatory response, which results in scar tissue formation (Badylak, 2007). Although the goal in the use of ECM scaffolds is the regeneration of normal tissue, most products available today result in varying degrees of regenerated and repaired (scarred) tissue.

The products presented here are used primarily for wound management. However, multiple acellular products, both allogeneic and xenographic, are used for surgical indications such as hernia repair, breast reconstruction, and other reconstructive surgeries (Table 19-4).

Allogeneic ECM Scaffolds

AlloDerm (LifeCell, Branchburg, NJ, USA) is an acellular dermal matrix derived from cadaveric human skin. It has a distinct basement membrane side and a dermal side. AlloDerm is available in multiple sizes and thicknesses. The orientation of AlloDerm into a defect and the thickness used depend on what is being treated (e.g., hernia vs soft tissue defect); therefore the package insert

TABLE 19-4	Acellular Products Used in Tissue Reconstruction and Hernia Repair
Product	**Manufacturer**
Acellular Human Dermis	
AlloDerm	LifeCell (Branchburg, NJ, USA)
Bard AlloMax Surgical Graft	Davol (Cranston, RI, USA)
DermaMatrix Acellular Dermis	Synthes CMF (West Chester, PA, USA)
FlexHD Acellular Hydrated Dermis	Ethicon (Piscataway, NJ, USA)
Acellular Porcine Dermis	
Bard CollaMend Implant	Davol
Permacol Biologic Implant	Covidien (Mansfield, MA, USA)
Strattice	LifeCell
XenMatrix	Brennen Medical (St. Paul, MN, USA)
Porcine Small Intestinal Submucosa	
Surgisis Soft Tissue Graft	Cook Biotech (West Lafayette, IN, USA)
Surgisis ES Soft Tissue Graft	Cook Biotech
Surgisis Gold Hernia Repair Graft	Cook Biotech
Surgisis IHM Inguinal Hernia Matrix	Cook Biotech
Acellular Bovine Fetal Dermis	
SurgiMend	TEI Biosciences (Boston, MA, USA)
Bovine Pericardium	
Tutopatch	RTI Biologics (Alachua, FL, USA)
Veritas Collagen Matrix	Synovis (St. Paul, MN, USA)

should be checked for application instructions. AlloDerm has been studied for treatment of multiple surgical defects and wound repair procedures. No randomized controlled trials have examined the use of AlloDerm in chronic wound care.

Cymetra (LifeCell) is an injectable, micronized particulate form of AlloDerm. Only case reports and case series on the use of Cymetra in chronic wounds unresponsive to conventional therapy have been published. Although these cases are interesting and appear to indicate that Cymetra stimulates healing in chronic ulcers, no randomized controlled trials have compared this product to standard care in the treatment of chronic wounds. Therefore no strong conclusions regarding its efficacy can be made.

GraftJacket regenerative tissue matrix (Wright Medical Technology, Arlington, Tenn., USA) is essentially the same product as AlloDerm. Unlike AlloDerm, GraftJacket is meshed and is available in only two sizes and one thickness for chronic wound care. GraftJacket is applied to clean, debrided ulcers with the dermal reticular side against the wound bed. It should cover the entire wound and be sutured or stapled in place. GraftJacket

must be kept moist with mineral oil–soaked gauze packing, which is used to ensure that the product does not dry out and maintains good contact with the wound base. The dressing is left in place for 5 days without being disturbed and then changed every 3 to 5 days after that. Two small pilot studies have demonstrated enhanced healing of diabetic foot ulcers compared to control (Brigido et al, 2004; Brigido, 2006). A study of 86 patients with diabetic foot ulcers demonstrated complete healing at 12 weeks in 67% of patients treated with GraftJacket versus 46% in the control group ($p = .03$) (Reyzelman et al, 2009).

GraftJacket Xpress (Wright Medical Technology) is essentially the same product as Cymetra. It is processed by LifeCell for Wright Medical and is marketed for the treatment of wounds with depth. The cover dressing should maintain a moist environment and apply gentle pressure to keep the matrix in place. It should be left in place for 3 to 5 days and then changed as needed to manage exudate. No randomized controlled trials have examined the use of GraftJacket Xpress in the treatment of chronic wounds.

Xenographic ECM Scaffolds

Oasis Wound Matrix (Healthpoint, Fort Worth, Tex., USA) is derived from porcine small intestinal submucosa (SIS). It has been examined in numerous preclinical studies, in the clinical treatment of soft tissue defects, wounds, and hernias, and in urologic, gynecologic, and orthopedic reconstructive surgeries (Badylak, 2007; Cook Biotech, 2010; Hodde et al, 2005). In a prospective randomized controlled trial, 55% of 120 patients with venous ulcers healed at 12 weeks compared to 34% in the control group ($p < .02$) (Mostow et al, 2005). In clinical practice, Oasis should be applied to clean, debrided wounds that are free of infection, cut slightly larger than the wound, secured with Steri-strips, glue, staples, or sutures, and then moistened with normal saline. A nonadherent contact layer is then applied, and the cover dressing is based on the amount of exudate. Foam dressings work well to absorb exudate and provide local compression to maintain good contact of the Oasis to the wound bed. Secondary dressings may be changed as needed, but any remnants of the Oasis, which may appear as an amber gelatinous material in the wound, should be left undisturbed. Additional Oasis can be reapplied weekly as needed.

MatriStem (Medline Industries, Mundelein, IL., USA) is derived from porcine urinary bladder. There are no published studies of the use of MatriStem in chronic wound care. While animal studies indicate potential for this product to stimulate tissue regeneration (Gilbert et al, 2008; Nieponice et al, 2006), clinical trials in chronic wounds are needed to establish efficacy. It may be used in the clinical setting in the same fashion as Oasis.

Unite Biomatrix (Synovis Orthopedic and Woundcare, Irvine, Calif., USA) is derived from decellularized equine pericardium. It is re-hydrated and cut 2 to 4 mm larger than the wound size so that it will slightly overlap the edges and then is secured with the clinician's method of choice. Stapling the product in place is ideal. A nonadherent contact layer should then be applied, covered with a gauze bolster or foam dressing to ensure good contact of the product with the wound bed. Mineral oil should not be used to moisten this product. Silver dressings can be used to decrease bacterial counts. The initial cover dressing should be left undisturbed for 5 days, and then subsequent dressings can be changed every 3 to 7 days as needed. If exudate is low, the outer aspect of Unite Biomatrix may dry out, but the product will maintain a moist interface at the wound surface. Unite Biomatrix should not be removed from the wound; the edges can be trimmed as they lift. There are case reports and case series on the use of this product in multiple types of chronic wounds (Mulder and Lee a-c, 2009), but no randomized controlled trials have been published.

PriMatrix (TEI Biosciences, Boston, Mass., USA) is derived from fetal bovine dermis and is processed to preserve the natural structure and biologic properties of its native collagen. It should be applied with either side down to clean, debrided wounds, with a 1-mm overlap onto surrounding skin, and then secured with the clinician's choice of fixation. It can be fenestrated for heavily draining wounds. After application, PriMatrix should be covered with a nonadherent contact layer and then moist dressings, based on the amount of exudate. There are no published reports or studies testing the efficacy of PriMatrix in the care of patients with chronic wounds.

Mediskin and *E-Z Derm* (Brennen Medical, St. Paul, Minn., USA) are porcine xenografts that have been used for years as temporary coverage of burns, surgical wounds, and partial- and full-thickness wounds of variable etiologies (Davis and Arpey, 2000). They are applied to freshly debrided wounds and left in place for 1 to 2 weeks. During that period, the underlying tissue granulates and, frequently upon removal of the xenograft, a split-thickness skin graft is immediately applied. No large randomized controlled trials have demonstrated the efficacy of xenografts in the treatment of chronic wounds.

Biosynthetic ECM Scaffolds

Biobrane (UDL Laboratories, Sugar Land, Tex., USA) consists of a very thin sheet of semi-permeable silicone bonded to nylon fabric. It has been used for over 25 years in the treatment of superficial burns and has good data supporting its use for this indication (Whitaker et al, 2008). Because if its ease of use, Biobrane may be particularly useful in pediatric burn care (Mandal, 2007).

Biobrane should be applied to freshly debrided, non-infected wounds with the dull fabric side down and then secured with staples, sutures, or tape. It should be covered firmly with a gauze bolster to prevent movement of the dressing for 24 to 36 hours. The gauze dressing should be removed at 24 to 36 hours for assessment and again at 48 to 72 hours. Adherence of Biobrane is the goal. After 72 hours, if the Biobrane is loose or fluid or purulence is present under the dressing, the Biobrane may need to be removed, the tissue debrided, and a new piece of Biobrane applied if no infection is present. Once there is good adherence after 3 days, then the secondary dressings can be removed and the patient can resume normal activity and bathing as desired. Biobrane should be removed once the underlying tissue is healed, usually 7 to 14 days later. Removal should be delayed if excessive pain or bleeding occurs when attempting to take the Biobrane off an apparently healed area. Further studies are needed before wide use of Biobrane can be recommended in chronic wound care.

Integra Dermal Regeneration Template (IDRT) (Integra Life Sciences, Plainsboro, NJ, USA) is a bi-layered product composed of an outer semi-permeable silicone sheet and an inner ECM scaffold. The outer layer provides protection from bacterial invasion and significant fluid loss. The inner layer facilitates cell migration and tissue ingrowth, which leads to dermal regeneration, usually within 2 to 3 weeks of application. As the neodermis is formed, the ECM matrix of IDRT degrades. Once the new dermis is present, the silicone layer is removed and a very thin autograft can be applied, if required. There are no randomized controlled trials of IDRT in the treatment of chronic wounds.

Integra Bilayer Matrix Wound Dressing (BMWD) (Integra Life Sciences) is the exact same product as Integra Dermal Regeneration Template but is renamed for use and marketing in chronic wound care; therefore, available data are the same for both products. BMWD is available meshed or unmeshed in various sizes. Wounds should be thoroughly debrided and meticulous hemostasis achieved prior to application of BMWD. The BMWD is rinsed in normal saline for 1 to 2 minutes prior to application and applied to the wound bed with the ECM matrix side down. All air bubbles and wrinkles should be eliminated from the dressing to achieve intimate contact of the product with the wound. It then should be secured with either staples or sutures. An antimicrobial dressing should be applied next, consisting of a silver product, silver nitrate 0.5% soaks, or mafenide acetate 5% soaks, followed by a bulky pressure dressing and a compression bandage. Alternatively, negative pressure wound therapy can be used over meshed BMWD to hold it in place. Dressings over the product should be changed every 2 to 3 days or more often if needed to manage exudate or to remoisten antimicrobial dressings. Any blood or fluid accumulation under the dressing should be gently aspirated or wicked away with a gauze pad (if a meshed product is not being used, the silicone layer should be incised). Generally, the matrix will be completely vascularized in about 3 weeks, as evidenced by blanching of the underlying tissue when gentle pressure is applied to the BMWD. At this point, the silicone can be removed, and a thin autograft can be applied. Conversely, the underlying wound may completely heal within 3 to 4 weeks. At the point of healing, the silicone portion of the product will start to loosen and can be removed.

Integra Matrix Wound Dressing (Integra Life Sciences) is the ECM matrix without the silicone covering and is used alone or with BMWD for deeper wounds. When used alone, the Integra Matrix Wound Dressing should be applied in a similar fashion as noted for the BMWD and covered with a nonadherent contact layer, followed by an antimicrobial dressing and a pressure dressing. Postapplication care is the same for both products.

Integra Flowable Wound Matrix (Integra Life Sciences) has the same ingredients (minus the silicone layer) as the other Integra products; however, the ECM matrix is provided in a syringe as dry granules that are hydrated with saline prior to use. It has the same indications as BMWD, but its use focuses on application to wounds with deep tunnels or undermining. It is available for one-time use in a 3-cc syringe. It is injected directly into wounds with depth and/or undermining until the wound is filled and then is covered with a dressing of choice to hold the matrix in place and absorb exudate. Dressing change frequency is based on the amount of exudate. There are no published studies on Integra Flowable Wound Matrix in chronic wound care.

Synthetic ECM Scaffolds

Hyalomatrix PA (Fidia Advanced Biopolymers, Abano Terme, Italy) is a bilayered product consisting of a thin moisture vapor permeable silicone sheet adhered to a nonwoven pad composed entirely of the benzyl ester of hyaluronic acid (Hyaff 11). It does not contain any animal-derived products. When the Hyaff contacts the wound bed, it provides a scaffold for cell attachment and migration, and the silicone backing maintains a moist wound bed and protects against bacterial contamination (Price et al, 2006). The Hyaff degrades over time as host tissue infiltrates the matrix. Case series have been published on the use of Hyalomatrix PA in deep partial-thickness burns and diabetic foot ulcers (Gravante et al, 2007; Caravaggi et al, 2009). It is intended for one-time use and is indicated for the treatment of most chronic wounds, partial- and full-thickness burns, surgical wounds, and traumatic wounds. Hyalomatrix PA is widely used in Europe. It received 510K clearance by the FDA in 2007 but is not yet marketed in the United States.

SUMMARY

The days of simply covering a wound with a moisture-retentive dressing and treating the underlying pathology are over for recalcitrant, nonresponsive wounds. When a wound does not improve with optimal care within 2 to 4 weeks of treatment, the use of adjunctive modalities such as skin substitutes and ECM scaffolds should be considered by the clinician. However, in contemplating the use of these products, many of which are expensive and may not be reimbursed by insurance companies, clinicians must review the available data to ensure that the cost is worth any potential benefit. Many of these products do not have strong data supporting their use in chronic wound care, and clinicians cannot hope for payers to provide reimbursement without scientific evidence of efficacy. Wound care clinicians must encourage manufacturers to provide this evidence in the form of randomized controlled clinical trials. When used in conjunction with good care, these products may increase the probability of ultimate wound closure.

REFERENCES

Ågren MS, Werthén M: The extracellular matrix in wound healing: a closer look at therapeutics for chronic wounds, *Int J Low Extrem Wounds* 6:82-97, 2007.

Allam RC: Micronized, particulate dermal matrix to manage a non-healing pressure ulcer with undermined wound edges: a case report, *Ostomy Wound Manage* 53:78-82, 2007.

Badylak SF: The extracellular matrix as a biologic scaffold material, *Biomaterials* 28:3587-3593, 2007.

Banta MN et al: Healing of refractory sinus tracts by dermal matrix injection with Cymetra, *Dermatol Surg* 29:863-866, 2003.

Bastidas N et al: Acellular dermal matrix for temporary coverage of exposed critical neurovascular structures in extremity wounds, *Ann Plast Surg* 62:410-413, 2009.

Becker S et al: Alloderm versus DermaMatrix in immediate expander-based breast reconstruction: a preliminary comparison of complication profiles and material compliance, *Plast Reconstr Surg* 123:1-6, 2009.

Beele H et al: A prospective multicenter study of the efficacy and tolerability of cryopreserved allogenic human keratinocytes to treat venous leg ulcers, *Int J Low Extrem Wounds* 4:225-233, 2005.

Bindingnavele V et al: Use of acellular cadaveric dermis and tissue expansion in postmastectomy breast reconstruction, *J Plast Reconstr Aesthet Surg* 60:1214-1218, 2007.

Branski LK et al: Longitudinal assessment of Integra in primary burn management: a randomized pediatric clinical trial, *Crit Care Med* 35:2661-2662, 2007.

Brigido SA: The use of an acellular dermal regenerative tissue matrix in the treatment of lower extremity wounds: a prospective 16-week pilot study, *Int Wound J* 3:181-187, 2006

Brigido SA et al: Effective management of major lower extremity wounds using an acellular regenerative tissue matrix: a pilot study, *Orthopedics* 27:s145-s149, 2004.

Britton-Byrd BW et al: Early use of allograft skin: are 3-day microbiologic cultures safe? *J Trauma* 64:816-818, 2008.

Candage R et al: Use of human acellular dermal matrix for hernia repair: friend or foe? *Surgery* 144:703-709, 2008.

Caravaggi C et al: Hyaff 11-based autologous dermal and epidermal grafts in the treatment of noninfected diabetic plantar and dorsal foot ulcers, *Diabetes Care* 26:2853-2859, 2003.

Caravaggi C et al: Safety and efficacy of a dermal substitute in the coverage of cancellous bone after surgical debridement for severe diabetic foot ulceration, *EWMA J* 9:19-22, 2009.

Cavorsi J et al: Best-practice algorithms for the use of a bilayered living cell therapy (Apligraf) in the treatment of lower-extremity ulcers, *Wound Rep Regen* 14:102-109, 2006.

Clark RAF et al: Tissue engineering for cutaneous wounds, *J Invest Dermatol* 127:1018-1029, 2007.

Cook Biotech: Cook Biotech reference page, available at http://www.cookbiotech.com/technology.php, accessed May 9, 2010.

Davis DA, Arpey CJ: Porcine heterografts in dermatologic surgery and reconstruction, *Dermatol Surg* 26:76-80, 2000.

Ehrenreich M, Ruszczak Z: Update on tissue-engineered biological dressings, *Tissue Eng* 12:2407-2424, 2006.

Eisenberg M, Llewelyn D: Surgical management of hands in children with recessive dystrophic epidermolysis bullosa: use of allogeneic composite cultured skin grafts, *Br J Plast Surg* 51:608-613, 1998.

Esposito M et al: Enamel matrix derivative (Emdogain) for periodontal tissue regeneration in intrabony defects, *Cochrane Database Syst Rev* 19(4):CD003875, 2005.

Falanga V, Sabolinski M: A bilayered living skin construct (Apligraf) accelerates complete closure of hard-to-heal venous ulcers, *Wound Rep Regen* 7:201-207, 1999.

Falanga V et al: Rapid healing of venous ulcers and lack of clinical rejection with an allogeneic cultured human skin equivalent, *Arch Dermatol* 134:293-300, 1998.

Frame JD et al: Use of dermal regeneration template in contracture release procedures: a multicenter evaluation, *Plast Reconst Surg* 113:1330-1338, 2004.

Gajiwala K, Gajiwala AL: Evaluation of lyophilized, gamma-irradiated amnion as a biological dressing, *Cell Tissue Bank* 5:73-80, 2004.

Gentzkow GD et al: Improved healing of diabetic foot ulcers after grafting with a living human dermal replacement, *Wounds* 11(3):77-84, 1999.

Gilbert TW et al: Repair of the thoracic wall with an extracellular matrix scaffold in a canine model, *J Surg Res* 147:61-67, 2008.

Gravante G et al: The use of Hyalomatrix PA in the treatment of deep partial-thickness burns, *J Burn Care Res* 28:269-274, 2007.

Griffiths M et al: Survival of Apligraf in acute human wounds, *Tissue Eng* 10:1180-1195, 2004.

Groos N et al: Use of an artificial dermis (Integra) for the reconstruction of extensive burn scars in children: about 22 grafts, *Eur J Pediatr Surg* 15:187-192, 2005.

Harris N: *Regenerative medicine–glossary*, London, 2008. PAS 84.

Hasegawa T et al: Intractable venous leg ulcer treated successfully with allogeneic cultured dermal substitute, *Scand J Plast Reconstr Surg Hand Surg* 41:326-328, 2007.

Haslik W et al: Management of full-thickness skin defects in the hand and wrist region: first long-term experiences with the dermal matrix Matriderm, *J Plast Reconstr Aesthet Surg* 63(2):360-364, 2010.

Heimbach DM et al: Multicenter postapproval clinical trial of Integra dermal regeneration template for burn treatment, *J Burn Care Rehabil* 24:42-48, 2003.

Helgeson MD et al: Bioartificial dermal substitute: a preliminary report of its use for the management of complex combat-related soft tissue wounds, *J Orthop Trauma* 21:394-399, 2007.

Hoang AM et al: Amelogenin is a cell adhesion protein, *J Dent Res* 81:497-500, 2002.

Hodde JP et al: An investigation of the long-term bioactivity of endogenous growth factor in Oasis Wound Matrix, *J Wound Care* 14:23-25, 2005.

Hrabchak C et al: Biological skin substitutes for wound cover and closure, *Expert Rev Med Devices* 3:373-385, 2006.

Horch RE et al: Tissue engineering of cultured skin substitutes, *J Cell Mol Med* 9:592-608, 2005.

Humphries LK, Mansavage VL: Quality control in tissue banking-ensuring the safety of allograft tissues, *AORN J* 84:385-398, 2006.

Kagan RJ et al: Human skin banking, *Clin Lab Med* 25:587-605, 2005.

Kamolz LP et al: Tissue engineering for cutaneous wounds: an overview of current standards and possibilities, *Eur Surg* 40:19-26, 2008.

Kesting MR et al: The role of allogenic amniotic membrane in burn treatment, *J Burn Care Res* 29:907-916, 2008.

Kumar RJ et al: Treatment of partial-thickness burns: a prospective, randomized trial using TransCyte, *ANZ J Surg* 74:622-626, 2004.

Lee LF et al: Integra in lower extremity reconstruction after burn injury. *Plast Reconstr Surg* 121:1256-1262, 2008.

Letendre S et al: Pilot trial of Biovance collagen-based wound covering for diabetic ulcers, *Adv Skin Wound Care* 22:161-166, 2009.

Levy D et al: Cymetra: a treatment option for refractory ulcers, *Wounds* 16:359-363, 2004.

Lipkin S et al: Effectiveness of bilayered cellular matrix in healing of neuropathic diabetic foot ulcers: results of a multicenter pilot trial, *Wounds* 15:230-236, 2003.

Lobmann R et al: Autologous human keratinocytes cultured on membranes composed of benzyl ester of hyaluronic acid for grafting in nonhealing diabetic foot lesions: a pilot study, *J Diabetes Complicat* 17(4):199-204, 2003.

Mandal A: Paediatric partial-thickness scald burns—is Biobrane the best treatment available? *Int Wound J* 4:15-19, 2007.

Marston WA et al: The efficacy and safety of Dermagraft in improving the healing of chronic diabetic foot ulcers, *Diabetes Care* 26:1701-1705, 2003.

Marston WA et al: Initial report of the use of an injectable porcine collagen-derived matrix to stimulate healing of diabetic foot wounds in humans, *Wound Rep Regen* 13:243-247, 2005.

Martin BR et al: Outcomes of allogenic acellular matrix therapy in treatment of diabetic foot wounds: an initial experience, *Int Wounds J* 2:161-165, 2005.

Mermet I et al: Use of amniotic membrane transplantation in the treatment of venous leg ulcers, *Wound Rep Regen* 15:459-464, 2007.

Metcalfe AD, Ferguson MWJ: Tissue engineering of replacement skin: the crossroads of biomaterials, wound healing, embryonic development, stem cells and regeneration, *J R Soc Interface* 4:413-437, 2007.

Misra S et al: Results of AlloDerm use in abdominal hernia repair, *Hernia* 12:247-250, 2008.

Mostow EN et al: Effectiveness of an extracellular matrix graft (Oasis Wound Matrix) in the treatment of chronic leg ulcers: a randomized clinical trial, *J Vasc Surg* 41:837-843, 2005.

Muangman P et al: Complex wound management utilizing an artificial dermal matrix, *Ann Plast Surg* 57:199-202, 2006.

Mulder G, Lee D: Case presentation: xenograft resistance to protease degradation in a vasculitic ulcer, *Int J Low Extrem Wounds* 8:157-161, 2009a.

Mulder G, Lee D: A retrospective clinical review of extracellular matrices for tissue reconstruction: equine pericardium as a biological covering to assist with wound closure, *Wounds* 21:254-261, 2009b.

Mulder G, Lee D: Use of equine derived pericardium as a biological cover to promote closure of a complicated wound with associated scleroderma and Raynaud's Disease, *Wounds* 21:297-301, 2009c.

Munster AM et al: Acellular allograft dermal matrix: immediate or delayed epidermal coverage? *Burns* 27:150-153, 2001.

Nataraj C et al: Extracellular wound matrices: novel stabilization and sterilization method for collagen-based biologic wound dressings, *Wounds* 19:148-156, 2007.

Navrátilová Z et al: Cryopreserved and lyophilized cultured epidermal allografts in the treatment of leg ulcers: a pilot study, *J Eur Acad Dermatol Venereol* 18:173-179, 2004.

Nieponice A et al: Reinforcement of esophageal anastomoses with an extracellular matrix scaffold in a canine model, *Ann Thorac Surg* 82:2050-2058, 2006.

Niezgoda JA et al: Randomized clinical trial comparing Oasis Wound Matrix to Regranex Gel for diabetic ulcers, *Adv Skin Wound Care* 18:258-266, 2005.

Noordenbos J et al: Safety and efficacy of TransCyte for the treatment of partial-thickness burns, *J Burn Care Rehabil* 20:275-281, 1999.

Patton JH et al: Use of human acellular dermal matrix in complex and contaminated abdominal wall reconstructions, *Am J Surg* 193:360-363, 2007.

Pollak RA et al: A human dermal replacement for the treatment of diabetic foot ulcers, *Wounds* 9(1):175-183, 1997.

Price RD et al: A comparison of tissue-engineered hyaluronic acid dermal matrices in a human wound model, *Tissue Eng* 12:3001-3011, 2006.

Purdue GF et al: A multicenter clinical trial of a biosynthetic skin replacement, Dermagraft-TC, compared with a cyropreserved human cadaver skin for temporary coverage of excised burn wounds, *J Burn Care Rehabil* 118:52-57, 1997.

Reyzelman A et al: Clinical effectiveness of a acellular dermal regenerative tissue matrix compared to standard wound management in healing diabetic foot ulcers: a prospective, randomized multicentre study, *Int Wound J* 6:196-208, 2009.

Roberts C, Mansbridge J: The scientific basis and differentiating features of Dermagraft, *Can J Plast Surg* 10(Suppl A):6A-13A, 2002.

Robson MC et al: Guidelines for the treatment of venous ulcers, *Wound Rep Regen* 14:649-662, 2006.

Romanelli M et al: Amelogenin, an extracellular matrix protein, in the treatment of venous leg ulcers and other hard-to-heal wounds: experimental and clinical evidence, *Clin Interv Aging* 3:263-272, 2008a.

Romanelli M et al: Effect of amelogenin extracellular matrix protein and compression on hard-to-heal venous leg ulcers: follow-up data, *J Wound Care* 17:17-18, 20-23, 2008b.

Rosales MA et al: Gamma-irradiated human skin allograft: a potential treatment modality for lower extremity ulcers, *Int Wound J* 1:201-206, 2003.

Ryssel H et al: The use of MatriDerm in early excision and simultaneous autologous skin grafting in burns—a pilot study, *Burns* 34:93-97, 2008.

Ryssel H et al: Matriderm in depth-adjusted reconstruction of necrotizing fasciitis defects, *Burns*, 2010 Apr 12 [Epub ahead of print].

Schurr MJ et al: Phase I/II clinical evaluation of StrataGraft: a consistent pathogen-free human skin substitute, *J Trauma* 66:866-874, 2009.

Schwarze H et al: Suprathel, a new skin substitute, in the management of donor sites of split-thickness skin grafts: results of a clinical study, *Burns* 33:850-854, 2007.

Schwarze H et al: Suprathel, a new skin substitute, in the management of partial-thickness burn wounds: results of a clinical study, *Ann Plast Surg* 60:181-185, 2008.

Shores JT et al: Skin substitutes and alternatives: a review, *Adv Skin Wound Care* 20:493-508, 2007.

Silverstein G: Dermal regeneration template in the surgical management of diabetic foot ulcers: a series of five cases, *J Foot Ankle Surg* 45:28-33, 2006.

Steed DL et al: Guidelines for the treatment of diabetic ulcers, *Wound Rep Regen* 14:680-692, 2006.

Still J et al: The use of a collagen sponge/living cell composite material to treat donor sites in burn patients, *Burns* 29:837-841, 2003.

TEI Biosciences: TEI Biosciences wound management page, available at http://www.teibio.com/WoundManagementSpeciality.aspx, accessed May 9, 2010.

Topol BM et al: Immediate single-stage breast reconstruction using implants and human acellular dermal tissue matrix with adjustment of the lower pole of the breast to reduce unwanted lift, *Ann Plast Surg* 61:494-499, 2008.

Tufaro AP, Buck DW, Fischer AC: The use of artificial dermis in the reconstruction of oncologic surgical defects, *Plast Reconstr Surg* 120:638-646, 2007.

Uccioli L: A clinical investigation on the characteristics and outcomes of treating chronic lower extremity wounds using the TissueTech Autograft System, *Int J Low Extrem Wounds* 2:140-151, 2003.

Vanscheidt W et al: Treatment of recalcitrant venous leg ulcers with autologous keratinocytes in fibrin sealant: a multinational randomized controlled clinical trial, *Wound Rep Regen* 15:308-315, 2007.

van Winterswijk PJ, Nout E: Tissue engineering and wound healing: an overview of the past, present, and future, *Wounds* 19:277-284, 2007.

Veves A et al: Graftskin, a human skin equivalent, is effective in the management of noninfected neuropathic diabetic foot ulcers, *Diabetes Care* 24:290-295, 2001.

Vowden P et al: The effect of amelogenins (Xelma) on hard-to-heal venous leg ulcers, *Wound Rep Regen* 14:240-246, 2006.

Vowden P et al: Effect of amelogenin extracellular matrix protein and compression on hard-to-heal venous leg ulcers, *J Wound Care* 16:189-195, 2007.

Wainwright D et al: Clinical evaluation of an acellular allograft dermal matrix in full-thickness burns, *J Burn Care Rehabil* 17:124-136, 1996.

Whitaker IS et al: A critical evaluation of the use of Biobrane as a biologic skin substitute: a versatile tool for the plastic and reconstructive surgeon, *Ann Plast Surg* 60:333-337, 2008.

Winters CL et al: A multicenter study involving the use of a human acellular dermal regenerative tissue matrix for the treatment of diabetic lower extremity wounds, *Adv Skin Wound Care* 21:375-381, 2008.

Woodley DT et al: Burn wounds resurfaced by cultured epidermal autografts show abnormal reconstitution of anchoring fibrils, *JAMA* 259:2566-2571, 1998.

Yonezawa M et al: Clinical study with allogeneic cultured dermal substitutes for chronic leg ulcers, *Int J Dermatol* 46:36-42, 2007.

Young RR: Pioneer's startlingly innovative biologics portfolio, *Orthop This Week* 3(36):1-2, 2007.

20

Molecular and Cellular Regulators

Gregory Schultz

OBJECTIVES

1. Describe the importance of adhesion and the migration of leukocytes in inflammation.
2. Distinguish between growth factors and cytokines.
3. Identify important processes in wound healing that are regulated by growth factors, cytokines, proteases, or hormones.
4. Describe the molecular environment that growth factors need to promote wound healing.
5. For each growth factor family, list one member, a key target cell, one main action, and one therapeutic use.
6. Describe the molecular differences among acute healing wounds and chronic nonhealing wounds.
7. Correlate the application of the principles of wound bed preparation with the removal of wound healing barriers.

At the cellular level, the complex process of the healing of skin wounds involves platelets, leukocytes, epidermal cells, fibroblasts, and vascular endothelial cells. At the molecular level, many growth factors, cytokines, proteases, and hormones regulate most of the key actions of cells during wound healing, such as the directed movement of cells into a wound (chemotactic migration), replacement of damaged epidermal and dermal cells (mitosis), growth of new blood vessels (neovascularization), formation of scar tissue (synthesis of extracellular matrix proteins), and remodeling of scar tissue (proteolytic turnover of extracellular matrix proteins) (Bennett and Schultz, 1993a, 1993b). Any condition that disrupts the normal actions of these molecular regulators in wounds will directly disrupt healing and promote the establishment and maintenance of chronic wounds (Mast and Schultz, 1996; Tarnuzzer and Schultz, 1996). By identifying abnormalities in the actions of molecular regulators in chronic wounds, therapies can be designed that will reestablish an environment that permits molecular regulators to function normally and achieve healing.

BIOLOGIC ROLES OF CYTOKINES AND GROWTH FACTORS

Growth factors are polypeptide proteins produced by the body to regulate division, proliferation, and growth of cells by binding to receptors on the cell surface. Specifically, proliferation and differentiation of nonimmune system cells are regulated primarily by growth factors. In contrast, cytokines are protein molecules that primarily regulate the interactions between cells that participate in the immune response (Frenette and Wagner, 1996a, 1996b; Springer, 1990).

Cytokines are a unique family of growth factors that are small signaling proteins that mediate and regulate immunity, inflammation, and hematopoiesis. Produced in response to an immune stimulus, cytokines are secreted primarily from leukocytes. Cytokines function at very low concentration and act over short distances. After the cytokines bind to specific membrane receptors, second messengers are triggered that signal the cell to alter its behavior by increasing or decreasing membrane proteins, proliferation, and secretion of molecules. The same cytokine may be secreted by different types of cells, and the same cytokine may act on several different cell types.

General Phases of Wound Healing

The phases of wound healing are hemostasis, inflammation, proliferation and repair, and remodeling. There is considerable temporal overlap of these phases of healing, and the entire process lasts for several months. Immediately after injury the process of blood clotting is initiated by activation of a proteolytic cascade, which ultimately converts fibrinogen into fibrin. As the fibrin molecules self-associate into a weblike net, red blood cells (RBCs) and platelets become entrapped. The aggregate of fibrin, RBCs, and platelets quickly grows large enough to form a tampon that blocks an injured capillary and stops the flow of blood.

The process of blood clotting also induces platelet degranulation, which releases a burst of preformed growth factors stored in platelet granules. These include platelet-derived growth factor (PDGF), transforming growth factor-β (TGF-β), epidermal growth factor (EGF), and insulin-like growth factor-I (IGF-I). These growth factors initiate two major processes: inflammation and tissue repair. The growth factors released from platelets quickly diffuse from the wound into the surrounding tissues and attract leukocytes into the injured area (Bennett and Schultz, 1993a, 1993b).

ADHESION MOLECULES AND ADHESION RECEPTORS IN INFLAMMATION

The chemotactic attraction of leukocytes to a wound and the movement of leukocytes from the blood into wounded tissue (extravasation) involve expression and activation of adhesion molecules and adhesion receptors on leukocytes, platelets, and vascular endothelial cells. Cytokines and growth factors play key roles in these processes (Arai et al, 1990; Frenette and Wagner, 1996a, 1996b; Springer, 1990). Among the many types of adhesion molecules and receptors on the cell surface, four major families of transmembrane proteins stand out in the process of inflammation: integrins, selectins, cell adhesion molecules, and cadherins (Figure 20-1).

Integrins are glycoproteins composed of two different types of subunits, designated α and β. In simple terms, integrins are cellular receptors for extracellular matrix proteins, as shown with $\alpha_5\beta_1$, which is a receptor for fibronectin. A short amino acid sequence, such as arginine-glycine-aspartate (RGD), is often the site of recognition by the integrin receptor. Integrins are important because they are capable of generating signals inside cells when the integrin receptor binds to a specific extracellular matrix protein, in much the same way the insulin receptor generates intracellular signals, which regulate glucose transport into a cell when insulin binds to its cellular receptor. Expression of β_2 integrins is limited to leukocytes, whereas β_1 integrins are expressed on most cell types. β_1 integrins primarily bind to extracellular matrix components such as fibronectin, laminin, and collagens. (These substances are discussed in more detail in Chapter 4.)

Selectins are proteins that have a unique structure called a *lectin domain* at the distal end, which can bind specific carbohydrate groups of glycoproteins or mucins on adjacent cells. Thus, unlike other adhesion proteins, which recognize specific protein structures, selectins recognize and bind to carbohydrate ligands on leukocytes and vascular endothelial cells. E-selectin appears on endothelial cells after they have been activated by inflammatory cytokines, and P-selectin is stored in the

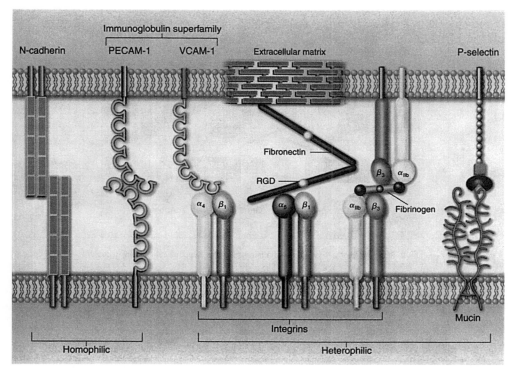

FIGURE 20-1 Four major classes of adhesion proteins and adhesion receptors embedded in a theoretic plasma membrane: integrins, selectins, cell adhesion molecules (platelet-endothelial cell adhesion molecule [PECAM-1] and vascular cell adhesion molecule VCAM-1]), and cadherins. (From Frenette PS, Wagner DD: Adhesion molecules. Part I, *N Engl J Med* 334:1526, 1996.)

α-granules of platelets and the storage granules of endothelial cells (Weibel-Palade bodies).

Cell adhesion molecules (CAMs) are members of the immunoglobulin superfamily of proteins. CAMs can bind to other CAMs or to integrins on cells. CAMs that are important in inflammation include the platelet-endothelial cell adhesion molecule (PECAM), vascular cell adhesion molecule (VCAM), and intercellular adhesion molecule-1 (ICAM-1).

Cadherins are important in establishing molecular links between adjacent cells, especially during embryonic development. They form zipperlike structures of dimers at specialized regions of contact between neighboring cells called *adherens junctions*. Cadherins are linked to the cytoskeleton through molecules called *catenins*, which associate with actin microfilaments.

During the process of extravasation of inflammatory cells into a wound, important interactions occur between blood vessels and blood cells (Arai et al, 1990; Frenette and Wagner, 1996a, 1996b; Springer, 1990). Initially, circulating leukocytes begin rolling on endothelial cells through the binding of glycoproteins expressed on their cell surface to selectins, transiently expressed by activated endothelial cells of venules (Figure 20-2). The binding affinity of selectins is relatively low but is enough to serve as a biologic brake, making leukocytes quickly decelerate by rolling on endothelial cells. While rolling, leukocytes can become activated by chemoattractants (cytokines, growth factors, or bacterial products). After activation, leukocytes firmly adhere to endothelial cells as a result of the binding between their β_2 class of integrins and ligands, such as VCAM and ICAM expressed on activated endothelial cells. Chemotactic signals present outside the venule induce leukocytes to squeeze between endothelial cells of the venule and migrate into the inflammatory center by using their β_1 class of integrins to recognize and bind to extracellular matrix components.

Adhesion and degranulation of platelets at sites of vascular injury also use a system of adhesion molecules and adhesion receptor proteins. Vascular injury immediately induces endothelial cells to release the contents of their storage granules (Weibel-Palade bodies), including the proteins P-selectin and von Willebrand factor. P-selectin promptly moves to the plasma membrane of endothelial cells, where it induces rolling of platelets on endothelial cells, and von Willebrand factor is quickly deposited on the exposed extracellular matrix, where it plays a crucial role in the adhesion of platelets to the damaged site.

Inflammatory Cell Proteases

When the inflammatory cascade is activated, neutrophils enter the wound initially, followed by macrophages. Neutrophils and macrophages become activated and engulf and destroy bacteria through their production of reactive oxygen species (super oxide anion, oxygen free radicals, or hydrogen peroxide). Activated neutrophils and macrophages also release several proteases, including neutrophil elastase (a serine type of protease), neutrophil collagenase (a matrix metalloproteinase type of protease designated MMP-8), and macrophage metalloelastase (MMP-12). These proteases play important, beneficial roles in initiating normal wound healing by removing (proteolytically degrading) damaged extracellular matrix components, which must be replaced by new, intact extracellular matrix molecules for wound

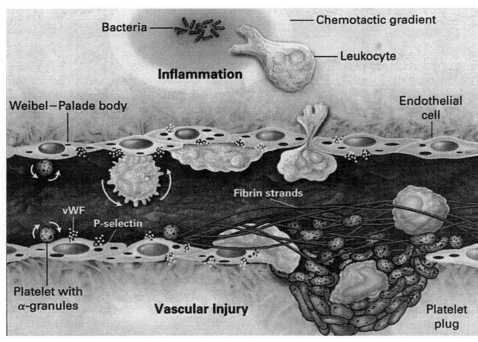

FIGURE 20-2 Interactions between blood cells and a stimulated or injured venule. (From Frenette PS, Wagner DD: Adhesion molecules. Part II: Blood vessels and blood cells, *N Engl J Med* 335:43, 1996.)

healing to proceed. These proteases also are important for enabling inflammatory cells to move through the basement membrane that surrounds capillaries.

Inflammatory Cell Cytokines and Growth Factors in Proliferation and Repair

The growth factors released by platelets diffuse away from a wound within a few hours, but they are replaced by growth factors and cytokines that are produced by neutrophils, macrophages, activated fibroblasts, vascular endothelial cells, and epidermal cells that are drawn into the wound area. For example, activated macrophages secrete several important cytokines, including tumor necrosis factor-α (TNF-α) and interleukin-1β (IL-1β), which have a variety of actions on different cells. TNF-α and IL-1β are potent inflammatory cytokines, which further stimulate inflammation. TNF-α also induces macrophages to produce IL-1β, which is mitogenic for fibroblasts and up-regulates expression of MMPs. Both TNF-α and IL-1β directly influence deposition of

collagen in the wound by inducing synthesis of collagen by fibroblasts and by up-regulating expression of MMPs. In addition, these cytokines down-regulate expression of the tissue inhibitors of metalloproteinases (TIMPs), which are the natural inhibitors of MMPs. Interferon-γ (IFN-γ), produced by lymphocytes attracted into the wound, inhibits fibroblast migration and down-regulates collagen synthesis (Table 20-1).

Inflammatory cells secrete other growth factors, including TGF-β, TGF-α, heparin-binding epidermal growth factor (HB-EGF), and basic fibroblast growth factor (bFGF). The growth factors secreted by macrophages continue to stimulate migration of fibroblasts, epithelial cells, and vascular endothelial cells into the wound. As the fibroblasts, epithelial cells, and vascular endothelial cells migrate into the site of injury, they begin to proliferate, and the cellularity of the wound increases. This begins the proliferative and repair phase, which often lasts several weeks. If the wound is not infected, the number of inflammatory cells in a wound begins to decrease after a few days. Other types of cells,

TABLE 20-1	Growth Factor Families		
Growth Factor Family	**Cell Source**	**Actions**	**Relevant Research**
Transforming growth factor-β (TGF-β$_1$, TGF-β$_2$, TGF-β$_3$)	Platelets Fibroblasts Macrophages	Fibroblast chemotaxis and activation ECM deposition Collagen synthesis TIMP synthesis MMP synthesis Reduces scarring Collagen synthesis Fibronectin synthesis	Chronic skin ulcers (Robson et al, 1995)
Platelet-derived growth factor (PDGF-AA, PDGF-BB, vascular endothelial growth factor)	Platelets Macrophages Keratinocytes Fibroblasts	Activation of immune cells and fibroblasts ECM deposition Collagen synthesis TIMP synthesis MMP synthesis Angiogenesis	Pressure ulcers (Robson et al, 1992a) Diabetic ulcers (Steed, Diabetic Ulcer Study Group, 1995)
Fibroblast growth factor (acidic FGF, basic FGF, keratinocyte growth factor)	Macrophages Endothelial cells Fibroblasts	Angiogenesis Endothelial cell activation Keratinocyte proliferation and migration ECM deposition	Pressure ulcers (Robson et al, 1992b) Second-degree burns (Fu et al, 1998)
Insulin-like growth factor (IGF-I, IGF-II, insulin)	Liver Skeletal muscle Fibroblasts Macrophages Neutrophils	Keratinocyte proliferation Fibroblast proliferation Endothelial cell activation Angiogenesis Collagen synthesis ECM deposition Cell metabolism	No published reports evaluating IGF-I for treatment of wounds
Epidermal growth factor (EGF, heparin-binding epidermal growth factor, transforming growth factor-α, amphiregulin, betacellulin)	Keratinocytes Macrophages	Keratinocyte proliferation and migration ECM deposition	Burns, donor sites (Brown et al, 1986, 1989) Venous ulcers (Falanga et al, 1992)
Connective tissue growth factor (CTGF)	Fibroblasts Endothelial cells Epithelial cells	Mediates action of TGF-βs on collagen synthesis	No published reports evaluating CTGF for treatment of wounds

ECM, Extracellular matrix; *MMP,* matrix metalloproteinase; *TIMP,* tissue inhibitor of metalloproteinase.

such as fibroblasts, endothelial cells, and keratinocytes, are drawn into the wound and begin to synthesize growth factors. Fibroblasts secrete IGF-I, bFGF, TGF-β, PDGF, and keratinocyte growth factor (KGF). Endothelial cells produce vascular endothelial cell growth factor (VEGF), bFGF, and PDGF. Keratinocytes synthesize TGF-α, TGF-β, and IL-1β. These growth factors continue to stimulate cell proliferation and synthesis of extracellular matrix proteins and to promote formation of new capillaries.

Remodeling Phase

After the initial scar forms, proliferation and neovascularization cease and the wound enters the remodeling phase, which can last for many months. During this last phase, a new balance is reached between the synthesis of extracellular matrix components in the scar and their degradation by metalloproteinases such as collagenase, gelatinase, and stromelysin. Fibroblasts synthesize a majority of the collagen, elastin, and proteoglycans that compose the dermal scar matrix. Fibroblasts also are a major source of the MMPs that degrade the scar matrix as well as their inhibitors, the TIMPs. They also secrete lysyl oxidase, an enzyme that covalently cross-links components of the extracellular matrix, such as collagen and elastin molecules, producing a stable extracellular matrix. Keratinocytes secrete much of the type IV collagen that re-forms the basement membrane, which separates the epidermal and dermal layers and forms the surface on which keratinocytes prefer to migrate.

Angiogenesis ceases and the density of capillaries decreases in the wound site as a result of programmed cell death (apoptosis) of the vascular endothelial cells. Eventually, remodeling of the scar tissue reaches equilibrium, although the mature scar is never as strong as uninjured skin.

CYTOKINES

Cytokines are produced extensively by activated T cells and macrophages, although nonimmune system cells such as keratinocytes and vascular endothelial cells also produce some cytokines. Studies have revealed that cytokines generally induce multiple biologic activities (pleiotropic) and that a single cytokine can act as both a positive signal and a negative signal, depending on the type of the target cell. Cytokines such as IL-1, IL-2, IL-3, IL-4, IL-5, IL-6, and IL-10, granulocyte-macrophage colony-stimulating factor (GM-CSF), granulocyte colony-stimulating factor (G-CSF), IFN-γ, and TNF-α are key mediators of immune and inflammatory responses. A cytokine is also referred to as a *lymphokine* (cytokine made by lymphocytes), *monokine* (cytokine made by monocytes), *chemokine* (cytokine with chemotactic action), and *interleukin* (cytokines made by one leukocyte and acting on other leukocytes). Two cytokines in particular, TNF-α and IL-1β, have activities that substantially influence skin wound healing through their ability to increase production of MMPs and suppress production of TIMPs. Table 20-2 lists the cytokines involved in wound healing along with cell source, biologic

TABLE 20-2	Cytokines Involved in Wound Healing	
Cytokine	Cell Source	Biologic Activity
Proinflammatory Cytokines		
TNF-α	Macrophages	PMN margination and cytotoxicity; collagen synthesis; provides metabolic substrate
IL-1	Macrophages Keratinocytes	Fibroblast and keratinocyte chemotaxis; collagen synthesis
IL-2	T lymphocytes	Increases fibroblast infiltration and metabolism
IL-6	Macrophages PMNs Fibroblasts	Fibroblast proliferation; hepatic acute-phase protein synthesis
IL-8	Macrophages Fibroblasts	Macrophage and PMN chemotaxis; keratinocyte maturation
IFN-γ	T lymphocytes Macrophages	Macrophage and PMN activation; retards collagen synthesis and cross-linking; stimulates collagenase activity
Antiinflammatory Cytokines		
IL-4	T lymphocytes Basophils Mast cells	Inhibition of TNF, IL-1, IL-6 production; fibroblast proliferation; collagen synthesis
IL-10	T lymphocytes Macrophages Keratinocytes	Inhibition of TNF, IL-1, IL-6 production; inhibits macrophage and PMN activation

IFN, Interferon; *IL,* interleukin; *PMN,* polymorphonuclear leukocyte; *TNF,* tumor necrosis factor.

activity, and their subclassification as proinflammatory or antiinflammatory.

Cytokines have not been investigated extensively in human wound healing studies. IL-1β was evaluated in a prospective, randomized, double-blind, placebo-controlled trial performed on 26 patients with Stage III and IV pressure ulcers (Robson et al, 1994). No statistically significant differences were seen in the percentage decrease of wound volumes between the treatment groups.

GROWTH FACTORS

Discovery, Purification, and Cloning of Growth Factors

Protein growth factors were discovered as a consequence of their ability to stimulate multiple cycles of cell growth (mitosis) when added to cultures of normal, quiescent cells. This process distinguishes growth factors from essential nutrients such as vitamins, cofactors, and trace minerals (e.g., selenium), which are required for metabolic processes but are not sufficient to initiate cell division by themselves. Both nutrients and growth factors are necessary for mitosis, but only growth factors can initiate mitosis of quiescent cells.

Based on the ability of growth factors to stimulate continuous mitosis of cells in culture, it is not surprising that many growth factors initially were isolated from medium conditioned by tumor cells. Other sources of growth factors included platelets, macrophages, and normal tissues that can proliferate rapidly, such as ovarian follicles and placenta. Although growth factors were present in minute quantities from these natural sources, tiny amounts eventually were purified using traditional biochemical methods. The amino acid sequences of the proteins were determined, which permitted cloning and sequencing of the growth factor genes. With the development of recombinant DNA technology, large amounts of synthetic human growth factors were produced from cultures of bacteria, yeast, or human cells that carried the gene for the growth factor. The availability of large amounts of the synthetic growth factors enabled research that led to a better understanding of the biologic roles of growth factors in wound healing and other physiologic processes, such as fetal development, aging, and cancer. Ultimately, this led to experiments that evaluated the effects of synthetic growth factors in animal wound healing models and eventually to clinical trials in patients.

Autocrine and Paracrine Action of Growth Factors

Growth factors are synthesized and secreted by many types of cells involved in wound healing, including platelets, inflammatory cells, fibroblasts, epithelial cells, and vascular endothelial cells. Moreover, growth factors usually act either on the producer cell (autocrine stimulation) or on adjacent cells (paracrine stimulation). In contrast to classic endocrine hormones, growth factors generally do not enter the bloodstream and act on cells at a great distance (Figure 20-3) (Barrientos et al, 2008).

Receptors

All peptide growth factors initiate their effects on target cells by binding to specific, high-affinity receptor proteins located in the plasma membrane of target cells (Fantl et al, 1993). Only cells that express the specific receptor protein can respond to the growth factor. Binding of the growth factor to its receptor activates a region of receptor protein called a *kinase domain*, which is located inside the cell (Figure 20-4). Kinase domains have the enzymatic ability to covalently transfer a phosphate group from the high-energy adenosine triphosphate (ATP) molecule to an amino acid, such as tyrosine, serine, or threonine, in a protein. The activated receptor

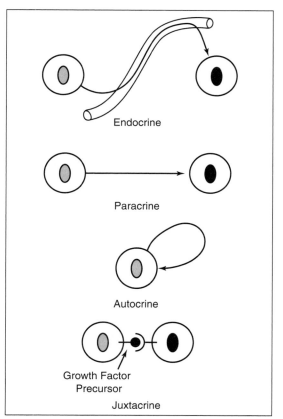

FIGURE 20-3 Growth factor action. Secreted growth factors act predominately by an autocrine (self-stimulation) or a paracrine (adjacent cells) pathway and usually not by classic endocrine pathways. Membrane-bound growth factors may also interact with adjacent cells by juxtacrine stimulation. (From Bennett NT, Schultz GS: Growth factors and wound healing: biochemical properties of growth factors and their receptors, *Am J Surg* 165:728, 1993.)

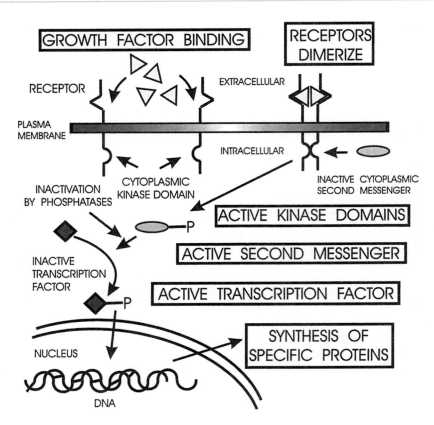

FIGURE 20-4 Growth factor receptor signal generation. Growth factors typically affect cells by binding to specific, high-affinity receptor proteins located in the plasma membrane of target cells, which then dimerize and activate tyrosine or serine/threonine kinase domains located in the cytoplasmic region of the receptor. The activated receptor then phosphorylates second messenger proteins, which frequently also are kinases that participate in a cascade of phosphorylation/activation steps that ultimately activate an RNA transcription factor, which selectively initiates synthesis of proteins that alters the behavior of the target cell. The second messenger system is turned off by enzymes called phosphatases that remove phosphate groups from proteins.

protein is the "first messenger" in the response system of a cell to a growth factor.

The activated receptor kinase domain then phosphorylates amino acids on a small number of specific cytoplasmic proteins. These cytoplasmic proteins become activated when phosphorylated and are the first in a series of "second messenger" proteins that eventually generate a response in the cell to the growth factor. Second messenger proteins also typically contain kinase domains that are activated when the proteins are phosphorylated. The activated cytoplasmic kinase proteins in turn phosphorylate other cytoplasmic proteins in a sequential cascade of phosphorylations and activations that eventually leads to activation of special proteins called *RNA transcription factors*. Activated RNA transcription factors bind with selected regions of the DNA to help initiate transcription of genes into messenger RNAs (mRNAs), which are translated into proteins that ultimately alter the functions of the target cell.

Another system of cytoplasmic proteins acts to turn off the transcription of genes that are turned on by growth factors. These proteins are called *phosphatases*. They remove the phosphate groups that were added to the amino acids of the second messenger kinase proteins and to the RNA transcription factors. Removal of the phosphate groups inactivates the second messenger proteins and the transcription factors. Thus the effects of growth factors on target cells require an integrated balance among receptor proteins, second messenger kinase proteins, RNA transcription factors, and phosphatases.

MAJOR FAMILIES OF GROWTH FACTORS

The first attempt to use growth factors to promote healing of human wounds was based on the concept that platelets contained numerous growth factors that were released at the time of injury. Furthermore, substantial amounts of activated platelet supernatant could be obtained from individual patients with chronic skin ulcers or from apheresis donors. This would permit patients to be treated with their own activated platelet supernatant or from carefully screened platelet donors. To test this concept, a U.S. Food and Drug Administration (FDA)-approved, randomized, controlled, multicenter, dose-response trial of topically applied activated platelet supernatant in 97 patients with a chronic, nonhealing diabetic wound was conducted (David et al, 1992; Holloway et al, 1993).

The use of placebo treatment, combined with good basic wound care, reduced wound area 77% and reduced wound volume 83% from baseline to final visit, although only 29% of the placebo group healed completely compared with 63% of the patients treated with platelet releasate. All healing parameters were significantly improved in the patients who were treated with all doses of platelet releasate. These results demonstrated the benefit of treatment of chronic diabetic wounds with a mixture of growth factors and proteins released from platelets. Table 20-1 presents an overview of the major families of growth factors, including those growth factors that have been shown to play roles in wound healing in animals or humans (not all known growth factors are included).

EGF Family

EGF was the first growth factor to be purified and biochemically characterized (Carpenter and Cohen, 1990). Other members of the EGF family that influence wound healing are TGF-α (Massague, 1990) and HB-EGF (Shigeki et al, 1992). Members of the EGF family are small single-chain proteins that bind to a common receptor protein (EGF receptor) that has tyrosine kinase activity and is expressed on almost all types of cells. Members of the EGF family have similar, but not identical, biologic effects on target cells. They are chemoattractants and mitogens for epidermal cells, fibroblasts, and vascular endothelial cells but are most effective for epidermal cells.

EGF and TGF-α are synthesized as membrane-bound precursors that are released by proteolysis in a wide range of cells, including cells of the lacrimal and salivary glands. EGF and TGF-α are present in saliva and tears, and data from many different types of experiments strongly suggest that EGF and TGF-α play important roles in both the normal turnover of epithelial cells of the gut and cornea and in the healing of wounds in these tissues. Specifically, in the skin, epidermal cells synthesize large amounts of TGF-α. Mice that lack TGF-α or EGF receptors have abnormal hair and skin architecture. Levels of EGF receptor are elevated in the leading edge of epidermal cells in burn wounds (Nanney and King, 1996). Specific inhibition of the EGF receptor delays healing of partial-thickness skin injuries in animals. HB-EGF is produced by macrophages and presumably is retained in a wound for longer periods than EGF or TGF-α because of reversible binding to heparin.

Current models of skin wound healing propose that TGF-α is the growth factor that is primarily responsible for the normal maintenance and turnover of epidermal cells of the skin. When a skin injury occurs, epidermal cell proliferation and migration are stimulated by TGF-α produced by epidermal cells; EGF produced by epithelial cells lining the hair follicles, sweat glands, and sebaceous glands; and HB-EGF produced by macrophages that enter the wound. In addition, fibroblasts surrounding the wound secrete KGF, a member of the fibroblast growth factor system, which exclusively promotes migration and mitosis of keratinocytes.

PDGF Family

The PDGF family comprises two major proteins, PDGF and VEGF, which influence wound healing (Heldin and Westermark, 1996). PDGF and VEGF share about 25%

amino acid sequence homology, and both are composed of two subunits that are covalently linked by disulfide bonds. PDGF has two different subunits (designated types A and B). Human platelets contain high levels of PDGF, and many types of human cells important in skin wound healing can secrete PDGF, including fibroblasts, vascular smooth muscle cells, and vascular endothelial cells.

PDGF and VEGF bind to different receptor proteins (both are tyrosine kinases) and stimulate different biologic actions. Two distinct PDGF receptors have been characterized. The PDGF-α receptor recognizes both α- and β-subunits of PDGF, whereas the PDGF-β receptor only recognizes the β-subunit of PDGF.

PDGF is a chemoattractant and mitogen primarily for fibroblasts, whereas VEGF is a chemoattractant and mitogen primarily for vascular endothelial cells. VEGF is one of the most effective angiogenic factors yet discovered, and synthesis of VEGF by vascular endothelial cells is increased by hypoxia.

TGF-β Family

The TGF-β family of proteins is the newest family to be discovered (Roberts and Sporn, 1996). Three distinct TGF-βs have been identified in humans: TGF-β_1, TGF-β_2, and TGF-β_3. All three are synthesized as inactive proteins that must be activated by proteolytic removal of a segment of the proteins. The TGF-βs are synthesized by a variety of cell types, including platelets, macrophages, lymphocytes, fibroblasts, bone cells, and keratinocytes, and nearly all nucleated cells have TGF-β receptors. Thus TGF-βs probably are the most broadly acting of all the families of growth factors.

Three different TGF-β receptor proteins have been identified and are designated type I, type II, and type III receptors. Although all three TGF-β isoforms bind to all three types of TGF-β receptors, they do not appear to have the same biologic effects on target cells. Two of the most important actions of TGF-βs in the context of skin wound healing are their ability to stimulate chemotaxis of inflammatory cells and to stimulate synthesis of extracellular matrix. Elevated, chronic production of TGF-β has been strongly implicated in nearly all fibrotic diseases, including hepatic cirrhosis, pulmonary fibrosis, kidney glomerulonephritis, and pelvic adhesions (Border and Noble, 1994). This has stimulated research into methods for inhibiting the action of TGF-β in vivo. For example, neutralizing antibodies to TGF-βs have been reported to reduce scar formation in rat skin incisions (Kurt et al, 1992; Shah et al, 1992, 1994).

Connective Tissue Growth Factor

TGF-β has been shown to induce synthesis of another important protein, connective tissue growth factor (CTGF) (Bradham et al, 1991; Frazier et al, 1996).

CTGF is a potent inducer of extracellular matrix synthesis, and much of the increase in extracellular matrix that occurs in the skin after treatment with TGF-β probably is due to the action of CTGF. Many human fibrotic diseases have been reported to contain elevated levels of CTGF protein (Ito et al, 1998; Kucich et al, 2001). Macrophages and fibroblasts, as well as epithelial cells, secrete CTGF. The receptor for CTGF has not been conclusively identified. No clinical studies of CTGF have been performed, but adding exogenous CTGF to stimulate healing of chronic wounds is logical. Conversely, inhibiting CTGF action by adding neutralizing antibodies or antisense oligonucleotides to wounds should reduce fibrosis.

FGF Family

Three proteins of the FGF family are thought to be important regulators of wound healing: acidic fibroblast growth factor (aFGF or FGF-1), basic FGF (bFGF or FGF-2), and keratinocyte growth factor (KGF or FGF-7) (Abraham and Klagsbrun, 1996). More than 30 synonyms have been reported in the literature describing proteins that eventually were shown to be either aFGF or bFGF. As their names imply, aFGF and bFGF are potent mitogens for fibroblasts that share many similar biochemical and biologic properties. The mechanism of release for aFGF and bFGF from cells is not clear.

FGFs have the ability to bind the glycosaminoglycan heparin and the proteoglycan heparan sulfate. When FGF is associated in the extracellular matrix and in basement membranes with heparan sulfate, it is protected from proteolytic degradation. The binding of FGF to heparin or to heparan sulfate proteoglycans in the membranes of cells results in a substantial increase in cell division. The activity of FGF appears to be regulated by the binding FGFs by heparin-containing components of the extracellular matrix.

FGFs appear to play major roles in wound healing. FGFs stimulate proliferation of the major cell types involved in wound healing, including fibroblasts, keratinocytes, and endothelial cells. FGFs and VEGF probably are the major angiogenic factors in wound healing. Many of the cells that respond to FGF also synthesize the peptide, including fibroblasts, endothelial cells, and smooth muscle cells.

KGF shares the ability to bind to heparin. In contrast to aFGF and bFGF, synthesis of KGF is restricted to fibroblasts, and KGF expression is rapidly up-regulated in fibroblasts after an injury (Werner et al, 1992). More importantly, KGF only stimulates mitosis of keratinocytes and not fibroblasts, as the receptor for KGF is not expressed by fibroblasts. This has led to the concept that KGF is a paracrine effector of epithelial cell growth.

Four FGF receptors have been identified—FGFR-1, FGFR-2, FGFR-3, and FGFR-4. However, the receptors differ in their ability to bind bFGF and KGF. Expression of different FGF receptor variants by cells may provide another method for regulating the response of cells to FGFs.

IGF Family

IGF-I and IGF-II have substantial amino acid sequence homology to proinsulin, and both are synthesized as precursor molecules that are proteolytically cleaved to generate active monomeric proteins of approximately 7,000 molecular weight. IGF-II is synthesized more prominently during fetal development, whereas IGF-I synthesis persists at high levels in many adult tissues, especially in the liver in response to stimulation by pituitary-derived growth hormone. Many of the biologic actions originally attributed to growth hormone, such as cartilage and bone growth, are mediated in part by IGF-I. However, combinations of growth hormone and IGF-I are more effective than either hormone alone.

Unlike other growth factors, IGF-I is present in substantial levels in plasma, which primarily reflects hepatic synthesis. High-affinity IGF-binding proteins reversibly bind almost all the IGF-I in plasma. Because the IGFs are inactive while bound to their binding proteins, the dynamic balance between free and bound IGFs has a substantial influence on the effects of IGF-I in wound healing. IGF-I also is found in high levels in platelets and is released during platelet degranulation. IGF-I is a potent chemotactic agent for vascular endothelial cells, and IGF-I released from platelets or produced by fibroblasts may promote migration of vascular endothelial cells into the wound area, resulting in increased neovascularization. IGF-I stimulates mitosis of fibroblasts and may act synergistically with PDGF to enhance epidermal and dermal regeneration.

IGF-I and IGF-II each has distinct receptor proteins. The IGF-I receptor is similar in structure to the insulin receptor. It consists of two α-subunits that contain the IGF-I binding site linked by disulfide bonds to the two β-subunits that contain the transmembrane and cytoplasmic regions with the tyrosine kinase domain. The IGF-I receptor binds IGF-I with high affinity, binds IGF-II with lower affinity, and binds insulin weakly. The IGF-II receptor is a monomeric protein that has no kinase activity but binds proteins that contain the sugar mannose-6-phosphate. The IGF-II receptor binds IGF-II with high affinity, binds IGF-I with low affinity, and does not bind insulin.

There are no published reports of clinical studies evaluating IGF-I treatment of wounds. However, IGF-I and growth hormone may act synergistically to promote wound healing. Two small double-blind, placebo-controlled studies showed improved healing with topical application of growth hormone to leg ulcers and systemic administration of growth hormone to severely burned pediatric patients (Gilpin et al, 1994; Rasmussen et al, 1991).

INTEGRATING GROWTH FACTORS INTO CLINICAL PRACTICE

PDGF has been approved by the FDA for treatment of diabetic foot ulcers. Although no growth factor has received approval for pressure ulcer treatment, national and international guidelines suggest considering PDGF use for pressure ulcers that are not responsive to comprehensive therapy and/or before surgical repair (EPUAP-NPUAP, 2009; Whitney et al, 2006). Efficacy data is insufficient for national and international guidelines to recommend the application of topical growth factors with other wound types. However, isolated reports (listed in Table 20-1) suggest potential usefulness (Hopf et al, 2006; Robson et al, 2006; Steed et al, 2006).

From a practical clinical perspective, whether manipulating the wound topically with growth factors or with semiocclusive dressings (as discussed in Chapter 18), the three principles of wound management remain the same and must be followed:

1. The underlying condition that caused the wound must be controlled or alleviated.
2. Cofactors that impair healing must be corrected. Similar to the concept of "barren soil," the cells in or adjacent to the wound must be properly prepared so that they can respond to stimulation by growth factors. For example, the cells must have adequate levels of oxygen, nutrients, and intact extracellular matrix components to be able to support cell mitosis, migration, and attachment.
3. A physiologic wound environment (both cellular and molecular) must be created for topical growth factors to be effective, also referred to as *wound bed preparation* (Schultz et al, 2003).

To create a physiologic wound environment, molecular imbalances that are common to chronic wounds (Box 20-1) and detrimental to healing must be corrected. Protease activity and levels may be one of the most important factors preventing chronic wounds from healing because the protease will degrade proteins that are essential for healing, such as growth factors, their receptors, and extracellular matrix proteins. Growth factors added to chronic wound fluids are quickly degraded by the proteases (MMPs and serine proteases such as neutrophil elastase) present in the fluid. Fortunately, levels of protease activity decrease in chronic wounds as they begin to heal (Figures 20-5 and 20-6).

Numerous interventions are available to facilitate wound bed preparation and the creation of a physiologic wound environment. The acronym "TIME" as described in Table 20-3 identifies clinical interventions that should be used. For example, sharp debridement to remove nonviable tissue may be necessary to convert the detrimental chronic wound environment into a pseudo-acute wound environment in which growth factors can function more effectively. Topical dressings designed to chemically bind to members of the MMP family (e.g., Promogran) will reduce protease levels in chronic wounds. An added benefit to sharp debridement is that it will remove any biofilm that is present. Biofilm is discussed in Chapter 16. Biophysical and biologic agents can be used to alter the wound environment and correct senescent cells. These agents are described in detail in Chapters 19 through 24.

BOX 20-1	Molecular Imbalances in Chronic Wounds

- Chronic wound fluid does not consistently stimulate growth (mitosis) of skin fibroblasts (Alper et al, 1985; Bucalo et al, 1993; Katz et al, 1991).
- Ratios of proinflammatory cytokines (tumor necrosis factor-α and interleukin-1β) and natural receptors are significantly increased (Harris et al, 1995; Mast and Schultz, 1996).
- Protease activity is significantly elevated (Bullen et al, 1995; Harris et al, 1995; Mast and Schultz, 1996; Nwomeh et al, 1998; Rogers et al, 1995; Tarnuzzer and Schultz, 1996; Yager et al, 1996, 1997).
- Cells may be unable to respond or may be senescent (Hopf et al, 2006; Robson et al, 2006; Steed et al, 2006; Whitney et al, 2006).

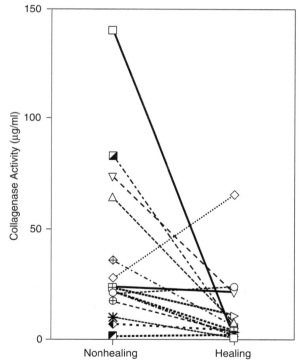

FIGURE 20-5 Protease levels in fluids from chronic venous ulcers before and after initiating healing. Protease activity was measured in fluids collected from nonhealing venous leg ulcers of 15 patients at the start of hospitalization and 2 weeks later, after the ulcers had clinical evidence of healing. Lines connecting the protease levels measured in the two samples from each patient (nonhealing and healing) indicate that protease activity tends to decrease as ulcers begin to heal. (From Schultz GS, Mast BA: Molecular analysis of the environment of healing and chronic wounds: cytokines, proteases and growth factors, *Wounds* 10:1F, 1998.)

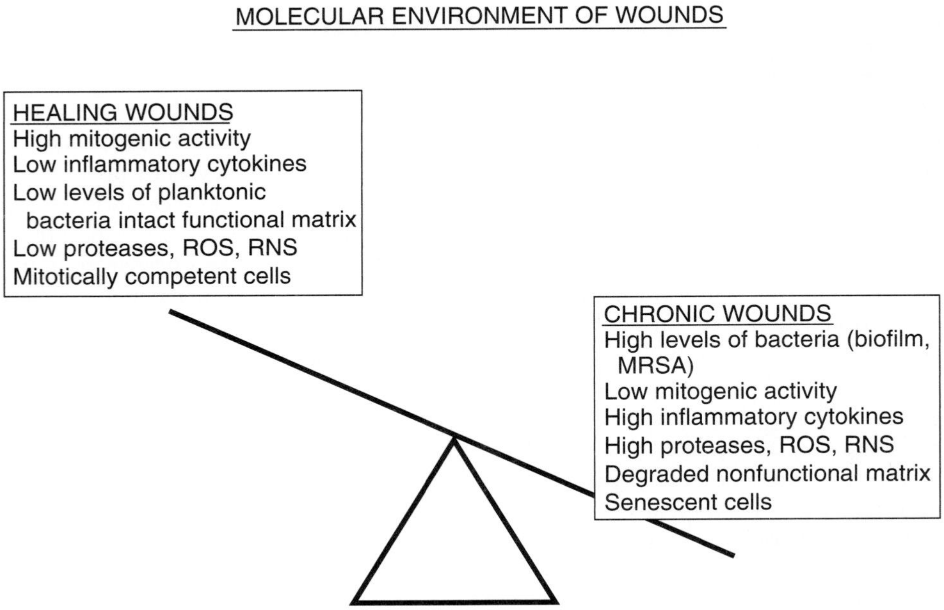

MOLECULAR ENVIRONMENT OF WOUNDS

HEALING WOUNDS
High mitogenic activity
Low inflammatory cytokines
Low levels of planktonic
  bacteria intact functional matrix
Low proteases, ROS, RNS
Mitotically competent cells

FIGURE 20-6 Imbalanced molecular environments of healing and chronic wounds.

CHRONIC WOUNDS
High levels of bacteria (biofilm,
  MRSA)
Low mitogenic activity
High inflammatory cytokines
High proteases, ROS, RNS
Degraded nonfunctional matrix
Senescent cells

TABLE 20-3	TIME: Principles of Wound Bed Preparation			
Clinical Observations	**Proposed Pathophysiology**	**WBP Clinical Actions**	**Effect of WBP Actions**	**Clinical Outcomes**
*T*issue nonviable or deficient	Defective matrix and cell debris impair healing	Debridement (episodic or continuous) • Autolytic, sharp, surgical, enzymatic, mechanical, or biologic agents	Restoration of wound base and functional extracellular matrix proteins	Viable wound base
*I*nfection or inflammation	High bacterial counts or prolonged inflammation ↑ Inflammatory cytokines ↑ Protease activity ↓ Growth factor activity	Remove infected foci Implement topical/systemic • Antimicrobials • Antiinflammatories • Protease inhibition	Low bacterial counts or controlled inflammation: ↓ Inflammatory cytokines ↓ Protease activity ↑ Growth factor activity	Bacterial balance and reduced inflammation
*M*oisture balance	Desiccation slows epithelial cell migration Excessive fluid causes maceration of wound margin	Apply moisture-balancing dressings Compression, negative pressure, or other methods for removing fluid	Restoration of epithelial cell migration, desiccation avoided Edema, excessive fluid controlled, maceration avoided	Moisture balance
*E*dge of wound (nonadvancing or undermined)	Nonmigrating keratinocytes Nonresponsive wound cells and abnormalities in extracellular matrix or abnormal protease activity	Reassess cause or consider corrective therapies • Debridement • Skin grafts • Biologic agents • Adjunctive therapies	Migrating keratinocytes and responsive wound cells Restoration of appropriate protease profile	Advancing edge of wound

TIME, Tissue, Infection, Moisture, Edge; *WBP,* Wound bed preparation.

SUMMARY

New products, including recombinant growth factors (PDGF) and biologically active, engineered artificial skin substitutes, are a direct result of our increased understanding of the molecular regulation of wound healing. However, these new products only function optimally when they are properly applied to wounds that are able to respond to them. For this high-priced technology to find broad application, it must ultimately be shown to have a significant positive effect (e.g., decreased duration of confinement, reduced cost of supplemental therapies, reduced amputation rate). The promise of growth factor therapy remains enormous but will require additional clinical investigations that are carefully conducted and properly designed. Thus the wound specialist must stay abreast of new discoveries in these areas of wound research to be able to effectively integrate these new advances into clinical practice.

REFERENCES

Abraham J, Klagsbrun M: Modulation of wound repair by members of the fibroblast growth factor family. In Clark RAF, editor: *The molecular and cellular biology of wound repair,* New York, 1996, Plenum Press.

Alper JC et al: The in vitro response of fibroblasts to the fluid that accumulates under a vapor-permeable membrane, *J Invest Dermatol* 84:513, 1985.

Arai K et al: Cytokines: coordinators of immune and inflammatory responses, *Annu Rev Biochem* 59:783, 1990.

Barrientos S et al: Growth factors and cytokines in wound healing, *Wound Rep Regen* 16:585, 2008.

Bennett NT, Schultz GS: Growth factors and wound healing: biochemical properties of growth factors and their receptors, *Am J Surg* 165:728, 1993a.

Bennett NT, Schultz GS: Growth factors and wound healing. II. Role in normal and chronic wound healing, *Am J Surg* 166:74, 1993b.

Border WA, Noble NA: Transforming growth factor-β in tissue fibrosis, *N Engl J Med* 10:1286, 1994.

Bradham DM et al: Connective tissue growth factor: a cysteine-rich mitogen secreted by human vascular endothelial cells is related to the SRC-induced immediate early gene product CEF-10, *J Cell Biol* 114(6):1285, 1991.

Brown GB et al: Enhancement of epidermal regeneration by bio-synthetic epidermal growth factor, *J Exp Med* 163:1319, 1986.

Brown GL et al: Enhancement of wound healing by topical treatment with epidermal growth factor, *N Engl J Med* 321:76, 1989.

Bucalo B et al: Inhibition of cell proliferation by chronic wound fluid, *Wound Rep Regen* 1:181, 1993.

Bullen EC et al: Tissue inhibitor of metalloproteinases-1 is decreased and activated gelatinases are increased in chronic wounds, *J Invest Dermatol* 104:236, 1995.

Carpenter G, Cohen S: Epidermal growth factor, *J Biol Chem* 265:7709, 1990.

David LS et al: Randomized prospective double-blind trial in healing chronic diabetic foot ulcers, *Diabetes Care* 11:1598, 1992.

European Pressure Ulcer Advisory Panel (EPUAP) and National Pressure ulcer Advisory Panel (NPUAP): *Prevention and treatment of pressure ulcers,* Washington DC, 2009, National Pressure Ulcer Advisory Panel.

Falanga V et al: Topical use of human recombinant epidermal growth factor (h-EGF) in venous ulcers, *Phlebology* 18:604, 1992.

Fantl WJ et al: Signaling by receptor tyrosine kinases, *Annu Rev Biochem* 62:453, 1993.

Frazier K et al: Stimulation of fibroblast cell growth, matrix production, and granulation tissue formation by connective tissue growth factor, *J Invest Dermatol* 107:404, 1996.

Frenette PS, Wagner DD: Adhesion molecules, blood vessels and blood cells, *N Engl J Med* 335:43, 1996a.

Frenette PS, Wagner DD: Molecular medicine, adhesion molecules, *N Engl J Med* 334:1526, 1996b.

Fu X et al: Randomised placebo-controlled trial of use of topical recombinant bovine basic fibroblast growth factor for second-degree burns, *Lancet* 352:1661, 1998.

Gilpin DA et al: Recombinant human growth hormone accelerates wound healing in children with large cutaneous burns, *Ann Surg* 220:19, 1994.

Harris IR et al: Cytokine and protease levels in healing and non-healing chronic venous leg ulcers, *Exp Dermatol* 4:342, 1995.

Heldin C, Westermark B: Role of platelet derived growth factor in vivo. In Clark RAF, editor: *The molecular and cellular biology of wound repair,* New York, 1996, Plenum Press.

Hopf HW et al: Guidelines for the treatment of arterial insufficiency ulcers, *Wound Repair Regen* 14(6):693-710, 2006.

Holloway GA et al: A randomized, controlled, multicenter, dose response trial of activated platelet supernatant, topical CT-102 in chronic, nonhealing, diabetic wounds, *Wounds* 5:198, 1993.

Ito Y et al: Expression of connective tissue growth factor in human renal fibrosis, *Kidney Int* 53:853, 1998.

Katz MH et al: Human wound fluid from acute wounds stimulates fibroblast and endothelial cell growth, *J Am Acad Dermatol* 25:1054, 1991.

Kucich U et al: Signaling events required for transforming growth factor–β stimulation of connective tissue growth factor expression by cultured human lung fibroblasts, *Arch Biochem Biophys* 395:103, 2001.

Kurt S et al: Transforming growth factor-β acts as an autocrine growth factor in ovarian carcinoma cell lines, *Cancer Res* 52:341, 1992.

Massague J: Trasforming growth factor alpha. A model for membrane anchored growth factors. *J Biol Chem* 265(35):21393-21396, 1990.

Mast BA, Schultz GS: Interactions of cytokines, growth factors, and proteases in acute and chronic wounds, *Wound Rep Regen* 4:411, 1996.

Nanney LB, King LE: Epidermal growth factor and transforming growth factor-α. In Clark RAF, editor: *The molecular and cellular biology of wound repair,* New York, 1996, Plenum Press.

Nwomeh BC et al: Dynamics of the matrix metalloproteinases MMP-1 and MMP-8 in acute open human dermal wounds, *Wound Rep Regen* 6:127, 1998.

Rasmussen LH et al: Topical human growth hormone treatment of chronic leg ulcers, *Phlebology* 6:23, 1991.

Roberts AB, Sporn MB: Transforming growth factor-β. In Clark RAF, editor: *The molecular and cellular biology of wound repair,* New York, 1996, Plenum Press.

Robson MC et al: Recombinant human platelet-derived growth factor-BB for the treatment of chronic pressure ulcers, *Ann Plast Surg* 29:193, 1992a.

Robson MC et al: The safety and effect of topically applied recombinant basic fibroblast growth factor on the healing of chronic pressure sores, *Ann Surg* 216:401, 1992b.

Robson MC et al: Safety and effect of topical recombinant human interleukin-1β in the management of pressure sores, *Wound Rep Regen* 2:177, 1994.

Robson MC et al: Safety and effect of transforming growth factor-B2 for treatment of venous stasis ulcers, *Wound Rep Regen* 3:157, 1995.

Robson MC et al. Guidelines for the treatment of venous ulcers, *Wound Repair Regen* 14(6):649-662, 2006.

Rogers AA et al: Involvement of proteolytic enzymes—plasminogen activators and matrix metalloproteinases—in the pathophysiology of pressure ulcers, *Wound Rep Regen* 3:273, 1995.

Schultz G et al: Wound bed preparation, a systemic approach to wound bed management, *Wound Rep Regen* 11(Suppl):1, 2003.

Shah M et al: Control of scarring in adult wounds by neutralising antibody to transforming growth factor beta, *Lancet* 339:213, 1992.

Shah M et al: Neutralising antibody to TGF-β1,2 reduces cutaneous scarring in adult rodents, *J Cell Sci* 107:1137, 1994.

Shigeki H et al: Structure of heparin-binding EGF-like growth factor, *J Biol Chem* 267:6205, 1992.

Springer TA: Adhesion receptors of the immune system, *Nature* 346:425, 1990.

Steed DL: Diabetic Ulcer Study Group: Clinical evaluation of recombinant human platelet-derived growth factor for the treatment of lower extremity diabetic ulcers, *J Vasc Surg* 21:71, 1995.

Steed DL et al: Guidelines for the treatment of diabetic ulcers, *Wound Repair Regen* 14(6):680-692, 2006.

Tarnuzzer RW, Schultz GS: Biochemical analysis of acute and chronic wound environments, *Wound Rep Regen* 4:321, 1996.

Werner S et al: Large induction of keratinocyte growth factor expression in the dermis during wound healing, *Proc Natl Acad Sci U S A* 89:6896, 1992.

Whitney J et al: Guidelines for the treatment of pressure ulcers, *Wound Repair Regen* 14(6):663-679, 2006.

Yager DR et al: Wound fluids from human pressure ulcers contain elevated matrix metalloproteinase levels and activity compared to surgical wound fluid, *J Invest Dermatol* 107:743, 1996.

Yager DR et al: Ability of chronic wound fluids to degrade peptide growth factors is associated with increased levels of elastase activity and diminished levels of proteinase inhibitors, *Wound Rep Regen* 5:23, 1997.

21

Negative Pressure Wound Therapy

Debra S. Netsch

OBJECTIVES

1. Compare and contrast two different types of negative pressure wound therapy (NPWT).
2. Discuss three mechanisms for the effects of NPWT on wound healing.
3. Describe three indications, contraindications, and precautions for NPWT.
4. Describe the application of NPWT, including in undermined or sinus areas.

Negative pressure wound therapy (NPWT) is the application of subatmospheric (negative) pressure to a wound through suction to facilitate healing and collect wound fluid (Campbell et al, 2008; Vikatmaa et al, 2008). The use of NPWT as an open wound therapy was developed during the 1940s in Germany (Vikatmaa et al, 2008). During the 1970s and 1980s, the concept was applied to the management of draining wounds, such as enteric fistulas, by placing a suction catheter or fenestrated drain tube on a moist gauze-covered wound bed, connecting the catheter to wall suction, and covering the wound (and exit site of the catheter) with a transparent adhesive dressing (Chariker et al, 1989; Irrgang and Bryant, 1984; Orringer et al, 1987). This technique was referred to as *closed suction wound drainage,* with the primary objective of containing drainage.

During the 1990s, NPWT was further explored by Morykwas et al (1997). A porous polyurethane foam was introduced as the filler dressing. Since that time, NPWT has evolved to worldwide acceptance in wound healing (Vikatmaa et al, 2008).

Today, several systems are available that provide NPWT (Table 21-1). The components of NPWT include a wound filler dressing, suction catheter, transparent cover dressing, suction source (i.e., pump) and collection container. Various wound filler dressings are now used: (1) open cell foam, (2) silicone tubing wrapped with gauze (either plain or antimicrobial), (3) honeycomb configured nonadherent matrix, and (4) non-woven superabsorbent polymer.

MECHANISM OF ACTION

NPWT expedites wound healing through the use of controlled subatmospheric pressure using the body's own defense mechanisms to enhance moist wound healing (Ubbink et al, 2008). Thus far, the mechanisms of action have been elucidated through animal and in vivo models (Saxena et al, 2004). Primary effects have been categorized as (1) edema reduction and fluid removal, (2) macro-deformation and wound contraction, and (3) micro-deformation and mechanical stretch perfusion. Secondary effects include increased angiogenesis, granulation tissue formation, and reduction in bacterial bioburden (Orgill et al, 2009).

Edema Reduction and Removal of Wound Fluid

Removal of exudate containing toxic cytokines, bacteria, and matrix metalloproteinases and reduction of interstitial edema is a primary benefit of NPWT (Ubbink et al, 2008). By reducing tissue edema, the compressive effects of edema upon the periwound vasculature are decreased, thereby improving tissue perfusion, delivery of nutrients, and uptake of oxygen culminating in the wound's ability to resist bacterial proliferation and microbial penetration (Orgill et al, 2009). A decrease in wound bacterial load was first described in the porcine model by Morykwas et al (1997). Three mechanisms have been theorized to address the reduced wound bioburden associated with NPWT: (1) removal of stagnant wound fluid, (2) direct

TABLE 21-1	NPWT Systems and Features*					
Brand Name and Company Website	Wound Filler	Canister Volume (ml)	Setting Variability	Pump Weight (lb) Settings (mm Hg)	Battery Life (hr)
Vacuum-Assisted Closure (V.A.C.)					
Kinetic Concepts, Inc. (http://www.kci1.com)					
VAC-ATS	Polyurethane black foam with multiple variations	500 or 1,000	Continuous and intermittent	12.3 lb 50–200 mm Hg	4
VAC-Freedom	Polyvinyl alcohol white foam	300		3.2 lb 50–200 mm Hg	12
VAC-Instill	Silver-impregnated polyurethane foam	500		14.5 lb 50–200 mm Hg	4
ActiVAC		300		2.4 lb 25–200 mm Hg	14
V1STA/EZCare					
Smith & Nephew (http://global.smith-nephew.com)					
V1STA	Available with drains of various sizes and shapes Filler dressing moist antimicrobial gauze	Small: 250 Large: 800	Adjustable by 1 mm Hg Adjustable by 10 mm Hg	4.3 lb 7.4 lb 40–200 mm Hg	Rechargeable 40
EZCare					
RENASYS					
Smith & Nephew (http://www.myrenasys.com)					
RENASYS EZ	Drains of various sizes and shapes available to be used with gauze filler	250 and 800	Continuous and intermittent	7.4 lb 40–200 mm Hg	40
RENASYS GO	Filler dressing option of either moist antimicro-bial gauze or open-pore foam	300 and 750		2.4 lb 40–120 mm Hg	20
Prospera PRO					
Prospera (http://www.prospera-npwt.com)					
PRO-II	Antimicrobial moist gauze with silicone drains of various sizes and shapes	800	High pressure: 40–80 mm Hg Low pressure: 30–40 mm Hg Continuous and intermittent Adjustable by 5 mm Hg	6.16 lb 40–80 mm Hg	
PRO-III		250		2.65 lb 40–80 mm Hg	
Engenex					
ConvaTec (http://www.convatec.com)					
Engenex	Biodome Easy Release or tunnel dressing	500	Continuous and intermittent	30–75 mm Hg	
ATMOS S 041					
ATMOS (http://www.atmosnpwt.com)					
S 041	Nonadherent gauze with drains of various sizes and shapes Filler dressing oil immulsing nonadhering gauze	800	Continuous and intermittent	4.2 lb Defaults at 80 mm Hg Settings are adjustable	24
NPD 1000					
Kalypto (http://www.kalyptomedical.com)					
NPD 1000	Adherent gasket with silver coated woven layer covering an absorbent dressing	No canister; dressing absorbs 50 cc's	Continuous and intermittent	8 ounces 40 – 125 mm Hg	3 weeks or more with use of Alkaline batteries

*This list is not all inclusive.
NPWT, Negative pressure wound therapy.

removal of bacteria from the wound bed, and (3) increased perfusion and thus increased immunity and oxygenation (Orgill et al, 2009). A porcine model study with daily biopsies revealed a reduction of *Staphylococcus aureus* from 10^8 to 10^5 by days 4 and 5 when the wound was treated with NPWT. In comparison, the moist saline dressing wound did not experience a decrease in *Staphylococcus* until day 11 (Banwell and Téot, 2003). Additional inconsistent reductions in bioburden have been reported. For example, NPWT has created a significant decrease in nonfermentative, gram-negative bacilli, but an increase in *S. aureus* was found in the NPWT wound (Moues et al, 2004). Removal and collection of wound exudate allow closed system containment that significantly reduces the frequency of dressing changes and exposure to external contaminants (Pham et al, 2006).

Macro-deformation and Wound Contraction

Intact skin and soft tissue have a natural tension that, when disrupted, causes skin and soft tissues to typically pull apart (separate). Distractive tissue forces may act to keep a wound open, with vectors that oppose contraction, thereby delaying healing. Negative pressure dressings can oppose these distractive soft tissue vectors (Franz et al, 2008). The application of suction allows contraction or pulling together of the wound edges, simulating the application of an abdominal binder. The pulling together of the wound edges (contraction) has allowed earlier healing, with delayed primary or secondary intention. This contraction process occurs three dimensionally through mechanical forces, thus allowing decreased wound volume symmetrically and facilitating faster wound closure (Orgill et al, 2009; Ubbink et al, 2008).

Micro-deformation and Mechanical Stretch

Histologic wound sections have demonstrated micro-deformations of the wound surface present with NPWT that is not present underneath occlusive dressings alone (Saxena et al, 2004). Mechanically, deformation results in fluid flow within the matrix and strain where the matrix cells are anchored. Thus, cells are subjected to both mechanical stretch mediated by their attachments to the matrix as well as shear stresses due to fluid flow. Fluid shear stresses are known to regulate cellular proliferation (Ubbink et al, 2008).

Wound surface micro-deformations seem to stimulate increased vascular growth. The stretching of the wound surface is hypothesized to stimulate cell division, proliferation, and angiogenesis (Orgill et al, 2004). In vivo models have demonstrated that cells respond to tension with directional growth and specific gene release (vascular endothelial growth factor) when mechanical tension has been applied (Orgill et al, 2004; Saxena et al, 2004). Saxena et al (2004) hypothesized that application of mechanical force initiates cellular response inducing a cascade of cellular proliferation, angiogenesis, and thus promotion of wound healing. The term *mechanotransduction* has been adopted to denote this cellular and physiologic response to mechanical strain (Orgill et al, 2009). In terms of the effect of NPWT on surrounding skin perfusion, it is hypothesized that increased perfusion occurs with the treatment, although the testing mechanism (laser Doppler) was criticized as being an indirect measure of blood flow (Morykwas et al, 2006; Orgill et al, 2009).

Morykwas et al (1997) reported an increase of more than 60% in granulation tissue formation using NPWT in comparison to moist gauze in porcine wounds. Numerous human studies have found increased and/or faster closure rates of wounds when treated with NPWT versus standard practice. Comparison of NPWT to standard compression therapy in primarily venous lower leg ulcerations revealed faster wound bed preparation (7 vs 17 days) and faster healing rates (29 vs 45 days) (Vuerstack et al, 2006). Faster granulation tissue coverage over diabetic foot wounds resulted in accelerated wound closure when NPWT was used (Blume et al, 2008).

INDICATIONS AND USES

NPWT is approved for use with chronic, acute, traumatic, subacute and dehisced wounds, partial-thickness burns, ulcers (e.g., diabetic or pressure), and flaps and grafts once nonviable tissue is removed. The modality is used clinically with wounds of all sizes and depths but most favorably in complicated deep wounds. It can be used with tunnels, undermining, or sinus tracts as long as the type of wound filler dressing used can be easily retrieved and is compatible with the chosen system. Granulation tissue has formed with NPWT over orthopedic hardware, tendons, and bone. NPWT can be used in the presence of wound infection or osteomyelitis only after appropriate debridement and antibiotics have been initiated (Andros et al, 2006).

Among national evidence-based guidelines for chronic wounds, NPWT is recommended for the treatment of nonhealing pressure ulcers and diabetic wounds when conventional therapies have failed (NPUAP-EPUAP, 2009; Steed et al, 2006; Whitney et al, 2006). The WOCN reports increased rates of healing associated with Stage III and IV pressure ulcers (WOCN, 2010). Arterial ulcer treatment guidelines note NPWT may have an adjunct role in the management of arterial ulcers (Hopf et al, 2006). Acute wound healing guidelines advocate NPWT to oppose distractive soft tissue vectors that may act to delay healing and keep an acute wound, especially an open abdominal wound (Franz et al, 2008). NPWT has been identified as a strong option for preparation and management of skin graft/flap (Gray and Peirce, 2004; Robson et al, 2006).

NPWT is used to promote wound healing of acute enteric fistulas and to promote closure of enterocutaneous fistulas if they have been explored and evaluated (i.e., for involved organs, abscesses, distal obstruction). Use in chronic enteric fistulas of nonsurgical candidates involves the promotion of wound healing. The wound is treated with NPWT while the enterocutaneous fistula is separated from the wound and the fistula effluent is contained separately from the NPWT system. Fistula effluent containment or management is not a recommended nor intended use of the vacuum-assisted closure (VAC) sponge method (Kinetic Concepts, Inc., San Antonio, Tex., USA). However suction of body fluids is noted as an indication for most NPWT systems using gauze wound filler dressing.

CONTRAINDICATIONS AND PRECAUTIONS

Although serious adverse events are rare (Gray and Peirce, 2004), the U.S. Food and Drug Administration (FDA) has released reports of six deaths and 77 injuries associated with NPWT (FDA, 2009). The contraindications and precautions for NPWT use are given in Checklist 21-1. NPWT is contraindicated in the presence of untreated osteomyelitis, necrotic tissue, exposed blood vessels, exposed organs, nonenteric or unexplored fistulas, and malignancy in the wound (select manufacturers). Precautions and close monitoring are indicated with the use of NPWT in the presence of treated infection, treated osteomyelitis, potential for hemorrhage, anticoagulation therapy, postsurgical malignancy excision, and poor patient compliance with supervision (Andros et al, 2006).

Debridement and appropriate antibiotics should be implemented prior to using NPWT in an infected wound or when osteomyelitis is present. It is essential that all infected and nonviable tissue or bone be debrided in conjunction with use of appropriate antibiotics prior to

---

CHECKLIST 21-1

Negative Pressure Wound Therapy: Contraindications and Precautions

Contraindications
- ✓ Untreated osteomyelitis
- ✓ Necrotic tissue
- ✓ Exposed blood vessels
- ✓ Exposed organs
- ✓ Nonenteric or unexplored fistulas
- ✓ Malignancy in the wound (select manufacturers)

Precautions and Close Monitoring
- ✓ Presence of treated infection
- ✓ Treated osteomyelitis
- ✓ Potential for hemorrhage
- ✓ Anticoagulation therapy
- ✓ Postsurgical malignancy excision
- ✓ Poor patient compliance

NPWT placement. Increased frequency of dressing changes to every 12 to 24 hours should be considered as well (Andros et al, 2006).

When the potential for hemorrhage exists, NPWT can be used but cautiously. If the patient's coagulation tests cannot be maintained within a therapeutic range, ecchymosis develops in the wound or periwound area or wound drainage becomes bloody, the pressure setting of the NPWT should be reduced (Andros et al, 2006). A less aggressive wound filler dressing, such as white polyurethane foam or nonadherent contact layer prior to wound filler dressing placement, may be indicated (Andros et al, 2006). Because NPWT associated bleeding occurred in all six deaths and 77 injuries reported to the FDA (FDA, 2009), it is critical that the potential for hemorrhage be thoroughly evaluated when considering NPWT.

Use of NPWT in the presence of malignancy is listed as a contraindication by most manufacturers (Andros et al, 2006). At least one product can be used for palliative care. A study on the use of NPWT in palliative care reported improved quality of life through reduced frequency of painful dressing changes and containment of exudate and odor (Ford-Dunn, 2006). Following surgical excision of the malignancy, NPWT can be implemented in the acute surgical wound to aid in closure.

The suction pump should be disconnected from the NPWT prior to defibrillation directly over the site, magnetic resonance imaging, or hyperbaric oxygen therapy. In the ischemic full-thickness rabbit ear wound model, NPWT alone increased wound healing, whereas the addition of hyperbaric oxygen therapy combined with NPWT did not further improve the results (Fabian et al, 2000).

CLINICAL APPLICATIONS

In at least two systematic reviews, NPWT has been reported to be a safe treatment, with rare reports of serious adverse events (Ubbink et al, 2008; Vikatmaa et al, 2008). In a systematic review of 25 studies (10 randomized controlled trials and two systematic reviews), Pham et al (2006) reported improved wound healing over conventional methods with few serious complications. In contrast, in the systematic review conducted and reported by Ubbink et al (2008), the authors found no clear evidence that NPWT outcomes were any different than those associated with moist wound healing dressings. Like all other topical therapies, the efficacy of NPWT is contingent upon correcting host cofactors (e.g., nutritional status, oxygenation, perfusion, pressure redistribution).

In general, NPWT relies upon the patient's cooperation with treatment for positive outcomes. NPWT can be difficult to use in situations where the patient is unable to consciously cooperate (e.g., due to dementia). In these cases, adequate supervision by the caregivers is necessary (Andros et al, 2006). Patient tolerability and thus compliance with NPWT can be difficult to achieve if dressing changes are difficult or painful. Box 21-1 offers interventions for reducing pain upon dressing removal (Gupta et al, 2004; NPUAP-EPUAP, 2009; Pham et al, 2006). Each system uses the same basic principles of negative pressure despite wound filler dressing differences. Although each company denotes the nuances of their product, more research is needed to compare effectiveness between different products and wound filler dressings. One in vivo study found that the pressure delivered with gauze and foam was very similar and concluded that the overall NPWT impact should be the same (Malmsjo et al, 2009). However, until research proves otherwise, current NPWT product selection should be based on features, availability, reimbursement, and cost (Campbell et al, 2008; Long and Blevins, 2009). Table 21-1 lists a variety of NPWT systems and features. Because most systems are rented, vendor customer service is another important consideration in the selection process.

Intermittent versus Continuous Suction

Suction can be delivered intermittently or continuously, most often continuously. Research suggests improved microvascular blood flow and granulation tissue formation with intermittent therapy compared to continuous therapy delivered at 125 mm Hg (WOCN, 2010). However, the potential loss of seal and subsequent backflow of wound fluid onto the wound, as well as the increased caregiver supervision required to monitor the intermittent therapy, increase the "work" of providing intermittent suction and consequently outweigh its benefits. Studies have shown that after pressures fall, reexpansion of sponge fillers can lead to tissue disruption and increased pain (Ahearn, 2009). Therefore, continuous therapy delivered at 125 mm Hg is most routinely used. In addition to the interventions listed in Box 21-1, lower levels of pressure (75–80 mm Hg) can be used to reduce pain without compromising effectiveness (Isago et al, 2003; NPUAP-EPUAP, 2009).

BOX 21-1 Reducing Pain upon Dressing Removal

- Instill normal saline to moisten wound filler dressing and allow it to loosen the wound filler dressing from granulation tissue (either with or without adherent cover dressing in place).
- Decrease pressure setting.
- Change from intermittent to continuous cycling.
- Use nonadherent contact layers (e.g., silicone mesh dressing, impregnated wide-mesh dressings).
- Instill topical diluted 1% lidocaine without epinephrine into wound filler dressing and/or use systemic analgesics per prescriber's directions.
- Change wound filler dressing to one less likely to allow granulation growth into dressing.
- Change type of NPWT system.

NPWT, Negative pressure wound therapy.

Topical Products Used in Conjunction with NPWT

Adjunct wound dressings (e.g., silver products, enzymatic debridement agents, impregnated wide mesh gauze, silicone mesh dressings, collagen wound dressings, skin substitutes, skin grafts), are frequently used in conjunction with NPWT despite limited to no research regarding their combined use. Instillation of fluids, including topical or antibiotic solutions, is commonplace, with the NPWT cycled or tubing clamped for short periods of time to hold the fluids at the wound site. Initial experiences with instillation of topical solutions in conjunction with NPWT indicate low bioburden maintenance in wounds. In addition, the use of topical or antimicrobial solutions or silver, including silver-coated polyurethane foam, also may provide improved bioburden reduction than NPWT alone (Orgill et al, 2009). As such, the combined use of NPWT with antimicrobial products (e.g., solutions, silver and impregnated gauze) may provide a mechanism for reducing the bioburden of the wound (Orgill et al, 2009).

Procedure Components

Once NPWT has been determined to be appropriate, the application procedure for most brands of NPWT are similar. However, it is important to follow the specific manufacturer's instructions. Application essentials are listed in Box 21-2 (Gupta et al, 2004).

Prepare the Skin. The sealant dressing requires an airtight seal to allow NPWT to function properly (Figures 21-1 and 21-2). Most air leaks can be prevented by (1) drying the periwound skin; (2) framing the periwound area with skin sealant, skin barrier, hydrocolloid, or transparent film dressing; and (3) filling uneven skin surfaces (e.g., creases, scars, and folds) with a skin barrier product (paste, strip, etc) or hydrocolloid to obtain an airtight seal. Contact dermatitis may result if suction is applied directly to the skin. This can be prevented by protecting skin near or under suction with a hydrocolloid or transparent film dressing framed under the vulnerable area (Gupta et al, 2004).

Fill Wound Depth, Undermining, Tunneling, or Sinus Tracts. Nonviable tissue should be removed and exposed structures (e.g., bone, surgical mesh, tendon) protected with a contact layer before applying the wound filler dressing. The brand of NPWT or specific wound filler dressing may need to be adjusted based on undermining, tunneling, or sinus tracts present. Infections from retained pieces of foam filler necessitating surgery and antibiotics has been reported by the FDA MedWatch (FDA, 2009). Therefore, it is imperative that products are selected, prepared, and used to ensure retrieval of the wound filler dressing. Undermining, tunneling, or sinus tracts should *not* be packed. The wound filler dressing should be gently placed all the way

---

BOX 21-2   NPWT Application Essentials

Preparation
1. Assessment of wound and periwound is initial step to NPWT application.
2. Debridement of eschar or slough, if present, should be performed for removal of devitalized tissue as a step in wound bed preparation.
3. Measurement of wound is necessary as key assessment of wound healing progression in addition for justification of continuation of NPWT with third-party payers.

Dressing
1. Cover exposed structures (e.g., bone, surgical mesh, tendon) with a nonadherent contact dressing (e.g., silicone or impregnated mesh).
2. Fill wound with wound filler dressing.
3. Cover with adherent dressing.
4. Mark on adherent dressing the number of wound filler pieces used.
5. Typically change entire dressing, including wound filler, every 48 hours or three times per week.

Suction
1. Place suction device per manufacturer's recommendations.
2. Connect suction device to suction mechanism.
3. Ensure that all clamps are open.
4. Turn on suction with settings ordered according to patient tolerance, type of wound, and underlying structures.
5. Verify pressure settings and maintenance of seal.
6. Change canister weekly unless wound drainage collection necessitates earlier changes.
7. Review need for suction at least 20 hours of every 24 hours with disruption no more than 2 hours at a time.

Documentation
1. Removal process: Ease of removal; wound filler dressing type and number of wound filler dressing pieces removed
2. Assessment process: Assessment of periwound skin, wound, exudate
3. Application process: Nonadherent dressing type and number of pieces, if used; wound filler dressing type and number of wound filler dressing pieces used; suction settings; patient's tolerance of procedure

NPWT, Negative pressure wound therapy.

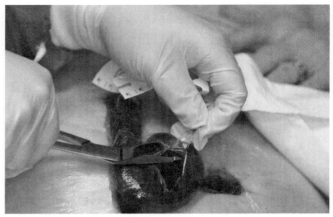

FIGURE 21-1 Negative pressure wound therapy foam placed and secured in wound. An opening is made to accommodate the suction. Note foam is bubbled up above skin level because suction not applied as yet. (Courtesy Debra S. Netsch.)

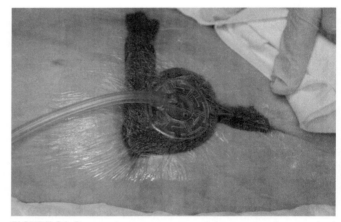

FIGURE 21-2 Negative pressure wound therapy dressing attached to suction; airtight seal achieved. (Courtesy Debra S. Netsch.)

---

into the undermined, tunneled, or sinus area. Then 1 to 2 cm of the wound filler dressing should be withdrawn from the opening of the undermined, tunneled, or sinus area. The higher pressures will collapse the undermined portion together and promote granulation of the undermined area from the inner most aspect of the wound towards the exterior surface. Progressively smaller amounts of wound filler should be used to allow for contraction and decrease in wound volume over time.

Bridge Multiple Wounds/Areas. If more than one wound/area requires NPWT, these areas can be Y-connected together to the same NPWT suction device. If a Y-connector is not feasible or available, these multiple areas can be "bridged together" (Figure 21-3). Bridging together is accomplished by using a wound

filler dressing for each wound/area and protecting the skin between the wound/area to prevent development of contact dermatitis from suction on intact skin. The filler dressing is applied over the protected skin between the wounds/areas, creating a bridge between them. The sealant dressing is applied over the bridged wounds/areas and the wound filler connecting or bridging the wounds/areas together. Thus this method allows the use of one NPWT suction device for more than one wound/area requiring NPWT (Gupta et al, 2004).

Prevent Pressure from Device/Tubes. Pressure ulcers associated with the device, and with the drainage tubing in particular, may develop primarily over a bony prominence. Prevention can be achieved by creating a path for the tubing and suction device that leads to an area without pressure points away from the wound. First lay down a dressing on the skin such as a hydrocolloid or transparent dressing to prevent suction from being applied directly to the skin. Over this lay a strip of the wound filler (Figure 21-4). The sealant dressing then is applied over the wound/area requiring NPWT, the

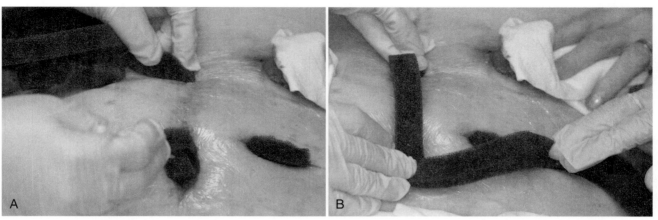

FIGURE 21-3 Bridging three wounds with one suction device instead of three. (Courtesy Debra S. Netsch.)

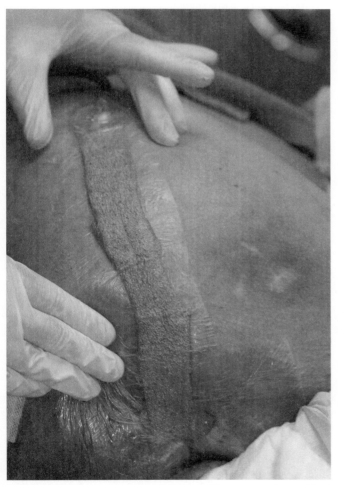

FIGURE 21-4 Patient lying on left side with pressure ulcer evident over right ischial tuberosity. Bridge created from ischial ulcer to position tubing and suction device on right lateral buttock to avoid vulnerable pressure points near ulcer. (Courtesy Julie Freyberg RN, BSN, CWOCN).

wound filler dressing trail, and the suction device as directed by the manufacturer (Gupta et al, 2004).

Maintain a Seal. Although many NPWT systems compensate for small air leaks, it is important that significant air leaks are found and sealed. Air leaks can be identified with the use of a stethoscope and repaired with a sealant dressing (e.g., transparent dressing). Although one or two additional layers of sealant dressing will repair large air leaks, multiple layers of transparent dressing will potentially reduce moisture vapor transmission and cause maceration of the wound and periwound area.

SUMMARY

Clinically, NPWT provides significant benefit to the management of the patient with an open abdominal wound or deep and highly exudative pressure ulcer and to preoperative wound preparation (Franz et al, 2008; NPUAP-EPUAP, 2009). NPWT as a wound healing modality is a significant addition to the current wound healing arsenal and should be considered an option for promoting wound healing (Pham et al, 2006). Well-designed randomized controlled clinical trials with standardized protocols are needed to further determine clinical outcomes and compare alternative NPWT systems (Gregor et al, 2008; Pham et al, 2006; Vikatmaa, 2008).

REFERENCES

Ahearn C: Intermittent negative pressure wound therapy and lower negative pressures—exploring the disparity between science and current practice: a review of the literature, *Ostomy Wound Manage* 55(6):22-28, 2009.

Andros G et al: Consensus statement on negative pressure wound therapy (VAC therapy) for the management of diabetic foot wounds, *Ostomy Wound Manage*, June(Suppl): S1-S32, 2006.

Banwell PE, Téot L: Topical negative pressure (TNP): the evolution of a novel wound therapy, *J Wound Care* 12(1):22-28, 2003.

Blume P et al: Comparison of negative pressure wound therapy using vacuum-assisted closure with advanced moist wound therapy in the treatment of diabetic foot ulcers. *Diabetes Care* 31(4):631-636, 2008.

Campbell P, Smith G, Smith J: Retrospective clinical evaluation of gauze-based negative pressure wound therapy, *Int Wound J* 5(2):280-286, 2008.

Chariker ME, Jeter KF, Tintle TE, Bottsford JE: Effective management of incisional and cutaneous fistulae with closed suction wound drainage, *Contemp Surg* 34:59-63, 1989.

Fabian T et al: The evaluation of subatmospheric pressure and hyperbaric oxygen in ischemic full-thickness wound healing, *Am Surg* 66(12):1136-1143, 2000.

Food and Drug Administration (FDA): *Negative pressure wound therapy (NPWT): preliminary public health notice*, available at http://www.fda.gov/Safety/MedWatch/SafetyInformation/Safety-AlertsforHumanMedicalProducts/ucm190704.htm, accessed November 13, 2009.

Ford-Dunn S: Use of vacuum assisted closure therapy in the palliation of a malignant wound, *Palliat Med* 20(4):477-478, 2006.

Franz MG et al: Guidelines to aid healing of acute wounds by decreasing impediments of healing, *Wound Rep Regen* 16(6):723-748, 2008.

Gray M, Peirce B: Is negative pressure wound therapy effective for the management of chronic wounds? *J Wound Ostomy Continence Nurs* 31(3):101-105, 2004.

Gregor S et al: Negative pressure wound therapy: a vacuum of evidence? *Arch Surg* 143(2):189-196, 2008.

Gupta S et al: Guidelines for managing pressure ulcers with negative pressure wound therapy, *Adv Skin Wound Care* 17(Suppl 2):1-16, 2004.

Hopf H et al: Guidelines for the treatment of arterial insufficiency ulcers, *Wound Repair Regen* 14(6):693-710, 2006.

Irrgang S, Bryant R: Management of the enterocutaneous fistula, *J Enterostomal Ther* 11(6):211-228, 1984.

Isago T et al: Effects of different negative pressures on reduction of wounds in negative pressure dressings, *J Dermatol* 30(8):596-601, 2003.

Long MA, Blevins A: Challenges in practice: options in negative pressure wound therapy. Five case studies, *J Wound Ostomy Continence Nurs* 36(2):202-211, 2009.

Malmsjo M et al: The physical properties of gauze and polyurethane open cell foam in negative pressure wound therapy, *Wound Rep Regen* 17(2):200-205, 2009.

Morykwas M et al: Vacuum-assisted closure: a new method for wound control and treatment: animal studies and basic foundation, *Ann Plast Surg* 38(6):553-562, 1997.

Morykwas M et al: Vacuum-assisted closure: state of basic research and physiologic foundation, *Plast Reconstr Surg* 117(Suppl):121S-126S, 2006.

Moues CM et al: Bacterial load in relation to vacuum-assisted closure wound therapy: a prospective randomized trial, *Wound Rep Regen* 12(1):11-17, 2004.

National Pressure ulcer Advisory Panel (NPUAP) and European Pressure Ulcer Advisory Panel (EPUAP): *Prevention and treatment of pressure ulcers*, Washington, DC, 2009, National Pressure Ulcer Advisory Panel.

Orgill D et al: Guidelines for treatment of complex chest wounds with negative pressure wound therapy, *Wounds* December(Supplement B):1-23, 2004.

Orgill D et al: The mechanisms of action of vacuum assisted closure: more to learn, *J Surg* 146(1):40-51, 2009.

Orringer JS, Mendeloff EN, Eckhauser FE: Management of wounds in patients with complex enterocutaneous fistulas, *Surg Gynecol Obstet* 165(1):79-80, 1987.

Pham C, Middleton P, Maddern G: The safety and efficacy of topical negative pressure in non-healing wounds: a systematic review, *J Wound Care* 15(6):240-250, 2006.

Robson M et al: Guidelines for the treatment of venous ulcers, *Wound Rep Regen* 14(6):649-662, 2006.

Saxena V et al: Vacuum-assisted closure: microdeformations of wounds and cell proliferation, *Plast Reconstr Surg* 114(5):1086-1096, 2004.

Steed D et al: Guidelines for the treatment of diabetic ulcers, *Wound Rep Regen* 14(6):680-692, 2006.

Ubbink DT et al: Topical negative pressure for treating chronic wounds, *Cochrane Database Syst Rev* 3:CD001898, 2008.

Vikatmaa P et al: Negative pressure wound therapy: a systematic review on effectiveness and safety, *Eur J Vasc Endovasc Surg* 36(4):438-448, 2008.

Vuerstack J et al: State of the art treatment of chronic leg ulcers: a randomized controlled trial comparing vacuum-assisted closure (V.A.C.) with modern wound dressings, *J Vasc Surg* 44(5):1029-1038, 2006.

Whitney J et al: Guidelines for the treatment of pressure ulcers, *Wound Rep Regen* 14(6):663-679, 2006.

Wound, Ostomy and Continence Nurses (WOCN) Society: *Guideline for prevention and management of pressure ulcers*, WOCN clinical practice guideline series #2, Glenview IL, 2010.

22

Hyperbaric Oxygenation

Craig L. Broussard

OBJECTIVES

1. List at least two indications for hyperbaric oxygen therapy.
2. List at least two contraindications for hyperbaric oxygen therapy.
3. Explain the physiologic effects of electrical hyperbaric oxygen therapy.

Hyperbaric oxygenation (HBO) is the systemic, intermittent administration of oxygen delivered under pressure. A hyperbaric environment exists when atmospheric pressure is greater than 1 atmosphere absolute (ATA) (Hammarlund, 1995). A medically significant hyperbaric exposure occurs when atmospheric pressure is increased to greater than 1.4 ATA or 10.2 pounds per square inch gauge pressure (psig) (Undersea and Hyperbaric Medical Society [UHMS], 1996). The typical HBO treatment takes place at a pressure of 2.0 to 2.5 ATA, or 14.7 to 22.0 psig. For HBO to occur, the patient must breathe 100% oxygen while physically exposed to the hyperbaric environment.

Just as wound care is not a subspecialty of HBO, neither is HBO a subspecialty of wound care. In addition to wound management, HBO is indicated for many other conditions, such as carbon monoxide poisoning, osteomyelitis, soft tissue radiation injury, and decompression sickness. Oxygen under pressure functions as a pharmacologic agent in that it has a therapeutic dose, a toxic dose, side effects, contraindications, interactions with other drugs, and incompatibilities with other drugs (Heimbach, 1998).

HISTORY

Much of what is known about the effects of hyperbaric treatment comes from observations and studies of caisson workers and divers. The first description of a pressurization vessel dates to 1662, when Henshaw used bellows to increase and decrease pressures to treat respiratory problems. The nineteenth century saw the advent of caisson workers for bridge construction and the subsequent description of caisson's disease (or decompression sickness), bubble theory, and oxygen toxicity by

Paul Bert in 1878 (Elliott, 1995). Eleven years later, Moir used recompression to treat decompression sickness in caisson workers building the Hudson River tunnel. The twentieth century also brought about extensive research and application of hyperbaric therapy for decompression sickness by the military. As we enter the twenty-first century, research is being conducted on a variety of disorders, including stroke, myocardial infarction, and autism.

Modern use of HBO to potentiate the effects of radiation in cancer patients began in 1955 (Kindwall, 1995). The National Academy of Science–National Research Council appointed a committee to review the physiologic basis for HBO in 1962. In 1966, this group published *Fundamentals of Hyperbaric Medicine,* which describes the physical and physiologic effects of HBO. However, it did not address clinical conditions treated with hyperbaric treatment (UHMS, 1996). The Undersea Medical Society (UMS) was founded in 1967 and was primarily devoted to diving and undersea medicine. The UMS became the Undersea and Hyperbaric Medical Society (UHMS) in 1986. The UHMS is the primary, worldwide source of information on hyperbaric and diving medicine. The purpose of the UHMS is to "improve the scientific basis of hyperbaric oxygen therapy, [and] promote sound treatment protocols and standards of practice" (UHMS, 2009).

PHYSIOLOGIC EFFECTS

The mechanical effect of HBO follows the physical law described by Boyle, which states that as pressure increases, volume decreases. Therefore, in the case of decompression sickness or air/gas embolism, hyperbaric treatment is used to decrease the size of the air bubble or embolism. Physiologic effects of HBO use the physical law described by Henry's law, which states that the amount of gas dissolved in a liquid is directly proportional to the partial pressure of the dissolved gas. As a result, oxygen tensions can be raised 10 to 13 times higher than oxygen breathed at ambient pressure (Hammarlund, 1995). With these increases in oxygen tension, oxygen acts as a drug and has several effects on wound healing (Table 22-1).

HBO increases the capacity of blood to carry and deliver oxygen to tissues. This hyperoxygenation occurs because oxygen is administered under pressure to the patient. Consequently, hyperbaric treatment significantly enhances oxygen delivery to compromised tissues, increases oxygenation to the tissues, and may restore perfusion to compromised areas. The increased capacity of blood to carry oxygen assists in the restoration of cellular function. The volumetric levels of diffusion achieved with HBO are two to three times those obtained under normobaric conditions.

Oxygen is a powerful vasoconstrictor and can be helpful in managing edema related to traumatic wounding or crush injuries. Although HBO may seem injurious in that it decreases blood supply to an injured area, the increase in diffusion of oxygen more than compensates for the decrease in circulation associated with vasoconstriction. The effect of HBO in blood is instantaneous, with a subsequent plateau in soft tissues approximately 1 hour after exposure. The effect of HBO declines steadily over 2 to 4 hours after exposure (Hammarlund, 1995).

INDICATIONS

The UHMS continuously reviews scientific data regarding the therapeutic benefit of HBO. It currently has designated the conditions or disease processes listed in Box 22-1 as indications for hyperbaric therapy (Gesell, 2008). HBO is the primary therapy for arterial gas embolism, carbon monoxide poisoning, and decompression sickness. When used for any other indication, hyperbaric therapy must be incorporated as part of the plan of care that includes appropriate clinical and surgical treatments (Cianci and Sato, 1994; Gesell, 2008; Hopf et al, 2006; Marx, 1995). The effects of HBO on wound healing and the mechanisms for those effects are listed in Table 22-1. Patient selection should focus on the origin and hypoxic nature of wound. For example, a pressure ulcer is best treated with pressure reduction; a hypoxic wound is best treated by maximization of oxygen to the wound. Indications specific to wound management recommended by national organizations and guidelines are listed in Table 22-2.

HBO may be considered for the treatment of patients with limb-threatening diabetic and vascular insufficiency wounds of the lower extremity (Hopf et al, 2006; Steed, et al, 2006; UHMS, 2010; Wound, Ostomy and Continence Nurses Society [WOCN Society], 2004, 2008). To meet Centers for Medicare Medicaid Services criteria, the lower extremity diabetic wound must be Wagner grade III or higher and not responsive to standard wound care, including assessment and correction of vascular insufficiency, maximization of nutritional status, optimization of glycemic control, debridement of nonvital tissue, and maintenance of moist wound healing with the use of topical dressings. Infection should be resolving, and the wound must be appropriately offloaded as described in Chapter 14. Transcutaneous oximetric values greater than 400 mm Hg during HBO exposure indicates a likely

TABLE 22-1	Effects and Mechanisms of Hyperbaric Oxygen Therapy on Wound Healing
Effect	**Mechanism**
Hyperoxygenation	Improved oxygen-carrying capacity Increased distance of diffusion Improved local tissue oxygenation Decreased vasoconstriction and local tissue edema Improved cellular energy metabolism
Improved growth factor expression	Up-regulation of platelet-derived growth factor receptor Increased angiogenesis Increased extracellular matrix formation and granulation tissue Enhanced epithelial cell proliferation and migration
Fibroblast proliferation	Increased collagen deposition Improved collagen cross-linking Increased production of fibronectin
Increased nitric oxide production	Enhanced neutrophil activity Enhanced macrophage activity Increased leukocyte-killing ability Enhanced effectiveness of antibiotics

BOX 22-1	Indications for Hyperbaric Oxygen Therapy

- Air/gas embolism*
- Carbon monoxide/cyanide poisoning*
- Decompression sickness*
- Crush injury, compartment syndrome, acute traumatic ischemia
- Clostridial myositis and myonecrosis (gas gangrene)
- Compromised skin grafts and/or flaps
- Exceptional blood loss
- Intracranial abscess
- Necrotizing soft tissue infections
- Delayed radiation injury (soft tissue and bony necrosis)
- Thermal burns
- Osteomyelitis (refractory)
- Enhancement of healing in selected problem wounds

*Primary therapy.
Adapted from Undersea and Hyperbaric Medical Society (UHMS): *Indications for Hyperbaric oxygen therapy*, available at http://www.uhms.org/Default.aspx?tabid=270. Accessed August 22, 2010.

TABLE 22-2	Wound-Related Indications for Hyperbaric Oxygen Therapy
Indication	**Source**
Thermal burns	UHMS (2010)
Acute traumatic ischemia	UHMS (2010)
Necrotizing infections	UHMS (2010)
Osteomyelitis refractory	UHMS (2010)
Delayed radiation injury (soft tissue and bony necrosis)	UHMS (2010)
Compromised skin grafts and/or flaps	UHMS (2010)
Selected problem wounds that fail to respond to established medical and surgical management	UHMS (2010)
Diabetic Wagner grade III or higher lower extremity wounds not responsive to established medical and surgical management	CMS (2002)
Diabetic limb-threatening lower extremity wound	WOCN Society (2004) WHS (Steed et al, 2006)
Arterial limb-threatening lower extremity wound	WOCN Society (2008) WHS (Hopf et al, 2006) Society for Vascular Surgery (Norgren et al, 2007)

UHMS, Undersea and Hyperbaric Medical Society; *WHS,* Wound Healing Society; *WOCN,* Wound, Ostomy and Continence Nurses.

successful outcome in the diabetic lower extremity wound. Transcutaneous oximetric values less than 15 mm Hg when breathing room air and less than 100 mm Hg during HBO exposure are predictive of wound healing failure (Broussard, 2003; Fife et al, 2002). Although it is understood that not all wounds heal, consideration for hyperbaric treatment should be given to those patients with lower extremity wounds when it is known that these wounds may not heal. Hyperbaric treatment could mean the difference between limb salvage, a transmetatarsal, below-the-knee or above-the-knee amputation with appropriate circulatory assessment, intervention, and preamputation preparation with HBO.

Crush injury, compartment syndrome, and acute traumatic ischemia benefit from hyperbarics because of the improved oxygen tension in tissue that is inadequately perfused because of a disruption of blood supply and edema associated with injury. HBO helps to decrease edema through its vasoconstrictive action. In addition, it helps to decrease reperfusion injury. The use of hyperbarics in these cases is emergent, and patients should be treated as early as possible for the best outcome.

Clostridial myonecrosis and necrotizing fasciitis are emergent conditions treated with surgical excision and HBO. Clostridial myonecrosis is an anaerobic bacterial infection where clostridial toxins cause tissue death in advance of the bacteria. HBO helps to neutralize the effects of the toxins and halts the progression of tissue

destruction. Necrotizing fasciitis is an acute bacterial infectious process that may include anaerobic and aerobic bacteria that act synergistically to cause rapid tissue destruction. Hyperbarics, as an adjunct to surgical intervention, improves oxygenation and may have a direct effect on anaerobic bacteria as well as improving neutrophil activity.

Chronic osteomyelitis occurs when repeated attempts of standard interventions have failed. It is thought that HBO improves available oxygen at the bone site to improve leukocyte killing ability through oxidative mechanisms. In addition, antibiotic activity may be enhanced. It is also thought that osteoclastic activity and osteogenesis are improved with the use of HBO.

Delayed radiation injury results from endarteritis and subsequent tissue hypoxia. There typically is a latent period of at least 6 months before the effects of delayed injury are seen. Injury may not be seen for many years and often is precipitated by injury or surgical procedures. HBO is used prophylactically before oromaxillary surgical procedures to prevent osteoradionecrosis. Soft tissue radiation injuries, including proctitis and cystitis, can be treated with HBO. The rationale for use of hyperbarics is induction of neovascularization in the irradiated area.

Compromised grafts and flaps benefit from HBO by facilitating increased distance of oxygen diffusion, thereby supporting the ischemic graft or flap. In addition, it now is believed that graft and flap failure may have a component of reperfusion injury that is overcome with the administration of HBO. Hyperbarics is not indicated in uncomplicated grafts or flaps, nor is it indicated in bioengineered tissues.

HBO has been and is being used for other disease processes and conditions (Box 22-2). Although the UHMS currently does not recognize the use of hyperbaric treatment in these instances, research continues and is providing support (Asamoto et al, 2000; Baugh, 2000; Bern et al, 2000; Carl et al, 1998; Gottlieb and Neubauer, 1988; Hughes et al, 1998; Ishihara et al, 2001; Jordan, 1998; Laden, 1998; Mayer et al, 2001; Mychaskiw et al, 2001; Neubauer, 1998; Nighoghossian and Trouillas, 1997; Pascual, 1995; Reillo and Altieri, 1996; Wallace et al, 1995). In a systematic review of the literature, the WOCN concluded there is insufficient evidence to support the use of HBO in the treatment of pressure ulcers (WOCN, 2010).

CONTRAINDICATIONS

Rigorous assessment of the patient must be completed to rule out contraindications to hyperbaric therapy (Box 22-3). Any air-filled cavity must be assessed. The gas law described by Boyle states that as pressure increases, volume decreases, and vice versa. This guides the practitioner to assess air-filled body cavities, such as ears and sinus cavities, and the patient's ability to equalize pressure to prevent barotrauma. A chest X-ray

BOX 22-2	Situations for Hyperbaric Oxygen Therapy Under Investigation

- Acute myocardial infarction
- Acute cerebrovascular accident
- Closed head injury
- Spinal cord injury
- Sickle cell crisis
- Rheumatic diseases
- Migraine/cluster headache
- Multiple sclerosis
- Radiation cystitis/proctitis
- Human immunodeficiency virus/acquired immunodeficiency syndrome
- Cerebral palsy
- Autism

examination will rule out trapping of air in the lungs. Patients with a history of seizure activity should be assessed for seizure control. Hyperbaric treatment is absolutely contraindicated for patients who have a history of receiving bleomycin because it increases the risk for oxygen toxicity. Hyperbaric treatment also is contraindicated for patients receiving cis-platinum, mafenide acetate (Sulfamylon), or disulfiram. Another absolute contraindication is an untreated pneumothorax. Relative contraindications to hyperbaric treatment include pregnancy, known malignancy, emphysema, pneumonia, bronchitis, and hyperthermia (Foster, 1992; Heimbach, 1998).

PROTOCOLS AND CLINICAL APPLICATION

Hyperbaric treatment protocols depend upon the specific disease process. The UHMS has outlined acceptable protocols for hyperbaric exposure. However, this

BOX 22-3	Contraindications to Hyperbaric Oxygen Therapy

Absolute Contraindications
- Untreated pneumothorax
- History of bleomycin
- Adriamycin
- Disulfiram
- Cis-platinum
- Sulfamylon (mafenide acetate)

Relative Contraindications
- Pregnancy
- Upper respiratory infection
- Emphysema with CO_2 retention
- Hyperthermia
- Seizure disorder
- Spherocytosis
- History of spontaneous pneumothorax
- History of optic neuritis
- History of surgery for otosclerosis

does not preclude physician preference and individualization to meet the patient's needs. Typically, a patient will receive a daily hyperbaric exposure five to seven times per week. The treatment will last for 90 minutes at 2.0 to 2.5 ATA. The patient generally receives 40 to 60 treatments. Continuous assessment of the patient's progress assists the physician in determining when the maximum benefit from HBO therapy has been reached (Gesell, 2008).

Staff Education and Certification

The UHMS and the American College of Hyperbaric Medicine (ACHM) offers certification and a method for physicians to set themselves apart as hyperbaric specialists (ACHM, 2009). The American Board of Medical Specialties offers an examination for hyperbaric medicine that requires completion of a fellowship in hyperbaric medicine (after a grandfather period expired in 2004). The Baromedical Nurses Association (BNA) provides guidance for providing nursing care in the hyperbaric environment. Nurses may obtain national certification in hyperbaric nursing through the Baromedical Nurses Association Certification Board (BNACB), an association that promotes the status and standards of baromedical nursing practice. Three levels of certification are available depending upon practice participation and educational background (BNA, 2009).

Methods and Chambers

To achieve a hyperbaric state, the patient is placed into either a monoplace chamber or a multiplace chamber. The monoplace chamber (Figure 22-1) has rapidly become the predominant chamber seen in outpatient settings. A monoplace chamber typically is compressed with oxygen. These chambers are rated for a maximum clinical pressurization of 44 psi, or 3 ATA. The major advantage of using monoplace chambers is that they are relatively inexpensive. The chamber can be placed anywhere an adequate gas supply

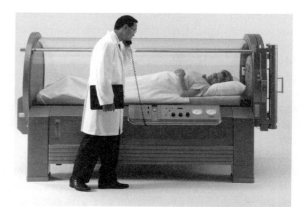

FIGURE 22-1 HBO Sechrist 3200 monoplace chamber. (Courtesy Sechrist Industries, Anaheim, Calif., USA.)

is available and can be housed in most areas without significant construction costs. Another advantage is that the monoplace chamber can be staffed by either a nurse or technician and a physician. Current reimbursement guidelines dictate that a physician must be available for the duration of a hyperbaric treatment.

Disadvantages of the monoplace chamber include the lack of direct patient contact and the difficulty involved in monitoring the patient other than visually. Methods are available to monitor electrocardiogram, arterial blood pressure, pulmonary artery pressure, wedge pressure, central venous pressure, cuff blood pressure, temperature, and transcutaneous partial pressure of oxygen ($TcPO_2$) monitoring. It also is possible to ventilate a patient in the monoplace chamber; however, most hyperbaric chambers that are integrated within an outpatient wound care clinic do not have the ability to provide support to the critically ill patient.

The multiplace chamber (Figures 22-2 and 22-3) allows a caregiver to enter the chamber with the patient. The caregiver, or *tender,* may be a technician, nurse, or physician. The multiplace chamber can accommodate multiple patients in a single treatment, or *dive.* The number of patients who can be treated simultaneously depends on the size of the chamber and whether the patients are ambulatory or chair- or bed-bound. The multiplace chamber can easily be equipped to handle the critically ill. The critically ill patient can be monitored the same as in the monoplace chamber. To breathe oxygen, the patient wears either a mask or a hood. The major disadvantages of the multiplace chamber are the cost and the housing of the chamber. The American Society of Mechanical Engineers (ASME) provides standards for pressure vessels for human occupancy (PVHO-2). The National Fire Protection Association (NFPA, 2002) sets forth construction requirements for the physical structure containing the chamber. A disadvantage of the multiplace chamber is the need to abort a multioccupant dive if a patient is unable to equalize pressure during pressurization. A final consideration

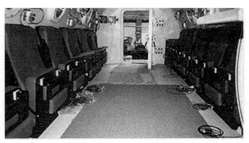

FIGURE 22-3 HBO Gulf Coast Multiplace Chamber, inside view. (Courtesy Gulf Coast Hyperbarics, Inc., Panama City, Fla., USA.)

of the multiplace chamber is staffing. The multiplace chamber requires a greater expenditure for staff than does the monoplace chamber. The multiplace chamber is staffed with a chamber operator, tender, nurse, and physician.

Patient Preparation and Safety

Two factors dictate the need to follow rigorous procedures for patient preparation and patient safety. The first factor is the nature of hyperbarics (i.e., atmospheric pressure changes). Patient instruction should include air equalization techniques to prevent aural or sinus barotrauma. The patient should be instructed not to hold his or her breath during ascent to prevent pneumothorax. The caregiver responsible for assessing the patient before treatment should assess breath sounds to prevent exposing the patient with compromised pulmonary status to the hyperbaric environment. A random blood sugar measurement before treatment should be obtained for all patients with diabetes because HBO can significantly lower blood sugar levels. Vital signs are obtained to assess for hypertension and hyperthermia. HBO is a potent vasoconstrictor and can predispose the patient to a hypertensive crisis; an oral temperature greater than 102°F (38.9°C) predisposes the patient to an oxygen toxicity seizure.

The second factor affecting patient preparation and safety is the pressurized high-oxygen environment. This is significant in any hyperbaric environment and is of extreme importance when the patient is pressurized in a 100% oxygen environment. This situation poses a significant fire safety issue. Although no clinical hyperbaric chamber fire has occurred in the United States, chamber fires that have occurred in other countries have resulted in death (Sheffied and Desautels, 1997). Patients should be instructed not to use products that have a petroleum or alcohol base before they go into the chamber. Checklist 22-1 provides a list of materials banned in the hyperbaric chamber. Cosmetic products such as hair spray, hair creams, lotions, Vaseline, deodorants, and perfumes must be removed before treatment. All skin care products pose a risk and should be removed prior to treatment. Only cotton linens and clothing are allowed into the chamber to decrease spark potential.

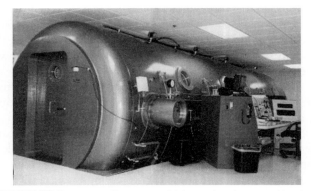

FIGURE 22-2 HBO Gulf Coast Multiplace Chamber, outside view. (Courtesy Gulf Coast Hyperbarics, Inc., Panama City, Fla., USA.)

CHECKLIST 22-1

Materials Banned from the Hyperbaric Chamber

✓ Cosmetic products, including the following:
- Hair spray
- Hair cream
- Skin care products, including lotions and barrier ointments
- Deodorant
- Perfume
- Lipstick
- Fingernail polish

✓ Petrolatum and products containing petrolatum and paraffin
✓ Mineral oil and products containing mineral oil
✓ Dressing products containing synthetic fibers (e.g., nylon)
✓ Elastic products (e.g., compression wraps)
✓ Any device with a battery (e.g., hearing aid)
✓ Dentures if patient at risk for seizure activity
✓ All jewelry
✓ Magnesium eyeglass frames

Prosthetics, including hearing aids, should be removed. Although glasses, contact lenses, and dentures are not absolutely contraindicated in the hyperbaric environment, they should be removed if the patient is at risk for seizure activity or has an altered mental condition (Hart, 1995; Larson-Lohr and Norvell, 2002; Weaver and Straas, 1991).

Side Effects

The most common side effect or complication of HBO is claustrophobia. Patients who experience claustrophobia should be reassured, and a tender should be present and in contact with the patient at all times. In the multiplace chamber, the tender can offer direct physical comfort. In the monoplace chamber, the tender should maintain both visual and verbal contact with the patient. Benzodiazepines offer relief of claustrophobia in most cases. Occasionally, a treatment is aborted and subsequent hyperbaric therapy is discontinued as a result of claustrophobia.

Aural barotrauma, referred to as an *ear squeeze,* will manifest as ear pain and may result in a hematoma to the tympanic membrane, hemorrhage in the middle ear, or tympanic rupture. If a patient experiences an ear squeeze, a myringotomy or placement of pressure equalization tubes may be necessary. Sinus barotrauma, or sinus squeeze, results in extreme sinus pain and may lead to hemorrhage of the sinus. The patient who comes for a hyperbaric treatment and has a congested nasal passage may benefit from nasal decongestant sprays before the treatment. Oral decongestants may be indicated for a more long-term approach (Capes and Tomaszewski, 1996; Kidder, 1995; Vrabec et al, 1998).

Visual acuity changes during hyperbaric therapy are not rare. Myopia may worsen after 20 or more hyperbaric exposures. Frequently, a patient who uses glasses

to correct presbyopia will find that he or she is able to read without corrective lenses. The exact mechanism behind these visual changes is not known. The patient who experiences a visual change should be instructed not to change prescription eyewear for 2 to 3 months after hyperbaric treatment because the visual change usually is temporary (Maki, 1996).

A physiologic anomaly, breath holding, or cessation of respiration can cause air to be trapped in the lungs. This trapped air can lead to a tension pneumothorax. Should this occur in a multiplace chamber, the patient can be recompressed and the pneumothorax corrected within the chamber before decompression of the chamber. In a monoplace environment, the patient should be recompressed to treatment depth until supplies, equipment, and personnel are available. Once the team and supplies are assembled, the patient should be decompressed and treated immediately upon removal from the chamber.

Seizure activity from oxygen toxicity, although ominous in appearance, is self-limiting and benign. The patient in the monoplace environment should be maintained at pressure until seizure activity has stopped. If the patient is breathing oxygen by mask or hood, the oxygen should be stopped and the patient placed on air. Once the seizure has stopped, the patient can be removed from the chamber. Generally, no further precautions or anticonvulsant medications are necessary for subsequent treatments. Patients with a known history of seizure or who are predisposed to seizure activity would benefit from periodic, scheduled discontinuation of oxygen breathing (air breaks) during the treatment (Clark, 1995).

TOPICAL OXYGEN IS NOT HBO

Various methods for providing topical oxygen have been created, including plastic chambers over a limb, continuous oxygen flow through a battery-operated system or a reservoir within a bandage, and gas dissolved or saturated within saline, gel, or foam (Hopf et al, 2006). Topical oxygen at the wound surface has been shown to enhance cytokine production and wound healing in normal animal studies (Fries et al, 2005). A limited number of case studies and clinical series suggest a benefit of topical oxygen in the treatment of a variety of ulcers (Edsberg et al, 2002; Gordillo and Sen, 2003; Heng et al, 2000a; Heng et al, 2000b; Kalliainen et al, 2003). However, until further rigorous studies are performed, there is insufficient evidence to recommend topical oxygen for the treatment of wounds (EPUAP-NPUAP, 2009; Hopf et al, 2006; Robson et al, 2006; WOCN, 2010).

Published information related to topical oxygen can be confusing when the modality is inaccurately labeled topical hyperbaric oxygen (THBO). Topical therapy literature further confuses the consumer by using HBO to demonstrate it's value. In fact, topical oxygen therapy is not HBO; the route of delivery and the mode of action are different. It is important to distinguish between the two modalities in order to clarify the discussion of efficacy (Hopf et al, 2006) and reimbursement; topical oxygen is not reimbursed for wound management (CMS, 2002).

Topical oxygen may produce transient, slight elevations in ambient pressure applied to the wound (as high as 1.03 ATA). The degree of pressure that can be applied is significantly limited by the possibility of occluding arterial inflow or venous outflow with high pressure. In contrast, HBO (systemic) is defined medically as the application of pressures greater than atmospheric to a patient who is entirely enclosed within the pressurized chamber, at pressures of 1.5 to 6 ATA (generally 2–3 ATA for wound-healing indications) (Hopf et al, 2006).

SUMMARY

Oxygen is a powerful and versatile agents used in many aspects of medicine. The therapeutic use of oxygen under pressure has been used for many years for multiple medical conditions including wound healing. Hyper-oxygenation of tissue, vasoconstriction, down regulation of inflammatory cytokines, up-regulation of growth factors and antibacterial effects of HBO can benefit patients with specific wound types. As with other biophysical modalities used in wound care today, more research is needed before expanding the list of indications.

REFERENCES

American College of Hyperbaric Medicine (ACHM): *Certification*, February 2, 2009, available at http://www.hyperbaricmedicine. org, accessed April 2, 2009.

Asamoto S et al: Hyperbaric oxygen (HBO) therapy for acute traumatic cervical spinal cord injury, *Spinal Cord* 38(9):538, 2000.

Baromedical Nurses Association (BNA): *Certification*, March 4, 2009, available at http://www.hyperbaricnurses.org/html/certification.html http://www.hyperbaricnurses.org/certification.html, accessed March 4, 2009.

Baugh MA: HIV: reactive oxygen species, enveloped viruses and hyperbaric oxygen, *Med Hypoth* 55(3):232, 2000.

Bern J et al: Use of hyperbaric oxygen chamber in the management of radiation-related complications of the anorectal region: report of two cases and review of the literature, *Dis Colon Rectum* 43(10):1435, 2000.

Broussard CL: Hyperbaric oxygenation and wound healing, *J Wound Ostomy Continence Nurs* 30(4):210, 2003.

Capes JP, Tomaszewski C: Prophylaxis against middle ear barotrauma in US hyperbaric oxygen therapy centers, *Am J Emerg Med* 14(7):645, 1996.

Carl UM et al: Treatment of radiation proctitis with hyperbaric oxygen: what is the optimal number of HBO treatments? *Strahlenther Onkol* 174(9):482, 1998.

Cianci P, Sato R: Adjunctive hyperbaric oxygen therapy in the treatment of thermal burns: a review, *Burns* 20(1):5, 1994.

Clark JM: Oxygen toxicity. In Kindwall EP, editor: *Hyperbaric medicine practice*, Flagstaff, Ariz., 1995, Best.

CMS: Program Memorandum Intermediaries/Carriers, Transmittal AB-02-183, *Coverage of Hyperbaric Oxygen (HBO) Therapy for the Treatment of Diabetic Wounds of the Lower Extremities*, Department of Health & Human Services, December 27, 2002. Available at: http://www.cms.gov/transmittals/downloads/AB02183.pdf.

Edsberg LE et al: Topical hyperbaric oxygen and electrical stimulation: exploring potential synergy, *Ostomy Wound Manage* 48(11):42-50, 2002.

Elliott DH: Decompression sickness. In Kindwall EP, editor: *Hyperbaric medicine practice*, Flagstaff, Ariz., 1995, Best.

European Pressure Ulcer Advisory Panal (EPUAP) and National Pressure ulcer Advisory Panal (NPUAP): *Prevention and treatment of pressure ulcers*, Washington, DC, 2009, National Pressure Ulcer Advisory Panel.

Fife CE et al: The predictive value of transcutaneous oxygen tension measurement in diabetic lower extremity ulcers treated with hyperbaric oxygen therapy: a retrospective analysis of 1144 patients, *Wound Rep Regen* 10:198, 2002.

Foster JH: Hyperbaric oxygen treatment contraindications and complications, *J Maxillofac Surg* 50(10):1081, 1992.

Fries RB et al: Dermal excisional wound healing in pigs following treatment with topically applied pure oxygen, *Mutat Res* 579(1-2):172-181, 2005.

Gesell LB: *Hyperbaric oxygen therapy indications*, ed 12, Durham, NC, 2008, Undersea and Hyperbaric Medical Society.

Gordillo GM, Sen CK: Revisiting the essential role of oxygen in wound healing, *Am J Surg* 186(3):259, 2003.

Gottlieb SF, Neubauer RA: Multiple sclerosis: its etiology, pathogenesis, and therapeutics with emphasis on the controversial use of HBO, *J Hyperbaric Med* 3(3):43, 1988.

Hammarlund C: The physiologic effects of hyperbaric oxygen. In Kindwall EP, editor: *Hyperbaric medicine practice*, Flagstaff, Ariz., 1995, Best.

Hart GB: The monoplace chamber. In Kindwall EP, editor: *Hyperbaric medicine practice*, Flagstaff, Ariz., 1995, Best.

Heimbach RD: Physiology and pharmacology of HBO_2. In Jefferson C, editor: *Davis Wound Care and Hyperbaric Medicine Center [Course]*, San Antonio, Texas, March 4, 1998, Hyperbaric Medicine Team Training, Southwest Texas Methodist Hospital and Nix Medical Center.

Heng MCY et al: Angiogenesis in necrotic ulcers treated with hyperbaric oxygen, *Ostomy Wound Manage* 46(9):18-32, 2000a.

Heng MCY et al: Enhanced healing and cost effectiveness of low pressure oxygen therapy in healing necrotic wounds: a feasibility study of technology transfer, *Ostomy Wound Manage* 46(3):52-62, 2000b.

Hopf HW et al: Guidelines for the treatment of arterial insufficiency ulcers, *Wound Repair Regen* 14(6):693-710, 2006.

Hughes AJ et al: Hyperbaric oxygen in the treatment of refractory haemorrhagic cystitis, *Bone Marrow Transplant* 22(6):585, 1998.

Ishihara H et al: Prediction of neurologic outcome in patients with spinal cord injury by using hyperbaric oxygen therapy, *J Orthop Sci* 6(5):385, 2001.

Jordan WC: The effectiveness of intermittent hyperbaric oxygen in relieving drug-induced HIV-associated neuropathy, *J Natl Med Assoc* 90(6):355, 1998.

Kalliainen LK et al: Topical oxygen as an adjunct to wound healing: a clinical case series, *Pathophysiology* 9(2):81-87, 2003.

Kidder TM: Myringotomy. In Kindwall EP, editor: *Hyperbaric medicine practice*, Flagstaff, Ariz., 1995, Best.

Kindwall EP: A history of hyperbaric medicine. In Kindwall EP, editor: *Hyperbaric medicine practice*, Flagstaff, Ariz., 1995, Best.

Laden G: HOT MI pilot study: hyperbaric oxygen and thrombolysis in myocardial infarction, *Am Heart J* 136(4 Pt 1):749, 1998.

Larson-Lohr V, Norvell H, editors: *Hyperbaric nursing*, Flagstaff, Ariz., 2002, Best.

Maki RD: Ophthalmic side effects of hyperbaric oxygen therapy, *Insight* 21(4):114, 1996.

Marx RE: Radiation injury to tissue. In Kindwall EP, editor: *Hyperbaric medicine practice*, Flagstaff, Ariz., 1995, Best.

Mayer R et al: Hyperbaric oxygen—an effective tool to treat radiation morbidity in prostate cancer, *Radiother Oncol* 61(2):151, 2001.

Mychaskiw G et al: In vitro effects of hyperbaric oxygen on sickle cell morphology, *J Clin Anesth* 13(4):255, 2001.

National Fire Protection Association: *NFPA 99: standard for health care facilities*, Quincy, Mass., 2002, Author.

Neubauer R: Hyperbaric oxygen therapy beats carbon monoxide poisoning, decompression sickness, broken bones, gangrene, multiple sclerosis, severe burns, *Bottom Line/Health* 12(5):13, 1998.

Nighoghossian N, Trouillas P: Hyperbaric oxygen in the treatment of the acute ischemic stroke: an unsettled issue, *J Neurol Sci* 150(1):27, 1997.

Norgren L et al: Inter-Society Consensus for the Management of Peripheral Arterial Disease (TASC II), *J Vasc Surg* 45(Suppl S): S5-S67, 2007.

Pascual J: Hyperbaric oxygen and relief of migraine and cluster headache, *J Neurosci* 27(4):261, 1995.

Reillo MR, Altieri RJ: HIV antiviral effects of hyperbaric oxygen therapy, *J Assoc Nurses AIDS Care* 7(1):43, 1996.

Robson MC et al: Guidelines for the treatment of venous ulcers, *Wound Repair Regen* 14(6):649-662, 2006.

Sheffield PJ, Desautels DA: Hyperbaric and hypobaric chamber fires: a 73-year analysis, *Undersea Hyperb Med* 24(3): 153-164, 1997.

Steed DL et al: Guidelines for the treatment of diabetic ulcers, Wound Rep Reg 14(6):680-692, 2006

Undersea and Hyperbaric Medical Society (UHMS): *Hyperbaric oxygen therapy: a committee report*, Kensington, Md., 1996. Author.

Undersea and Hyperbaric Medical Society (UHMS): *About the UHMS*, available at http://www.uhms.org/AboutUHMS/tabid/90/Default.aspx, accessed August 22, 2010.

Undersea and Hyperbaric Medical Society (UHMS): Indications for hyperbaric oxygen therapy. http://www.uhms.org/Default.aspx?tabid=270, accessed August 22, 2010.

Vrabec JT et al: Short-term tympanostomy in conjunction with hyperbaric oxygen therapy, *Laryngoscope* 108(8):1124, 1998.

Wallace DJ et al: Use of hyperbaric oxygen in rheumatic diseases: case report and critical analysis, *Lupus* 4(3):172, 1995.

Weaver LK, Straas MB, editors: *Monoplace hyperbaric chamber safety guidelines: report to the Hyperbaric Chamber Safety Committee of the Undersea and Hyperbaric Medical Society*, Kensington, Md., 1991, UHMS.

Wound, Ostomy and Continence Nurses (WOCN) Society: *Guideline for management of patients with lower extremity neuropathic disease*, WOCN clinical practice guideline series #1, Glenview IL, 2004.

Wound, Ostomy and Continence Nurses (WOCN) Society: *Guideline for management of patients with lower extremity arterial disease*, WOCN clinical practice guideline series #1, Glenview IL, 2008.

Wound, Ostomy and Continence Nurses (WOCN) Society: Guideline for the prevention and management of pressure ulcers, WOCN clinical practice guideline series #2, Glenview IL, 2010.

23

Electrical Stimulation

Rita A. Frantz

OBJECTIVES

1. Explain the physiologic effects of electrical stimulation.
2. List at least two indications for electrical stimulation.
3. List at least two contraindications for electrical stimulation.

Electrical stimulation is a physical wound care modality that uses the transfer of electrical current to tissues to support wound healing. Devices used for wound healing applications consist of a source of electrical current, a minimum of two wires or leads, and their corresponding electrodes (Figure 23-1). One lead is connected to the negative jack of the device and is the source of negatively charged electrons in an electrical circuit; this is referred to as the *cathode*. The other is connected to a positive jack on the device that serves as an electron depository for the flow of electrons in the electrical circuit; this is called the *anode*. Electrodes are attached to the patient end of the wires and placed on either the patient's wound bed or the adjacent skin. When the device is operating, a unidirectional current flows through this circuit, causing positively charged ions (Na^+, K^+, H^+) in the tissues and positively charged cells (activated neutrophils and fibroblasts) to migrate toward the cathode; negatively charged ions (Cl^-, $HCO_3^-P^-$ and negatively charged cells (epidermal, neutrophils, and macrophages) migrate toward the anode. To understand the basis of electrical stimulation as an adjunctive therapy for wounds, it is important to understand several terms. Table 23-1 provides definitions of relevant terms.

EFFECTS OF ELECTRICAL STIMULATION

In an effort to examine the entire body of evidence on electrical stimulation and chronic wound healing, Gardner et al (1999) conducted a meta-analysis of 15 studies that assessed the efficacy of electrical stimulation. Studies included in the meta-analysis were limited to randomized controlled trials (n = 9) and nonrandom controlled trials (n = 6). Meta-analysis procedures were applied to a total of 24 electrical stimulation samples (n = 591 wounds) and 15 control samples wounds (n = 212). The calculated average rate of healing for the electrical stimulation samples was 22% per week compared to 9% for the control samples. The net effect of electrical stimulation therapy was 13% per week, a 144% increase over the control rate. These data provide substantive evidence that electrical stimulation can produce substantial improvement in the healing of chronic wounds. The physiologic effects of electrical stimulation that contribute to its wound healing efficacy include galvanotaxic, stimulatory, antibacterial, blood flow, and tissue oxygenation.

The underlying physiologic effects of electrical stimulation are mediated by the endogenous bioelectric system in the human body and its response to positive and negative polarity. Several investigators have demonstrated the existence of transepithelial potentials on the skin surface (Barker et al, 1982; Illingsworth and Baker, 1980). These transepithelial potentials arise from Na channels on the mucosal surface of the skin that allow Na to diffuse from the area surrounding epidermal cells to the inside of the cells. As a result of the movement of Na from the skin surface to the interior of epidermal cells, the exterior of the skin maintains a variable level of negative electrical charge (Foulds and Barker, 1983). Jaffe and Vanable (1984) demonstrated that when the epidermis is injured, current flows as ions are transmitted through the tissue fluid between the damaged regions of the epidermis. This "current of injury" has a positive polarity, whereas the adjacent intact skin retains its negative polarity, producing a unidirectional force sufficient to attract reparative cells to the wound bed during the inflammatory and proliferative phases of healing (Vanable, 1989). Once reepithelialization has closed the wound, the current of injury disappears, suggesting that it does not play a role in the remodeling phase of healing. It is important to note that the flow of current out of the wound is blocked if the wound bed is allowed to desiccate and form a scab (Alvarez et al, 1983).

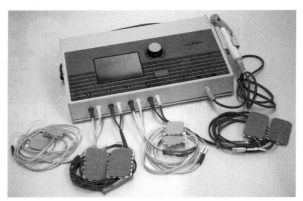

FIGURE 23-1 Example of a high-voltage pulsed current electrical stimulation device. (Courtesy Rich-Mar Corporation, Inola, Okla., USA.)

TABLE 23-1	Terms and Definitions for Electrical Stimulation
Terms	**Definitions**
Alternating current	Uninterrupted, bidirectional current flow
Amperage	Measure of rate of flow of current; expressed as amperes (A), milliamperes (mA), or microamperes (μA)
Amplitude	Maximum (peak) excursion of voltage or current pulse
Charge	Property of matter determined by proportion of electrons (negatively charged particles) contained by the matter; substance may be neutral, positively charged, or negatively charged; measured in units of coulombs (C) or microcoulombs (μC)
Current	Rate of flow of charged particles (ions or electrons); measured in units of amperes (A) or milliamperes (mA)
Direct current	Uninterrupted, unidirectional current flow
Frequency	Number of pulses delivered per unit of time; also termed *pulse rate;* frequency is the reciprocal of cycle time; usually measured as pulses per second (pps) or hertz (Hz); 0.1 Hz is on for 10 seconds, and a pulse of 1,000 Hz is on for 1 ms
Interpulse interval	Time between pulses when no voltage is applied and no current is flowing
Polarity	Property of possessing two oppositely charged electrodes in an electrical circuit (positive and negative); negative electrode (cathode) provides electrons in a circuit; positive electrode (anode) serves as depository to which electrons flow
Pulse duration	Time during which current is flowing
Voltage	Measure of force of flow of electrons through a conductor (wound tissue) between two or more electrodes; created by difference of charges between two electrodes (one with excess in relation to the other); electrodes are polarized in comparison to each other (negative electrode and positive electrode)
Waveform	Graphic representation of current flow; may be monophasic (current that deviates from isoelectric zero line in one direction and then returns to baseline) or biphasic (current that deviates above and below isoelectric zero line); may be symmetrical or asymmetrical

Galvanotaxic Effects

Positively and negatively charged cells are attracted toward an electric field of opposite polarity, a process termed *galvanotaxis*. Multiple in vitro studies have established that cells essential to tissue repair will migrate toward the anode or cathode created by an electric field within a tissue culture (Bourguignon and Bourguignon, 1987; Eberhardt et al, 1986; Orida and Feldman, 1982; Stromberg, 1988). Preliminary evidence from in vivo studies has demonstrated that electrical stimulation creates a similar galvanotaxic response. Eberhardt et al (1986) showed that treating wounds with electrical stimulation for 30 minutes increased the relative number of neutrophils in the wound exudate compared to control wounds. Using the pig model, Mertz et al (1993) treated experimentally induced wounds with two 30-minute sessions of monophasic pulsed current (PC) using varying polarity. They found that wounds initially treated with negative polarity (day 0) followed by positive polarity on days 1 to 7 showed 20% greater epithelialization compared to wounds that received only one type of polarity. In the wounds treated by alternating polarity daily (negative one day, positive the next), epithelialization was limited by 45%. Although the influence of polarity on cell migration in human wounds remains to be elucidated more completely, these findings suggest that bioelectric signals play a role in facilitating the phases of healing.

Stimulatory Effects on Cells

Basic science studies have shown that electrical current has a stimulatory effect on fibroblasts. Using the pig model, Cruz et al (1989) demonstrated the presence of significantly more fibroblasts in burn wounds treated with electrical stimulation than in controls. Alvarez et al (1983), also using the pig model, documented more fibroblasts and increased collagen synthesis in partial-thickness wounds, thus substantiating previous findings. Castillo et al (1995) found significant increases in collagen density with burn wounds in the rat model. The stimulatory effect of electrical current on fibroblasts, reported by Bourguignon and Bourguignon (1987), was observed when fibroblasts in culture increased DNA and protein (including collagen) synthesis in response to electrical stimulation. This effect was most noticeable near the negative electrode.

Blood Flow and Tissue Oxygen Effects

Accumulating evidence indicates that electrical stimulation exerts a positive influence on blood flow and localized tissue oxygen. Hecker et al (1985) showed that negative polarity increased blood flow in the upper extremity as measured by plethysmography. In a sample of patients diagnosed with Raynaud disease and diabetic polyneuropathy, Kaada (1982) demonstrated that application of distant, low-frequency transcutaneous electrical stimulation (TENS) produced pronounced and prolonged cutaneous vasodilation. Using skin temperature as a measurement of peripheral vasodilation, Kaada found a rise in the temperature of ischemic extremities from 71.6°F to 75.2°F (22°C–24°C), to 87.8°F to 93.2°F (31°C–34°C). The latency from stimulus onset to the abrupt rise in temperature averaged 15 to 30 minutes with a duration of response ranging from 4 to 6 hours. Kaada (1983) subsequently reported successful treatment of 10 patients with 19 leg ulcers, previously resistant to treatment, by applying a TENS device to the web space between the first and second metacarpals of the ipsilateral wrist. Using the burst mode, Kaada delivered 15 to 30 mA of pulsed direct current by the cathode for 30 to 34 minutes three times per day. He proposed that the remote application of electrical stimulation enhanced microcirculation in the tissues of the ipsilateral lower extremity, as demonstrated by the increase in toe temperature and ulcer healing. Based on findings from subsequent basic research, Kaada suggested that the improvement in tissue microcirculation was the result of activation of a central serotonergic link that inhibits sympathetic vasoconstriction (Kaada and Helle, 1984; Kaada et al, 1984).

Additional evidence of increased blood flow in wounds treated with electrical stimulation is provided by reports of increasing capillary density following implementation of this therapy. Fifteen venous leg ulcers, previously resistant to healing, were treated for 30 minutes daily for an average of 38 days (Junger et al, 1997). Using light microscopy to measure capillary density, they found densities increased from a prestimulation baseline of 8.05 capillaries/mm^2 to 11.55 capillaries/mm^2 following stimulation ($p < .039$). Transcutaneous oxygen in the periwound skin was noted to increase from 13.5 to 24.7 mm Hg.

Although research on the effects of electrical stimulation on wound oxygenation has been minimal, preliminary studies demonstrate that cutaneous oxygen can be improved with electrical stimulation. In separate studies, investigators showed that application of electrical stimulation improved cutaneous oxygen in the lower extremity of elderly patients, subjects with diabetes, and patients with spinal cord injuries (Gagnier et al, 1988; Peters et al, 1998). These works provide indirect evidence of the potential for electrical stimulation to increase wound oxygenation.

Antibacterial Effects

Evidence indicates that electrical stimulation has bacteriostatic and bactericidal effects on microorganisms that are known to infect chronic wounds (Daeschlein, 2007). In a study of 20 patients with burn wounds that had been unresponsive to conventional therapy for 3 months to 2 years, Fakhri and Amin (1987) showed a quantitatively lower level of organisms after treatment for 10-minute intervals twice weekly. This decrease in bacterial count was accompanied by epithelialization of the wound margins within 3 days of beginning electrical stimulation. Although the mechanism underlying the bactericidal or bacteriostatic effects remain unclear, the galvanotaxic effect on macrophages and neutrophils has been implicated (Eberhardt et al, 1986; Orida and Feldman, 1982). These studies suggest that the anodal attraction of neutrophils to tissue with high bacterial levels may be a primary mode of action, rather than destruction of pathogens by electrolysis or elevation of tissue pH. However, these studies used direct current, which is not as commonly used in wound management as the PC type (see section on types of electrical stimulation). It appears that the voltage required to produce an antibacterial effect with PC would create profound muscle contractions and therefore would not be applicable in clinical practice (Guffey and Asmussen, 1989; Kincaid and Lavoie, 1989; Szuminsky et al, 1994).

INDICATIONS AND CONTRAINDICATIONS

The U.S. Food and Drug Administration (FDA) has not yet approved any type of electrical stimulation device for wound healing. Consequently, devices cannot be marketed for this indication, although they can be marketed for other already approved indications, such as edema and pain, and subsequently used as off-label treatment of wound healing.

Among national guidelines disseminated by professional societies dedicated to wound care, recommendations related to electrical stimulation as therapy for chronic wounds vary considerably. The Wound, Ostomy and Continence Nurses (WOCN) Society reports electrical stimulation as being effective in enhancing the healing of recalcitrant Stage II pressure ulcers and the healing of Stage III and IV pressure ulcers (WOCN Society, 2010). In separate guidelines on treatment of pressure ulcers, diabetic foot ulcers, venous ulcers, and arterial ulcers, the Wound Healing Society states that electrical stimulation may be useful as adjuvant therapy to promote healing, but the society stops short of making specific recommendations for its use (Hopf et al, 2006; Robson et al, 2006; Steed, 2006; Whitney, 2006). Recently released guidelines on pressure ulcer treatment developed collaboratively by the National Pressure Ulcer Advisory Panel (NPUAP) and the European Pressure Ulcer Advisory Panel (EPUAP) report sufficient evidence exists to support the use of electromagnetic agents, including electrical stimulation, in the management of recalcitrant Stage II, as well as Stage III and IV pressure ulcers (NPUAP-EPUAP, 2009).

As is the case with most therapies, certain contraindications apply to use of electrical stimulation (Checklist 23-1). It should not be used when basal or squamous cell carcinoma is suspected in the wound or surrounding tissue, or when osteomyelitis is present. Patients with electronic implants, such as pacemakers, should not be treated with electrical stimulation. Electrical stimulation is also contraindicated for use over the heart or when iodine or silver ion residues are present in the wound.

TYPES OF ELECTRICAL STIMULATION

Although several electrotherapy modalities are cited in the literature, the two basic types of electrical current are direct current and alternating current. In general, alternating current is not used for wound treatment and is not described in this chapter. Direct current (DC) is characterized as a continuous and monophasic (unidirectional) in which the voltage does not vary with time. The parameters used to stimulate wound healing typically are 200 to 300 μA at a low voltage (<100 V). The polarity that is selected determines the direction of current flow delivered to the wound tissue, with positively charged ions migrating toward the negative electrode (cathode) and negatively charged ions migrating toward the positive electrode (anode). Small, older, clinical trials have demonstrated benefits from the use of DC with chronic wounds (Carley and Wainapel, 1985; Gault and Gatens, 1976). However, charged ions of Na^+ and Cl^- in the wound tissue move toward the cathode and anode, respectively, producing a chemical reaction with caustic end-products at the interface of electrode and tissue. In the case of the cathode, Na^+ reacts with H_2O to form NaOH and H_2, whereas the anode reacts with Cl^- and H_2O to form HCl and O_2. Even when DC is delivered at therapeutic doses, these products form at the electrode tissue interface, creating acid–base changes. If the dosage of DC is delivered at high amplitude over an extended period,

the acid–base changes lead to tissue irritation that varies in intensity from erythema to blistering due to electrochemical burning. This side effect can be diminished to some extent by using current amplitudes in the microamperage (μA) range.

PC Electrical Stimulation

Devices used to deliver the DC are also capable of delivering PC, a pattern or flow that has become the predominant type of electrical stimulation used for wound healing. Electrodes placed on the tissues deliver the PC as a series of pulses, with each pulse separated by a period in which no current is flowing. PC can be visually constructed as a waveform that plots amplitude and time.

Waveforms Patterns (Monophasic and Biphasic). Two waveforms patterns are available as PC (Figure 23-2). Monophasic (unidirectional) PC is the movement of current in one direction away from the isoelectric zero line. Monophasic (bidirectional) PC has been applied to clinical treatment of wounds using rectangular waveform (Feedar et al, 1991; Gentzkow et al, 1991, 1993; Junger et al, 1997) and twin-peak waveform of high voltage (Fitzgerald and Newsome, 1993; Griffin et al, 1991; Kloth and Feedar, 1988). Biphasic PC is the movement of current in two directions on either side of the isoelectric zero line. Biphasic PC is configured as charged particles moving above and below the isoelectric zero line in brief succession. The biphasic waveform may be symmetrical or asymmetrical with respect to the isoelectric zero line. The biphasic symmetrical waveform is characterized by amplitude, duration, and rate of rise and decays of current that are identical in relation to the isoelectric zero line. This creates a balanced electrical charge. In contrast, with the biphasic asymmetrical waveform, one or more of these elements of the current are unequal in relation to the isoelectric zero line. This produces waveforms that may be electrically balanced or unbalanced. Both biphasic symmetrical (Baker et al, 1996, 1997; Debreceni et al, 1995) and asymmetrical (Baker et al, 1996, 1997) waveforms have been studied as a modality for promoting wound healing.

Application and Administration Methods. Regardless of the waveform of PC selected for treatment, the electrodes are applied using one of two methods (Baker et al, 1996; Kloth and Feedar, 1988). The first method involves placing one electrode in direct contact with a clean, electrically conductive material (commonly a saline-moistened gauze dressing) that is positioned in the wound, while the second electrode is placed on intact skin approximately 15 to 30 cm from the wound edge. With the second method, the electrodes are positioned on the skin at the wound edges on opposite sides of the wound. The treatment protocol is similar whether the device is a low-voltage or a high-voltage stimulator. The pulse frequency is set to 100 pulses per second, with a current or voltage sufficient to produce a comfortable

---

CHECKLIST 23-1

Contraindications for Electrical Stimulation

- Placement of electrodes tangential to the heart
- Presence of cardiac pacemaker
- Placement of electrodes along regions of phrenic nerve
- Presence of malignancy
- Placement of electrodes over carotid sinus
- Placement of electrodes over laryngeal musculature
- Placement of electrodes over topical substances containing metal ions, exogenous iodine, povidone iodine, or mercurochrome
- Placement of electrodes over osteomyelitis

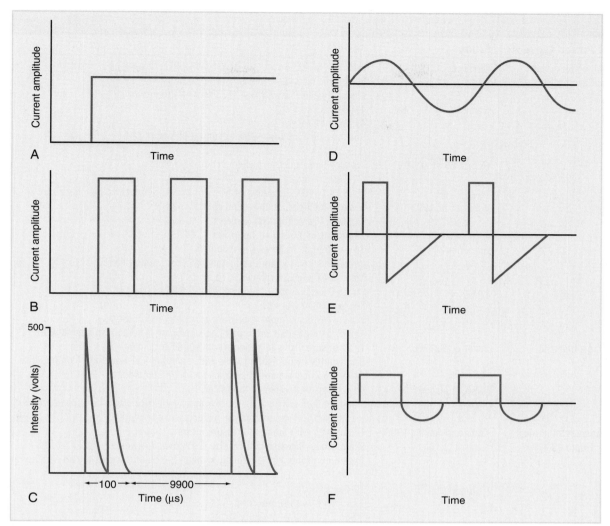

FIGURE 23-2 Waveforms used in electrical stimulation. **A,** Direct current. **B,** Monophasic pulsed current. **C,** Monophasic high-voltage pulsed current. **D,** Symmetrical biphasic pulsed current (balanced). **E,** Asymmetric biphasic pulsed current (balanced). **F,** Asymmetrical biphasic pulsed current (unbalanced). (Modified from Dyson M: Adjuvant therapies: ultrasound, laser therapy, electrical stimulation, hyperbaric oxygen and negative pressure therapy. In: Morison MJ, Ovington LG, editors: *Chronic wound care: a problem-based learning approach*, Edinburgh, Scotland, 2004, Mosby.)

tingling sensation or, in insensate skin, at a level just below the motor threshold (Feedar et al, 1991; Gentzkow et al, 1991, 1993; Griffin et al, 1991; Kloth and Feedar, 1988). The polarity is determined by the status of the wound and the specific cells that are to be targeted for migration into the wound (Bourguignon and Bourguignon, 1987). Treatments are administered for 1 hour, 5 to 7 days per week, and are continued as long as the wound is progressing toward closure.

Research identifies a range of electrical charge that has supported positive wound healing outcomes. This dosage of current, defined in microcoulombs (μC), is between 250 and 500 μC/s (Feedar et al, 1991; Gentzkow et al, 1991, 1993; Griffin et al, 1991; Junger et al, 1997; Kloth and Feedar, 1988). The evolution of electrical stimulation devices led to the evaluation of two different types of PC for treatment of chronic wounds: low-voltage amplitude and high-voltage ampli-

tude. Low-voltage amplitude devices deliver PC with either a monophasic or a biphasic waveform. Their pulse durations are relatively long, so low driving voltages (<150 V) are adequate. High-voltage amplitude devices provide only monophasic PC. Their pulses are of short duration (10–20 μs), so these devices must have a high driving voltage (>150 V). Each voltage type of electrical stimulation devices has been examined in clinical studies of wound healing (Table 23-2).

PAYMENT COVERAGE

Policies related to payment coverage for treatment of chronic wounds with electrical stimulation differ dramatically among third-party payers. In 2002, the Centers for Medicare and Medicaid Services (CMS) approved payment for electrical stimulation when used for treatment of chronic Stage III or Stage IV pressure

TABLE 23-2	Studies Using Pulsed Current Electrical Stimulation of Chronic Wounds	
Type of Pulsed Current	**Study**	**Results**
Low-voltage monophasic Example: Dermapulse®	Feedar et al, 1991	RCT 50 chronic wounds Weekly healing rate 14% vs 8.25% in control group
	Gentzkow et al, 1991	4-week RCT 40 pressure ulcers Healing rate 12.5% vs 5.8% in control group $p = .042$
	Gentzkow et al, 1993	7.3-week, prospective, baseline controlled study 61 pressure ulcers 55 (82%) of 61 showed improvement in two or more wound characteristics
	Wood et al, 1993	8-week, multisite, double-blind clinical trial 74 Stage II and III pressure ulcers 25 healed vs 31 in placebo group
	Junger et al, 1997	38-day trial of 15 venous leg wounds Wound history: 79 months of standard compression therapy Mean area decreased by 63% $(p < .01)$
	Junger et al, 2008	Prospective, placebo-controlled, double-blind study 39 venous leg wounds Wound history: 3 months of standard compression therapy Rapid, lasting reduction in pain, no significant difference in wound size
Low-voltage, biphasic	Baker et al, 1996	185 pressure ulcers in patients with spinal cord injury Significantly faster healing rates with asymmetrical waveform (compared to symmetrical waveform and microcurrent stimulation)
	Baker et al, 1997	80 subjects with diabetic foot ulcers Significantly faster healing rates with asymmetrical waveform (compared to symmetrical waveform and microcurrent stimulation)
High-voltage asymmetrical Example: Figure 23-1	Kloth and Feedar, 1988	16 subjects with Stage IV pressure ulcers Sham group: increase in ulcer size (29% over 7.4 weeks) Treatment group: 100% healing in mean period of 8 weeks (mean healing rate 44.8%)
	Griffin et al, 1991	20-day trial 17 subjects with spinal cord injury Stage II, III, and IV pressure ulcers Significant decrease in wound surface area by days 5, 15, 20 $(p < 0.05)$ vs placebo
	Alon et al, 1986	12 of 15 subjects with diabetic foot ulcers achieved closure in mean period of 2.6 months

RCT, Randomized controlled trial.

ulcers and for wounds of the lower extremity caused by arterial and venous insufficiency and diabetes, if no measurable improvement is evidenced after at least 30 days of standard wound therapy (CMS, 2002). In contrast, a health technology assessment of electrical stimulation as an adjuvant treatment of chronic wounds conducted by Blue Cross Blue Shield Association (Blue Cross Blue Shield, 2005) in April 2005 concluded that the available evidence does not demonstrate convincingly that electrical stimulation results in clinically significant improvement in the most relevant outcome—the percentage of patients whose wounds heal completely.

SUMMARY

The transfer of electrical stimulation to mainstream wound care practice continues to be variable and inconsistent. In addition to the lack of consensus regarding the strength of

evidence supporting the efficacy and payment for electrical stimulation, several system-level factors are barriers to implementation in practice. Many clinicians and wound specialists are unfamiliar with the therapy. Furthermore, many clinical settings do not have personnel with the necessary expertise to administer the treatment. Finally, the FDA has not approved any electrical stimulation device for wound healing (off-label use).

REFERENCES

Alon G et al: Diabetic ulcer healing using high voltage TENS, *Phys Ther* 66:775, 1986 (abstract).

Alvarez OM et al: The healing of superficial skin wounds is stimulated by external electrical current, *J Invest Dermatol* 81(2):144, 1983.

Baker L et al: Effect of electrical stimulation waveform on healing of ulcers in human beings with spinal cord injury, *Wound Rep Regen* 4(1):21, 1996.

Baker L et al: Effects of electrical stimulation on wound healing in patients with diabetic ulcers, *Diabetes Care* 20(3):405, 1997.

Barker A et al: The glabrous epidermis of cavies contains a powerful battery, *Am J Physiol* 11:R358, 1982.

Blue Cross Blue Shield Association: Electrical stimulation or electromagnetic therapy as adjunctive treatments for chronic skin wounds. Chicago IL: Blue Cross Blue Shield Association (BSBC) 2005:31.

Bourguignon G, Bourguignon L: Electric stimulation of protein and DNA synthesis in human fibroblasts, *FASEB J* 1(5):398, 1987.

Carley PJ, Wainapel SF: Electrotherapy for acceleration of wound healing: low intensity direct current, *Arch Phys Med Rehabil* 66(7):443, 1985.

Castillo E et al: The influence of pulsed electrical stimulation on the wound healing of burned rat skin, *Arch Med Res* 26(2):185, 1995.

Center for Medicare and Medicaid Services (CMS): *Medicare coverage issues manual (Transmittal 161)*, November 8, 2002, available at http://www.cms.gov/transmittals/downloads/R161C1M.pdf

Cruz N, Bayron F, Suarez A: Accelerated healing of full-thickness burns by the use of high-voltage pulsed galvanic stimulation in the pig, *Ann Plast Surg* 23(1):49, 1989.

Daeschlein G: Antibacterial activity of positive and negative polarity low-voltage pulsed current (LVPC) on six typical Gram-positive and Gram-negative bacterial pathogens of chronic wounds, *Wound Rep Regen* 15(3):399, 2007.

Debreceni L et al: Results of transcutaneous electrical stimulation (TNS) in cure of lower extremity arterial disease, *Angiology* 46(7):613, 1995.

Dyson M: Adjuvant therapies: ultrasound, laser therapy, electrical stimulation, hyperbaric oxygen and negative pressure therapy. In Morison MJ, Ovington LG, editors: *Chronic wound care: a problem-based learning approach*, Edinburgh, Scotland, 2004, Mosby.

Eberhardt A et al: Effect of transcutaneous electrostimulation on the cell composition of skin exudate, *Acta Physiol Pol* 37(1):41, 1986.

Fakhri O, Amin M: The effect of low-voltage electric therapy on the healing of resistant skin burns, *J Burn Care Res* 8(1):15, 1987.

Feedar J et al: Chronic dermal ulcer healing enhanced with monophasic pulsed electrical stimulation, *Phys Ther* 71(9):639, 1991.

Fitzgerald GK, Newsome D: Treatment of a large infected thoracic spine wound using high voltage pulsed monophasic current, *Phys Ther* 73(6):355, 1993.

Foulds I, Barker A: Human skin battery potentials and their possible role in wound healing, *Br J Dermatol* 109:515, 1983.

Gagnier KA et al: The effects of electrical stimulation on cutaneous oxygen supply in paraplegics, *Phys Ther* 68(5):835, 1988 (abstract).

Gardner S et al: The effect of electrical stimulation on chronic wound healing: a meta analysis, *Wound Rep Regen* 7(6):495, 1999.

Gault W, Gatens P: Use of low intensity direct current in management of ischemic skin ulcers, *Phys Ther* 56(3):265, 1976.

Gentzkow GD et al: Improved healing of pressure ulcers using Dermapulse®, a new electrical stimulation device, *Wounds* 3(5):158, 1991.

Gentzkow GD et al: Healing of refractory Stage III and IV pressure ulcers by a new electrical stimulation device, *Wounds* 5(3):160, 1993.

Griffin J et al: Efficacy of high voltage pulsed current for healing of pressure ulcers in patients with spinal cord injury, *Phys Ther* 71(6):433, 1991.

Guffey JS, Asmussen MD: In vitro bactericidal effects of high voltage pulsed current versus direct current against *Staphylococcus aureus*, *J Clin Electrophysiol* 1(1):5, 1989.

Hecker B et al: Pulsed galvanic stimulation: effects of current frequency and polarity on blood flow in healthy subjects, *Arch Phys Med Rehabil* 66(6):369, 1985.

Hopf HW, et al: Guidelines for the treatment of arterial insufficiency ulcers, *Wound Rep Regen* 14(6):693, 2006.

Illingsworth CM, Barker AT: Measurement of electrical currents emerging during the regeneration of amputated finger tips in children, *Clin Phys Physiol Meas* 1:87, 1980.

Jaffe L, Vanable J: Electric fields and wound healing, *Clin Dermatol* 2(3):34, 1984.

Junger M et al: [Treatment of venous ulcers with low-frequency pulsed current (Dermapulse): effect on cutaneous microcirculation], *Hautarzt* 48(12):879, 1997.

Junger M et al: Local therapy and treatment costs of chronic, venous leg ulcers with electrical stimulation (Dermapule®): a prospective, placebo controlled, double blind trial, *Wound Rep Regen* 16(4):480, 2008.

Kaada B: Vasodilation induced by transcutaneous nerve stimulation in peripheral ischemia (Raynaud's phenomenon and diabetic polyneuropathy), *Eur Heart J* 3(4):303, 1982.

Kaada B: Promoted healing of chronic ulceration by transcutaneous nerve stimulation (TNS), *VASA* 12(3):262, 1983.

Kaada B, Helle K: In search of mediators of skin vasodilation induced by transcutaneous nerve stimulation: IV. In vitro bioassay of the vasoinhibitory activity of sera from patients suffering from peripheral ischaemia, *Gen Pharmacol* 15(2):115, 1984.

Kaada B et al: Failure to influence the VIP level in the cerebrospinal fluid by transcutaneous nerve stimulation in humans, *Gen Pharmacol* 15(6):563, 1984.

Kincaid C, Lavoie K: Inhibition of bacterial growth in vitro following stimulation with high voltage, monophasic, pulsed current, *Phys Ther* 69(8):651, 1989.

Kloth L, Feedar J: Acceleration of wound healing with high voltage, monophasic, pulsed current, *Phys Ther* 68(4):503, 1988.

Mertz PM et al: Electrical stimulation: acceleration of soft tissue repair by varying the polarity, *Wounds* 5(3):153, 1993.

National Pressure Ulcer Advisory Panel (NPUAP) and European Pressure Ulcer Advisory Panel (EPUAP): *Prevention and treatment of pressure ulcers*, Washington, DC, 2009, National Pressure Ulcer Advisory Panel.

Orida N, Feldman J: Directional protrusive pseudopodial activity and motility in macrophages induced by extracellular electric fields, *Cell Motil* 2:243, 1982.

Peters EJG et al: The benefit of electrical stimulation to enhance perfusion in persons with diabetes mellitus, *J Foot Ankle Surg* 37(5):396, 1998.

Robson MC et al: Guidelines for the treatment of venous ulcers, *Wound Rep Regen* 14(6):649, 2006.

Steed DL: Guidelines for treatment of diabetic ulcers, *Wound Rep Regen* 14(6):680, 2006.

Stromberg BV: Effects of electrical currents on wound contraction, *Ann Plast Surg* 21(2):121, 1988.

Szuminsky NJ et al: Effect of narrow, pulsed high voltages on bacterial viability, *Phys Ther* 74(7):660, 1994.

Vanable JW Jr: Integumentary potentials and wound healing. In Borgan RB, et al, editors: *Electric fields in vertebrate repair*. New York, 1989, Alan R. Liss.

Whitney J: Guidelines for treatment of pressure ulcers, *Wound Rep Regen* 14(6):663, 2006.

Wound, Ostomy and Continence Nurses Society (WOCN Society): *Guideline for the prevention and management of pressure ulcers*, WOCN clinical practice guideline series #2, Glenview, IL, 2010.

Wood J et al: A multicenter study on the use of pulsed low-intensity direct current for healing chronic Stage II and Stage III decubitus ulcers, *Arch Dermatol* 129(8):199, 1993.

24

Ultraviolet Light and Ultrasound

Renee Cordrey

1. List at least one indication each for ultraviolet-C, high-frequency ultrasound, and low-frequency ultrasound use.

2. List at least two contraindications for each modality.
3. Explain the mechanism of action for each modality.

The use of physical agents can support wound healing through mechanical action or by their effect on tissue function. Common modalities include ultraviolet (UV) light and ultrasound. Each of these tools offers parameter options that have different impacts. Selective use of these devices may reduce wound bioburden, facilitate wound debridement, or speed granulation and reepithelialization.

ULTRAVIOLET LIGHT

UV light is a simple-to-use modality that may be a valuable tool in addressing wound bioburden, especially in this era of resistant organisms. Specialized lamps generate UV light. Hot quartz mercury vapor lamps produce UV-A and UV-B. Cold quartz lamps create UV-C. These lamps are generally easier to use, and treatment may be started immediately, without a warm-up or cool-down period (Figure 24-1).

UV light consists of the portion of the electromagnetic spectrum that is at a higher frequency than visible light. The wavelength ranges from 320 to 400 nm for UV-A, 290 to 320 nm for UV-B, and 185 to 290 nm for UV-C. UV light has long been used for treatment of many skin conditions, including psoriasis (Kirke et al, 2007; Lapidoth et al, 2007) and acne vulgaris. In recent decades, usage for those conditions has declined due to the advent of more topical and systemic treatments and the increased awareness of the potential damage from UV radiation. However, UV-C has seen a resurgence in the care of chronic wounds.

Physiologic Effects

UV light does not heat tissue. Instead, it is believed to alter cellular function, increase cell wall permeability through altering the shape of proteins, stimulate production of

various chemicals such as prostaglandins and arachidonic acid, and increase the production of adenosine triphosphate (Camp et al, 1978). The erythema that results increases local vasodilation, tissue oxygenation, and histamine release. Earlier studies using high doses of UV report increases in epithelialization and epithelial cell turnover (Freytes et al, 1965; Wills et al, 1983), increased granulation tissue growth and tissue perfusion at lower doses (Ramsay and Challoner, 1976), stimulated growth factor release (James et al, 1991), and increased autolysis (Kloth, 1995). However, these older studies used a different standard of care for comparison than exists today. Therefore, whether UV enhances wound healing in conjunction with advanced wound healing approaches is not known.

Each form of UV has different effects on tissue. UV-A and UV-B are nonionizing. They are both found environmentally, as they pass through the atmosphere. UV-A produces a mild erythema, whereas UV-B elicits a stronger erythematous response while it penetrates the epidermis. The impact of UV-A can be increased with the use of oral psoralens, a photosensitizing agent, before treatment. UV-A penetrates several millimeters into the skin, the deepest of the three forms. UV-B produces hyperplasia of the dermis and stratum corneum 3 days after treatment and has been used to toughen scars (Parrish et al, 1981).

UV-C is mutagenic but is not linked to skin cancers for several reasons: (1) UV-C only penetrates the most superficial layers of the epidermis; (2) the superficial layers of epidermis are sloughed often enough to prevent development of neoplasms; and (3) naturally occurring UV-C is blocked by the atmosphere before it reaches the earth's surface. However, as wound treatment exposes the more permanent healing tissue, and not the epidermis, to UV-C radiation, the long-term cancer risk is unknown. UV-C is recognized to be germicidal, which has come to be the primary use for UV treatment.

Copyright © 2011, Elsevier Inc.

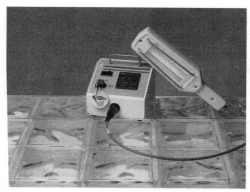

FIGURE 24-1 Ultraviolet light. (Courtesy National Biological Corporation, Twinsburg, Ohio, USA.)

Other evidence suggests that UV-C can increase epithelialization, increase epithelial cell turnover (Freytes et al, 1965), increase granulation tissue growth and tissue perfusion at lower doses (Ramsay and Challoner, 1976), stimulate growth factor release (James et al, 1991), and increase autolysis (Kloth, 1995; Spielholz and Kloth, 2000).

The bacteriocidal effects of UV have been recognized for more than a century (Gates, 1928). UV-C has been demonstrated to kill methicillin-resistant *Staphylococcus aureus* (MRSA) and vancomycin-resistant enterococcus (VRE) in vitro in 90 seconds (Conner-Kerr et al, 1999). The mechanism of action is theorized to be inhibition of DNA synthesis (Hall and Mount, 1981). Another in vitro study (Sheldon et al, 2005) found MRSA eradication with use of UV-C, with an even greater impact on *Pseudomonas*. A case series by Thai et al (2002) demonstrated reduced bacterial counts and more rapid healing with UV-C use, although treatment was not standardized and there was no control, which limit the ability to connect use of UV to the improvements observed. Thai et al (2005) later studied the effect of one 180-second UV-C treatment session on semiquantitative swab culture results of 22 patients whose chronic ulcers contained high levels of bacteria and exhibited signs of infection. Types of wounds included pressure, venous, diabetic, and arterial etiologies. Results showed a statistically significant reduction of the predominant bacteria and significant reductions of MRSA and *S. aureus*.

Indications and Use

Because of its antimicrobial effects, UV-C is sometimes used in operating rooms in place of laminar flow to reduce surgical infections (Ritter et al, 2007). Following a systemic review, Reddy et al (2008) did not recommend UV treatment of pressure ulcers. However, international guidelines for treatment of pressure ulcers (EPUAP-NPUAP, 2009) advocate the consideration of UV-C treatment in the short term for pressure ulcers that do not respond to traditional therapies or as adjunctive therapy

to reduce bioburden in clean, critically colonized Stage III and IV pressure ulcers. Pressure ulcer guideline recommendations related to UV are based on expert opinion and small in vitro and in vivo studies (Conner-Kerr et al, 1998, 1999; Thai et al, 2005). The guideline further states that UV should not be used in the absence of additional appropriate therapies due to insufficient evidence to draw definitive conclusions (EPUAP-NPUAP, 2009).

A common protocol involves the application of petrolatum to the periwound and a towel or sheet drape to the surrounding areas to prevent UV absorption. Limited evidence supports periwound UV treatment for promoting wound closure. The lamp is kept 1 inch from the wound, perpendicular to the skin surface. Treatment is provided for 90 to 120 seconds. Treatment should be discontinued when the bioburden is adequately reduced. Both the patient and the clinician must wear UV-blocking eye protection. Even if a person does not look directly at the light, the waves may bounce off surfaces and reflect into the eye, causing damage.

Contraindications and Precautions

Safe and effective dosage of UV-C may vary based on the distance from the light source, the intensity of the light source, and the size of the treated area. UV-C has a very low risk of causing burns. Contraindications, precautions, and conditions that can be exacerbated by UV treatment (especially with UV-A or UV-B over large areas of the body) vary according to the source (Box 24-1). Conditions and medications requiring the clinician to use caution when applying UV treatment are listed in Box 24-2 (Cameron, 2008; Michlovitz and Nolan, 2005).

BOX 24-1   Contraindications and Conditions Exacerbated by Ultraviolet (UV) Light Therapy

Absolute Contraindications
- History of skin cancer
- Systemic lupus erythematosus
- Fever
- Radiation therapy anywhere on body within previous 3 months
- Sarcoidosis
- Treatment over eye
- Presence of erythema from last UV treatment

Conditions That Can Be Exacerbated by UV Treatment (Especially UV-A or UV-B Over Large Areas of Body)
- Pulmonary tuberculosis
- Cardiac disease
- Renal disease
- Hepatic disease
- Human immunodeficiency virus/acquired immunodeficiency syndrome
- Hyperthyroidism
- Diabetes
- Herpes simplex infection

- Acute eczema or dermatitis
- Radiation therapy more than 3 months earlier
- Photosensitivity
- Human immunodeficiency virus/acquired immunodeficiency syndrome
- Use of photosensitizing medication (may shorten treatment time or preclude treatment altogether)
  - Psoralens (intentionally given to increase susceptibility to UV-A)
  - Tetracycline
  - Sulfonamides
  - Quinolones
  - Gold medications for rheumatoid arthritis
  - Thiazide diuretics
  - Diphenhydramine
  - Oral contraceptives
  - Phenothiazines

ULTRASOUND

Ultrasound is a term used to describe sound waves greater than 20,000 Hz, the upper limit of human hearing. Three forms of ultrasound are commonly used: 1–3.3 MHz, 40 kHz, and 25 kHz. Each has distinct uses.

Traditional High-Frequency Ultrasound (1.0–3.3 MHz)

Traditional clinical therapeutic applications use a frequency of 1 or 3.3 MHz. The user may elect to use a duty cycle. This parameter results in pulsing of the current, with periods of wave production followed by quiet periods. A 20% duty cycle is most commonly used, in which the sound waves are on for 1 ms and then off for 4 ms. Heat is produced but is dispersed so quickly that no temperature change occurs in the tissue. Ultrasound has been used to promote soft tissue healing for more than 6 decades, primarily for orthopedic conditions. More recently, that use has extended to wound healing.

An ultrasound device consists of the control unit and the hand-held sound head, or *transducer* (Figure 24-2). The user is able to control the intensity (amount of power used), whether the waves are continuous or pulsed, the duration of treatment, and, on some units, the wavelength. The device runs electricity through a crystal in the sound head, causing the crystal to vibrate through a reverse piezoelectric effect. These vibrations create sound waves that pass through the sound head membrane and into the tissue. These waves elicit both thermal and nonthermal effects.

Physiologic Effects. Nonthermal effects are attributed to cavitation and acoustic microstreaming. Stable cavitation is the vibration of tiny bubbles within the

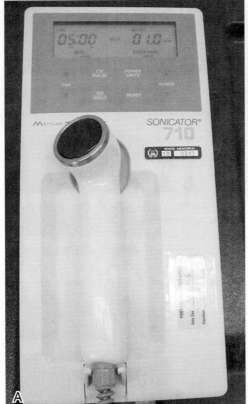
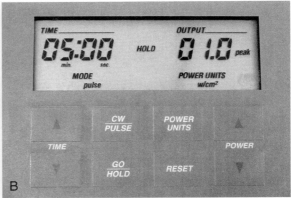

FIGURE 24-2 A, Ultrasound device. **B,** Close-up of ultrasound parameter settings. (Courtesy Renee Cordrey.)

interstitial spaces. With microstreaming, current eddies form around gas bubbles that are near vibrating particles. In addition, streaming stimulates the movement of fluid within and between cells. Some investigators believe that using ultrasound in a water bath stimulates wound debridement through acoustic streaming of the water itself. These nonthermal effects occur with pulsed and continuous ultrasound. The resulting forces stimulate an inflammatory response in wounds (Young and Dyson, 1990a). Pulsed ultrasound has been shown to stimulate fibroblast proliferation and macrophage phagocytic activity in vitro (Young & Dyson, 1990b; Zhou et al, 2004, 2008). However, peak benefit occurred after 20 minutes of treatment, which is longer than is usually acceptable by the clinician providing the treatment. Other effects of ultrasound include leukocyte adhesion, and increased fibrinolysis, permeability of cell membranes and skin, mast cell degranulation, and production of growth factors and nitric oxide (Ennis et al, 2007; Stanisic et al, 2005; Young and Dyson, 1990b).

The thermal effects of continuous ultrasound stimulate an increase in local circulation that disperses heat and increases cell metabolism (Taskan et al, 1997). Increases in macrophage activity, protein synthesis by fibroblasts, and angiogenesis occur (Young & Dyson, 1990a). As a result, wounds may progress through the inflammatory phase more quickly (Demir et al, 2004), or acute inflammation may be reinitiated if healing has stalled. Other work has found increased tensile strength and collagen deposition after ultrasound treatments (Byl et al, 1993; Demir et al, 2004).

Protocol and Clinical Application. Based on theory and in vitro research, ultrasound should have a significant impact on wound healing. However, in the more complex in vivo environment, this expectation has not borne out. Treatment time and sound head movement pattern have not always been modified appropriately to accommodate wound size and the effective radiating area of the transducer. Ultrasound treatment is commonly combined with other modalities, which also may influence study results. Robertson and Baker (2001) identified eight randomized clinical trials addressing ultrasound. Seven of the studies were rejected because of inadequate controls, inadequate analysis, inadequate treatment details, insufficient sample size, or use of multiple interventions. More current studies continue to omit full descriptions of parameters and technique. Therefore, no standard protocol for ultrasound exists and its application to clinical practice is difficult.

In general, low-intensity ultrasound has ranged from 0.1 to 0.3 W/cm^2, medium-intensity ultrasound from 0.3 to 1.2 W/cm^2, and high-intensity ultrasound from 1.2 to 3.0 W/cm^2. Time of treatment varies from 1 to 10 minutes, and transducer frequency has run between 0.3 and 3 MHz. Frequency of treatment has ranged between 1 and 5 days per week, and treatment duration has ranged from 2 weeks through wound closure. Most of these studies used periwound techniques, although Peschen et al (1997) used a water immersion technique. Most studies used pulsed ultrasound, possibly because of the risks of thermal heating in a person with sensory, vascular, or cognitive compromise.

Indications. International pressure ulcer guidelines recommend considering the use of high-frequency ultrasound as an adjunct for treatment of infected pressure ulcers. This recommendation is based on expert opinion and a randomized study conducted in 1985 of 40 patients with Stage I and II pressure ulcers (EPUAP-NPUAP, 2009; McDiarmid et al, 1985). Other than for treatment of infection, pressure ulcer research on high-frequency ultrasound points to a lack of benefit. Two randomized controlled trials demonstrated no difference in healing rates (McDiarmid et al, 1985; ter Reit et al, 1996). A meta-analysis combining the two studies strengthened that conclusion with a stronger sample size (Flemming and Cullum, 2001). Although some trials did show a small improvement in the ultrasound group, the sample sizes were too small to reach statistical significance. Selkowitz et al (2002) conducted a single-subject baseline–ultrasound–sham trial on a Stage III coccyx ulcer using low-intensity pulsed ultrasound. The baseline period had the greatest healing rate and the sham the poorest, although this result may be attributed to natural variation as a wound heals. The Cochrane Library review of ultrasound for pressure ulcers concluded that there was no evidence supporting the efficacy of ultrasound (Baba-Akbari Sari et al, 2006). The WOCN reports similar conclusions (WOCN, 2010).

Outcomes of venous ulcers have been largely inconclusive, often lacking statistical significance, although they do trend toward effectiveness (Al-Kurdi et al, 2008; Flemming and Cullum, 2001; Robson, 2006; Wound, Ostomy and Continence Nurses [WOCN] Society, 2005). Several studies using both high-intensity and low-intensity pulsed ultrasound have found no significant difference in the percentage of wounds that closed during the treatment period compared to sham treatment (Eriksson et al, 1991; Luckstead and Coursey, 1995). Studies that showed improvement with ultrasound lacked sufficient description of the baseline data to properly evaluate the results, had poor follow-up, or had significant differences between groups (e.g., wound size) that could lead to the differences in findings (Johannsen, 1998; Peschen et al, 1997). Taradaj et al (2008) found that patients with venous ulcers healed equally well with compression plus venous surgery, pulsed ultrasound, or both compared to compression alone. However, patients had self-selected into the surgery or nonsurgery group, and the ultrasound was delivered in a warm water bath with the leg in a dependent position. Both of these factors could alter the findings.

Contraindications and Precautions. The sound head must be kept in constant motion. If the sound head stays in place for even 0.1 ms, standing waves and banding may occur. A *standing wave* occurs when the sound wave reflects off tissue back onto itself. The resulting interference wave is twice as strong as the original wave, which increases tissue heating and potentially leads to burning. *Banding* is the separation of cells and plasma within the blood vessels. This action causes irreversible damage to the endothelial linings of the vessel walls.

Contraindications are related to the thermal and non-thermal effects of ultrasound. Ultrasound must not be used over the eyes, the heart, the carotid sinuses, a pregnant uterus, or the exposed central nervous system (e.g., over a laminectomy site). The inflammatory and metabolic effects of ultrasound contraindicate its use in situations where they would be harmful, such as areas of active bleeding, active infection, over breast or other silicone implants, over malignancies, and in the presence of thrombophlebitis. Ultrasound should not be used over pacemakers, active epiphyseal plates, the reproductive organs, or orthopedic cement or plastic components (because the increased reflection of sound waves overheats local tissue).

A lower-intensity nonthermal setting should be used with wounds on a limb with arterial insufficiency because heat dispersion is compromised and the increased metabolic demands cannot be met. Results from a small clinical trial involving patients with ischemic wounds revealed a statistically significant improvement in partial wound healing after 12 weeks of treatment with low frequency ultrasound (Kavros et al, 2007). However, because of insufficient studies, the Wound Healing Society stipulates thermal ultrasound is contraindicated in ischemic areas and is not recommended for treatment of arterial ulcers (Hopf et al, 2006).

The clinician must exercise good judgment when deciding whether to use ultrasound. Ultrasound may often be used in the presence of a contraindication if the treatment location is remote to the site of contraindication. For example, ultrasound may be used on a foot wound despite the presence of a cardiac pacemaker, total hip replacement, or pregnancy because of the localized effects of ultrasound. Caution should be used around superficial bones because periosteum heats and burns easily from reflection off the bone. The clinician should be especially vigilant when thermal ultrasound is used in a person with sensory or cognitive deficits because the patient is not able to provide feedback relating to tissue heating. Ultrasound may be used with caution in an area of acute inflammation if the benefits outweigh the risks of increasing inflammation.

Noncontact Low-Frequency Ultrasound (40 kHz)

A new ultrasound technique has become available. Low-frequency ultrasound, also called *acoustic pressure therapy* or *noncontact kilohertz ultrasound,* is a noncontact method (Figures 24-3 and 24-4). Low-frequency ultrasound has been found to have two primary benefits: wound size reduction and bioburden reduction (Ennis et al, 2007;

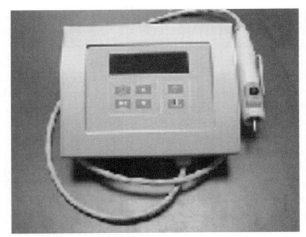

FIGURE 24-3 Ultrasound MIST control unit. (Courtesy Celleration, Eden Prairie, Minn., USA.)

Kavros and Schenck, 2007; Lai and Pittelkow, 2007). The device vaporizes saline into microdroplets (60 μm), which are then propelled to the wound bed via 40-kHz ultrasonic waves, with an intensity of 1.5 W/cm². Microstreaming and cavitation, which are thought to be the primary sources of any healing impact from ultrasound, are more common with kilohertz ultrasound (Ennis et al, 2007; Kavros and Schenck, 2007).

Because low-frequency ultrasound is a relatively new modality, published evidence is limited. Two studies conducted with a proprietary ultrasound device (MIST, Celleration, Eden Prairie, Minn., USA) demonstrated increased venous insufficiency ulcer closure with 30-kHz ultrasound at 0.1 W/cm² (Peschen et al, 1997; Weichenthal et al, 1997). One randomized, double-blind trial of 55 patients with diabetic foot wounds showed a 40.3% closure rate with low-frequency ultrasound compared to 13.3% with standard wound care (*p* = .0366). One retrospective study by Bell and Cavorsi (2008) found improvements in granulation tissue percentage, periwound maceration, and exudates volume after initiating low-frequency ultrasound treatments in mixed chronic

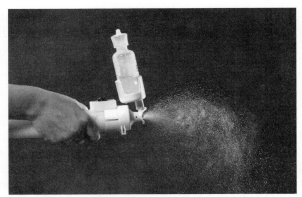

FIGURE 24-4 Demonstration of saline vaporized into microdroplets using the ultrasound MIST handset. (Courtesy Celleration, Inc., Eden Prairie, Minn., USA.)

wounds. Conversely, two studies conducted by Ennis et al (2005, 2006) reported adverse events when low-frequency ultrasound was used on diabetic foot ulcers (pain, erythema, blister, edema, ulcer enlargement) and no statistically significant improvement in 29 chronic lower extremity wounds of various etiologies.

International pressure ulcer guidelines, however, recommend considering the use of noncontact low-frequency (40-kHz) ultrasound spray for treatment of clean recalcitrant Stage III and IV pressure ulcers. These recommendations are based on expert opinion and previously reported studies (EPUAP-NPUAP, 2009). The limited number of controlled clinical trials on human chronic ulcers led Ramundo and Gray (2008) to conclude that low-frequency ultrasound may be beneficial at removing necrotic tissue, but the evidence still is inconclusive.

Ultrasonic Low-Frequency Debridement (22.5, 25, 35 kHz)

The third form of ultrasound is ultrasonic debridement. Use of this approach has been reported in the literature as pilot studies or case reports of effective removal of debris in a contaminated wound or necrosis in chronic leg ulcers (Breuing et al, 2005; King et al, 1996; McDonald and Nichter, 1994; Tan et al, 2007). At kilohertz frequencies, ultrasound is effective at fibrinolysis of the wound surface without causing damage to underlying granulation tissue (Stanisic et al, 2005). Softer fibrinous slough with a higher water content has been reported as being more responsive to ultrasonic debridement compared to drier, tougher fibrinous tissue (Tan et al, 2007).

A variety of probes are available, selected according to the wound surface to be treated. Saline is dripped over the end of the probe as it moves across the wound bed, with 25-kHz ultrasound generating fine gas-filled bubbles that pass to the wound. Unstable cavitation results in destruction of the bubbles at the wound surface, supporting debridement. Although the ultrasound intensity can be adjusted and the treatment often is painless or minimally pain-inducing, some patients may benefit from a topical anesthetic or pain medication before treatment. International pressure ulcer guidelines recommend considering the use of low-frequency ultrasound for debridement of soft necrotic tissue (not eschar) (EPUAP-NPUAP, 2009).

SUMMARY

UV and ultrasound therapies have long been in existence and used for wound healing, with varying results. Well-controlled human clinical trials are needed to further define the mechanism of action and efficacy of these therapies. As we learn more about how these modalities affect the healing process, these classic tools have the potential to become important additions to the arsenal of wound interventions.

REFERENCES

Al-Kurdi D et al: Therapeutic ultrasound for venous leg ulcers, *Cochrane Database Syst Rev* 1:CD001180, 2008.

Baba-Akbari Sari A et al: Therapeutic ultrasound for pressure ulcers, *Cochrane Database Syst Rev* 3:CD001275, 2006.

Bell AL, Cavorsi J: Noncontact ultrasound therapy for adjunctive treatment of nonhealing wounds: retrospective analysis, *Phys Ther* 88:1517-1524, 2008.

Breuing KH et al: Early experience using low-frequency ultrasound in chronic wounds, *Ann Plast Surg* 55(2):183-187, 2005.

Byl N et al: Incisional wound healing: a controlled study of low and high dose ultrasound, *J Ortho Sports Ther* 18(5):619, 1993.

Cameron MH: *Physical agents in rehabilitation: from research to practice*, ed 3, Philadelphia, 2008, WB Saunders.

Camp RD et al: Irradiation of human skin by short wavelength ultraviolet radiation (100–290 nm) (u.V.C): increased concentrations of arachidonic acid and prostaglandines E2 and F2alpha, *Br J Clin Pharmacol* 6(2):145, 1978.

Conner-Kerr TA et al: The effects of ultraviolet radiation on antibiotic-resistant bacteria in vitro, *Ostomy Wound Manage* 44(10):50, 1998.

Conner-Kerr TA et al: UVC reduces antibiotic-resistant bacterial numbers in living tissue, *Ostomy Wound Manage* 45(4):84, 1999.

Demir H et al: Comparison of the effects of laser and ultrasound treatments on experimental wound healing in rats, *J Rehabil Res Dev* 41(5):721, 2004.

Ennis WJ et al: Ultrasound therapy for recalcitrant diabetic foot ulcers: results of a randomized, double-blind, controlled, multicenter study, *Ostomy Wound Manage* 51(8):24-39, 2005.

Ennis WJ et al: Evaluation of clinical effectiveness of MIST ultrasound therapy for the healing of chronic wounds, *Adv Skin Wound Care* 19(8):437-446, 2006.

Ennis WJ et al: A biochemical approach to wound healing through the use of modalities, *Clin Dermatol* 25:63-72, 2007.

Ericksson S et al: A placebo controlled trial of ultrasound therapy in chronic leg ulceration, *Scand J Rehab Med* 23(4):211, 1991.

European Pressure Ulcer Advisory Panel (EPUAP) and National Pressure Ulcer Advisory Panel (NPUAP): *Treatment of pressure ulcers: quick reference guide*, Washington DC, 2009, National Pressure Ulcer Advisory Panel.

Flemming K, Cullum N: Systematic reviews of wound care management: (5) beds; (6) compression; (7) laser therapy, therapeutic ultrasound, electrotherapy and electromagnetic therapy, *Health Tech Assess* 5(9):1, 2001.

Freytes HA et al: Ultraviolet light in the treatment of indolent ulcers, *South Med J* 58:223, 1965.

Gates F: Discussion and correspondence on nuclear derivatives and the lethal action of ultraviolet light, *Science* 68:479, 1928.

Hall JD, Mount DW: Mechanisms of DNA replication and mutagenesis in ultraviolet-irradiated bacteria and mammalian cells, *Prog Nucl Acid Res Mol Biol* 25:53, 1981.

Hopf HW, et al: Guidelines for the treatment of arterial insufficiency ulcers, *Wound Repair Regen* 14:693-710, 2006.

James LV et al: Transforming growth factor alpha: in vivo release by normal human skin following UV irradiation and abrasion, *Skin Pharmacol* 4:61-64, 1991.

Johannsen F AN Gam, et al: Ultrasound therapy in chronic leg ulceration: a meta-analysis, *Wound Repair Regen* 6:121-126, 1998.

Kavros SJ, Schenck EC: Use of noncontact low-frequency ultrasound in the treatment of chronic foot and leg ulcerations: a 51 patient analysis, *J Am Podiatr Med Assoc* 97(2):95-101, 2007.

Kavros SJ et al: Treatment of ischemic wounds with noncontact, low-frequency ultrasound: the Mayo Clinic experience, 2004–2006, *Adv Skin Wound Care* 20(4):221-226, 2007.

King WW et al: Debridement of burn wounds with a surgical ultrasonic aspirator, *Burns* 22(4):307-309, 1996.

Kirke SM et al: A randomized comparison of selective broadband UVB and narrowband UVB in the treatment of psoriasis, *J Invest Dermatol* 127:1641-1646, 2007.

Kloth LC: Physical modalities in wound management: UVC, therapeutic heating and electrical stimulation, *Ostomy Wound Manage* 41(5):18, 1995.

Lai JY, Pittelkow MR: Physiological effects of ultrasound mist on fibroblasts, *Int J Dermatol* 46(6):587-593, 2007.

Lapidoth M et al: Targeted UVB phototherapy for psoriasis: a preliminary study, *Clin Exp Dermatol* 32:642-645, 2007.

Luckstead A, Coursey RD: Consumer perceptions of pressure and force in psychiatric treatments, *Psychiatr Serv* 46:146, 1995.

McDiarmid T et al: Ultrasound and the treatment of pressure sores, *Physiotherapy* 71:66, 1985.

McDonald WS, Nichter LS: Debridement of bacterial and particulate-contaminated wounds, *Ann Plast Surg* 33(2):142-147, 1994.

Michlovitz SL, Nolan TP Jr: *Modalities for therapeutic intervention*, ed 4, Philadelphia, 2005, FA Davis.

Parrish JA et al: Cumulative effects of repeated subthreshold doses of ultraviolet radiation, *J Invest Dermatol* 76(5):356, 1981.

Peschen M et al: Low-frequency ultrasound treatment of chronic venous leg ulcers in an outpatient therapy, *Acta Derm Venereol* 77(4):311, 1997.

Ramsay CA, Challoner AV: Vascular changes in human skin after ultraviolet irradiation, *Br J Dermatol* 94(5):487, 1976.

Ramundo J, Gray M: Is ultrasonic mist therapy effective for debriding chronic wounds? *J Wound Ostomy Continence Nurs* 35(6):579-583, 2008.

Reddy et al: Treatment of pressure ulcers: a systematic review, *JAMA* 300(22):2647-2662, 2008.

Ritter MA et al: Ultraviolet lighting during orthopaedic surgery and the rate of infection, *J Bone Joint Surg* 89:1935-1940, 2007.

Robertson VJ, Baker KG: A review of therapeutic ultrasound: effectiveness studies, *Phys Ther* 81(7):1339, 2001.

Robson MC: Guidelines for the treatment of venous ulcers, *Wound Repair Regen* 14:649-662, 2006.

Selkowitz DM et al: Efficacy of pulsed low-intensity ultrasound in wound healing: a single-case design, *Ostomy Wound Manage* 48(4):40, 2002.

Sheldon JL et al: The effects of salt concentration and growth phase on MRSA solar and germicidal ultraviolet radiation resistance, *Ostomy Wound Manage* 51(1):36, 2005.

Spielholz NI, Kloth LC: Electrical stimulation and pulsed electromagnetic energy: differences in opinion, *Ostomy Wound Manage* 46(5):8, 2000.

Stanisic MM et al: Wound debridement with 25 kHz ultrasound, *Adv Skin Wound Care* 18(9):484-490, 2005.

Tan J et al: A painless method of ultrasonically assisted debridement of chronic leg ulcers: a pilot study, *Eur J Vasc Endovasc Surg* 33:234-238, 2007.

Taradaj J et al: The use of therapeutic ultrasound in venous leg ulcer: a randomized, controlled clinical trial, *Phlebology* 23:178-183, 2008.

Taskan I et al: A comparative study of the effect of ultrasound and electrostimulation on wound healing in rats, *Plast Reconstr Surg* 100(4):966, 1997.

Thai TP et al: Ultraviolet light C in the treatment of chronic wounds with MRSA: a case study, *Ostomy Wound Manage* 48(11):52, 2002.

Thai TP et al: Effect of ultraviolet light C on bacterial colonization in chronic wounds, *Ostomy Wound Manage* 51(10):32, 2005.

ter Reit G et al: A randomized clinical trial of ultrasound in the treatment of pressure ulcers, *Phys Ther* 76(12):1301, 1996.

Weichenthal M et al: Low-frequency ultrasound treatment of chronic venous ulcers, *Wound Rep Regen* 5(1):18, 1997.

Wills EE et al: A randomized placebo-controlled trial of ultraviolet light in the treatment of superficial pressure sores, *J Am Geriatr Soc* 31(3):131, 1983.

Wound, Ostomy and Continence Nurses (WOCN) Society: *Guideline for management of patients with lower extremity venous disease*, WOCN clinical practice guideline series #1, Glenview IL, 2005.

Wound, Ostomy and Continence Nurses (WOCN) Society: *Guideline for the prevention and management of pressure ulcers*, WOCN clinical practice guideline series #2, Glenview IL, 2010.

Young S, Dyson M: Effect of therapeutic ultrasound on the healing of full-thickness excised lesions, *Ultrasonics* 28:175, 1990a.

Young S, Dyson M: Macrophage responsiveness to therapeutic ultrasound, *Ultrasound Med Biol* 16:809, 1990b.

Zhou S et al: Molecular mechanisms of low intensity pulsed ultrasound in human skin fibroblasts, *J Biol Chem* 279(52):544639, 2004.

Zhou S et al: Low intensity pulsed ultrasound accelerates macrophage phagocytosis by a pathway that requires actin polymerization, Rho, and src/MAPKs activity, *Cell Signal* 20:695-704, 2008.

Critical Cofactors

25

Wound Pain: Impact and Assessment

Diane L. Krasner

OBJECTIVES

1. Describe the different types of pain experienced by the patient with a wound.
2. Describe the physiologic effect of pain.
3. List the indicators of pain in the conscious and unconscious patient.
4. Describe two methods for assessing wound pain.
5. Identify the common and unique features of three wound pain models.
6. Discuss the effects of wound pain on quality of life.

General pain concepts, as well as wound pain-specific concepts, guidelines, and research are essential underpinnings for all wound care clinicians because painful wounds are so ubiquitous. McCaffery first defined pain in 1972 in her pioneering nursing research in this field as "whatever the experiencing person says it is and exists whenever he says it does" (McCaffery and Pasero, 1999). Today this definition poses a clinical dilemma in the case where an individual is unable to communicate (e.g., patient with severe dementia) and is not able to verbalize his or her pain. However, the inability to communicate verbally does not negate the possibility that an individual is experiencing pain and is in need of appropriate pain-relieving treatment (European Wound Management Association [EWMA], 2002; World Union of Wound Healing Societies [WUWHS], 2004). With McCaffery as co-chair, the International Association for the Study of Pain (IASP) and the American Pain Society (APS) subsequently redefined pain as "an unpleasant sensory and emotional experience associated with actual or potential tissue damage, or described in terms of such damage" (McCaffery and Pasero, 1999). The National Advisory Council on Aging (2002) describes pain management as "the elimination or control of pain, with a goal of restoring comfort, quality of life, and the capacity to function as well as possible given individual circumstances and the source of pain."

This chapter discusses pain-related concepts, perception, and consequences of wound pain as well as physiology, classification, assessment of pain, and an introduction to wound models. Chapter 26 provides a detailed discussion of pain management.

PERCEPTIONS ABOUT PAIN

A patient's expectation of pain can be largely dependent on his or her cultural and ethnic background, social support system, medical history, and prior pain experience (Morris, 1991). When a patient cannot communicate in the language of the care provider, effective management of his or her pain becomes more difficult and often leads to undertreatment. Erroneous assumptions and perceptions on the part of the provider about pain tolerance based on traits such as age, gender or ethnic background, can result in inadequate analgesia (Lasch, 2002). However, studies indicate that when patients control their own analgesia (e.g., with patient-controlled analgesia pumps), patients self-administer similar doses for similar injuries independent of race or cultural background. Health care providers must be aware of obstacles such as language and cultural barriers and use more care and time in assessing and treating such patients. Interventions that alter a patient's expectation of pain may positively affect the pain experienced by that patient.

A long-held myth in wound care is that venous ulcers and pressure ulcers are not painful. Ironically, in a study of patients with venous ulcers, patients often did not request pain medication because they expected their wounds to be painful (Krasner, 1997). Therefore health care professionals often do not even assess for venous ulcer pain, which then contributes to the undertreatment of venous ulcer pain. In a study conducted by Dallam et al (1995) involving 132 patients with pressure ulcers, 68% reported some type of wound pain, yet only

2% were given analgesics for pressure ulcer pain within 4 hours of pain measurement.

In a 2008 review of the literature on pain with pressure ulcers, reported pain prevalence ranged from 37% to 100%, and ulcer stage was reported to most consistently affect pain (Girouard et al, 2008). In 2009, the National Pressure Ulcer Advisory Panel (NPUAP) published a systematic literature review and white paper on pressure ulcer pain advocating the importance of pressure ulcer pain and the need for further research in all populations across all settings (Pieper et al, 2009).

In a qualitative study of nurses providing care to patients with a pressure ulcer who experienced pain, nurse generalists and advanced practice nurses were asked to reflect and write a story about the phenomenon of caring for the patient with wound pain (Krasner, 1996). Text analysis of the reflections from the 42 participants revealed three patterns of responses by the caregivers. By examining and understanding these patterns of response and the examples of behaviors relative to each response, valuable insight can be gained into the delivery of more sensitive care that is patient focused rather than wound focused.

The first pattern of response is described as "nursing expertly." With this type of response, the nurse uses a set of skills and behaviors that make a qualitative difference in the patient's care. Skills commonly used include (1) read the pain, (2) attend to the pain, and (3) acknowledge the presence of or potential for pain (i.e., empathize with the patient). "Reading" the pain is a critical aspect of assessing for the presence of pain that extends beyond simply asking patients if they are experiencing pain. It is the recognition of signs associated with pain, such as increased anxiety, sweating, bulging eyes, increased respirations, and exaggerated movement in bed. Unfortunately, these signs are easily overlooked by the caregiver when the patient is nonverbal. Attending to the pain indicates that the nurse has taken steps to control pain with medications, positioning, distraction, and so on. Acknowledging the presence of pain or the potential for an intervention or procedure to trigger pain demonstrates empathy for the patient and creates an opportunity to discuss the nature of the pain and identify strategies to minimize or relieve the pain. Empathic care for the patient with pain is demonstrated by using a slower pace in performing procedures, conducting dressing changes in a gentle fashion, allowing short "breaks" during painful procedures, providing careful explanations for every step of the procedure, providing words of encouragement, and offering a menu of pain control interventions.

The second pattern of caregiver response reported in the study is to actually "deny the pain." In this type of response, the caregiver essentially fails to recognize or treat pain and leaves the patient to deal with the pain alone. Ultimately, to "deny the pain" is associated with the care provider who is trying to cope with personally uncomfortable situations, such as those in which the provider feels powerless, feels as though nothing else can be done to ameliorate the patient's pain, or feels that the situation is "not the best" but is acceptable and somewhat expected. Three key behaviors exhibited by the nurse are typical of this pattern of response. (1) Assuming pain does not exist. This behavior is common, along with the erroneous but previously held belief that venous and pressure ulcers are not painful despite the twinges of pain or other verbal or nonverbal signs the patient would manifest. (2) Ignoring the patient's cries of pain. This behavior could be characteristic of situations where the patient continues to report the presence of pain with a dressing change or sharp debridement despite the analgesic given. (3) Avoidance of personal failure. This behavior is characterized by the nurse who simply avoids interacting with the patient or limits the extent of contact with the patient because the patient continues to experience discomfort and all possible interventions for this patient have been exhausted.

The third and final pattern of response observed by this group of nurses was to "confront the challenge of pain" as exemplified by coping with the frustrations and "being with" the patient. A central benefit to this type of response by the nurse is the insight gained into the meaning of the pain experience to the patient. For example, the challenge of the pain may be triggered more by anxiety rather than pain. This insight then can be used to develop a more individualized plan of care. A hermeneutic phenomenologic study by Kohr and Gibson (2008) suggests that although nurses want to do the right thing and protect the patient from physical and psychic wound pain, many barriers to optimal pain management exist.

CONSEQUENCES OF WOUND PAIN

Wound pain negatively affects quality of life and impacts physiologic processes, including oxygenation and infection control. Unfortunately, many patients with a wound suffer these negative consequences because undertreatment of patients with chronic wound pain is far too common.

Quality of Life

Chronic pain has been well documented to affect a patient's physical, psychological, and spiritual well-being and social concerns. Patients experience lack of sleep, fatigue, anxiety, depression, and fear of future pain. Chronic pain increases caregiver burden and greatly affects roles and relationships (Ferrell, 2005). Patients with wounds are at high risk for acute and chronic pain that tends to be moderately severe to severe in intensity. Uncontrolled pain is considered the most significant predictor of impaired quality of life (Dallam et al, 1995; Szor and Bourguignon, 1999). Pressure ulcer pain, specifically, affects activities of daily living because the pain could limit the patient's mobility and ability to reposition, thus increasing the risk for wound deterioration (Popescu and Salcido, 2004).

Specific to venous ulcer pain, Hofman et al (1997) found that for 69% of the patients in their study, pain was "the worst thing about having an ulcer," disrupting sleep and negatively affecting quality of life. Previous studies reported similar findings in patients with venous ulcers (Phillips et al, 1994; Walshe, 1995). Using a Heideggerian hermeneutic phenomenologic approach, Krasner (1997, 1998a, 1998b) described the experience of patients with venous ulcer pain. The common pattern that emerged from the study was "carrying on despite the pain." Eight themes provide a glimpse at the impact of venous ulcer pain on quality of life and activities of daily living were identified (Box 25-1).

Physiologic

Wound pain that is inadequately treated can lead to poor wound healing and increased infection rates. These negative sequelae occur first because pain impedes the patient's ability to tolerate wound care and second because pain may cause or worsen wound hypoxia. Poor pain control impedes the care provider's ability to cleanse, dress, and debride the wound, all of which are required for healing. When pain is poorly controlled, patients frequently refuse debridement and cleansing and postpone needed dressing changes. These factors increase the risk of infection and allow wounds to stagnate.

Acute pain increases circulating catecholamines, including epinephrine and, leads to peripheral vasoconstriction, decreased perfusion of blood to the skin and extremities, and, consequently, reduced oxygen availability in the tissues (Franz et al, 2008). As tissue oxygen decreases, leukocyte activity is progressively impaired so that bacteria have a greater likelihood of remaining viable and cause wound infections (Hopf and Holm, 2008). To function properly (i.e., to remove cellular debris and kill bacteria in the wound), leukocytes require oxygen. A major mechanism by which leukocytes kill bacteria is oxidative bacterial killing. The membrane-bound enzyme phagosomal oxygenase or primary oxidase converts oxygen to superoxide, which itself is bactericidal. Superoxide is then converted to multiple other bactericidal oxidants within the phagosome, including hydrogen peroxide, hypochlorite (bleach), and hydroxyl radical (Allen et al, 1997). An hypoxic wound environment will further impair wound healing by disrupting fibroblast activity and angiogenesis, thereby impacting negatively on collagen synthesis and migration and the delivery of oxygen to the wound cells.

PAIN PHYSIOLOGY

Although pain is a subjective experience, objective physiologic mechanisms control how pain is initiated, transmitted, and perceived. The objective neural response to a painful stimulus (e.g., at the wound) is called *nociception*. Nociception is defined as the detection of impending or actual tissue damage and is accomplished by specialized sensory nerve terminals (nociceptors) derived from Aδ (delta) and C fibers. All nerve endings in the epidermis are considered nociceptors (Popescu and Salcido, 2004). When cells are damaged, chemicals are released, triggering the nerve fibers to transmit the pain impulses along nerve sheaths to the spinal cord. The spinal cord transmits the information to the brain, where it is centrally processed. Synaptic junctions in the spinal cord and brain will either attenuate or amplify the pain signal and thus affect how the intensity of the pain signal will be perceived or interpreted.

In addition to the actual tissue injury that triggers the pain episode, psychological, physical, emotional, and cultural factors as well as the patient's expectations collectively define an individual's pain experience. Thus the same type of injury in two different individuals often generates a very different pain experience in terms of severity, quality, and impact (Turk, 1993). Reported pain may appear to be either less than expected or excessive given the degree of tissue injury. Distress out of proportion to the injury is often ascribed to anxiety as well as "catastrophizing" (Sullivan and Neish, 1999; Sullivan et al, 1998).

Catastrophizing is significantly correlated with mood and personality variables such as depression, fear of pain, coping strategies, and state and trait anxiety (Rosenstiel and Keefe, 1983; Sullivan et al, 1995). These variables have been shown to be important predictors of the pain experience. Preoperative levels of anxiety and catastrophizing can be predictive of postoperative pain intensity. A study by Granot and Ferber (2005) found that moderately anxious surgical patients are at greater risk for developing greater postoperative pain.

BOX 25-1	"Carrying on Despite the Pain": Eight Themes

Key Themes
Responses
- Expecting pain with the ulcer
- Feeling frustrated

Practical Knowledge
- Swelling = pain
- Not standing

Common Experiences
- Interfering with the job
- Starting pain all over again: painful debridements

Shared Meanings
- Having to make significant life changes
- Finding satisfaction in new activities

From Krasner D: *Carrying on despite the pain: living with painful venous ulcers: a Heideggerian hermeneutic analysis* (doctoral dissertation), Ann Arbor, Mich., 1997, University of Michigan.

CLASSIFICATIONS

Types of pain may vary by wound type and underlying etiology. For example, pain associated with lower extremity wounds can be related to claudication, to nocturnal or rest pain from ischemia (arterial disease) or increased edema (venous), to neuropathy (neuropathic). The types of pain typical of lower extremity ulcers (i.e., arterial, venous, neuropathic) are described in the lower extremity wounds section of this text.

Before initiating pain management interventions (either pharmacologic or nonpharmacologic), the type of wound pain that is being experienced and the source of that pain must be determined. Interventions then can be tailored to the patient's needs and effective outcomes achieved. Pain experts categorize pain into two types: nociceptive and neuropathic.

Nociceptive (Acute) Pain

Nociceptive pain, also referred to as *acute pain*, is the normal processing of the pain impulse. It serves to alert the individual to ongoing or impending injury. Acute pain usually is consistent with the degree of tissue injury; hence, greater tissue injury translates into greater pain sensation. Acute pain can be subclassified as operative, procedural, incident, and background pain (Figure 25-1) (World Union of Wound Healing Societies [WUWHS], 2004). Nociceptive pain typically is well localized, constant, and time limited (pain resolves when the painful procedure ends) and often has an aching or throbbing quality.

The persistence of severe, inadequately treated acute pain can lead to anatomic and physiologic changes in the nervous system (Woolf and Salter, 2000). The ability of neural tissue to change in response to repeated incoming stimuli, a property known as *neuroplasticity*, can lead to the development of chronic, disabling neuropathic pain (Cohen et al, 2004). Opioids are commonly used to manage nociceptive pain.

Neuropathic Pain

Neuropathic pain results from damaged or malfunctioning nerve fibers. Nerves can be compressed by a tumor, strangulated by scar tissue, or inflamed by infection. Unlike acute pain, neuropathic pain is not an indication of impending tissue injury; rather, neuropathic pain is an indication that sensory nerves are malfunctioning. Common in chronic wounds, neuropathic pain is often described as burning; it also may have "electric shock-like" qualities.

Neuropathic pain may be visceral or somatic in origin. *Visceral pain* stems from organs or the gastrointestinal tract. Visceral pain is often described as diffuse and gnawing or cramping and poorly localized (Hader and Guy, 2004). The neural signal crosses into the spinal cord at vagal ganglia and at dorsal root ganglia. This type of pain is commonly seen in conjunction with injuries to internal organs, as occurs with appendicitis, myocardial ischemia, pneumonia, or gastric ulcers (Hader and Guy, 2004). *Somatic pain* originates from the bone, joints, muscles, skin, and connective tissue. As with acute pain, somatic pain is described as a throbbing, well-localized pain. The pain sensation from a wound usually is somatic and can be further subdivided according to the source of the pain.

Numerous pathologic responses to pain may be seen and can result from inadequately treated pain, excessive inflammation, and other pathophysiologic processes. Chronic wound pain, as occurs with a pressure or

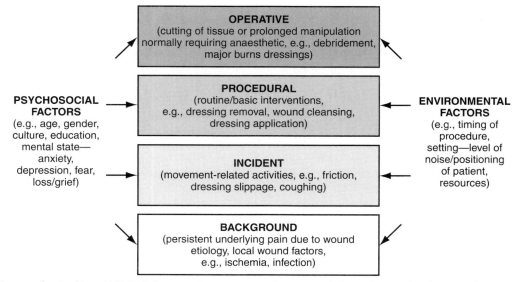

FIGURE 25-1 Causes of pain. (From IASP Task Force on Taxonomy. Merskey H, Bogduk N, editors: *Classification of chronic pain: descriptions of chronic pain syndromes and definitions of pain terms*, ed 2, Seattle, Wash., 1994, IASP Press.)

venous ulcer, is commonly characterized by hyperalgesia (increased response to a normally painful stimulus) and allodynia (pain due to a stimulus that normally does not provoke pain). In the presence of hyperalgesia, any touch to the wound surface or surrounding skin, regardless of how gentle, may be interpreted as painful. Allodynia is present when gentle cleansing of the periwound skin triggers a pain episode. Hyperalgesia and allodynia are responsible for the pain that is "out of proportion" to the stimulus (Popescu and Salcido, 2004). Thus routine dressing changes and periwound skin care become excruciating.

Typically, the pathologic process that initiated the neuropathic pain is not fully reversible. However, with appropriate management of the pathologic process, neuropathic pain can be reduced. Neuropathic pain often responds to antiseizure and antidepressant medications rather than opioids.

Mixed Nociceptive/Neuropathic

Mixed category pain results from a complex mixture of nociceptive and neuropathic factors. Although the nervous system initially may malfunction, tissue injury resulting from this malfunction triggers the release of inflammatory mediators. Venous ulcer pain has been reported to be a combination of nociceptive and neuropathic pain, a finding that has important ramifications for medicating for pain using polypharmacy (Krasner 1997, 1998a, 1998b).

ASSESSMENT

The goal to control wound pain is to reduce or eliminate pain so that patients can resume and perform their activities. In cognitively impaired patients, the goal is to maximize their comfort and enhance their quality of life. A systematic and thorough assessment of wound pain is an essential first step. Most regulatory agencies, such as the Centers for Medicare and Medicaid (CMS), state departments of health, and The Joint Commission require systematic assessment and documentation of pain, pain relief measures, and their efficacy.

The patient's pain experience does not correlate with visible wound manifestations, and there is no direct relationship between pathology and the intensity of pain (Turk, 1993). Although superficial wounds with multiple exposed nerves may be intensely painful (because sensory nerve endings are most numerous in the dermis), some patients may not experience intense pain from these wounds. Conversely, subcutaneous tissue contains few sensory nerves, so deep wounds with destruction of dermis would be expected to be less painful. In fact, necrotic and deep subcutaneous tissues can be debrided many times without application of significant analgesia, whereas debridement of wound edges or debridement that disturbs the wound edges (as occurs when pulling

adherent eschar) may be extremely painful. Consequently, assessment of pain based upon wound depth is not appropriate and may be flawed. In general, wounds become less painful as they begin active healing. The mechanism is not clear but probably involves decreased inflammation, covering of exposed nerve endings, and decreased wound ischemia and hypoxia.

In practice, assessment and documentation of pain are inconsistent. Hollinworth (1995) reported inadequate pain management and poor accountability and inadequate or uninformed assessment, management, and documentation of pain at wound dressing changes. Nurses failed to assess pain verbally or to use pain assessment tools. Instead, pain was assessed based on nurses' experience or on nonverbal patient indicators. In a cross-sectional quantitative study of 132 patients with pressure ulcer pain, Dallam et al (1995) found that 59% reported having pain of some type; however, only 2% were given analgesics for the pain (within 4 hours of interview). In a study of venous ulcer healing and pain in current and former users of injected drugs, researchers found many of these patients were denied adequate pain control based upon their history. Researchers concluded that providers need to listen to patient concerns about pain medication and, with the patient, determine the best medication protocol (Pieper 1994; Pieper et al, 1998).

Many factors must be assessed to adequately manage wound pain: pain history, etiology, condition of the wound, topical wound care, type of pain, and source of wound pain. Pain assessment should include an assessment of body language and nonverbal cues (e.g., change in activity, loss of appetite, guarding, grimacing, moaning) (Feldt, 2000; NPUAP-EPUAP, 2009). Furthermore, because the condition of the wound greatly affects wound pain and the wound condition is frequently changing, pain assessment must be done regularly, with wound manipulations and dressing changes as well as performed on a routine daily basis. Pain is assessed by its type: nociceptive, neuropathic, or intrinsic (chronic noncyclic); procedural (acute noncyclic); or incident (acute cyclic). With this detailed assessment, appropriate pain control measures can be identified.

Pain History

A pain history should provide sufficient detail to characterize the nature of the pain and factors that affect the patient's pain experience. A pain history may be difficult to obtain when the patient is experiencing referred pain or when the pain is nonspecific.

Self-Report Pain Intensity Scales

Self-report is the most reliable indicator of the existence and intensity of acute pain (APS, 2008). Numerous pain assessment tools are available to quantify the severity of pain and measure the effectiveness of pain control interventions. Intensity-of-pain scales range from simple visual analogue scales to complex multidimensional, multipage instruments. For example, visual analogue scales measure only one dimension of the pain phenomenon at a time (e.g., intensity, from "no pain" to "worst possible pain"), using words, numbers, faces, or other culturally congruent objects (e.g., coins or poker chips). Examples of these scales are provided in Figure 25-2. Visual analogue scales are particularly useful in clinical practice for use with patients who are in active pain and do not have the capacity to complete a long, arduous questionnaire. A systematic review of 164 articles found single-item pain intensity ratings to be valid and reliable (Jensen, 2003).

More complex pain assessment tools, such as the McGill Pain Questionnaire (Melzack, 1975), and its modifications, such as the Dartmouth Pain Questionnaire (Corson and Schneider, 1984), measure a quality of the pain experience, such as functional limitation or impact on quality of life, in addition to pain intensity. These descriptive scales are used primarily in clinical research and specialized pain clinics.

Observational Pain Intensity Scales

Nonverbal and cognitively impaired individuals are at risk for poor pain management due to lack of pain assessment. Between 40% and 60% of long-term care residents do not use the analgesics and pain relief medications ordered for them (Horgas and Tsai, 1998; Kaasalainen et al, 1998). Unfortunately, instead of frequently offering *as needed* pain medications, caregivers tend to interpret *as needed* to mean "when the patient asks for it" (Feldt, 2000). Of course, verbalization of pain or requesting pain medication is unlikely to occur in the nonverbal or cognitively impaired patient.

The cognitively impaired individual has difficulty finding the words to describe discomfort or has impaired executive skills, which limits the ability to correlate a number on a pain scale with the sensation of pain or to interpret the "crying face" of a scale as an indication of "severe" pain (Wynne et al, 2000). However, patients manifest several observational behaviors when they are in pain (Weiner et al, 1999).

The Pain Assessment in Advanced Dementia (PAINAD) scale is presented in Table 25-1. Endorsed for use in

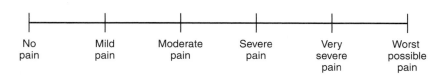

Simple Descriptive Pain Intensity Scale[1]

No pain — Mild pain — Moderate pain — Severe pain — Very severe pain — Worst possible pain

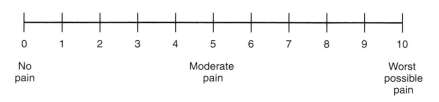

0-10 Numeric Pain Intensity Scale[1]

0 1 2 3 4 5 6 7 8 9 10

No pain — Moderate pain — Worst possible pain

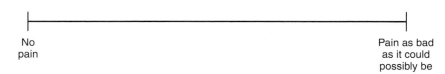

Visual Analog Scale (VAS)[2]

No pain — Pain as bad as it could possibly be

FIGURE 25-2 Three examples of pain intensity scales as published by the Agency for Healthcare Research and Quality. (From Bergstrom N et al: *Treatment of pressure ulcers*, Clinical Practice Guideline #15, AHCPR Publication No. 95-0622, Rockville, Md., 1994, US Department of Health and Human Services, Public Health Service.)

[1] If used as a graphic rating scale, a 10 cm baseline is recommended.

[2] A 10 cm baseline is recommended for VAS scales.

TABLE 25-1	Pain Assessment in Advanced Dementia (PAINAD) Scale			
Items*	0	1	2	Score
Breathing independent of vocalization	Normal	Occasional labored breathing Short period of hyperventilation	Noisy labored breathing Long period of hyperventilation Cheyne-Stokes respirations	
Negative vocalization	None	Occasional moan or groan Low-level speech with a negative or disapproving quality	Repeated troubled calling out Loud moaning or groaning	
Facial expression	Smiling or inexpressive	Sad Frightened Frown	Facial grimacing	
Body language	Relaxed	Tense Distressed pacing Fidgeting	Rigid Fists clenched Knees pulled up Pulling or pushing away Striking out	
Consolability	No need to console	Distracted or reassured	Unable to console, distract, or reassure	
			Total†	

Breathing

1. Normal breathing is characterized by effortless, quiet, rhythmic (smooth) respirations.
2. Occasional labored breathing is characterized by episodic bursts of harsh, difficult, or wearing respirations.
3. Short period of hyperventilation is characterized by intervals of rapid, deep breaths lasting a short time.
4. Noisy labored breathing is characterized by negative sounding respirations on inspiration or expiration. They may be loud, gurgling, or wheezing. They appear strenuous or wearing.
5. Long period of hyperventilation is characterized by an excessive rate and depth of respirations lasting a considerable time.
6. Cheyne-Stokes respirations are characterized by rhythmic waxing and waning of breathing from very deep to shallow respirations with periods of apnea (cessation of breathing).

Negative Vocalization

1. None is characterized by speech or vocalization that has a neutral or pleasant quality.
2. Occasional moan or groan is characterized by mournful or murmuring sounds, wails, or laments. Groaning is characterized by louder than usual inarticulate involuntary sounds, often abruptly beginning and ending.
3. Low-level speech with a negative or disapproving quality is characterized by muttering, mumbling, whining, grumbling, or swearing in a low volume with a complaining, sarcastic, or caustic tone.
4. Repeated troubled calling out is characterized by phrases or words being used over and over in a tone that suggests anxiety, uneasiness, or distress.
5. Loud moaning or groaning is characterized by mournful or murmuring sounds, wails, or laments that are much louder than usual volume. Loud groaning is characterized by louder than usual inarticulate involuntary sounds, often abruptly beginning and ending.
6. Crying is characterized by an utterance of emotion accompanied by tears. There may be sobbing or quiet weeping.

Facial Expression

1. Smiling is characterized by upturned corners of the mouth, brightening of the eyes, and a look of pleasure or contentment. Inexpressive refers to a neutral, at ease, relaxed, or blank look.
2. Sad is characterized by an unhappy, lonesome, sorrowful, or dejected look. There may be tears in the eyes.
3. Frightened is characterized by a look of fear, alarm, or heightened anxiety. Eyes appear wide open.
4. Frown is characterized by a downward turn of the corners of the mouth. Increased facial wrinkling in the forehead and around the mouth may appear.
5. Facial grimacing is characterized by a distorted, distressed look. The brow is more wrinkled, as is the area around the mouth. Eyes may be squeezed shut.

Body Language

1. Relaxed is characterized by a calm, restful, mellow appearance. The person seems to be taking it easy.
2. Tense is characterized by a strained, apprehensive, or worried appearance. The jaw may be clenched (exclude any contractures).
3. Distressed pacing is characterized by activity that seems unsettled. A fearful, worried, or disturbed element may be present. The rate may be faster or slower.
4. Fidgeting is characterized by restless movement. Squirming about or wiggling in the chair may occur. The person might be hitching a chair across the room. Repetitive touching, tugging, or rubbing body parts may be observed.
5. Rigid is characterized by stiffening of the body. The arms and/or legs are tight and inflexible. The trunk may appear straight and unyielding (exclude any contractures).

TABLE 25-1 | **Pain Assessment in Advanced Dementia (PAINAD) Scale—cont'd**

6. Fists clenched is characterized by tightly closed hands. They may be opened and closed repeatedly or held tightly shut.
7. Knees pulled up is characterized by flexing the legs and drawing the knees up toward the chest. An overall troubled appearance may be seen (exclude any contractures).
8. Pulling or pushing away is characterized by resistiveness upon approach or to care. The person may try to escape by yanking or wrenching himself or herself free or shoving you away.
9. Striking out is characterized by hitting, kicking, grabbing, punching, biting, or other form of personal assault.

Consolability
1. No need to console is characterized by a sense of well-being. The person appears content.
2. Distracted or reassured by voice or touch is characterized by a disruption in the behavior when the person is spoken to or is touched. The behavior stops during the period of interaction with no indication that the person is distressed.
3. Unable to console, distract, or reassure is characterized by the inability to soothe the person or stop a behavior with words or actions. No amount of comforting, verbal or physical, will alleviate the behavior.

*See the description of each item in the lower part of the table.
†Total scores range from 0 to 10 (based on a scale from 0 to 2 for five items), with a higher score indicating more severe pain (0 = "no pain" to 10 = "severe pain").
From Warden V et al: Development and psychometric evaluation of the pain assessment in advanced dementia (PAINAD) scale, *J Am Med Dir Assoc* 4:9, 2003, excerpted from Frampton K: Vital sign #5, *Caring for the Ages* 5(5):26, 2004.

long-term care by the American Medical Directors Association (AMDA), the PAINAD scale is an easy-to-use, five-item observational instrument. Items to assess are breathing, negative vocalization, facial expression, body language, and consolability. Each item is rated on a scale from 0 to 2 based on descriptions for each score category. Total scores range from 0 to 10, with a higher score indicating severe pain (Warden et al, 2003).

Options for assessing pain in the nonverbal pediatric patient include the FLACC and CRIES observational scales (Tables 25-2 and 25-3). The FLACC (face, legs, activity, crying, consolability) scale provides a rating between 0 and 10 and was designed and validated for use with children between the ages of 2 months and 7 years. However, some practitioners have used the FLACC scale with adults who are unable to communicate their pain (Merkel et al, 1997). The CRIES (Crying; Requires O_2; Increasing vital signs; Expression; Sleepless) pain scale, originally created to assess postoperative pain in the neonate, is reportedly effective for use in neonates up to age 6 months (Krechel and Bildner, 1995). Each category is scored on a scale from 0 to 2, total scores range between 0 and 10 (Krechel and Bildner, 1995).

WOUND PAIN CARE MODELS

Wound pain care models assist the clinician in addressing pain through every aspect of wound management. The value of these models is that they go beyond simply listing all possible strategies for controlling wound pain. Rather, these models guide the clinician through a logical, systematic, and thorough assessment of the wound (i.e., etiology and related interventions, topical wound condition and the related interventions, and type of pain) so that interventions can be selected based upon the patient's type and source of pain.

TABLE 25-2 | **FLACC Pain Scale for Children 2 Months to 7 years**

Category	Scoring		
	1	*2*	*3*
Face	No particular expression or smile	Occasional grimace or frown, withdrawn, disinterested	Frequent to constant quivering chin, clenched jaw
Legs	Normal position or relaxed	Uneasy, restless, tense	Kicking, or legs drawn up
Activity	Lying quietly, normal position, moves easily	Squirming, shifting back and forth, tense	Arched, rigid or jerking
Cry	No cry (awake or asleep)	Moans or whimpers; occasional complaint	Crying steadily, screams or sobs, frequent complaints
Consolability	Content, relaxed	Reassured by occasional touching, hugging or being talked to, distractible	Difficult to console or comfort

From Merkel S et al: The FLACC: a behavioral scale for scoring postoperative pain in young children, *Pediatr Nurse* 23(3):293-297, 1997.

TABLE 25-3	CRIES Pain Scale for Neonates (0–6 Months)

Crying

0   No crying, or crying but not high pitched
1   High pitched but infant consolable
2   Inconsolable

Requires O$_2$
Babies experiencing pain manifest decreased oxygenation. Consider other causes of
    hypoxemia (e.g., oversedation, atelectasis, pneumothorax).
0   No oxygen required; oxygen saturation >95%
1   ≤30% supplemental oxygen required to keep oxygen saturation >95%
2   >30% supplemental oxygen required to keep oxygen saturation >95%

Increased vital signs
Take BP last because process may awaken the child, making mean assessments difficult.
0   Both HR and mean BP is unchanged or is less than baseline
1   HR or mean BP is increased ≤20% from baseline level
2   HR or BP is increased >20% over baseline level

Expression
Facial expression most often associated with pain is a grimace, which may be characterized by
    brow lowering, eyes squeezed shut, deepening nasolabial furrow, or open lips and mouth.
0   No grimace present
1   Grimace alone is present
2   Grimace and non-cry vocalization grunt is present

Sleepless
Scored based on infant's state during the hour preceding this recorded score.
0   Child has been continuously asleep
1   Child has awakened at frequent intervals
2   Child has been awake constantly

BP, Blood pressure; *HR,* heart rate.
From Krechel SW, Bildner J: CRIES: a new neonatal postoperative pain measurement score-initial testing of validity and reliability, *Paediatr Anaesth* 5:53-61, 1995.

The Chronic Wound Pain Experience (CWPE) model (Krasner, 1995) was empirically and inductively derived. It can be used to assist with establishing a plan of care for pain control (Figure 25-3). The CWPE model introduces a classification scheme tailored specifically to pain associated with wounds:

1. Noncyclical acute wound pain: a single episode of pain (e.g., pain that occurs with sharp debridement)
2. Cyclic acute wound pain: acute wound pain that recurs as a result of repeated treatments (e.g., pain that occurs with dressing changes)
3. Chronic wound pain: persistent, continuous pain that occurs without manipulation of the wound

Each type of pain has a menu of pain control options appropriate for that type of pain. The CWPE model assumes that most patients with chronic wounds experience all three types of pain at some time, although not necessarily simultaneously. It also recognizes that some patients may not experience or may not be able to indicate pain. Others may not experience one of the pain types because of the particular course of their treatment or disease (e.g., the patient who has never had sharp debridement may never experience noncyclical acute wound pain). Another assumption is that many commonly held beliefs about wound pain might lack validity

(e.g., patients with diabetes do not experience wound pain in the presence of neuropathy).

The Wound Associated Pain (WAP) model (Woo and Sibbald, 2009) guides the clinician through the process of addressing underlying causes of the wound and patient-centered concerns, including anxiety and depression, and providing appropriate local wound care as well as systemic strategies that address associated pain. The key components are (1) patient-centered concerns, (2) wound etiology, and (3) local wound factors (Figure 25-4). Authors demonstrated pain reduction after the model was used to manage 111 subjects with chronic leg and foot ulcers. Using an 11-point numerical rating scale, the average level of pain was reduced from 6.3 at week 0 to 2.8 at week 4 (*p* < .001).

The Wound Pain Management (WPM) model was developed by an international advisory panel of eight members in 2003 and updated in 2008. The WPM model guides the clinician in identifying the correct wound diagnosis and related prevention and treatment strategies. Next, the model presents five wound conditions (devitalized tissue, colonization/infection, inflammation, exudate/edema, periwound skin) with corresponding prevention and treatment strategies. Parameters and examples to facilitate a complete pain assessment are then listed. Finally, a menu of local and systemic treatment options is

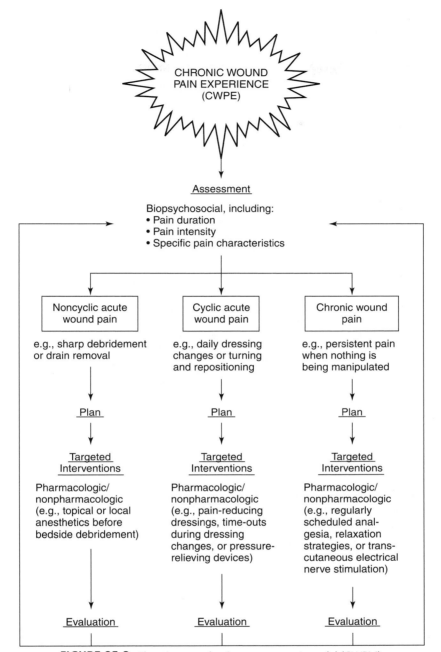

FIGURE 25-3 Chronic wound pain management model (CWPM).

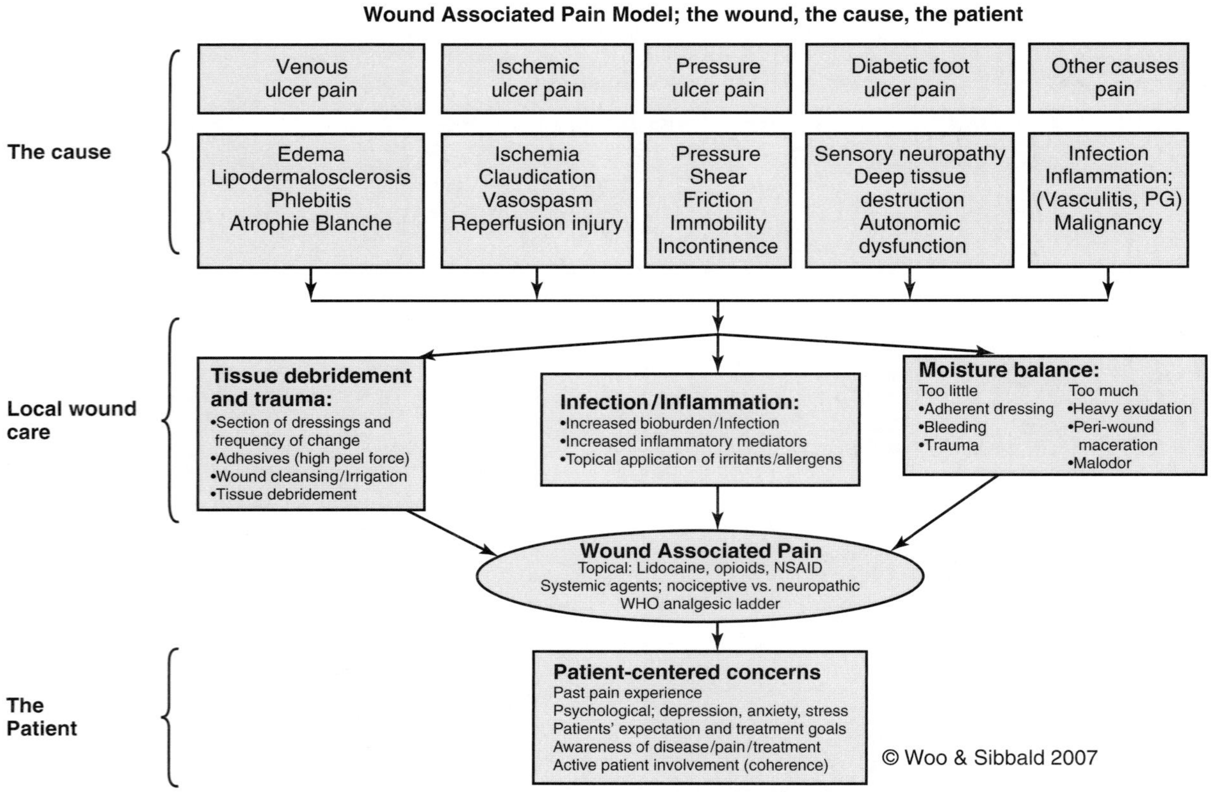

Wound Associated Pain Model; the wound, the cause, the patient

FIGURE 25-4 Wound associated pain model: the wound, the cause, the patient. (From Woo KY, Sibbald RG: The improvement of wound-associated pain and healing trajectory with a comprehensive foot and leg ulcer care model, *J Wound Ostomy Continence Nurs* 36(2):184-191, 2009.)

provided. However, to date this model has not been published in a peer-reviewed journal. It is available online through the manufacturer who supported the project (Fogh et al, 2008).

SUMMARY

Accurately conceptualizing wound pain leads to proficiency in clinical assessment and management of wound pain. Managing wound pain improves patient quality of life and patient satisfaction.

> *To cure—occasionally.*
>
> *To relieve—often.*
>
> *To comfort—always.*
>
> — *Hippocrates*

REFERENCES

Allen DB et al: Wound hypoxia and acidosis limit neutrophil bacterial killing mechanisms, *Arch Surg* 132(9):991, 1997.

American Pain Society (APS): *Principles of analgesic use in the treatment of acute and cancer pain*, ed 5, Glenview, Ill., 2008, Author.

Bergstrom N et al: *Treatment of pressure ulcers*, Clinical Practice Guideline #15, AHCPR Publication No. 95-0622, Rockville,

Md., 1994, US Department of Health and Human Services, Public Health Service.

Cohen SP et al: Pain management in trauma patients, *Am J Phys Med Rehabil* 83:142, 2004.

Corson J, Schneider M: The Dartmouth pain questionnaire: an adjunct to the McGill pain questionnaire, *Pain* 19:59, 1984.

Dallam L et al: Pressure ulcer pain: assessment and quantification, *J Wound Ostomy Continence Nurs* 22(5):211, 1995.

European Wound Management Association (EWMA): *Position document: pain at wound dressing changes*, 2002, Medical Education Partnership, available at http://www.ewma.org, accessed September 25, 2005.

Feldt KS: Improving assessment and treatment of pain in cognitively impaired nursing home residents, *Ann Long-Term Care* 8(9):36, 2000.

Ferrell B: Ethical perspectives on pain and suffering, *Pain Manage Nurs* 6(3):83, 2005.

Fogh K et al: *The Wound Pain Management Model (WPM)*, 2008, available at http://www.woundcare.coloplast.com/EEndCom/Woundcare/Homepage.nsf/0/cf42a4d4bcadb4a4c125740f00425d76/$FILE/Wound%20Pain%20Management%20Model.pdf, accessed January 17, 2010.

Franz MG et al: Guidelines to aid healing of acute wounds by decreasing impediments of healing, *Wound Rep Regen* 16:723-748, 2008.

Girouard K et al: The symptom of pain with pressure ulcers: a review of the literature, *Ostomy Wound Manage* 54(5):30, 2008.

Granot M, Ferber SG: The roles of pain catastrophizing and anxiety in the prediction of postoperative pain intensity: a prospective study, *Clin J Pain* 21:439, 2005.

Hader CF, Guy J: Your hand in pain management, *Nurs Manage* 35(11):21, 2004.

Hofman D et al: Pain in venous leg ulcers, *J Wound Care* 6(5): 222-224, 1997.

Hollinworth H: Nurses' assessment and management of pain at wound dressing changes, *J Wound Care* 4(2):77, 1995.

Hopf HW, Holm J: Hyperoxia and infection, *Best Pract Res Clin Anaesthesiol* 22:553, 2008.

Horgas AL, Tsai PF: Analgesic drug prescription and use in cognitively impaired nursing home residents, *Nurs Res* 47:235, 1998.

IASP Task Force on Taxonomy. Merskey H, Bogduk N, editors: *Classification of chronic pain: descriptions of chronic pain syndromes and definitions of pain terms*, ed 2, Seattle, Wash., 1994, IASP Press.

Jensen MP: The validity and reliability of pain measure in adults with cancer, *J Pain* 4(1):2-21, 2003.

Kaasalainen S et al: Pain and cognitive status in the institutionalized elderly: perceptions & interventions, *J Gerontol Nurs* 24(8): 24-31, 1998.

Kohr R, Gibson M: Doing the right thing: using hermeneutic phenomenology to understand management of wound pain, *Ostomy Wound Manage* 54(4):52, 2008.

Krasner D: The chronic wound pain experience: a conceptual model, *Ostomy Wound Manage* 41(3):20, 1995.

Krasner D: Using a gentler hand: reflections on patients with pressure ulcers who experience pain, *Ostomy Wound Manage* 42(3):20, 1996.

Krasner D: *Carrying on despite the pain: living with painful venous ulcers: a Heideggerian hermeneutic analysis* (doctoral dissertation), Ann Arbor, Mich., 1997, University of Michigan.

Krasner D: Painful venous ulcers: themes and stories about living with the pain and suffering, *J Wound Ostomy Continence Nurs* 25(3):158, 1998a.

Krasner D: Painful venous ulcers: themes and stories about their impact on quality of life, *Ostomy Wound Manage* 44(9):38, 1998b.

Krechel SW, Bildner J: A new neonatal postoperative pain measurement score. Initial testing of validity and reliability, *Paediatr Anaesth* 5:53-61, 1995.

Lasch KE: Culture and pain, *Pain Clin Updates* 10(5), 2002, available at http://www.iasp-pain.org/PCU02-5.html.

McCaffery M, Pasero C: *Pain clinical manual*, ed 2, St Louis, 1999, Mosby.

Merkel SL et al: A behavioral scale for scoring postoperative pain in young children, *Pediatr Nurse* 23(3):293-297, 1997.

Melzack R: The McGill pain questionnaire: major properties and scoring methods, *Pain* 1:277, 1975.

Morris DB: *The culture of pain*, Berkeley, 1991, University of California Press.

National Advisory Council on Aging: Stop the pain. In: *Expression: Bulletin of the National Advisory Council on Aging*, 15(3), 2002.

National Pressure ulcer Advisory Panal (NPUAP) and European Pressure Ulcer Advisory Panal (EPUAP) and prevention and treatment of pressure ulcers. Washington DC: National Pressure Ulcer Advisory Panel; 2009.

Phillips T et al: A study of the impact of leg ulcers on quality of life: financial, social and psychologic implications, *J Am Acad Dermatol* 31(1):49, 1994.

Pieper B: A retrospective analysis of venous ulcer healing in current and former drug users of injected drugs, *J Wound Ostomy Continence Nurs* 23(6):291, 1994.

Pieper B et al: Pain associated with venous ulcers in injecting drug users, *Ostomy Wound Manage* 44(11):54, 1998.

Pieper B et al: Pressure ulcer pain: a systematic literature review and National Pressure Ulcer Advisory Panel white paper, *Ostomy Wound Manage* 55(2):16, 2009.

Popescu A, Salcido RS: Wound pain: a challenge for the patient and the wound care specialist, *Adv Skin Wound Care* 17(1):14, 2004.

Rosenstiel AK, Keefe FJ: The use of coping strategies in chronic low back pain patients: relationship to patient characteristics and current adjustment, *Pain* 17:33, 1983.

Sullivan MJL, Neish N: The effects of disclosure on pain during dental hygiene treatment: the moderating role of catastrophizing, *Pain* 79:155, 1999.

Sullivan MJL et al: The pain catastrophizing scale: development and validation, *Psychol Assess* 7:524, 1995.

Sullivan MJL et al: Catastrophizing, pain, and disability in patients with soft-tissue injuries, *Pain* 77:253, 1998.

Szor JK, Bourguignon C: Description of pressure ulcer pain at rest and at dressing change, *J Wound Ostomy Continence Nurs* 26(3):115, 1999.

Turk DC: Assess the person, not just the pain, *Pain Clinical Updates* 1(3), 1993, available at http://www.iasp-pain.org.

Walshe C: Living with a venous leg ulcer: a descriptive study of patients' experiences, *J Adv Nurs* 22:1092, 1995.

Warden V et al: Development and psychometric evaluation of the pain assessment in advanced dementia (PAINAD) scale, *J Am Med Dir Assoc* 4:9, 2003.

Weiner DK et al: Chronic pain-associated behaviors in the nursing home: resident versus caregiver perception, *Pain* 80:577, 1999.

Woo KY, Sibbald RG: The improvement of wound-associated pain and healing trajectory with a comprehensive foot and leg ulcer care model, *J Wound Ostomy Continence Nurs* 36(2):184-191, 2009.

Woolf CJ, Salter MW: Neuronal plasticity: increasing the gain in pain, *Science* 288:1765, 2000.

World Union of Wound Healing Societies (): Principles of best practice: minimising pain at wound dressing-related procedures. A consensus document, London, 2004, MEP, available at http://www.wuwhs.org/datas/2_1/2/A_consensus_document_-_ Minimising_pain_at_wound_dressing_related_procedures.pdf, accessed January 17, 2010.

Wynne CF et al: Comparison of pain assessment instruments in cognitively intact and cognitively impaired nursing home residents, *Geriatr Nurs* 21:20, 2000.

26

Managing Wound Pain

Harriet W. Hopf, Dag Shapshak, and Scott Junkins

OBJECTIVES

1. State three strategies for managing procedural wound pain.
2. State three strategies for managing nonprocedural wound pain.
3. Describe the pharmacologic options for treating wound pain.

Although not all wounds are painful, in general most acute and chronic wounds cause moderate to severe pain. Management of this pain can be challenging. Given a thoughtful approach and modern pharmacologic and nonpharmacologic interventions, most patients can achieve an acceptable level of pain control. The first step in any patient is identifying and measuring the degree, site, and type of pain; a step that guides the appropriate treatment of pain (see Chapter 25). This chapter presents approaches to preventing and managing acute and chronic wound pain.

NONPHARMACOLOGIC PAIN CONTROL

Many nonpharmacologic pain control measures are essential when caring for a patient with a wound. A simple and effective intervention is acknowledging a patient's pain and making a commitment to the patient to address the pain. Explaining the potential harmful effects of pain on healing, along with a careful explanation of how to manage pain, will help to shape the patient's expectations as well as increase the individual's sense of control. Both of these strategies may reduce the pain experienced (Acute Pain Management Panel [APMP], 1992). Additional interventions related to pain control begin with controlling and reducing procedural pain or cyclic acute pain through appropriate and conscientious topical care.

Wound Cleansing

Avoiding cytotoxic topical agents (e.g., antiseptics, antimicrobials), harsh chemicals, and highly concentrated agents for wound cleansing can significantly reduce wound pain. In general, use of these agents should be avoided unless the wound warrants such intervention (e.g., traumatic wound) and the patient has been adequately anesthetized (van Rijswijk, 1999).

Wound cleansing can also be used as a strategy for reducing wound pain. The buildup of exudate in a wound bed can cause pressure and pain. Pain can be relieved by removing exudate with gentle flushing, low-pressure irrigation, or, in selected patients, cautious use of whirlpool.

Periwound Skin Care

Eroded or denuded wound margins can contribute significantly to the pain experienced by the patient with a wound (National Pressure Ulcer Advisory Panel [NPUAP]-European Pressure Ulcer Advisory Panel [EPUAP], 2009). Use of skin sealants on intact skin can prevent painful denuding of skin or skin stripping. Use of ointments or skin barriers on open areas can prevent and/or minimize the pain secondary to damaged wound margins.

Debridement

Although many factors are considered when a method of debridement is selected, pain is a frequently neglected consideration. Regardless of the method of debridement selected, pain assessment and management must be considered. Wet-to-dry dressing changes for debridement (nonselective and painful) should be avoided. Using autolysis for debridement, when feasible and appropriate, can significantly reduce the pain associated with debridement (NPUAP-EPUAP, 2009; Robson et al, 2006; Whitney et al, 2006).

Conservative or surgical sharp debridement provokes acute noncyclical pain, which leads patients to ask the clinician to stop the debridement unless they are given additional analgesia or anesthesia (Briggs and Nelson, 2003; Evans and Gray, 2005; Hansson et al, 1993). When sharp debridement is indicated, pharmacologic interventions are an important consideration and are described in detail later in this chapter.

Inflammation and Edema

Inflammation and edema contribute to wound pain, so any measures that reduce inflammation and edema likely will provide pain relief. This includes elevation of edematous extremities, appropriate edema-reducing dressings and devices (e.g., compression bandaging and sequential compression pumps), and systemic medications.

Support and Positioning

Binders, splints, body positioners, and other devices that stabilize a wound can significantly reduce pain, especially pain related to mobilization. Care must be taken to fit these devices properly so that the wound dressing is appropriately accommodated and increased pressure on the wound does not result. However, certain medical devices, such as immobilizers and negative pressure therapy devices, can become a source of pain. Various methods can be used to reduce that pain, including pressure relief and use of nonadherent dressings at the device–wound interface (NPUAP-EPUAP, 2009).

Positioning patients for comfort and off their wound can reduce pain at the wound site. If this is not possible, judicious use of support surfaces can offer pain relief to bed- or chair-bound patients. Individuals should be encouraged to request a "time-out" during any procedure that causes pain. Patients should be premedicated, if needed, prior to activities that cause or trigger pain. Using lift sheets (to lift and move) instead of draw sheets (that drag) to move patients in bed prevents friction and shear, which can cause painful injuries to the skin and deeper tissues (NPUAP-EPUAP, 2009).

Wound Dressings

Many commercially available moisture-retentive dressings are designed for the care of wounds. The main analgesic efficacy of these products appears to stem from their ability to keep the wound moist and protected from the environment, reduce inflammation, and stimulate healing. Moisture-retentive dressings have at least some capacity to reduce pain associated with wounds (NPUAP-EPUAP, 2009; Steed et al, 2006; Whitney et al, 2006). Thus, dressings can be selected with the aim of reducing pain in a particular patient. The most effective dressing will depend on patient factors such as volume of exudate, condition of surrounding skin, wound depth, and necrotic tissue. Dry, wet-to-dry, or wet-to-damp dressings are not moisture retentive and consequently are the most painful. As the gauze dehydrates, it tends to become attached to the wound surface and, along with damaging new granulation tissue, is painful to remove (NPUAP-EPUAP, 2009; Robson et al, 2006; Whitney et al, 2006). The trauma that patients must endure then is multiplied because wet-to-damp or dry dressing must be changed three times per day.

The patient with a wound often dreads the dressing change procedure, which is cyclic in nature. Box 26-1 lists several interventions for pain control during dressing changes. Dressings should be selected that will, upon removal, minimize the degree of sensory stimulus to the wound area (European Wound Management Association [EWMA], 2002).

PHARMACOLOGIC INTERVENTIONS

The World Health Organization (WHO) Pain Clinical Ladder, a three-step analgesic ladder approach for the treatment of cancer pain, can also been used to guide the treatment of nonmalignant pain (Boxes 26-2 and 26-3 and Figure 26-1). This approach uses a combination of pain control medications based on assessment of pain intensity. If pain persists after reassessment, the ladder guides the clinician in adding a medication or combination of medications to effectively control pain (McCaffery and Portenoy, 1999). Pharmacologic interventions can be topical, subcutaneous or perineural injectable, or systemic (McCaffery and Beebe, 1989; McCaffery and Portenoy, 1999).

Topical Medications

Topical analgesics are commonly used before debridement or before manipulation inside the wound margins, which includes wound packing or application of materials that contact the wound. These medications usually are in the form of a jelly, cream, or ointment, although liquid forms and patches are available. They generally include

---

BOX 26-1	Interventions for Pain Reduction During Dressing Changes

- Minimize degree of sensory stimulus (e.g., drafts from open windows, prodding and poking).
- Allow patient to perform own dressing changes.
- Allow "time-outs" during painful procedures.
- Schedule dressing changes when patient is feeling best.
- Give an analgesic and then schedule dressing change for time of drug's peak effect.
- Soak dried dressings before removal.
- Avoid use of cytotoxic cleansers.
- Avoid aggressive packing.
- Minimize number of dressing changes.
- Prevent periwound trauma.
- Position and support wounded area for comfort.
- Consider using low-adhesive or nonadhesive dressings.
- Offer and use distraction techniques (e.g., headphones, TV, music, warm blanket).

BOX 26-2 World Health Organization Analgesic Ladder (see Figure 26-1)

Step 1

Patients with mild to moderate pain should be treated with a non-opioid analgesic, which should be combined with an adjuvant drug if an indication for one exists.

For example: Nonsteroidal antiinflammatory drugs, acetylsalicylic acid, acetaminophen.

Step 2

Patients who have limited opioid exposure and moderate to severe pain or who fail to achieve adequate relief after a trial of a nonopioid analgesic should be treated with an opioid conventionally used for moderate pain.

For example: Step 1 medications plus codeine, tramadol, and so forth.

Step 3

Patients who have severe pain or who fail to achieve adequate relief after appropriate administration of drugs in step 2 of the analgesic ladder should receive an opioid conventionally used for severe pain.

For example: Step 1 medications and morphine (discontinue step 2 medications).

Note: Unrelieved pain should raise a red flag that attracts the clinician's attention.

From McCaffery M, Portenoy RK: Overview of three groups of analgesics. In McCaffrey M, Pasero C, editors: *Pain clinical manual*, ed 2, St. Louis, 1999, Mosby.

BOX 26-3 Examples of Opioid, Nonopioid, and Adjuvant Medications

Opioids
- Codeine
- Dolophine (Methadone)
- Fentanyl
- Hydromorphone (Dilaudid)
- Levorphanol
- Morphine
- Oxycodone
- Tramadol

Combination Medications
- Percocet (oxycodone/acetaminophen)
- Lortab, Vicodin, Norco (hydrocodone/acetaminophen)

Nonopioids
- Aspirin
- Acetaminophen
- Nonsteroidal antiinflammatory drugs (NSAIDs)

Adjuvant Medications
- Tricyclic antidepressants
- Anticonvulsants
- Systemic local anesthetics
- Topical anesthetics

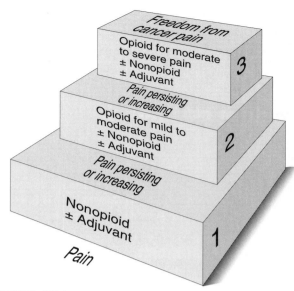

FIGURE 26-1 World Health Organization analgesic ladder for cancer pain. (From the World Health Organization, 2010.)

lidocaine or another local anesthetic with sodium channel receptor blockade activity. Topical anesthetics require at least 15 to 30 minutes to reach optimal analgesic states. Although lidocaine preparations have been widely available and safely used for years, topical use of these preparations in open wounds is considered off label in the United States. Topical lidocaine products should be used with caution, especially with large wounds, to avoid systemic absorption and potential neurologic and/or cardiovascular manifestations.

The most commonly used topical analgesics include 2% and 4% lidocaine jelly, which act on only the superficial layer of tissue and can inactivate exposed wound pain receptors. The strongest evidence base for the effectiveness of topical analgesics in wound care is associated with eutectic mixture of local anesthetics (EMLA) cream (Astra Pharmaceutics, Wayne, Pa., USA), which contains lidocaine and prilocaine. It is applied 30 to 60 minutes before debridement under occlusion with a film dressing. Instructions for use of EMLA cream are given in Box 26-4 (Evans and Gray, 2005; Hansson et al, 1993).

BOX 26-4 Application of Eutectic Mixture of Local Anesthetics (EMLA) Cream

- 10 g EMLA can safely cover a surface area of approximately 100 cm^2.
- Apply directly to wound.
- Cover with plastic or transparent wrap for 20 minutes.
- If pain is not managed after 20 minutes, increase time to 45 to 60 minutes.

Data from Evans E, Gray M: Do topical analgesics reduce pain associated with wound dressing changes? *J Wound Ostomy Continence Nurs* 32(5):287, 2005.

Topical anesthetic patches also may be useful. Examples include the Synera patch and the Lidoderm (lidocaine) patch. The Synera patch incorporates 70 mg of lidocaine and 70 mg of tetracaine, thus providing fairly rapid onset (20–30 minutes) and prolonged duration (up to hours). The patch is self-warmed, which facilitates drug delivery and may improve wound perfusion, although this has not specifically been studied using the Synera patch (Sawyer et al, 2009).

Subcutaneous or Perineural Injectable Medications

Injectable medications (subcutaneous or perineural) frequently contain the same type of active drug that is found in the topical analgesic formulations (local anesthetics such as lidocaine). However, these medications are in solution and are designed to be injected into the soft tissue. These medications include lidocaine or longer-acting agents (e.g., bupivacaine, tetracaine). Epinephrine can be added to these medications to cause vasoconstriction, increasing the duration of action as well as decreasing bleeding. Epinephrine is contraindicated for use in distal areas such as hands and feet because of the risk of necrosis from interruption of blood supply. Epinephrine is generally avoided in wounds due to concern of impairing blood supply, although it may be useful in extremely vascular wounds. Injectable local anesthetics can be used for either field or regional blockade.

A *field blockade* is accomplished by injecting local anesthetic adjacent to or directly into the wound margins, encircling the entire area. It blocks transmission of pain signals that are carried in the superficial cutaneous nerves that supply the wound area. At times, injection within the wound edges is less painful. If tolerated, however, the block is generally more effective when the injection is made outside the wound margins. Inflammation in the wound may inactivate or reduce the activity of the local anesthetic.

A *regional* or *nerve block* is accomplished by injecting local anesthetic into an often singular, proximal location where the larger nerve bundles are contained. Examples of regional blocks include not only digital, wrist, and ankle blocks but also other larger, more proximal nerves. Brachial plexus blockade and blockade of lower extremity nerves in the popliteal fossa may provide larger areas of coverage. Regional blocks require more training but are useful in the management and debridement of wounds that either cross many dermatomes or cover a large area that is supplied by many separate proximal nerves, or in patients with severe periwound hyperalgesia. Ultrasound or nerve stimulator guidance often is used to improve accuracy and avoid complications of nerve blockade.

Selective blockade of the sympathetic nervous system may reduce pain and improve healing. Stellate ganglion and lumbar sympathetic blocks can be used for upper and lower extremity sympathetic blockade, respectively. These interventions may optimize blood flow and oxygen delivery while relieving sympathetically mediated pain. Trauma and inflammation may increase sympathetic tone and up-regulate α-receptors in the wound, leading to sympathetically maintained pain in lower extremity ulcers (McLachlan et al, 1993). These procedures usually are performed using fluoroscopic X-ray guidance. The goal of these blocks is not temporary relief but long-term blockade, so they often use an alcohol-based medication to permanently inactivate nerve transmission of the painful area to the spinal cord (Hopf et al, 1997). Spinal cord stimulation is another method for effective long-term sympathetic blockade (Graber and Lifson, 1987; Wu et al, 2008). All nerve blocks can be done safely in an outpatient clinic by properly trained personnel who monitor appropriately for the degree of sedation required.

Systemic Medications

The goal of systemic medication administration as a pain control strategy is not to stop pain signal transmission from the wound but to alter the response of the central nervous system (CNS) to that pain signal. Whether the medication is given intravenously, subcutaneously, transcutaneously, or orally, many pain management choices are available when utilizing systemic pain control (Tables 26-1 through 26-3). These include nonsteroidal antiinflammatory drugs (NSAIDs), opioids (e.g., morphine, methadone, oral lidocaine, acetaminophen, partial μ-receptor agonists (e.g., tramadol), anticonvulsants (e.g., gabapentin [Neurontin]), antidepressants, and

TABLE 26-1	Recommended Starting Doses (and Equivalence) for Opioid Treatment of Intrinsic Wound Pain	
PO/PR (mg)	**Analgesic**	**IV or IM (mg)**
30	Morphine	1–5 IV or 5–10 IM
6	Hydromorphone (Dilaudid)	0.2–0.6 or 1.5
20	Methadone	10–20
Not recommended	Meperidine (Demerol)	10–30 or 100*
60	Codeine	30–60
5–10	Oxycodone (Percocet)	N/A

PO, by mouth; PR, per rectum; IV, intravenous; IM, intramuscular.
*Meperidine should not be used for analgesia because normeperidine, a metabolite, may accumulate. Seizures are common when high doses (1,000 mg in 1 day or 600 mg/day for several days) are given. Meperidine is more likely to cause dependence than other clinically used opioids.
Acute Pain Management Panel (APMP): *Acute pain management: operative or medical procedures and trauma,* Clinical practice guideline, AHCPR Publication No. 92-0032, Rockville, Md., 1992, US Department of Health and Human Services, Public Health Service.

TABLE 26-2 | **Agents Appropriate for Sedation/Analgesia for Procedures in Adults**

Agent	Dose (IV)	Frequency
Diazepam	1–2 mg	q3–10min
Lorazepam	0.05 mg/kg (max 4 mg)	One time
Midazolam	0.25–1 mg	q1–5min
Fentanyl	Loading dose up 1 μg/kg, then 12.5–50 μg	q5-10min
Meperidine	12.5–25 mg	q2–15min
Morphine	1–3 mg	q2–15min
Droperidol	0.625–1.25 mg	q5–10min

clonidine (central α_2-adrenergic agonist that reduces sympathetic outflow) (Veith et al, 1984). These medications act on different target locations to combat the perception of pain. For example, predominantly neuropathic pain is more responsive to antidepressants and anticonvulsants than to NSAIDs and opioids (Wound, Ostomy and Continence Nurses [WOCN] Society, 2004). Some medications (e.g., NSAIDs) can also act by secondary means to reduce pain; that is, besides their direct analgesic properties, they reduce inflammation in the wound area, leading to a decrease in pain.

Combining several analgesic agents often is more successful than using a single agent. Drugs may act additively or synergistically. This may allow a reduction in the required dose of each agent, thus potentially reducing side effects while providing equal or even superior analgesia (Hopf and Weitz, 1994). A patient with mixed nociceptive and neuropathic pain will require a combination of analgesics and antidepressants or anticonvulsants.

Because of their potency and reliable analgesic action, opioids are a mainstay of pain management in both acute and chronic settings. One of the actions of opioids is stimulation of receptors in the central and peripheral nervous system that down-regulate both the afferent response to pain as well as central pain perception. Gabapentin (Neurontin) is an excellent drug for treating neuropathic pain, as occurs in patients with diabetic neuropathy. It often is effective for wound pain probably because of the neuropathic nature of much wound pain. The maximum recommended dose is 900 mg by mouth three times daily, but wound pain frequently responds to the lowest dose range of 100 to 200 mg three times daily. Other agents that may be beneficial in the treatment of neuropathic pain include tricyclic antidepressants and pregabalin.

Further research is necessary to confirm which strategies or groups of strategies optimize pain relief and for which type of pain. For example, will applying a topical anesthetic compress before sharp debridement be more effective for this type of acute noncyclical pain than taking an oral pain medication? Around-the-clock medications might be most effective for continuous chronic wound pain. Applying pain-reducing dressings or selecting pressure-reducing devices may prove to reduce acute cyclic pressure ulcer pain more effectively than pharmacologic measures.

TABLE 26-3 | **Pharmacologic Interventions for Neuropathic Pain**

Type of Pain	Medication
Dysesthesia	Capsaicin cream topically applied tid to qid; may take 3 weeks for effect to be seen Gabapentin Selective serotonin reuptake inhibitor (e.g., fluoxetine, paroxetine) Serotonin and noradrenergic reuptake inhibitors (e.g., venlafaxine) Dextromethorphan syrup Tricyclic antidepressant (e.g., imipramine, amitriptyline)
Paresthesia	Anticonvulsant (e.g., carbamazepine, Tegretol, phenytoin) Analgesic (e.g., Tramadol)
Muscular pain	Muscle relaxant (e.g., metaxalone, baclofen [Lioresal], tizanidine by mouth)
General neuropathic pain	Analgesics (e.g., lidocaine [Lidoderm] patch) Gabapentin Hemorrheologic agent (e.g., pentoxifylline [Trental]) Diuretic (e.g., furosemide, metolazone, bumetanide); may diminish pain with reduction in vasodilation Platelet inhibitor, cilostazol (Pletal) Bisphosphonate (e.g., pamidronate) Aldose reductase inhibitor (e.g., fidarestat, sorbinil) Antithromboembolitic therapy (e.g., heparin, warfarin, acetylsalicylic acid, antiinflammatory drugs) Clopidogrel (Plavix)

Addiction Concerns

The degree of pain that a patient experiences and reports often is influenced by the patient's fear of addiction. A common social and medical problem is drug and alcohol abuse, and treating painful wounds can be especially difficult in patients who abuse these substances. Because patients who are addicted to alcohol or drugs can exhibit tolerance to CNS depressants and opioids, higher dosages of analgesic medications may be required. In addition, liver and kidney disease associated with alcohol or other drug abuse may alter the metabolism and excretion of opioids and other analgesics. Tolerance and altered metabolism along with variability in recent drug use by the patient and attitudes among health care providers toward addicted patients are factors that make designing an effective analgesic regimen for these patients difficult.

Furthermore, opioid-addicted patients may exhibit a tendency for hyperalgesia, in which patients experience a greater intensity of pain than expected for a given wound. When treating these individuals, the fundamental principle of pain management is the same as it is for other patients: complaints of pain should be taken seriously and treated aggressively (Cohen et al, 2004). Intravenous drug abusers may require higher doses of analgesics to obtain similar degrees of pain relief because of the development of opioid cross-tolerance. Careful consideration of adjunctive medications or interventions may be useful in this patient population.

The history of opioid prescribing has been particularly variable. Patients have commonly been undertreated with opioid pain medications when opioids were indicated (Owen et al, 1990). However, recent data show some alarming trends in prescription drug misuse and abuse over the past 10 years. In 2009, the American Pain Society detailed the guidelines for opioid prescribing. The risks and benefits of opioid therapy should be carefully weighed and continually assessed in each patient (Chou et al, 2009). Although the fear of becoming addicted is generally unfounded—less than 0.1% of patients receiving opioids for acute pain become addicted—safe prescribing methods and monitoring of therapy are important (APMP, 1992). Medication contracts between patient and prescriber, urine drug screenings, and periodic monitoring of prescriptions filled can be vital in maintaining adherence to medical management.

Because patients frequently take inadequate doses of opioids because of their fear of addiction, they should be reassured and encouraged to use the drugs appropriately. When the doses are inadequate because of side effects, different opioids should be tried and adjunct agents added to reduce the required opioid dose. Referral to a pain medicine specialist may be warranted if pain is poorly controlled or is refractory to appropriate dose escalation, interventions are needed, or comprehensive, multidisciplinary treatment is needed. Pain relief, safety, and active monitoring for medication misuse should be the cornerstones of opioid therapy.

Potential Complications of Medical Pain Management

Medications are rarely benign. Almost every drug has an associated set of potential side effects that can be inconvenient or harmful to the patient. The *Physician's Desk Reference* lists every reported side effect for each medication, but certain sets of complications are commonly encountered in the setting of analgesic control. The most powerful systemic analgesic agents are opioids; they have the most acutely serious side effects, including sedation and respiratory depression.

Whenever opioids are given, attention must be given to avoiding excess sedation and respiratory depression. This is particularly true when opioids are given to manage procedural pain. Most health care facilities recognize five categories of sedation (Table 26-4). However, these categories are artificially drawn because sedation is a continuum. Sedation is different from simple pain control; sedation implies that the medications are given

TABLE 26-4	Categories of Sedation	
Level	Category	Definition
1	No sedation	
2	Minimal or light sedation	Patient responds normally to verbal commands. Patient's ventilatory and cardiac functions are unaffected.
3	Moderate or conscious sedation	Patient responds purposefully to verbal commands. Patient's spontaneous ventilation is adequate.
4	Deep sedation	Patient cannot be easily aroused. Patient can respond purposefully following repeated or painful stimulation. Patient has increased probability of respiratory or hemodynamic compromise.
5	Anesthesia	Most often performed in operating room. Patient is not arousable by painful stimulation.

to specifically facilitate the ability to perform a painful procedure. The use of analgesics or sedatives solely to provide analgesia and/or allay anxiety (as occurs during dressing changes) but with no intention of performing a procedure is not considered sedation. Nonetheless, such drugs must be used with caution because respiratory depression and sedation can be induced whenever these drugs are used. Box 26-5 lists prescribing principles developed by the American Geriatrics Society Panel on Persistent Pain in Older Persons (2002) for chronic pain management in the long-term care setting.

A patient receiving light or greater sedation requires constant monitoring, which includes, at a minimum, cardiac monitoring, pulse oximetry, and direct supervision by a provider not involved in performing the procedure. When a patient is being managed using sedation, the most serious common complication is respiratory depression. Therefore, the sedation should be performed only in a setting where a medical practitioner is available who can provide a definitive airway and handle the complications of ventilatory and/or circulatory collapse. Whenever patients are given analgesics for procedural pain, consideration should be given to monitoring, and hospital guidelines should always be followed.

Potential side effects of opioid medications should be discussed at the initiation of therapy. High-dose and/or long-term opioid therapy may place patients at higher risk for hormonal disturbances (decreased testosterone) or sleep disorders. Respiratory depression is the most serious side effect. Other less serious but common side effects include nausea, vomiting, constipation, urinary retention, and pruritus. All patients receiving opioids should be given stool softeners and counseled on ways to prevent constipation, including increased fluid and fiber intake. Antiemetic medications, changing to a different opioid, or limiting opioid dose by using nonopioid analgesics (e.g., NSAIDs) can manage nausea and vomiting. Pruritus can be managed with diphenhydramine or other antihistamines.

Side effects of NSAIDs include stomach pain, ulcers, gastrointestinal bleeding, renal impairment; allergies, and platelet inhibition (Buckley and Brogden, 1990). Side effects of acetaminophen are few, but overdoses (>4–6 g/day) can result in acute fulminant liver failure. Care should be exercised when using opioid–acetaminophen combinations, especially those with relatively low-potency opioids and high-dose acetaminophen (500 mg per tablet), such as Vicodin (hydrocodone–acetaminophen). Acetaminophen is a powerful adjunct, so it should be used when possible. For tolerant patients, it should be given separately as an around-the-clock drug to reduce the risk of liver injury. More potent opioids (e.g., oxycodone, hydromorphone [Dilaudid], morphine, methadone) should be selected as well to reduce the number of doses required daily.

Side effects of antiepileptics and antidepressants include sedation, which usually resolves with continued use. These drugs can be started as a bedtime dose for several days to allow acclimatization.

Side effects of clonidine include sedation and dry mouth (acclimatization is rapid). It can decrease blood pressure and heart rate but rarely causes hypotension or bradycardia. Clonidine is available as a transdermal patch, which allows constant plasma levels and improved compliance. Usually the lowest dose (no. 1 or 2 patch) is sufficient. Clonidine may reduce opioid requirements in tolerant patients (Flacke et al, 1987). It often increases perfusion and oxygenation in patients with hypoxic wounds because of their excess sympathetic tone or peripheral vascular disease, which may also reduce pain (Hopf et al, 1996).

BOX 26-5	Principles that Guide Chronic Wound Pain Management

Manage intrinsic (background) pain with medications provided on a routine schedule.

Manage break-through pain with fast-acting medications as required (PRN).

Consider the following regarding route of administration:
- Use the least invasive route first (i.e., administer medications orally, when feasible).
- Use topical patches or creams when oral medications are insufficient.

Analgesic dose should be titrated to an effective level, starting with a low dose and advancing slowly.

Reassessment of background pain as well as procedural or incident pain should be ongoing and treatment individualized per patient need.

Monitor elderly patients closely for undesirable effects.

American Geriatrics Society Panel on Persistent Pain in Older Persons: The management of persistent pain in older persons, *J Am Geriatr Soc* 50(S6):1, 2002.

SUMMARY

Managing pain associated with the presence of a wound not only enhances the cellular and molecular activities of wound healing but also enhances the patient's ability to participate in activities essential to healing. Pharmacologic agents need to be selected and titrated to the type and severity of pain. Nonpharmacologic interventions are also important to prevent exacerbation of pain.

REFERENCES

Acute Pain Management Panel (APMP): *Acute pain management: operative or medical procedures and trauma*, Clinical practice guideline, AHCPR Publication No. 92-0032, Rockville, Md., 1992, US Department of Health and Human Services, Public Health Servcie.

American Geriatrics Society Panel on Persistent Pain in Older Persons: The management of persistent pain in older persons, *J Am Geriatr Soc* 50(S6):1, 2002.

Briggs M, Nelson EA: Topical agents or dressings for pain in venous leg ulcers, *Cochrane Database Syst Rev* 1:CD001177, 2003.

Buckley MM, Brogden RN: Ketorolac: a review of its pharmacodynamic and pharmacokinetic properties, and therapeutic potential, *Drugs* 39(1):86, 1990.

Chou R et al: Clinical guidelines for the use of chronic opioid therapy in chronic noncancer pain, *J Pain* 10(2):113-30, 2009.

Cohen SP et al: Pain management in trauma patients, *Am J Phys Med Rehabil* 83:142, 2004.

European Wound Management Association (EWMA): *Position document: pain at wound dressing changes*, 2002, Medical Education Partnership, available at http://www.ewma.org, accessed September 25, 2005.

Evans E, Gray M: Do topical analgesics reduce pain associated with wound dressing changes or debridement of chronic wounds? *J Wound Ostomy Continence Nurs* 32(5):287-290, 2005.

Flacke JW et al: Reduced narcotic requirement by clonidine with improved hemodynamic and adrenergic stability in patients undergoing coronary bypass surgery, *Anesthesiology* 67:11-19, 1987.

Graber JN, Lifson A: The use of spinal cord stimulation for severe limb-threatening ischemia: a preliminary report, *Ann Vasc Surg* 1(5):578-582, 1987.

Hansson C et al: Repeated treatment with lidocaine/prilocaine cream (EMLA) as a topical anaesthetic for the cleansing of venous leg ulcers. A controlled study, *Acta Derm Venereol* 73(3):231-233, 1993.

Hopf HW Weitz S: Postoperative pain management, *Arch Surg* 129(2):128-132, 1994.

Hopf HW et al: Clonidine increases tissue oxygen in patients with local tissue hypoxia in non-healing wounds, *Wound Rep Regen* 4(1):A129, 1996.

Hopf HW et al: Percutaneous lumbar sympathetic block increases tissue oxygen in patients with local tissue hypoxia in non-healing wounds, *Anesth Analg* 84:S305, 1997.

McCaffery M, Beebe A: *Pain: clinical manual for nursing practice*, St. Louis, 1989, Mosby.

McCaffery M, Portenoy RK: Overview of three groups of analgesics. In McCaffery M, Pasero C, editors: *Pain clinical manual*, ed 2, St. Louis, 1999, Mosby.

McLachlan EM et al: Peripheral nerve injury triggers noradrenergic sprouting within dorsal root ganglia, *Nature* 363(6429):543, 1993.

National Pressure Ulcer Advisory Panal (NPUAP) and European Pressure Ulcer Advisory Panel (EPUAP): *Prevention and treatment of pressure ulcers*, Washington DC, 2009, NPUAP.

Owen H et al: Postoperative pain therapy: a survey of patients' expectations and their experiences, *Pain* 41:303, 1990.

Robson MC et al: Guidelines for the treatment of venous ulcers, *Wound Repair Regen* 14(6):649-662, 2006.

Sawyer J et al: Heated lidocaine/tetracaine patch (Synera, Rapydan) compared with lidocaine/prilocaine cream (EMLA) for topical anaesthesia before vascular access, *Br J Anaesth* 102(2):210-215, 2009.

Steed DL et al: Guidelines for the treatment of diabetic ulcers, *Wound Repair Regen* 14(6):680-692, 2006.

van Rijswijk L: Wound pain. In McCaffery M, Pasero C, editors: *Pain clinical manual*, ed 2, St. Louis, 1999, Mosby.

Veith RC et al: Dose-dependent suppression of norepinephrine appearance rate in plasma by clonidine in man, *J Clin Endocrinol Metab* 59:151, 1984.

Whitney J et al: Guidelines for the treatment of pressure ulcers, *Wound Repair Regen* 14(6):663-679, 2006.

Wound, Ostomy and Continence Nurses (WOCN) Society: *Guideline for management of wounds in patients with lower-extremity neuropathic disease*, WOCN Clinical Practice Guideline Series #3, Glenview Ill., 2004, Author.

Wu M et al: Putative mechanisms behind effects of spinal cord stimulation on vascular diseases: a review of experimental studies, *Auton Neurosci* 138(1-2):9-23, 2008.

27

Nutritional Assessment and Support

Nancy A. Stotts

OBJECTIVES

1. Compare and contrast the pathophysiology and clinical manifestations of protein malnutrition, protein-calorie malnutrition, and obesity.
2. Identify how starvation without injury differs from the metabolic response to starvation with injury.
3. Distinguish between the purpose of a nutrition screening tool and a nutrition assessment tool.
4. Compare and contrast nutritional assessment using Subjective Global Assessment and the Mini Nutritional Assessment.
5. Describe anthropometric and laboratory data that can be used to evaluate whether nutritional support is adequate to support healing.
6. Identify the role of nutrients in wound healing, including requirements for calories, protein, zinc, and vitamin C.

Nutrition is fundamental to normal cellular integrity as well as tissue repair and regeneration. Carbohydrates, proteins, fat, minerals, vitamins, and fluids are required in sufficient amounts to meet nutritional requirements for these basic processes. Individual needs vary depending on the underlying nutritional status, metabolic rate, and concomitant biologic demands (e.g., diabetes, heart failure, pneumonia, renal failure).

Wound healing is an anabolic process that requires specific nutrients to fuel the biochemical processes in healing (e.g., zinc is required for hydroxylation of proline in collagen formation) (Arnold and Barbul, 2006; Demling, 2009). Although adequate nutrition is important for all patients, it is of particular importance for the patient with a wound to prevent severe or prolonged depletion of nutrients that can impact healing (Arnold and Barbul, 2006). A patient with a wound may lose as much as 100 g of protein per day through wound exudate (Pompeo, 2007). Furthermore, once malnourished, the tube-fed patient in long-term care may require 3 to 4 weeks or longer before protein stores normalize (Pompeo, 2007).

MALNUTRITION

Nationwide, the prevalence of malnutrition in all hospitals is estimated at between 20% and 50% (Norman et al, 2008), and as many as 69% of patients experience further deterioration of nutritional status during their hospitalization. This prevalence is particularly alarming because malnutrition is associated with increased morbidity (25%) and mortality (5%) in patients with acute or chronic disease as well as longer hospitalization and higher treatment costs compared to patients without malnutrition. Risk factors for malnutrition are listed in Checklist 27-1.

Malnutrition is a state in which nutritional deficiency or an imbalance of energy, protein, and other nutrients causes measureable adverse effects on tissue, body structure, body function, and clinical outcome. Malnutrition can be classified as undernutrition or overnutrition, which is caused by a deficit or excess of nutrients in the diet, respectively. Table 27-1 lists the causes and manifestations of the various types of malnutrition.

Undernutrition

Undernutrition occurs because intake of macronutrients or micronutrients is inadequate or the individual is unable to absorb or metabolize nutrients that are ingested. Undernutrition most often is related to disease or infirmity (Norman et al, 2008). Some patients are admitted to the hospital with undernutrition due to underlying disease. Others develop undernutrition during hospitalization as a result of decreased intake, the hypermetabolic response

CHECKLIST 27-1
Risk Factors for Malnutrition

✓ Hypermetabolism
✓ Weight loss
✓ Decreased appetite
✓ Therapeutic dietary restriction
✓ Inability to buy or prepare food
✓ Lack of teeth or poorly fitting dentures
✓ Inability to feed self
✓ Food intolerance (e.g., as occurs with chemotherapy)
✓ Alterations in ingestion, digestion, absorption, metabolism
✓ Change in pattern or variety of food ingested
✓ Nausea, vomiting, anorexia, diarrhea
✓ Limited income
✓ Social isolation

that accompanies acute injury and inflammation, or secondary to illness or treatment (e.g., diarrhea, wound drainage).

Undernutrition is generally divided into protein-calorie malnutrition and protein malnutrition. Protein-calorie malnutrition is sometimes called *protein-energy malnutrition* or *marasmus,* and protein malnutrition is known as *kwashiorkor.* Protein-calorie malnutrition is more often seen in developed countries rather than in underdeveloped countries. It affects both adults and children. Protein-calorie malnutrition reflects the inadequate intake, absorption, or metabolism that occurs in persons with chronic illnesses, such as cancer and chronic heart failure, as well as acute and traumatic injury. Severe weight loss, muscle wasting, and loss of adipose tissue characterize protein-calorie malnutrition (Heimburger, 2008).

In contrast, protein malnutrition occurs in persons in whom sufficient protein is not ingested, absorbed, or metabolized. It is often seen in patients with chronic disease, such as chronic obstructive pulmonary disease, heart failure, and cancer (Heimburger, 2008). It also is seen in third world countries where protein sources are scarce.

The phenomenon of rapidly occurring protein-calorie malnutrition has been termed *mixed protein-calorie malnutrition,* or *marasmus-kwashiorkor.* It has an acute onset and is common in acutely ill persons and in those who are hospitalized. Understanding the processes that take place during malnutrition provides a rationale for use of specific assessment parameters and prescription of specific nutrients.

Starvation. Starvation occurs when caloric intake is inadequate to meet metabolic needs. The classic picture of someone who is starved is the individual who has inadequate intake, is in an unstressed state, and is hypometabolic (Heimburger, 2008). Initially with inadequate intake, compensatory processes are initiated to meet the glucose needs of essential tissues (e.g., brain, white blood cells). Glycogen that is stored in the liver is mobilized for energy; however, stores are small and are exhausted in less than 24 hours. Subsequently, glucose needed for cellular activities is formed by the catabolism of protein in muscle and tissues. Protein is not stored in the body, so when protein is used for gluconeogenesis, functional muscle and organs are destroyed and weight loss is rapid. Weight loss occurs from both the breakdown of protein and the osmotic diuresis that allows for excretion of the byproducts of protein metabolism in the urine.

If inadequate intake persists, compensatory processes allow fat to become the primary energy source and for protein to be used at a much slower rate (Heimburger, 2008). The brain adapts and uses ketones from fat metabolism for energy, the muscle releases less protein, and the kidneys recycle the end-products of protein metabolism for glucose. Over time, the basal metabolic

TABLE 27-1	Causes and Manifestations of Malnutrition	
Type of Malnutrition	**Cause**	**Manifestations**
Protein-calorie malnutrition (marasmus)	Inadequate protein and energy	Gradual weight loss resulting in underweight, then progressive cachexia Visceral protein levels preserved Immune function well preserved
Protein malnutrition (kwashiorkor)	Inadequate protein intake and adequate energy intake	Well-nourished appearance Rapid onset with loss of visceral proteins Skeletal muscle mass well preserved Edema
Mixed protein-calorie malnutrition (marasmus-kwashiorkor)	Inadequate protein and energy intake	Common in hospitalized patients Acute onset Presents with rapid weight loss, fat and muscle wasting, rapid decline in visceral proteins
Obesity	Excessive energy intake	Body mass index >30 Large waist size

rate decreases and weight loss is slowed. Protein is converted to glucose for use by only a few tissues (e.g., red blood cells, fibroblasts, renal medulla). Serum protein measures decline gradually (Glasgow and Hermann, 2006).

When fat stores are depleted, protein again becomes the primary energy source and is rapidly depleted. Skeletal muscle size rapidly decreases, and serum protein levels fall. If treatment is not prompt, death will ensue. Table 27-2 compares the type and manifestations of various types of starvation.

Stress and Starvation. Injury causes stress, catecholamine release, and increased metabolic rate. The degree of hypermetabolism is directly related to the severity of injury. For example, severe burns cause a greater increase in metabolic rate than uncomplicated surgery (Demling, 2009). The inflammatory response is elicited concomitantly. Cortisol released from the adrenal cortex enhances protein catabolism, amino acid mobilization, and hepatic glucose production (Heimburger, 2008). Cytokines, including tumor necrosis factor, transforming growth factor-β, and interleukin-1 and interleukin-6, contribute to the stress response. While insulin levels are elevated, insulin resistance prevents anabolism. During this period of hypermetabolism, caloric needs increase, and protein requirements increase disproportionately. Hypermetabolic demands decrease gradually, and, if no additional insult occurs, metabolic needs return to baseline within 10 to 14 days of the acute injury.

In the injured but healthy person, inadequate intake for 5 to 7 days usually is not a problem. Surgical patients are an excellent example. A combination of hypermetabolism and starvation occurs due to inadequate intake. The hypermetabolic response is a physiologic response to injury and results in increased energy needs. At the same time, patients initially are provided with intravenous fluids containing 5% glucose (about 200 calories per liter). This administration spares protein but is not able to meet metabolic needs. As oral intake resumes, caloric intake is less than normal, and auto-catabolism occurs to meet metabolic needs. These patients usually have a brief but rapid decrease in weight. When they return to adequate caloric intake, they regain the lost weight (Heimburger, 2008). If the cause of the stress is not resolved, additional stresses occur (e.g., infection) or the individual's intake does not meet metabolic needs, the patient is set up for a downward spiral.

Overnutrition

Overnutrition results in obesity, which is defined as a body mass index (BMI) >30. The prevalence of obesity in the United States has risen in the last 40 years from 13% to 27% of the adult population. A greater proportion of women than men are obese, and the frequency of obesity is especially high among African Americans, Native Americans, Native Hawaiians, and Hispanics (U. S. Preventive Services Task Force, 2003).

Obese patients may develop problems related to wound healing, such as delayed wound healing, dehiscence, and infection. They often have concomitant medical problems, including diabetes, hypertension, and poor oxygenation from pulmonary restrictive disease (Wilson and Clark, 2004). In addition, because adipose tissue is not as well perfused as muscular tissue, the obese patient is at increased risk for delayed healing and infection. Mobility may be a problem, placing the obese patient at risk for pneumonia, deep venous thrombosis, and pressure ulcers.

The excess weight of an obese patient does not necessarily reflect adequate nutritional health. Protein deficiency as well as deficiencies of vitamins and minerals

TABLE 27-2	Manifestations of Starvation
Type of Starvation	**Manifestations**
Brief: Protein is primary energy source.	Increased nitrogen in urine Increased urine output Rapid weight loss Decreased muscle mass
Prolonged: Fat becomes primary energy source. Protein is spared.	Slow weight loss Slow loss of muscle mass Increased urinary ammonia Decreased urinary nitrogen
Premorbid: Protein becomes primary energy source. Ends with exhaustion of protein or nutritional support to reverse the process.	Cachectic appearance Rapid weight loss Decreased arm muscle circumference and skinfold measures Increased creatinine/weight index Increased urinary urea Decreased serum proteins (albumin, transferrin, prealbumin) Decreased immune capacity (decreased lymphocyte count, anergy to recall antigens)

may be present. Unfortunately, nutritional evaluation of the obese person is often incorrectly deferred simply because his or her weight is so much more than normal (Gallagher and Gates, 2003). However, the obese person with a wound *needs* exogenous nutrients to heal, and his or her diet must be individualized to meet the patient's needs.

SCREENING AND ASSESSMENT

In a healthy state, people ingest sufficient carbohydrates, protein, fat, vitamins, minerals, and fluids to meet nutritional needs and maintain a positive nitrogen balance. Wound healing requires additional nutrients. Because malnutrition is so prevalent in the hospital setting and is associated with significant morbidity and mortality, it is wise to screen patients for possible malnutrition upon admission; ideally it should be done in tandem with the admission assessment. In contrast to screening, nutritional assessment is conducted by a dietitian or a member of the nutrition support team. Nutritional assessment involves a systematic process of collecting, verifying, and interpreting data on the patient's nutritional status and forms the basis for nutritional interventions (National Pressure Ulcer Advisory Panel [NPUAP] and European Pressure Ulcer Advisory Panel [EPUAP], 2009). Sample screening and assessment forms discussed in this section are provided in Appendix B.

Screening for Possible Malnutrition

Nutrition *screening* identifies the patient who is (1) not at risk and therefore is not in need of a nutritional assessment, (2) at potential risk for malnutrition, or (3) possibly undernourished. The latter two are indications of the need for a nutritional *assessment* by a registered dietician (Anthony, 2008; NPUAP-EPUAP, 2009). For the hospitalized patient, nutritional screening provides baseline data on a person's nutritional status and should be done at admission or as early as possible following admission (Green and Watson, 2006; NPUAP-EPUAP, 2009). Many screening tests for possible malnutrition are used in patient care, but few have been validated. According to the NPUAP-EPUAP (2009) Pressure Ulcer Prevention and Treatment Clinical Practice Guideline, the nutritional screening tool should be validated, reliable, relevant to the desired patient group, applicable to different health care settings, able to detect undernutrition and overnutrition, and quick and easy to use. The two screening tools recommended by the NPUAP-EPUAP as being the most accurate and readily available for the general hospital and inpatient population are the Malnutrition Screening Tool (MST) and the Short Nutritional Assessment Questionnaire (SNAQ) (Kruizenga et al, 2005) (see Appendix B). Composed of questions that are most predictive of malnutrition, these tools are easy to implement. According to the NPUAP-EPUAP guideline, each health care setting

should have a policy on nutritional screening and frequency. The policy should indicate that the patient who is screened as being at risk for malnutrition should be referred to a registered dietician or nutritional support team for a nutritional assessment.

Assessment of Nutritional Status

A nutritional *assessment* is indicated for the patient who is obese, has a coexisting wound, or is screened as being at a potential risk for malnutrition. Nutritional assessment is designed to confirm the presence or absence of malnutrition and to measure the extent of existing malnutrition. Although the nurse may be instrumental in gathering the data used in a nutritional assessment, assimilation of the data into an assessment requires a referral to a dietician or a multidisciplinary nutrition support team (dieticians, nurses, pharmacists, physicians). With the implementation of interventions, the patient's response should be monitored closely, often daily. Reassessments are recommended every week, with changes in the patient's condition, and with any significant weight loss. For individuals in home care, it is important to be vigilant to changes in patient status and weight. Significant weight loss is defined as weight loss of 5% or greater within 30 days or 10% or greater within 180 days (NPUAP-EPUAP, 2009).

Assessment of nutritional status involves compiling a constellation of data: relevant patient history and physical (e.g., weight change, diet, edema), anthropometric measures, and biochemical laboratory data. No single parameter (e.g., weight, serum protein level) is a valid or reliable marker of nutritional status. Furthermore, many assessment parameters commonly used are affected by other conditions, such as inflammation, renal failure, dehydration, cancer, and pregnancy. However, research is ongoing to determine which parameters provide the most reliable and accurate representation of the malnourished state.

Nutritional status is sometimes evaluated entirely based on data from the patient's history and physical. In these situations, the admission assessment should sequence the history taking so that significant dimensions reflective of nutritional status are clustered. This information can be used to direct the physical examination, laboratory work, and referrals. Checklist 27-2 lists the parameters to address in the patient history.

The physical examination is performed after the history is taken. Although no single physical finding is diagnostic of malnutrition, many different signs and symptoms are associated with specific nutritional alterations, such as coarse hair or thin skin (Seidel et al, 2008). Signs and symptoms associated with nutritional alterations are listed in Table 27-3. However, these findings correlate with other conditions, such as disease process, medication side effects, metabolic alterations, and age-related changes (Heimburger, 2008). Often the physical

CHECKLIST 27-2
Parameters to Address in a Patient History

✓ Chief complaint
✓ Present illness(es)
✓ General health
✓ Major adult illnesses
✓ Childhood illnesses
✓ Prior surgery
✓ Functional limitations
✓ Emotional status
✓ Social history
✓ Personal history
✓ Home condition
✓ Environment
✓ Review of systems

assessment findings can be used to confirm concerns or suspicions derived from the data obtained from the patient's history or the laboratory work. For patients at risk of, or with, early malnutrition, the physical findings for malnutrition may be subtle or absent because some signs do not appear until the malnutrition becomes advanced. With overt malnutrition, anthropometric changes often are key findings. Obese patients are especially difficult to evaluate because their weight may mask the skeletal muscle wasting of malnutrition (Gallagher and Gates, 2003).

Nutritional Assessment Instruments. Nutritional assessment instruments are used to capture various pieces of data that collectively will provide an index on the patient's nutritional status. The ideal nutritional assessment instrument should be sensitive to early changes and specific enough to identify only nutritional causes of the measure; it should be corrected with nutritional intervention, and correction of its values should result in a positive outcome (Barbosa-Silva, 2008; Keith, 2008). In addition, the approach/instrument should be easy to use, readily implemented by various members of the team, and possess sufficient reliability and validity to accurately identify any problems (NPUAP-EPUAP, 2009).

The Subjective Global Assessment (SGA) (see Appendix B), first described in 1982, is a widely used assessment tool with clearly delineated assessment parameters obtained through a focused history (weight change, dietary intake, gastrointestinal symptoms, functional capacity, coexisting disease) and physical examination (subcutaneous fat, muscle wasting, ankle and sacral edema, ascites). Once the SGA is completed, the patient is classified as well nourished (grade A), moderately malnourished or suspected of being malnourished (grade B), or severely malnourished (grade C) (Keith, 2008). The SGA has been reported to consistently predict malnutrition better than objective measures (transferrin, delayed hypersensitivity, skin fold measures, creatinine height index). Originally created for the surgical patient, the validity and reliability of the SGA have been demonstrated in diverse patient populations, including children, the elderly, and patients undergoing dialysis. When the SGA is combined with serum albumin, prediction of malnutrition was more consistent than with either measure alone (Detsky et al, 1994). Although the SGA is a clinically effective and simple tool for nutrition assessment, the grading of malnutrition is subjective and best conducted by a trained clinician.

The Mini Nutritional Assessment (MNA) is a reliable and valid 18-item tool that combines screening with assessment. The MNA consists of anthropometric, general, dietary, and subjective assessments, has been used in a variety of health care settings, and has been shown to detect malnutrition before changes in weight or serum protein levels, especially in an elderly population (Bauer et al, 2008). From a cross-sectional study of elderly patients with pressure ulcers, Langkamp-Henken et al (2005) concluded that use of the MNA was advantageous over serum protein levels for screening or assessment.

Recently the new MNA-Short Form (see Appendix B) has been validated as a stand-alone screening tool; requiring less time to complete and being more user friendly, the MNA-Short Form has become the preferred form for clinical practice (Kaiser et al, 2009). Furthermore, it has been demonstrated that when BMI is not available, the calf circumference is a valid alternative.

Anthropometric Measures. Anthropometric measures are easy to perform and are pivotal in the evaluation of nutritional status. The most commonly used anthropometric parameters are height, weight, and head circumference (children only). Less frequently used are mid-arm muscle circumference and skinfold measurements (Table 27-4).

Weight is the cornerstone in the diagnosis of malnutrition and can be used alone or in relation to height or frame size. Box 27-1 lists examples of weight-related indicators of malnutrition. Weight is often considered in relation to height. Recent tables for interpretation of these parameters are based on the National Research Council data on weight and height, the dietary guidelines, and

TABLE 27-3	Physical Findings Associated with Nutritional Deficiencies	
Site	**Signs and Symptoms**	**Nutritional Deficit**
Skin	Cracking	Protein
	Petechiae	Vitamin C
	Scaling	Vitamin A
Hair	Corkscrew hairs	Vitamin C
	Easily pluckable hair	Protein
Muscles	Weakness	Protein, calories
Mouth	Bleeding	Vitamins A, C, K
	Atrophic tongue	Protein, iron

TABLE 27-4	Anthropometric Measures	
	Measures	**Condition Measure Reflects**
Common measures	Height and weight (body mass index)	Overnutrition, undernutrition
	Head circumference	Undernutrition
Less frequently used measures*	Mid-arm circumference	Muscle stores
	Skinfold measurements	Fat stores

*Measures performed by dietician.

BMI. The BMI is calculated by dividing weight (in kilograms) by height (in meters) squared and most often is used to determine whether people are underweight or overweight. BMI is a predictor of morbidity and mortality (Gallagher and Gates, 2003; U.S. Preventive Services Task Force, 2003). BMI is not always perfectly correlated with fat distribution; therefore, it should be considered in conjunction with other assessment findings (Evans, 2005). Also, the Centers for Disease Control and Prevention (CDC) advise that age and gender can affect the relationship between BMI and body fat, as women and older persons have a greater proportion of fat than do men and younger persons.

Head circumference is used in children to evaluate their growth. Measurements are compared with tables of norms, allowing head size to be classified in percentiles. Chronic undernutrition results in delayed growth of the head, and its identification and treatment are important so that permanent damage does not occur (Mascarenhas et al, 1998). Although the test measures are performed primarily by dieticians, it is important to understand what the test measures mean in order to appreciate the relevance of the findings.

Arm muscle circumference and skinfold measurements initially were used in underdeveloped countries and obtained with only the most basic of instruments to evaluate the nutritional status of the population (Jeliffe, 1966). Standards exist in the United States for specific age groups and for a limited number of minority populations (Frisancho, 1984; Gray and Gray, 1979; Marshall

et al, 1999). *Mid-upper arm circumference* is a measure of muscle mass, bones, and skin. It is used to calculate *mid-arm muscle circumference* as a measure of lean body mass (Heimburger, 2008). A decrease in arm muscle mass occurs with protein and calorie deficiencies (see Table 27-4 for anthropometric measures).

Fat stores are measured with skinfold measures. A skinfold caliper is used to evaluate skinfold thickness. The triceps site is most frequently used; other sites include the scapula, waist, and triceps. Fat stores do not change rapidly, so skinfold thickness is not a sensitive measure of malnutrition. Dieticians, advanced practice nurses, and the nutritional support team may perform arm muscle circumference and skinfold measurements, with low scores indicative of undernutrition.

Laboratory Data. There is no ideal laboratory test for malnutrition. Levels of serum proteins (albumin, prealbumin, transferrin, retinol binding protein) are commonly used as biochemical indicators of malnutrition. Serum proteins are synthesized primarily by the liver and vary considerably in their turnover rates. It is generally assumed that the shorter the turnover rate, the more directly the protein reflects nutritional status. Unfortunately, these proteins are associated with numerous conditions that blur or confuse the interpretation of their serum levels. Table 27-5 lists the plasma protein measures frequently used to evaluate protein status, normal values, and factors that affect these proteins (Demling, 2009; Dwyer 2008).

Serum proteins are visceral proteins that comprise a small portion of the body's total protein pool. Additional visceral proteins include erythrocytes, granulocytes, lymphocytes, and other solid tissue organs. Serum proteins are negative acute phase proteins or reactants during the inflammatory response. Inflammatory processes such as acute or chronic infection, surgery, trauma, and burns trigger a systemic response referred to as the *acute phase response*. The serum levels of most proteins either increase or decrease during the acute phase response. Serum proteins that decrease levels during inflammation are called *negative acute phase reactants* (e.g., albumin and prealbumin) and are expected to return to normal as the inflammatory process resolves. Positive acute phase reactants are proteins that increase levels during times of stress because they are essential for the immune response. C-reactive protein, fibrinogen, protein S, and fibronectin

BOX 27-1	Weight Indicators of Malnutrition

Weight loss in last 6 months
- <5% = mild loss
- 5%–10% = moderately severe loss
- >10% = severe loss

Body Mass Index (BMI)
- <18.5 kg/m^2 = underweight
- 18.5 – 24.9 kg/m^2 = normal weight
- 25.0 – 29.9 kg/m^2 = overweight
- ≧30 kg/m^2 = obese

Weight <90% ideal body weight = malnutrition

From Evans E: Nutritional assessment in chronic wound care, *J Wound Ostomy Continence Nurs* 32(5):317-320, 2005.

TABLE 27-5	Plasma Protein Levels		
Visceral Protein	**Malnutrition**	**Normal**	**Factors Affecting Reliability**
Serum albumin	<3.5 g/dl	3.5–5.0 g/dl	Inflammation, dehydration, overhydration
Serum prealbumin	<19.5 mg/dl	19.5–35.8 mg/dl	Inflammation, dehydration, overhydration
Transferrin	<100 mg/dl	230–390 mg/dl	Iron deficiency

are examples of positive acute phase reactants. Because of its ability to change quickly with changing conditions, the positive acute phase reactant C-reactive protein is a commonly used marker for the presence of inflammation (Banh, 2006).

In addition to inflammation, hydration status will affect serum protein levels. For example, when the patient is dehydrated, serum albumin and prealbumin levels will be falsely elevated, which could be erroneously interpreted as normal values. Conversely, when the patient is overhydrated, serum protein levels will be falsely low, which could be erroneously interpreted as malnutrition. Serum proteins are also affected by medications, impaired liver function, and circadian rhythm (Banh, 2006).

Historically, albumin was used as a measure of nutritional status and probably is the most frequently measured of the laboratory parameters. Albumin has a long half-life (17–21 days) and is not sensitive to rapid changes in nutritional status, and albumin levels fall only late during the course of prolonged and premorbid starvation (Demling, 2009; Heimburger, 2008). As a negative acute phase protein influenced by many factors, serum albumin is not an appropriate measurement for use in the diagnosis of either recent or mild to moderate malnutrition; it is a carrier protein and primarily helps to maintain oncotic pressure.

Transferrin has a shorter half-life than albumin (8–10 days) and a smaller body pool. Its major function is iron transport. Usually about one third of the body's transferrin is bound to iron. Therefore, iron status influences transferrin levels such that iron deficiency, which frequently occurs with protein-calorie malnutrition, stimulates hepatic synthesis, resulting in very high transferrin levels. At the other extreme, certain types of anemia may trigger depressed transferrin levels (Demling, 2009; Stotts and Bergstrom, 2004). Transferrin level is not sufficiently sensitive or specific to be a meaningful measurement of nutritional status.

Prealbumin, also known as *thyroxin-binding prealbumin* or *transthyretin,* is a transport protein for thyroxine and vitamin A (Evans, 2005). It is affected by many of the same factors that affect albumin. However, because of its short half-life (2 days), prealbumin is expected to reflect decreased intake of protein or calories more rapidly and respond quickly when exogenous nutrients are provided. Prealbumin has been used as a measure of nutritional status because it is believed to reflect not only what has been ingested but also what the body has been able to absorb, digest, and metabolize.

Less commonly measured is retinol-binding protein, a plasma protein with a very short half-life (12 hours) and very low serum levels. It participates in the transport of vitamin A, and its response follows that of prealbumin. Although it has a theoretic advantage over other plasma proteins by virtue of its short half-life, its low normal values and the technical difficulties associated with its measurement limit its usefulness compared to other measures of nutrient status (Evans, 2005; Langemo et al, 2006).

The use of serum proteins as a marker for nutritional status is increasingly controversial. Serum albumin and prealbumin may not correlate well with clinical observations of nutritional status (NPUAP-EPUAP, 2009; Shenkin, 2006). In addition, serum concentrations of these proteins may not be markers of undernutrition or caloric repletion; rather, they are indicators of morbidity and mortality (Fuhrman et al, 2004; Myron et al, 2007). Currently, guidelines to aid healing of acute wounds by decreasing impediments of healing (Franz et al, 2008) recommend monitoring weight and prealbumin and albumin levels to identify patients who are malnourished and in need of nutritional support because obesity and malnutrition increase the risk of postoperative complications.

Creatinine levels have been used for more than 20 years in nutritional support settings to evaluate lean body mass. Creatinine gives an indirect measure of skeletal muscle mass and is a measure of long-term protein status (Demling, 2009). Creatinine assessment is complex because the patient must have normal renal function and urinary output, have the ability to accurately collect a 24-hour urine sample, be adequately hydrated, and not be on prolonged periods of bedrest or a recent high-protein meal.

Nutritional status also is evaluated using a 24-hour urine creatinine excretion divided by normal creatinine for height, producing a creatinine height index. An index of 40% to 60% reflects minimal protein depletion, whereas an index less than 40% indicates severe nutrition depletion. Age-specific tables are used to interpret the findings.

Nitrogen balance also is used to evaluate whether the patient's diet is providing sufficient protein. Nitrogen intake and loss from the body are carefully regulated and, under normal nutritional circumstances, closely approximate each other so that nitrogen turnover is in balance. Anabolism and repair require positive nitrogen balance. Negative nitrogen balance is a reflection of catabolism or inadequate ingestion.

The immune system is highly sensitive to protein status because protein is a major constituent of immune system components such as antibodies and lymphocytes. Consequently, gross tests of immune function, such as total lymphocyte count, also reflect protein status. Lymphocytes constitute a variable percentage of the circulating white blood cells and are reported in a white blood cell differential. The total lymphocyte count is calculated by multiplying the percentage of lymphocytes by the white cell count. The normal level ranges from 1,500 to 3,000 cells/mm^3. Below-normal levels may be a reflection of malnutrition; however, the total lymphocyte count may also be depressed due to chemotherapy, autoimmune diseases, stress, and infection, including human immunodeficiency virus (Stotts and Bergstrom, 2004).

NUTRIENT NEEDS FOR HEALING

Body composition can be conceptualized as having two components: fat mass and fat-free mass (Demling, 2009). The majority of the body is fat, which acts as a calorie reservoir. Fat is a calorie-dense substrate, with 9 calories per gram of fat. When the body's intake of calories is greater than expenditure, fat forms and weight increases. In times of need, fat is catabolized and weight loss occurs.

In contrast, the fat-free compartment, or lean body mass, is composed primarily of protein and water. The protein portion is located primarily in muscles, red blood cells, connective tissues, and organs, including the skin, which is the largest of the body's organs. Healing requires protein synthesis (Demling, 2009). When energy requirements exceed intake, even for short periods, body protein is broken down to meet metabolic need; the protein in this situation is used for energy rather than for anabolism. Protein has less than half the calories of fat (4 calories per gram); when it is catabolized, weight loss is rapid. Also, because protein is not stored in the body, catabolism of protein results in loss of functional tissue (muscle, organs), which is referred to as *muscle wasting*.

Normal healing requires adequate protein, fat, and carbohydrates, as well as vitamins and minerals. When intake, absorption, or metabolism of nutrients does not meet metabolic requirements, biochemical changes occur that have implications for healing (e.g., impaired fibroplasia). However, these changes often occur without clinical manifestations, although they may be detected with appropriate tests (e.g., low zinc levels, below-normal prealbumin levels). Severe changes must occur before signs and symptoms of impaired healing due to malnutrition are manifest (e.g., dehiscence). In part, the wound receives the biologic priority of muscle

catabolism, which provides substrates that preferentially allow repair of injured tissues. This protection is tightly tied to the percentage of lean body mass. When more than 15% of lean body mass is lost, impaired healing is seen. At 30% loss of lean body mass, more severe alterations in healing occur (e.g., dehiscence). With 40% loss of lean body mass, death occurs, often due to pneumonia (Demling, 2009).

The best data about nutritional requirements for healing come from the surgical and pressure ulcer literature (Demling, 2009; Heimburger, 2008; NPUAP-EPUAP, 2009; Posthauer, 2006a, 2006b). Energy needs usually are based on a modification of the Harris-Benedict equation, which takes into account the person's age, gender, height, and weight; the modification portion of the equation considers the individual's stress and activity. This equation provides a good starting point for determining nutritional therapy. The alternative is to perform indirect calorimetry; however, that approach usually is reserved for patients who are hypermetabolic from sepsis or trauma in whom body weight cannot accurately be determined and those who are being weaned from a ventilator (precise prescription in order to avoid excess CO_2 production and delay weaning) (Heimburger, 2008). Once caloric needs are determined, protein, fat, and carbohydrate as well as vitamin and mineral distributions are planned.

Calories

The range of normal calories administered is broad and is based on a multitude of factors. Usual caloric needs are 20 to 35 calories per kilogram of body weight. Lower estimates are used for patients with chronic illness who are chronically starved, whereas higher estimates are used, for those who are hypermetabolic and have significant injuries (Bistrian and Driscoll, 2008; Posthauer, 2006b). With injury, more calories and substrates are needed for healing than in an uninjured state. About 50% to 60% of an individual's caloric needs are met through carbohydrates, 20% to 25% through protein, and the remainder from fat (Posthauer, 2006b).

Protein

Protein needs are disproportionally increased after injury, and a protein deficiency can prolong a person's healing time (Arnold and Barbul, 2006). In adults, 15% of lean body weight is composed of protein, of which 3% (approximately 300 mg) is turned over daily during normal protein metabolism. Most of this protein is reused in the synthesis of new proteins, and some is lost through excretion. The recommended daily allowance (RDA) of protein for a healthy person is 0.8 g of protein per kilogram per 24 hours; protein needs with injury may increase to 1.25 to 1.5 g kilogram per day (Demling, 2009; NPUAP-EPUAP, 2009). Older adults often are protein deficient because they have proportionally greater daily protein requirements than younger persons; at the same time, their intake of protein often is inadequate. During times of limited intake, the older adult is at especially high risk for undernutrition (Green and Watson, 2006).

Proteins are made of amino acids, which are necessary to generate acute phase proteins, including collagen and proteoglycans, and are essential for wound healing, hormonal and immune balance, and muscle health. With stress, two amino acids, arginine and glutamine, become conditional essential amino acids because the body's ability to produce these amino acids cannot meet the increased need (Posthauer, 2006b).

Arginine

Arginine is converted to ornithine, a precursor to praline and subsequent collagen formation. In animal models, arginine decreases nitrogen loss and stimulates immune function, wound breaking strength and collagen formation; it also facilitates wound healing by augmenting the release of the anabolic hormones insulin, insulin-like growth factors, glucagon, prolactin, and various growth factors (Posthauer, 2006b; Stechmiller et al, 2005; Thompson and Fuhrman, 2005). The clinical effect and cost benefit of arginine supplementation on healing chronic wounds in humans has not been studied; the current state of evidence for arginine is with animal models and artificially induced surgical wounds in healthy humans (Arnold and Barbul, 2006; Stechmiller et al, 2005). Therefore dietary supplementation for the patient with a wound is considered to be premature.

Glutamine

As one of the most abundant amino acids in the body, glutamine helps preserve the functional integrity of the intestinal brush border. It is used to synthesize nonessential fatty acids and the nucleotide units of RNA and DNA. With stress, glutamine levels diminish (≤ 400 μmol/L), thereby compromising the integrity of the immune system. Replacement is important to reduce the risk of systemic sepsis. By stimulating growth hormone, glutamine enhances immune system function. Normal glutamine levels of 600 μmol/L or higher facilitate intact immunologic function. The patient with a major wound has a glutamine requirement of 0.3 to 0.4 g per kilogram per day (Demling, 2009).

Carbohydrates

Carbohydrates provide a significant portion of nutrients. Carbohydrate is turned to glucose, which is available immediately for ATP formation and provides the energy for phagocytosis and collagen development. Glucose levels must be kept within normal limits to facilitate healing; excessive levels result in impaired healing. Glucose is important to prevent the use of protein as an energy source.

Fats

Fats are important for development and stability of cell membranes (both intracellular and cell wall). Fats also participate actively in various aspects of the inflammatory response to injury and thus in healing. The type of fat ingested determines the type of prostaglandins produced. Omega-3 fatty acids favor prostaglandin (PG) E_3 and leukotrienes; they participate in inflammation, vasoconstriction, and platelet aggregation. Omega-6 fatty acids facilitate protection from inflammation and immunosuppression by generating a preponderance of PGE_1 and PGE_2, vasodilators, and antiinflammatory agents (Arnold and Barbul, 2006).

Vitamins

All of the vitamins are needed for tissue repair and regeneration because of their various functions in normal cellular metabolism. Table 27-6 lists the role of various nutrients in healing. Vitamins A and C are especially critical for healing. Vitamin A is fat soluble and is important in various steps of collagen deposition. Collagen is the most important component in scar formation and in maintaining wound closure. In persons treated with corticosteroids, vitamin A is an important antagonist; it reverses all the effects of corticosteroids except for their impairment of contracture (Heimburger, 2008).

Vitamin C is a water-soluble vitamin, is a cofactor in collagen formation, and is important to fibroplasia. It enables complement to perform its functions. Vitamin C works synergistically with vitamin E to prevent oxidative cell damage. Lack of vitamin C can result in impaired collagen formation. When vitamin C intake ceases, the stores become depleted within 2 to 3 months (Arnold and Barbul, 2006).

Minerals

Among the minerals, zinc, copper, and iron have received the most attention in the context of wound healing. Zinc is important because of its role in protein synthesis, enzyme systems, immune competence, and collagen formation (Heimburger, 2008). Zinc supplementation enhances collagen formation in patients with zinc deficiency. In persons with normal zinc levels, supplementation has not been shown to alter healing (Posthauer, 2006b). Supplementation should be based on serum deficits, and treatment should be limited to 7 to 10 days. Supplementation in those who are not in need may result in disruption of normal phagocytic activity and cause copper deficiency. Copper deficiency may result in weaker scar tissue and decreased tensile strength, predisposing the person to dehiscence. Iron is important in hemoglobin for oxygen transport. Persons with anemia who are not able to compensate for low oxygen with increased circulation rates may experience

TABLE 27-6	Role of Nutrients in Wound Healing
Nutrient	**Role in Healing**
Protein	Angiogenesis
	Collagen synthesis/remodeling
	Wound contraction
	Immune function
	Precursor to nitric oxide
Carbohydrate	Energy source
	Protein sparing
	Angiogenesis
Fat	Cell walls
	Intracellular structures
	Inflammation
Vitamin A*	Epithelialization
	Angiogenesis
	Inflammatory response
B vitamins	Cofactor in enzymes
	Immune response
	Synthesis of macronutrients
Vitamin C	Collagen synthesis
	Capillary wall integrity
	Fibroblast function
	Immune function
	Antioxidant
Vitamin D*	Calcium metabolism
Vitamin E*	Antioxidant
Vitamin K*	Coagulation
Copper	Cross-linking collagen
Iron	Collagen formation
	Immune function
	Oxygen transport
Zinc	Collagen formation
	Protein synthesis
	Cell membrane stability
	Immune function

*Fat soluble.

impaired collagen formation and ineffective phagocytic activity.

Electrolytes

Water and balanced electrolytes are the sea in which the various nutrients function. Adequate hydration and electrolytes provide the physiologic space in which nutrients and oxygen are transported to the site of injury so that healing can occur. The usual rule for fluid is at least 1,500 cc per 24 hours, with most receiving fluids based on the equation 30 ml per kilogram body weight (Dwyer, 2008). The exception to this rule is people with heart or renal failure, for whom the recommendation is 25 ml/kg or replacement of fluid losses; loss of wound fluid or treatment with an air fluidized bed may increase the patient's fluid requirement needs (Posthauer, 2006a, 2006b). Evaluation of hydration status is an integral part of nutritional assessment (Posthauer, 2006a). Table 27-7 lists laboratory measures of hydration.

TABLE 27-7	Laboratory Measures of Adequate Hydration	
Laboratory Test	**Underhydration**	**Normal Values**
Serum sodium	>150 mEq/L	130–150 mEq/L
Osmolality	>295 mOsm/L	285–295 mOsm/L
BUN	Elevated	7–23 mg/dl
BUN-Creatinine ratio	>25:1	10:1
Urine specific gravity	>1.028	1.003–1.028

BUN, Blood urea nitrogen.

NUTRITIONAL SUPPORT

Depending on the health care system, the appropriate action when a patient is screened and assessed as being malnourished or at risk for malnutrition is referring the patient to a dietician, notifying the physician of the findings, or calling the nutritional support team. A sequence of events for providing nutritional support is summarized in Box 27-2.

Nutritional needs are dependent on many variables, including age, gender, height, weight, presence of severe wasting or obesity, current disease state, and severity of illness. Additional nutrient needs are present when the patient has a wound due to loss of protein and fluid from the wound as well as the increased demands required to support the wound healing process. When the patient is

BOX 27-2	Sequence of Events for Nutritional Support

1. Screen nutritional status of all patients upon admission (skip and move to assessment if patient is obese or has a wound)
2. Nutritional assessment of patients at risk for malnutrition:
   - All patients with a wound
   - Obese patients
   - Patients screened to be at risk for malnutrition
3. Estimate nutritional requirements
4. Compare nutrient intake with estimated requirements
5. Provide appropriate nutrition intervention based on nutritional requirements
6. Provide sufficient nutrients
   - 30–35 kcal per kilogram of body weight per day
   - 1.25–1.5 g of protein per kilogram per day
   - 1 ml of fluid intake per kcal per day
   - 1,600–2,000 retinol equivalents of vitamin A
   - 100–1,000 mg of vitamin C
   - 15–30 mg of zinc
   - 200% of recommended dietary allowance of the B vitamins
   - 20–30 mg of iron
   - 0.3–0.4 g of glutamine per kilogram per day
   - Daily multivitamin and mineral supplement
7. Monitor intake to ensure patient is meeting nutritional requirements
8. Monitor and evaluate nutritional outcomes, with reassessment of nutritional status at frequent intervals while individual is at risk

at risk for pressure ulcers as identified by the nutrition subscale of the Braden scale, supplementation of dietary intake may be warranted (Whitney et al, 2006).

Most diets are a combination of protein, carbohydrate, fat, vitamins, and minerals, so deficiencies of individual nutrients are uncommon. Increased intake or supplements are needed if the patient is undernourished or is at risk for pressure ulcer formation. Protein intake should be sufficient to support growth of granulation tissue (Whitney et al, 2006). Goals of nutritional support for the patient who is at risk or who has an existing wound are to provide a minimum of 30 to 35 kcal per kilogram of body weight per day, with 1.25 to 1.5 g per kilogram per day of protein and 1 ml per kilocalorie per day of fluid intake (NPUAP-EPUAP, 2009; Whitney et al, 2006).

Vitamins and mineral supplements should be provided if deficiencies are detected or suspected. Daily vitamin and mineral needs are increased to 1,600 to 2,000 retinol equivalents of vitamin A, 100 to 1,000 mg of vitamin C, 15 to 30 mg of zinc, 200% of the RDA of the B vitamins, and 20 to 30 mg of iron. A daily multivitamin and mineral supplement is recommended (Bistrian and Driscoll, 2008; Posthauer, 2006b). Research has demonstrated no acceleration in healing with supplemental vitamin A or C or zinc (Whitney et al, 2006). Arginine has been found to have no impact on the rate of healing in patients with a pressure ulcer.

Anabolic steroids have been recommended and demonstrated to be useful in supporting healing in some populations by stimulating increased protein buildup and weight gain (Demling, 2009). Approved by the U.S. Food and Drug Administration in the 1960s for treatment of severe weight loss due to chronic infections, severe trauma, or failure to thrive without a pathophysiologic reason, anabolic steroids have been used to treat severe malnourishment and wasting syndrome typical with human immunodeficiency virus and acquired immunodeficiency syndrome–related conditions and burns. The anabolic steroid oxandrolone (Oxandrin, Bio-Technology General Corporation, Iselin, NJ, USA), a testosterone analogue, has been shown to decrease catabolism and significantly attenuate lost lean mass with severe wounds. Androgens influence wound healing by increasing collagen deposition and facilitating leukocyte migration and monocyte adhesion to enhance the inflammatory response. Shortened healing times have also been reported with human growth hormone, another anabolic steroid (Oh and Phillips, 2006). Estrogen has been reported to have antiinflammatory properties, decreasing elastase activity so that fibronectin degradation is decreased and collagen content deposition is increased, particularly in estrogen-deficient women. However, estrogen therapy increases the risk of endometrial hyperplasia and cancer and has been observed to adversely affect the quality of scar formation (Oh and Phillips, 2006).

The preferred route of nutritional support is oral, and, whenever possible, the gastrointestinal tract should be used for feeding. A person who is receiving oral feeding should be counseled to select foods that contain protein. Foods high in protein, including milk, eggs, cheese, tuna fish, and meat, should be encouraged. Supplemental snacks, including pudding, peanut butter and crackers, protein bars, and ice cream, are other sources of protein.

If the patient's intake is not adequate with oral feeding, then one of the various approaches to the gastrointestinal tract used for tube feedings should be considered to supplement or supplant the oral feeding. As with other patient populations, use of specialized nutritional support (tube feeding or parenteral nutrition) is based on the likelihood that prevention or treatment protein-calorie malnutrition will increase the possibility of recovery, mitigate infection, improve healing, or shorten hospital stay (Bistrian and Driscoll, 2008). For a portion of those who are malnourished, weight loss and debilitation are inevitable consequences of disease that will lead to death, and the outcomes cannot be changed with nutritional support. However, in those in whom nutritional support can enhance outcomes, early nutritional evaluation and initiation of therapy support positive outcomes (Bistrian and Driscoll, 2008). When the gastrointestinal tract cannot be used, parenteral nutrition is the route of choice. At times a combination of peripheral parenteral nutrition and oral intake may be used.

SUMMARY

Nutritional assessment and support play important roles in wound healing. All patients with wounds should undergo evaluation of their nutritional status. A thorough nutritional assessment should reveal the risk for or presence of malnutrition and provide the necessary information to develop an individualized nutritional plan of care. The nutritional status should be evaluated at baseline and at regular intervals to determine the effectiveness of the nutritional plan.

REFERENCES

Anthony PS: Nutrition screening tool for hospitalized patients, *Nutr Clin Pract* 23(4):373-382, 2008.

Arnold M, Barbul A: Nutrition and wound healing, *Plast Reconstr Surg* 117(7 Suppl):42S-58S, 2006.

Banh L: Serum proteins as markers of nutrition: what are we treating? *Pract Gastroenterol* 29(10):46-64, 2006.

Barbosa-Silva MC: Subjective and objective nutritional assessment methods: what do they really assess? *Curr Opin Clin Nutr Metab Care* 11(3):248-254, 2008.

Bauer JM et al: The Mini Nutritional Assessment—its history, today's practice, and future perspectives, *Nutr Clin Pract* 23(4):388-396, 2008.

Bistrian BR, Driscoll DF: Enteral and parenteral nutrition therapy. In Fauci AS et al, editors: *Harrison's principles of internal medicine*, ed 17, New York, 2008, McGraw-Hill.

Demling RH: Nutrition, anabolism, and the wound healing process: an overview, *Eplasty* 9:e9, 2009.

Detsky AS et al: The rational clinical examination. Is this patient malnourished? *JAMA* 271(1):54-58, 1994.

Dwyer J: Nutritional requirements and dietary assessment. In Fauci AS et al, editors: *Harrison's principles of internal medicine*, ed 17, New York, 2008, McGraw-Hill.

Evans E: Nutritional assessment in chronic wound care, *J Wound Ostomy Continence Nurs* 32(5):317-320, 2005.

Franz MG et al: Guidelines to aid healing of acute wounds by decreasing impediments of healing, *Wound Repair Regen* 16(6):723-748, 2008.

Frisancho AR: New standards of weight and body composition by frame size and height for assessment of nutritional status of adults and the elderly, *Am J Clin Nutr* 40(4):808-819, 1984.

Fuhrman MP et al: Hepatic proteins and nutrition assessment, *J Am Diet Assoc* 104:1258-1264, 2004.

Gallagher S, Gates JL: Obesity, panniculitis, panniculectomy, and wound care: understanding the challenges, *J Wound Ostomy Continence Nurs* 30(6):334-341, 2003.

Glasgow SC, Hermann VM: Surgical metabolism and nutrition. In Doherty GM, Way LW, editors: *Current surgical diagnosis and treatment*, ed 12, York, 2006, McGraw-Hill.

Gray GE, Gray LK: Validity of anthropometric norms used in the assessment of hospitalized patients, *JPEN J Parenter Enteral Nutr* 3(5):366-368, 1979.

Green SM, Watson R: Nutritional screening and assessment tools for older adults: literature review, *J Adv Nurs* 54(4):477-490, 2006.

Heimburger DC: Malnutrition and nutritional assessment. In Fauci AS et al, editors: *Harrison's principles of internal medicine*, ed 17, New York, 2008, McGraw-Hill.

Jeliffe DB: *The assessment of nutritional status of the community*, WHO Monograph No. 53, Geneva, Switzerland, 1966, World Health Organization.

Kaiser MJ et al: Validation of the mini nutritional assessment short-form (MNA®-SF: a practical tool for identification of nutritional status, *Journal Nutrition, Health & Aging* 13(9):782-788, 2009.

Keith JN: Bedside nutrition assessment past, present and future: a review of the Subjective Global Assessment, *Nutr Clin Pract* 23(4):410-416, 2008.

Kruizenga HM et al: Development and validation of a hospital screening tool for malnutrition: the short nutritional assessment questionnaire (SNAQ), *Clin Nutr* 24(1):75-82, 2005.

Langemo D et al: Nutritional considerations in wound care, *Adv Skin Wound Care* 19(6):297-298, 300, 303, 2006.

Langkamp-Henken B et al: Mini nutritional assessment and screening scores are associated with nutritional indicators in elderly people with pressure ulcers, *J Am Diet Assoc* 105(10):1590-1596, 2005.

Marshall JA et al: Indicators of nutritional risk in a rural elderly Hispanic and non-Hispanic white population: San Luis Valley health and aging study, *J Am Diet Assoc* 99(3):315, 1999.

Mascarenhas MR et al: Nutritional assessment in pediatrics, *Nutrition* 14(1):105, 1998.

Myron JA et al: Clinical indications for plasma protein assays: transthyretin (prealbumin) in inflammation and malnutrition, *Clin Chem Lab Med* 45(3):419-426, 2007.

National Pressure Ulcer Advisory Panel (NPUAP) and European Pressure Ulcer Advisory Panel (EPUAP): *Prevention and treatment of pressure ulcers*, Washington DC, 2009, NPUAP.

Norman K et al: Prognostic impact of disease-related malnutrition, *Clin Nutr* 27(1):5-15, 2008.

Oh DM, Phillips TJ: Sex hormones and wound healing, *Wounds* 1(1), 2006. available at http://www.woundsresearch.com/article/5190, accessed January 25, 2010.

Pompeo M: Misconceptions about protein requirements for wound healing: results of a prospective study, *Ostomy Wound Manage* 53:30, 2007.

Posthauer ME: Hydration: does it play a role in wound healing? *Adv Skin Wound Care* 19(2):74-76, 2006a.

Posthauer ME: The role of nutrition in wound care, *Adv Skin Wound Care*, 19(1):43-52, 2006b.

Seidel HM et al, editors: *Mosby's guide to physical assessment*, Philadelphia, 2008, Mosby.

Shenkin A: Serum prealbumin: is it a marker of nutritional status or of risk of malnutrition? *Clin Chem* 52(12):2177-2179, 2006.

Stechmiller JK et al: Arginine supplementation and wound healing, *Nut Clinical Practice* 20: 52-61, 2005.

Stotts NA, Bergstrom N: Measuring dietary intake and nutritional outcomes. In Frank-Stromborg M, Olsen SJ, editors: *Instruments for health-care research*, ed 3, Sudbury, Mass., 2004, Jones and Bartlett.

Thompson C, Fuhrman MP: Nutrients and wound healing: still searching for the magic bullet, *Nutr Clin Pract* 20(3):331-347, 2005.

U.S. Preventive Services Task Force: *Screening for obesity in adults: recommendations and rationale*, Rockville, Md., 2003, Agency for Healthcare Research and Quality, available at http://www.ahrq.gov/clinic/3rduspstf/obesity/obesrr.htm.

Whitney J et al: Guidelines for the treatment of pressure ulcers, *Wound Repair Regen* 14:663-679, 2006.

Wilson JA, Clark JJ: Obesity: impediment to postsurgical wound healing, *Adv Skin Wound Care* 17(8):426-435, 2004.

28

Perfusion and Oxygenation

JoAnne D. Whitney

OBJECTIVES

1. Identify and describe two factors that impair perfusion and related wound repair processes.
2. Describe the microcirculation and tissue oxygen characteristics of the wound environment.
3. Discuss the effects of an activated sympathetic nervous system on the wound repair processes.
4. Differentiate among the roles of wound tissue oxygen and arterial oxygen in wound repair.
5. Describe four interventions to increase tissue oxygen or improve wound healing.

A great deal has been learned over several decades about tissue repair and the importance of perfusion and oxygenation to healing, although much of that information has not been applied widely in daily clinical practice. Recognition is growing that inadequate wound healing and complications, such as surgical site infection, of acute wounds likely have their origins early in the initial inflammatory response and early in the healing process, when tissue breaking strength is low and physiologic responses may not be optimal (Dubay and Franz, 2003).

Classic and recent evidence serves as a guide to understanding the importance of adequate blood flow to peripheral tissues with an adequate oxygen supply so that optimal healing and resistance to infection for acute and chronic wounds may occur. This chapter addresses factors that influence perfusion and local wound oxygenation during wound repair, including autonomic nervous system activation, fluids, supplemental oxygen, pain, stress, hypothermia, obesity, and tobacco use. The efficacy of interventions for modifying these factors to achieve better wound tissue perfusion and healing responses are discussed in light of current evidence.

IMPACT OF OXYGEN AND PERFUSION IN WOUND HEALING

The critical roles of oxygen in healing are summarized in Table 28-1. Oxygen fuels the cellular functions essential to the repair process; therefore the ability to perfuse the tissues and the availability of oxygen (partial pressure of oxygen [PO_2]) to the local wound area are critical to wound healing. The processes of tissue repair that require oxygen include oxidative bacterial killing and resistance to infection, collagen synthesis and fibroplasia, angiogenesis, and epithelialization (Hartmann et al, 1992; Hopf and Rollins, 2007; Hunt, Ellison, and Sen, 2004; Hunt and Aslam, 2004; Sen, 2003).

Tissue oxygen levels are dependent on both perfusion status and oxygen content of the blood. However, because wounds remove only 1 ml of oxygen per each 100 ml of blood perfusing the tissues, compromised perfusion is more likely to jeopardize wound healing than is compromised oxygenation secondary to pulmonary conditions (Waldorf and Fewkes, 1995). Tissues that are adequately perfused are often able to heal even if the blood is poorly oxygenated or the patient is anemic. In fact, anemia usually does not significantly affect repair unless the hematocrit drops below 20% (Stotts and Wipke-Tevis, 1996). Arterial oxygen levels are not necessarily reflective of tissue oxygen delivery. Although PaO_2 of 90 mm Hg in a healthy volunteer breathing room air maintains a wound PO_2 of 50 mm Hg or greater, the postoperative patient experiencing autonomic nervous system activation or periodic desaturation will exhibit predictably low oxygen levels within the wound. This observation led to an approach of adrenergic activation as an etiology for wound hypoxia (West, 1990).

Wound Tissue Hypoxia

Wound tissue hypoxia occurs to some extent at the time of injury in everyone, regardless of their age or state of health (Silver, 1980). Incisions closed during elective surgery under the best of aseptic conditions appear to have the fewest reparative obstacles to healing. However, any tissue injury disrupts vascular and therefore oxygen supply. All wounds are relatively hypoxic at the center, in the range from 0 to 5 mm Hg (Niinikoski et al,

TABLE 28-1	Important Roles of Oxygen in Wound Healing
Event in Wound Healing	**Specific Role of Oxygen**
Inflammation: Bacteria control	Oxygen is substrate for enzymatic step for leukocyte production of reactive oxygen species (superoxide and other oxidants) during phagocytosis
Proliferation: Angiogenesis	Local tissue hypoxia and oxidants induce release of growth factors that stimulate angiogenesis
Proliferation: Collagen synthesis and cellular export	Oxygen with adequate vitamin C is required for enzymatic hydroxylation of procollagen to form triple helical, mature collagen structure for export from fibroblasts Production and release of collagen are necessary for tissue strength
Proliferation: Epithelialization	Oxygen and growth factors are needed for generation of new epithelium

1972; Silver, 1969). After oxygen leaves the red blood cells in the capillaries, it diffuses into the wound space. The driving force of diffusion is partial pressure. In wounds, damage to the microvasculature, vasoconstriction, and intravascular fluid overload markedly increase intercapillary distances (Hunt and Hopf, 1997).

Local oxygen tension influences wound healing and bacterial control in several ways. Initial injured tissue is hypoxic, a state that acts as a stimulus for repair. The one potentially beneficial effect of moderate hypoxia is enhanced stimulus to neoangiogenesis (Wilson and Clark, 2003; Zamboni et al, 2003). However, prolonged and decreased local wound oxygen (tissue hypoxia) is a major contributor to wound complications (Goodson et al, 1979; Jönsson et al, 1988; Knighton et al, 1984). A main role of oxygen during repair is that of controlling bacteria within the wound site. During repair, production of reactive oxygen species by leukocytes for phagocytosis is needed prior to rebuilding tissue (Hopf and Rollins, 2007; Hunt, Ellison, and Sen, 2004). Oxidant production by leukocytes requires molecular oxygen and the presence of tissue oxygen levels of 45 to 80 mm Hg up to 300 mm Hg (Allen et al, 1997). In addition to their role in controlling bacteria, reactive oxygen species serve other roles in healing, which include acting as chemical signals and mitogens for fibroblasts and other cells, inducing cellular adhesion in neutrophils and macrophages, and cellular expression of growth factors that are critical for repair (Sen, 2003). Vascular endothelial growth factor that stimulates angiogenesis is one of the growth factors released in response to hypoxia and reactive oxygen species production (Hunt and Aslam, 2004). Through these processes, reactive oxygen species act to help coordinate the tissue repair process.

FACTORS THAT ALTER PERFUSION AND OXYGENATION

Pain and Stress

Cannon (1970) revealed the mechanisms that activate the autonomic nervous system to respond to stress. He directly observed the constriction of blood vessels in peripheral tissues during stress in animals. The mediators of the sympathetic and adrenal response to stress

(epinephrine and norepinephrine) induced profound vasoconstriction in subcutaneous and skin blood vessels supplying peripheral tissues (Rowell, 1986). Sympathetic activation in the postoperative period is a function of the severing of afferent nerves, hypovolemia, fear, pain, and cold rather than anesthesia (Halter et al, 1977). Catecholamine levels may remain elevated for days after surgery (Derbyshire and Smith, 1984; Halter et al, 1977), and concentrations vary with the length and severity of surgery (Chernow et al, 1987). Norepinephrine is increased threefold in the early postoperative hours (Derbyshire and Smith, 1984), peaking with the patient's first expression of pain (Niinikoski et al, 1972). Increased levels of circulating catecholamines, including epinephrine, triggered by pain and stress lead to peripheral vasoconstriction, decreased perfusion of blood to the skin and extremities, and, consequently, reduced oxygen availability in the tissues (Franz et al, 2008; Jensen et al, 1985). Evidence of how stress and pain limit perfusion has been demonstrated by infusion of exogenous epinephrine in healthy subjects. In a study designed to mimic the body's response to stress, increasing levels of epinephrine decreased the level of subcutaneous tissue oxygen 45%, whereas heart rate and arterial PO_2 did not markedly change (Jensen et al, 1985).

Hypothermia

Adverse consequences of perioperative body heat loss are significant and include prolonged hypothermia and postanesthesia recovery, longer postoperative warming time, shivering and thermal discomfort, reduced antibody and cell-mediated responses, reduced tissue oxygen peripherally, and increased incidence of wound infections (Reynolds et al, 2008). The effects of temperature on the amount of vasomotor tone primarily determine cutaneous capillary blood flow. Cooling increases norepinephrine affinity to α-adrenergic receptors on vascular smooth muscle. This augments the response of cutaneous vessels to autonomic activation, which increases constrictive vessel tensions up to fivefold (Vanhoutte et al, 1981).

Hypothermia-induced vasoconstriction has decreased subcutaneous oxygen tension in anesthetized volunteers (FiO_2 0.6 mm Hg) to a mean of 50 mm Hg (Sheffield et al, 1992). Furthermore, a lower blood temperature shifts the oxyhemoglobin curve to the left, thereby increasing the amount of oxygen carried in the blood but decreasing the amount of oxygen released (Severinghaus, 1958). This effect may exacerbate tissue hypoxia induced by peripheral vasoconstriction.

Virtually all anesthetic agents are vasodilators and may cause a rapid initial decrease in core temperature (1°C–2°C) during the first hour after induction of anesthesia (Sessler, 1993). Internal redistribution of body heat from core to periphery is exacerbated by conductive and evaporative losses as a result of visceral exposure in a cold environment (Roe, 1971). Rapid initial body heat loss can be limited by heating the operating room and aggressive preoperative warming (Morris, 1971). Preinduction warming may nearly prevent rapid initial body heat loss (Hynson and Sessler, 1992).

Perioperative shivering in the elderly, although rare, is dangerous because oxygen demand may increase by 400% to 500% (Bay et al, 1968). This drastic increase in oxygen demand increases cardiac workload. Increased oxygen consumption has been shown to coincide with core decrements of 0.3°C to 1.2°C (Roe et al, 1966). Prolonged postoperative hypothermia is associated with increased mortality (Slotman et al, 1985) and myocardial ischemia (Frank et al, 1993).

Tobacco

Smoking is associated with poor wound outcomes in part through the catecholamine-mediated vasoconstrictive effects of nicotine, increases in carbon monoxide that reduce blood oxygen content, and effects on immune and proliferative cell function that reduce repair (Gottrup, 2004; Warner, 2005). Vasoconstrictive effects resulting in significant decreases in tissue oxygen tension occur after a single cigarette is smoked, and tissue oxygen requires an hour to return to baseline levels (Jensen et al, 1991). Reductions in tissue oxygen translate clinically into lower amounts of collagen production and reduced wound strength (Jorgensen et al, 1998). Based on multiple studies and reviews demonstrating an association between smoking and wound-related problems, including infection and poor wound healing, all patients with wounds should be advised to abstain from smoking.

Smoking is the single most predictive factor of wound complications in patients undergoing elective hip or knee replacement (Moller et al, 2003). Forty-seven percent of patients undergoing abdominoplasty who smoked had wound complications compared to 14.7% of those who did not smoke (Manassa et al, 2003). At least one study has shown that 2 weeks of abstinence is inadequate to limit wound-related problems, whereas a minimum of 3 to 4 weeks of abstinence has been associated with reduced incisional wound infection and improved wound healing (Kuri et al, 2005; Sorensen et al, 2003). Due to the reductions in tissue oxygen supply when a person smokes, the substantial time needed for levels to recover, and the multiple clinical studies documenting the significance of smoking as a factor that impairs healing, the Wound Healing Society recommends that patients stop smoking at least 3 to 4 weeks before elective surgery and that they not resume smoking in the postoperative period (Franz et al, 2008).

Obesity

Wound healing problems are more likely to occur in patients who are overweight, which is a growing national problem. More than 72 million Americans are considered obese (body mass index [BMI] ≥30), representing an obesity rate of 34% in adults older than age 20 years (Ogden et al, 2007). Individuals who are severely obese often suffer from a number of related health problems that potentially impact healing: type 2 diabetes, hypertension, coronary artery disease, sleep apnea, venous stasis disease, lower extremity ulcers, osteoarthritis, urinary incontinence, gastroesophageal reflux disease, fatty liver, cholelithiasis, and depression (Mun et al, 2001).

Obesity as a single factor is an independent predictor of surgical site infection (Harrington et al, 2004). Regardless of the surgical procedure, the incidence of postsurgical wound complications, such as infection and wound dehiscence, are higher in patients with obesity compared to those of normal weight (Franz et al, 2008). Postsurgical wound complication rates of patients with obesity have been reported to be as high as 15% to 22% (Fried et al, 1997; Israelsson and Jönsson, 1997; Myles et al, 2002; Vastine et al 1999; Winiarsky et al, 1998).

Several studies document low oxygen levels associated with obesity. Abdominal tissue oxygen tension is reported to be negatively associated with the percentage of fat as measured by body composition dual-energy X-ray absorptiometry, with obese subjects found to have lower adipose tissue capillary density (Pasarica et al, 2009). In surgical populations, patients with BMI greater than 30 kg/m^2 who had undergone abdominal surgery had significantly lower tissue oxygen readings compared to those with BMI less than 30 kg/m^2 (Fleishmann et al, 2005; Kabon et al, 2004). Tissue oxygen levels measured in patients with obesity fell below normal, even with administration of supplemental oxygen, and were within a range associated with increased surgical site infection risk.

Because of the increased vulnerability to wound complications, extra vigilance and measures to ensure peripheral perfusion must be taken with patients who are obese, including increased FiO_2 during the perioperative period unless contraindicated by patient condition, maintenance of normothermia, and adequate fluid resuscitation. Higher oxygen concentrations may be needed in order to maximize tissue levels. In addition, larger doses of prophylactic antibiotics may be needed because of evidence indicating that decreasing serum and tissue concentrations fall below therapeutic levels as BMI increases (Anaya and Dellinger, 2006). Obesity is addressed in greater detail in Chapter 35.

INTERVENTIONS TO IMPROVE PERFUSION AND OXYGEN

Wound tissue oxygen delivery may be impaired unless conditions of diminished peripheral perfusion are anticipated and corrected. Factors most likely to adversely affect perfusion to the wound bed include hypovolemia, hypotension, factors producing vasoconstriction (e.g., cold, sympathetic stimulation), vascular disease, and edema. Correction of adrenergic vasoconstrictive stimuli, particularly cold, pain, and volume loss, elevates tissue PO_2 and leads to fewer postoperative infections (Hopf et al, 1997; Kurz et al, 1996). The degree of regional tissue perfusion regulates the supply of oxygen and therefore is the prime determinant of the competency of wound healing. Strategies for optimizing perfusion by addressing specific sympathetic nervous system activators are described in this section and listed in Table 28-2. As previously described, pain management is a critical strategy for improving perfusion and oxygenation. Techniques for pain control are described in Chapter 26.

Warming

Aggressive intraoperative warming and rapid postoperative warming are effective modalities for minimizing the risks of prolonged hypothermia (Hynson and Sessler, 1992). Sympathetic vasoconstriction can be overcome by warmth to provide uncomplicated healing. In a large study combining intraoperative and postoperative warming, wound infection rates were reduced by 60% (Kurz

et al, 1996). Maintenance of normothermia during surgery and in the immediate recovery period is defined as sustaining a minimum core temperature of 36.5°C. In patients undergoing colorectal surgery, a temperature higher than 36°C immediately after surgery is recommended as one of the metrics for documenting optimal care for prevention of surgical infection (Bratzler and Hunt, 2006). Warming prior to and after surgery may also provide benefit and should be considered. Fewer wound infections (13% vs 27%) were observed within 8 weeks of elective abdominal surgery in patients who were warmed for 2 hours prior to and after surgery in addition to the standard warming of all patients during the operation (Wong et al, 2007).

Local Warming. Local wound temperature modification using controlled warming improves blood flow directly to sites of injury and may benefit healing. Multiple small clinical studies examining local warming with chronic wounds (pressure, venous, diabetic, arterial) suggest benefits that include increased transcutaneous wound oxygen, less pain, and fewer infections (Puzziferri et al, 2001; Whitney and Wickline, 2003). Surgical sites with local warming have shown significantly higher tissue oxygen in the immediate recovery period and on the first postoperative day (Plattner et al, 2000) and fewer wound related complications compared with systemic warming or no warming (Melling et al, 2001; Whitney et al, 2004). Although these studies suggest benefits of local warming, more rigorous research is needed to confirm these benefits as well as the best methodology (i.e., temperature, duration, frequency) for maximizing them.

Supplemental Oxygen

A growing number of researchers have suggested that increased fraction of inspired oxygen (FiO_2) be routinely prescribed for postoperative patients during the first few

TABLE 28-2	Interventions to Reduce Factors that Impair Perfusion and Oxygenation
Factor	**Examples of Interventions**
Hypothermia	Provide active warming to maintain perioperative normothermia Provide postoperative warming and warm blankets Prevent heat loss and shivering Apply socks, slippers, sweaters, blankets
Pain	Provide analgesia and nonpharmacologic measures (e.g., repositioning, relaxation for pain control) (see Chapter 26)
Fear/stress	Provide patient teaching to reduce fear related to procedures or knowledge deficits Administer medications as needed to reduce anxiety and fear
Pharmacologic	If possible, avoid medications that activate the sympathetic nervous system (e.g., beta-blockers) Avoid high-dose α-adrenergic agonists
Smoking	Encourage minimum of 4 weeks' abstinence before surgery until incision is healed Refer to tobacco cessation program and encourage successful completion
Obesity	Increase FiO_2 perioperatively unless contraindicated Maintain normothermia and fluid balance Realize larger doses of prophylactic antibiotics may be needed

days after surgery to increase oxygen delivery to the reparative site. Relatively low levels of supplemental oxygen (28%) in the first 24 to 36 postoperative hours have been shown to increase tissue oxygen tension in patients undergoing below-the-knee amputation and cervical laminectomy procedures (Butler et al, 1987; Whitney et al, 2001). This practice is especially emphasized in patients undergoing lengthy abdominal or pelvic procedures. However, it is important to recognize that correcting tissue hypoxia requires more than simply providing increased FiO_2 to increase arterial saturation (SaO_2) and arterial PO_2. Wound PO_2 may remain unchanged even while the patient is breathing additional oxygen if other important clinical factors are not also addressed. In a study of patients who underwent general surgery, approximately 30% had reduced tissue oxygen tension levels despite adequate urine output and arterial oxygen levels (Chang et al, 1983). This is a result of early postoperative compartmental fluid shifts, in which kidney perfusion is restored at the expense of peripheral vasculature vasoconstriction.

HBO is recommended for specific clinical conditions and wound types; however, evidence is insufficient to recommend topical oxygen at the wound surface for wound healing (Hopf et al, 2006; National Pressure Ulcer Advisory Panel [NPUAP] and European Pressure Ulcer Advisory Panel [EPUAP], 2009; Robson et al, 2006). Topical oxygen at the wound surface and hyperbaric oxygen (HBO) are discussed in Chapter 22.

Volume Support

Jönsson et al (1987) demonstrated that tissue oxygen levels in general surgery patients could be corrected with infusion of fluids and that a fluid bolus of 250 ml of normal saline was sufficient in most cases. In well-perfused patients, tissue oxygen pressure continues to rise as PaO_2 rises. Findings of subsequent clinical studies in which supplemental fluids were provided perioperatively have produced mixed results of tissue PO_2 change and wound infection related to increasing fluids. In patients undergoing abdominal and colon surgeries, those who received aggressive fluid repletion (defined as maintenance levels of 16–18 ml/kg/hr during surgery and 1 hour postoperatively, or for the first 24 postsurgical hours, for an average 1.1-L increase above standard fluids) showed significantly higher wound PO_2 than did patients who received standard fluids (Arkilic et al, 2003; Hartmann et al, 1992). Higher levels of collagen deposition were associated with the increased fluids and improved wound oxygen status (Hartmann et al, 1992). Testing of fluid supplementation in randomized clinical trials has not shown benefit in terms of reducing surgical site infection. Fewer postsurgical complications, including wound dehiscence, were reported in a randomized clinical trial of 152 cases of elective intraabdominal surgeries in patients randomized to restricted versus liberal fluid repletion protocols (Nisanevich et al, 2005). Kabon et al (2004) reported no

significant differences in wound infection rates in their randomized clinical trial comparing small versus large perioperative fluid management in a trial of more than 200 elective colon surgeries. The fluid protocols in each study are not directly comparable, and neither study documented tissue oxygen levels in response to fluid, so interpretation of these differing findings is difficult. At present, data suggest that fluid supplementation as a single intervention is not sufficient to reduce wound infections or improve clinical healing outcomes.

Volume Support Combined with Supplemental Oxygen

Supporting the critical relationship between vascular volume and tissue oxygen, fluid repletion along with supplemental oxygen has been shown to effectively raise wound PO_2. This was demonstrated in a randomized trial of 500 patients, half of whom received 80% oxygen during surgery compared to 30% for the other half. All patients were aggressively hydrated during surgery at a rate of 15 ml/kg/hr and after surgery at a rate of 3.5 ml/kg/hr for the first 24 hours and 2 ml/kg/hr for the subsequent 24 hours. Patients in the higher oxygen group had significantly higher tissue oxygen levels and fewer wound infections (Greif et al, 2000). The clinical findings of the studies on hydration and supplemental oxygen support the practices of ensuring patients are well hydrated and provided oxygen to support wound healing. It is recommended that supplemental oxygen be given in the presence of good peripheral perfusion during surgery and for 24 to 48 hours postoperatively for infection control as well as for support of collage synthesis and healing (Chikungwa and Jönsson, 2002; Hopf and Holm, 2008).

The optimal dosage and duration of supplemental oxygen and the optimal fluid replacement rates needed to achieve healing and to prevent complications have yet to be determined. Among 300 patients undergoing colorectal surgery, fewer postoperative wound infections were documented in a trial of 80% versus 30% oxygen provided during surgery and for only 6 hours postoperatively (Belda et al, 2005). Fluids were given at a rate of 15 ml/kg/hr during surgery and then decreased to 3 ml/kg/hr during the first 6 postoperative hours. However, other studies testing 80% versus 30% oxygen given perioperatively to 165 general surgery patients and to women undergoing cesarean delivery did not confirm these findings in terms of wound infection rates (Gardella et al, 2008; Pryor et al, 2004). Method and protocol differences in the studies (e.g., patient populations, diagnosis of infection, volume of fluid replacement, antibiotic use) may explain the variation in outcomes (Kabon and Kurz, 2006). The conflicting results illustrate the need for additional studies to elucidate dosage (as only 30% and 80% oxygen concentrations were tested in the earlier studies), timing during the perioperative period that would be most beneficial, standardization of fluid replacement, and the patient populations that are most likely to benefit from this intervention.

Combining More Than Two Interventions

Combining the interventions of fluid repletion, oxygen support and warming, and pain control seems warranted given the existing evidence. Hypovolemia is a powerful physiologic vasoconstrictor. Therefore volume replacement and oxygen therapy must coincide with postoperative warming to benefit peripheral perfusion and tissue oxygen supply. Core temperature is not a clinically useful indicator in this equation. Skin surface temperatures do correlate with fingertip blood flow; a forearm-minus-fingertip difference of 4°C defines a state of peripheral vasoconstriction. However, this method is not commonly used in practice (Rubinstein and Sessler, 1990).

In a prospective randomized trial that combined interventions, aggressive postoperative warming and pain control increased the wound PO_2 to 70 mm Hg within 4 to 6 hours, a level nearly equal to that found in normal volunteers (West, 1994). In addition, the actively rewarmed patients who had undergone lengthy abdominal surgeries were given a 1-L fluid bolus to replace fluids lost as urine during the diuresis, which commonly accompanies hypothermia and vasoconstriction. These same interventions have been applied to trauma patients who have demonstrated improved regional perfusion but only after warming and adequate fluid resuscitation (Knudson et al, 1997). Patients who are warm, well perfused, and oxygenated rarely develop wound infections (Hopf and Holm, 2008; Hopf et al, 1997).

Patient Education

The knowledgeable provider uses theory-based assessment and a coordinated therapeutic plan to optimize wound care within the context of a larger plan, including patient teaching and necessary follow-up. Patients in acute care settings require instruction on wound care, fluid replacement, avoidance of dehydration, cessation of tobacco use, and practical ways to conserve body heat. Unfortunately, this instruction frequently occurs at a time when the patient is fatigued and somewhat overwhelmed by the entire surgical experience. In this case, teaching is best done succinctly and should be reinforced by providing the patient or family member with written guidelines. Follow-up of the patient's understanding and emphasis on healthy postoperative behaviors at clinic appointments reinforce initial teaching.

Cigarette smoking and obesity are particularly deleterious to wound repair because of their affects on both perfusion and oxygenation. Studies indicate a higher incidence of wound infection, dehiscence, and delayed healing among smokers and obese individuals compared nonsmokers and nonobese individuals. Therefore patients should be counseled regarding the negative effect of smoking and obesity and should be offered programs and resources as needed to address these lifestyle choices or addictions (Fleishmann et al, 2005; Kabon et al, 2004; Manassa et al, 2003; Sorensen et al, 2003; Stotts and Wipke-Tevis, 1996).

MEASURING THE RESPONSE

Although low periwound oxygen is an initial feature of most wounds, continued and unexplained hypoxia is of particular importance. Wound healing is proportional to local oxygen tension. Transcutaneous oxygen tension is a useful, noninvasive way to assess the adequacy of tissue oxygenation near a wound or suture line in relationship to FiO_2 (Figure 28-1). Defining the contribution of hypoxia in the context of the recent history of the patient and time from wounding clarifies the reason for low wound PO_2. Tests can be conducted to reveal the responsiveness of the wound to factors such as local warming, vasodilating drugs, oxygen therapies, sympathetic blockade, positioning, pain, and anxiety management. For example, during an oxygen challenge (e.g., breathing increased, controlled oxygen via face mask) in the absence of vasoconstriction, significant oxygen diffusion into the capillary-perfused wound edge will occur. Simple, effective, and conservative corrective therapy then can be initiated. Because improved wound PO_2 is a real measure of wound healing progress, serial measurements of damaged tissue can be obtained during the course of healing.

SUMMARY

Wound oxygen is a clinically valid and reliable index that responds more rapidly to intravascular fluid shifts than do blood pressure and pulse. When adequate oxygen is available for wound fibroblasts, collagen formation and wound tensile strength can be achieved. Collagen maturation then continues for months after wounding. From the onset of injury, any degree of interference to oxygen delivery will proportionately compromise reparative processes and increase susceptibility to infection (Hunt and Dunphy, 1979). Therefore supportive care for the patient with a wound must include measures to enhance perfusion. "Standard" interventions to enhance tissue perfusion

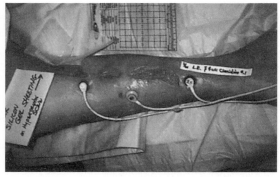

FIGURE 28-1 Recording transcutaneous oxygen tension near a lower leg wound.

include measures to prevent hypothermia and hypovolemia, reduce pain and anxiety, and eliminate edema. Approaches requiring further study include routine use of supplemental oxygen, local warming of the wound, use of epidural anesthetic blockade to increase blood flow in the microcirculation, and use of angiogenic growth factors for the management of ischemic wounds (Quirinia and Viidik, 1998; Veering and Cousins, 2000; Wu and Mustoe, 1995).

REFERENCES

Allen DB et al: Wound hypoxia and acidosis limit neutrophil bacterial killing mechanisms, *Arch Surg* 132(9):991-996, 1997.

Anaya DA, Dellinger EP: The obese surgical patient: a susceptible host for infection, *Surg Infect (Larchmt)* 7(5):473-480, 2006.

Arkilic CF et al: Supplemental perioperative fluid administration increases tissue oxygen pressure, *Surgery* 133(1):49-55, 2003.

Bay J et al: Factors influencing arterial PO_2 during recovery from anaesthesia, *Br J Anaesth* 40(6):398-407, 1968.

Belda FJ et al: Supplemental perioperative oxygen and the risk of surgical wound infection: a randomized controlled trial, *JAMA* 294(16):2035-2042, 2005.

Bratzler DW, Hunt DR: The surgical infection prevention and surgical care improvement projects: national initiatives to improve outcomes for patients having surgery, *Clin Infect Dis* 43(3):322-330, 2006.

Butler CM et al: The effect of adjuvant oxygen therapy on transcutaneous PO_2 and healing in the below-knee amputee, *Prosthet Orthot Int* 11(1):10-16, 1987.

Cannon WB: *Bodily changes in pain, hunger, fear and rage: an account of recent researches into the function of emotional excitement*, College Park, Md, 1970, McGrath.

Chang N et al: Direct measurement of wound and tissue oxygen tension in postoperative patients, *Ann Surg* 197(4):470-478, 1983.

Chernow B et al: Hormonal responses to graded surgical stress, *Arch Intern Med* 147(7):1273, 1987.

Chikungwa MT, Jönsson K: The need for perioperative supplemental oxygen, *Cent Afr J Med* 48(5-6):72-74, 2002.

Derbyshire D, Smith G: Sympathoadrenal responses to anaesthesia and surgery, *Br J Anaesth* 56:725, 1984.

Dubay DA, Franz MG: Acute wound healing: the biology of acute wound failure, *Surg Clin North Am* 83:463, 2003.

Fleischmann E et al: Tissue oxygenation in obese and non-obese patients during laparoscopy, *Obes Surg* 15:813, 2005.

Frank SM et al: Unintentional hypothermia is associated with postoperative myocardial ischemia: the Perioperative Ischemia Randomized Anesthesia Trial Study Group, *Anesthesiology* 78:468, 1993.

Franz MG et al: Guidelines to aid healing of acute wounds by decreasing impediments of healing, *Wound Repair Regen* 16(6):723-748, 2008.

Fried M et al: Bariatric surgery at the 1st Surgical Department in Prague: history and some technical aspects, *Obes Surg* 7:22, 1997.

Gardella C et al: High-concentration supplemental perioperative oxygen to reduce the incidence of postcesarean surgical site infection: a randomized controlled trial, *Obstet Gynecol* 112(3):545-552, 2008.

Goodson WH 3rd et al: Wound oxygen tension of large vs small wounds in man, *Surg Forum* 30:92-95, 1979.

Gottrup F: Oxygen in wound healing and infection, *World J Surg* 28:312, 2004.

Greif R et al: Supplemental perioperative oxygen to reduce the incidence of surgical-wound infection, *N Engl J Med* 342:161, 2000.

Halter JB et al: Mechanism of plasma catecholamine increases during surgical stress in man, *J Clin Endocrinol Metab* 45(5):936, 1977.

Harrington G et al: Surgical-site infection rates and risk factor analysis in coronary artery bypass graft surgery, *Infect Control Hosp Epidemiol* 25(6):472-476, 2004.

Hartmann M et al: Effect of tissue perfusion and oxygenation on accumulation of collage in healing wounds, *Eur J Surg* 158:521, 1992.

Hopf HW, Holm J: Hyperoxia and infection, *Best Pract Res Clin Anaesthesiol* 22(3):553-569, 2008.

Hopf HW, Rollins MD: Wounds: an overview of the role of oxygen, *Antioxid Redox Signal* 9(8):1183-1192, 2007.

Hopf HW et al: Wound tissue oxygen tension predicts the risk of wound infection in surgical patients, *Arch Surg* 132:997, 1997.

Hopf HW et al: Guidelines for the treatment of arterial insufficiency ulcers, *Wound Repair Regen* 14(6):693-710, 2006.

Hunt TK, Aslam RS: Oxygen 2002: wounds, *Undersea Hyperb Med* 31(1):147-153, 2004.

Hunt TK, Dunphy JE: *Fundamentals of wound management*, New York, 1979, Appleton Century Crofts.

Hunt TK, Ellison EC, Sen C: Oxygen: at the foundation of wound healing—introduction. *World J Surg* 28:291, 2004.

Hunt TK, Hopf H: Wound healing and wound infection: what surgeons and anesthesiologists can do, *Surg Clin North Am* 77:587, 1997.

Hynson JM, Sessler DI: Intraoperative warming therapies: a comparison of three devices, *J Clin Anesth* 4:194, 1992.

Israelsson LA, Jönsson T: Overweight and healing of midline incisions: the importance of suture technique, *Eur J Surg* 163:175, 1997.

Jensen JA et al: Epinephrine lowers subcutaneous wound oxygen tension, *Curr Surg* 42(6):472, 1985.

Jensen JA et al: Cigarette smoking decreases tissue oxygen, *Arch Surg* 126:1131, 1991.

Jönsson K et al: Assessment of perfusion in postoperative patients using tissue oxygen measurements, *Br J Surg* 74:263, 1987.

Jönsson K et al: Oxygen as an isolated variable influences resistance to infection, *Ann Surg* 208:783, 1988.

Jorgensen et al: Less collagen production in smokers, *Surgery* 123:450, 1998.

Kabon B, Kurz AL: Optimal perioperative oxygen administration, *Curr Opin Anaesthesiol* 19(1):11-18, 2006.

Kabon B et al: Obesity decreases perioperative tissue oxygenation, *Anesthesiology* 100(2):274-280, 2004.

Knighton DR et al: Oxygen as an antibiotic: the effect of inspired oxygen on infection, *Arch Surg* 119:199, 1984.

Knudson MM et al: Use of tissue oxygen tension measurements during resuscitation from hemorrhagic shock, *J Trauma* 42:608, 1997.

Kuri M et al: Determination of the duration of preoperative smoking cessation to improve wound healing after head and neck surgery, *Anesthesiology* 102:892, 2005.

Kurz A et al: Perioperative normothermia to reduce the incidence of surgical-wound infection and shorten hospitalization, *N Engl J Med* 334:1209, 1996.

Manassa EH et al: Wound healing problems in smokers and nonsmokers after 132 abdominoplasties, *Plast Reconstr Surg* 111:2082, 2003.

Melling AC et al: Effects of preoperative warming on the incidence of wound infection after clean surgery: a randomized controlled trial, *Lancet* 358:876, 2001.

Moller AM et al: Effect of smoking on early complications after elective orthopaedic surgery, *J Bone Joint Surg* 85:178, 2003.

Morris RH: Influence of ambient temperature on patient temperature during intraabdominal surgery, *Ann Surg* 173:230, 1971.

Mun EC et al: Current status of medical and surgical therapy for obesity, *Gastroenterology* 120:660, 2001.

Myles et al: Obesity as an independent risk factor for infections morbidity in patients who undergo cesarean delivery, *Obstet Gynecol* 100:959, 2002.

National Pressure Ulcer Advisory Panel (NPUAP) and European Pressure Ulcer Advisory Panel (EPUAP): *Prevention and treatment of pressure ulcers*, Washington, DC, 2009, NPUAP.

Niinikoski J et al: Oxygen tensions in human wounds, *J Surg Res* 12:77, 1972.

Nisanevich V et al: Effect of intraoperative fluid management on outcome after intraabdominal surgery, *Anesthesiology* 103:25-32, 2005.

Ogden CL et al: *Obesity among adults in the United States—no change since 2003–2004. NCHS data brief no 1.* Hyattsville, Md, 2007, National Center for Health Statistics.

Pasarica M et al: Reduced adipose tissue oxygenation in human obesity: evidence for rarefaction, macrophage chemotaxis, and inflammation without an angiogenic response, *Diabetes* 58(3):718-725, 2009.

Plattner O et al: The influence of two surgical bandage systems on wound tissue oxygen tension, *Arch Surg* 135(7):818-822, 2000.

Pryor KO et al: Surgical site infection and the routine use of perioperative hyperoxia in a general surgical population, *JAMA* 291:79, 2004.

Puzziferri N et al: Local warming increases oxygenation and decreases pain in ischemic ulcers, *Wound Repair Regen* 9(2):146, 2001.

Quirinia A, Viidik A: The effect of recombinant basic fibroblast growth factor (bFGF) in fibrin adhesive vehicle on the healing of ischaemic and normal incisional skin wounds. *Scand J Plast Reconstr Surg Hand Surg* 32:9, 1998.

Reynolds L at al: Perioperative complications of hypothermia, *Best Pract Res Clin Anaesthesiol* 22:645, 2008.

Robson MC et al: Guidelines for the treatment of venous ulcers, *Wound Repair Regen* 14(6):649-662, 2006.

Roe CF: Effect of bowel exposure on body temperature during surgical operations, *Am J Surg* 122:13, 1971.

Roe CF et al: The influence of body temperature on early postoperative oxygen consumption, *Surgery* 60:85, 1966.

Rowell LB: *Human circulation: regulation during physical stress*, New York, 1986, Oxford University Press.

Rubinstein EH, Sessler DI: Skin-surface temperature gradients correlate with fingertip blood flow in humans, *Anesthesiology* 73:541, 1990.

Sen CK: The general case for redox control of wound repair, *Wound Repair Regen* 11:431, 2003.

Sessler DI: Perianesthetic thermoregulation and heat balance in humans, *FASEB J* 7(8):638-644, 1993.

Severinghaus J: Oxyhaemoglobin dissociation curve correction for temperature and pH variation in human blood, *J Appl Physiol* 12:485, 1958.

Sheffield CW et al: Thermoregulatory vasoconstriction decreases subcutaneous oxygen tension in anesthetized volunteers, *Anesthesiology* 77:A96, 1992.

Silver IA: The measurement of oxygen tension in healing tissue, *Prog Resp Res* 3:124, 1969.

Silver IA: The physiology of wound healing. In Hunt T, editor: *Wound healing and wound infection: theory and surgical practice*, New York, 1980, Appleton-Century-Crofts.

Slotman GJ et al: Adverse effects of hypothermia in postoperative patients, *Am J Surg* 49:495, 1985.

Sorensen LT et al: Abstinence from smoking reduces incisional wound infection: a randomized controlled trial, *Ann Surg* 238:1, 2003.

Stotts NA, Wipke-Tevis D: Co-factors in impaired wound healing, *Ostomy Wound Manage* 42(2):44-6, 48, 50-54, 1996.

Vanhoutte PM et al: Local modulation of adrenergic neuroeffector interaction in the blood vessel well, *Physiol Rev* 61:151, 1981.

Vastine VL et al: Wound complications of abdominoplasty in obese patients, *Ann Plast Surg* 42:34, 1999.

Veering BT, Cousins MJ: Cardiovascular and pulmonary effects of epidural anaesthesia, *Anaesth Intensive Care* 28:620, 2000.

Waldorf H, Fewkes J: Wound healing, *Adv Dermatol* 10:77-96, 1995.

Warner DO: Preoperative smoking cessation. How long is long enough? *Anesthesiology* 102:883, 2005.

West JM: Wound healing in the surgical patient: influence of the perioperative stress response on perfusion, *AACN Clin Issues Crit Care Nurs* 1(3):595, 1990.

West JM: *The effect of postoperative forced-air rewarming on subcutaneous tissue oxygen tension and wound healing in hypothermic abdominal surgery patients*, San Francisco, 1994, University of California, San Francisco.

Whitney JD, Wickline MM: Treating chronic and acute wounds with warming: review of the science and practice implications, *J Wound Ostomy Continence Nurs* 30(4):199-209, 2003.

Whitney JD et al: Tissue and wound healing effects of short duration postoperative oxygen therapy, *Bio Res Nurs* 2:206, 2001.

Whitney JD et al: Warming surgical wounds: effects on healing and wound complications, *Wound Rep Regen* 12:A8, 2004.

Wilson JA, Clark JJ: Obesity: impediment to wound healing, *Crit Care Nurs Q* 26(2):119-132, 2003.

Winiarsky R et al: Total knee arthroplasty in morbidly obese patients, *J Bone Joint Surg Am* 80:1770, 1998.

Wong PF et al: Randomized clinical trial of perioperative systemic warming in major elective abdominal surgery, *B J Surg* 94:421, 2007.

Wu L, Mustoe TA: Effect of ischemia on growth factor enhancement of incisional wound healing. *Surgery* 117, 570, 1995.

Zamboni et al: Hyperbaric oxygen and wound healing, *Clin Plast Surg* 30:67, 2003.

29

Noncompliance, Nonadherence, or Barriers to a Sustainable Plan?

Denise P. Nix and Ben Peirce

OBJECTIVES

1. List potential barriers to achieving a sustainable wound management plan.
2. Describe interventions to prevent or minimize barriers.
3. Provide examples of factors associated with impaired activity that may be mistaken for patient noncompliance.
4. Summarize The Joint Commission standards related to patient education.
5. Identify strategies to improve education materials and methods.

Historically, the term *noncompliant* has been used to describe the patient who, for whatever reason, does not adapt to interventions deemed necessary by health care providers. Nurses' descriptions of behaviors from noncompliant patients have ranged from passive resistance and lack of motivation to overt refusal and deliberate interference with care (Hallett et al, 2000). However, patients who have been labeled noncompliant report a lack of understanding of why or what they were supposed to do, or an inability to perform prescribed interventions (Edwards et al, 2002).

This gap in perception leads to obvious questions about the noncompliance label, which has been described as an arrogant term suggesting that the patient's job is to do what he or she is told to do by the health care provider (Rappl, 2004; van Rijswijk, 2004). In recent years, the term *noncompliance* has been replaced with the more politically correct term *nonadherence* or *inability to perform self-care* (Seley, 2009). Regardless of terminology, however, misperceptions remain; the patient did not comply with the plan. The wound specialist's role is to critique the plan of care (rather than the patient). This chapter presents important factors to address in order to formulate a sustainable wound management plan designed to achieve mutually agreed upon goals.

SIGNIFICANCE

In the United States in 2005, 133 million Americans had at least one chronic disease (Ogden et al, 2007). Medical care of chronic diseases accounts for more than 75% of the nation's $1.4 trillion in medical care costs (National Center for Chronic Disease Prevention and Health Promotion, 2009). Economic costs related to medication noncompliance are as high as $100 billion annually in health care and lost productivity and up to $8.5 billion annually in preventable clinic visits and hospitalizations (Durso, 2001). The Wound, Ostomy and Continence Nurses (WOCN) Society (2003) estimated that $2.2 to $3.6 billion was spent annually for the care of pressure ulcers and cited noncompliance as one of the causes of the 13% to 56% recurrence rate. Recurrence rates for venous leg ulcers are reported to be as high as 70% (Robson et al, 2006). The most important intervention to prevent recurrence, graduated compression, is associated with noncompliance (Furlong, 2001; Phillips, 2001; Wipke-Tevis and Sae-Sia, 2004). Similarly, a 59% recurrence rate is reported with diabetic foot ulcers (Steed et al, 2006), and the offloading and footwear options critical to prevention are associated with noncompliance (Armstrong et al, 2005; Wu et al, 2008).

BARRIERS TO A SUSTAINABLE WOUND MANAGEMENT PLAN

When planned interventions are not completed and goals are not met, the best question is not, "What's wrong with the patient?" Rather, we should be asking, "What's wrong with the plan?" The patient and care team together must reevaluate the goals to determine if they are patient centered and realistic and then identify actual or potential barriers to achieving a sustainable plan. Ideally, this process should occur while the initial plan of care is being developed so that barriers can be minimized or eliminated at the onset. This section discusses potential and actual barriers. Possible interventions to prevent or minimize each barrier are listed in Table 29-1.

Inappropriate Goals

Outcomes improve when patients are involved in setting the goals that affect their lives (Masspro, 2008). In order to facilitate a sustainable plan of care, health care professionals need a paradigm shift from a directive, paternalistic style to a more collaborative interactive style in which problems, treatment goals, and management stratagems are defined together (Heisler et al, 2002). Identification and consideration of patient preferences and actions are central to evidence-based decision making (DiCenso et al, 2005).

The goal of wound healing as a standard for all patients is unrealistic and often is inappropriate (Whitney et al, 2006). For example, a patient who is malnourished and does not care to receive enteral or elemental feedings will not achieve the goal of wound healing. Once the patient understands that wound healing is unrealistic, he or she may decide to reconsider supplemental feedings or may aim for a goal that keeps him or her at home, avoid hospital admission, control symptoms (e.g., odor, exudate),

TABLE 29-1	Interventions to Prevent or Minimize Barriers to a Sustainable Wound Management Plan
Barrier	**Intervention**
Inappropriate goals	Collaborate with patient; make sure goals are mutual
	Set goals based on best evidence
	Ensure goals are clearly written and understood
	Explain interventions needed to accomplish goals before patient commits to the goal
	Provide guidance by breaking goals into intermediate steps
	Adjust goals as needed for changes in assessment parameters
Depression, pain, anxiety	Be aware that many patients with depression will not ask for help
	Appropriate pain assessment and management (see Chapters 25 and 26)
	Address aspects of wound management that trigger or exacerbate depression, pain, or anxiety
	Collaborate with social services and physician for appropriate referrals
Cognitive impairment, complicated regimens, impaired dexterity	Simplify procedures
	Divide procedures into easier intermediate steps
	Choose dressings that require fewer changes
	Choose products that are easy to use
	Use combination products to minimize steps
	Encourage use of memory aids and assistive devices when indicated
	Clearly label supplies
	Dispense appropriate number of supplies
	Collaborate with occupational therapy
Impaired activity and mobility	Prescribe compression that is compatible with appropriate shoe wear
	Prescribe offloading devices compatible with wheelchair and home environment
	Adapt clinical environment to accommodate patients with mobility impairment (low examination tables, closer parking)
	Be aware of wound management recommendations that may hinder mobility
	Prescribe sitting program compatible with employment and parenting needs
	Facilitate home care when appropriate
Financial barriers, lack of social/environmental resources	Collaborate with social services
	Identify payer and reimbursement sources
	Learn prices of products and less expensive alternatives
	Learn resources and available funds available to patients with low income
	Financial guidance for prioritizing
Skepticism	Address concerns immediately
	Be honest about risk versus benefits of recommended interventions
	Respect and incorporate life experiences
	Do not minimize concerns
	Recommend a second opinion
	Provide alternative interventions (and goals as needed)
Knowledge deficit	Develop education plan that matches developmental phase, cognitive and physical abilities, and educational and cultural background (see Boxes 29-2 and 29-3)
	Use multiple methods of educational methods and tools (see Table 29-3)

and enhance quality of life as defined by the patient. In other cases, the treatment may produce added discomfort or risk for the patient (Whitney et al, 2006). For example, bed rest for a patient with an ischial tuberosity wound may put the patient at risk for pneumonia due to prolonged immobility. The resulting deconditioning may lead to falls during transfers, causing a vicious cycle with broken bones and more immobility.

Wound healing potential must be based on the most current evidence and communicated in such a way that the patient and family understand (e.g., a patient with peripheral vascular disease with an ankle–brachial index <0.5 requires revascularization for healing to occur; venous insufficiency requires compression for wound healing to occur; pressure ulcer healing is not realistic without pressure relief, nutrition support, and management of urinary or fecal incontinence). When healing is no longer realistic, the plan of care should be revised to focus on goals that support the patient's comfort and his or her need and desire for socialization.

Goals are prioritized into short- and long-term goals. Short-term goals focus on the most pressing issues, such as pain control, infection prevention, and dressing changes. Long-term goals focus on disease management and fostering independence. Discharge goals vary by practice setting. Crucial decisions, such as the patient being able to return to home and live alone, rest on the outcome of learning. The minimum performance necessary for the patient to function must be identified, and progress toward this level must be communicated.

In order to integrate interventions needed for optimal healing, the patient must face multiple adaptations to accommodate the wound as well as the underlying disease. To understand the range of adaptations facing the patient, the wound specialist must know the impact of the wound on the patient's life. The National Family Caregivers Association estimates that family caregivers provide approximately 75% of the home care in the United States (Turnbull, 1999). Hence, to achieve a sustainable plan of care, education and goal setting must include families and caregivers. The wound specialist must help the patient and family determine their goals based on what the patient and family are able and willing to do to achieve those goals. This can be accomplished only if decisions are based on full disclosure and an understanding of relevant information.

Depression, Pain, and Anxiety

A systemic review of the impact of wounds and of quality of life underscored the number of problems, such as pain, sleeplessness, social isolation, loneliness, and job loss, that can lead to anxiety and depression (Herber et al, 2007). The National Institute of Mental Health estimates that 14.8 million adults in the United States suffer from depression. This constitutes 6.7% of the

population at any given time. Up to 80% of patients with depression are untreated or undiagnosed. Many patients with depression will not ask for help, have difficulty performing activities of daily living, and may be unable to follow through with agreed upon interventions (Kessler et al, 2005). A quality-of-life survey conducted by Hyland et al (1994) reported that patients spent an average of 1.5 to 2 hours thinking about their wounds. Whether a patient experiences depression prior to developing a wound or becomes depressed because of the profound challenges the wound presents, the patient's perception related to quality of life should be assessed.

Cognitive Impairment

Cognitive impairment may be an obvious barrier to achieving a sustainable treatment plan; however, the presence of cognitive impairment can be subtle. It is important to review past medical records and speak with family members so that cognitive deficits can be identified and the plan of care adjusted accordingly. In many settings, occupational therapy and speech therapy can assist in identifying cognitive deficits and can assist the wound specialist in developing a plan of care that incorporates the unique learning needs of the patient. Memory aids and reminders have shown effectiveness in medication compliance studies (Durso, 2001).

Complicated Regimens

Complicated regimens present considerable room for error and confusion, especially in the presence of impaired cognition, mobility, or dexterity. Interventions must be described in as few steps as possible. If multiple steps are required, combination products can simplify the process (Nix and Ermer-Seltun, 2004). Dispensing appropriate amounts of supplies and clearly labeling them simplifies the procedure for the patient. Combining interventions with routines already established (e.g., meal times) will increase the likelihood of success.

Impaired Dexterity

The wound specialist must have the expertise and resources available to design a plan of care that accommodates the individual with impaired dexterity. For example, many combination dressings and products eliminate the need for cutting tape. Practice and return demonstrations are critical for the patient with impaired dexterity. Often the patient has learned to compensate for impaired dexterity and just needs an easy-to-apply product or an assistive device (Phillips, 2001). Because impaired dexterity can significantly affect procedure time, selecting dressings that require fewer changes may be more realistic and sustainable.

Impaired Activity and Mobility

Impaired activity and mobility affect the patient's ability to accomplish many important activities needed for disease management and wound healing. Unfortunately, these challenges are not always understood by the health care system and lead to inaccurate assumptions about noncompliance (Box 29-1). The extent to which impaired activity and mobility affect a patient's life must be explored thoroughly before realistic goals and interventions can be put in place. For example, the wound specialist must be aware of the many interventions (e.g., sitting restrictions) and devices (e.g., bulky compression and high-profile support surfaces) that actually can create an activity or mobility deficit for the patient (Armstrong et al, 2001, 2003; Furlong, 2001; Phillips, 2001; Rappl, 2004; Wipke-Tevis and Sae-Sia, 2004). Patients have reported losing their jobs or retiring early because of immobility secondary to a wound or treatment for a wound (Ashford et al, 2000; Brod, 1998; Herber et al, 2007; Phillips et al, 1994).

Lack of Finances and Available Resources

The financial impact of a wound to a patient and family ranges from lack of productivity to early retirement and job loss. For persons who are elderly, are chronically ill,

BOX 29-1 | **Activity/Mobility Issues that Contribute to Inaccurate Assumptions About Noncompliance**

Transportation to Clinic
- Patient misses clinic appointments due to unreliable transportation
- Transfer method to vehicle causes friction and shear
- Amount of time sitting in vehicle is not compatible with sitting restrictions
- Parking at the clinic is too expensive, does not accommodate vehicle, or is located too far away for patient to get to appointment on time or at all

Mobility
- Mobility deficits limit patient's ability to shop and prepare meals to meet nutrition plan
- Wound care devices prescribed for patient are too difficult to apply and remove
- Compression prescribed for patient prohibits patient from wearing an appropriate shoe for safe ambulation or exercise
- Sitting limitations threaten patient's ability to maintain employment or parental rights
- Offloading boots and cushions prescribed for patient do not fit properly in patent's wheelchair

Transfer Method
- Profile of prescribed chair cushion is not compatible with home furniture and makes transfers too difficult or unsafe
- Resources are unavailable for Hoyer lift transfers, and sliding board transfers cause friction or shear

or are in a low-income bracket, as much as 31% of their total income may be spent on health care. Patients cut corners with health care in order to afford rent or food (Lantz, 2003). Financial barriers are frequently cited as a reason for failing to fill or pick up medication prescriptions (Durso, 2001). Treatment decisions should be made, bearing in mind what is financially reasonable for the patient as well as the less expensive alternatives. It is important to be aware of the payer source as well as the patient's out-of-pocket expenses for noncovered items, transportation, and loss of pay due to time missed from work.

The wound specialist needs to understand the logistics of obtaining equipment and other resources to ensure proper patient care. This is especially important between care settings so that the patient is discharged only after the appropriate equipment is ready at the next care setting. Resources may not be available due to a lack of funds or support from friends and family because of a variety of reasons (e.g., distance or family dynamics). Although finances are a powerful risk factor, they can be a powerful motivator as well. For example, a family member or patient who is not ready to learn a dressing change may become motivated when he or she learns there will be out-of-pocket expense for another care setting or home care.

Skepticism and Mistrust

Patients can become skeptical as they are inundated with information from sources that are credible and others that are misleading or inaccurate. Patients can quickly access a plethora of information on the Internet. However, some Internet sources are extremely helpful, whereas others, if followed, can sabotage the plan of care. Criteria can be applied to assess the credibility of information on the Internet (see Table 1-7). The wound specialist should respectfully discuss this information with the patient. Becoming defensive or dismissing the patient's concerns will leave the patient feeling alienated. Such interactions can damage the trust between patient and caregiver. The patient should have his or her concerns addressed and should be encouraged to obtain a second opinion, if desired.

Potential or Actual Side Affects. People make decisions and agree to interventions based on what they know. If they are uninformed about the side effects or do not understand the impact these side effects may have on their life, patients may develop mistrust and skepticism, may choose to discontinue an activity, or may not modify their behavior. A 2007 study found that the typical Medicare beneficiary saw two primary care physicians and five specialists annually; pharmacies and diagnostic facilities are not included in these numbers. Patients with several chronic conditions visited as many as 16 physicians in a year (Pham et al, 2007). These data underscore the importance of a holistic assessment that includes concurrent medications and therapies for the patient. Studies have shown that people are less likely to adopt behaviors or implement interventions that have unpleasant side effects (Armstrong et al, 2005; Furlong, 2001; Phillips, 2001; Wipke-Tevis and Sae-Sia, 2004; Wu et al, 2008).

Ineffective Care Transitions

Care transitions are defined as patient transfers between locations or levels of care with the same location. Examples include patients transferring from a hospital to their home after surgery while needing continued wound care; or a patient living at home with a chronic wound and being referred by their primary care provider to an outpatient wound clinic. Patients with wounds associated with complex conditions often require care by numerous providers within and between care settings. One study found that patients with chronic conditions see eight different physicians in a year (Coleman, 2003). As patients transition between providers, details of the patient's wound management plan can be omitted or communicated incompletely (Bodenheimer, 2008), which then becomes a barrier to effective care. Inefficient care transitions also reduce patient satisfaction and waste valuable resources. Care transitions are most effective: when patients understand what to expect in the next location and have input in their wound management plan, when receiving clinicians have complete information from the sending clinicians, and when clinicians in a community work together to understand the requirements and capabilities of each others' care settings (Bodenheimer, 2008).

Knowledge Deficit

Because full disclosure and understanding of relevant information are critical to decision making and goal setting, lack of knowledge probably is one of the most common barriers associated with a failed plan of care. Box 29-2 summarizes The Joint Commission standards for patient education (Canobbio, 2006).

Patient education begins with an assessment of what the patient needs to know to achieve recovery and return of function. Once the assessment is made, the wound specialist must help the patient understand enough about the wound, underlying disease, and treatment options to make informed decisions. Each treatment option must be explained in terms of processes, outcomes, probabilities, and tradeoffs (e.g., length of life vs quality of life, cost vs benefit). Table 29-2 lists key questions and information needed to address the essential issues so that the patient, family, and caregivers can make informed decisions.

It is estimated that 50% of medical information is lost immediately after a patient speaks with a health professional (So et al, 2003). Therefore education assessment and techniques must take into consideration all the

---

BOX 29-2	**Summary of The Joint Commission Statements for Patient Education Standards**

- Provide patient and family/significant other with information that will enhance their knowledge and skills necessary to promote recovery and improve function.
- Encourage patient participation in decision making, and include family in the teaching process.
- Assess the patient's learning needs, abilities, preferences, and readiness to learn.
- Consider cultural and religious practices, emotional barriers, desire and motivation to learn, physical and cognitive limitations, language barriers, and financial implications of care choices.
- Educate patients about safe and effective use of medications according to law and their needs.
- Educate patients about safe and effective use of equipment and supplies.
- Educate patients about potential drug–foods interaction and provide counseling on nutrition and modified diets.
- Inform patients about access to additional resources in the community.
- Inform patient about when and how to obtain further treatment the patient may need.
- Provide discharge instructions to patient and those responsible for providing continuing care.
- Educate patient regarding self-care activities as appropriate.

From Canobbio MM: *Mosby's handbook of patient teaching,* ed 3, St. Louis, 2006, Mosby/Elsevier.

---

factors that may influence the patient's ability, motivation, and readiness to learn (Checklist 29-1). The educational assessment and plan may require a team approach as described in Chapter 1. For example, speech therapy and occupational therapy can provide vital assessment input for communication, language, and physical and cognitive limitations as well as techniques to incorporate for successful teaching and learning. The education plan must be age appropriate, taking into account principles of adult learning (Knowles et al, 1998) (Box 29-3) and features of development that impact coping and learning strategies for children as described in Chapter 36.

Providing ample time for patient teaching has always been a challenge. With shorter hospital stays, the wound specialist must take even more care to develop a variety of strategies to ensure the patient's educational needs are identified and that progress toward meeting these needs is communicated to providers in the next care setting. In acute care, the education plan begins at admission and must be incorporated into routine care, as convenient, during frequent daily encounters (Canobbio, 2006). For example, skin inspection can be taught during the patient's bath. Protection of skin surrounding wounds and moist wound healing can be discussed during dressing changes. Each time a patient is repositioned, pressure ulcer prevention strategies can be taught and reinforced. Information may need to be limited to the skills and behaviors necessary for the patient to learn before

TABLE 29-2	Decision-Making Template for Treatment Options	
Required Element	**Key Patient Questions**	**Information Provided**
Clinical condition reported	What are the characteristics of my diagnosis/disease/disorder?	Details of clinically important subgroups
Patient decision situation	What are the different ways this disorder can be treated?	Options for surgical treatments, medical treatments, watchful waiting, contemporary therapies
For Each Treatment Option		
Treatment process	What kind of treatment is it? How much time does it involve? What do I have to do to undergo this treatment?	Mode and duration of treatment, nature of patient involvement
Outcomes and probabilities	What are the chances of improvement over the next x days/weeks/months/years or over my lifetime?	Rates for different outcomes over various times, absolute number improved, improvement rates
	What kinds of side/toxic effects can occur, and what are the chances of each?	Rates for different side effects
Value tradeoffs	What are the tradeoffs between length and quality of life? If length of life is not affected, what are the tradeoffs among the inconveniences, costs, chances of side effects, etc., in order to gain a benefit such as symptom relief? Where can I get descriptions of other patients' experiences?	Material for clarification of values

From Holmes-Rovner M et al: Patient choice modules for summaries of clinical effectiveness: a proposal, *BMJ* 322:664-667, 2001.

CHECKLIST 29-1
Educational Assessment

✓ Age and developmental phase
✓ Cognitive abilities
✓ Physical abilities (activity, mobility, dexterity)
✓ Educational background
✓ Life experiences that may influence learning
✓ Cultural and religious practices
✓ Language skills
✓ Occupation
✓ Finances and financial implications of care choices
✓ Type of health care coverage and discharge plan
✓ Support from family and friends
✓ Pain, anxiety, and depression
✓ Learning needs and readiness to learn

discharge and information needed to establish mutually agreed upon goals.

Printed materials are an economical use of time if they are well designed and match the learner's reading and literacy levels. Educational methods must be sensitive to the culture of patients who will be using them, addressing their lifestyles and using cultural language and symbols they understand (Redman, 2007). Approximately half of the population in the United States struggles with basic reading skills. For many persons, the materials available are written at a higher level than they can understand, sometimes as many as five grades higher than the school level the patient has completed (Redman, 2007). Techniques that improve readership, comprehension, and memory of printed materials are summarized in Table 29-3 (Buxton, 1999).

Research suggests that combining educational methods leads to better outcomes (Redman, 2007). Focus group have given high ratings to use of video vignettes combined

with discussions because they could relate to the situations presented, and the videos stimulated important discussions (Anderson and Funnell, 1999). A meta-analysis examining the effectiveness of interventions to improve patient compliance found that education combined with behavioral therapies were very effective for teaching coping strategies (Roter et al, 1998). A prospective, randomized study of 28 patients with burn injury compared instructional methods with adherence to dressing changes and hypertrophic scar formation. The standard group received a written handout and verbal rationale for their dressing changes, whereas the enhanced group received a written handout, verbal rationale, and a video presentation. Results revealed that the enhanced group had a statistically significant $(p < .001)$ improved adherence with dressing changes and less hypertrophic scar formation (So et al, 2003).

BOX 29-3	Principles of Adult Learning

1. Adults want to know why they should learn.
   - Adults are motivated to put time and energy into learning if they know the benefits of learning and the costs of not learning.
2. Adults need to take responsibility.
   - Adult learners perceive themselves as being in charge of their lives and decisions and need to be seen as capable.
3. Adults bring experience to learning.
   - Adults define themselves by their experiences and need to have their experiences valued and respected. Experiences can give deeper meaning to new ideas and skills or may lead to bias.
4. Adults are ready to learn when the need arises.
   - Adults learn when they choose to learn, usually when they perceive a need to learn.
5. Adults are task oriented.
   - Education often is subject centered, and adults need education that is task centered.

Data from Knowles MS et al: *The adult learner,* Houston, 1998, Gulf Publishing.

TABLE 29-3	Techniques to Improve Health Education Materials	
Do		**Don't**

Direct Readers to the Message

• Use arrows, underlines, bold type, boxes, white space, and bullets to direct readers' eyes to the key messages.	• Use italics, all capital letters, or screens of color over text. • Require reader to look in many directions on the page to read copy and find the message.

Select an Easy-to-Read Typeface

• Use 10- to 14-point type size. • Use a typeface with serifs in the body copy (e.g., Times Roman).	• Go below 10-point type size for good readers and 12-point for poor readers. • Mix typefaces or use more than three sizes of print on one page. • Use white letters on black background.

Create Easy-to-Read Copy

• Use columns that are 40 to 50 characters wide, left justified. • Use lots of white space. Consider question-and-answer or bullets rather than paragraphs. • Use highly contrasting colors for text and background, such as black on white or cream. • Use the same dark color for headings and body copy or colors with similar intensity.	• Break margins with illustrations or other graphics. If required, break only the right margin. • Use light or unusual ink colors, such as red, green, or orange.

Create Clear Visuals

• Convey one key message per visual. Print the message in a caption. • Make the message easy to grasp at a glance. • Show only the "desired" way to act. • Use realistic drawings, photos, or humanlike figures. • Use visuals with which the audience can identify.	• Add any visuals simply to decorate the material. • Include any details or background in the visual that are not required to communicate the message. • Use highly stylized or abstract graphics. • Portray blood cells and other body parts as cartoon characters.

Adapted from Buxton T: Effective ways to improve health education materials, *J Health Educ* 30(1):47, 1999. From Redman BK: *The practice of patient education,* ed 10, St. Louis, 2006, Mosby/Elsevier.

SUMMARY

The wound management team must be guided by an underlying philosophy that care providers work in partnership with the patient to develop a sustainable plan of care based upon mutually agreed upon goals. Identifying and addressing actual or potential barriers to achieving a sustainable plan may improve the ability to achieve care plan goals, decrease recurrence rates, and, if appropriate, maximize the potential for wound healing. The wound specialist is in a pivotal position to avoid mislabeling patients as noncompliant. At a minimum, a complete assessment and documentation of interventions addressing the barriers to achieving a sustainable plan should be completed before such a conclusion can be reached.

REFERENCES

Anderson RM, Funnell MM: Theory is the cart, vision is the horse: reflections on research in diabetes patient education, *Diabetes Educ* 25:43, 1999.

Armstrong DG et al: Off-loading the diabetic foot wound: a randomized clinical trial, *Diabetes Care* 24(6):1019, 2001.

Armstrong DG et al: Activity patterns with diabetic foot ulceration: patients with active ulceration may not adhere to a standard pressure off-loading regimen, *Diabetes Care* 26(9):2595, 2003.

Armstrong DG et al: Evaluation of removable and irremovable cast walkers in the healing of diabetic foot wounds: a randomized controlled trial, *Diabetes Care* 28(3):551-554, 2005.

Ashford RL et al: Perception of quality of life by patients with diabetic foot ulcers, *Diab Foot* 3:150-155, 2000.

Bodenheimer T: Coordinating care—a perilous journey through the health care system, *N Engl J Med* 358(10):1064-1071, 2008.

Brod M: Quality of life issues in patients with diabetes and lower extremity ulcers: patients and caregivers, *Qual Life Res* 7(4):365-372, 1998.

Buxton T: Effective ways to improve health education materials, *J Health Educ* 30(1):47 1999.

Canobbio MM: *Mosby's handbook of patient teaching*, ed 3, St Louis, 2006, Mosby.

Coleman EA, Falling through the cracks: challenges and opportunities for improving transitional care for persons with continuous complex care needs. *J Am Geriatr Soc* 2003 Apr;51(4):549, 2003.

DiCenso A et al: *Evidenced-based nursing: a guide to clinical practice*, St. Louis, 2005, Elsevier Mosby.

Durso S: Technological advances for improving medication adherence in the elderly, *Ann Long-Term Care* 9(4):43, 2001.

Edwards LM et al: An exploration of patients' understanding of leg ulceration, *J Wound Care* 11(1):35, 2002.

Furlong W: Venous disease treatment and compliance: the nursing role, *Br J Nurs* 10(11Suppl):S18, 2001.

Hallett CE et al: Community nurses' perceptions of patient 'compliance' in wound care: a discourse analysis, *J Adv Nurs* 32(1):115-123, 2000.

Heisler M et al: The relative importance of physician communication, participatory decision-making, and patient understanding in diabetes self-management, *J Gen Intern Med* 17:243, 2002.

Herber OR et al: A systematic review on the impact of leg ulceration on patients' quality of life, *Health Qual Life Outcomes* 5:44, 2007.

Holmes-Rovner M et al: Patient choice modules for summaries of clinical effectiveness: a proposal, *BMJ* 322:664-667, 2001.

Hyland ME et al: Quality of life of leg ulcer patients: questionnaire and preliminary findings, *J Wound Care* 3:294-298, 1994.

Kessler RC et al: Prevalence, severity, and comorbidity of twelve-month DSM-IV disorders in the National Comorbidity Survey Replication (NCS-R), *Arch Gen Psychiatry* 62(6):617-627, 2005.

Knowles MS et al: *The adult learner*, Houston, 1998, Gulf Publishing.

Lantz M: Economic noncompliance in the treatment of depression: when the patient can't afford prescription drugs, *Clin Geriatr* 11(09):18-22, 2003.

Medicare Quality Improvement Organization for Massachusetts (Masspro): *A systems approach to quality improvement in home health: planned care: self-management support in home healthcare*, 2008, available at http://www.masspro.org/HH/CPIM/docs/tools/Plnd%20Cre%20Wkbk%20rev2_FNL.pdf, accessed May 26, 2009.

National Center for Chronic Disease Prevention and Health Promotion: *Chronic diseases and health promotion*, 2009, available at http://www.cdc.gov/nccdphp/overview.htm, accessed February 3, 2010.

Nix D, Ermer-Seltun J: A review of perineal skin care protocols and skin barrier product use, *Ostomy Wound Manage* 50(12):59, 2004.

Ogden CL, Carroll MD, McDowell MA, Flegal KM. *Obesity among adults in the United States—no change since 2003–2004*. NCHS data brief no 1. Hyattsville, MD: National Center for Health Statistics; 2007. Available from: http://www.cdc.gov/nchs/data/databriefs/db01.pdf [PDF-366KB]

Pham HH et al: Care patterns in Medicare and their implications for pay for performance, *N Engl J Med* 356:1130-1139, 2007.

Phillips T: Current approaches to venous ulcers and compression, *Dermatol Surg* 27:611, 2001.

Phillips T et al: A study of the impact of leg ulcers on quality of life: financial, social, and psychologic implications, *J Am Acad Dermatol* 31:49-53, 1994.

Rappl L: Non-compliance: adding insult to injury, *Ostomy Wound Manage* 50(5):6, 2004.

Redman BK: *The practice of patient education: a case study approach*, ed 10, St Louis, 2007, Mosby.

Robson MC et al: Guidelines for the treatment of venous ulcers, *Wound Repair Regen* 14(6):649-662, 2006.

Roter DL et al: Effectiveness of interventions to improve patient compliance: a meta-analysis, *Med Care* 36:1138, 1998.

Seley JJ: Noncompliance verses diabetes self care: are we still playing the blame game? *Diabetes Health*, June 19, 2009, available at http://www.diabeteshealth.com/read/2009/06/18/6248/non-compliance-vs—diabetes-self-care—are-we-still-playing-a-blame-game/#share, accessed February 3, 2010.

So K et al: Effects of enhanced patient education on compliance with silicone gel sheeting and burn scar outcome: a randomized prospective study, *J Burn Care Rehabil* 24(6):411, 2003.

Steed DL et al: Guidelines for the treatment of diabetic ulcers, *Wound Repair Regen* 14(6):680-692, 2006.

Turnbull G: The dollars and sense of patient teaching, *Ostomy Wound Manage* 45(3):16, 1999.

van Rijswijk L: Non-compliance no more, *Ostomy Wound Manage* 50(1):6, 2004.

Whitney J et al: Guidelines for the treatment of pressure ulcers, *Wound Repair Regen* 14(6):663-679, 2006.

Wipke-Tevis D, Sae-Sia W: Caring for vascular leg ulcers, *Home Healthcare Nurse* 22(4):237, 2004.

Wound, Ostomy and Continence Nurses (WOCN) Society: *Guideline for management of pressure ulcers*, WOCN Clinical Practice Guideline Series #2, Glenview IL, 2003.

Wu SC et al: Use of pressure offloading devices in diabetic foot ulcers, *Diabetes Care* 31(11):2118-2119, 2008.

Acute and Traumatic Wounds

30

Intrinsic Diseases and Uncommon Cutaneous Wounds

Ruth A. Bryant

OBJECTIVES

1. Differentiate between staphylococcal scalded skin syndrome and toxic epidermal necrolysis (TEN) and between graft-versus-host disease (GVHD) and pyoderma gangrenosum in terms of manifestations and etiology.
2. Describe the process of tissue damage and treatment options for vasculitis, calciphylaxis, epidermolysis bullosa (EB), GVHD, frostbite, and TEN.
3. Discriminate among the patient populations at risk for calciphylaxis, frostbite, TEN, and extravasation.

4. Compare and contrast the role of debridement in necrotizing fasciitis, TEN, extravasation, and frostbite.
5. Describe the distinguishing features of a chronic wound with malignant transformation.
6. Identify four conditions that require a tissue biopsy for diagnosis.

Many less common skin lesions exist, some of which are life threatening. This chapter discusses atypical ulcerations that often are intrinsic to another disease. These lesions are rare but are associated with significant morbidity and mortality. When a wound does not "fit" the pattern of more common skin lesions or the wound is unresponsive to appropriate treatment, uncommon cutaneous wounds should be considered. The wound specialist should be familiar with the clinical manifestations of these less common conditions to facilitate early detection and prompt referral for appropriate medical management. In many situations, early detection is essential to arrest the underlying pathology and to prevent progression of ulcerations, infection, sepsis, and death.

INFECTIOUS ETIOLOGY

Staphylococcal Scalded Skin Syndrome

Staphylococcal scalded skin syndrome (SSSS) is a superficial blistering skin disorder caused by the exfoliative toxins of some strains of *Staphylococcus aureus*. Initially an infection is present most commonly in the oral or nasal cavities, neck, axillae, groin, or umbilicus (King and de Saint Victor, 2009). The toxins produced by the infecting organism are transferred through the bloodstream to a site remote from the original infection where significant erythema will develop, followed by

separation of the superficial epidermis (i.e., desquamation). The primary lesions are superficial bullae. Secondarily, lesions develop superficial scales. The skin may have a sandpaper feel. Significant pain is unusual for SSSS and, if present, suggests another diagnosis, such as toxic epidermal necrolysis (TEN), a drug-induced necrosis of the epidermis.

Although SSSS has been reported in adults, it most commonly occurs in healthy children 6 years or younger and in neonates (Habif et al, 2005; King and de Saint Victor, 2009). Mortality in children is very low (1%–5%) unless SSSS is associated with sepsis or a coexisting serious medical condition. SSSS, when it develops in adults, occurs in adults who are chronically ill, immunocompromised, or with renal failure. The mortality rate in adults is substantial (50%–60%), although this may be attributable to the overall health status of the adults rather than the SSSS (King and de Saint Victor, 2009).

Suspicious sites (nose, eyes, ears, throat, vagina) should be swabbed for microbial cultures to confirm the diagnosis. Bullae from the primary lesion usually yield cultures that are negative for bacteria. A frozen section of sloughing skin is needed to differentiate SSSS from a drug-induced skin reaction (TEN). Full-thickness epidermal necrosis is inconsistent with SSSS and suggests a drug-induced process.

Once SSSS is diagnosed, treatment consists of supportive care and elimination of the primary infection.

Debridement and antibiotics are essential to manage the infection. Topical management of the desquamated skin should address exudate management, pain control, and maintenance of a moist environment. Foam dressings, superabsorbent dressings, sheet hydrogels, and alginates are preferred dressing options; adhesives should be avoided. Steroids may worsen immune function, and nonsteroidal antiinflammatory drugs (NSAIDs) should be avoided because they potentially can reduce renal function (King and de Saint Victor, 2009). When massive tissue loss is apparent, the wound should be managed according to the principles for burn therapy as outlined in Chapter 32.

Toxic Shock Syndrome

Toxic shock syndrome is caused by a toxin produced by certain types of *Staphylococcus* bacterial infections. The most common pathogen for this serious infection is *S. aureus*. Acute onset consists of a widespread macular erythematous eruption (within 1–3 days) that extends to include the soles of the feet and the palms of the hands. Desquamation of the skin is highly characteristic of toxic shock syndrome. It occurs 10 days to 3 weeks after onset and primarily includes the fingertips and plantar surfaces of the palms and feet. Additional clinical manifestations include edema of the hands and feet (50%), petechiae (27%), conjunctival injection (85%), oropharyngeal hyperemia (90%), and genital hyperemia (100%) (Habif et al, 2005).

Diagnosis is based on a constellation of symptoms: fever (>102°F), hypotension, rash progressing to desquamation, and mucosal membrane involvement (mouth, eyes, vagina). In addition, the condition must be multisystem as evidenced by impaired functioning of at least three organs (muscular, gastrointestinal, central nervous system, renal, hepatic, hematologic, cardiopulmonary, metabolic) (Habif et al, 2005; Smith, 2008). A skin biopsy is indicated to exclude TEN as a diagnosis.

The goal of treatment of toxic shock syndrome is preventing organ damage through supportive care and aggressive antibiotic therapy; the mortality rate of toxic shock syndrome ranges from 3% to 12% (Habif et al, 2005). Local wound management is based on wound needs (e.g., exudate absorption), and topical dressings should be nonocclusive and nonadhesive.

Necrotizing Fasciitis

Necrotizing fasciitis is an uncommon but serious subcutaneous tissue infection that spreads rapidly along the superficial fascial plane. The overall mortality rate from this very rapidly spreading condition is variable: 20% in pediatric cases and anywhere from 6% to 73% in adults (Anaya and Dellinger, 2007). Necrotizing fasciitis is characterized by widespread necrosis of the fascia and deep subcutaneous tissue, with thrombosis of nutrient vessels and sloughing of overlying tissue (Plate 59). It usually occurs in the extremities after a minor operation or injury. The clinical markers of necrotizing fasciitis are a rapidly spreading erythema in the skin around the wound and subcutaneous crepitus that may be visible on radiograph. Additional signs of necrotizing fasciitis are pain (considered to be out of proportion for the extent of the skin damage), swelling at the site of the wound, chills, fever, and toxemia. The skin may initially appear normal over the cellulitis, but as the infectious process compromises blood supply the skin becomes erythematous, edematous, and reddish-purple to patchy blue gray. Bullae form within 3 to 5 days from onset and progress to necrosis of the skin, sloughing, and frank cutaneous gangrene (Anaya and Dellinger, 2007). Tendon sheaths and muscle will liquefy when infected; in the operating room, "dishwater fluid" is the hallmark of liquefactive necrosis.

Necrotizing fasciitis can be detected by its dramatic clinical presentation and by probing the wound. When the affected area is probed with a hemostat through a limited incision, the instrument passes easily along a plane of superficial to deep fascia. This examination helps to distinguish necrotizing fasciitis from cellulitis. This infection is most often polymicrobial with group A streptococci or *S. aureus* predominating. A subset of necrotizing soft tissue infections caused by *Clostridium* species are monomicrobial and associated with a significantly worse prognosis (Anaya and Dellinger, 2007).

The presence of necrotizing fasciitis requires aggressive surgical debridement; any nonviable or questionably viable tissue must be removed. Because the infection spreads subcutaneously, a wound may need to be extended to allow access to and debridement of all necrotic tissue (Attinger et al, 2006). Despite aggressive local control, necrotizing fasciitis has a 24% to 50% mortality rate secondary to persistent wound sepsis or systemic sepsis (Martin et al, 2008). Local wound care consists of close monitoring for further dissection, which indicates progression of the infection. Topical dressing recommendations are largely based on expert opinion or preference. Dressings should be used that meet the needs of the wound (e.g., fill dead space, absorb exudate), allow for frequent monitoring of the wound, and are nonadhesive and nonocclusive.

SPIDER BITES

Only 60 of the 20,000 species of spiders in the world are capable of inflicting a bite, and only four can cause significant injury; evidence of that tissue damage is documented for only two spiders: the brown recluse and the black widow. The brown recluse spider is one of five species of spiders within the genus *Loxosceles*. This spider is about the size of a U.S. quarter, is yellow to brown in color, and has a distinctive fiddle-shaped mark on its back (Rhoads, 2007). The brown recluse spider usually is shy and nocturnal. It tends to avoid humans and seek shelter in abandoned or infrequently used buildings, attics, and basements. Bites generally occur when a person disturbs a pile of wood or rocks, moves boxes that have been stored, or dresses in clothes that have been stored for a long period of time. The most common site for a *Loxosceles* spider bite is on the extremities, but they also can occur on the buttocks or genitalia.

The venom of the brown recluse spider is a mixture of enzymes that destroy cellular membranes, resulting in damage to the surrounding skin, fat, nerves, and blood vessels. Manifestations of a brown recluse spider bite can range from small lesions with erythema to full-thickness necrotic wounds (known as necrotic arachnidism). Fewer than 10% of patients develop severe skin necrosis or other systemic reaction (e.g., loxoscelism, which is characterized by fever, nausea, hemolysis, and thrombocytopenia) (Schwartz, 2009; Zeglin, 2005). Severity of the reaction depends on the amount of venom injected, the site of the bite, and host susceptibility. However, it is the accumulation of activated neutrophils that is responsible for the cutaneous necrosis (Schwartz, 2009). Accumulation of neutrophils occurs 24 to 72 hours before skin necrosis and ulceration. The very young, the elderly, and individuals in poor physical condition are at highest risk for serious illness from a spider bite.

After a spider bite, the person may experience a mild burning sensation or may experience no discomfort at all. Within 6 to 12 hours, itching, pain, a central papule, and erythema may develop. Wounds that progress usually begin to do so within 48 to 72 hours of the bite. As the tissue damage progresses, the characteristic "red, white, and blue" sign of a brown recluse bite develops; the sign consists of a ring of blanched skin (due to vasoconstriction) surrounded by erythema with gray-to-red-purple bullae at the site of the bite (Schwartz, 2009; Zeglin, 2005) (Plate 60). Severe necrosis is more likely when the bite is located in an area with significant adipose tissue, such as the thighs and buttocks. When the bite remains localized with a central blister, resolution occurs within 3 weeks. Severe bites that develop necrosis heal over a 2- to 3-month time span (Rhoads, 2007).

The standard treatment of spider bite lesions is (1) thorough cleansing, (2) rest, (3) application of ice, (4) compression, and (5) elevation. Oral antiinflammatory medications, an antihistamine, and tetanus vaccine also may be given. If cellulitis appears to be developing, an antibiotic such as erythromycin is indicated (Zeglin, 2005). Treatment of severe necrotic lesions is controversial; however, the goals are to (1) maintain skin integrity, (2) prevent spread of infection, and (3) maintain circulatory status. The following interventions are indicated (Smith et al, 1997): (1) ice pack on the affected area (no heat) to lessen tissue damage, (2) empiric antibiotics to treat cellulitis, (3) NSAIDs to relieve inflammation and pain, (4) tetanus toxoid, and (5) nonocclusive topical dressings to provide a moist environment, fill dead space, and absorb exudate. The site should be monitored for signs of deterioration and cellulitis (Rhoads, 2007).

Patients with severe and rapidly progressing lesions may be given dapsone (Avlosulfon) therapy, which is an inhibitor of neutrophil function. However, it must be administered within hours of a bite to be effective. By inhibiting the spread of neutrophils, dapsone is believed to minimize tissue necrosis (Zeglin, 2005). However, dapsone can have multiple moderate to severe adverse effects. Alternative interventions include hyperbaric oxygenation, nitroglycerin patches, electric shock therapy, and heparin therapy, although no evidence is conclusive for the effectiveness of these treatments. Systemic reactions and complications from the bite of a recluse spider include renal failure and coagulation disorders such as thrombocytopenia and disseminated intravascular coagulopathy (Zeglin, 2005).

PYODERMA GANGRENOSUM

Pyoderma gangrenosum (PG) is a chronic neutrophilic inflammatory disease that most likely represents an aberrant immune response to an as yet unidentified antigen; alterations of neutrophils and interleukins through action of tumor necrosis factor (TNF)-α cytokines have been reported (Brooklyn et al, 2006). The pathogenesis of PG may be related to abnormal T-cell responses and production of a powerful proinflammatory cytokine (TNF-α) (Reguiaĩ and Grange, 2007). Histologically, the presence of numerous polymorphonuclear leukocytes creates a dense infiltrate of the dermis that can extend from the superficial dermis to the subcutaneous tissue.

These painful lesions have been associated with underlying systemic diseases, such as inflammatory bowel disease in 30% of cases and rheumatoid arthritis with seropositive increase of the rheumatoid factor in 25% of cases (Box 30-1). Approximately 40% to 50% of cases occur in patients with no known associated systemic disease and are idiopathic (Snyder, 2008; Wollina, 2007). When PG accompanies a systemic disease, it does not necessarily parallel the underlying disease and instead be triggered by trauma (Paparone et al, 2009).

PG has several different manifestations, but generally these extremely painful lesions begin with a nodule, pustule, or bulla that develops significant induration and

---

BOX 30-1	Systemic Diseases Associated with Pyoderma Gangrenosum

- Ankylosing spondylitis
- Rheumatoid arthritis
- Sarcoidosis
- Chronic active hepatitis
- Inflammatory bowel disease
- Monoclonal gammopathies
- Myeloma

erythema and proceeds to ulceration. The three clinically distinct variations of PG are classic, atypical, and peristomal. The most common presentation is the classic ulcerative form. This particular variation is characterized by ulcers that usually occur on the lower extremities but may also occur on the abdomen, genitalia, trunk, head, and neck. It is commonly associated with inflammatory bowel disease (particularly Crohn's disease) and rheumatoid arthritis and may occur before, during, or after the disease (Callen and Jackson, 2007).

Atypical PG is commonly associated with myeloproliferative disease, refractory anemias, and myelogenous leukemia (Callen and Jackson, 2007). These are superficial ulcerations or deep erosions primarily located on the hands, arms, face, head, or neck that begin as pustules and extend into plaques. This particular variation of PG is commonly misdiagnosed as cellulitis.

Peristomal PG consists of lesions around a stoma commonly associated with inflammatory bowel disease. These lesions are similar to those typical of classic PG. Although rare, extracutaneous manifestations of PG can involve the lungs, bones, cornea, liver, spleen, heart, skeletal muscles, and central nervous system (Callen and Jackson, 2007).

Common characteristics of the ulcerative PG lesion include irregularly shaped wound edges that are elevated and violaceous (Plate 61). Ulcers are exudative and extremely tender. The wound base is often filled with yellow slough and/or islands of necrosis; wound edges are undermined. A band of erythema may extend from the wound edge, which defines the direction in which the ulcer will extend. Healing may be present along one edge of the ulcer while enlargement occurs along another edge. Ulcers heal slowly and leave an atrophic, irregular scar. A common and notable characteristic of PG is a phenomenon known as *pathergy*, which is the abnormal and exaggerated inflammatory response to noxious stimuli. Patients often report the lesion developing after minor trauma, such as a bump against a piece of furniture. Minor trauma preceding the development of the ulcer is an important piece of information to obtain during the patient interview (Paparone et al, 2009).

PG is difficult to diagnose; it is essentially a diagnosis by exclusion. It can be misdiagnosed as venous, arterial, neuropathic disease, vasculitis (i.e., polyarteritis nodosa), thrombophilic disease (livedoid vasculitis, antiphospholipid syndrome), neoplasia (squamous cell carcinoma, cutaneous lymphoma, metastatic carcinoma), or infection (cellulitis, herpes, cutaneous tuberculosis) (Callen and Johnson, 2007). Diagnosis is based on clinical manifestations and a thorough examination in which other ulcerative skin disorders (e.g., vasculitis, infections) and psychosomatic illnesses have been excluded. A history and physical examination, skin biopsy for histology and microbiology, and an investigation for an associated illness constitute a thorough workup (Box 30-2). The histopathologic findings are not specific for PG; however, they are

---

BOX 30-2 | **Proposed Diagnostic Criteria for Pyoderma Gangrenosum**

Major Criteria
1. Rapid[a] progression of painful[b] necrolytic cutaneous ulcer[c] with irregular, violaceous, undermined border
2. Exclusion of other causes of cutaneous ulceration

Minor Criteria
1. History suggestive of pathergy[d] or clinical finding of cribriform scarring
2. Systemic diseases associated with pyoderma gangrenosum[e]
3. Histopathologic findings (sterile dermal neutrophilia ± mixed inflammation ± lymphocytic vasculitis)
4. Treatment response (rapid response to systemic glucocorticoid treatment)[f]

[a]Characteristic margin expansion of 1 to 2 cm/day, or 50% increase in ulcer size within 1 month.
[b]Pain usually out of proportion to size of ulceration.
[c]Typically preceded by papule, pustule, or bulla.
[d]Ulcer development at sites of minor cutaneous injury.
[e]Inflammatory bowel disease, polyarthritis, myelocytic leukemia, or preleukemia.
[f]Generally responds to dosage of 1–2 mg/kg/d, with 50% decrease in size within 1 month.
Adapted from Su WPD et al: Pyoderma gangrenosum: clinicopathologic correlation and proposed diagnostic criteria, *Int J Dermatol* 43:790–800, 2004. From Callen JP, Jackson JM: Pyoderma gangrenosum: an update, *Rheum Dis Clin North Am* 33:793, 2007.

---

supportive of the disease. A biopsy of the ulcer is essential, even though it may enlarge the size of the ulcer through the process of pathergy. The biopsy must be obtained from the erythematous margin of the wound for accurate histopathologic findings, which will assist in ruling out vasculitic, vasoocclusive, and infectious causes (Callen and Jackson, 2007). Laboratory tests for antineutrophilic cytoplasmic antibodies (ANCAs) and antiphospholipid antibodies (anticardiolipin antibodies, lupus anticoagulant, rapid plasma reagin [RPR]) are important to exclude other diseases that could account for these lesions. The diagnosis of PG is reached only after this workup is complete.

Treatment of PG consists of a combination of systemic therapy and local wound care. Of the several treatments that have been used to manage PG, the most consistent, effective results have been obtained with immunosuppression with corticosteroids and cyclosporine. Large, orally administered doses of prednisolone (60–120 mg) are given daily until the disease is under control as demonstrated by the reduction in pain and presence of granulation tissue. Although PG is not an infectious disease process, it can be complicated by infections. In fact, patients may receive treatment with antibiotics for cellulitis and may not improve because an initial biopsy was not obtained (Callen and Jackson, 2007; Wollina, 2007). Dapsone has been useful in controlling the wound bioburden, particularly during the diagnostic workup. Researchers are reporting the effectiveness of anti–TNF-α therapy for PG associated with inflammatory bowel disease, with complete ulcer healing within 7 to 21 days (Reguiaï and Grange, 2007).

Topical wound management should address wound needs, which include exudate management, protection from trauma, a moist wound environment, and pain control. Typically, management of the wound is necessary before its cause is known. Because of the extreme pain that typifies PG, nonadhesive dressings are preferred. Debridement is achieved only through autolysis and regression of the disease process itself. Aggressive sharp debridement is contraindicated because it will lead to extension of the disease through the process of pathergy. In fact, local care should be delivered with great caution because of the tendency for pathergy to occur. Skin grafts also are to be avoided due to pathergy (Paparone et al, 2009). Antibacterial topical dressings are often warranted to manage the wound bioburden and potential secondary bacterial infections (Callen and Jackson, 2007).

VASCULITIS AND CONNECTIVE TISSUE DISORDERS

Vasculitis comprises a group of disorders that have in common the pathologic features of inflammation of the blood vessels, endothelial swelling, and necrosis. Vessels of any size can be affected, so any organ or system may be involved, resulting in a wide array of symptoms and clinical presentations. Vasculitis ulcers usually are the sign of a complex process and may indicate a systemic disorder such as rheumatoid arthritis or lupus. However, vasculitis ulcers also can occur as a primary condition (Anderson, 2008; Armitage and Roberts, 2004). Most vasculitic syndromes are believed to have an immunologic etiology.

The size of the vessels involved (large, medium, or small) helps to characterize the skin manifestations. When a small vessel is affected, pinpoint areas of bleeding may develop, and small red or purple spots on the skin (petechiae) may appear, particularly on the legs. Inflammation of larger vessels causes the vessel to swell, producing a nodule that may be palpated. Blood flow will be impaired when the lumen of the blood vessel becomes narrowed or occluded from the edema; thus islands of ischemia or necrosis will develop on the skin, and the tips of digits may become cold or ischemic.

Specific diseases that may have vasculitis as a prominent feature include rheumatoid arthritis, systemic lupus erythematosus, polyarteritis nodosa, hypersensitivity vasculitis, Wegener granulomatosis, Sjögren syndrome, cryoglobulinemia, scleroderma, and dermatomyositis (Hunter et al, 2002; Rubano and Kerstein, 1998).

The general signs and symptoms of vasculitis are fever, myalgias, arthralgias, and malaise. Patients sometimes describe a vague, flulike illness. Peripheral neuropathy may be present. Other symptoms depend on the organ involved, which is determined by the specific disease. For example, cryoglobulinemic vasculitis likely will be associated with renal and skin problems, Wegener granulomatosis may lead to respiratory as well as renal involvement, and the vasculitis associated with Sjögren syndrome attacks the brain, lungs, and skin (Jennette and Falk, 1997).

Cutaneous features of vasculitis can vary depending on the disease, but certain characteristics are common. The lesions can range from erythematous, nonblanching macules and/or nodules to hemorrhagic vesicles and palpable purpura, to necrotic lesions and ulceration. Skin biopsy is critical and is best taken from early lesions. Two or three sites might be needed to obtain the correct diagnosis (Roenigk and Young, 1996). Skin ulcers associated with vasculitis are frequently located on the lower extremities, making them difficult to distinguish from venous ulcers (Plate 62).

The goal of treatment of vasculitis ulcers is control of the underlying disease process. Bed rest and administration of antihistamines, corticosteroids, and immunosuppressive agents often are necessary (Hunter et al, 2002). Plasmapheresis might be necessary in cases associated with circulating immune complexes. Topical therapy includes debridement of necrotic tissue, prompt identification and treatment of infection, maintenance of a moist wound base, absorption of excess exudate, packing of any dead space, insulation, and protection from further trauma.

The various vasculitis syndromes have many similarities but also have specific differences unique to some of the diseases. The unique features of rheumatoid arthritis, systemic lupus erythematosus, and polyarteritis nodosa are listed in Table 30-1.

Drug-Induced Vasculitis

In approximately 10% of patients with vasculitis, the cause is a drug reaction rather than a disease process. Drug-induced vasculitis usually is confined to the skin and appears about 1 week after administration of the drug. The drug binds to serum proteins, causing an immune-complex vasculitis (Jennette and Falk, 1997). The typical presentation is purpura and ulceration involving the lower extremities. Once systemic disease has been ruled out, treatment involves removal of the precipitating drug and symptomatic treatment. Antihistamines and NSAIDs are most often prescribed. Corticosteroids may be added for more severe symptoms. Wound care is based on wound needs, and ulcers resolve spontaneously once the drug is removed.

EPIDERMOLYSIS BULLOSA

Epidermolysis bullosa (EB) is the name given to a group of similar skin conditions with various defects in the epidermal basement membrane. Manifestations include a tendency to develop blisters and erosions in the skin,

TABLE 30-1	Characteristics of Skin Lesions with Vasculitic Disorders	
Vasculitic Disorder	**Description**	**Ulcer Characteristics**
Rheumatoid arthritis	Not well understood Associated with high levels of rheumatoid factor (RF) (Ikeda et al, 1998; Yamamoto et al, 1995) Evidence of venous insufficiency (McRorie et al, 1998) Limited ankle movement contributes to poor calf muscle pump function and may place patient at risk for venous ulcer development	Begin as palpable purpura and ecchymosis May progress to ulceration Shallow, well-demarcated, painful, slow to heal May require addition of compression therapy (McRorie et al, 1998)
Systemic lupus erythematosus (SLE)	Chronic immune disorder Characterized by periods of exacerbation and remission Affects multiple organs (skin, serosal surfaces, central nervous system, kidneys) and red blood cells Circulating immune complexes and autoantibodies cause tissue damage and organ dysfunction No single cause; influenced by environment, host immune responses, hormones Common symptoms include fatigue, weight loss, fever, malaise Butterfly rash (facial edema over cheeks, nose) is typical Potential manifestations include seizures, hemiparesis, pericarditis, pleuritis, renal failure, nausea, vomiting, abdominal pain, arthralgias	Present as palpable purpura Progress to ulceration Occur on malleolar area Present as round lesions with erythematous borders Wound may have atrophy and loss of pigmentation
Polyarteritis nodosa (PAN)	Medium- and small-vessel vasculitis Necrotizing arteritis affecting small- and medium-sized arteries of most organs Involved organs commonly include kidney, liver, intestine, peripheral nerves, skin, muscle Characterized by fresh and healing lesions Clinical manifestations include anorexia, weight loss, fever, fatigue Organ-specific manifestations include abdominal pain, myalgia, arthralgia, paresthesia Subcutaneous painful nodules of lower extremities may develop	Skin involvement occurs in approximately 40% of patients Lesions have "punched out" appearance Painful Lesions may begin as purpura with urticaria before progressing to ulceration May have "starburst" pattern extending from ulcer Painful subcutaneous nodules present

and sometimes in mucous membranes, after mild mechanical trauma (Ly and Su, 2008). EB is most often inherited, although there is a noninherited form (EB acquisita). There are many types of EB, and symptoms can range from mild, seasonal blistering to life-threatening skin erosions (Schober-Flores, 2003). EB can affect every epithelial structure in the body, including the eyelids, conjunctivae, corneas, bowels, skin, and gums.

Inherited EB is rare, affecting 100,000 people, mostly children (Pillay, 2008). It is classified as one of three types: EB simplex, junctional EB, and dystrophic EB. At least 23 distinctive phenotypes of EB have been identified. Differences between the three types are based on ultrastructural levels of the skin within which the blisters develop. Immunofluorescence or electron microscopic studies of skin specimens are most reliable in establishing the diagnosis. Distinctive characteristics of EB are listed in Box 30-3.

Extracutaneous manifestations—gastrointestinal, ophthalmologic (corneal abrasions and ulcerations), skeletal (osteoporosis due to decreased weight bearing), genitourinary (obstructive uropathy, immunoglobulin A nephropathy) and cardiac—are common. Chronic anemia may be present due to blood loss from open wounds and poor nutritional intake (Pillay, 2008). The severity of these manifestations varies with the category of EB as well as the subtype within that category. Gastrointestinal complications are a major source of symptoms and morbidity for all EB patients. The most severe problems are associated with the oropharynx, esophagus, and proximal gut. The use of eating utensils and the passage of foods result in the formation of bullae that rupture, erode, and heal with scar formation. Strictures are inevitable, and nutritional problems develop.

Anemia is another major problem with EB and is multifactorial in origin. Poor nutrition resulting from painful oral blisters and esophageal strictures precipitates a deficiency in iron, trace metals, and protein, which contributes to anemia. Protein and blood are also lost through the chronic skin lesions typical of junctional EB and dystrophic EB.

The patient with EB is deprived of an epidermal barrier to bacterial invasion. *Staphylococcus aureus* and other pathogens often colonize the chronic, nonhealing wound. Sepsis is a serious complication, especially in infants. Judicious use of topical antibiotics is warranted to decrease bacterial flora and minimize the risk of soft tissue infection. Silver sulfadiazine cream is contraindicated in

BOX 30-3	Characteristics of Epidermolysis Bullosa by Category

Epidermolysis Bullosa Simplex (EBS)
- Intraepidermal blisters
- Heals without scar formation
- Nails and teeth normal
- Occasional cutaneous blistering
- Autosomal dominant trait

Junctional Epidermolysis Bullosa (JEB)
- Autosomal recessive trait
- Blisters form at lamina lucida (between epidermis and basement membrane)
- Several subtypes with distinct clinical manifestations

Recessive Dystrophic Epidermolysis Bullosa (RDEB)
- Dystrophic scarring is distinctive feature that serves as clinical marker
- Separation at basement membrane zone deep to basement membrane
- Recessive inheritance
- Blister formation results from even minimal mechanical trauma
- Blisters may be hemorrhagic
- Blisters eventually rupture to form slow-to-heal superficial ulcers that continue to be exposed to minimal mechanical trauma
- Healing always involves scarring, so skin has atrophic and wrinkled appearance
- Elbows, knees, hands, feet are sites of repeated trauma
- Predisposes patient to squamous cell cancer

Dominant Dystrophic EB (DDEB)
- Formation of blisters below basement membrane
- Autosomal dominant inheritance
- Trauma-induced blisters form at birth or shortly thereafter
- Blisters heal with scar formation but usually are less extensive than in recessive form
- Predisposes patient to squamous cell cancer

newborns younger than 8 weeks because of the increased risk for kernicterus (Caldwell-Brown et al, 1992). Topical antibiotics should not be used as a lubricating ointment because they are for use with open lesions only. In the presence of cellulitis, systemic antibiotics are required (Marinkovich and Pham, 2009). Close monitoring of lesions and bacteriologic studies is imperative.

The primary objective in the care of patients with EB is promoting healing and preventing trauma (Pillay, 2008; Schober-Flores, 2003). Nursing considerations include wound care, nutrition, education, pain control, and social support. Wound healing ability is often compromised in patients due to malnutrition, anemia, increased wound bioburden, and loss of protective functions of the skin (Pillay, 2008). Special precautions to minimize cutaneous trauma during select clinical procedures are listed in Table 30-2. Interventions such as the routine use of convoluted foam on pad rails, sheepskin, an air-fluidized support surface, and joint protectors is important. Low-adherence foam dressings or thin hydrocolloids may be appropriate for protecting the patient's hands or feet. However, if these dressings are used,

they should be left in place and allowed to fall off rather than being removed and reapplied on a regular basis.

There is no single approach to wound care for managing EB lesions; rather, interventions should strive to achieve key objectives: containing exudate, avoiding trauma, preventing infection, and maintaining a moist environment (Denyer, 2010; Schober-Flores, 2003). Only nonadherent dressings should be used, and they should be secured with roll gauze, tubular gauze, or a stockinette. Fenestrated, nonadherent dressings can be used so that wound moisture can pass through the fenestrations and be trapped by the cover dressing. Ointments can be applied over the fenestrated layer when trying to reduce wound bioburden. Creative dressing techniques often are necessary for difficult locations, such as the digits or face particularly to prevent fusion of digits (Denyer, 2010). To avoid sensitization, the use of topical antibiotics is not recommended in the absence of very strong evidence of an infection. When infection is suspected (i.e., presence of increased drainage, odor, or wound pain), antimicrobial dressings (silver or Iodosorb) are appropriate. Vesicles or bullae should be lanced and drained to prevent extension through defectively bound skin layers (Denyer, 2010; Pillay, 2008). Temporary skin substitutes and bioengineered skin hold a great deal of promise for this dangerous disease. Clinical trials also are underway to investigate the therapeutic potential of bone marrow or cord blood transplantation for EB and results thus far are encouraging (Kiuru et al, 2010; Wagner et al, 2009).

Pruritus is a common problem with EB and is the source of new blister formation and breakdown of healing wounds (Pillay, 2008). Moisturizers (e.g., emollients) and oral antipruritics are often indicated. Atrophic scarring and contractures are common and result in fusion of digits (i.e., mitten deformity or pseudosyndactyly), which requires repeat surgical release of contractures (Fine et al, 2005). Additional complications include squamous cell cancer, which is almost inevitable, so constant monitoring with aggressive skin surveillance is essential (Pillay, 2008). Additional information about this disease is available from the Dystrophic Epidermolysis Bullosa Research Association of America (DebRA, 141 Fifth Avenue, New York, NY 10010; 212-995-2220; http://www.debra.org).

CALCIPHYLAXIS

Calciphylaxis, also known as calcific uremic arteriolopathy, is an extremely rare disorder that occurs in up to 5% of dialysis-dependent patients (Rogers and Coates, 2008). It is characterized by indurated, necrotic lesions with a violaceous discoloration (Plate 63). A significant feature of this condition is severe pain that is refractory to common analgesics. Initially, the lesions are serpiginous, indurated plaques with surrounding pallor or ecchymosis. The lesions progress to subcutaneous nodules and ulcerations that eventually become gangrenous. Subsequent infection and gangrene contribute to the high mortality rate (up to 80%) associated with the

TABLE 30-2	Special Precautions to Minimize Cutaneous Trauma to Patients with Dystrophic Epidermolysis Bullosa During Select Clinical Procedures
Procedure	**Suggestions**
Blood pressure monitoring	Apply dressing under blood pressure cuff.
Electrocardiogram monitoring	Use nonadhesive plastic film (e.g., Omiderm (Taureon, The Netherlands), which does not interfere with electrical conduction) as a barrier between patient's skin and adhesive of electrode pads.
Urine collections (young children)	Wring out cloth diaper; do not apply urine bags containing adhesives.
Blood drawing	To cleanse skin, allow alcohol or Betadine swab to remain in place for 5 min without rubbing; place tourniquet over padding to protect skin; or apply direct pressure on vein using thumb in parallel position to skin.
Parenteral therapy	Cut piece of extra thin hydrocolloid dressing into horseshoe shape and put dressing with adhesive backing side in contact with skin. Start intravenous (IV) line between legs of horseshoe bandage and tape tubing onto dressing. Secure IV with roller gauze, or place snug-fitting piece of tube gauze (e.g., Bandnet) on extremity adjacent to IV and secure with tape to tube gauze.
Preoperative preparations (operating room, table, surgical drapes, surgical scrubs)	Operating room table should be well padded. Sheepskin covered by table-sized burn pad (e.g., Exu-Dry [Smith & Nephew, St. Petersburg, Fl], which has double layer of meshed material to minimize friction) is advised. If positioning with pillows is necessary for patient with joint contractures, place Exu-Dry pad between pillow and patient's skin. Place sterile sheets of nonadherent mesh (e.g., Exu-Dry Mesh, N-Terface [Winfield Laboratories, Inc., Richardson, Tx]) under sterile drapes to protect exposed skin from friction. Fold mesh over edge of drape and secure with clamps. Adhesive drapes are contraindicated. Apply antimicrobial solution to surgical site and allow to remain on skin for 5 minutes, then irrigate to rinse. Repeat this process three times.
Mask-delivered anesthesia	Protect skin on face from possible shearing by using nonadherent foam, which adheres to any damp surface and is easily removed by rewetting; or apply copious amount of petrolatum to face before applying mask.

From Caldwell-Brown D et al: Nursing aspects of EB: a comprehensive approach. In Lin AN, Carter DM, editors: *Epidermolysis bullosa: basic and clinical aspects*, New York, 1992, Springer Verlag.

disease (Rogers and Coates, 2008). A distinctive finding with calciphylaxis is intact peripheral pulses because blood flow distal to or deeper than the necrosis remains intact. This clinical assessment is critical in distinguishing the disease from other forms of peripheral vascular disease. No blood tests are available to confirm the diagnosis of calciphylaxis.

Histologically, microvascular calcifications of the intima layer of the arteriole (and occasionally the media layer) are found. These calcifications precipitate a narrowing of the lumen, and arterial thrombosis is also occasionally observed. However, complete occlusion of the arteriole seldom develops. The primary cause of the accompanying ischemia is hyperplasia, another histologic change that occurs within the intimal lining of the arteriole. The combination of microvascular calcification of the media layer and hyperplasia within the intima of arterioles with a diameter of approximately 0.04 to 0.1 mm is considered a histologic marker for calciphylaxis. These findings assist in differentiating this disease from peripheral arterial occlusion. Arteriole hyperplasia and microvascular calcification have also been reported in patients with normal renal function who have diabetes, multiple myeloma, breast cancer with hypercalcemia, or primary parathyroidism (Hafner et al, 1995; Khafif et al, 1990). Clotting disorders (e.g., protein C, protein S, and antithrombin III deficiency)

must be excluded because these conditions result in similar skin lesions (Rogers and Coates, 2008).

The etiology of calciphylaxis is unknown. Elevated calcium and phosphate products increase mortality due to vascular disease; their effect on the cause of calciphylaxis is not established (Rogers and Coates, 2008). Protein C functional deficiency that precipitates thrombosis in small blood vessels has been studied as a risk factor for calciphylaxis, although this deficiency is not consistently found (Hafner et al, 1995).

Treatment of calciphylaxis is neither universally standardized nor necessarily effective. Prompt recognition and treatment yield the best results. Systemically, normalization of abnormal calcium and phosphorus levels is warranted. Severe hyperparathyroidism may be managed pharmacologically or surgically. Fine and Fontaine (2008) reported a sharp decrease in the incidence of calciphylaxis in dialysis patients with use of less calcium salts in dialysis solutions. Sodium thiosulfate (administered by either intravenous or intraperitoneal infusion) has been reported to be beneficial by acting as a chelator of cations, converting the insoluble tissue deposits of cations (e.g., calcium) into more soluble cations (Rogers and Coates, 2008). Antibiotics should be given to treat wound infection and prevent sepsis. Historically, most individuals who develop calciphylaxis require limb amputation and reconstructive surgery.

Topical wound management should address specific wound needs: fill dead space, provide physiologic environment, and absorb exudate. Aggressive debridement is indicated to reduce the potential for wound infection; increased patient survival has been reported with aggressive early debridement (Rogers and Coates, 2008). The severity of wound-related pain should be assessed regularly, and control measures for pain should be implemented routinely and during wound procedures. Applications of split-thickness skin grafts have been successful (Snyder et al, 2000).

EXTRAVASATION

The role of the wound care specialist in caring for the patient with an extravasation is to provide consultation in the management of the resulting wound. Initial interventions required upon extravasation of a chemotherapeutic agent are provided by the oncology staff as guided by best evidence (Sauerland et al, 2006; Wickham et al, 2006). Therefore the wound care specialist is not expected to be familiar with each medication, irritant potential, or immediate postextravasation intervention specific to each medication. However, the wound care specialist may be consulted for wound management once tissue damage is evident. This section will address risk factors, prevention, assessment, and treatment of extravasation injury.

Extravasation is the inadvertent leakage of a drug or solution into surrounding tissue (Sauerland et al, 2006). It generates a reaction in the surrounding tissues that ranges from swelling to an inflammatory reaction and irritation to tissue necrosis (Polovich et al, 2005). In most situations, leakage of intravenous fluids or medications into surrounding tissues is innocuous. The spectrum of cutaneous reactions depends upon whether the solution that leaked is a nonvesicant, an irritant, or a vesicant. Nonvesicant extravasation creates swelling but no tissue damage. An irritant solution induces an inflammatory reaction but no persistent tissue damage. Nonpharmacologic interventions, such as elevation and applying either cold or warm cloths, are sufficient to reduce swelling and discomfort.

In contrast, extravasation of a vesicant results in blistering and progressive tissue destruction. Vesicants may be nonantineoplastic agents (hyperosmolar solutions, vasopressor agents, antibiotics) but most commonly are antineoplastic agents (Table 30-3). Vesicants cause tissue damage by either binding to DNA within cells or interfering with mitosis. When the vesicant binds with DNA and the cells dies, the drug is released into surrounding tissue and binds to more DNA. This process repeats a chain of events such that the area of tissue damage continues to widen. The vesicant then interferes with mitosis, causes tissue damage, and results in cell death but to a lesser degree than expected with DNA-binding chemicals. It is important for the wound specialist to be aware of the potential for significant local reactions caused by nonantineoplastic agents because these medications are administered to many patients in a variety of health care settings.

The incidence of extravasations with antineoplastic infusions ranges from 0.1% to 6% of peripheral infusions and 0.3% to 4.7% of implanted venous access port infusions (Sauerland et al, 2006). This discrepant incidence probably reflects the challenges in measuring the incidence of extravasation. The extent of tissue damage is determined by several factors: drug concentration, amount infiltrated, duration of tissue exposure, extravasation site, and timeliness of postextravasation intervention. Ulcer formation at the extravasation site of a cytotoxic agent may be delayed for several days or weeks as a result of diffusion of the drug into adjacent tissue. Subsequent tissue damage and the formation of slough will progress over several weeks and months (Plate 64).

TABLE 30-3	Common Vesicants	
DNA-Binding Agents	**Non–DNA-Binding Agents**	**Nonantineoplastic Vesicants**
Anthracycline Agents	Vinca Alkaloids	Hyperosmotic Solutions
Doxorubicin	Vincristine	Concentrated electrolyte solutions
Daunorubicin	Vinblastine	Agents altering intracellular pH
Idarubicin	Vindesine	(sodium bicarbonate)
Mitoxantrone	Vinorelbine	Vasopressors
		Phenytoin
Antitumor antibiotics	Taxane agents	Aminophylline
Mitomycin	Paclitaxel	Mannitol
Bleomycin	Docetaxel	Chloramphenicol
Doxorubicin		Nafcillin
Alkylating agents		Oxacillin
Mechlorethamine		Vancomycin
Platinum analogs		

Prevention

One of the most important steps in preventing extravasation is patient education so that the patient is aware of the signs and symptoms to report and the risk of extravasation, particularly when receiving antineoplastic medications. With patient education, patients are empowered to help prevent and detect harmful extravasation. Guidelines to prevent extravasation developed by the Oncology Nursing Society further emphasize the value of patient education (Polovich et al, 2005; Smith, 2009).

Recognizing patients at risk for extravasation, along with the risk profile of the medications, can signal the need for precautions that will decrease the occurrence of extravasation injuries. All departments in which vesicants are given must have written guidelines for handling vesicant agents, procedures to detect and treat acute extravasation, and an extravasation kit that contains all the necessary materials and drugs for treating extravasation should it occur (Polovich et al, 2005).

Factors that place a patient at risk for extravasation are patient factors, agent-related factors, clinician factors, and device-related factors (Box 30-4) (Ener et al, 2004; Sauerland et al, 2006). Age, both young and old, is recognized as one of the most significant risk factors because of the condition of blood vessels and skin structure. Any condition that masks inflammation will similarly mask the early warning signs of pending extravasation (e.g., pain and erythema) and therefore make the patient more vulnerable to extravasation (e.g., patient who is immunosuppressed). In addition, erythema is difficult to identify in darkly pigmented skin and pain is difficult to identify in infants and individuals with paralysis or impaired communication.

BOX 30-4	Risk Factors for Extravasation Injury

Patient Factors
- Impaired ability to communicate pain (confusion, debilitation)
- Age (very young or old)
- Inadequate veins
- Compromised circulation

Agent-Related Factors
- Vesicant potential
- Volume infiltrated
- Concentration
- Repeated use of same vein for administration of vesicant

Device-Related Factors
- Inadequately secured intravenous needle or catheter
- Undesirable intravenous site location (antecubital fossa, dorsum of hand)
- Metal needles and large-gauge catheters for peripheral access sites

Clinician-Related Factors
- Knowledge
- Skill
- Interruptions or distractions

Assessment

Prevention of extravasation injuries includes a thorough assessment of the patient, the venous access, and related risk factors, and knowledge of the vesicant potential of the drug. Vesicant agents should be given only through a newly established line. Infusions should be halted at the first sign of discomfort, altered infusion flow, lack of blood return, or local reaction.

During administration of vesicants, the injection site must be monitored closely for sudden swelling, stinging, burning, palpable subcutaneous fluid, bleb formation, pain, and redness. Induration, or obvious ulcer formation, is not an immediate manifestation, and visual inspection cannot determine the potential for or extent of tissue impairment (Polovich et al, 2005). Lack of blood return may suggest extravasation but alone is not always an indicator. Because extravasation can occur without symptoms, periodic reassessment of the injection site after completion of the infusion is warranted. Late indicators of extravasation include localized erythema, inflammation, blanching, induration, vesicle formation, ulceration, and tissue sloughing. However, tissue damage and sloughing may continue for up to 6 months (Froiland, 2007).

Extravasation must be distinguished from other local reactions, such as venous flare and recall. Venous flare is a self-limiting localized hypersensitivity response that involves the development of an erythematous streak along the course of the vein with pruritus, patchy erythema, and/or urticaria. Venous flare occurs in approximately 3% of antineoplastic agent infusions, does not have the serious sequelae of extravasations, and disappears within 30 minutes (Polovich et al, 2005).

Interventions

Early intervention after extravasation can lessen the severity of tissue injury. It is estimated that one third of all extravasations will produce ulceration in the absence of therapy (Ener et al, 2004). Treatment of extravasation of chemotherapy or biotherapy agents should be guided by best evidence (Polovich et al, 2005; Wickham et al, 2006, 2007). Standard interventions are as follows: (1) disconnect the intravenous (IV) tubing from the IV device; (2) leave the needle in place; (3) attach a 1- to 3-ml syringe to the IV device and aspirate residual drug from the IV; (4) avoid pressure on the site; (5) apply cold or heat (depending upon the extravasant) as indicated by published evidence and institutional policy; and (6) elevate the involved extremity for 24 hours (Polovich et al, 2005).

Antidotes for the extravasation of cytotoxic agents are used to neutralize the chemicals in the tissues. The use of antidotes is largely empirical, although guidelines are available through the Oncology Nursing Society (Polovich et al, 2005; Schulmeister 2009).

Manufacturers may be a source of recommendations for the medications they offer. The U.S. Food and Drug Administration (FDA) has approved one drug specifically for extravasations, Totect (TopoTarget USA), which is administered as an IV infusion into anthracycline extravasations. Hyaluronidase and sodium thiosulfate are often used as antidotes but are not approved by the FDA for this use (Schulmeister, 2009). Other antidotes have been reported in the literature (topical dimethylsulfoxide, granulocyte-macrophage colony-stimulating factor, dexrazoxane), but evidence is limited (Schulmeister, 2009; Wickham et al, 2006). Hyaluronidase is also an antidote for several antibiotics, total parenteral nutrition, calcium, potassium, and high-concentration dextrose. Additional interventions that have been used include making stab incisions in the involved tissue, flushing with normal saline, and placing drains (Wickham et al, 2006).

Topical Wound Care. During follow-up, the site should be monitored closely for 24 hours, then at 1 week, 2 weeks, and as indicated for pain, redness, swelling, ulceration, and necrosis. Depending upon the patient's overall health and immune status, more frequent monitoring of the site may be needed if necrosis and ulceration develop. A referral to a plastic surgeon may be warranted if a large volume of vesicant was extravasated or the area and depth of tissue damage was significant (Polovich et al, 2005). However, routine surgical excision is not warranted because not all vesicant extravasations will cause tissue ulceration (Polovich et al, 2005; Wickham et al, 2006). Surgical debridement may be indicated for extensive tissue damage or overwhelming infection. Surgical intervention, such as skin grafting, often is necessary to achieve wound closure (Polovich et al, 2005; Wickham et al, 2006).

Topical care of extravasation wounds should be dictated by the characteristics of the wound. Key objectives for topical care include absorption of exudate, removal of nonviable tissue, prevention of infection, elimination of dead space, and pain management. As the extent of tissue damage is revealed, the characteristics of the wound will change and the local wound care choices will require modification. The area should be protected from shear and trauma; a transparent dressing can be applied to protect the intact surrounding skin (Froiland, 2007). Hydrogels or hyperosmolar gauze can be used to promote autolysis of slough and necrotic tissue.

Documentation and close follow-up with appropriate consultations are highly recommended. Photographic documentation of the extravasation may be mandated by institutional policy. It is important to record the date and time of the infusion, when extravasation was noted, the size and type of catheter, the drug and amount of drug administered, and the estimated amount of extravasated solution (Polovich et al, 2005; Wickham et al, 2006).

IMMUNE REACTIONS

Toxic Epidermal Necrolysis

TEN is a rare but severe exfoliating disorder characterized by epidermal sloughing at the dermal–epidermal junction. It is caused primarily by reaction to medication (Plate 65). Milder variants include erythema multiforme and Stevens-Johnson syndrome (SJS). The Severe Cutaneous Adverse Reaction (SCAR) classification system (Box 30-5) differentiates SJS from TEN based on total body surface area (TBSA) affected. SJS involves epidermal loss of less than 10% of TBSA, whereas TEN involves greater than 30% TBSA. From 10% to 30% TBSA affected is described as SJS/TEN overlap (French, 2006; Garra and Turner, 2009). Based on seven known adverse prognostic factors, the SCORTEN severity of illness scale (Table 30-4) is used to stratify severity of illness and predict mortality of TEN (Endorf et al, 2008; Trent et al, 2004). The average mortality of SJS is 1% to 5%, whereas the average mortality of TEN is 25% to 35%. Death usually results from overwhelming sepsis.

Both SJS and TEN are characterized by epidermal detachment. Mucosal tissue is also affected in greater than 90% of the patients with TEN. The lesions affect the mouth, eyes, respiratory tract, and genitourinary tract and tend to be very painful. Mucosal tissue is much less common with SJS. Both SJS and TEN occur in adults and children.

BOX 30-5	Severe Cutaneous Adverse Reaction (SCAR) Classification System

Erythema Multiforme (EM)
- Typically round targets with three different zones and well-defined borders
- Most prominent on distal portions of extremities (acral distribution)
- Less than 1% of total body surface area involved

Stephens-Johnson Syndrome (SJS)
- Widespread irregularly shaped erythematous or purpuric macules
- Blistering occurs on all or part of macule
- Confluence of lesions and epidermal detachment is limited, involving less than 10% of total body surface area

Overlap SJS and Toxic Epidermal Necrolysis (TEN)
- Same as SJS above
- 10%–29% of body surface area involved

TEN "with Spots"
- Blisters become more confluent, resulting in detachment of epidermis and erosions on greater than 30% of total body surface area
- Mucosal surfaces usually involved

TEN "without Spots"
- Widespread large erythematous areas with no discrete lesions (macules or blisters)
- Epidermal detachment involves greater than 10% of total body surface area

TABLE 30-4	SCORTEN Clinical Scoring System for Predicting Outcome in Toxic Epidermal Necrolysis	
Clinical–Biologic Parameter	**Individual Score**	
	Yes	*No*
Age >40 years	1	0
Malignancy	1	0
Tachycardia (>120/min)	1	0
Initial surface of epidermal detachment >10%	1	0
Serum urea >10 mmol/L	1	0
Serum glucose >14mmo/L	1	0
Bicarbonate <20 mmol/L	1	0
SCORTEN (Sum of Individual Scores)	**Predicted Mortality (%)**	
0–1	3.2	
2	12.1	
3	35.3	
4	58.3	
≥5	90	

From Bastuji-Garin S et al: SCORTEN: a severity-of-illness score for toxic epidermal necrolysis, *J Invest Dermatol* 115:149-153, 2000.

TEN is a T-cell–mediated immune reaction similar to graft-versus-host disease (GVHD) (Endorf et al, 2008). The epidermal necrolysis that occurs appears to be due to massive keratinocyte cell death via apoptosis caused by activation of cellular immunity, including cytotoxic lymphocytes and natural killer cells (French, 2006; Garra and Turner, 2009). The most common medications associated with SJS and TEN are antibiotics and anticonvulsants, but more than 100 drugs, including oxicam, NSAIDs, allopurinol, antiretroviral medications, and corticosteroids, also are associated (Clennett and Hosking, 2003; Endorf et al, 2008; Garra and Turner, 2009). Of the antibiotics, sulfonamides are most strongly associated with SJS/TEN; aminopenicillins, quinolones, cephalosporins, tetracyclines, and imidazole antifungals have also been identified (French, 2006). Less commonly, herpes virus, hepatitis A, immunizations, and bone marrow or solid organ transplantation have been associated with TEN (Garra and Turner, 2009). Symptoms typically appear within the first 14 days of starting the antibiotic and within the first 2 months of taking anticonvulsants. Within hours the skin becomes painful.

Shortly before clinical skin manifestations (1–3 days), the patient may experience a phase of fever and malaise resembling a viral illness. Skin lesions initially appear on the trunk but then spread to the neck, face, and upper arms. The palms and soles can be affected. An irregularly shaped erythematous, dark red, or purpuric macular rash typically develops, and the macules gradually coalesce. Mucosal manifestations may include sloughing of stratified epithelium in the upper respiratory tract, mouth, vagina, anal canal, and eyes. These mucosal lesions in conjunction with the macular rash are strongly suspicious of TEN (French, 2006). As epidermal involvement progresses, the macular lesions take on a translucent gray hue that can occur rapidly (hours) or over several days (Hockett, 2004). As the epidermis necroses, it begins to separate from the dermis, and the macular lesions evolve into flaccid blisters. Slight thumb pressure applied to intact skin next to blisters causes the skin to wrinkle and slide laterally, which indicates a positive Nikolsky sign (top layers of skin slip away from lower layers when slightly rubbed), a hallmark sign for TEN (Endorf et al, 2008; French, 2006; Garra and Turner, 2009). Large sheets of skin are sloughed, exposing fragile, bleeding dermis.

Diagnosis of TEN is made by performing two full-thickness punch biopsies taken from a border of intact epidermis surrounding bullous lesions. Necrosis of the epidermis is an essential component in making the definitive diagnosis (Endorf et al, 2008). The differential diagnosis for TEN includes distinction from SSSS, which is distinguished by skin biopsy, and GVHD of the skin, which is distinguished by history.

Treatment of the patient with TEN requires prompt cessation of suspicious medications and supportive care (Endorf et al, 2008). The standard of care for the patient with TEN is transfer to a burn center to best manage the complex and life-threatening complications, such as temperature regulation, electrolyte disturbances, significant nutrition needs, and propensity to wound or skin infections (Clennett and Hosking, 2003; Endorf et al, 2008; Smith, 2007). Delay in transfer of patients to a burn center has been associated with increased mortality (Endorf et al, 2008). In general, systemic corticosteroids are not recommended, enteral rather than parenteral nutrition is recommended, intravenous administration of immunoglobulin G may be beneficial but should be sucrose free, empiric prophylactic antibiotics are not recommended, and ophthalmologic consultation to manage ocular manifestations of TEN is recommended (Endorf et al, 2008).

The goal of wound care is preventing infection so that the epithelial cells can resurface the exposed dermis. Sloughed epidermis can be debrided, but a temporary skin substitute (biologic or biosynthetic) or antimicrobial dressings (silver or antibiotic impregnated) should be applied to exfoliated areas; these are discussed in detail in Chapter 19. Sulfa-based topical antibiotics are contraindicated because sulfonamides are strongly associated with TEN.

Graft-versus-Host Disease

After allogeneic bone marrow transplantation (bone marrow from another individual), the transferred immunocompetent cells have the potential to produce a severe reaction in the transplant patient. Clinically, acute GVHD occurs early after transplantation (<100 days). Chronic GVHD occurs after 100 days following transplantation. Risk factors that predispose the bone marrow transplantation patient to GVHD include recipient age (>40 years), recipient history of blood transfusions, the conditioning regimen, the prophylaxis protocol, and the number of T cells infused (Alcoser and Burchett, 1999; Sullivan, 1999).

GVHD affects the skin, gut, and liver. It is a clinical diagnosis that cannot be confirmed by laboratory findings (Antin and Deeg, 2005). In the skin, cutaneous manifestations include a maculopapular rash that usually begins on the palms and then spreads to the face, arms, shoulders, and ears (Plate 66). These manifestations may be asymptomatic, pruritic, or painful. In severe cases, generalized erythema, bullae, and desquamation may be present. GVHD may have the appearance of SSSS, a drug reaction, or TEN. A skin biopsy is beneficial to differentiate among these three possibilities (Sullivan, 1999; Antin and Deeg, 2005).

Treatment of GVHD requires a combination of immunosuppressant and antiviral medications. To stimulate adequate neutrophil levels with these treatment regimens, granulocyte-colony–stimulating factor is also given. Topical wound care requires attention to infection control, maintenance of a physiologic wound environment, and pain management. Adhesive occlusive dressings are seldom desirable. Topical wound management should be determined collaboratively with input and discussion from the marrow transplantation team. More detailed information about this disease is available from additional resources (Ferrara et al, 2005; Ringden, 2005; Thomas et al, 1999). Increasing use of autologous bone marrow stem cells for treatment of cancer patients after lethal irradiation is greatly reducing the incidence of GVHD.

FROSTBITE

Frostbite is a cold-related injury resulting from prolonged exposure to subfreezing temperatures. Skin can freeze at 28°F (−2°C) when no wind is present (Mohr et al, 2009). Wind decreases the amount of time required for skin to freeze. For example, exposed skin freezes within 1 hour when the temperature is 0°F (−18°C) and the wind is 10 mph. However, the skin will freeze in only 30 minutes at the same temperature when the wind is 20 mph. Therefore heat loss is accelerated by wind speed, a concept known as wind chill temperature. A wind chill temperature of −40°F will result in tissue freezing within minutes (Mohr et al, 2009). In general, frostbite is a condition of morbidity, not mortality. However, when frostbite is combined with hypothermia or wound-related sepsis, death is possible.

Risk factors for frostbite are listed in Box 30-6. The majority of frostbite patients are male (80%), and 20% have been reported to be homeless (Mohr et al, 2009). Not all cold exposure results in tissue freezing (i.e., frostbite). The spectrum of cold injury is given in Table 30-5.

Extent of tissue damage is influenced by several factors: (1) susceptibility of specific body tissues to cold, (2) rate of cooling, (3) lowest tissue temperature achieved, (4) duration of cold exposure, (5) duration of ischemia, and (6) rewarming condition (Mohr et al, 2009; Twomey et al, 2005). Although skin freezes more quickly with lower temperatures, the speed of freezing does not impact on the degree of irreversible damage; rather, the extent of damage is related to the length of time the tissue remained frozen. Ultimately, tissue damage occurs as a result of tissue freezing and tissue reperfusion (Mohr et al, 2009; Murphy et al, 2000).

When freezing is slow (as occurs with frostbite), *extra*cellular ice crystals are formed; when freezing is quick (as occurs with flash freeze injury), *intra*cellular

---

BOX 30-6 | **Risk Factors for Frostbite**

- Intoxication (alcohol or drugs decrease awareness of cold and impair judgment; alcohol inhibits shivering and causes cutaneous vasodilation)
- Psychiatric illness (e.g., individuals with schizophrenia may have impaired ability to assess tissue cooling or comprehend cold injury)
- Neuropathy
- People who are inexperienced with or new to cold climates
- Homelessness
- Individuals stranded in the cold
- Cold-weather rescuers, soldiers, people who work in the cold
- Winter and high-altitude athletes
- Use of nicotine or other vasoconstrictive drugs
- Inadequate or constrictive clothing
- Underlying conditions (e.g., malnutrition, infection, peripheral vascular disease, atherosclerosis, arthritis, diabetes, thyroid disease, previous cold injury)

and *extra*cellular crystals are formed, and cells lyse. Flash freeze injuries occur after contact with cold surfaces or volatile liquids. Cellular damage, vascular injury, and resulting thrombosis are key mechanisms in the pathophysiologic process of frostbite injury (Twomey et al, 2005).

Rapid rewarming is recommended because it results in less irreversible damage to the tissue. Blood flow is restored quickly, without vasospasm or clot formation. Within 20 minutes, venous stasis develops and progresses retrograde through the capillary bed to the arterioles. When arterial inflow to the capillary bed is unchanged, edema develops. Although vascular permeability and edema are inevitable, rapid rewarming results in less irreversible damage to the extremity (Mohr et al, 2009). During the ensuing reperfusion, the damaged endothelial lining of the affected blood vessels release inflammatory mediators (prostaglandins, thromboxanes, bradykinin, histamine) that cause additional edema formation. Ischemic injury to the affected tissue is progressive as a result of (1) capillary compression from increasing edema, (2) stagnation of blood in the vessels, (3) vessel occlusion caused by shedding of damaged endothelium into the blood vessels, and (4) thrombus formation due to the thrombogenic nature of the exposed basement membrane in blood vessels.

Within 6 to 24 hours of rewarming, blisters develop due to the accumulation of extravasated fluid under the detached epidermis. Little or no fluid in the blister implies poor blood flow. Clear blister fluid contains high levels of prostaglandin and thromboxane, which result in vasoconstriction, leukocyte adherence, and platelet aggregation, factors known to intensify dermal ischemia. Blister fluid may also contain blood, which indicates the superficial dermis is damaged and thus more serious tissues damage has occurred than with a clear fluid blister.

Classification of Skin Injury

Initially frozen skin has the same appearance: cold, white, and firm to touch. The digits, ears, nose, and exposed facial skin are the most commonly injured. To classify the severity of the frostbite, the tissue must first thaw, and even then the extent of skin damage will not be apparent for 10 days or more (Mohr et al, 2009). Frostbite injuries can be classified by degree of injury as defined in Table 30-6. Superficial frostbite includes first- and second-degree frostbite injuries, which generally heal. Deep frostbite includes third- and fourth-degree injuries, which are associated with tissue loss and chronic disability. Hemorrhagic bullae located proximally on the limb and distal tissue that remains cold, ischemic, and insensate are indicators of poor prognosis (Mohr et al, 2009).

TABLE 30-5	Spectrum of Cold Injury
Frostnip	Mild cold injury Completely reversible Skin pallor, numbness Typical on face, hands No ice crystal formation, no tissue damage Warmed tissue becomes hyperemic; decreased sensation or tingling may persist for weeks
Chilblain (Pernio)	Results from repeated exposure to near-freezing temperatures No ice crystal formation Skin has violaceous color with plaques or nodules May experience pain and pruritus with cold exposure Usually located on face, anterior lower leg, hands, feet
Frostbite	Occurs when tissues freeze slowly and form extracellular ice crystals Injuries are circumferential and progress distal to proximal Potentially reversible
Flash freeze	Extremely rapid cooling and formation of intracellular ice crystals Mechanism is contact with cold metals (handles) or volatile liquids Rapid onset, almost never circumferential

TABLE 30-6	Classification System for Frostbite Injury
Degree of Injury	**Classification**
First	Superficial injury Intact sensation Normal to hyperemic skin color No blister formation on rewarming Transient mild burning, stinging, throbbing Desquamation but no tissue loss
Second	Superficial injury Edema may be substantial Blisters filled with clear or milky fluid within 24 hours of injury
Third	Deep injury that results in hemorrhagic blister Blood-filled blisters that progress to black eschar over weeks Blisters are located deeper in dermis and more proximal Skin color is violaceous, soft, or boggy Does not blanch to palpation Initially no pain then progresses to shooting, throbbing, and burning pain
Fourth	Results in full-thickness, cyanotic skin appearance Full-thickness damage affects muscles, tendons, bone Edema forms proximal, not distal, to involved area and becomes line of demarcation between viable tissue and full-thickness infarction Distal parts undergo mummification over weeks

Management of Frostbite

Similar to burns, treatment of frostbite may occur in a variety of health care settings. The phases or levels of care required for frostbite depend on the severity of the injury. Initial care generally is given at the location at which the injury occurs and addresses life-threatening conditions. Wet clothing should be replaced with dry, soft clothing to minimize further heat loss. The affected area should not be rubbed with warm hands due to risk for further injury. Alcohol or sedatives should not be given because they may enhance heat loss. Rewarming of the affected area should be initiated as soon as possible *unless* there is a danger of refreezing. If refreezing is a risk, get to shelter before attempting to rewarm at the scene. Walking on frostbitten feet can cause tissue chipping or fracture. The affected body part should be wrapped in a blanket for protection during transport.

Emergency department care first addresses life-threatening conditions, such as fluid resuscitation to enhance blood flow and tissue perfusion. Rapid rewarming of the affected body part is attempted using water or wet packs at 40°C to 42°C with a mild antibacterial soap. Warmer temperatures or dry heat should be avoided due to risk for thermal injury. Thawing usually takes 20 to 40 minutes and is complete when the distal tip of the affected area blanches with pressure. Associated dislocations are reduced as soon as thawing is complete. Fractures are managed conservatively until post thaw edema has resolved. The only indication for early surgical intervention is debridement of necrotic tissue and fasciotomy in the case of compartment syndrome. Hemorrhagic blisters are left intact to reduce risk of infection in the injured extremity (Mohr et al, 2009). Once thawed, the injury is kept in sterile nonadherent dressings, elevated, and splinted when possible. Clear fluid blisters usually are aspirated to remove the prostaglandins and thromboxane and thus prevent further dermal damage.

Weeks can pass before frostbitten tissue demarcates to reveal viable and nonviable tissue. Therefore any decision about amputation should be delayed as long as possible. The goals of management for frostbite include salvaging as much tissue as possible, achieving maximal return of function, optimizing nutrition for healing, and preventing sepsis. Box 30-7 gives the standard protocol for frostbite care. Thrombolytic therapy is also used within 24 hours postwarming to correct the underlying pathology (thrombi formation) leading to delayed tissue necrosis. The goals of topical wound care are maintaining a moist wound environment, protecting the skin from further cold-related damage, and reducing bacterial bioburden (Varnado, 2008). Light compression may be used to manage edema. Splints are indicated to maintain proper immobilization of limbs and range of motion exercises to prevent long-term contractures. Neuropathic pain is common and challenging to alleviate.

BOX 30-7	Standard Protocol for Frostbite Care

- Rapid rewarming with water at 104°F–108°F (40°C–42°C)
- Tetanus prophylaxis
- Narcotic analgesics
- Ibuprofen
- Antibiotics
- Topical aloe vera
- Limb elevation
- No ambulation until edema resolved
- No smoking
- Daily hydrotherapy

Data from Mohr WJ et al: Cold injury, *Hand Clin* 25(4):481-496, 2009.

PRIMARY MALIGNANT AND MALIGNANT TRANSFORMATION WOUNDS (MARJOLIN ULCER)

Malignancies can develop on the skin as a wound (the primary malignant wound), and wounds of any etiology can develop a malignancy (malignant transformation wounds). In general, malignancies that present as ulcers often go misdiagnosed for a long time because practitioners mistake them for nonmalignant ulcers. An increase in the frequency of skin cancers and the malignant transformation of wounds is anticipated as the population of people who have received a transplant and/or who are immunosuppressed increases (Alexander, 2009; Snyder et al, 2003).

Examples of primary malignant wounds include Kaposi sarcoma, lymphoma, melanoma, basal cell carcinoma, and squamous cell carcinoma. Primary malignant wounds have a rapid onset and develop in many locations of the skin, frequently on sun-exposed areas that have not undergone radiotherapy (Snyder et al, 2003). Basal cell carcinoma arises from the epidermal basal cells and has a very low metastatic potential. Primary squamous cell cancer arises from the keratinizing epidermal cells and can metastasize and grow very quickly.

Chronic wounds are susceptible to developing squamous cell carcinoma. Of chronic wounds, 1.7% will undergo malignant degeneration, most commonly squamous cell carcinoma. Marjolin originally reported the problem in chronic burn wounds; however, this malignant transformation has also been observed in venous ulcers, in pressure ulcers, in sinus tracts secondary to osteomyelitis and fistulas, and in scar tissue. Among trauma patients, burn patients are at the highest risk for malignant transformation of chronic wounds. Marjolin ulcers present as flat indolent white/pearly lesions with indurated and elevated margins (Ethridge et al, 2007). They have a malodorous exudate and can be mistaken for infection.

Any clinical cause for suspicion, such as raised borders, unusual wound base, unexplained pain, changes in shape or color, previous history, or family history of skin cancer, requires referral for biopsy. Ulcers or lesions that

TABLE 30-7	Characteristics of Skin Lesions with Blood Dyscrasias		
Blood Dyscrasia	**Pathology**	**Ulcer Characteristics**	**Treatment**
Sickle cell anemia	Sickled blood cells are rigid May clump together, occluding microcirculation Damage to endothelium leads to thrombus formation (Eckman, 1996) Altered vasomotor response can lead to rise in capillary pressure and edema formation (Mohan et al, 1997)	Exact etiology of ulceration is unclear Located on lower leg near malleolus May be single or multiple Can range significantly in size Ulcers are well defined, vary in depth, have raised borders (Eckman, 1996; Roenigk and Young, 1996) Tend to be heal slowly High recurrence rate (Eckman, 1996)	Control of edema (compression therapy and/or bed rest) Systemic management of underlying disease process (address anemia either pharmacologically or by transfusion) Debridement Prevention of infection Protection from trauma Pain management Moist wound healing (e.g., with hydrocolloids [Cackovic et al, 1998; Chung et al, 1996; Eckman, 1996])
Thalassemia	Microcytic anemia common in people of Mediterranean descent	Etiology related to decreased hemoglobin and increased iron loading, making patients more susceptible to trauma	Blood transfusions and iron chelation therapy Topical care based on wound needs and moist wound healing principles Emphasis on insulating wound to prevent hypothermia Protect wound from further trauma

do not respond to optimal therapy also warrant a referral for biopsy (Snyder et al, 2003). Biopsy technique is critical to cancer detection. It is recommended that wounds be biopsied from multiple sites (i.e., at 12, 6, 3, and 9 o'clock positions) and from multiple depths (e.g., 2, 4, and 6 mm). The biopsy sites should be recorded because rebiopsy is indicated if the wound does not respond as expected to treatment (Snyder, 2006).

BLOOD DYSCRASIAS

Two types of blood dyscrasias may lead to chronic leg ulceration: sickle cell anemia and thalassemia. Their etiologies, ulcer characteristics, and treatments are summarized in Table 30-7.

SUMMARY

Although the wound specialist is not expected to be proficient in the overall care of patients with the unusual pathologies described in this chapter, the management of the resulting complex cutaneous wounds requires astute observation, close monitoring, and adherence to the principles of wound healing. As with other chronic wounds, the goals of treatment for these types of wounds range from healing to palliation to symptom management. Collaboration with the multidisciplinary team (medical staff, surgeons, nursing staff, physical therapy, dieticians) is essential to identifying these rare complications early during onset and implementing interventions that are timely and appropriate to minimize tissue damage and maximize healing.

REFERENCES

Alcoser PW, Burchett S: Bone marrow transplantation, *Am J Nurs* 99(6):26, 1999.

Alexander S: Malignant fungating wounds: key symptoms and psychosocial issues, *J Wound Care* 18(8):325-329, 2009.

Anaya DA, Dellinger EP: Surgical infections and choice of antibiotics. In Townsend CM Jr et al, editors: *Sabiston textbook of surgery*, Philadelphia, 2007, WB Saunders.

Anderson I: Mixed aetiology: complexity and comorbidity in leg ulceration, *Br J Nurs* 17(15):S17-S23, 2008.

Antin JH, Deeg HJ: Clinical spectrum of acute graft-vs-host disease. In Ferrara JF, Cooke KR, Deeg HJ, editors: *Graft-vs-host disease*, ed 3, New York, 2005, Marcel Dekker.

Armitage M, Roberts J: Caring for patients with leg ulcers and an underlying vasculitic condition, *Br J Community Nurse* Suppl:S16-S22, 2004.

Attinger CE et al: Clinical approach to wounds: debridement and wound bed preparation including the use of dressings and wound-healing adjuvants, *Plast Reconstr Surg* 117(7 Suppl): 72S-109S, 2006.

Bastuji-Garin S et al: SCORTEN: a severity-of-illness score for toxic epidermal necrolysis, *J Invest Dermatol* 115:149-153, 2000.

Brooklyn T et al: Diagnosis and treatment of pyoderma gangrenosum, *BMJ* 333(7560):181-184, 2006.

Cackovic M et al: Leg ulceration in the sickle cell patient, *J Am Coll Surg* 187(3):30, 1998.

Caldwell-Brown D et al: Nursing aspects of EB; a comprehensive approach. In Lin AN, Carter DM, editors: *Epidermolysis bullosa: basic and clinical aspects*, New York, 1992, Springer-Verlag.

Callen JP, Jackson JM: Pyoderma gangrenosum: an update, *Rheum Dis Clin North Am* 33:787-802, 2007.

Chung C et al: Leg ulcers in patients with sickle cell disease, *Adv Wound Care* 9(5):46, 1996.

Clennett S, Hosking G: Management of toxic epidermal necrolysis in a 15-year-old girl, *J Wound Care* 12(4):151-154, 2003.

Denyer JE: Wound management for children with epidermolysis bullosa, *Dermatol Clin* 28(1):257-264, 2010.

Eckman J: Leg ulcers in sickle cell disease, *Hematol Oncol Clin North Am* 10(6):1333, 1996.

Endorf FE et al: Toxic epidermal necrolysis clinical guidelines, *J Burn Care Res* 29(5):706-712, 2008.

Ener RA et al: Extravasation of systemic hemato-oncological therapies, *Ann Oncol* 15:858, 2004

Ethridge RT et al: Wound healing. In Townsend CM Jr, et al (eds): *Sabiston textbook of surgery*, Philadelphia, 2007, WB Saunders.

Ferrara JF et al (eds): *Graft-vs-host disease*, ed 3, New York, 2005, Marcel Dekker.

Fine A, Fontaine B: Calciphylaxis: the beginning of the end? *Perit Dial Int* 28(3):268-270, 2008.

Fine JD et al: Pseudosyndactyly and musculoskeletal contractures in inherited epidermolysis bullosa: experience of the National Epidermolysis Bullosa Registry, 1986-2002, *J Hand Surg Br* 30(1):14-22, 2005.

French LE: Toxic epidermal necrolysis and Stevens Johnson syndrome: our current understanding, *Allergol Int* 55(1):9-16, 2006.

Froiland K: Extravasation injuries: implications for WOC nursing, *J Wound Ostomy Continence Nurs* 34(3)299-302, 2007.

Garra GP, Turner ED: *Toxic epidermal necrolysis*, 2009, available at http://emedicine.medscape.com/article/787323-overview, accessed January 29, 2010.

Habif TP et al: *Skin disease: diagnosis and treatment*, ed 2, St. Louis, 2005, Mosby.

Hafner J et al: Uremic small-artery disease with medial calcification and intimal hyperplasia (so-called calciphylaxis): a complication of chronic renal failure and benefit from parathyroidectomy, *J Am Acad Dermatol* 33:954, 1995.

Hockett KC: Stevens-Johnson syndrome and toxic epidermal necrolysis, *Clin J Onc Nurs* 8(1):27-30, 2004.

Hunter JAA et al: *Clinical dermatology*, Oxford, 2002, Blackwell Science.

Ikeda E et al: Rheumatoid vasculitis in a patient with seronegative rheumatoid arthritis, *Eur J Dermatol* 8(4):268, 1998.

Jennette J, Falk R: Small-vessel vasculitis, *N Engl J Med* 337(21):1512, 1997.

Khafif RA et al: Calciphylaxis and systemic calcinosis: collective review, *Arch Intern Med* 150:956, 1990.

King RW, de Saint Victor PR: *Staphylococcal scalded skin syndrome*, 2009, available at http://emedicine.medscape.com/article/788199-overview, accessed January 28, 2010.

Kiuru M et al: Cell therapy for recessive dystrophic epidermolysis bullosa, *Dermatol Clin* 28(1):371-382, 2010.

Ly L, Su JC: Dressings used in epidermolysis bullosa blister wounds: a review, *J Wound Care* 17(11):482-492, 2008.

Marinkovich MP, Pham N: *Epidermolysis bullosa*, 2009, available at http://emedicine.medscape.com/article/1062939-overview, accessed February 8, 2010.

Martin DA et al: Necrotizing fasciitis with no mortality or limb loss, *Am Surg* 74(9): 809-812, 2008.

McRorie E et al: The relevance of large-vessel vascular disease and restricted ankle movement to the aetiology of leg ulceration in rheumatoid arthritis, *Br J Rheumatol* 37(12):1295, 1998.

Mohan J et al: Postural vasoconstriction and leg ulceration in homozygous sickle cell disease, *Clin Science* 92:153, 1997.

Mohr WJ et al: Cold injury, *Hand Clin* 25(4):481-496, 2009.

Murphy JV et al: Frostbite: pathogenesis and treatment, *J Trauma* 48:171-178, 2000.

Paparone PP et al: Post-traumatic pyoderma gangrenosum, *Wounds* 21(4):89-94, 2009.

Pillay E: Epidermolysis bullosa. Part 1: causes, presentation and complications, *Br J Nurs* 17(5):292-296, 2008.

Polovich M et al: *Chemotherapy and biotherapy guidelines and recommendations for practice*, ed 2, Philadelphia, 2005, Hanley and Belfus.

Reguiaï A, Grange F: Therapy in pyoderma gangrenosum associated with inflammatory bowel disease, *Am J Clin Dermatol* 8(2):67-77, 2007.

Rhoads J: Epidemiology of the brown recluse spider bite, *J Am Acad Nurse Pract* 19(2):79-85, 2007.

Ringden O: Introduction to graft-versus-host disease, *Biol Blood Marrow Transplant* 11(2 Suppl 2):17-20, 2005.

Roenigk H, Young J: Leg ulcers. In Young J, Olin J, Bartholomew J, editors: *Peripheral vascular diseases*, ed 2, St Louis, 1996, Mosby.

Rogers NM, Coates PTH: Calcific uraemic arteriolopathy: an update, *Curr Opin Nephrol Hypertens* 17:629-634, 2008.

Rubano J, Kerstein M: Arterial insufficiency and vasculitides, *J Wound Ostomy Continence Nurs* 25(3):147, 1998.

Sauerland C et al: Vesicant extravasation. Part I: Mechanisms, pathogenesis, and nursing care to reduce risk, *Onc Nursing Forum* 33(6):1134-1141, 2006.

Schober-Flores C: Epidermolysis bullosa: the challenges of wound care, *Dermatol Nurse* 15(2):141, 2003.

Schulmeister L: Vesicant chemotherapy extravasation antidotes and treatments, *Clin J Oncol Nurs* 13(4):395-398, 2009.

Schwartz RA: *Spider envenomation, brown recluse*, 2009, available at http://www.emedicine.com/DERM/topic598.htm, accessed June 29, 2009.

Smith DB et al: Brown recluse spider bite, *J Wound Ostomy Continence Nurs* 24(3):137, 1997.

Smith DS: *Toxic shock syndrome*, 2008, available at http://www.nlm.nih.gov/medlineplus/ency/article/000653.htm, accessed January 29, 2010.

Smith LH: Toxic epidermal necrolysis, *Clin J Oncol Nurs* 11(3):333-336, 2007.

Smith LH: National patient safety goal #13: patients' active involvement in their own care: preventing chemotherapy extravasation, *Clin J Oncol Nurs* 13(2):233-234, 2009.

Snyder R: Skin cancers and chronic wounds. In Norman R, editor: *Handbook of geriatric dermatology*, New York, 2006, Cambridge University Press.

Snyder RJ: "Immunopathic" ulcers. *Podiatr Manage* 185-188, 2008.

Snyder RJ et al: Calciphylaxis and its relation to end-stage renal disease: a literature review and case presentation, *Ostomy Wound Manage* 46(10):40-47, 2000.

Snyder RJ et al: Epidermoid cancers that masquerade as venous ulcer disease, *Ostomy Wound Manage* 49(4):63, 2003.

Sullivan KM: Graft-versus-host disease. In Thomas ED et al, editors: *Hematopoietic cell transplantation*, ed 2, Malden, Mass, 1999, Blackwell Science.

Thomas ED et al: *Hematopoietic cell transplantation*, ed 2, Malden, Mass, 1999, Blackwell Science.

Trent JT et al: Use of SCORTEN to accurately predict mortality in patients with toxic epidermal necrolysis in the United States, *Arch Dermatol* 140:890-892, 2004.

Twomey JA et al: An open-label study to evaluate the safety and efficacy of tissue plasminogen activator in treatment of severe frostbite, *J Trauma* 59:1350-1355, 2005.

Varnado M: Frostbite, *J Wound Ostomy Continence Nurs* 35(3):341-346, 2008.

Wagner JE, et al: Adult stem cells for treatment of recessive dystrophic epidermolysis bullosa (RDEB), *J Invest Dermatol* (S1); (129):S55, 2009.

Wickham R et al: Vesicant extravasation. Part II: Evidence-based management and continuing controversies, *Oncol Nurs Forum* 33(6):1143-1150, 2006.

Wickham R et al: Letters to the editor. Readers share comments and questions about extravasation management, *Oncol Nurs Forum* 34(2):275-280, 2007.

Wollina U: Pyoderma gangrenosum—a review, *Orphanet J Rare Dis* 2:19, 2007.

Yamamoto T et al: Skin manifestations associated with rheumatoid arthritis, *J Dermatol* 22(5):324, 1995.

Zeglin D: Brown recluse spider bites, *Am J Nurs* 105(2):64-68, 2005.

Traumatic Wounds: Bullets, Blasts, and Vehicle Crashes

John Christopher Graybill, Alexander Stojadinovic,
David R. Crumbley, and Eric Elster

OBJECTIVES

1. Identify the five most common war wounds.
2. Describe critical components of acute management of traumatic wounds.
3. List three initial assessments of a traumatic wound.
4. Define compartment syndrome.

Traumatic wounds result from any foreign body impact that results in tissue damage. Their etiology can vary widely: bullet or projectile wounds, blasts, industrial accidents, falls, and car crashes. Modern care for the trauma patient has its origins in military medicine. Practices developed to treat war injuries have been modified and refined to address civilian trauma. War injuries tend to be exaggerations of civilian injuries. For example, an M16 or AK-47 round causes significantly more damage than a 22 and 45 round, even though the mechanism is largely the same. For this reason, this chapter emphasizes treatment of war wounds. Although the severity of injury may be different, the principles guiding wound care remain the same. Box 31-1 lists the components of traumatic wound care.

ETIOLOGY OF WAR WOUNDS

Weapon-related injuries are of two basic types: those resulting from small arms fire and those resulting from explosive munitions. Small arms fire includes pistols, rifles, and machine guns. Explosive munitions include mines, grenades, mortars, missiles, bombs, and improvised explosive devices (IEDs). Regardless of the mechanism of injury, extremity wounds have compromised the majority of wounds among U.S. and U.K. soldiers since World War I, followed by head and neck, thoracic, and abdominal injuries (Burris et al, 2004).

Bullet Wounds

Small arms fire a projectile (aka, a bullet) at an object. When in motion, a projectile compresses the air in front of it and creates a shockwave. The shockwave contacts an object prior to the projectile. The shockwave can injure hollow viscera, such as the lungs, bowel, and eardrums. The shockwave also can knock a victim against surrounding objects. However, the shockwave is not known to cause direct injury to solid tissue.

Upon contact with tissue, a projectile creates two cavities: a permanent cavity and a temporary cavity. The temporary cavity is much larger than the permanent cavity. Elastic tissue such as muscle, fat, and connective tissue will expand and rebound, leaving only the permanent cavity. Nonelastic tissue, such as bone, will fracture secondary to the temporary cavity (Burris et al, 2004).

Further damage is caused by two additional aspects of bullets. When traveling through tissue, bullets fragment after several centimeters. This increases the diameter of the injured tissue beyond the diameter of the bullet. Bullets also yaw, or tumble. When in contact with tissue, bullets rotate 180 degrees. This tumbling greatly increases the damage by a round. Bullets that yaw earlier cause more damage. Higher-velocity bullets cause more damage than lower-velocity rounds, but yaw and fragmentation more heavily influence the amount of damage inflicted (Burris et al, 2004). Common misconceptions regarding bullets are that bullets yaw in flight, that bullets with a full metal jacket do not fragment, and that exit wounds are larger than entrance wounds.

Explosive Munitions (Ballistic, Blast, and Thermal)

Explosive munitions come in a large variety and inflict damage in multiple ways. The three types of damage inflicted by most explosive munitions are ballistic, blast,

BOX 31-1	Components of Traumatic Wound Care

- Stabilization of injured patient via acute trauma life support (ATLS) protocol is first step in traumatic wound care.
- Wound treatment is same regardless of etiology, although etiology may help practitioner discover concurrent occult injuries.
- Blood vessels, nerves, and bones must be covered with soft tissue if exposed in a wound to prevent further injury.
- Surgical debridement, low-to-intermediate pressure pulsatile lavage irrigation, and negative pressure therapy using vacuum-assisted closure repeated every 48–72 hours until wound closure or coverage are the hallmarks of traumatic wound care.
- Negative pressure dressings facilitate healing, decrease patient stress, and reduce provider time commitments.
- Optimizing the wound base includes reducing bacterial load and improving blood supply.
- Wound closure may occur through a variety of techniques based on size and location. Techniques for soft tissue wounds include: primary closure, secondary intention, muscle and fasciocutaneous flaps, skin grafting, and skin substitutes.
- Techniques to close open abdominal wounds (used alone or in combination): primary fascial closure, delayed fascial closure, component separation, planned ventral hernia, and serial abdominal closure.
- Systemic disease, the inflammatory response, and poor nutrition adversely affect wound closure; normalization of physiology, provision of adequate nutrition, and treatment of local or systemic infection are integral parts of wound healing.
- Chronic wounds are treated by converting the wound to an acute wound and treating it accordingly.
- Amputation is necessary for limb injuries when limb salvage is impossible, treatment of life-threatening injuries precludes prompt treatment of severe limb injuries, and limb ischemia time exceeds 6 hours.
- Tetanus vaccination should be standard practice for all patients with traumatic wounds.

and thermal. Depending on a person's distance from an explosion, they can be exposed to any or all of these elements.

Ballistic injuries can be sustained far away from the blast. They are caused by flying fragments, whether it is the shell casing of a grenade, the ball bearings in an antipersonnel bomb, or the random dirt and debris from the area near an explosion. Different weapons are designed to propel fragments of different masses and velocities. Most explosive munitions have been designed to disperse fragments evenly. However, some weapons are shaped to fire fragments in a particular direction.

Blast injuries are caused by the sonic shockwave produced by the explosion. The shockwave typically has a much smaller range than ballistic damage. As with bullets, the shockwave can inflict damage to hollow organs. Explosions produce a much larger shockwave than bullets. Therefore, injuries resulting from a body being thrown against an object are much more common. Thermobaric devices are designed to cause much larger

shockwaves. During the initial explosion, these devices disperse a volatile substance such as fuel vapor. The fuel vapor then ignites and produces a longer and more powerful secondary explosion. This technology is frequently used in "bunker-busting" devices (Buchanon, 2006).

Thermal injuries of varying thickness are the third type of injury inflicted by a blast. This damage is done only at the site of the explosion. Different types of explosive munitions have been developed for different uses. There are a wide variety of grenades. Fragmentary grenades are antipersonnel tools that inflict injuries primarily through ballistic damage. Concussion grenades are designed to inflict blast damage. An incendiary grenade disperses hot chemicals to cause thermal injuries.

Three types of antipersonnel land mines predominate. *Static* land mines are planted and activated when stepped on. These mines commonly result in traumatic amputations. Further injury is caused by the fragments that are driven up between fascial planes. *Bounding* land mines bounce 1 to 2 m after being stepped upon. They then spray fragments, which enable them to injure multiple targets simultaneously. *Horizontal spray* land mines propel fragments in one direction and typically are remotely or tripwire activated.

Several types of antiarmor devices exist. A shaped charge is designed to direct an explosion at a target. People in an armored vehicle can be injured by two types of fragments: fragments from the charge and spall, which is debris knocked off the armor plating. Some vehicle interiors are coated with Teflon as an antispall liner. Teflon can burn and produce toxic fumes if the thermal damage from the explosion is significant. Rocket-propelled grenades (RPGs) and tube-launched, optically tracked, wire-guided (TOW) missiles are two types of shaped charges. An explosively formed projectile (EFP) is a specialized shaped charge that is commonly used by insurgents in Iraq. Kinetic energy rounds are aerodynamically shaped pieces of metal, usually depleted uranium or tungsten. Depleted uranium has a hypothetical risk of heavy metal toxicity, but the risks surrounding fragment removal exceed the risk of heavy metal toxicity, so removal is not recommended (Buchanon, 2006). Two common types of kinetic energy rounds are armor-piercing, fin-stabilized, discarding sabots (APFSDS) and high-explosive, antitank (HEAT) shells. Antitank mines are similar to land mines except the former are more powerful and are designed to disable vehicles. In Iraq and Afghanistan, the most common antitank mine is the IED or roadside bomb.

Vehicle Crashes

Vehicle crashes are yet another type of injury. Although some soft tissue injury may be due to penetrating trauma, much of the damage sustained is due to blunt trauma. Closed head injuries, fractures, cardiac contusions, pneumothoraces, spinal cord injuries, and spleen and liver injuries typically result from blunt trauma. Most of these blunt injuries are deceleration injuries. Organs in hollow cavities (brain, heart, abdominal viscera) are injured by contacting soft tissue or shearing off of ligaments and vessels. Traumatic brain injury and traumatic aortic rupture are two frequently fatal deceleration injuries. Crush injuries may result when a patient is trapped in a vehicle following a crash. The lower extremities and pelvis are particularly vulnerable in car crashes.

ACUTE MANAGEMENT OF TRAUMATIC WOUNDS

Advanced Trauma Life Support

The acute management of traumatic wounds is a component of the Advanced Trauma Life Support (ATLS) guidelines. Treatment of any wounded patient should follow these guidelines. Failure to recognize and correct life-threatening problems early postinjury will make wound care meaningless. ATLS guidelines emphasize an organized and methodical approach to trauma. A brief overview of ATLS guidelines is given here, but a more comprehensive review can be found in most general surgery texts. Anyone caring for acutely traumatized patients should take the ATLS course offered by the American College of Surgeons.

Any trauma can be managed using the ABCDE method: airway, breathing, circulation, disability, and exposure. The airway and breathing components of the ATLS guidelines emphasize that a person who is not able to breathe cannot oxygenate his or her tissues. This situation quickly leads to tissue ischemia, organ failure, and death. Priority should be given toward securing the patient's airway. If the patient is unconscious, has an altered consciousness, or has injuries that compromise the airway, a temporary airway (e.g., nasopharyngeal tube, oropharyngeal tube, cricothyroidotomy) should be established until a definitive airway (e.g., endotracheal tube or tracheostomy tube) can be placed. Next, any injuries that prevent respiration should be addressed immediately. This includes simple or tension pneumothorax, or hemothorax. All are addressed with a tube thoracostomy (chest tube).

Once a person is able to oxygenate and ventilate, attention should be given to circulation. Organs and tissue that are not perfused will become ischemic. Beyond the obvious risk of death, ischemia has profound negative effects on wound healing. Ischemia results in larger wounds, longer healing times, and higher incidences of wound failure and infection. Some of the problems that can compromise circulation include cardiac tamponade, shock, and bleeding. Cardiac tamponade can be treated emergently by pericardiocentesis. In trauma, shock (the inability to maintain end-organ perfusion) is predominantly secondary to hemorrhage, but a patient also may present with neurogenic shock, septic shock, cardiogenic shock, or adrenal insufficiency.

Control of Bleeding. Hemorrhagic shock is treated by first resuscitating the patient with crystalloid solutions (e.g., 0.9% NaCl or lactated ringers solution) and then blood products. Second, the source of bleeding is identified and controlled. A significant portion of trauma-related bleeding is internal. Fatal internal bleeding can occur in the thorax, abdomen, pelvis, and long bones (e.g., femur). Identification of bleeding source requires knowledge of the mechanism of injury and the use of various imaging modalities or surgical exploration. If a patient is hemodynamically unstable, surgical correction of the bleeding is necessary. Once bleeding control has been established, the patient can be assessed for neurologic disability and treated accordingly. The patient's clothing should be removed to ensure that no injury has been overlooked. The management of trauma is team oriented and multidisciplinary, and several steps of the ATLS guidelines may progress simultaneously depending on the resources of the hospital.

To control hemorrhage, direct pressure should be the initial therapy. Direct pressure is noninvasive, requires no supplies other than a hand, and prevents further damage to the injured vessel and other tissue. When a wound is too large or the bleeding is too brisk, control of bleeding can be attempted with a tourniquet. A tourniquet circumferentially applies pressure proximal to damaged, bleeding tissue. The pressure is transferred to the underlying vessels, causing occlusion of the arteries and veins. Tourniquets are more effective than direct pressure in stopping hemorrhage. They can be purchased or constructed out of something as simple as a belt or a bed sheet.

Tourniquet use comes at a price, however. When applied, hypoperfusion and subsequent ischemia occur to all tissue distal to the point of compression. Prolonged tourniquet use (as short as 90 minutes) can result in ischemia, compartment syndrome, and nerve damage. Use for more than 6 hours can result in limb loss (Beekley et al, 2008; Kam et al, 2001). Therefore, tourniquet use is traditionally not recommended for civilian extremity trauma in the United States. Traumatic hemorrhage typically requires definitive surgical correction.

However, in a combat theater, multiple factors may lead to delayed casualty evacuation. Environmental (e.g., sandstorms), geographic (e.g., mountain ranges), and tactical (e.g., ongoing combat) factors can delay evacuation for hours, if not days. Among combat fatalities, 30% to 40% result from hemorrhage (Perkins et al, 2008). In patients who are not killed immediately, hemorrhage is the most preventable cause of death. ATLS protocol should be followed as strictly as field capabilities allow. Placement of a tourniquet can temporarily halt bleeding, allowing perfusion of crucial organs and survival until an adequate surgical facility can be reached. Recent research derived from U.S. experiences in Iraq and Afghanistan suggests tourniquets are safe and limb loss is low when tourniquets are applied judiciously (Beekley et al, 2008; Kragh et al, 2009).

Upon the patient's arrival to an operating room, tourniquets should be removed and the patient's wounds explored for sites of bleeding. Blind clamping of vessels can lead to ischemia of healthy tissue and therefore should be avoided. Damaged vessels can be addressed with ligation or graft repair depending on the structure and degree of collateral flow. If external bleeding occurs where a tourniquet cannot be applied (e.g., axial areas) or if a tourniquet inadequately stops hemorrhage, a hemostatic dressing can be applied. Table 31-1 lists examples and descriptions of hemostatic agents and dressings (Kozen et al, 2008; Neuffer et al, 2004; Perkins et al, 2008; Pusateri et al, 2003; Rhee et al, 2008).

Immunization

Once a patient has been stabilized, tetanus prophylaxis should be administered. Tetanus, a disease characterized by intense muscle contractions and autonomic dysfunction, is caused by a toxin produced by the anaerobic bacteria *Clostridium tetani*. These contractions can be fatal if they affect the diaphragm (Wood, 2004). Wounds necessitating tetanus prophylaxis include wounds older than 6 hours, those with significant contamination or associated necrotic or ischemic tissue, puncture wounds, stab and gunshot wounds, and wounds resulting from burns or frostbite (Wood, 2004). Patients who were immunized within the last 5 years or have received a tetanus booster during this time period may be exempt. Due to the significant contamination of war wounds and the difficulties in verifying medical records in a combat environment, many trauma surgeons recommend immunizing all wounded patients (Anaya and Dellinger, 2007).

Irrigation and Assessment

Once a patient's life- and limb-threatening injuries have been addressed, it is appropriate to start wound care. Regardless of the etiology, traumatic wounds almost always occur in a nonsterile environment. Therefore, by definition, traumatic wounds are contaminated by debris and foreign objects from the surrounding environment. Many weapons are designed to embed foreign objects in their targets. Explosive munitions displace large volumes of dirt and debris upon detonation. To treat a traumatic wound, you must first assess the nature and extent of wounding, including size, depth, and nerve, bone, or blood vessel exposure. Irrigation of the wound with sterile saline or water facilitates proper assessment and removes gross debris and contaminants and chemicals that could lead to further tissue injury (National Pressure Ulcer Advisory Panel [NPUAP] and European Pressure Ulcer Advisory Panel [EPUAP], 2009).

Coverage and Repair of Vital Structures

There are three types of nerve injury. *Neuropraxia,* the most minor nerve injury, is a conduction block of the nerve. These injuries are common in blunt trauma and compartment syndrome. Function lost secondary to neuropraxia usually returns in 3 months. *Axonotmesis* is an intermediate injury to the nerve that results from damage to the axon. The surrounding endoneurium and perineurium remain intact. The damaged axon will undergo wallerian degeneration (degeneration of axon distal to the injury) but then slowly grow back (about 1 cm/month). Most function will return following this type of injury. Both neuropraxia and axonotmesis will heal without specific intervention. The most severe type of nerve injury is *neurotmesis,* or complete transaction of the nerve. If the injury is secondary to penetrating

TABLE 31-1	Examples of Hemostatic Agents and Dressings		
Component	**Brand Name**	**Manufacturer**	**Formulation**
Zeolite	QuikClot	Z-Medica	Powders and beads Zeolite is a mineral
Gelatins	Gelfoam FloSeal	Pharmacia Upjohn Baxter Health Care	Absorbable foam dressing Absorptive granules
Collagen	Avitene	CR Bard	Sponge
Microporous polysaccharides	TraumaDEX BioHemostat	Bleed-X Hemodyne	Plant-based powder Absorptive granules in a dressing Derived of volcanic rock
Chitosan-derived from shrimp shells	Celox HemCon ChitoFlex ChitoGauze	SAM Medical HemCon Medical Technologies	Granular powder or gauze dressing Patch or bandage Impregnated packing Impregnated gauze
Fibrin sealant	Tisseel VH Crosseal	Baxter Health Care	Tissue adhesive
Polyethylene glycol	CoSeal		Tissue adhesive
Cyanoacrylate	Dermabond	Ethicon	Tissue adhesive

trauma, it usually can be repaired. Neurotmesis secondary to gunshot wounds have a less favorable outcome. The gunshot wound results in thermal and shockwave injuries in addition to the penetrating injury, making functional recovery after surgical repair less likely. Optimally, a nerve should be repaired with a tension-free anastomosis. If this cannot be done because of a substantial defect in the nerve, grafting can be attempted. Autologous nerve grafting, usually using a patient's sural nerve as the donor, is the most common technique. Autologous vein grafts also can be used to guide regenerating nerves over defects. The timing of nerve repair depends on the degree of contamination and the need for subsequent operations to the same wound. Regardless of the degree of injury, an exposed nerve should be covered with soft tissue (Peterson and Lehman, 2008). The exposed nerve is at higher risk for infection and iatrogenic injury during subsequent surgery. A nerve that is allowed to heal without soft tissue coverage becomes highly susceptible to even minor blunt trauma.

Traumatic wounds may contain open fractures that need to be reduced and stabilized. Open fractures are at risk for infection, bleeding, increased soft tissue damage, delayed union, and nonunion. Bone infections (osteomyelitis) are difficult to treat because of the density of the bone and the paucity of adjacent blood vessels supplying the cortical bone. After the wound is irrigated and debrided, open fractures are stabilized, either temporarily or definitively. Depending on the fractured bone, fixation can be achieved by a variety of methods, most commonly screw and/or plate fixation for periarticular fractures and intramedullary nails or external fixators for diaphyseal fractures. After fixation, open fractures require soft tissue coverage with either local tissue or transferred flaps. This typically is performed at a subsequent, definitive operation. Because coverage often cannot be performed at the initial operation due to contamination, infection, or physiologic reasons, a sterile dressing is placed over the bone until a later time when surgery can be performed under more favorable conditions (Smith et al, 2008).

A wound should be explored for exposed traumatized blood vessels. Similar to nerves, exposed vessels are at risk for infection and iatrogenic injury during subsequent operations. Furthermore, any compromise to the blood supply compromises all the tissue it supplies. Medium and large arteries that supply an area of soft tissue without adequate collateral flow require repair around the time of injury. Examples include the superficial femoral, common femoral, and brachial arteries. Due to the presence of collateral veins, most major veins can be ligated following injury. If needed, repair can be performed using a variety of techniques, depending on the vessel and degree of injury. Most exposed vessels in open wounds will occur in the extremities. Repair of these vessels is by autologous or prosthetic graft. In the acute setting, a patient may be too unstable to tolerate a long operation. If this is the case and the patient has a large defect to a vessel supplying a limb, a temporary vascular shunt can be placed to maintain blood flow to the limb until definitive vascular repair can be achieved. Once a patient is able to tolerate a longer operation, the injured vessel should be repaired with an autologous vein graft, typically the saphenous vein, or an artificial conduit such as polytetrafluoroethylene. In most cases an autologous vein graft is preferred over an artificial graft because of superior patency rates. Next, consideration should be given to coverage of the exposed vessel. In addition to the risks of infection and iatrogenic injury, vessel walls will desiccate, erode, and possibly disrupt if wounds are allowed to heal without coverage. Coverage of a blood vessel can be provided by myocutaneous flap or fasciocutaneous flap. When the wound is too large for flap coverage or is too contaminated for a viable flap, an extraanatomic bypass of the injured vessel should be performed, directing a graft to route the blood vessel around the wound in an uninjured tissue plane. When an injured vessel is being repaired, the graft should be similarly routed through uninjured well-perfused tissue planes (Frykberg and Schinco, 2008).

Debridement

Once a wound has been irrigated copiously and assessed, all nonviable tissue should be debrided to prevent its negative effects to the wound bed (see Chapter 17). For the patient with a traumatic wound, the continued presence of nonviable tissue poses significant threats systemically by releasing toxic oxygen radicals, chemokines, cytokines, electrolytes, myoglobin, and other muscle breakdown products. These molecules lead to deleterious inflammatory responses that are exacerbated by resuscitation, leading to systemic inflammatory responses such as systemic inflammatory response syndrome (SIRS), compensatory antiinflammatory response syndrome (CARS), and multiorgan dysfunction syndrome (MODS). The SIRS response can become a maladaptive and hypermetabolic physiologic state that leads to prolonged healing times, poor wound healing, and a myriad of other complications. CARS is the body's attempt at compensating for SIRS. This compensation also is maladaptive, leading to increased infectious morbidity. MODS is the end result of an exaggerated or prolonged SIRS response, which is characterized by multisystem organ failure and high morbidity and mortality rates. Further injury caused by necrotic tissue includes kidney damage secondary to myoglobin released by necrotic muscle. Lysis of cells releases a large volume of electrolytes and metabolic products. Of particular concern is hyperkalemia, which can lead to fatal cardiac dysrhythmias.

Although some surgeons advocate the use of bedside wound exploration for smaller wounds, most traumatic wounds should be irrigated and debrided in the operating room to minimize patient discomfort and allow for adequate exploration. If the patient requires an operation for a traumatic injury, irrigation and debridement of the wound can take place during the operation once the patient is stable and all life-threatening injuries have been addressed.

Fasciotomy

Fasciotomies are performed for compartment syndrome or prophylactically for patients at risk for compartment syndrome. Compartment syndrome occurs following a crush injury or vascular injury with subsequent reperfusion in a closed fascial space, usually an extremity, although the abdomen and pelvis also can be involved. Tissue edema following injury places increased pressure directly on capillaries, resulting in decreased perfusion and ischemia. Additionally, external pressure on veins reduces capillary flow and further diminishes perfusion (Clayton et al, 1977). If ischemia continues, permanent nerve damage, renal failure, and loss of limb can ensue. Unlike open wounds, compartment syndrome has a more occult presentation. Symptoms include pain, paresthesias, paresis, poikilothermia, and pallor of the affected extremity. An absence of pulses may be noted in an affected limb but typically is a late finding. Compartment pressure can be measured using a needle attached to a Stryker Intra-compartmental Pressure Monitor System (Stryker Instruments, Kalamazoo, Mich., USA) or a modified arterial line kit. Elevated pressure mandating treatment is either compartment pressure greater than 30 mm Hg or compartment pressure 35 mm Hg less than arterial diastolic pressure (Browner and DeAngelis, 2007; Losken and Schaefer, 2008). Treatment involves surgical decompression of compartments by incising the surrounding deep investing muscular fascia (fasciotomy). In trauma, fasciotomies are performed prophylactically in patients at risk for compartment syndrome (e.g., those with severe crush injuries with or without prolonged ischemia). Once the fasciotomy is performed, subacute management of the open wound begins.

SUBACUTE MANAGEMENT OF TRAUMATIC WOUNDS

Usually, the degree of contamination, the severity of the wound, and the local and systemic inflammatory response to the critically ill state of the wounded patient do not allow for wound closure after initial evaluation, irrigation, and debridement because care must be focused on lifesaving procedures, ensuring adequate airway and ventilation, stopping blood loss, and preventing further organ injury. Therefore, wound bed preparation and wound closure are planned during the subacute phase of traumatic wound management.

Serial Irrigation and Debridement

Although a wound bed may appear to be free of necrotic tissue after initial debridement, repeat evaluation during subacute management may reveal additional necrosis. Patients with traumatic wounds tend to have physiologic, immunologic, and nutritional derangements that predispose them toward infection. On a local level, wounds are predisposed to colonization. Therefore, traumatic wounds typically require serial irrigation, evaluation, and debridement. Traditionally, open traumatic wounds are evaluated on a daily or twice-daily basis.

Debridement should be performed using an atraumatic surgical technique (Attinger et al, 2006). Examples include sharp dissection and bipolar cautery, which allow for minimal destruction of underlying, healthy tissue. Healthy tissue is well vascularized and bleeds. Other hallmarks of viable tissue depend on the tissue type. Healthy fascia appears white and glistens. Fat is bright yellow. Viable muscle can be recognized by the 4 Cs: red Color, Contraction upon stimulation with forceps or electrocautery, strong Consistency, and Capacity to bleed (Volgas, 2007). Most bleeding resulting from surgical debridement can be stopped with direct pressure. If direct pressure is inadequate, suture ligation or pinpoint electrocautery can be used.

Reevaluation of a traumatic wound with repeat irrigation and debridement should occur at least twice per week even if no grossly necrotic or nonviable tissue is noted in the wound bed (Attinger et al, 2006). As wound healing progresses, the extent of debridement needed decreases. Once a bed of granulation tissue is present throughout the wound, debridement may no longer be needed. At this point, wound irrigation and the use of negative pressure dressings can maintain the bacterial load at sufficiently low levels.

Many traumatic wounds have exposed bone. Although radiographs and magnetic resonance imaging are the standard techniques for diagnosing osteomyelitis, the presence of exposed bone in a wound is associated with up to a 66% chance of osteomyelitis (Brothers et al, 1998; Grayson et al, 1995). Infected or nonviable bone is friable and should be debrided. Curettes, Cobb elevators, and rongeurs are sharp surgical instruments typically used for bone debridement. Once bone has been adequately debrided, it should be covered with soft tissue (Attinger et al, 2006). Occasionally, adjacent tissue can be sutured over the defect. Otherwise, a rotational or free myocutaneous flap is needed. In cases where anatomic or physiologic restrictions contraindicate a flap procedure or ongoing infection is suspected, bone will granulate. Secondary intention is suboptimal because granulation is slow and takes several weeks. Early flap reconstruction is associated with shorter hospital stays for patients with traumatic wounds (Stanec et al, 1993).

Should a traumatic wound become infected, the infection can travel very quickly along fascial planes, a condition known as *necrotizing fasciitis* (see Chapter 30). Tendon necrosis or infection can be difficult to manage. Overzealous debridement of a tendon can lead to loss of muscle function. Care should be taken to preserve as much healthy tissue as possible. If the paratenon surrounding the tendon requires debridement, the tendon must be kept moist to prevent desiccation and necrosis. Because infection can quickly spread along tendons, small incisions should be made in the healthy tendon or muscle proximal and distal to the infected or necrotic tissue. Small tendons may require sacrifice if they become infected. Larger tendons should be preserved as much as possible. Reconstruction of certain large tendons (e.g., Achilles tendon) is possible using pedicle or free flaps (Attinger et al, 2006).

Following debridement, irrigation or pulse lavage (see Chapter 17) should be performed to remove bacteria and loose debris. Tangential hydrosurgery is a new technique that combines irrigation and debridement. A device called the Versajet (Smith & Nephew, Cambridge, United Kingdom) debrides tissue by shooting a stream of water across a small gap. The stream is very high pressure, up to 15,000 psi. The high-pressure stream creates a vacuum that pulverizes surrounding necrotic tissue, removes it from the wound bed, and preserves adjacent healthy tissue. Depending on the softness of the tissue, the pressure level can be adjusted. A separate pulse lavage step is not needed when this step is used (Granick et al, 2007; Klein et al, 2005).

Dressings

After the wound is irrigated and debrided, the wound should be covered with a sterile dressing. Different types of dressings perform different functions (Stojadinovic et al, 2008). In acute traumatic wounds, two major types of dressings are typically used. The traditional dressing is the wet-to-dry dressing; however, due to a variety of factors (see Chapter 18), wet-to-dry dressings have fallen out of favor. For heavily colonized wounds, wet-to-dry dressings may still be used, utilizing sodium hypochlorite (Dakin's solution) instead of water or saline. Sodium hypochlorite is a bleach that is bactericidal but has cytotoxic effects on healthy cells (Wilson et al, 2005). Depending on the degree of colonization, either half-strength or quarter-strength Dakin's solution can be used until the level of contamination decreases.

Negative pressure wound therapy (NPWT) between 75 and 150 mm Hg is the most commonly used dressing for traumatic wounds. NPWT is described in detail in Chapter 21. NPWT removes effluent from the wound. Less effluent results in less wound edema and faster healing. Negative pressure dressings are occlusive, preventing contamination of the wound by additional bacteria or debris. The therapy is believed to stimulate granulation

tissue by promoting capillary growth. Intermittent instead of continuous negative pressure has been shown to further increase the rate of granulation tissue formation (Lindstedt et al, 2008; Ubbink et al, 2008).

Different variants of wound filler dressings can be used for NPWT. A silver-impregnated sponge is available for infected wounds or for wounds with a heavy bacterial load. Silver ions are bacteriocidal and have potency against multidrug-resistant bacteria, such as methicillin-resistant *Staphylococcus aureus*, vancomycin-resistant *Enterococcus*, and *Pseudomonas aeruginosa* (Tredget et al, 1998; Yin et al, 1999). Because the standard sponge adheres to the wound base, a nonadherent sponge was developed. The nonadherent sponge is moist and works like the standard sponge except that it does not microdebride. Use of the nonadherent sponge is reserved for wounds that contain structures such as tendons, where adherence is detrimental and moisture is required. Due to the high expense of the nonadherent sponge, an alternative method involves placing impregnated gauze, such as Xeroform (Tyco Healthcare/Kendall, Greenwood, South Carolina) or Adaptic (Johnson & Johnson Wound Management, New Brunswick, New Jersey) overtop of the vulnerable structure. Some surgeons use this technique overtop of skin grafts to take advantage of increased capillary growth while preventing graft removal. Two randomized control trials demonstrated decreased graft loss (Llanos et al, 2006) and improved cosmetic outcome (Moisidis et al, 2004) when negative pressure dressings were placed over grafts.

For small, shallow wounds not amenable to NPWT, numerous alternative dressings may be used (see Chapters 16, 18, and 19). Dressings that reduce bacterial load and microdebride are generally preferred for traumatic wounds.

Antibiotic Beads

An additional adjunct that has been used for treatment of traumatic wounds with open fractures has been antibiotic cement or beads. Osteomyelitis is hard to treat due to the difficulty in achieving therapeutic levels of antibiotics in bone. Treatment generally requires 6 or more weeks of intravenous antibiotics. As an adjunct to systemic antibiotics, several German orthopedic surgeons placed antibiotics in bone cement used for hip arthroplasty (Buchholz and Engelbrecht, 1970). A reduction in postoperative arthroplasty infections was noted, leading to more widespread use of antibiotic-impregnated bone cement. Antibiotic-impregnated beads subsequently were developed for temporary placement at sites of bone debrided for osteomyelitis. The beads are created by mixing bone cement powder, typically polymerized polymethylmethacrylate (PMMA), with powdered antibiotics prior to adding liquid methylmethacrylate to make the adhesive cement. Before hardening, the beads can be threaded on a permanent suture to facilitate removal. Only a few antibiotics are available in powdered form, limiting the choice to aminoglycosides, vancomycin, and β-lactams (Wininger and Fass, 1996).

In traumatic wounds with open fractures, antibiotic beads have been used to decrease the bacterial load of the wound. In a study of 1,085 patients with compound limb fractures requiring debridement and stabilization, 845 received gentamicin-impregnated antibiotic beads plus systemic antibiotics versus 240 treated with systemic antibiotics alone. The rate of infection decreased from 12% to 3.7% in the group that received the beads (Ostermann et al, 1995). Due to the high incidence of multidrug-resistant Acinetobacter infections in U.S. soldiers with traumatic wounds sustained in Iraq and Afghanistan, antibiotic beads have become a frequently used method for treating and preventing osteomyelitis.

Wound Closure

The timing of wound closure is a clinical decision. The goal of closure is to protect the underlying tissue, restore the innate immunologic barrier of skin, and provide a cosmetically acceptable outcome. Although most healthy wounds will granulate and close by secondary intention, surgical closure reduces the duration of closure, produces a cosmetically superior appearance, decreases the need for wound care resources, and decreases the time burden on the patient. Timing is paramount to wound closure. Improper timing of closure leads to dehiscence and failure. Dehiscence results when a closed wound reopens. Failure includes dehiscence but also may include failure of a wound to accept a graft (e.g., skin graft). Currently, no laboratory tests or imaging modalities can predict the optimal time for wound closure. Providers are forced to rely on clinical factors, including wound appearance and patient physiology, as well as their own clinical experience. Due to the large number of traumatic wounds cared for by the U.S. Navy and Army Medical Corps, work is being done to describe the molecular mechanisms dictating wound failure.

Current criteria used to determine timing of wound closure include the patient's general condition, injury location, adequacy of perfusion, and gross appearance of the wound bed. Factors related to the patient's general condition include nutritional and nonspecific systemic inflammatory parameters. Relevance of injury location and visual assessment of the wound, such as the appearance of granulation tissue, are subjectively determined by the surgeon. However, considerable interobserver variability exists in wound assessment.

Once a wound has a base of healthy granulation tissue without evidence of infection, the wound can be closed. Several techniques are used to close traumatic wounds. As previously stated, secondary intention is one method. Secondary intention involves the growth of skin overtop of a granulated wound from the wound edge. No surgical intervention is necessary for secondary intention; however, the long duration (several months), resources needed (wound dressings), and cosmetic outcome do not favor its use, especially for large traumatic wounds.

For wounds with healthy skin edges, primary or delayed primary closure can be attempted. The term *delayed* refers to the time lapse between initial wound care and the time of closure. Delayed primary closure involves approximating the edges of a wound and fixating them together. Multiple methods for fixating skin exist, including skin adhesives, sutures, and staples. Each method along with selection, application, removal, and incision care considerations are described in Chapter 34. Regardless of the mechanism used, skin closures should be under low tension. High-tension closures result in failure and dehiscence.

Occasionally, larger wounds cannot be surgically closed due to unacceptably high tension, so a skin graft must be considered. As previously discussed, the provider must first analyze a wound for exposed bone, nerve, or blood vessel. If one of these structures appears in the wound base, a muscle, myocutaneous, or fasciocutaneous flap should be used for cover. Coverage protects nerves and vessels from subsequent trauma and bone from skin erosion. As described in Chapter 33, many types of tissue flaps exist, including pedicle flaps, rotational flaps, and free flaps. Choice of flap type and procedure usually requires an experienced plastic surgeon. Flaps, especially free flaps, require frequent monitoring in the first 48 hours to ensure adequate perfusion. Most flaps also contain a segment of skin. If the flap does not, a skin graft may be performed once the flap is viable and secure. Skin grafts are described in Chapter 32.

Several artificial skin substitutes have been developed (see Chapter 19). Although none of these substitutes can replace an autograft, they can promote graft acceptance. These products, in combination with vacuum-assisted closure devices, have proven useful in wounds with exposed tendon, allowing for granulation over tendon and eventual skin grafting (Helgeson et al, 2007).

Open Abdomen

Visceral swelling results secondary to trauma and is caused by massive cytokine release, increased vascular permeability, and loss of fluid to the interstitial space, most notably following resuscitation. Although the swelling typically resolves in 1 to 2 weeks, the bowel becomes so large that the abdominal wall cannot be reapproximated. Closure of the abdominal wall also can be difficult if a trauma results directly in a large soft tissue defect, or a "loss of domain."

Regardless of the cause, closure of the abdomen is necessary to contain and protect the viscera, prevent desiccation of the bowel, and prevent peritonitis. Multiple techniques have been developed to close the abdomen. The simplest method is primary fascial closure. To close an abdomen by primary fascial closure, a component separation is performed. Component separation dissects skin off the anterior rectus sheath and incises the external oblique fascia, allowing for increased mobilization of the fascia and closure (Ramirez et al, 1990). To reduce the amount of dissection needed and resultant large soft tissue flaps, laparoscopic versions of this procedure have been developed (Milburn et al, 2007; Rosen et al, 2007). A serious shortcoming of these techniques is the limited mobilization obtained by component separation, usually 10 to 16 cm (Shestak et al, 2000). The other major drawback is the high rate of ventral hernia formation, typically 5% to 10% (Lowe et al, 2000; Shestak et al, 2000). For these reasons, other techniques have been developed to close the abdomen.

One technique is the planned ventral hernia. In this technique, an absorbable mesh is used to close the fascial defect. Once the mesh granulates, a split-thickness skin graft is placed over the wound. Over time, the mesh is absorbed and a ventral hernia results. The ventral hernia is then surgically repaired 6 to 12 months after the trauma (Fabian et al, 1994; Jernigan et al, 2003; Weinberg et al, 2008). Due to the high rate of enterocutaneous fistula formation (approximately 8% of patients) and the need for future major abdominal surgeries, this technique is less popular than delayed fascial closure.

Delayed fascial closure involves placement of a negative pressure dressing over the open abdomen until bowel swelling reduces enough to allow closure by component separation and/or a mesh. Decreased adhesions between the abdominal wall and bowel have been noted. A negative pressure dressing is created by placing a plastic sheet or towel over the viscera and under the abdominal wall. The dressing is placed over the towel and is covered by an occlusive dressing. The dressing is connected to negative pressure. Every 2 to 3 days, the dressing is changed until abdominal closure is reasonable (Argenta et al, 2006; Bee et al, 2008; Morykwas et al, 1997; Schecter et al, 2006). Complications are decreased with this method and include fistula (5%), bowel obstruction (2%), and abscess formation (4%) (Barker et al, 2007).

Another technique used to close open abdomens is serial abdominal closure (Kafie et al, 2003). Serial abdominal closure requires placement of a temporary mesh in the open abdomen. As bowel edema lessens, the mesh loosens. During serial operations, the central portion of the loose mesh is cut and the edges are sewn together. Eventually, the residual mesh is removed and the abdomen is closed (Barker et al, 2007; Vertrees et al, 2008).

A variety of rotational and free muscle flaps have been used to cover large abdominal wounds. Muscle flaps typically are used when ostomies, drain sites, and multiple prior procedures have distorted or destroyed the normal anatomic planes. The rectus abdominis and tensor fascia lata are the two most commonly used muscles for flaps (Mathes et al, 2000).

Combination techniques have been attempted. For soldiers with large abdominal wounds resulting from blast injuries in Iraq and Afghanistan, a combined technique called "early-delayed fascial closure" has been described. The method combines delayed fascial closure, serial abdominal closure, and use of temporary and permanent meshes (Vertrees et al, 2008).

Choice of closure technique is largely based on anatomic factors, complication rates, and surgeon's experience and preference. Technique choice should emphasize protecting the bowel, closing the abdominal wall in a timely manner to allow rehabilitation, and preventing complications such as enterocutaneous fistulas and recurrent hernias.

Amputation

Extremely severe blast and crush injuries may result in mangled extremities with unsalvageable wounds. In these situations, amputation may be the only viable option. The decision to amputate can be extremely difficult due to the resulting cosmetic, functional, and psychological defects. Reasons to amputate include prolonged limb ischemia, irreparable peripheral nerve injury with no hope of meaningful limb rehabilitation, and presence of concurrent life-threatening injuries. Usually, the need to amputate is fairly straightforward. However, in a subset of trauma patients the duration of limb ischemia or degree of nerve injury may cause a surgeon to attempt limb salvage when amputation is warranted. Due to increased patient mortality rates and high hospital costs associated with failed efforts at limb salvage, a series of different limb injury scoring systems have been developed. One system is the Mangled Extremity Severity Score (MESS). MESS ranks the degree of soft tissue/skeletal injury, limb ischemia, shock, and age. A score of 7 correlates with a need to amputate (Johansen et al, 1990). Other scoring systems include the Limb Salvage Index (LSI), Predictive Salvage Index (PSI), Hannover Fracture Scale-97 (HFS-97), and Nerve Injury, Ischemia, Soft-Tissue Injury, Skeletal Injury, Shock, and Age of Patient Score (NISSSA). Two large studies evaluated the utility of these scoring systems. In a large prospective study, Bosse et al (2001) found that none of these scores could accurately predict limb salvage potential. A retrospective study by Ly et al (2008) found that no available scoring system was predictive of functional recovery of patients undergoing limb salvage.

The results of the Lower Extremity Assessment Project (LEAP) have been released. LEAP is a prospective, observational study conducted over 2 years in eight level 1 trauma centers. Although patients undergoing either limb salvage or amputation experienced a high number of complications, a significantly increased incidence of complications was noted in the limb salvage group (37.7% vs 24.8%) (Harris et al, 2009).

Over the past 7 years in U.S. military medical facilities, we have cared for more than 850 service members with amputation returning from Operations Iraqi Freedom and Enduring Freedom. Among the amputees, 88% have sustained blast injuries. Other amputations are sustained secondary to multiple gunshot wound and motor vehicle crash-related wounds, which can be nearly as bad. Approximately 20% of amputees have lost more than one limb. About 60% have sustained significant soft tissue wounds over other areas of the body. In prior conflicts, a significant number of these patients would have died, but improvements in medical knowledge and evacuation time have resulted in better outcomes. As a result, substantial improvements have been made in limb prostheses and physical rehabilitation.

Approximately 80% of combat-related amputations are performed within the zone of injury and therefore typically require delayed closure and results in frequent wound healing problems. Over the past year we have seen an increasing number of individuals returning after 1 or more years of living with a limb that went through multiple salvage procedures but just was not functioning at the level desired by the individuals, so they were presenting for an elective amputation (n = 51).

Due to increasing progress in prosthesis design and limb reconstruction (including areas such as hand transplantation) and faster patient evacuation times, limb salvage will continue to be a complex decision. Patients should be made aware, however, that they can have meaningful recoveries following amputation.

Heterotopic Ossification

Heterotopic ossification is the formation of lamellar bone in nonosseous tissue. Multiple events have been associated with its formation, including traumatic amputation, spinal cord trauma, severe head injuries, total hip arthroplasty, thermal or electrical burns, acetabular or elbow fractures, familial disorders, and neoplasm. Heterotopic ossification is a source of pain, causes breakdown of overlying skin, and interferes with prosthesis fitting and use (Potter et al, 2006).

Heterotopic ossification in the extremities remains a common complication in the setting of high-energy wartime extremity trauma. Recent literature suggests that the incidence may be higher than previously reported, particularly in blast-injured amputees and in those in whom the definitive amputation was performed within the zone of injury. A 63% incidence has been noted in the residual limbs of US soldiers injured in Iraq and Afghanistan (Potter et al, 2007).

An area of concern regarding heterotopic ossification and high-energy long bone fractures is the method of definitive fixation. Heterotopic ossification is a known complication of both external fixation as well as internal fixation. Because heterotopic ossification formation may result following muscle injury that occurs during surgical fixation, it is possible that in the with multiple injuries patient, internal fixation carries an increased risk of developing heterotopic ossification compared to definitive external fixation, especially when definitive internal fixation is delayed.

Prophylaxis against ectopic bone formation is well established in patients undergoing arthroplasty and operative treatment of acetabular fractures. Local radiation therapy and nonsteroidal antiinflammatory drugs (NSAIDs) have been found to reduce the incidence of heterotopic ossification. After a severe trauma, many patients are too unstable to undergo radiation therapy and have contraindications against NSAID use, including renal failure and increased bleeding risks. In a combat zone, providing radiation is logistically difficult (Potter et al, 2006, 2007).

Surgical excision is a mainstay of treatment. However, in amputees, excision may require limb revision. In most patients with heterotopic ossification, ectopic bone is removed once it has matured and become symptomatic. Orthopedic surgeons in the U.S. military have found that early excision results in faster recovery times and quicker prosthesis rehabilitation (Forsberg et al, 2008; Potter et al, 2006, 2007).

SUMMARY

When a wound occurs as a result of trauma, numerous patient care issues must be addressed emergently, such as airway stabilization, adequacy of cardiovascular function, and hemostasis. Tourniquets or hemostatic dressings are often needed to arrest bleeding. Once the patient is stabilized, the wound cleansing can begin so that a complete wound assessment can be obtained. Traumatic wounds are contaminated with environmental debris and may contain open fractures. Aggressive, prompt surgical debridement is generally needed to remove nonviable tissue and prevent extension of necrosis. Due to the life-threatening nature of most traumatic wounds, wound closure may not take place until the patient is stabilized. Many options exist for wound closure, and it is desirable to close the wound as soon as possible once clean granulation tissue is present.

REFERENCES

Anaya DA, Dellinger EP: Surgical infections and choice of antibiotics. In Townsend CM Jr et al editors: *Sabiston textbook of surgery*, Philadelphia, 2007, WB Saunders.

Argenta LC et al: Vacuum-assisted closure: state of clinic art, *Plast Reconstr Surg* 117(7 Suppl):127S-142S, 2006.

Attinger CE et al: Clinical approach to wounds: debridement and wound bed preparation including the use of dressings and wound-healing adjuvants, *Plast Reconstr Surg* 117(7 Suppl):72S-109S, 2006.

Barker DE et al: Experience with vacuum-pack temporary abdominal wound closure in 258 trauma and general and vascular surgical patients, *J Am Coll Surg* 204(5):784-792, 2007.

Bee TK et al: Temporary abdominal closure techniques: a prospective randomized trial comparing polyglactin 910 mesh and vacuum-assisted closure, *J Trauma* 65(2):337-342, 2008.

Beekley AC et al: Prehospital tourniquet use in Operation Iraqi Freedom: effect on hemorrhage control and outcomes, *J Trauma* 64(2 Suppl):S28-S37, 2008.

Bosse MJ et al: A prospective evaluation of the clinical utility of the lower-extremity injury-severity scores, *J Bone Joint Surg Am* 83A(1):3-14, 2001.

Brothers TE et al: Magnetic resonance imaging differentiates between necrotizing and non-necrotizing fasciitis of the lower extremity, *J Am Coll Surg* 187(4):416-421, 1998.

Browner BD, DeAngelis JP: Emergency care of musculoskeletal injuries. In Townsend CM Jr et al, editors: *Sabiston textbook of surgery*, Philadelphia, 2007, WB Saunders.

Buchanon BJ: *Gunpowder, explosives, and the state: a technological history*, Aldershot, 2006, Ashgate Publishing, p. 425.

Buchholz HW, Engelbrecht H: [Depot effects of various antibiotics mixed with Palacos resins]. *Chirurg* 41(11):511-515, 1970.

Burris DG et al: *Emergency war surgery*, ed 3, Washington DC, 2004, Borden Institute.

Clayton JM et al: Tissue pressure and perfusion in the compartment syndrome, *J Surg Res* 22(4):333-339, 1977.

Fabian TC et al: Planned ventral hernia. Staged management for acute abdominal wall defects, *Ann Surg* 219(6):643-650, 1994.

Forsberg JA et al: Correlation of procalcitonin and cytokine expression with dehiscence of wartime extremity wounds, *J Bone Joint Surg Am* 90(3):580-588, 2008.

Frykberg ER, Schinco MA: Peripheral vascular injury. In Feliciano DV et al, editors: *Trauma*, New York, 2008, McGraw-Hill.

Granick MS et al: Comparison of wound irrigation and tangential hydrodissection in bacterial clearance of contaminated wounds: results of a randomized, controlled clinical study, *Ostomy Wound Manage* 53(4):64-66, 68-70, 72, 2007.

Grayson ML et al: Probing to bone in infected pedal ulcers. A clinical sign of underlying osteomyelitis in diabetic patients, *JAMA* 273(9):721-723, 1995.

Harris AM et al: Complications following limb-threatening lower extremity trauma, *J Orthop Trauma* 23(1):1-6, 2009.

Helgeson MD et al: Bioartificial dermal substitute: a preliminary report on its use for the management of complex combat-related soft tissue wounds, *J Orthop Trauma* 21(6):394-399, 2007.

Jernigan TW et al: Staged management of giant abdominal wall defects: acute and long-term results, *Ann Surg* 238(3): 349-355, 2003.

Johansen K et al: Objective criteria accurately predict amputation following lower extremity trauma, *J Trauma* 30(5):568-572, 1990.

Kafie FE et al: Serial abdominal closure technique (the "SAC" procedure): a novel method for delayed closure of the abdominal wall, *Am Surg* 69(2):102-105, 2003.

Kam PC et al: The arterial tourniquet: pathophysiological consequences and anaesthetic implications, *Anaesthesia* 56(6):534-545, 2001.

Klein MB et al: The Versajet water dissector: a new tool for tangential excision, *J Burn Care Rehabil* 26(6):483-487, 2005.

Kozen et al: An alternative hemostatic dressing: comparison of CELOX, HemCon, and QuikClot, *Acad Emerg Med* 15(1):74-81, 2008.

Kragh JF Jr et al: Survival with emergency tourniquet use to stop bleeding in major limb trauma, *Ann Surg* 249(1):1-7, 2009.

Lindstedt S et al: Evaluation of continuous and intermittent myocardial topical negative pressure, *J Cardiovasc Med* 9(8):813-819, 2008.

Llanos S et al: Effectiveness of negative pressure closure in the integration of split thickness skin grafts: a randomized, double-masked, controlled trial, *Ann Surg* 244(5):700-705, 2006.

Losken A, Schaefer TG: Reconstructive surgery after trauma. In Feliciano DV et al, editors: *Trauma*, New York, 2008, McGraw-Hill.

Lowe JB et al: Endoscopically assisted "components separation" for closure of abdominal wall defects, *Plast Reconstr Surg* 105(2):720-729, 2000.

Ly TV et al: Ability of lower-extremity injury severity scores to predict functional outcome after limb salvage, *J Bone Joint Surg Am* 90(8):1738-1743, 2008.

Mathes SJ et al: Complex abdominal wall reconstruction: a comparison of flap and mesh closure, *Ann Surg* 232(4):586-596, 2000.

Milburn ML et al: Laparoscopically assisted components separation technique for ventral incisional hernia repair, *Hernia* 11(2):157-161, 2007.

Moisidis E et al: A prospective, blinded, randomized, controlled clinical trial of topical negative pressure use in skin grafting, *Plast Reconstr Surg* 114(4):917-922, 2004.

Morykwas MJ et al: Vacuum-assisted closure: a new method for wound control and treatment: animal studies and basic foundation, *Ann Plast Surg* 38(6):553-562, 1997.

National Pressure Ulcer Advisory Panel (NPUAP) and European Pressure Ulcer Advisory Panel (EPUAP): *Prevention and treatment of pressure ulcers*, Washington DC, 2009, NPUAP.

Neuffer MC et al: Hemostatic dressings for the first responder: a review, *Mil Med* 169(9):716-720, 2004.

Ostermann PA et al: Local antibiotic therapy for severe open fractures. A review of 1085 consecutive cases, *J Bone Joint Surg Br* 77(1):93-97, 1995.

Perkins JG et al: Massive transfusion and nonsurgical hemostatic agents, *Crit Care Med* 36(7 Suppl):S325-339, 2008.

Peterson SL, Lehman TP: Upper extremity injury. In Feliciano DV et al, editors: *Trauma*, New York, 2008, McGraw-Hill.

Potter BK et al: Heterotopic ossification in the residual limbs of traumatic and combat-related amputees, *J Am Acad Orthop Surg* 14(10 Spec No.):S191-S197, 2006.

Potter BK et al: Heterotopic ossification following traumatic and combat-related amputations. Prevalence, risk factors, and preliminary results of excision, *J Bone Joint Surg Am* 89(3):476-486, 2007.

Pusateri AE et al: Advanced hemostatic dressing development program: animal model selection criteria and results of a study of nine hemostatic dressings in a model of severe large venous hemorrhage and hepatic injury in swine, *J Trauma* 55(3):518-526, 2003.

Ramirez OM et al: "Components separation" method for closure of abdominal-wall defects: an anatomic and clinical study, *Plast Reconstr Surg* 86(3):519-526, 1990.

Rhee P et al: QuikClot use in trauma for hemorrhage control: case series of 103 documented uses, *J Trauma* 64(4):1093-1099, 2008.

Rosen MJ et al: Laparoscopic versus open-component separation: a comparative analysis in a porcine model, *Am J Surg* 194(3): 385-389, 2007.

Schecter WP et al: Open abdomen after trauma and abdominal sepsis: a strategy for management, *J Am Coll Surg* 203(3): 390-396, 2006.

Shestak KC et al: The separation of anatomic components technique for the reconstruction of massive midline abdominal wall defects: anatomy, surgical technique, applications, and limitations revisited, *Plast Reconstr Surg* 105(2):731-738, 2000.

Smith WR et al: Lower extremity. In Feliciano DV et al, editors: *Trauma*, New York, 2008, McGraw-Hill.

Stanec Z et al: High-energy war wounds: flap reconstruction, *Ann Plast Surg* 31(2):97-102, 1993.

Stojadinovic A et al: Topical advances in wound care, *Gynecol Oncol* 111(2 Suppl):S70-S80, 2008.

Tredget EE et al: A matched-pair, randomized study evaluating the efficacy and safety of Acticoat silver-coated dressing for the treatment of burn wounds, *J Burn Care Rehabil* 19(6):531-537, 1998.

Ubbink DT et al: A systematic review of topical negative pressure therapy for acute and chronic wounds, *Br J Surg* 95(6): 685-692, 2008.

Vertrees A et al: Modern management of complex open abdominal wounds of war: a 5-year experience, *J Am Coll Surg* 207(6): 801-809, 2008.

Volgas DA: Care of the soft tissue envelope In Stannard JP et al, editors: *Surgical treatment of orthopaedic trauma*, New York, 2007, Thieme Medical Publishers, p. 976.

Weinberg JA et al: Closing the open abdomen: improved success with Wittmann Patch staged abdominal closure, *J Trauma* 65(2):345-348, 2008.

Wilson JR et al: A toxicity index of skin and wound cleansers used on in vitro fibroblasts and keratinocytes, *Adv Skin Wound Care* 18(7):373-378, 2005.

Wininger DA, Fass RJ: Antibiotic-impregnated cement and beads for orthopedic infections, *Antimicrob Agents Chemother* 40(12):2675-2679, 1996.

Wood MJ: Toxin-mediated disorders: tetanus, botulism, and diphtheria. In Cohen J et al, editors: *Infectious diseases*, Philadelphia, 2004, Mosby.

Yin HQ et al: Comparative evaluation of the antimicrobial activity of ACTICOAT antimicrobial barrier dressing, *J Burn Care Rehabil* 20(3):195-200, 1999.

32

Burns

Jill Evans

OBJECTIVES

1. Identify the three phases of burn care and discuss the goals of each phase.
2. Discuss the causes of burns, including thermal, chemical, and electrical injuries.
3. Identify how the three zones of tissue damage relate to the depth of the burn wound.
4. Compare and contrast the severity of burn trauma using the following terminology: superficial, superficial partial-thickness, deep partial-thickness, and full-thickness burns.
5. Describe three methods commonly used to calculate the total body surface area of a burn.

6. Describe the advantages and disadvantages of at least four topical burn care products or dressings.
7. Describe the indications and techniques for escharotomy, fasciotomy, tangential excision, and skin grafting.
8. Distinguish among indicators for managing the patient with a burn in the outpatient setting, the inpatient setting, and a specialized burn care facility.
9. Identify three principles of managing burn wounds in an outpatient setting.

Patients with burn injuries present with unique, complex care needs that require the collaboration and expertise of a multidisciplinary team consisting of physicians, nurses, physical and occupational therapists, a pharmacist, nutrition specialist, case manager, and social worker. In addition to topical wound care needs, the patient is at risk for systemic complications associated with the absence of large amounts of epidermis and/or dermis (e.g., edema, wound infection).

Beyond the patient's physical needs, all burn team members must be aware of the psychological impact of acute injury, the phases of recovery from a burn injury, and the long-term rehabilitation needs of the patient. Throughout the United States, a number of specialized burn centers are dedicated to the management of the patient with a burn and other conditions that require care similar to burn care. In a facility that does not provide this type of specialized care, it is crucial that the wound specialist facilitate referral immediately. Box 32-1 lists the criteria for burn center referral.

EPIDEMIOLOGY

It is estimated that more than one million burn injuries occur each year in the United States, with more than 500,000 annual emergency department visits and more than 50,000 hospital admissions (American Burn Association, 2007). The majority of these injuries involve burns of less than 10% of the total body surface area (TBSA). Flame burns and scalds from hot liquids account for almost 70% of reported cases; almost half of these injuries occur in the home (American Burn Association, 2008). The National Burn Repository 2007 Report (American Burn Association, 2008), which includes data on more than 181,836 burn cases from 73 U.S. burn centers, further identifies characteristics of burn-injured patients. Nearly 70% of all burn victims are male; mean age of all reported cases is 35 years; and 12% of all burn injuries occur in children younger than 5 years and 14% in patients 60 years and older. The mortality rate for these patients is 4% to 5%.

TYPES OF BURN INJURY

Burns result from thermal, electrical, and chemical injuries. Inhalation injury occurs frequently and is the most common accompanying injury seen in patients with burns.

Thermal (Flame, Scald, and Contact)

Thermal. Thermal burns are the most common cause of burn injuries. They result from exposure to flames, scalds from hot liquids, and contact with hot objects. The severity of injury is related to the temperature and duration of contact. *Flame* burns commonly involve

BOX 32-1	Criteria for Burn Center Referral

- Partial-thickness burns >10% of total body surface area
- All full-thickness burns
- Burns that involve the face, hands, feet, genitalia, perineum, major joints
- Electrical burns, including lightning injury
- Chemical burns
- Inhalation injury
- Presence of preexisting medical disorders that could complicate management, prolong recovery, or affect mortality
- Patients with concomitant trauma in whom the burn poses the greatest risk of morbidity or mortality
- Burned children in hospitals without qualified personnel or equipment to care for children
- Patients who require special social, emotional, or long-term rehabilitative intervention

Adapted from American Burn Association: Guidelines for the operations of burn centers, *J Burn Care Rehabil* 28(1):134-141, 2007.

exposure to fire, with ignition of clothing, outdoor trash, and brush fires frequently involving use of an accelerant (Wibbenmeyer et al, 2003).

House fires are another significant cause of flame burn injury and are associated with the additional risk of smoke inhalation injury. Smoke inhalation injury is present in approximately 10% to 20% of patients admitted to burn centers (Palmieri, 2007). In 2006, fire departments in the United States responded to 412,500 home fires, which resulted in 2,580 nonfirefighter deaths and 12,925 injuries. In 2005, residential fires caused nearly $7 billion in property damage (Karter, 2009). Most fatalities at fire scenes are caused by inhalation of smoke with toxic compounds (Palmieri, 2007). The combustion of household items, such as carpeting and furniture, generates a number of gases, including carbon monoxide, hydrogen cyanide, ammonia, aldehydes, sulfur dioxide, and isocyanates (Prien and Traber, 1988). Carboxyhemoglobin levels greater than 50% are often found in patients with such exposure. Administration of 100% oxygen should be initiated as soon as possible (American Burn Association, 2005).

Inhaled hot air (temperatures >150°C) causes heat injury to respiratory epithelia (Palmieri, 2007). Tissue edema can occur very rapidly to the upper airway and may cause airway obstruction. The patient with burns to the face, singed nasal and facial hair, edema of the tongue or pharynx, and increased respiratory rate should be monitored closely for airway obstruction due to edema. Intubation with mechanical ventilation may be necessary to provide adequate oxygenation until the edema resolves.

Scald. Most *scald* injuries occur in the kitchen or bathroom of the home and are associated with cooking (food and grease spills) and hot water exposure (Evans et al, 2006; Lowell et al, 2008). Temperatures up to 45°C (113°F) may be tolerated for relatively long periods without injury, but as few as 10 seconds of exposure to water at 70°C can result in full-thickness injury in adults (Carrougher, 1997; Jordan and Harrington, 1997). At the temperature of most home water heaters (60°C [140°F]), tissue destruction in a child can occur in less than 5 seconds; only 1 second in an infant (Helvig, 1993).

Contact. *Contact* burns can occur in the home or in the workplace. They frequently occur on the hands, face, and upper body as the object is touched. Common causes of contact burns include oven doors, fireplace screens, space heaters, clothing and curling irons, cookware, and hot machinery and containers (Alden et al, 2006; Hunt et al, 2000; Wibbenmeyer et al, 2003). Children younger than 5 years are at particular risk for scald and contact injuries due to a limited ability to recognize and respond appropriately to danger. The elderly have predisposing factors associated with age that put them at risk for burn injury, including reduced reaction times, decreased dexterity, decreased mobility, inaccurate risk assessment, and impaired senses (Redlick et al, 2002). Working adults are at risk for scald and contact burns; exposure to hot objects or substances are the second leading cause of burn injury in the workplace (Hunt et al, 2000).

Electrical

Electrical injuries account for 4% of burn center admissions (American Burn Association, 2008). It is estimated that as many as 50,000 injuries and 1,000 deaths from electrical causes occur each year in the United States. The American Burn Association (2005) estimates that the risk of being struck by lightning is 1:280,000; lightning injuries kill 80 to 100 people in the United States every year. Tissue injury results when electrical energy is converted into thermal or heat energy. The extent of injury to the body when it becomes part of an electrical current is determined by the (1) strength and type of current, (2) pathway of flow, (3) local tissue resistance, and (4) duration of exposure (American Burn Association, 2005). Various tissues of the body have different resistances to current flow; once electrical contact is made with the skin and resistance is overcome, the body acts as a volume conductor as current flows through the body part (Luce, 2000). Bone has a very high resistance, which allows current to flow along the surface of the bone. Adjacent deep muscle tissue is damaged while superficial muscle and the skin surface remain viable.

Classification of electrical injuries is divided into four categories: high voltage (>1,000 V), low voltage (<1,000 V), lightning strikes, and electric arc without passage of current through the body. The highest incidence of injuries are work related and high voltage, with the primary victims being young men (Arnoldo et al, 2004). Electrical injuries in children are generally low voltage, occur in the home, and involve contact with electrical appliances or frayed cords or placement of objects into electrical outlets. Because of the mechanism of injury, electrically injured patients are at risk for concomitant blunt trauma, soft tissue injuries, and thermal (flame or flash) burns (American Burn Association, 2005). Electrical injuries may also result in potentially fatal cardiac dysrhythmias. Practice guidelines for the management of electrical injuries recommend an electrocardiogram be performed on all patients who sustain either high- or low-voltage electrical injuries (Arnoldo et al, 2006).

Chemical (Alkalis, Acids, and Organic Compounds)

Chemical burns account for 3% of burn unit admissions (American Burn Association, 2008), with approximately 60,000 people seeking medical treatment each year. Chemical injuries often are smaller in size than thermal burns but are more likely to be full thickness in depth (Winfree and Barillo, 1997).

The severity of chemical burns is related to the agent of exposure, duration of contact, and agent's concentration, volume, and mechanism of action. Tissue damage continues after initial exposure until the chemical is removed or inactivated (diluted) with irrigation. In general, neutralization of the agent with another chemical is not recommended unless the exact mechanism is known because the reaction may generate more heat and result in further tissue destruction (American Burn Association, 2005). Health care providers must protect themselves from exposure by using universal precautions and eye protection while caring for the chemical-injured patient. The American Burn Association (2005) identifies the common causes of chemical injury as alkalis, acids, and organic compounds.

Alkalis are commonly found in oven and drain cleaners, fertilizers, industrial cleaners, and cement and concrete. Alkalis damage tissue by liquefaction necrosis and protein denaturation, which allows for deeper spread of the chemical into tissues and a more severe injury. *Acids* are found in bathroom cleansers, rust removers, acidifiers for home swimming pools, and industrial drain cleaners. Acids damage tissue by coagulation necrosis and protein precipitation, which usually limits the depth and spread of tissue damage (Winfree and Barillo, 1997). *Organic compounds,* such as phenols and petroleum products (gasoline, diesel fuel, and creosote), can be responsible for systemic toxicity as well as contact chemical burns. Organic compounds cause cutaneous damage as a result of their fat solvent action and, once absorbed, can produce toxic effects on the pulmonary, renal, and hepatic systems (American Burn Association, 2005).

Health care providers must have a high degree of suspicion of lower airway injury related to inhalation of noxious chemicals that are products of combustion (Monafo, 1996). Chemical inhalation may cause sloughing of the airway-lining epithelium, mucus secretion, inflammation, atelectasis, and airway obstruction. Clinical evolution is delayed from 1 to 3 days after exposure (Palmieri, 2007). Treatment requires ventilatory support, meticulous pulmonary toilet, and general critical care management.

EVALUATION OF BURN INJURY

Zones of Tissue Damage

Determining burn depth can be difficult for even the most experienced burn care provider. Immediately following injury, burns may appear superficial but declare themselves to be deeper by post-burn day 3 (Gibran and Heimbach, 2000). The phrase zones of tissue damage describes the extent of the injury from the deepest or most severely damaged area to the superficial or outermost area. The three zones of tissue damage are zone of coagulation, zone of stasis, and zone of hyperemia (Jackson, 1953). The *zone of coagulation* is the area of greatest damage, is closest to the heat source, and is characterized by coagulation of cells. The *zone of stasis* surrounds the zone of coagulation and involves the vascular system in the area. Thrombosis and vasoconstriction cause transient dermal ischemia. Circulation will return if the area is adequately perfused and protected from further damage from infection, desiccation, and mechanical stress during transfers and repositioning. The *zone of hyperemia* is the outermost area. Usually no cellular death occurs because this area is only minimally damaged. Cells in this zone recover in 7 to 10 days. The area is reddened because of vasodilation and inflammation. The zone of hyperemia is similar to a superficial partial-thickness burn.

Severity of the Burn Wound

Treatment of the burn wound is based on the depth, extent, and severity of the injury. The depth of the injury is based on the number of cells injured or destroyed. With the exception of the fourth degree, the traditional classification of burns as first, second, and third degree has largely been replaced by the more descriptive designations of superficial, superficial partial-thickness, deep partial-thickness, and full-thickness injury (Figure 32-1). Most burns are not uniform in depth; the edges may be more shallow than the central aspect. The severity of the burn can deteriorate in certain circumstances and become more severe, a process known as *wound conversion*. Risk factors for wound conversion are similar to factors that impair other acute and chronic wounds (e.g., oxygenation, infection, mechanical trauma, malnutrition).

Calculation of Body Surface Area Burned

Three methods are used to determine the extent of a burn injury: (1) Lund-Browder chart (Figure 32-2), (2) rule of nines, and (3) hand method. The Lund-Browder

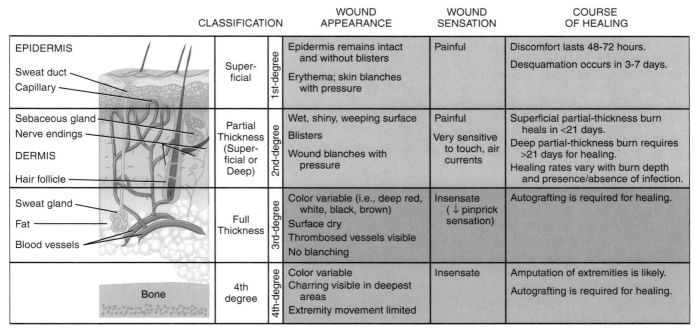

	CLASSIFICATION		WOUND APPEARANCE	WOUND SENSATION	COURSE OF HEALING
EPIDERMIS Sweat duct Capillary	Superficial	1st-degree	Epidermis remains intact and without blisters Erythema; skin blanches with pressure	Painful	Discomfort lasts 48-72 hours. Desquamation occurs in 3-7 days.
Sebaceous gland Nerve endings DERMIS Hair follicle	Partial Thickness (Superficial or Deep)	2nd-degree	Wet, shiny, weeping surface Blisters Wound blanches with pressure	Painful Very sensitive to touch, air currents	Superficial partial-thickness burn heals in <21 days. Deep partial-thickness burn requires >21 days for healing. Healing rates vary with burn depth and presence/absence of infection.
Sweat gland Fat Blood vessels	Full Thickness	3rd-degree	Color variable (i.e., deep red, white, black, brown) Surface dry Thrombosed vessels visible No blanching	Insensate (↓ pinprick sensation)	Autografting is required for healing.
Bone	4th degree	4th-degree	Color variable Charring visible in deepest areas Extremity movement limited	Insensate	Amputation of extremities is likely. Autografting is required for healing.

FIGURE 32-1 Burn injury classification according to depth of injury. (Adapted from Black JM, Hawks JH: *Medical-surgical nursing: clinical management for positive outcomes,* ed 8, St. Louis, 2009, WB Saunders.)

chart is the most accurate method for estimating burn extent in patients of all ages (Mertens et al, 1997). The Lund-Browder chart is completed at admission to determine fluid requirements and is repeated after 72 hours to recalculate any areas of burn injury that may have extended. The rule of nines is based on 11 anatomic regions of the body representing 9% (or multiples of 9%) of TBSA. The rule of nines must be modified for use in children because it does not accurately reflect body surface area in children younger than 15 years (Deitch and Rutan, 2000). The hand method of determining the extent of a burn injury is useful for estimating small, scattered burns. The patient's hand, including the fingers, represents approximately 1% of TBSA (American Burn Association, 2005). The TBSA burned is expressed as a percentage and helps estimate the extent of the injury for diagnosis, treatment, prognosis, and statistical analysis.

Referral Criteria

The American Burn Association has categorized burns as minor, moderate, and major (Table 32-1) and has defined the criteria for burn center referral (see Box 32-1). Patients with major burn injuries or those who meet the criteria identified in Box 32-1 require treatment in a specialized center. A burn center is a facility with a burn physician as director and a highly trained, multidisciplinary staff dedicated to caring for the patient with burns (American Burn Association, 2007).

PATHOPHYSIOLOGY OF BURN INJURY ON THE BODY

Inflammatory mediators released from the damaged cells at the site of the burn (e.g., arachidonic acid metabolites, oxidants, histamine, serotonin, kinins, other vasoactive amines) cause increased capillary permeability not only at the site of injury but throughout the body (Ahrns, 2004; Jordan and Harrington, 1997). Although capillary permeability returns to normal roughly 18 to 24 hours after injury, the initial body response is a dramatic outpouring of fluids, electrolytes, and protein into the interstitial space, which creates intravascular volume deficits. The release of fluids through the hyperpermeable capillaries and the increased capillary pressure combine to create local or systemic edema. The body responds with a classic hemodynamic response: an almost immediate fall in cardiac output, metabolic rate, oxygen consumption, and blood pressure, along with ongoing fluid imbalance and cellular shock, for 3 to 7 days. In patients with a burn wound of at least 15% to 20% TBSA, hypovolemic shock develops quickly unless interventions are started (Lim et al, 1998).

The fluid and electrolyte imbalance that immediately results following a burn injury dominates postburn care priorities and poses potential complications to the pulmonary, cardiovascular, and renal systems. The shift of protein from the intracellular space and vascular compartment into the interstitial space causes numerous potential complications, such as edema, pulmonary edema, blister formation, weeping of fluid,

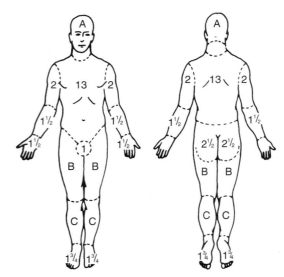

FIGURE 32-2 The Lund-Browder chart for estimating burn extent. Areas represent percentages of body surface area that vary according to age. The accompanying table indicates the relative percentages of these areas in various stages of life. (From Sabeston DC Jr, editor: *Textbook of surgery: the biographical basis of modern surgical practice,* ed 11, Philadelphia, 1977, WB Saunders.)

Relative percentages of areas affected by growth
(age in years)

	0	1	5	10	15	Adult
A: Half of head	$9\frac{1}{2}$	$8\frac{1}{2}$	$6\frac{1}{2}$	$5\frac{1}{2}$	$4\frac{1}{2}$	$3\frac{1}{2}$
B: Half of thigh	$2\frac{3}{4}$	$3\frac{1}{4}$	4	$4\frac{1}{4}$	$4\frac{1}{2}$	$4\frac{3}{4}$
C: Half of leg	$2\frac{1}{2}$	$2\frac{1}{2}$	$2\frac{3}{4}$	3	$3\frac{1}{4}$	$3\frac{1}{2}$

Second degree _____ and
Third degree _____ =
Total percent burned _____

TABLE 32-1	American Burn Association Categories of Burn Injury		
Minor Burns	**Moderate Burns**	**Major Burns**	
Adults: 15% TBSA	Adults: 15%–25% TBSA, mixed partial/full thickness	All patients: >25% TBSA	
Children and elderly: 10% TBSA	Children <10 years or adults >40 years: 10%–20% TBSA	Children <10 years or adults >40 years: 20% TBSA	
<2% TBSA full-thickness burns not involving cosmetic or functional risk or impairment of face, ears, eyes, feet, hands, perineum	< 10% TBSA full-thickness burns not involving cosmetic or functional risk or impairment of the face, ears, eyes, feet, hands, perineum	>10% TBSA full-thickness burns	
		All burns of face, eyes, ears, hands, or perineum, especially if functional or cosmetic impairment exists	
		All high-voltage electrical burns	
		All burns with inhalation injury or major trauma	
		Poor-risk patients	

TBSA, Total body surface area.

hypovolemia, hypoproteinemia, tachycardia, increased capillary pressure, vasoconstriction of the microcirculation, decreased central venous pressure, and decreased urinary output. Sodium, magnesium, calcium, and phosphorus loss can occur directly through open burn wounds (Supple, 2004). Potassium is released from damaged cells, triggering hyperkalemia and metabolic acidosis.

Loss of skin integrity causes increased fluid and heat loss through the wound. Evaporative fluid loss caused by loss of skin integrity is 4 to 20 times the normal rate, which contributes to hypovolemia; this fluid loss continues until all the wounds are closed. Hypothermia should be prevented rigorously throughout the phases of recovery. The patient with burn injury has an increased thermal neutral point so that exposure to low temperatures results in an increase in the patient's metabolic rate (Jordan and Harrington, 1997). Restoration and maintenance of intravascular volume with fluid similar to that which is lost in the tissues are essential aspects of burn management.

Patients with burn injuries of 20% or greater TBSA will experience a hypermetabolic response with elevated catecholamine, glucocorticoid, and glucagon levels and decreased insulin level requiring nutritional support for optimal recovery (Mertens et al, 1997). The increase in metabolic rate causes an increase in protein catabolism, gluconeogenesis, and lipolysis. This response is characterized by increased heat loss, negative nitrogen balance, and weight loss (Carrougher, 1997). The severity and duration of hypermetabolic activity are directly proportional to the extent of injury. The peak occurs in the first 2 weeks and slowly returns to normal with closure of the wound. Elevated catecholamines, decreased bowel perfusion, and increased gastric secretions place the burn patient at risk for paralytic ileus, intestinal mucosal atrophy, decreased nutrient absorption, Curling stress ulcer (Supple, 2004), and impaired ability to function as a bacterial barrier (Rutan TC, 1998).

PHASES OF BURN CARE

Burn care is divided into three overlapping phases of recovery: emergent, acute/wound care, and rehabilitation. The emergent phase is the first 72 hours after injury. The acute/wound care phase begins when the patient has been stabilized. Goals of this period include healing partial-thickness wounds, grafting full-thickness wounds, and preventing complications. Wound management during the acute phase consists of debridement, daily wound care, and surgical interventions for wound closure. The rehabilitation phase begins when wound healing is complete and focuses on restoring or maximizing the patient's functional capacity. This phase may last several years and deals with functional and cosmetic problems associated with contractures and scar tissue formation.

Emergent Phase

As with any trauma victim, the initial assessment of the patient with a burn injury includes the primary and secondary surveys. The primary survey (conducted out in the field) includes advanced burn life support as outlined by the American College of Surgeons Committee on Trauma (American Burn Association, 2005). The guidelines include the ABCDE assessment: airway, breathing, circulation, disability, and exposure and evaluation.

The secondary survey is initiated after immediate resuscitative measures are established and includes a complete physical assessment and medical history. Because care is based on the mechanism, location, and severity of the injury, as much information as possible regarding the incident should be obtained, such as whether the injury occurred in an enclosed space, chemicals were involved, and the victim lost consciousness. Aspects of the patient's medical history (e.g., preexisting disease, medications, allergies, alcohol or drug use, immunization status) influence management decisions (American Burn Association, 2005).

Care during the emergent phase centers on emergency management and stabilization and on wound assessment/diagnosis. The first 24 hours is devoted to fluid resuscitation, ventilatory management, and establishing the hemodynamic stability of the patient. During this phase, the depth and extent of the wound are estimated in order to calculate the severity of the injury and fluid resuscitation needs. For a small burn (see Table 32-1), the development of edema is immediate, rapid, limited to the wound site, and peaks within 8 to 12 hours (Ahrns, 1999). Intravascular fluid losses associated with small burns can be managed with oral replacement at 150% of calculated maintenance rate. Intravenous supplementation can be used if the patient has difficulties meeting the oral intake goal.

Large burns reach maximum edema within 12 to 24 hours postinjury. The goal of fluid resuscitation is to maintain adequate tissue and vital organ perfusion while preventing complications associated with inadequate or excessive fluid therapy (American Burn Association, 2005). If fluid resuscitation is inadequate, hypovolemia will progress and acute renal failure will occur. The amount of fluid for replacement depends on the extent and depth of the burn and the patient's age and medical history. Many fluid resuscitation formulas exist, and most are based on the percent of TBSA burned, body weight, or a combination of both. According to the American Burn Association, fluid resuscitation, regardless of solution type or estimated need, should be titrated to maintain urine output of approximately 0.5 to 1.0 ml/kg/hr in adults and 1.0 to 1.5 ml/kg/hr in children. Increased volume requirements can be anticipated in patients with full-thickness injury, inhalation injury, and delay in resuscitation (Pham et al, 2008). Adequacy of resuscitation is determined by urinary output, mental status, peripheral temperature, systolic blood pressure, heart rate, and base deficit (Sheridan, 2002).

Early initiation of enteral feeding is recommended for nutritional support of the patient with a burn (Gottschlich et al, 2002; McDonald et al, 1991; Raff et al, 1997a and 1997b) to prevent stress ulcers, increase intestinal blood flow, preserve gastrointestinal function, and minimize bacterial translocation from the gut as a result of mucosal atrophy (Andel et al, 2001; Raff et al 1997a and 1997b; Supple, 2004). The parenteral route has no clear advantage and is used only in patients with prolonged ileus or selected patients on mechanical ventilation (Tassiopoulos, 1999).

Nearly all burn centers report supplementing vitamins and/or minerals (Graves et al, 2009). Dosage guidelines established by the National Advisory Group/American Medical Association are appropriate for burn-injured patients unless symptoms of deficiency occur. Because zinc deficiencies are well documented in burn-injured patients, supplemental zinc as well as vitamin C often are required (Sicoutris and Holmes, 2006). Nutrition assessment and support is discussed in great detail in Chapter 27.

This phase ends when capillary permeability begins to normalize and the patient begins to diurese the large volume of fluid given for resuscitation, usually around post-burn day 4.

Wound Stabilization. Wound intervention during the emergent phase involves cleansing, debridement, and prevention of obstructed blood flow from edema and eschar formation. The usual burn wound care given during this period follows patient stabilization and involves cleansing the areas with a nonirritating detergent and rinsing with warm water. The environment should be warmed to prevent hypothermia. Loose necrotic or devitalized tissue is lightly debrided, and large intact bullae (>2 cm) are opened. Small, frequent doses of intravenous analgesics are provided for pain control. Full-thickness wounds usually are dressed with a topical antimicrobial agent; systemic prophylactic antibiotics are not routinely used unless specific organisms have been identified (Jordan and Harrington, 1997).

Escharotomy. Deep partial-thickness or full-thickness burns that are circumferential, or nearly circumferential, to an extremity may require an escharotomy to relieve pressure. Edema and eschar formation can obstruct venous return and lead to decreased arterial blood flow. Early identification of extremities at risk and serial examination are essential; monitoring should include temperature, pliability, voluntary motion, pain with passive motion, changes in the quality of pulses, and delayed capillary refill. The escharotomy is a linear incision through the full-thickness wound dividing the eschar. The incision is only as deep as necessary to separate the eschar. Full-thickness eschar lacks nerve endings, so pain is minimal, although small doses of narcotics and anxiolytics are given intravenously to control background pain and anxiety. This procedure can be done at the bedside with a sterile field and scalpel or electrocautery to control the small amount of bleeding that occurs (Jordan and Harrington, 1997). Midmedial and midlateral incisions are designed to completely section the eschar while preventing injury to underlying superficial structures. The structures most at risk during escharotomy are the brachial artery in the upper arm, the ulnar nerve at the elbow, the superficial peroneal nerve at the knee, and the neurovascular bundles and extensors of the digits (Sheridan, 2002). The escharotomy incision wounds are dressed with a topical agent.

Similarly, deep circumferential burns to the chest and/or abdomen may restrict the expansion needed for breathing and adequate ventilation. Frequent assessment of the adequacy of chest expansion, quality of respirations, oxygenation, and mental status of the patient is essential. Circumferential chest burns require an escharotomy placed in the anterior axillary line bilaterally. If there is significant extension of the burn onto the adjacent abdominal wall, the incisions should be extended to this area and connected by a transverse incision along the costal margin (American Burn Association, 2005).

Fasciotomy. When the burn injury extends to the muscle, as occurs with a high-voltage electrical injury or skeletal trauma, edema develops beneath the fascia and muscle compartment, which precipitates tissue ischemia and nerve damage. A fasciotomy, or surgical incision of the fascia, then is necessary. This procedure is conducted in the operating room under general anesthesia.

Pain Control and Emotional Support. Initially, during the hypermetabolic phase, opioids such as morphine sulfate are best administered for pain control in small, frequent doses. Patient-controlled analgesia devices are effective in the delivery of opioids and allow the patient a sense of control. Supplemental pain control measures (e.g., morphine, benzodiazepines, acetaminophen with codeine, acetaminophen, nonnarcotic medications such as nonsteroidal antiinflammatory drugs) are necessary to control background or procedural pain. Anxiolytic agents are commonly given to augment pain medications. The use of diversionary activities, imagery, and relaxation, particularly during dressing changes, are frequently used to assist patients with coping during stressful procedures (Davis and Sheely-Adolphson, 1997). Self-reported pain rating tools and anxiety scores are of great value to the burn team because they indicate the degree of relief achieved from the patient's perspective (see Chapter 25).

Acute/Wound Care Phase

Care of the burn wound is a priority of the acute/wound care phase. Goals of this phase are to heal partial-thickness wounds, graft full-thickness wounds, and prevent complications such as infection. Wound cleansing and debridement, in conjunction with the appropriate topical agent, dressing, or skin replacement, are required to prevent infection and promote wound healing.

Initially, wound care is dependent on the location, extent, and depth of the wound. The management of burn injuries can differ significantly based on injury location, joint involvement, small BSA burns as opposed to large BSA burns, and partial as opposed to full-thickness burns (see Figure 32-1 and Table 32-1). Factors that influence the care plan may include age of the patient, pain and anxiety management, and ability of the patient and/or caregiver to participate in daily care.

Hydrotherapy. Team members in the burn unit often perform gentle cleansing, debridement, and wound assessments during hydrotherapy. The patient is medicated for pain and anxiety prior to the procedure, so this is an ideal time for physical and occupational therapists to perform range-of-motion exercises and functional evaluations. Diversionary activities such as music or videos are often used to assist with patient coping. For the pediatric patient, the child life specialist is invaluable in providing developmentally appropriate activities while role modeling supportive behaviors to caregivers.

Bioburden Management. Consequences of burn wound infection include conversion of partial-thickness wounds to full-thickness wounds, increased nutritional requirements, delays in healing, and increased scar and contracture formation (Greenfield and McManus, 1997). The most common organisms responsible for infection in the burn-injured patient are gram positive. Group A *Staphylococcus* infections are a threat to skin graft survival. Other gram-positive microorganisms of concern are group A β-hemolytic *Streptococcus* and *Enterococcus* species. Both *Staphylococcus aureus* and *Enterococcus* have increasing levels of antibiotic resistance. *Pseudomonas aeruginosa* continues to be the primary gram-negative pathogen of concern, especially in burn centers that do not routinely practice early wound excision and grafting. *P. aeruginosa* typically is a later-developing infection and is becoming less frequent, and with later onset, as a result of aggressive wound closure techniques. Gram-negative bacteremia has been associated with mortality up to 50% higher than that predicted on the basis of the severity of the burn injury (Greenfield and McManus, 1997).

Nonbacterial sources of infection include yeast, fungus, and virus (e.g., herpes). Candida wound infections are uncommon in burn patients and are seen most frequently in patients with large burns who receive broad-spectrum antibiotics for treatment of other infections. Fungi, particularly *Aspergillus* species, are commonly found on burn wounds. Fungi can be found throughout the environment, including the air, nonsterile wound supplies, and laundry items. Fungal infections are treated with topical antifungal agents, systemic amphotericin B, and, if necessary, surgical excision of the infected tissue (Greenfield and McManus, 1997). A viral infection in the patient with a burn injury usually is localized. Herpetic infections most commonly occur in healing or recently healed partial-thickness burns. Assessment and management of bacterial bioburden, including descriptions and indications for topical antimicrobials, are described in Chapter 16.

Topical Antimicrobials. Topical antimicrobials are indicated for deep burns that cannot undergo early excision and wound closure but are not proved necessary for shallow burns, donor sites, and meshed skin grafts (Franz et al, 2008). The ideal topical antimicrobial for the patient with the burn should (1) have a broad spectrum of activity, (2) have minimal systemic absorption, (3) not delay wound healing, (4) penetrate eschar well, (5) be painless upon application, and (6) be inexpensive (Patel et al,

2008). Because no single product meets all of these criteria, an antimicrobial should be chosen based on the individual patient and the wound needs. The following section briefly discusses the topical antimicrobials used most commonly used with burns.

Silver Sulfadiazine. Silver sulfadiazine (Silvadene, Aventis Pharmaceuticals, Bridgewater, NJ; Thermazene, Kendall Company, Mansfield, MA) probably is the most frequently used prophylactic topical antimicrobial for burn care. It is active against both gram-positive and gram-negative organisms and fungus. Silver sulfadiazine, which is available as a 1% cream, is easy to apply without pain on application and has a relatively low toxicity (Honari, 2004). Silver sulfadiazine can cause a transient leukopenia, which resolves after the first week even with continued use.

Silver Antimicrobial Dressings. Silver antimicrobial dressings provide a broad spectrum of antimicrobial and bactericidal coverage, including vancomycin-resistant enterococcus, methicillin-resistant *S. aureus, P. aeruginosa,* and Candida. Ionic silver dressings are available in many forms and discussed in Chapters 16 and 18. Some of these dressings are contraindicated for particular burn injuries, so it is essential to check the manufacturer's information for indications and contraindications.

Mafenide Acetate. Mafenide acetate (Sulfamylon, Bertek Pharmaceuticals, Morgantown, WV) is a suspension cream with broad-spectrum activity against gram-positive and gram-negative organisms, including *P. aeruginosa.* Mafenide penetrates burn eschar well, so it is useful when infection is suspected (Honari, 2004) or vascular supply is minimal (Jordan and Harrington, 1997). Mafenide is a potent carbonic anhydrase inhibitor. Metabolic acidosis is a frequent side effect when mafenide is used on burns greater than 25% TBSA. Other adverse effects include pain on application to partial-thickness burns and a maculopapular rash. A 5% solution also is available and is approved for use as a prophylactic agent applied as a soak to fresh autografts (Maggi et al, 1999). Some burn centers rotate the use of silver sulfadiazine and mafenide acetate cream with each dressing change. This alternating therapy provides the advantages of both agents while minimizing side effects (McManus, 1996).

Bacitracin/Neomycin/Polymyxin. Bacitracin/neomycin/polymyxin are nontoxic and moisturizing and can be reapplied one to five times daily, so they are useful for facial and perineal burns. Bacitracin alone has mild antimicrobial activity against gram-positive bacteria, so the addition of neomycin and polymyxin B bolsters gram-negative coverage (Patel, et al, 2008).

Temporary Skin Substitutes. Temporary skin substitutes (biologic, synthetic, biosynthetic, or bioengineered dressings) are effective with partial-thickness burns while the patient is awaiting epithelialization and with excised full-thickness burns while the patient is awaiting skin graft closure. As explained in Chapter 19, when skin is replaced by a material from a source other than the patient, the material will not provide permanent wound closure and eventually will be rejected. However, the product can maintain a wound free of infection until epithelialization or permanent wound closure occurs (Franz et al, 2008). Additional benefits include a reduction on heat and water loss from the wound, less pain as sensory nerve terminals are covered, fewer dressing changes required, and increased patient participation with therapies and activities critical to recovery (Delatte et al, 2001). Ideally the product will not be rejected until after the host has established a healthy epithelial wound bed. Descriptions, components, indications, and contraindications of each of the skin substitutes are given in Chapter 19. The following section briefly discusses the types of skin substitutes most appropriate for burns based on severity and location.

Biobrane. Biobrane (Bertek Pharmaceuticals) is used for the management of superficial partial-thickness wounds, as donor site dressing, and on excised burns that do not have eschar. Biobrane readily conforms to surface irregularities, so it can be placed on the joints, face, and trunk, thus promoting an early return to activities of daily living. Biobrane is also available as a preformed glove for use on partial-thickness burns to the hand.

BGC Matrix. BGC Matrix (Brennan Medical, St. Paul, MN) wound dressing is useful for the management of partial-thickness burns and donor sites. As the BGC Matrix dressing becomes dry and well adhered to the wound, the dressing becomes quite stiff, which limits its use over joints and on the face and neck; these same properties make it ideal as a donor site dressing because it does not easily become dislodged from the donor site as the patient resumes activity (Delatte et al, 2001).

Allograft. Allograft, harvested from human donors, is considered to be the gold standard for excised burns when no donor sites are available. However, supply may be limited, and, as with any human donor situation, there is a potential for disease transmission. Some burn centers report rejection of allograft in as few as 5 to 9 days (Hansbrough et al, 1997).

Xenograft. Xenograft (heterograft, pigskin) is used primarily as a dressing for partial-thickness burns that are not expected to require skin grafting. Xenograft is easier to obtain but is not as effective as allograft when used as a temporary dressing with excised wounds because it does not establish vessel-to-vessel connections. When xenograft is rejected, it undergoes vascular necrosis and it sloughs, which creates more subgraft bacteria compared with allograft (Pruitt, 1997).

Dermal Matrix Substitutes. Dermal matrix substitutes are useful for treatment of large, full-thickness BSA burns. Examples include Integra (Integra LifeSciences Corporation, Plainsboro, NJ, USA) and Alloderm (LifeCell Corp., Branchburg, NJ, USA). When used in conjunction with thin autografts, dermal replacements may decrease the amount of scar tissue formation, which improves the elasticity and flexibility of healed burn by allowing more normal ingrowth of the body's own vascular cells and tissues (Paul, 2008).

Surgical Excision and Autograft Closure. Early eschar excision and graft closure is recommended for deep burn wounds to decrease risk of infection, improve survival, and initiate healing. Exceptions include (1) special areas such as the hands and face where improved outcomes from early excision and closure have not been demonstrated and (2) patients at the extremes of age or with comorbid conditions for whom early excision and grafting would impose significant insult (i.e., inhalation injury) (Franz et al, 2008).

In general, if the burn is greater than 30% TBSA, graft closure is done in stages because the operative process of excision and harvesting skin involves blood loss and is physiologically stressful, and donor sites need time to heal before they are reused. When an excised burn is so large that donor sites for split-thickness skin grafts are insufficient, nonimmunogenic cultured epidermal autograft (Epicell, Genzyme Tissue Repair, Cambridge, MA) can serve as a permanent skin replacement without fear of rejection (Franz et al, 2008). A temporary skin graft can be used to cover the wound and protect it from infection while awaiting the cultured epidermal autograft.

Split-thickness skin grafts are the most commonly used autografts. The skin is harvested using a guarded dermatome, which controls the thickness of the graft (usually 0.008–0.0012 inch thick), and includes the epidermis and a thin layer of dermis. Split-thickness skin grafts may be used as sheets or meshed to provide expansion (Mozingo, 1998). Sheet grafts provide a better functional and cosmetic result and are commonly used on the face, hands, feet, neck, and joints. Postoperatively, sheet grafts may collect serous drainage or blood, which can lift the graft from the wound bed, causing graft loss. Frequent assessment identifies the presence of excess fluid or hematoma, which can be removed by aspiration or rolling of a cotton-tipped applicator to the surface of the graft to remove collected fluid.

For large BSA burns, skin grafts are meshed to allow more wound coverage with fewer donor sites. After the skin is harvested, it is guided through a mechanical meshing device (Jordan and Harrington, 1997). The meshed graft is secured with staples or sutures and then covered with a nonadherent inner layer to prevent shearing. Fluff gauze moistened with a topical antimicrobial, such as 5% Sulfamylon or triple antibiotic solution is placed to prevent desiccation. If the graft is applied to an extremity or joint, splints are fitted at this time to maintain a position of function while engraftment occurs. The dressing usually is left in place for 4 to 7 days before changing, at which time the graft is inspected and redressed. The dressing is changed daily until the graft is sufficiently stable to remain open to air, usually in about 2 weeks. Physical and occupational therapy can be resumed after 5 to 7 days, starting with passive range-of-motion exercises and progressing at an individual rate depending on the area grafted and the patient's condition. Splinting continues to areas at risk for contracture.

Split-thickness skin graft donor sites heal by epithelialization, which is facilitated in a moist environment. Advanced wound care dressings are more effective than simple impregnated gauze dressings at accelerating healing and decreasing pain in skin graft donor sites. The small differences in improvement must be balanced with the differences in cost and patient comfort (Franz et al, 2008). As with most wounds, dressing selection is dependent on the characteristics of the wound (donor site location, size, proximity to other wounds). Healing of donor sites in a timely manner is especially important in patients with large BSA burns who will need reharvesting to obtain full wound coverage. It may be prudent to consider the administration of human growth hormone or the testosterone analogue oxandrolone to enhance healing of the donor site because both of these agents have been shown to significantly decrease weight and nitrogen loss and increase healing rates (Demling, 1999).

Full-thickness skin grafts are obtained by surgically excising the entire thickness of the donor skin to the level of the subcutaneous tissue, resulting in grafts 0.025 to 0.030 inch thick. Transfer of the entire dermal layer is accomplished, which makes the graft durable and less prone to contracture. Full-thickness skin grafts are limited to use for small full-thickness burns and are frequently used in reconstructive surgery. The full-thickness skin graft donor site is a full-thickness wound, which usually is closed by primary suturing or split-thickness grafting (Mozingo, 1998).

Pain and Psychological Support. During each of the phases of burn recovery, the patient with a burn faces numerous sources of anxiety and types of pain: exposure of nerve endings, inflammation, edema, dressing changes, debridement, insertion of intravenous lines, blood draws, invasive monitoring procedures, physical and occupational therapy, and surgical procedures (Byers et al, 2001). Pain and anxiety may lead to prolongation of the stress response following injury, which could potentially delay wound healing and lengthen recovery time (Monafo, 1995). Chapters 25 and 26 discuss pain as a critical cofactor in wound healing and provide valuable information related to understanding, assessing, and managing pain.

Initially, during the hypermetabolic phase, opioids such as morphine sulfate are best administered in small, frequent doses. Patient-controlled analgesia devices are effective in the delivery of opioids and allow the patient a sense of control. Supplemental pain control measures (morphine, benzodiazepines, acetaminophen with codeine, acetaminophen, nonnarcotic medications such as nonsteroidal antiinflammatory drugs) are

necessary to control background or procedural pain (Davis and Sheely-Adolphson, 1997).

Pediatrics. Although children experience the same physical stress as adults during burn recovery, their behavioral responses can be quite different and are related to their stage of development. Behavioral responses typically include anxiety, agitation, anger, conditioned fear, and regression. Causes of psychological and emotional distress include separation anxiety, repeated painful procedures, and loss of control and independence (Adcock et al, 1998). Specific interventions are listed in Box 32-2.

The incidence of attention deficit hyperactivity disorder is estimated to be as high as 20% in children admitted to burn centers (Mangus et al, 2004). This should be addressed throughout the phases of burn recovery to optimize participation in the recovery process (Sheridan, 2007). Acute stress syndrome and posttraumatic stress syndrome also should be assessed for and anticipated, as up to 30% of burn-injured children may develop significant symptoms (Ehde et al, 2000; Stoddard et al, 2006).

Abuse and Neglect. Approximately 10% of child abuse cases involve burning, and up to 20% of pediatric burn admissions involve abuse or neglect (Ruth et al, 2003). Burn care providers must understand the assessment and interventional processes related to suspected abuse and neglect cases. Knowledge of individual institutions' protocols governing the management of these cases is key to maintaining patient safety and obtaining optimal outcomes. Primary responsibility for initial assessments, communications with law enforcement, and initiation of specific interventions may involve nursing or medical staff, specialized teams for abuse and neglect, and social services (Doctor, 1998). Similar considerations are applicable to adult patients who have been deliberately injured. Stone et al (1970) identified criteria for burn injuries that are suspicious for abuse or neglect (Box 32-3).

Rehabilitation Phase

The goal of the rehabilitation phase is to restore or maximize the patient's functional capacity. This rehabilitation phase begins once wound healing is complete and

---

BOX 32-2 | **Interventions for Psychological Support of the Pediatric Burn Patient**

- Encourage parents and family to be present during hospitalization.
- Role model supportive behaviors.
- Isolate painful procedures to a particular place and identify the child's room as a "safe zone."
- Allow older children some control and choices regarding wound care and therapy.
- Provide preparation before and assistance with coping during painful procedures.
- Make appropriate resources available to children who may show long-term adjustment issues.

BOX 32-3	Nonaccidental Burn Criteria

- Multiple hematomas or scars in various stages of healing
- Concurrent injuries or evidence of neglect (e.g., malnutrition)
- History of prior hospitalization for "accidental" trauma
- Unexplained delay between time of injury and first attempt to obtain medical attention
- Burns appear older than the alleged time of the accident
- Account of accident not compatible with age and ability of patient
- Adults in charge allege that there are no witnesses to the "accident" and that the child was merely discovered to have been burned
- Relatives other than parents bring injured child to the hospital
- Burn is attributed to the action of a sibling or other child (this can, in fact, happen)
- Injured child is excessively withdrawn, submissive, or overly polite or does not cry during painful procedures
- Scalds on hands or feet, often symmetrical, appear to be full thickness in depth, suggesting extremities were forcibly immersed and held in hot liquid
- Isolated burns of buttocks that could hardly be produced by accidental means in children

may last several weeks to several years, depending on the extent and severity of the burn injury. Skin- and wound-related complications that manifest after healing, such as scarring, contractures, and itching, require management during the rehabilitation phase.

Excessive Scarring, Contractures, and Itch. Excessive scarring is rare in burn injuries that heal within 21 days (Franz et al, 2008). Patients with deep burn, children, young adults, and patients with darkly pigmented skin are at particular risk (Engrav et al, 2007). Two types of scarring are seen post-burn injury. *Hypertrophic* scars are red, raised, painful, itchy, and lack elasticity. Hypertrophic scars remain within the boundary of the original injury, regress with time, and are more frequently seen following burn injury. *Keloids* are firm, fibrous nodules that extend beyond the original wound margin and are often hyperpigmented (Mafong and Ashinoff, 2000).

Excessive scar formation and treatment modalities are described in Chapter 4 and Table 4-3. The exact pathophysiology of scar formation and the mechanism of action of these treatment modalities are not known. Treatments most frequently used with burn scars alone or in combination include pressure garments, hydrogel or silicone sheeting, corticosteroid injections, surgical excision, and laser.

Scar contracture is the primary cause of functional deficits in the patient with a burn. A contracture is essentially a shortening of a scar over a joint surface that limits joint mobility (Leman and Ricks, 1994). A study by Schneider et al (2006) identified contractures as developing in more than one third of hospitalized burn-injured patients by the time of discharge. The

shoulder was the most frequently affected joint (38%), followed by the elbow (34%) and the knee (22%). Patients at risk for contracture development included those with longer lengths of stay, higher percent BSA burns, and inhalation injury. Early wound closure, mechanical splinting for stretch and position, and diligent range-of-motion exercise of the site are essential components of burn wound care to limit scar and contracture development (Jordan and Harrington, 1997).

Treatment of post-burn injury scarring can last several months to years. Compliance with the treatment plan may be difficult to achieve because patients find pressure garments uncomfortable and confining. It is important to instruct patients and caregivers that any treatment of hypertrophic or keloid scars is aimed at minimizing the scars. Complete normalization of the skin to preburn appearance and texture may not be possible. In a meta-analysis of excessive scarring treatments, the mean amount of improvement to be expected was only 60% (Franz et al, 2008).

Patients recovering from burn injuries experience itching from a variety of sources. Histamines released during the inflammatory phase of healing cause itch, particularly in large BSA burns that take longer to heal. Infection also prolongs healing time and causes excess production of collagen in the wound, which leads to hypertrophic scarring and an increased amount of itch. Itching can be a side effect of the morphine used to manage burn pain (Matheson et al, 2001). Itching in a burn wound usually begins within 2 weeks of the injury and may last for an extended period. Current treatment of itching includes a combination of oral or topical antihistamines, topical doxepin hydrochloride, a potent histamine receptor antagonist (Gibran et al, 2007), skin moisturizers, and pressure garments (Bell and Gabriel, 2009).

Discharge Planning. The main goal of treatment throughout all phases of recovery is functional return of the patient to preburn lifestyle or as close to that lifestyle as is reasonably possible. The patient with a burn injury is identified as a candidate for discharge when wound healing is progressing; nutritional intake is adequate to support continued healing; pain, itching, and infection are controlled with medications by mouth; and the patient and/or caregiver have demonstrated competence in wound care and exercises. The discharge process is similar for major and minor burns and should incorporate five major areas of patient/caregiver education: (1) wound management, (2) pain and itch relief, (3) exercises, (4) scar maturation, and (5) emotional support for the patient and family.

An individualized plan of care that addresses age-specific needs is necessary for each patient with a burn injury (Rutan RL, 1998). The discharge goal for pediatric patients is social reintegration. Appropriate objectives to be met prior to discharge include the following:

1. The child will achieve an age-appropriate level of functioning.
2. The child and caregiver will understand the processes of injury and recovery.
3. The child will begin to integrate a new body image.

Many burn centers offer school reentry programs that provide psychosocial support for the child and education about the burn recovery process for teachers and classmates. Camps for children with a history of severe burn injury, staffed by burn care professionals, provide the opportunity for the child to meet and socialize with other children with burns. The camp is a safe environment for building self-esteem.

Goals for discharge planning for the adult patient with a burn injury often focus on return to work. Employment equates with life satisfaction, provides an identity, and allows for financial independence. Collaboration with a vocational rehabilitation counselor often is necessary for a successful outcome. The discharge plan for the elderly patient with a burn injury must take into consideration that the injury may have resulted from a chronic degenerative or physical process. Involvement of family members or other caregivers who can assist with wound care and activities of daily living are of particular importance (Rutan RL, 1998).

OUTPATIENT BURN MANAGEMENT

The American Burn Association injury severity grading system classifies burn injuries as minor, moderate, or severe. Many minor and moderate burn injuries now are treated on an outpatient basis only. Over the 10-year period from 1998 to 2007, the average length of hospital stay for burn-injured patients has decreased from 11 days to 7 days (American Burn Association, 2008). Factors that may influence the shift to outpatient care include a desire to decrease health care costs, reduction in the risk of nosocomial infections, psychological benefits of home care, increasing numbers of outpatient surgical procedures, direct referrals to burn clinics for care (Moss, 2004), and new developments in wound dressings. It is estimated that 90% of burn-injured patients who receive medical care do so on an outpatient basis (Peck et al, 2007).

Assessment of the outpatient includes history of injury, medical history, psychosocial and economic assessments, and evaluation of the location, extent, depth, and severity of the burn injury. Although most minor and some moderate burn injuries can receive appropriate care on an outpatient basis, hospital admission should be considered if factors that influence the patient's safety or the patient's ability to heal are identified in the assessment. Inpatient care may be required if the cause of injury is suspected of being not accidental, the presence

of chronic disease would prolong wound healing, resources are lacking to provide daily care or return to clinic, the location of the burn impairs ability to provide self-care and perform activities of daily living, or wound care/therapy needs are such that pain cannot adequately be controlled with oral medication (Moss, 2004).

The goals for the patient with a burn who is treated in the outpatient setting include wound protection, timely wound healing, adequate pain control, and rapid rehabilitation with return to school or work (Moss, 2004). Wound care in the outpatient setting begins with gentle cleansing with mild soap and water to remove devitalized skin and debris. Appropriate pain medication by mouth is generally used for small burns seen in the clinic setting. If extensive debridement is required, additional medications for pain and anxiety will be needed, and this is best performed in the more controlled setting of the emergency department or inpatient burn unit. Controversy exists as to whether to shave the hair surrounding a wound or to unroof intact blisters (Moss, 2004). Often, small blisters to the palms, fingers, or soles of the feet are left intact if they do not limit range of motion, whereas larger blisters (>2 cm) are debrided (Honari, 2004).

Individual assessments of the extent and depth of the wound and the size, location, and fragility of the blisters will dictate treatment. Wound care and dressings should be kept as simple as possible while the wound is kept clean, moist, and protected. In addition to selecting a dressing that meets the needs of the wound, priorities include patient comfort, mobility, and activity. Evaluation of the risk for functional impairment is performed at this time by the physical or occupational therapist, and the appropriate splinting or exercises are implemented.

Patient and/or caregiver education is vital to successful outpatient management. Explanations regarding the depth of the wound and demonstration of appropriate wound care techniques and dressing application should be given in conjunction with written instructions. Instructions should include information specific to the wound, signs and symptoms of infection, therapy schedule, activity restrictions, nutrition, pain management, and how to contact the burn team for assistance (Moss, 2004).

Initial follow-up visits may range in frequency from daily to weekly, based on factors identified in the initial assessment and including the extent and depth of the burn and the ability of the patient or caregiver to adequately perform daily care and monitor the wound. Once healing occurs, intermittent visits continue until the scar maturation process has ended, as evidenced by a mature scar that is soft, supple, of normal color, and without contractures (Moss, 2004). As the wound heals, patients are instructed on side effects of burn injury that may occur: excessive scarring, itching, sleep disturbances, discomfort associated with pressure garments, splinting, and exercise, and color and texture changes to the skin. Newly healed burn wounds are more sensitive to ultraviolet light, so the need for protection in the form of a sunscreen with a sun protection factor (SPF) of 30 and for covering the area with clothing should be incorporated into the teaching plan. Appropriate referrals for support and counseling should be made in a timely manner for patients experiencing distress related to psychological symptoms.

SUMMARY

Whether involved in the care of a patient with massive tissue loss or a minor burn, the wound care specialist must be familiar with the principles of initial assessment, management based on the type and severity of injury, and prevention of complications. Knowledge of the phases of recovery and the associated therapeutic and psychosocial needs of the patient contributes to optimal outcomes.

REFERENCES

Adcock RJ et al: Psychologic and emotional recovery. In Carrougher GJ, editor: *Burn care and therapy,* St. Louis, 1998, Mosby.

Ahrns KS: Initial resuscitation after burn injury: therapies, strategies, and controversies, *AACN Clin Issues* 10(1):46, 1999.

Ahrns KS: Trends in burn resuscitation: shifting the focus from fluids to adequate endpoint monitoring, edema control, and adjuvant therapies, *Crit Care Nurs Clin North Am* 16(1):75, 2004.

Alden NE et al: Contact burns: is further prevention necessary? *J Burn Care Rehabil* 27(4):472-475, 2006.

American Burn Association: *Advanced burn life support course,* Chicago, 2005, Author.

American Burn Association: Guidelines for the operations of burn centers, *J Burn Care Rehabil* 28(1):134-141, 2007.

American Burn Association: *National burn repository 2007 report,* Chicago, 2008, Author.

Andel H et al: Impact of early high caloric duodenal feeding on the oxygen balance of the splanchnic region after severe burn injury, *Burns* 27(4):389-393, 2001.

Arnoldo BD et al: Electrical injuries: a 20-year review, *J Burn Care Rehabil* 25(6):479, 2004.

Arnoldo B et al: Practice guidelines for the management of electrical injuries, *J Burn Care Rehabili* 27(4): 439-447, 2006.

Bell PL, Gabriel V: Evidence based review for the treatment of post-burn pruritus, *J Burn Care Rehabil* 30(1):55-61, 2009.

Black JM, Hawks JH: *Medical-surgical nursing: clinical management for positive outcomes,* ed 8, St. Louis, 2009, WB Saunders.

Byers JF et al: Burn patients' pain and anxiety experiences, *J Burn Care Rehabil* 22(2):144, 2001.

Carrougher GJ: Management of fluid and electrolyte balance in thermal injuries: implications for perioperative nursing practice, *Semin Periop Nurs* 6(4):201, 1997.

Davis ST, Sheely-Adolphson P: Burn management. Psychosocial interventions: pharmacologic and psychologic modalities, *Nurs Clin North Am* 32(2):331, 1997.

Deitch EA, Rutan RI: The challenges of children: the first 48 hours, *J Burn Care Rehabil* 21(5):424, quiz 431, discussion 423, 2000.

Delatte SJ et al: Effectiveness of beta-glucan collagen for treatment of partial-thickness burns in children, *J Pediatr Surg* 36(1):113, 2001.

Demling RH: Comparison of the anabolic effects and complications of human growth hormone and the testosterone analog, oxandrolone, after severe burn injury, *Burns* 25(3):215, 1999.

Doctor M: Abuse through burns. In Carrougher GJ, editor: *Burn care and therapy,* St. Louis, 1998, Mosby.

Ehde DM et al: Post-traumatic stress symptoms and distress 1 year after burn injury, *J Burn Care Rehabil* 21(2):105, 2000.

Engrav LH et al: Hypertrophic scar, wound contraction and hyper-hypopigmentation, *J Burn Care Rehabil* 28(4):593-596, 2007.

Evans J et al: Your patients may be at risk: preventing pediatric burn injuries, *J SC Med Assoc* 102:17-18, 2006.

Franz MG et al: Guidelines to aid healing of acute wounds by decreasing impediments of healing, *Wound Repair Regen* 16(6):723-748, 2008.

Gibran NS, Heimbach DM: Current status of burn wound pathophysiology, *Clin Plast Surg* 27(1):11, 2000.

Gibran NS et al: Cutaneous wound healing, *J Burn Care Rehabil* 28(4):577-579, 2007.

Gottschlich MM et al: The 2002 Clinical Research Award. An evaluation of the safety of early vs delayed enteral support and effects on clinical, nutritional, and endocrine outcomes after severe burns, *J Burn Care Rehabil* 23(6):401, 2002.

Graves MS et al: Actual burn nutrition care practices: an update, *J Burn Care Rehabil* 30(1):77-82, 2009.

Greenfield E, McManus AT: Infectious complications: prevention and strategies for their control, *Nurs Clin North Am* 32(2):297, 1997.

Hansbrough JF et al: Clinical trials of a biosynthetic temporary skin replacement, Dermagraft-transitional covering, compared with cryopreserved human cadaver skin for temporary coverage of excised burn wounds, *J Burn Care Rehabil* 18(1 Pt 1):43, 1997.

Helvig EI: Pediatric burn injuries, *AACN Clin Issues* 4(2):433, 1993.

Honari S: Topical therapies and antimicrobials in the management of burn wounds, *Crit Care Nurs Clin North Am* 16(1):1, 2004.

Hunt JP et al: Occupation-related burn injuries, *J Burn Care Rehabil* 21(4):327, 2000.

Jackson D: The diagnosis of the depth of burning, *J Br Surg* 40:588, 1953.

Jordan BS, Harrington DT: Management of the burn wound, *Nurs Clin North Am* 32(2):251, 1997.

Karter MJ: *Fire loss in the United States 2008,* Quincy, Mass, 2009 (rev. Jan 2010), National Fire Protection Association.

Leman CJ, Ricks N: Discharge planning and follow-up burn care. In Richard RL, Staley MJ, editors: *Burn care and rehabilitation principles and practice,* Philadelphia, 1994, FA Davis.

Lim JJ et al: Rapid response: care of burn victims, *AAOHN J,* 46(4):169-178, quiz 179-180, 1998.

Lowell G et al: Preventing unintentional scald burns: moving beyond tap water, *Pediatrics* 122(4):799-804, 2008.

Luce EA: Electrical burns, *Clin Plast Surg* 27(1):133, 2000.

Mafong EA, Ashinoff R: Treatment of hypertrophic scars and keloids: a review, *Aesthet Surg J* 20(2):114, 2000.

Maggi SP et al: The efficacy of 5% Sulfamylon solution for the treatment of contaminated explanted human meshed skin grafts, *Burns* 25(3):237, 1999.

Mangus RS et al: Burn injuries in children with attention deficit/hyperactivity disorder, *Burns:*30:148-150, 2004.

Matheson JD et al: The reduction of itch during burn wound healing, *J Burn Care Rehabil* 22(1):76, discussion 75, 2001.

McDonald WS et al: Immediate enteral feeding in burn patients is safe and effective, *Ann Surg* 213:177, 1991.

McManus WF Jr: Thermal injuries. In Feliciano D, Moore EE, Mattox KL, editors: *Trauma,* Stamford, Conn, 1996, Appleton & Lange.

Mertens DM et al: Outpatient burn management, *Nurs Clin North Am* 32(2):343, 1997.

Monafo WW: Physiology of pain, *J Burn Care Rehabil* 16(3 Pt 2):345, 1995.

Monafo WW: Initial management of burns, *N Engl J Med* 335(21):1581, 1996.

Moss LS: Outpatient management of the burn patient, *Crit Care Nurs Clin North Am* 16(1):109, 2004.

Mozingo DW: Surgical management. In Carrougher GJ, editor: *Burn care and therapy,* St. Louis, 1998, Mosby.

Palmieri TL: Inhalation injury: research progress and needs, *J Burn Care Rehabil* 28(4):549-554, 2007.

Patel PP et al: Topical antimicrobials in pediatric burn wound management, *J Craniofac Surg* 19(4):913-922, 2008.

Paul CN: Skin substitutes in burn care, *Wounds* 20(7):203-205, 2008.

Peck MD et al: Invited critique: national study of emergency department visits for burn injures, 1993-2004, *J Burn Care Rehabil* 28(5):691-693, 2007.

Pham TN et al: American Burn Association practice guidelines burn shock resuscitation, *J Burn Care Rehabil* 29(1):257-266, 2008.

Prien T, Traber DL: Toxic smoke compounds and inhalation injury—a review, *Burns Incl Therm Inj* 14:451-460, 1988.

Pruitt BA Jr: The evolutionary development of biologic dressings and skin substitutes, *J Burn Care Rehabil* 18(1 Pt 2):S2, 1997.

Raff T et al: The value of early enteral nutrition in the prophylaxis of stress ulceration in the severely burned patient, *Burns* 23(4):313, 1997a.

Raff T et al: Early intragastric feeding of seriously burned and long-term ventilated patients: a review of 55 patients, *Burns* 23(1):19, 1997b.

Redlick F et al: A survey of risk factors for burns in the elderly and prevention strategies, *J Burn Care Rehabil* 23(5):351; discussion 341, 2002.

Rutan RL: Physiologic response to cutaneous burn injury. In Carrougher GJ, editor: *Burn care and therapy,* St. Louis, 1998, Mosby.

Rutan TC: Discharge planning. In Carrougher GJ, editor: *Burn care and therapy,* St. Louis, 1998, Mosby.

Ruth GD et al: Outcomes related to burn-related child abuse: a case series, *J Burn Care Rehabil* 24(5):318, discussion 317, 2003.

Sabeston DC Jr, editor: *Textbook of surgery: the biographical basis of modern surgical practice,* ed 11, Philadelphia, 1977, WB Saunders.

Schneider JC et al: Contractures in burn injury: defining the problem, *J Burn Care Rehabil* 27(4):508-514, 2006.

Sheridan RL: Burns, *Crit Care Med* 30(11 Suppl):S500, 2002.

Sheridan RL: Burns at the extremes of age, *J Burn Care Rehabil* 28(4):580-585, 2007.

Sicoutris CP, Holmes JH: Fire and smoke injuries, *Crit Care Nurs Clin North Am* 18(3):403-417, xi, 2006.

Stoddard FJ et al: Acute stress symptoms in young children with burns, *J Am Acad Child Adoles Psychiatry* 45:87-93, 2006.

Stone N et al: Child abuse by burning, *Surg Clin North Am* 50:1419-1424, 1970.

Supple KG: Physiologic response to burn injury, *Crit Care Nurs Clin North Am* 16(1):119, 2004.

Tassiopoulos AK: Nutritional support of the patient with severe burn injury, *Nutrition* 15(11-12):956, 1999.

Wibbenmeyer LA et al: Population-based assessment of burn injury in southern Iowa: identification of children and young-adult at-risk groups and behaviors, *J Burn Care Rehabil* 24(4):192, 2003.

Winfree J, Barillo DJ: Burn management. Nonthermal injuries, *Nurs Clin North Am* 32(2):275, 1997.

Reconstructive Surgery

Joyce M. Black and Steven B. Black

Surgical intervention for chronic wounds is seldom the first choice. In general, much local care of the wound has preceded any decision for surgery. However, some chronic wounds deteriorate and require emergent operative management, and some wounds reach a point in the healing trajectory where surgery is indicated to aid wound closure. This chapter addresses the wounds that benefit by operative treatment, decisions about operative care, and care of the patient and the wound before and after surgery.

HISTORY OF SURGERY FOR WOUNDS

Wounds, mostly resulting from trauma, have existed since the beginning of man. The Edwin Smith Papyrus, which was written more than 5,000 years ago, is the oldest known surgical treatise. It contains 142 different references to the management of sores and wounds. Surgical management of wounds is nearly as old. Hippocrates said, "He who wishes to be a surgeon should go to war." His words highlight the relationship of surgical advances and war-related injury. Modern reconstructive surgery had its beginnings with traumatic injury, at a time when the nose was cut off as a form of punishment. In Italy during the sixteenth century, noses were reconstructed using the skin of the inner upper aspect. This flap is known as the Tagliacozzi flap. Modern plastic surgery came into its own during World War II when the sulfa antibiotic allowed many wounded soldiers to survive their injuries, and consequently they required reconstructive surgery. Today, surgery remains an important aspect of wound care, and advances in surgical options continue to be made.

SURGICAL DECISION MAKING

Assessment of the Patient

A comprehensive patient assessment is required to determine the risk-to-benefit ratio and the type of surgical procedure indicated. The patient's condition forms the primary aspect of the risk portion of the risk-to-benefit ratio. Although it is always ideal to have a closed wound, the patient must be able to tolerate anesthesia, surgery, blood loss, and postoperative restrictions. An estimation of anesthetic risk, such as the American Society of Anesthesiologists (ASA) classification, provides an objective measure of relative risk for surgery. The patient must be able to tolerate the pain and immobility following surgery, and the facility must be willing to keep the patient as long as the surgeon deems necessary for safe healing.

Assessment of the Wound

Planning surgery requires an understanding of the wound in terms of causative factors and missing or needed tissue. Information concerning these two issues must guide the selection of the most appropriate surgical option.

Causative Factors. What caused the wound? Is the wound acute or chronic? Acute traumatic wounds may be missing fragments of skin, but with removal of these devitalized tissues and mobilization of surrounding skin, the laceration may be closed primarily. If the wound is chronic, can the factors contributing to the chronic nature of the wound be corrected? The underlying etiology of the wound must be corrected or minimized (e.g., pressure) and cofactors treated (e.g., infection, malnutrition) before healing can ensue. For example, the wound complicated by an ischemic process will require improvement of blood flow in order to heal. Likewise, an ischial pressure ulcer will not heal if the patient continues to sit on the ulcer. Surgical reconstruction of wounds in which the causative factor has not been addressed is not likely to succeed (Franz et al, 2008; WOCN 2010).

Missing/Needed Tissue. When planning surgical reconstruction of a wound, a full understanding of exactly what tissues are missing is needed in order to reconstruct the area for restoration of both form and function. If a wound lacks only skin, replacing the skin (skin graft) may be a reasonable option, provided other patient conditions are well managed. However, simply putting skin on a wound without controlling infection, ischemia, or pressure is a doomed enterprise. Frequently, tissue padding (e.g., subcutaneous tissue and muscle) is needed to protect a bony prominence from recurrent breakdown, so a flap containing these elements would be necessary.

SELECTION OF WOUND CLOSURE METHOD

Selecting a method of closure depends on a holistic assessment that considers the needs and goals of the patient. A common set of decision-making steps (e.g., the reconstructive ladder) serves as a guide for plastic and reconstructive surgery (Figure 33-1). The simplest method that accomplishes the patient's goals usually is the first choice. In addition to the complexity of the surgery, consideration is given to the morbidity that would be created for the donor site. For example, if a person lost a thumb, transplantation of the great toe to replace the thumb would be considered; however, the thumb would not be used to replace a great toe.

When considering donor site morbidity for pressure ulcer surgery, it is important to keep in mind that tissues usually can be moved or donated only once. Therefore, the choice of which tissue to use is important. Surgeons try to select donor areas that will not interfere with future potential flap donor sites, especially in patients with paraplegia or quadriplegia because this patient population often requires more than one operation during their lifetime. Large wounds of the entire perineum in patients with paralysis may require removal of the leg and filleting of the tissues to form an adequately sized flap of muscle and skin that will sufficiently close the wound. This situation is a dramatic example of donor site morbidity.

Surgical wound closure can be achieved using a number of techniques, such as linear closure, secondary healing, skin grafts, skin substitutes, and tissue flaps. Many factors are considered when determining the optimum wound closure technique. When little tissue is missing, the skin is sufficiently pliable and the wound is considered to be clean, a linear closure (i.e., approximating the wound edges and securing with suture) is a reasonable choice.

Secondary healing (i.e., letting a wound heal by scar tissue formation) is the simplest method of healing and a logical selection for a clean Stage II pressure ulcer. The ongoing risk of infection in the deeper open wound, however, may prompt a decision for surgical closure to speed healing. Similarly, some partial-thickness wounds (e.g., burn on the hand) create significant morbidity due to the contractile scars that form during healing. In these situations, skin grafting would be warranted to close the wound.

Skin grafts (i.e., sections of intact epidermis and upper layer of the dermis) can be removed from the patient's donor site and transferred to cover shallow, vascularized wounds. Split-thickness skin grafts can be placed as entire pieces of skin or meshed to promote drainage of wound exudate and contouring to the skin surface. Skin grafts also can be full thickness, but only where vascularity in the donor site is sufficient to heal full-thickness grafts.

Skin grafts provide superficial coverage but do not replace deeper tissue layers, such as subcutaneous tissue and muscle; thus they are unable to provide the padding needed to protect bony prominences from recurrent breakdown. Therefore, skin grafts are rarely, if ever, used in the surgical management of pressure ulcers, except to close donor sites from flaps containing multiple layers of tissue. Skin grafts are commonly used to manage burn wounds and are described in greater detail in Chapter 32. Skin grafts have also been used in the management of venous ulcers (Robson et al, 2006).

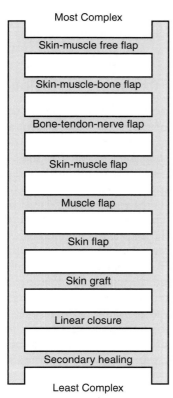

Most Complex

- Skin-muscle free flap
- Skin-muscle-bone flap
- Bone-tendon-nerve flap
- Skin-muscle flap
- Muscle flap
- Skin flap
- Skin graft
- Linear closure
- Secondary healing

Least Complex

FIGURE 33-1 Reconstructive ladder.

Skin substitutes can be used to close a wound. The skin substitute can be epidermis only, dermis only, or both. Epidermal skin substitutes are composed of keratinocytes, take 2 to 3 weeks to "grow," and are generally used when the patient does not have sufficient healthy skin graft donor sites available. Dermal substitutes are composed of fibroblasts embedded in a "matrix" material that provides a scaffolding for cellular and capillaries migration. Epidermal replacements and extracellular matrix scaffolds are discussed in Chapter 19.

Tissue Flaps

Tissue flaps involve the transfer of skin and underlying structures (e.g., subcutaneous tissue, fascia, muscle) to fill and pad a defect that will resist pressure once healed. Flaps differ from skin grafts in that they carry their own blood supply with them. The native nutrient vessels are moved along with the flap or are reestablished (microsurgery) once the flap is transferred. Maintaining this blood supply is a crucial aspect of flap survival. Tissue flaps are either local or distant (free).

Local flaps are most commonly used for pressure ulcers (WOCN, 2010). They are categorized by the anatomic structures they encompass, the method used to move the flap, or the method used to perfuse the flap (Box 33-1).

Anatomic Structures. Skin flaps are portions of skin moved from their usual location to cover a defect. Skin flaps are generally not used for pressure ulcer repair because they do not have enough padding or blood supply (provided by underlying muscle) to sustain pressure once the patient is sitting again.

Fasciocutaneous flaps include portions of the epidermis, dermis, and subcutaneous tissue supported by the underlying fascia. Fasciocutaneous flaps do provide padding and superficial coverage.

Myocutaneous (also called musculocutaneous) flaps involve rotation of all soft tissue layers (skin, subcutaneous tissue, fascia, muscle). These flaps provide optimal coverage for bony prominences and therefore are frequently used in the surgical reconstruction of

pressure ulcers and other full-thickness wounds. Myocutaneous flaps carry along with them the native arterial and venous blood supplies to the muscle and the overlying skin. Because these flaps must survive on their original blood flow, they have limited reach. When the flaps are pulled or stretched beyond their limits, the blood vessels also are stretched and are not able to perfuse the flaps. Therefore postoperative monitoring of arterial inflow and venous outflow are important for flap survival.

The area of potential reach for each muscle flap is now known. For example, the biceps femoris muscle (one of the lateral hamstring muscles) is supplied with blood via arteries from the profunda femoris. The flap has an arc of rotation that can cover defects of the ischium and groin.

Methods Used to Move the Flap

Flaps can be classified according to the surgical technique used to transport them to the recipient site as advancement flaps and rotation flaps. *Advancement* flaps involve elevation of the tissue to be transferred, undermining of the wound edges, and advancement of the tissue into the defect. Advancement flaps are useful in areas with significant redundant skin that can stretch. *Rotation* flaps are used to fill defects adjacent to the donor tissue. A flap is outlined on three sides, the tissue is elevated, and the flap is rotated into the defect. The donor site may be closed surgically or may require a split-thickness skin graft for closure. *Transposition* flaps are rotation flaps that are moved across normal skin to fill a defect (as opposed to being directly adjacent to the defect).

Methods of Retaining Perfusion

The perfusion of the flap is important in the design of the flap. All flaps of tissue carry with them a blood supply (unlike a skin graft). *Random flaps* depend on the dermal and subdermal vessels for their blood supply. Because these vessels are small, the blood supply to these flaps is tenuous. *Axial flaps* are designed to include an artery, which increases vascularity and the chances for flap survival. These vessels nourish the flap until new collateral capillary systems are established between the flap and the wound bed. Common axial flaps include the pectoralis flap to reconstruct the neck following radical neck surgery and the tensor fascia lata flap used to close ischial pressure ulcers. When tissue is not available locally, it can sometimes be brought in using a free flap. This type of operation is performed less commonly because it requires microvascular surgical techniques. In this approach, the donor tissue along with its blood supply is completely removed from the donor site and transferred to the recipient site. The artery and vein that supply the flap are attached by microvascular techniques

---

BOX 33-1	Categories of Surgical Tissue Flaps

Local flaps
    Classified by anatomic structures:
- Skin flap
- Fasciocutaneous
- Myocutaneous or musculocutaneous flap

    Classified by method used to move flap:
- Advancement flap
- Rotation flap
- Transposition flap

    Classified by methods of retaining perfusion:
- Random flap
- Axial flap

Distant (free) flaps

to vessels near the wound. These types of flaps can be used to repair wounds of the head and neck, breast, or lower third of the leg. For example, recalcitrant venous ulcers with severe lipodermatosclerosis may benefit from free flap transfer by allowing wide excision of diseased tissue and replacing it with healthy tissue with its own microvasculature and uninjured venous valves (Robson et al, 2006).

Tissue Expansion

An additional surgical option for wound closure is tissue expansion to stretch tissue, including skin near the wound, which then can be moved into the wound bed. Silicone expanders, or hollow pouches, are placed surgically into the subcutaneous or submuscular tissue layer in an area adjacent to the defect. Sterile fluid is injected into the expander at routine intervals until the pouch is fully expanded. This process induces expansion of the overlying tissue layers. When there is sufficient tissue to provide coverage of the defect, the expander is removed and the wound is closed. The stretched tissue then can be closed primarily or moved to cover the defect. For example, a scalp wound with alopecia may be treated with tissue expanders placed alongside the bare area to expand the hair-bearing scalp. Once fully expanded, the bare area is excised and the expanded hair-bearing tissue moved to cover the defect.

NONOPERATIVE CONDITIONS

Although it is important to know how to perform any given operation, it is equally important to know when not to operate. This discussion centers on the most common problems that rule out the use of surgical intervention; other conditions also may exist.

A pressure ulcer in a malnourished patient should not be repaired until the underlying malnutrition is controlled and the patient is anabolic again (WOCN, 2010). If malnutrition is a volitional decision, then surgery should not be an option. If the pressure ulcer did not heal due to malnutrition, then the surgical wound will not heal for the same reason. A typical flap doubles or triples the surface area of the wound the body must heal (the donor site wound also must heal now).

Recalcitrant venous insufficiency ulcers require a bed of well-oxygenated granulation tissue to nourish a skin graft. If the edema cannot be controlled or the patient is unable to wear an external compression device, a skin graft will not survive.

Calciphylaxis is due to ischemia in the skin from vascular calcification. It is most commonly seen in patients with renal failure, hypercalcemia, and hyperphosphatemia. Lesions usually develop on the legs and begin as areas of mottled skin that progress into painful, firm areas of necrosis. Surgery, if considered, usually consists of debridement of the lesion to prevent sepsis.

However, until the underlying problems are controlled, the wounds often reappear.

Stable eschar on the heel frequently presents a nonoperative condition. Stable eschar is dry, hard, and firmly attached to the underlying skin; indications of an infection (induration, erythema, pain) are absent. Stable eschar on the heels should be left intact, not debrided and not softened. Slowly, the eschar will release at the edges as the underlying tissue heals while the eschar forms a barrier to protect underlying relatively ischemic tendon and bone. The loose eschar then can be trimmed. Moistening or softening the eschar encourages invasion of bacteria. Removal of the eschar exposes the fat pad, which can desiccate and expose the calcaneus.

Operative closure of the ischemic wound is contraindicated. Performing debridements on lower extremity ischemic wounds often will make the wound larger with little hope of healing. Unless arterial inflow can be reestablished, the wound is best left alone. Local wound care for ischemic wounds, such as arterial wounds, includes protection and coverage with dressing material that is easily removed.

Inability to adhere to postoperative care requirements can be a significant deterrent to healing of a surgical wound. If the patient cannot remain off the flap, consume adequate calories, and control fecal and/or urinary contamination of the incision, the skin graft or flap likely will fail. It is important to keep in mind that only a given number of flap options can be used in a lifetime. Once a muscle is used, it cannot be used again. Therefore the decision to operate should be made only after the patient is adequately educated regarding the interventions necessary postoperatively to reduce complications and prevent recurrence. A recent review of 227 flaps to close ischial pressure ulcers reported 88 recurrences (39%). Recurrence was highest in patients who were younger than 45 years, had low albumin and elevated hemoglobin A1C (Keys, et al, 2010).

URGENT OPERATIVE CONDITIONS

Traumatic Wounds

Patients with traumatic wounds must undergo a thorough assessment to be certain they do not have major vessel, nerve, or tendon injury; therefore the examination must be completed before the administration of local anesthetics. The wound is closed primarily when possible, without creating donor site morbidity, for example, pulling the lower eyelid down and exposing the eye because the lid cannot close. Facial wounds require small sutures to avoid excess scar formation. The timing of suture removal is dependent on the anatomic location. For example, sutures on the face are generally removed sooner than sutures on the lower leg or buttocks. Linear wound closure as well as suture removal method, timing, and technique are described in Chapter 34.

When patients are severely injured, their wound issues may come second priority to tending to airway, breathing, and circulation. Clean wounds should be dressed with normal saline gauze and, if possible, closed within 12 to 24 hours. After that time, they are considered contaminated. Operative closure should be a delayed primary closure, or the wound should be allowed to heal secondarily, with scar revision at a later date. Chapter 31 further discusses the care of patients with traumatic wounds.

Abscess

An abscess is a local collection of pus and sometimes blood. Abscesses are incised and drained. The remaining cavity may require packing to prevent healing from occurring at the surface before healing occurs in the deeper tissues.

Gangrene

Wet gangrene develops from a sudden interruption in blood supply, as occurs with burns, freezing, hematoma, or injury that becomes infected, or from primary infection of tissues from certain bacteria. Wet gangrene from any organism can quickly spread into surrounding tissues as a result of the bacteria and destroy muscle and other tissues. The patient has pain and fever. The tissue becomes discolored, blistered, and boggy and may have crepitus if the wound is infected with gas-forming organisms such as *Clostridium perfringens* (formerly known as *Clostridium welchii*). Frequently no line of demarcation exists between normal and infected tissue. Anaerobic infections can develop into gas gangrene within 1 to 2 days, and if the patient develops bacteremia, the mortality rate is 20% to 25%. If the gangrene is recognized and treated early and aggressively, nearly 80% of patients will survive (Laor et al, 1995). Surgery for wet gangrene includes radical removal of infected tissues or amputation. Hyperbaric oxygen therapy may also be used. Spreading gangrene is a surgical emergency. The wounds from these operations can be large and deep, with extensive areas of tissue loss.

In contrast, *dry* gangrene develops slowly from progressive loss of arterial supply, commonly in the extremities. A coagulative necrosis develops, and the tissue becomes black, dry, scaly, and greasy. A clear line of demarcation exists between viable and gangrenous tissue. The body will slowly slough the gangrenous tissue at the line of demarcation. Surgery may not be needed unless the area becomes infected. Although the gangrene is not painful at this stage, it likely was painful earlier in the process because of ischemia, and adjacent compromised tissue may exhibit ischemic pain. Dry gangrene should be covered with dry dressings and the tissue not moistened to prevent conversion to wet gangrene. An area of dry gangrene should never be soaked.

Necrotizing Fasciitis

Necrotizing fasciitis is a rapidly spreading, inflammatory infection of the deep fascia, with secondary necrosis of the subcutaneous tissues. The causative bacteria may be aerobic or anaerobic. Frequently, the cause is two synergistic bacteria that thrive in the hypoxic tissues. Because of the common presence of gas-forming organisms, subcutaneous air is classically described in necrotizing fasciitis. Pain out of proportion to the physical findings is a hallmark sign. The infection spreads along the fascial plane. These infections can be difficult to recognize in their early stages, but they rapidly progress to septic shock and organ failure. Emergency aggressive surgical debridement is required to remove all the necrotic tissue. Empiric broad-spectrum intravenous antibiotics are used until culture findings are known; however, the shock does not improve until the involved tissue is debrided.

Hyperbaric oxygen is an important adjunct to treatment where available. Efem (1993) conducted a randomized clinical trial comparing customary treatment of Fournier gangrene (a form of necrotizing fasciitis) to topical dressings with honey. Forty-one consecutive cases of gangrene were randomly assigned to wound debridement or daily application of honey. Wounds treated with honey had less odor, edema, and drainage. No deaths occurred in the group treated with honey; their hospital stay was one-half week longer. Manuka honey contains antimicrobial properties, and its use in wound care is of increasing interest.

PREOPERATIVE MANAGEMENT

Reducing Cofactors

When the care team has the luxury of time, improving the patient's underlying condition will improve surgical wound healing (Franz et al, 2008). Many comorbid conditions can delay healing of both chronic and acute surgical wounds. Some of the most common conditions that require correction in this patient population (perfusion, oxygenation, bioburden, corticosteroids, diabetes, malnutrition, nicotine) are discussed in detail within chapters throughout this text. Fecal and urinary diversions are rarely needed to obtain a healed wound. Use of a bowel program or catheterization can divert urine and fecal material without the need for additional surgery (Whitney et al, 2006).

Spasms and Contractures. Patients with paraplegia, quadriplegia, or other neurologic diseases have spasms that can lead to friction damage or traction on the incision, which can cause dehiscence. Spasms and fixed contractures also may limit postoperative positioning and leave patients at risk for development of new pressure ulcers. Management of muscle spasm and contractures should begin preoperatively and continue until the wound is completely healed (Whitney et al, 2006).

Social Support. Closure of pressure ulcers with flaps is technically possible in many cases. However, maintaining a closed wound is difficult unless the patient has a social network that can encourage adherence to postoperative restrictions and promote a lifetime of self care (National Pressure Ulcer Advisory Panel [NPUAP] and European Pressure Ulcer Advisory Panel [EPUAP], 2009). A retrospective review by Schryvers et al (2000) of 168 patients with pressure ulcers revealed that the majority of patients were paraplegic, unemployed men who had a low level of education. Most lived alone or with family but were independent in self-care. They concluded that securing a safe home for placement following rehabilitation is crucial to the outcome. Therefore the ability of the individual to return home safely should be known prior to surgery. Kierney et al (1998) achieved a very low 19% ulcer recurrence rate by combining efforts of plastic surgery and physical medicine. In their experience, social service assistance is provided to each individual. The individual's wheelchair, wheelchair cushion, and other mechanical devices are assessed prior to surgery.

Wound Bed Preparation

Successful closure of any wound requires a clean, perfusing wound bed. Excisional debridement helps prepare the wound bed that is likely to heal either by acute wound healing methods or by attachment of surgically transferred tissues. A recurring criticism of sharp and surgical debridement is that it is nonselective so that viable as well as nonviable tissue are removed. Although this statement is true from a broad-brush perspective, most surgical debridements are done until the wound bed is clean and bleeding. Even though some layers of viable tissue may be sacrificed, there is a greater likelihood of removing all nonviable tissue, senescent cells, and avascular biofilm protective to bacteria (see Chapter 16). Newer debridement instruments can actually debride in thin layers less than 1 mm thick. Techniques for wound debridement are discussed in Chapter 17.

Although the exact mechanism of action is unproven, it appears that negative pressure applied to the wound bed reduces surrounding tissue edema allowing new, enriched blood to flow into the wound. The pull on the tissues also stimulates granulation tissue growth allowing definitive closure to occur earlier than usual. The removal of wound exudate reduces the colonization on the wound surface. Negative pressure wound therapy (NPWT) is especially useful for accelerating the process of wound bed preparation for flaps, treating dehisced wounds, and preparing wounds for delayed linear closure (Fife et al, 2004; Robson et al, 2006).

OPERATIVE MANAGEMENT

International pressure ulcer guidelines recommend surgical consultation for operative repair in individuals with Stage III or IV pressure ulcers that are not closing with conservative treatment and for individuals who desire more rapid closure of the ulcer (NPUAP-EPUAP, 2009). Pressure ulcer excision and closure are commonly completed with patients under general anesthesia, even in those with paralysis, to reduce spastic and reflexic muscle movement as well as to control their vasomotor instability. Blood loss is anticipated, and patients should have blood typed and cross-matched for intraoperative administration.

Sacral Ulcers

The sacrum is the most common location for pressure ulcers. Large skin defects in the sacral area are not uncommon and can be associated with even larger areas of undermining. Fortunately, these ulcers rarely are deep. Ostectomy of the sacral prominence is necessary if bone is infected. Coverage is most commonly obtained with a large myocutaneous or fasciocutaneous flap (Figure 33-2).

Greater Trochanteric Ulcers

Ulcers on the greater trochanter are seen in patients, many of whom have severe contractures and can only lie on their sides. The tensor fasciae latae myocutaneous flap is the workhorse of ulcer covering in this region. It is most commonly designed as a transposition flap with a large resultant dog-ear (Figure 33-3). V-Y advancement (see following section on ischial ulcers for description of V-Y flap) and rotation of the tensor fasciae latae flap often give an excellent functional and better esthetic result. Other flaps include the rectus femoris myocutaneous flap and random bipedicle or unipedicle fasciocutaneous flaps.

Ischial Ulcers

Ischial ulcers occur from prolonged erect sitting without changes in position and are most common in patients with lower limb paralysis. Usually a small skin wound with a large cavity beneath the surface is present. The ischial tuberosity is the pressure point and is always involved. Ischial ostectomy is avoided if the bone is not infected because this procedure distributes the body weight is distributed onto the perineum, and the resulting ulcers are very difficult to manage.

Many options for flaps to cover ischial ulcers exist, including the tensor fascia latae (see Figure 33-3). The hamstring V-Y myocutaneous flap can be used for patients with recurrent ulcerations in extremely large defects. This flap is particularly valuable for layer defects because thorough dissection yields 10 to 12 cm of

FIGURE 33-2 Sacral ulcers can be closed with a gluteus maximus myocutaneous flap. **A,** Gluteus muscle is identified using landmarks (indicated by X) of the ischial tuberosity and the posterior iliac spine. **B,** Small segment of the muscle is rotated into the wound and is fed by the superior gluteal artery. **C,** Muscle is divided and moved into the wound. The wound is closed primarily with a long incision to avoid tension. (From Cohen S: Pressure sores. In McCarthy J, editor: *Plastic surgery,* Philadelphia, 1990, WB Saunders.)

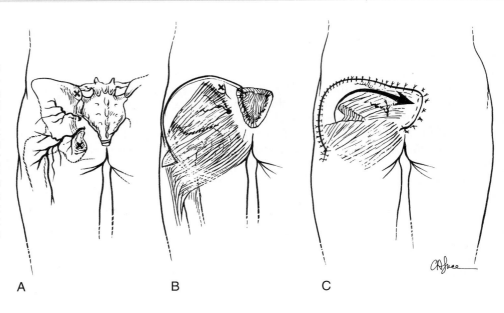

A   B   C

FIGURE 33-3 Ischial and trochanteric ulcers can be closed using a tensor fascia latae flap. **A,** Muscle is found on the lateral thigh and fed by the femoral circumflex artery, which enters at the superior anterior iliac spine. **B,** Advantage of the flap is the long muscle and skin cover. **C,** Arc of rotation can provide coverage for both ischial and trochanteric ulcers. (From Cohen S: Pressure sores. In McCarthy J, editor: *Plastic surgery,* Philadelphia, 1990, WB Saunders.)

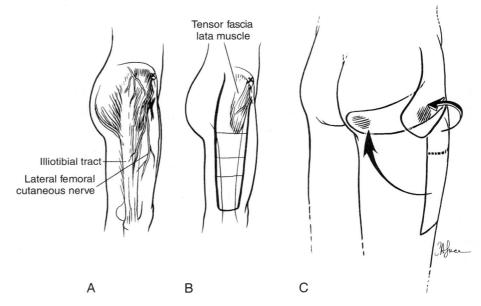

A   B   C

advancement. It is called a *V-Y flap* because the flap is raised with V-shaped incisions and then closed as a Y. This flap is well vascularized by segmental perforators from the hamstrings originating from the deep femoral artery. However, because the origins and insertions of the muscles are severed, this flap cannot be used in an ambulatory patient. Additional myocutaneous flaps for ischial ulcer closure include the rectus abdominis flap and the gracilis flap.

The gluteus maximus muscle flap offers a large amount of well-vascularized tissue with which to fill the defect. Even in the patient with a spinal cord injury, significant muscle mass still exists. Skin closure of the donor site can be obtained by linear closure in some cases or by a separate, inferiorly based fasciocutaneous rotation flap.

Ischial ulcers in paralyzed patients are difficult wounds. The recurrence of ulcers in this population can be high. The acute surgical wound can be delayed in healing and the psychosocial components in the patient can lead to recurrence. Krause and Broderick (2004) reported that the odds of having a recurrent pressure ulcer were reduced with a healthy lifestyle, being employed, and having a positive social network.

Multiple Pressure Ulcers

Extensive ulcerations of the sacrum, trochanters, and ischium are not uncommon, particularly in paralyzed patients. Amputation of a lower limb and use of the skin and muscle from the thigh, called a *total thigh flap,* has sometimes been necessary to provide enough tissue to close these extensive multiple wounds. Before surgery, urologic evaluation is completed because of the frequency of urinary infection. Urinary diversion may be required. Fecal diversion (temporary colostomy) also may be necessary. Common complications after surgery include hemorrhage and infection. Prolonged immobilization on special pressure redistribution beds is needed postoperatively, or these flaps will fail.

POSTOPERATIVE MANAGEMENT

Skin Grafts

Survival of skin grafts depends on revascularization of the grafted skin. Initially the skin survives because of the plasma on the wound surface. Within 72 hours, new vessels should traverse the graft and change it to a pink color. The change in color of the grafted skin signifies what is called a *take* and often is expressed as a percentage of take or adherence to the wound bed that occurs through the ingrowth of new capillaries and fibrin bands. For example, a split-thickness skin graft is reported to have a 90% take after 72 hours when the first dressing is changed.

The two factors most commonly associated with skin graft failure are (1) failure to adequately immobilize the graft, which is critical to revascularization, and (2) infection. One of the most common clinical problems after lower extremity skin grafting is failure to prevent edema in the wound bed. The patient must keep the skin graft site elevated for at least 72 hours. All too often, the patient tries to get to the bathroom quickly or to sit briefly on the edge of the bed, and the grafted site becomes engorged with blood despite stented dressings and wraps. Clear instructions are imperative.

NPWT is sometimes used over skin grafts to promote adherence. Although the actual mechanism of action is not known, it is likely that NPWT immobilizes the graft and reduces edema in the wound bed. The graft must be meshed for NPWT to be effective. The NPWT sponge cannot be placed directly on the graft, so fine mesh gauze usually is placed directly on the graft site. Constant suction must be applied for 72 hours. If NPWT fails to function, the surgeon should be notified before the vacuum on the device is reestablished.

Once the graft has taken, the site is dry and prone to pruritus, dermatitis, or folliculitis. These conditions occur because sweat and oil glands are located in the deep dermis and are not transferred with partial-thickness skin grafts. Patients must be taught to develop lifelong strategies to protect and moisturize the skin.

The donor site for the split-thickness skin graft is a partial-thickness wound, which heals by reepithelialization. Donor sites require protection for healing. Usual covers for donor sites include transparent films, fine mesh gauze, Xeroform, and an ointment containing castor oil, balsam of Peru, and trypsin. A small study of 36 patients showed that the ointment led to healing in an average of 11 days (Carson et al, 2003). In 1998, a review of healing rates, infection rates, and pain levels found that transparent film was the most efficacious cover for donor sites, leading to healing in an average of 9.47 days (Rakel et al, 1998).

Flaps

After flap surgery the patient is placed on a specialty bed that provides pressure redistribution and eliminates shear (e.g., low air-loss bed or air-fluidized bed). A minimum requirement is 10 days on a specialty bed; however, the time a patient is on the specialty bed varies by surgeon and the take of the flap. There are few studies examining the outcomes of one bed to another following flap surgery (Finnegan et al, 2008). Taking the patient off the bed or having the patient sit too early are common causes of flap injury or failure. The flap should not be pulled while the patient is being turned or is being slid to the edge of the bed because the edges of the flap can be pulled apart. Therefore, the use of turning sheets is imperative. Closed suction drainage devices are used in the wound and undermined areas until drainage is minimal to reduce the risk of hematoma and infection.

Mobility and exposure to pressure are gradually increased, beginning 3 to 5 weeks after the procedure, with careful monitoring of skin and suture lines (Ahluwalia, et al, 2010; Keys, et al, 2010). Padding for the seating surface (chair or wheelchair) should be provided after surgery to reduce the risk of ischemia. If the patient is wheelchair dependent, the seat cushion should be assessed before use. Inadequate pressure redistribution might have been the cause of the ulceration and will recur if the seat cushion is not revised or replaced. The patient should be reeducated on methods for reducing skin pressure and for monitoring skin daily for early signs of breakdown. Methods used by paraplegics to transfer from bed to chair (e.g., slide boards) should be discouraged until the flap is fully healed.

Complications include flap necrosis due to spasm or stretch of the feeding blood vessels to the flap. The tissue appears pale and is cool or cold. Assessment of the vascular status of a flap can be improved by having two nurses examine the flap together at shift change to establish a baseline appearance.

Separation of the suture line can occur. Suture line tension often is aggravated by moving or pulling forces. Seldom is surgery performed to close the dehisced area; most often the open area is allowed to heal secondarily.

The most common complication is recurrence of the ulcer. Early recurrences are due to mobilizing the patient too much and too early, which frequently is done in an effort to reduce hospital length of stay. Late recurrences are often due to failure to change the previous lifestyle behaviors that caused the first ulcer. Support, equipment, and educational needs must be addressed and in place before patient discharge to facilitate adaptation (see Chapter 29) and prevent reoccurrence. Flaps are not as resilient as native tissue, and periods of time sitting on the flaps must be limited in duration for the patient's lifetime. Remember that only a few flap sites are available for reconstruction of any given area; once they are all used, the prognosis is grim.

SUMMARY

Many surgical wound closure techniques are available. However, surgical closure of wounds is not a panacea and is not appropriate for all wounds or all patients. The success of surgical wound closures is contingent upon management of several issues, such as the causative factors of the wound, the type of tissue missing and needed, the patient's general physiologic condition, the type of wound closure technique selected, preoperative nutritional status, postoperative care, and lifestyle behaviors.

REFERENCES

Ahluwalia R et al: The operative treatment of pressure wounds: a 10 year experience in flap selection, *International Wound Journal* 7(2):103-106, 2010.

Carson SN et al: Using a castor oil-balsam of Peru-trypsin ointment to assist in healing skin graft donor sites, *Ostomy Wound Manage* 49(6):60, 2003.

Cohen S: Pressure sores. In McCarthy J, editor: *Plastic surgery,* Philadelphia, 1990, WB Saunders.

Efem SEE: Recent advances in the management of Fournier's gangrene: preliminary observations, *Surgery* 13(2):200-204, 1993.

Fife CE et al: Healing dehisced surgical wounds with negative pressure wound therapy, *Ostomy Wound Manage* 50(4A):28, 2004.

Finnegan M et al: Comparing the effectiveness of a specialized alternating air pressure mattress replacement system and an air-fluidized integrated bed in the management of post-operative flap patients: a randomized control pilot study, *J Tissue Viability* 17(1):2-9, 2008.

Franz, M et al: Guidelines to aid healing of acute wounds by decreasing impediments of healing, *Wound Repair Regen* 16:723-748, 2008.

Keys, K. et al: Multivariate predictors of failure after flap coverage of pressure ulcers. *Plastic and Reconstructive Surgery* 125; 1725-1734, 2010

Kierney PC et al: Results of 268 pressure sores in 158 patients managed jointly by plastic surgery and rehabilitation medicine, *Plast Reconstr Surg* 102(3):765-772, 1998.

Krause J, Broderick L: Patterns of recurrent pressure ulcers after spinal cord injury: identification of risk and protective factors 5 years or more after onset, *Arch Phys Med Rehabil* 85(8):1257-1264, 2004.

Laor E et al: Outcome prediction in patients with Fournier's gangrene, *J Urol* 154(1):89-92, 1995.

National Pressure Ulcer Advisory Panel (NPUAP) and European Pressure Ulcer Advisory Panel (EPUAP): *Prevention and treatment of pressure ulcers*, Washington DC, 2009, NPUAP.

Rakel BA et al: Split-thickness skin graft donor site care: a quantitative synthesis of the research, *Appl Nurs Res* 11(4):174, 1998.

Robson MC et al: Guidelines for the treatment of venous ulcers, *Wound Repair Regen* 14(6):649-662, 2006.

Schryvers OI et al: Surgical treatment of pressure ulcers: 20-year experience, *Arch Phys Med Rehab* 81(12):1556-1562, 2000.

Whitney J et al: Guidelines for the treatment of pressure ulcers, *Wound Repair Regen* 14(6):663-679, 2006.

Wound, Ostomy and Continence Nurses (WOCN) Society: *Guideline for prevention and management of pressure ulcers*, Glenview, IL, 2010.

34

Surgical Wounds and Incision Care

JoAnne D. Whitney

OBJECTIVES

1. Discuss current issues related to surgical wound infection and recommendations made by national collaboratives or evidence-based guidelines to address these problems and improve outcomes.
2. Compare intrinsic and extrinsic (modifiable) patient characteristics associated with surgical wound healing complications or infection.
3. Identify wound assessment characteristics comparing the ASEPSIS method of evaluating wounds with Centers for Disease Control and Prevention–defined characteristics for surgical site infection.
4. Identify evidence-based measures for surgical wounds, including dressings, topical treatment, and care of sutures, staples, and tissue adhesives.
5. Discuss three aspects of care or evaluation for patients with surgical wounds and how they can help to promote healing and prevent complications of healing.

Approximately 30 million surgeries are performed each year in the United States (Centers for Disease Control and Prevention [CDC], 2009). Although surgical procedures have become less invasive through the development and use of arthroscopic and laparoscopic techniques, many surgeries still are performed through open incisions. Even the less invasive surgical approaches create an incision and an acute wound requiring a normal physiologic wound healing response (see Chapter 4). Surgical wounds that heal within an expected time frame and without complications are considered acute wounds (Franz et al, 2008). In caring for the patient with a surgical wound, a major goal is preventing complications such as surgical site infection (SSI) and wound healing failure through careful surveillance and interventions. Surveillance is largely accomplished through patient evaluation for risk factors and assessment of the surgical wound for signs of disruption in healing. Interventions are targeted toward reducing modifiable risk factors associated with healing complications, providing systemic and environmental support to facilitate healing to the greatest extent possible. Box 34-1 lists the 11 impediments to surgical wound healing addressed in the guidelines (Franz et al, 2008), many of which are addressed in detail in chapters throughout this text.

SURGICAL WOUND CLOSURE

The goal of wound healing is to reestablish tissue integrity and function with a cosmetically acceptable result and to prevent infection. These are also the goals of wound closure. Surgical wounds are closed primarily or are left open for either delayed primary closure or healing by secondary intention (see Figure 4-2). Primary wound closure is the fastest method for facilitating wound healing (Hollander, 2003). However, wounds with greater than 10^5 bacteria per gram of tissue should not be closed (Franz et al, 2008). In these cases, wounds are often left open and then closed on a delayed schedule, but ideally within a few days, once bacterial load is reduced below critical levels and the wound bed is healthy and can support healing. Primary repair should approximate (Plate 67), but not strangulate, the incision (Franz et al, 2008). Incisions are approximated with sutures, staples, adhesive tapes, and skin adhesives to provide support and stability to tissues until healing has progressed and an acceptable degree of wound tensile tissue strength is reestablished.

Sutures and Staples

Multiple techniques and suture materials are available for closing an incision. National guidelines state that the type of suture material used does not matter, as

---

BOX 34-1	Impediments to Surgical Wound Healing

- Inadequate wound perfusion
- Presence of nonviable tissue
- Wound hematoma or seroma
- Infection or increased tissue bioburden
- Mechanical factors during wound repair
- Systemic immunodeficiencies
- Cancer and cancer treatment factors
- Systemic conditions, diabetes mellitus, obesity, malnutrition
- Burn injuries
- External agents (e.g., tobacco, drugs)
- Excessive scar formation

---

long as the primary repair is anatomic and perfused (Franz et al, 2008). The choice of suture technique depends on the type and anatomic location of the wound, the thickness of the skin, the degree of tension, and the desired cosmetic result. For example, absorbable sutures are used to close tissues deeper than the epidermis and to provide tissue support, relieve skin tension, and reduce wound dead space (Hollander, 2003). Continuous sutures are recommended for closure of laparotomy fascial incisions; however, the type of suture does not affect healing. Current evidence indicates that external or internal retention sutures do not prevent dehiscence and that dehiscence is more likely associated with other factors such as comorbidities (e.g., trauma and wound contamination) (Franz et al, 2008). Staples are commonly used to close the epidermis with acceptable healing and cosmetic result and no increase in infection (Hollander, 2003).

Sutures should be removed within 1 to 2 weeks of their placement, depending on the anatomic location: 3 to 5 days for the face; 7 to 10 days for scalp, chest, fingers, hand, and lower extremity; and 10 to 14 days for the back, forearm, and foot (Hollander, 2003; Wu, 2006). Sutures left in too long can lead to suture marks, local tissue reaction, and scarring. Premature suture removal places the wound at risk for reopening (Hollander, 2003; Wu, 2006). With the appropriate equipment, suture and staple removal is not difficult. The suture should be gently grasped by the knot and elevated slightly with forceps. One side of the suture is cut at skin level. With the forceps still grasping the knot, the suture is gently pulled toward the wound or suture line until the suture material is completely removed (Wilson et al, 2000).

Skin Adhesives

Tissue adhesives and derivatives of cyanoacrylate and other materials that add strength and flexibility have been used for several years for lacerations and other types of wound closure. A Cochrane review of eight randomized trials enrolling 630 patients compared adhesives to suture used for incision closure and identified no differences in rates of dehiscence or infection (Coulthard et al, 2002). The authors also noted that evaluation of adhesives in patients with healing risk factors and for wounds with high tension requires additional study because these subpopulations were excluded from the trials that were reviewed, therefore the comparative effectiveness is not known. Skin adhesives are not recommended for use with complex lacerations having wound edges that are difficult to approximate (Hollander, 2003). No removal is required for adhesives, although some cannot be exposed to water. Ointments should be avoided because they may loosen the adhesive and cause wound dehiscence (Hollander, 2003). Tissue adhesives slough off 5 to 10 days after they are applied.

Steri-Strips. Wound closure tapes, or Steri-Strips, are reinforced microporous surgical adhesive tape. Steri-Strips are used to provide extra support to a suture line when running subcuticular sutures are used or after sutures are removed. Wound closure tapes may reduce spreading of scar if they are kept in place for several weeks after suture removal. Often they are used with a tissue adhesive. These tapes are rarely used for primary wound closure (Wilson et al, 2000).

SURGICAL WOUND ASSESSMENT

Clinically, there is no single, standard, widely accepted method for assessing healing of acute wounds. Deposition of collagen in the wound begins immediately in the inflammatory phase and peaks during the proliferative phase, approximately 4 to 21 days after wounding. Sufficient synthesis of collagen early during the healing process is critical to successful repair. Wound dehiscence is most likely to occur fairly early after surgery (by postoperative day 5 to 8) in patients in whom normal physiologic healing responses, such as collagen synthesis, lag. However, a method for direct observation of collagen production in acute wounds has not been validated, thus the term *healing ridge* is not mentioned in the acute wound guidelines and has been deleted from Outcome and Assessment Information Set (OASIS) documentation requirements (Whitney et al, 2008; WOCN, 2010).

ASEPSIS Scoring Tool

Acute wound complications can be evaluated on the basis of specific parameters using the ASEPSIS scoring tool. ASEPSIS is an acronym for seven wound assessment parameters that are described within the tool and presented in Box 34-2. The ASEPSIS tool is the most frequently used quantitative tool for surgical wound evaluation (Bruce et al, 2001) and offers a scale for evaluating surgical wounds with greater objectivity and ability to be reproduced. The ASEPSIS method was originally developed in cardiac surgery patients to evaluate characteristics of the surgical incision associated with infection (Wilson et al, 1986a). In a validation study, ASEPSIS was reported to

BOX 34-2	ASEPSIS Scoring Tool for Evaluating Acute Wound Complications

Instructions for use: The surgical wound site is observed (if possible for the first 5 postoperative days) and the wound characteristics scored according to the proportion of the wound affected and the presence of the characteristic. Additional points are added based on factors such as antibiotic treatment specifically for wound infection. Daily points for characteristics and any additional factors are added for the final wound score and are interpreted according to the category of infection as shown in the table.

Total Score: Category of Infection

0. 0–10: Satisfactory healing
1. 11–20: Disturbance of healing
2. 21–30: Minor wound infection
3. 31–40: Moderate wound infection
4. >40: Severe wound infection

ASEPSIS Wound Score

Wound Characteristic	Proportion of Wound Affected (%)					
	0	<20	20–39	40–59	60–79	≥80
Serous exudate*	0	1	2	3	4	5
Erythema*	0	1	2	3	4	5
Purulent exudate*	0	2	4	6	8	10
Separation of deep tissue*	0	2	4	6	8	10

	Criteria and Points			Score
	Additional treatments†			
A	Antibiotics = 10	Drainage of pus (local anesthesia) = 5	Debridement of wound (general anesthesia) = 10	
S	Serous discharge = sum of daily scores (0–5 points possible each day)			
E	Erythema = sum of daily scores (0–5 points possible each day)			
P	Purulent exudate = sum of daily scores (0–10 points possible each day)			
S	Separation of deep tissue = sum of daily scores (0–10 points possible each day)			
I	Isolation of bacteria† = 10			
S	Stay as inpatient prolonged over 14 days† = 5			
			Total Score	

*Indicates factors that are scored only on days 0–5 of the first 7 postoperative days.
†Indicates factors that are scored and added to the total score once.

be as sensitive and significantly more specific compared to other clinical indicators of wound problems or to wound assessments made using standard definitions of wound infections (Wilson et al, 1990). Interrater reliability of 0.96 has been reported in patients undergoing general surgery (Byrne et al, 1989). Similar reliability has been shown for sternal and leg wounds of patients after cardiac surgery (Wilson et al, 1986b). Topaloglu et al (2008) noted statistically significant correlations between preoperative wound infection risk indices and ASEPSIS scores. The authors of this study reported ASEPSIS was easy to use, repeatable, and effective as an infection surveillance method. Summed scores over wound assessments performed each day for the first 5 postoperative days indicate severity of infection or complication.

Impediments to Surgical Wound Healing

Although ongoing assessment of the surgical wound is critical, identifying impediments to healing is important so that they may be minimized or eliminated when possible. Box 34-1 lists impediments to surgical wound healing (Franz et al, 2008). Most (perfusion and smoking, nonviable tissue, infection, mechanical factors, obesity, diabetes, malnutrition, and burn injuries) are discussed in great detail in chapters throughout this text.

Hematoma or Seroma. The occurrence of hematoma or seroma in surgical wounds has increased because of greater clinical use of anticoagulants and prophylactic treatments now recommended and implemented for deep vein thrombosis (Franz et al, 2007). When detected, hematoma or seroma requires intervention for removal by needle aspiration or prophylactic drainage (Franz et al, 2008). The presence of fluid collections, seromas, or hematomas delays healing in acute wounds through mechanisms of pressure and ischemia to the wound edges and adjacent tissues (Franz et al, 2008).

Surgical Wound Infection. Infections in surgical wounds are a concern, with 500,000 reported each year and high associated costs in terms of mortality, morbidity, and economic expenditures (Anderson et al, 2008). Surgical wound infection has been termed *surgical site infection* (SSI). Many definitions of SSI exist, and much data on how SSI is measured and monitored are available. In the United States, a large database created by the National Surgical Surveillance Initiative (NSSI) and available through the CDC is considered the most accurate data available (Bruce et al, 2001). CDC criteria for diagnosing various types of SSIs are widely accepted; the criteria are listed in Table 34-1. Infections of episiotomies, newborn circumcision sites, burns, and stitch abscesses are not classified as SSIs (Mangram et al, 1999).

TABLE 34-1	CDC Criteria for Incisional and Deep/Organ Space Infection		
Superficial SSI	**Deep Incisional SSI**	**Organ/Space SSI**	
Purulent damage	Purulent damage	Purulent damage	
Positive wound culture	Incision dehisces or is opened by physician when patient has one of the following: fever, local pain, tenderness (unless site is culture-negative)	Positive wound culture	
At least one of the following: signs or symptoms of infection, pain, or tenderness, local swelling, redness, heat	Abscess or other evidence of infection found on examination, X-ray study, histopathology	Abscess or other evidence of infection found on examination, X-ray study, histopathology	
Superficial incision is deliberately opened by a surgeon unless incision culture is negative			
Diagnosis by surgeon or attending physician	Diagnosis by surgeon or attending physician	Diagnosis by surgeon or attending physician	

CDC, Centers for Disease Control and Prevention; *SSI*, surgical site infection.
Modified from Mangram AJ et al: Guideline for prevention of surgical site infection, *Infect Control Hosp Epidemiol* 20(4):252, 1999, available at http://www.cdc.gov/ncidod/dhqp/pdf/guidelines/SSI.pdf, accessed January 25, 2010.

SSIs occur within 30 days of surgery or within 1 year if an implant has been inserted and the infection involves the site of surgery. SSI is an incision infection or an organ/space infection (Mangram et al, 1999). *Superficial incision infection* involves only skin and subcutaneous tissue at the incision. *Deep incision infection* involves the deep tissues, including the muscles and fascia. *Infection of the organ/spaces* involves organs or body cavities that were manipulated during surgery.

In 2002, the Centers for Medicare & Medicaid Services commissioned the Surgical Infection Prevention Collaborative. Through intensive work efforts, the Surgical Infection Prevention Collaborative and then the Surgical Care Improvement Project (consisting of several, multiagency cooperatives) produced guidelines for preventing surgical wound infection (Bratzler and Houck, 2004; Bratzler and Hunt, 2006). SSI prevention targets the perioperative period and has led to specific, evidence-supported guidelines for antibiotic choice and administration, hair removal, glucose control, and normothermia (for colon surgeries). For surgical wounds for which prophylactic antibiotics are used, administration within 60 minutes of surgery and choice of antibiotic consistent with published guidelines are recommended to attain effective tissue concentration (Anderson et al, 2008; Mangram et al, 1999).

Table 34-2 lists both intrinsic and extrinsic risk factors for SSI that have been identified in several studies. Risk factors that occurred in more than one study include diabetes, age extremes, obesity, malnutrition, ascites, low hematocrit, steroid use, smoking, and remote infection (Anderson et al, 2008; Barie, 2002; Haridas and Malangoni, 2008; Kompatscher et al, 2003; Malone et al, 2002; Mangram et al, 1999; Smith et al, 2004; Sorensen et al, 2005).

Further analysis shows that important factors were different for superficial infections (previous operation, prolonged duration of surgery, low albumin, chronic obstructive pulmonary disease) compared to deep and organ space infections (low albumin, previous operation). These data highlight some new factors that convey risk and emphasize that risk profiles are likely to vary for superficial versus deeper surgical infections (Haridas and Malangoni, 2008).

A number of risk factors are irreversible, but several may be modified through patient advisement and modification of aspects of perioperative care. Understanding who is at risk for SSI provides an opportunity to increase surveillance so that early detection can occur and timely intervention can be initiated.

Systemic Conditions. Perhaps the single most advantageous action that can be taken to minimize SSI risk is to prevent postoperative hyperglycemia. Hyperglycemia, defined as whole blood glucose level greater than 200 mg/dl, in the 48 hours after surgery is associated with diminished wound strength and significant reduction in the phagocytic ability of neutrophils (Goodson, 1979; Latham et al, 2001).

Recommendations for patients with cardiovascular disease and for wound healing of acute wounds advocate for protocol-based, aggressive glycemic control to achieve individualized target blood glucose levels, generally in the range from 80 to 180 mg/dl (Franz et al, 2008). Some researchers suggest a narrower range from 80 to 120 mg/dl maintained by insulin infusion protocol as the ideal target in order to reduce deep sternal wound infections (Kramer et al, 2008). Consistent themes for best care are careful monitoring and control of diabetes perioperatively and extending well into the postoperative period to optimize the healing environment during the months of collagen remodeling.

Obesity is an independent predictor of SSI (Harrington et al, 2004). Increased body mass index, intraabdominal fat, and subcutaneous fat are significantly associated with

TABLE 34-2	Risk Factors for Surgical Site Infection		
Intrinsic		**Extrinsic**	
Existing disease	Chronic obstructive pulmonary disease Congestive cardiac failure Diabetes Peripheral vascular disease Skin disease in surgical area	Presurgical factors	Current surgery through previous incision Emergency surgery Previous surgery Hair removal
Additional factors	Age Ascites Chronic inflammation Excessive alcohol use Hypercholesterolemia Hyperglycemia Hypoxemia Low albumin Low hemoglobin or hematocrit Malnutrition Nicotine use Prior surgical site radiation Remote infection Skin carrier of staphylococcus Steroid or other immunosuppressive medications	Perioperative factors	Estimated blood loss $\geq$500 ml Hypothermia Blood products Surgery $\geq$2 hours

surgery-related complications, including wound infection (Tsukada et al, 2004). A number of retrospective and prospective studies in cardiac, general, and gynecologic surgery populations have documented an increased risk for SSI in patients who are obese (Israelsson and Jonsson 1997; Myles et al, 2002; Vastine et al, 1999; Winiarsky et al, 1998). Regardless of the type of surgical procedure performed, the incidence of postsurgical wound complications in patients who are overweight, obese, or morbidly obese compared to those of normal weight is high, with reported rates of 15% to 22%. In an observational study of 1,211 patients undergoing total hip replacement, morbid obesity was significantly associated with prolonged wound drainage and, in turn, with higher risk for (42%) and rates of SSI (Patel et al, 2007).

Factors that can be clinically evaluated and optimized in patients with obesity have been identified. In patients with obesity, perfusion and oxygenation of the surgical wound is more likely to be compromised. Therefore, interventions that ensure adequate blood flow and oxygen delivery, such as increased perioperative FiO_2 (80% oxygen) and systemic warming to maintain normothermia, are important (see Chapter 28). Control of hyperglycemia in the perioperative period, provision of adequate doses of prophylactic antibiotics to maintain therapeutic serum and tissue levels (double the standard dose if weight is greater than 220 lb or body mass index is 35 or higher), closure of the subcutaneous tissue layer when its depth is greater than 2 cm, and laparoscopic surgery when possible are additional recommendations to decrease SSI in obese patients (Anaya and Dellinger, 2006; Walsh et al, 2009).

TOPICAL INCISION CARE

Regardless of their origin, wounds progress through the same phases of the reparative process—inflammation, angiogenesis, fibroplasia and matrix deposition, and epithelialization—in order to heal. Knowledgeable assessment of the patient's surgical incision site include evaluation of the primary dressing, epithelial resurfacing, wound closure, and local changes at the wound site that may signal infection. All healing incisions should be protected from sun exposure to prevent permanent hyperpigmentation (Ship and Weiss, 1985). General components of topical incision care are listed in Box 34-3 and described in this section.

Dressings provide initial protection, exudate absorption, and thermal insulation for acute wounds. Studies evaluating dressings that provide a moist, occlusive, or

BOX 34-3	Topical Incision Care

1. Keep incisions dry without prolonged exposure to moisture (including topical antibiotics and moisture).
2. Maintain original postoperative dressing for 48–72 hours (cleanse incision with sterile saline and use aseptic technique for changing dressings if needed in first 48 hours).
3. After 48–72 hours, patient may shower if suture line is closed with no drainage
4. Timing of suture or staple removal depends on wound location:
   - 3–5 days face
   - 7–10 days for scalp, chest, fingers, hand, lower extremity
   - 10–14 days for the back
5. Protect surgical wound incision from exposure to sun.

semiocclusive environment compared to standard dry absorbent gauze postsurgical dressings find no difference in the incidence of SSI for wounds after cardiac, vascular, or gastrointestinal surgeries, in patient comfort, or in cost (Shinohara et al, 2008; Vogt et al 2007; Wynne et al, 2004). For the secondary outcome of cost, dry absorbent dressings were reported to be less expensive (Vogt et al, 2007; Wynne et al, 2004), although Shinohara et al (2008) found hydrocolloid dressings were less costly. None of the studies found differences in comfort between dressing types. Of interest, some data suggest that dressings that provide some level of pressure or compression may actually impede local tissue perfusion (Plattner et al, 2000). This finding was based on the observation that wounds covered with dressings that provide some level of pressure had tissue oxygen levels 12 mm Hg lower than wounds with less constrictive covers. In the interest of supporting oxygen delivery to acute wounds, avoiding extra pressure over the wound seems prudent unless required for hemostasis.

Surgical dressings usually are removed 48 to 72 hours following injury, which is consistent with CDC guidelines for prevention of SSIs (Mangram et al, 1999) and with guidelines from the United Kingdom (Leaper et al, 2008). Aseptic technique for dressing changes and use of sterile saline if needed for cleansing are recommended within the 48-hour time frame (Leaper et al, 2008). If the wound is closed and dry after 48 hours, patients may shower.

Use of topical antibiotics on closed surgical incisions is not supported by current evidence and is not recommended by recent guidelines (Franz et al, 2008; Leaper et al, 2008). A trial comparing no ointment, paraffin, and mupirocin ointment on excised and sutured skin lesions (n = 562 wounds) reported no differences in wound infection rate and, interestingly, significantly fewer scar complications in the patients treated without any ointment (Dixon et al, 2006).

Resurfacing of the wound closed by primary intention occurs within 2 to 3 days after wounding because of the presence of intact epithelial appendages, such as hair follicles, and the relatively short distance that cells in the interrupted epithelial tissue must traverse. Although the incisional wound does not have the structural integrity (tensile strength) to withstand force at this time, by postoperative day 2 or 3, the incision is "sealed" and impenetrable to bacteria. However, many patients prefer that the wound remain covered. As healing evolves, some incisions begin to itch as a result of wound contraction or simply dry skin. Desire to view the surgical scar is personal. The presence of a dressing allows patients to gradually incorporate changes in body image. Although an incisional dressing may no longer be necessary once epithelial cells have resurfaced the wound, a soft dressing placed over the suture line often limits local irritation and provides additional comfort and support, particularly as the patient begins to wear regular clothing.

SUMMARY

A significant number of surgeries are performed annually in the United States and globally. Surgical wound complications include failure to heal, as occurs with dehiscence or hernia, and SSI. Wound assessment for indications of healing complication and infection surveillance are important in the first 3 to 4 weeks postsurgery in order to detect problems quickly and provide therapy as well as to capture accurate rates and level of severity of SSIs. A number of factors contribute to surgical wound complications, and some of these factors can be modified in advance of surgery. Other interventions are critical to monitor and modify during the perioperative procedure. National safety initiatives, quality reporting measures, and evidence-based guidelines for acute wounds offer new insights into risk and strategies to decrease wound healing failure following surgery.

REFERENCES

Anaya DA, Dellinger EP: The obese surgical patient: a susceptible host for infection, *Surg Infect* 7:473, 2006.

Anderson DJ et al: Strategies to prevent surgical site infections in acute care hospitals, *Infect Control Hosp Epidemiol* 29:S51, 2008.

Barie PS: Surgical site infections: epidemiology and prevention, *Surg Infect* 3:59, 2002.

Bratzler DW, Houck PM: Antimicrobial prophylaxis for surgery: an advisory statement from the National Surgical Infection Prevention Project, *Clin Infect Dis* 38:1706, 2004.

Bratzler DW, Hunt DR: The surgical infection prevention and surgical care improvement projects: national initiatives to improve outcomes for patients having surgery, *Clin Infect Dis* 43:322, 2006.

Bruce J et al: The quality of measurement of surgical wound infection as the basis for monitoring: a systematic review, *J Hosp Infect* 49:99, 2001.

Byrne D et al: Postoperative wound scoring, *Biomed Pharm* 43:669, 1989.

Centers for Disease Control (CDC): Surgical site infection, 2009, available at *http://www.cdc.gov/ncidod/dhqp/FAQ_SSI.html*, accessed June 19, 2009.

Coulthard P et al: Tissue adhesive for closure of surgical incisions, *Cochrane Database Syst Rev* (3):CD004287, 2002.

Dixon AJ et al: Randomized clinical trial of the effect of applying ointment to surgical wounds before occlusive dressing, *Br J Surg* 93:937, 2006.

Franz MG et al: Optimizing healing of the acute wound by minimizing complications, *Curr Prob Surg* 44:679, 2007.

Franz MG et al: Guidelines to aid healing of acute wounds by decreasing impediments of healing, *Wound Repair Regen* 16:723, 2008.

Goodson W: Wound healing and the diabetic patient, *Surg Gynecol Obstet* 149:600, 1979.

Haridas M, Malangoni MA: Predictive factors for surgical site infection in general surgery, *Surg* 144:496, 2008.

Harrington G et al: Surgical-site infection rates and risk factor analysis in coronary artery bypass graft surgery, *Infect Control Hosp Epidemiol* 25:472, 2004.

Hollander JE: Wound closure options. In Singer AJ, Hollander JE, editors: *Lacerations and acute wounds: an evidence-based guide*, Philadelphia, 2003, FA Davis.

Israelsson LA, Jonsson T: Overweight and healing of midline incisions: the importance of suture technique, *Eur J Surg* 163:175, 1997.

Kompatscher P et al: Comparison of the incidence and predicted risk of surgical site infection after breast reconstruction, *Anesth Plast Surg* 27(4):308, 2003.

Kramer R et al: Glycemic control and reduction of deep sterna wound infection rates, *Arch Surg* 143:451, 2008.

Latham RL et al: The association of diabetes and glucose control with surgical-site infections among cardiothoracic surgery patients, *Infect Cont Hosp Epidemiol* 22:607, 2001.

Leaper D et al: Prevention and treatment of surgical site infection: summary of NICE guidance, *BMJ* 337:a1924, 2008.

Malone DL et al: Surgical site infections: reanalysis of risk factors, *J Surg Res* 103(1):89, 2002.

Mangram AJ et al: Guideline for prevention of surgical site infection, *Infect Cont Hosp Epididemiol* 20:247, 1999.

Myles TD et al: Obesity as an independent risk factor for infections morbidity in patients who undergo cesarean delivery, *Obstet Gynecol* 100:959, 2002.

Patel VP et al: Factors associated with prolonged wound drainage after primary total hip and knee arthroplasty, *J Bone Joint Surg Am* 89:33, 2007.

Plattner O et al: The influence of two surgical bandage systems on wound tissue oxygen tension, *Arch Surg* 135:818, 2000.

Shinohara T et al: Prospective evaluation of occlusive hydrocolloid dressing versus conventional gauze dressing regarding the healing effect after abdominal operations: randomized controlled trial, *Asian J Surg* 31(1):1-5, 2008.

Ship AG, Weiss PR: Pigmentation after dermabrasion: an avoidable complication, *Plast Reconstr Surg* 75:528, 1985.

Smith RL et al: Wound infection after elective colorectal resection, *Ann Surg* 239(5):599, 2004.

Sorensen LT et al: Risk factors for tissue and wound complications in gastrointestinal surgery, *Ann Surg* 241:654, 2005.

Topaloglu S et al: Correlation of risk and postoperative assessment methods in wound surveillance, *J Surg Res* 146:211, 2008.

Tsukada K et al: Body fat accumulation and postoperative complications after abdominal surgery, *Am Surg* 70:347, 2004.

Vastine VL et al: Wound complications of abdominoplasty in obese patients, *Ann Plast Surg* 42:34, 1999.

Vogt DC et al: Moist wound healing compared with standard care of treatment of primary closed vascular surgical wound: a prospective randomized controlled study, *Wound Repair Regen* 15:624, 2007.

Walsh C et al: Prevention and management of surgical site infections in morbidly obese women, *Obstet Gynecol* 113:411, 2009.

Whitney J et al: Guidelines for the treatment of pressure ulcer, *Wound Repair Regen* 14(6):663-679, 2008.

Wilson APR et al: A scoring method (ASEPSIS) for postoperative wound infections for use in clinical trials of antibiotic prophylaxis, *Lancet* 1(8476):311, 1986a.

Wilson APR et al: Repeatability of ASEPSIS wound scoring method, *Lancet* 849:1208, 1986b.

Wilson APR et al: The use of the wound scoring method "ASEPSIS" in postoperative wound surveillance, *J Hosp Infect* 16(4):297-309, 1990.

Wilson JL et al: A systematic approach to laceration repair. Tricks to ensure the desired cosmetic result, *Postgrad Med* 107(4): 77-83, 87-88, 2000.

Winiarsky R et al: Total knee arthroplasty in morbidly obese patients, *J Bone Joint Surg Am* 80:12, 1770, 1998.

Wound, Ostomy and Continence Nurses (WOCN) Society: *Wound Ostomy Continence Nurses Society guidance on Oasis-C integumentary items*, 2009, available at http://www.wocn.org/pdfs/GuidanceOASIS-C.pdf, accessed January 25, 2010.

Wu TL: Plastic surgery made easy. Simple techniques for closing skin defects and improving cosmetic results, *Aust Fam Physician* 35:492, 2006.

Wynne R et al: Effect of three wound dressings on infection, healing comfort, and cost in patients with sternotomy wounds: a randomized trial, *Chest* 125(1):43-49, 2004.

SECTION VIII

Special Patient Populations

35

Skin Care Needs
of the Obese Patient

Susan Gallagher Camden

OBJECTIVES

1. Define obesity.
2. Describe necessary accommodations in the physical environment for the obese patient.
3. Identify risk factors for three common skin complications in the obese patient population.
4. Discuss two common pulmonary complications in the obese patient population.

Sixty-seven percent of Americans are overweight, more than one third of all Americans are obese, and 3% to 10% (at least eight million) are morbidly obese (Anaya and Dellinger, 2006; Ogden et al, 2007). Morbid obesity, once a rare occurrence in America, has essentially quadrupled since the 1980s (Camden, 2009). Studies suggest a substantial increase in obesity among all age, ethnic, racial, and socioeconomic groups (Lanz et al, 1998). In the early 1960s, only one fourth of Americans were overweight; today more than two thirds of U.S. adults are overweight, as are 25% of U.S. children. Worldwide, the number of individuals who are overweight or obese, which totals nearly two billion, now exceeds the number of those suffering from starvation (Aronne and Isoldi, 2008; Barrios and Jones, 2007).

Obesity has an economic, physical, and emotional impact on our patients. Americans spend close to $117 billion on obesity-related health problems, and $33 billion is spent annually in attempts to control or lose weight. Despite efforts at weight loss, Americans continue to gain weight, with obesity reaching epidemic proportions. Obesity is a factor in 5 of the 10 leading causes of death (Knudsen and Gallagher, 2003) and is considered the second most common cause of preventable death in the United States (Fox, 1995). In addition to the physiologic costs, some authors argue that obesity is associated with emotional conditions such as situational depression, altered self-esteem, and social isolation (Charles, 1987). However, others argue that society's response to the obese person (i.e., prejudice and discrimination) leads to these emotional conditions (Gallagher et al, 2004).

Major comorbidities associated with obesity include type 2 diabetes, cardiovascular disease, hypertension, sleep apnea or obesity hypoventilation syndrome, and lipid disorders, including the metabolic syndrome. Other associated conditions include malnutrition, immobility, and depression. These comorbidities affect the morbidly obese patient disproportionately, and at a younger age. Diagnosis in the obese patient is difficult and procedures are technically more complicated, which ultimately places the obese patient at a disadvantage (Kral et al, 2000). In addition, many hospitals, clinics, and home care settings are not prepared to meet the needs of the obese patient group because of inadequate equipment and insufficient personnel to accommodate the needs of the larger patient, factors known to contribute to the patient's risk of mechanical skin damage due to pressure, shear, or taping. However, advances in information, intervention, equipment, and education have helped reduce some of these risks (Gallagher et al, 2004).

DEFINING OBESITY

Obesity is defined as a body mass index (BMI) of 30 or greater; morbid obesity is defined as BMI greater than 40 (Box 35-1). *Bariatrics* is a term derived from the Greek word *baros* and refers to the practice of health care relating to the treatment of obesity and associated conditions. The American Society for Metabolic and Bariatric Surgery (2001) defines obesity as a lifelong, progressive, life-threatening, genetically related, multifactorial disease of excess fat storage with multiple comorbidities. Others describe obesity simply as the

BOX 35-1	Body Mass Index Categories
Underweight	<18.5
Normal weight	18.5–24.9
Overweight	25–29.9
Obesity	≥30

Source: National Heart, Lung, and Blood Institute, Bethesda, Md.

excessive accumulation of body fat, which manifests as slow, steady, progressive increase in body weight. However, recent discoveries suggest that obesity is more than simply overeating or lack of control. Genetics, gender, physiology, biochemistry, neuroscience, and cultural, environmental, and psychosocial factors influence weight and its regulation (Ludwig and Pollack, 2009). The National Institutes of Health regards obesity simply as a diagnostic category that represents a complex and multifactorial disease (Kuczmarski et al, 1994). However, obesity is most recently viewed as a chronic, multifactorial condition.

Misunderstandings about the etiologies of obesity are common among health care providers. For example, obesity has long been perceived as a problem of self-discipline. Such misunderstandings can fuel prejudice and discrimination. In a culture that worships thinness, obese patients experience discrimination in schools, the workplace, and health care settings (Puhl & Heuer, 2009). As early as 1997, health care clinicians were often noted as biased against the larger patient (Thone, 1997).

Prejudice and discrimination pose barriers to care regardless of practice setting or professional discipline. The overwhelming misunderstanding of obesity likely interferes with preplanning efforts, access to services, and resource allocation. This misunderstanding is not universal but is pervasive enough to pose obstacles, and clinicians interested in making changes will need to recognize these barriers (Camden et al, 2008).

ALTERED SKIN FUNCTION

In the obese person, a greater percentage of centralized and cutaneous adiposity is responsible for a number of changes in skin physiology and comorbidities that directly affect the skin. For example, the obese individual must perspire more efficiently when overheated in order to cool the body adequately due to the difference in the weight to skin ratio of the obese. Thus, the skin barrier function of the skin is altered to have increased transepidermal water loss than in skin with less adiposity. Dry skin is characteristic of obesity as a consequence of a fundamentally altered epidermal barrier. Levels of androgens, insulin, growth hormone, and insulin-like growth factors frequently are elevated, triggering sebaceous gland activity, altered skin pH, and an increased prevalence of inflammatory or noninflammatory papules, pustules, nodules, or cystonodules over the head, face, neck, back, or arms (Pokorny, 2008).

UNIQUE NEEDS

Common problems associated with the obese patient that interfere, at least potentially, with skin integrity include pressure ulcers, intertrigo, incontinence-associated dermatitis (IAD), and foot dysfunction. Risk factors, manifestations, and prevention and management are described in Chapters 5, 7, 14, and 15 however, unique aspects occur in the obese patient population.

Pressure Management

Pressure ulcers typically occur over a bony prominence and develop because of the inability to adequately offload the pressure; this is particularly true among very heavy patients. To compound this problem, friction and pressure can exist in locations unique to the obese person (Pokorny, 2008). Atypical or unusual pressure ulcers can result from tubes or catheters, an ill-fitting chair or wheelchair, or pressure within skin folds or over a point of contact not typically observed among nonobese patients (Camden, 2008).

Tubes and catheters can burrow into skin folds and ulcerate the skin surface. Pressure from side rails and armrests not designed to accommodate a larger person can cause pressure ulcers on the patient's hips. Patients often develop pressure injury over the buttocks rather than over the sacrum, an area that frequently is the point of maximum contact with the surface because of the obese patient's atypical body configuration. Shearing/pressure damage can develop lateral to the gluteal cleft over the fleshy part of the buttocks due to insufficient repositioning or transfer onto a stretcher or the operating room table. Interventions to prevent these types of mechanical injuries are listed in Table 35-1.

Bariatric beds with a pressure redistribution mattress will reduce the risk of pressure ulcers, promote patient independence, improve clinical outcomes, decrease staff workload, and help control unnecessary costs (Mathison, 2003). As described in Chapter 9, bariatric support surfaces are available in foam, air, gel, and water. They offer features with or without microclimate and moisture control that include low-friction covers. These devices are extremely useful for reducing friction and shear as well as dissipating moisture. In addition to benefiting the patient, bariatric beds provide specific features that impact on the staff and facility as listed in Table 35-2 (Kramer and Gallagher, 2004). The support surface with lateral rotation therapy, often regarded as the standard of care for certain pulmonary situations, can ensure sufficient repositioning for a very large patient whose need for frequent turning may otherwise pose a realistic challenge (Camden, 2008). Despite the value of rotation therapy in the prevention and treatment of skin injury among obese patients, additional precautions to prevent

TABLE 35-1	Prevention of Unique Features of Skin Damage in the Obese Patient	
Causative Factor	**Unique Feature in Obese Patient**	**Prevention Intervention**
Pressure	Tubes and catheters burrow into skin folds	Reposition tubes and catheters every 2 hours
		Place tubes so that patient does not rest on them
		Use tube and catheter holders
	Pressure between skin folds or under large breasts	Reposition large abdominal panniculus every 2 hours to prevent pressure injury beneath panniculus
		Physically reposition pannus off suprapubic area every 2 hours
		Use side-lying position with pannus lifted away from underlying skin surface, allowing air flow to regions
		Reposition breasts every 2 hours
	Pressure ulcer on hips or lateral thighs from side rails and armrests	Use properly sized bariatric equipment
	Pressure injury occurs in slightly lateral fleshy areas of the buttocks rather than midline (directly over the sacrum) because it is difficult to prevent excess skin on buttocks from being folded and compressed when repositioning the patient.	Bariatric support surface
		Proper repositioning
		Trapeze
		Establish, communicate, and implement safest transfer and positioning method to prevent shear that can be used during handoffs.
Moisture-associated skin damage (e.g., intertrigo)	Excess perspiration to more efficiently cool the body when overheated	Use cotton clothing (particularly undergarments)
	Redundant skin creating skin folds	Maintain weight
		Avoid tight clothing
	Severe pruritus, burning, local pain between skin folds	Avoid corticosteroids and antibiotics
		Burrow solution (aluminum acetate) soak applied for 15–20 minutes twice per day to soothe and dry affected area

friction and shear are well advised. The patient should be fitted to the appropriately sized surface with correct pressure settings, and frequent assessments for skin changes must be implemented (Gallagher, 2002). For a listing of various bariatric surfaces, see Table 9-1.

Skin Fold Management

Moisture-associated skin damage, pressure, and intertrigo can develop between skin folds of the obese patient. Common sites include the inner thighs, axilla, underside of breasts, and panniculus. Pressure from the weight of the pannus over the suprapubic area or breasts against the chest wall and upper abdomen are sufficient to cause skin breakdown (see Color Plate 68).

Because the obese patient experiences increased perspiration and sebum production and a change in skin pH, the barrier function of the skin is compromised. In addition, coexisting conditions in the obese patient that will further increase in the risk of moisture-associated skin damage and intertrigo include diabetes mellitus, immunosuppression, infection, chronic corticosteroid, and antibiotic use. Intertrigo (inflammation within cutaneous folds) can become an intertriginous infection with bacterial, viral, or fungal organisms alone or in combination. Clinical manifestations of intertrigo in this patient population include scaling, erythema and small pustules. Patients often complain of itching or burning that can progress to fissures and maceration. In the face of associated pruritus, patients may scratch the skin surface, further compromising skin integrity and leading to a secondary bacterial invasion. Not surprisingly,

many obese patients indicate they are constantly battling mild candidiasis in skin folds. When an individual is hospitalized, moisture from urine, perspiration, or wound drainage exacerbates this chronic but otherwise mild condition.

Knowing the obese patient is at risk for moisture-associated skin damage and intertrigo, preventive interventions should be implemented upon admission. In addition to the interventions presented in Box 5-4, prevention strategies unique to the obese patient are presented in Table 35-1.

Not all intertrigo is a fungal infection. As with all wound and skin care interventions, the area must be reassessed within a reasonable amount of time after the treatment plan is implemented to determine the effectiveness of that intervention. If the condition does not improve within 24 hours or the skin condition continues to deteriorate, a bacterial, viral, or fungal infection may develop, particularly when the skin is broken or denuded. This could progress to cellulitis or sepsis if left untreated, so further evaluation is necessary and the primary care provider should be notified. Topical antimicrobials dressings, such as silver-impregnated textile products, may be appropriate at this point.

Incontinence-Associated Dermatitis

Increased BMI has a direct association with urinary incontinence and is a risk factor for urinary incontinence independent of age (Engel et al, 1991). Sleep apnea, another condition associated with obesity, can lead to decreases in oxygen tension and relative central nervous

TABLE 35-2	Benefits of Bariatric Beds Features for Patient, Care Staff, and Facility		
Feature	**Patient Benefit**	**Staff Benefit**	**Cost Benefit/Risk Reduction**
600- to 1,000-lb capacity	Safely supports weight Eliminates fear of bed breaking	Reduces risk of injury during care	Reduces risk of patient injury (and possible litigation) if bed breaks Reduces risk of worker's compensation injury
Integrated scale	Safety Retained dignity More accurate than portable, under-mattress scales	Less time consuming than using a loading dock More accurate	Reduces risk of inappropriate treatment due to inaccurate weights
Expandable	Enhances patient participation by providing sufficient room in bed for proper repositioning	Bed width is a safe surface distance to prevent back injuries from overreaching Reduces risk of nosocomial pressure ulcer development from railings, skin fold pressure	Reduces risk of worker's compensation injury Reduces risk for litigation and citations from regulating agencies for nosocomial pressure ulcers
Trendelenburg/reverse Trendelenburg	Decreases friction on back when "boosting"	Helps with gravity-assisted "boosting" for fewer lifting injuries	Reduces risk of worker's compensation injury
Cardio-Chair	Increases mobility Decreases cardiac and pulmonary decomposition Facilitates faster recovery	Facilitates patient mobility Decreases staff lifting Simplifies transfers	Reduces risk of worker's compensation injury Reduces length of stay by decreasing effects of immobility
Trapeze	Increases mobility Facilitates patient independence Decreases friction on skin Facilitates deep breathing and pulmonary hygiene	Decreases staff lifting Facilitates mobility Reduces risk for nosocomial pressure ulcer development	Reduces length of stay by decreasing effects of immobility or staff injury Reduces risk of worker's compensation injury Reduces risk for litigation and citations from regulating agencies for nosocomial pressure ulcers
Therapeutic mattress with microclimate control	Redistributes pressure appropriately to reduce risk of mechanical trauma (pressure, shear, friction) Facilitates moisture evaporation to reduce moisture entrapment in skin folds and sweating	Eases transfers and turning of patients Saves additional linen changes due to adequate control of perspiration Reduces risk for nosocomial pressure ulcer development	Reduces risk of worker's compensation injury Reduces risk for litigation and citations from regulating agencies for effects of immobility Reduces length of stay by decreasing nosocomial pressure ulcers

Data from Kramer K, Gallagher S: WOC nurses as advocates for patients who are morbidly obese: a case study promoting use of bariatric beds, *J Wound Ostomy Continence Nurs* 31(1):276, 2004; Whittemore A et al: Specialized staff and equipment for weight loss surgery patients: best practice guidelines, *Obes Res* 13:283-289, 2005.

system hypoxia, both of which cause increased excitability of autonomic neurons and thus trigger urgency. Continuous positive pressure ventilation has been reported to improve symptoms associated with urinary incontinence, such as urgency and enuresis (Steers and Suratt, 1997).

Many otherwise continent persons develop short-term acute incontinence when they are physically dependent in a health care setting. This condition may occur because of medication, delays in locating a caregiver to place the patient on the bedpan, or simply because the patient cannot access a commode in time to prevent an incontinent episode. Additional barriers to maintaining continence include inadequate staffing, negative attitudes by the staff (Rose, 2006), and reluctance on the part of the patient to

ask for assistance. Patients need to be reminded that the goal of health care providers is to serve their needs. Maintaining clean, dry skin is the objective, and if the patient needs assistance in this effort, caregivers are available to help.

After each incontinent episode, the entire affected area should be cleansed with a no-rinse incontinence cleanser, dried, and appropriate skin sealant or moisture barrier applied. Table 5-4 and Box 5-4 list strategies and products used for the prevention and management of incontinence-associated skin damage. Patients report that drying the buttocks and the perineal area, and between folds with an institutionally approved blow dryer on the cool setting is more comfortable than towel drying. This technique may be less traumatic to the outermost layer of skin. An important potential barrier to the staff's ability to provide adequate perineal care is the lack of properly fitting gloves; health care facilities must provide elbow length gloves for the staff caring for the bariatric patient. If IAD develops despite preventive efforts, the skin care protocol must be reassessed and updated to include a moisture barrier ointment, skin barrier paste or barrier strip, external fecal pouch, or internal fecal device, all of which are described in Chapter 5.

Foot Dysfunction

Because the feet carry a person's entire weight, heavier individuals are prone to wear-and-tear injuries. Some activities can create loads on the feet as much as four times the body's weight. In addition, foot pain could signal other serious medical conditions, such as arthritis, nerve and circulatory disorders, and diabetes.

Among the obese population, foot discomfort or dysfunction requires prompt attention. Foot pain can discourage an obese patient from seeking outpatient wound care or ongoing diabetes follow-up due to ambulation and transportation difficulties. Accommodations in the physical environment that promote patient safety and comfort may overcome some of these obstacles (Checklist 35-1); however a podiatry consultation is also warranted when foot discomfort is reported. When the joints of the feet are involved, medication, physical therapy, exercise, orthotics, braces, specially designed shoes, and surgery are among the tools that can be used to restore feet to as near-normal function as possible (Medical Network, 2004).

CHECKLIST 35-1

Accommodations in Physical Environment for the Obese Patient

✓ Large blood pressure cuff
✓ Long needles
✓ Larger tracheostomy ties
✓ Longer abdominal binders
✓ Large gowns/drapes
✓ Elbow-length gloves for incontinence cleanup
✓ Beds wide enough for effective repositioning
✓ Support surfaces
✓ Overhead trapeze to facilitate repositioning
✓ Bariatric lifts for safely moving the patient
✓ Bedside commode (appropriate size)
✓ Wide wheelchair with pressure-reducing cushion
✓ Walker with proper support
✓ Size-friendly art and magazines
✓ Larger clinic examination tables anchored to floor with adequate step
✓ Sturdy, armless chairs for clinic waiting rooms
✓ Air displacement lateral transfer devices
✓ Mechanical lifts with provisions for limb band, pannus sling, turning band, lithotomy band

---

THE SURGICAL EXPERIENCE

The surgical experience predisposes the patient to skin injury due to intraoperative mechanical factors (shear, friction, and pressure) and postoperative factors (immobility, pain, sedation, fear of falling, and inadequate staffing). In addition, the obese patient is at increased risk for impaired healing of the surgical incision as well as complications from the anesthesia and from the surgical procedure itself (e.g., cardiovascular, respiratory complications) that can further jeopardize wound healing (Bamgbade et al, 2007).

Addressing Mechanical Threats to Skin Integrity

Although the patient may be awake and alert shortly after surgery, extra personnel and supportive equipment are required to transfer the patient, particularly to prevent shearing injury or placing undue stress on the incision. Early activity is encouraged to decrease the chances of immobility-related complications. Using bariatric equipment that will convert into a chair will facilitate achieving early mobilization. Deconditioning can occur very rapidly in the obese patient when mobilization after surgery is delayed, thus increasing the risk for skin and wound-related complications. A physical therapy consultation within 24 hours of an intensive care unit admission may be valuable to (1) evaluate for and demonstrate immobility-related equipment and (2) provide passive and active exercises to slow deconditioning. The larger patient typically has several comorbid conditions, so postoperative recovery can be complicated and require close monitoring. However, it is important to assess and reassess the skin frequently (at least every 8 hours) so that potential complications can be prevented or identified and interventions applied early (Davidson and Callery, 2001). This can be challenging due to the patient's size and postoperative slumber but, in today's environment of best practice zero tolerance for nosocomial pressure ulcers, cannot be overlooked or postponed. Preplanning for the obese patient by having proper bariatric equipment and appropriate staffing available is essential to providing competent, safe postoperative care.

After surgery, the obese patient seems to breathe more easily when the bed is at 30 degrees because this position reduces the weight of the abdominal adipose tissue pressing against the diaphragm (Lasater-Erhard, 1995). The challenge in terms of skin care is that the patient who fears shortness of breath may refuse repositioning from the 30-degree, semi-Fowler position, thus placing the patient at risk for sacral pressure injury. Introducing pressure redistribution early in the admission may reduce some of this risk, along with patient and clinical education designed to improve awareness about the risk. An appropriate bariatric support surface and trapeze should be in place to reduce shear on the sacrum and adequately redistribute pressure. The patient should be encouraged to offload and shift his or her weight at regular intervals, including reducing the head of bed when possible, to prevent prolonged pressure to the sacrum. Similarly, the lower back should be monitored frequently for signs of friction or shear.

Incisions and Sutured Wounds

Obesity is associated with a higher incidence of wound complications, such as surgical site infection and wound dehiscence (Anaya and Dellinger, 2006; Bamgbade et al, 2007; Franz et al, 2008). A significant contributing factor is hypoperfusion of adipose tissue due to the higher ratio of tissue mass to capillaries in adipose tissue. The resulting decreased oxygen tension in adipose tissue is essentially inadequate to meet the oxygen needs of the healing surgical incision (Anaya and Dellinger, 2006). Additional factors that contribute to the increased rate of surgical site infections in the obese patient include perioperative hyperglycemia (obesity is associated with insulin resistance and hyperglycemia), prolonged operative time (operative time is an independent predictor of surgical site infection), and suboptimal doses of prophylactic antibiotics to achieve therapeutic tissue concentrations (Anaya and Dellinger, 2006). In addition to optimizing tissue oxygen tension as discussed in Chapters 28 and 34, Anaya and Dellinger recommend tight perioperative glucose control, larger doses of prophylactic antibiotics to maximize serum and tissue concentrations intraoperatively, and performance of laparoscopic operations whenever feasible.

Incised and sutured wounds are expected to create a watertight seal within 48 hours; however, wound healing can be delayed in some obese patients due to malnutrition if the patient has a diet that lacks essential vitamins and nutrients. When the incision is within a skin fold, wound healing can be delayed due to moisture entrapment and bioburden in the skin fold. A well-placed and well-constructed stoma will be critical to prevent postoperative peristomal and stoma complications that can be aggravated by irregularities in abdominal topography (Gallagher and Gates, 2004).

To reduce the occurrence of abdominal wound separation, a surgical binder can be used to support the surgical incision. The binder should rest no higher than 4 cm below the xiphoid process and should allow 2.5 cm of space between the skin and binder to avoid constricting the chest wall and hampering ventilation. Binders are especially important when the patient ambulates. Some patients find the binders so comfortable that they ask to leave the binder on at all times. Regular and routine skin assessments of the area under the binder are important to monitor for signs of early pressure-related breakdown.

Hypoventilation Syndrome and Sleep Apnea

Morbidly obese patients tend to have pulmonary problems, two in particular: obesity hypoventilation syndrome and sleep apnea. Obesity hypoventilation syndrome is an acute respiratory condition in which the weight of fatty tissue on the rib cage and chest prevents the chest wall from expanding fully. Because patients are unable to breathe in and out fully, ventilatory insufficiency can occur (Gallagher, 2004).

Sleep apnea usually occurs when the patient is asleep in the supine position. The weight of the excess fatty tissue in the neck causes the throat to narrow, severely restricting or even cutting off breathing for seconds or even minutes at a time. Breathing can be made easier by keeping the patient in the semi-Fowler position, which takes some of the pressure off the diaphragm. Mobilizing the patient as early as possible also will help. At home, many patients manage the problems of nighttime sleep apnea by using a continuous positive airway pressure machine (Shinohara et al, 1997). However, in the health care setting, some patients use bilevel positive airway pressure for a short time after extubation.

Tracheostomy Care

If long-term ventilatory support becomes necessary, performing a tracheostomy can be especially challenging if the trachea is buried deep within fatty tissue. A large wound may be needed in order to locate the trachea. This larger wound can lead to complications such as bleeding, infection, or damage to the surrounding tissue. Postoperative tracheostomy care, therefore, must include steps to protect the peristomal skin, manage the tracheostomy, and contain wound drainage. Locally, a nonadhesive absorptive wound dressing is appropriate. Compounding the potential skin-related problems associated with a tracheostomy in the obese patient is the inadequacy of standard-sized tracheostomy tubes for use in patients with larger necks. In addition, narrow cloth tracheostomy ties can burrow deep within the folds of neck, further damaging the skin. Wider tracheostomy tie material should be used to accommodate the obese patient. When additional pressure relief is needed under the tracheostomy tie, padding such as a gauze or foam dressing can be applied between the skin and the tie.

NUTRITIONAL CONSIDERATIONS

Research suggests that 7% to 12% of the obese population in general is malnourished (Moize et al, 2003). Macronutrients and micronutrients have long been recognized as essential in skin integrity and wound healing among all individuals but especially in those at risk, such as obese patients, whose nutritional status may be compromised because of repeated dieting and weight cycling, simple misunderstanding of proper nutrition, or weight loss surgery. Weight loss surgery is a metabolic surgery designed to produce malnutrition. Energy deficit occurs due to decreased food intake, food intolerance, and nutrient malabsorption. The goal in weight loss surgery or any weight loss program is to achieve monitored weight loss without adverse complications. However, nutritional deficiencies and their consequences can occur if additional unforeseen events occur, such as injury to the skin and wound development. Critically ill obese individuals are already at risk for inflammatory issues that predispose them to sepsis at a rate greater than that of their lean peers. This becomes especially problematic in the face of protein deficiencies because protein malnutrition leads to even more severe inflammation and increased overall morbidity.

The malabsorptive procedures performed for purposes of weight loss carry the risk of interfering with absorption of iron, calcium, and the fat-soluble vitamins, such as vitamins A, D, E, and K. Chapter 27 discusses the role and dietary sources of these nutrients; Table 27-6 lists their specific relevance to the wound repair process.

QUALITY IMPROVEMENT

Even with good education, clinical skills, and motivation, the delivery of safe, effective skin and wound care still can be extremely challenging. In managing the skin care needs of the obese patient, preplanning for equipment is an essential first step (see Checklist 35-1). However, it simply is not sufficient to adequately prevent the costly, predictable complications that occur in caring for obese patients and their skin. A comprehensive, interdisciplinary patient care approach is necessary to provide safe patient care in a timely, cost-effective manner but also to prevent caregiver injury. This approach should include (1) a bariatric task force, (2) a criteria-based protocol, which includes preplanning equipment, (3) competencies/skill set, and (4) outcome measurement efforts.

Bariatric Task Force

The bariatric task force is an interdisciplinary quality improvement effort designed to address ongoing issues and ideas. The value of an interdisciplinary approach cannot be overlooked. Pharmacists, physical/occupational and respiratory therapists, physicians, clinical nurse specialists, the wound specialist, and others are essential in planning care. Each member of the team brings a unique and important perspective and should attend sensitivity training by a nationally accredited body. The entire health care team must be diligent in caring for the morbidly obese patient.

Criteria-Based Protocol

Health care facilities, regardless of where care is delivered, should have a plan in place for the special skin care needs of the morbidly obese patient. This could include resources such as equipment or clinical experts. A criteria-based protocol is simply preplanning based on specifically designated criteria. The patient's weight, BMI, body width, and clinical condition serve as such criteria (Gallagher, 2002). Actual weight is particularly useful because breakage, failure to function properly, or patient or caregiver injury can occur if the weight limit of equipment is exceeded. Body width is described as the patient's body at his or her widest point, which could be at the hips, the shoulders, across the belly when side-lying, or ankle-to-ankle. Furthermore, any clinical condition that interferes with mobility, such as pain, sedation, fear, or resistance to participating in care, places the patient at risk. Criteria-based protocols should be designed to meet the needs of the patient by ensuring access to resources, such as specialty equipment and clinical experts, in a timely, cost-effective manner (Gallagher et al, 2004).

Communication and timing are critical to prevent the costly, predictable, and often preventable complications associated with caring for very complex patients. Although sometimes difficult to arrange, a face-to-face interdisciplinary conference, which is planned within 24 hours of admission or service, may prevent costly intervention later. Consider including the patient's significant other because this person may offer insight into the patient's special needs. Documentation of meetings, individual goals, and corresponding intervention may protect the institution from risk. This level of accountability also outlines more fully each clinician's responsibilities and, when the timing is right, smoothes the transition from one health care setting to another.

Competency Skill Sets

Minimizing the challenges that basic care of the obese patient can present is simple. Typically straightforward tasks such as patient repositioning and urinal placement can require several staff members and various skills to accomplish these tasks safely and effectively. Education to ensure basic skills or competencies is imperative. In creating the bariatric care program, initially a survey to the staff can be used to determine their actual learning needs. Members of the bariatric task force can serve as a pool of experts to develop lesson plans and education addressing identified clinical needs. For example, when clinicians are seeking information on caregiver safety, a physical/occupational therapist, nurse expert, risk manager, and patient member of the task force could develop a 1-hour module to teach these skills.

Outcomes Measurement

In order to ensure the success of a comprehensive bariatric program, it is essential to monitor and collect relevant and appropriate outcomes. Patient and staff satisfaction, safety, and unexpected or adverse outcomes are among the issues that should be monitored.

SUMMARY

With obesity on the rise, wound care providers are increasingly responsible for managing the needs of this complex patient population. Although equipment is a helpful adjunct to care, it is never a substitute for care. Numerous resources are available. Compiling these resources in the form of a comprehensive bariatric care plan may ensure the most favorable outcome. The obese patient poses many care challenges, and it is in the interest of health care organizations to meet these skin and wound care challenges in a clinically, ethically, and legally sound manner.

REFERENCES

American Society for Metabolic and Bariatric Surgery: *Rationale for the surgical treatment of morbid obesity*, 2001, available at www.asmbs.org, accessed March12, 2009.

Anaya DA, Dellinger EP: The obese surgical patient: a susceptible host for infection, *Surg Infect* 7:473-480, 2006.

Aronne LJ, Isoldi KK: Mechanisms that influence body weight regulation. In Rosenthal RR, Jones DB, editors: *Weight loss surgery: a multidisciplinary approach*, Malvern, Penn, 2008, Matrix Medical Communications.

Bamgbade OA et al: Postoperative complications in obese and nonobese patients, *World J Surg* 31:556-560, 2007.

Barrios L, Jones DB: Healthcare economics of weight loss surgery, *Bariatr Times* 4(8):1, 16-17, 20-21, 2007.

Camden SG: Pressure ulcers, CMS and patients of size, *Bariatr Times*, 5(12):1, 8-13, 2008.

Camden SG: Childhood obesity looms large, *Nurs Manage* 40(2):25-32, 2009.

Camden SG, Brannan S, Davis P: Best practices for sensitive care and the obese patient: task report, *Bariatr Nurs Surg Patient Care* 3(3):189-196, 2008.

Charles S: Psychological evaluation of morbidly obese patients, *Gastroenterol Clin North Am* 16(3):41-47, 1987.

Davidson J, Callery C: Care of the obesity surgery patient requiring immediate-level care or intensive care, *Obesity Surg* 11:93-97, 2001.

Engel BT et al: Prevalence incidence and correlates of urinary incontinence in healthy middle aged women, *J Urol* 46(5):1255, 1991.

Fox HR: Discrimination: alive and well in the United States, *Obesity Surg* 5:352, 1995.

Franz MG et al: Guidelines to aid healing of acute wounds by decreasing impediments of healing, *Wound Repair Regen* 16(6):723-748, 2008.

Gallagher S: Obesity and the skin care in the critical care area, *Crit Care Nurs Q* 25(1):69, 2002.

Gallagher S: Bariatrics: considering mobility, patient safety, and caregiver injury. In Charney W, Hudson A, editors: *Back injury among healthcare workers*, Baton Rouge, La., 2004, Lewis Publishers.

Gallagher S, Gates J: Challenges of ostomy care and obesity, *Ostomy Wound Manage* 50(9):38, 2004.

Gallagher S et al: Preplanning protocols for skin and wound care in obese patients, *Adv Skin Wound Care* 17(8):436, 2004.

Knudsen AM, Gallagher S: Care of the obese patient with pressure ulcers, *J Wound Ostomy Continence Nurs* 30:111, 2003.

Kral JG et al: Perioperative risk management in obese patients. In Deitel M, editor: *Surgery for the morbidly obese patient*, North York, Canada, 2000, FD-Communications.

Kramer K, Gallagher S: WOC nurses as advocates for patients who are morbidly obese: a case study promoting use of bariatric beds, *J Wound Ostomy Continence Nurs* 31(1):276, 2004.

Kuczmarski RJ et al: Increasing prevalence of overweight among US adults. The National Health and Nutrition Examination surveys, 1960 to 1991, *JAMA* 272(3):205-211, 1994.

Lanz P et al: Socioeconomic factors, health behavior and mortality, *JAMA* 279(2):1703, 1998.

Lasater-Erhard M: The effect of patient position of arterial oxygen saturation, *Crit Care Nurs Q*, 15:31, 1995.

Ludwig DS, Pollack HA: Obesity and the economy, *JAMA* 301(5):533-535, 2009.

Mathison CJ: Skin and wound care challenges in the hospitalized morbidly obese patient, *J Wound Ostomy Continence Nurs* 30(2):78-83, 2003.

Medical Network: Foot problems: foot problems as symptoms and warning signs, 1999-2001, 2004, available at http://www.nlm.nih.gov/medlineplus/ency/article/003183.htm, accessed June 28, 2010.

Moize V et al: Obese patients have inadequate protein intake related to protein status up to 1 year following Roux-en-Y gastric bypass, *Obes Surg* 13:23-28, 2003.

Ogden CL et al: *Obesity among adults in the United States—no change since 2003-2004, NCHS brief data no. 1*, Hyattesville, Md., 2007, National Center for Statistics.

Pokorny ME: Lead in: skin physiology and disease in the obese patient, *Bariatr Nurs Surg Patient Care* 3(2):125-128, 2008.

Puhl RM, Heuer CA: The stigma of obesity: a review and update, *Obesity* 17(5):941-964, 2009.

Rose M: Nurse staffing requirements for care of morbidly obese patients in the acute care setting, *Bariatr Nurs Surg Patient Care* 1:115-120, 2006.

Shinohara E et al: Visceral fat accumulation as an important risk factor for obstructive sleep apnea syndrome in obese subjects, *J Intern Med* 241:11, 1997.

Steers WD, Suratt PM: Sleep apnea as a cause of daytime and nocturnal enuresis, *Lancet* 349(9069):1604, 1997.

Thone RR: *Fat: a fate worse than death*, New York, 1997, Harrington Park Press.

Whittemore A et al: Specialized staff and equipment for weight loss surgery patients: best practice guidelines, *Obes Res* 13:283-289, 2005.

36

Skin Care Needs of the Pediatric and Neonatal Patient

Part I: The Pediatic Patient   *Part II: The Neonate*

Teri Coha   Annette B. Wysocki, Ruth A. Bryant, and Denise P. Nix

OBJECTIVES

1. Define the terms infancy, neonate, premature, and micropreemie.
2. Identify skin, risk, and pain assessment tools designed for pediatric patients.
3. Discuss special considerations for neonatal skin care, including bathing and use of cleansers, antiseptics, and emollients.
4. List risk factors for skin breakdown in pediatric patients.
5. Describe common pediatric skin conditions and age-specific interventions.
6. Identify wound care products that can be used for pediatric patients.
7. Describe assessment tools and prevention strategies.

Pediatrics is a branch of medicine that deals with the care of infants, children, adolescents, and young adults. It is a specialty derived from the idea that children are not simply little adults but have their own special developmental and health needs. Similarly, neonatology has evolved into the specialty care of the premature infant, who has special physical and developmental needs unique from those of the full-term infant. This chapter addresses the skin and wound care needs of the pediatric patient-followed by the unique needs of the neonate.

PART I: THE PEDIATRIC PATIENT Teri Coha

Infants and children experience alterations in skin integrity related to congenital conditions, poor nutrition, severe illnesses, surgical procedures, and trauma. Box 36-1 lists factors and conditions that place the pediatric patient at risk for skin breakdown. Infants and children born with congenital anomalies often require surgical intervention. Children with anorectal or urinary tract malformations may need a colostomy, ileostomy, or urostomy, any of which places them at risk for developing peristomal skin issues. Children with swallowing difficulties and those with significant caloric needs that cannot be met with oral feedings alone require a gastrostomy tube, another potential source of skin breakdown. Incontinence-associated dermatitis (i.e., diaper rash) is a common problem in children after closure of an ostomy and in children who have diarrhea associated with short bowel syndrome or cancer treatments. Additionally, although more common in adults, pressure ulcers can develop in children. The wound care nurse plays an essential role in the management of children and can significantly impact the child's experience by minimizing the frequency of dressing changes with the use of advanced wound care products and by reducing the use of adhesives with creative methods of securing dressings. Although children vary significantly in size, the availability of a large number of dressings or multiple sizes of products is not necessary. A few key products can fulfill all requirements because most dressings can be cut to fit the needs of the pediatric patient.

COMMON PEDIATRIC CONDITIONS

Infants and children who require fecal or urinary stomas are at risk for wound dehiscence and peristomal skin breakdown. When the corrective surgery is completed and the stoma is closed, incontinence-associated

BOX 36-1	Risk Factors for Pediatric Skin Breakdown

- Neurologic deficits (affect mobility, ability to sense pain and communicate pain)
- Changes in height and weight with growth (may develop new pressure points with medical equipment such as wheelchairs and orthotic devices)
- Medications that alter body's ability to heal or increase likelihood of skin breakdown (chemotherapeutic agents, immunosuppressive medications)
- Alterations in nutrition, particularly feeding disorders requiring gastrostomy tube
- Factors that impair perfusion (edema, vasopressors)
- Medical equipment that limits position and mobility (extracorporeal membrane oxygenation, dialysis catheters)
- Medical devices that require adhesives to secure or that can cause pressure (endotracheal, nasogastric, vascular access tubes; bilevel positive airway pressure masks; monitoring equipment; electrodes)
- Prolonged hospitalization in intensive care unit
- Frequent or prolonged exposure to urine and/or stool
- Congenital anomalies requiring surgery
- Obesity

dermatitis is a frequent problem. The most common malformations and diseases that may require a stoma are described here.

Necrotizing enterocolitis is primarily a disease of premature infants who have started feedings. It is believed to result from decreased blood flow to the vascular system of the bowel and the inability of the premature infant to defend against bacterial toxins in the intestine. Infection and inflammation develop and evolve into segments of intestinal necrosis that usually are confined to the small intestine. Initially infants are managed with bowel rest, antibiotics, and total parenteral nutrition. Surgical intervention may be necessary for infants who do not respond to medical management and for those in whom bowel perforation occurs. During the operation, necrotic sections of bowel are removed. Necrotic bowel may be interspersed with segments of normal bowel, so multiple stomas may be brought through one incision in an attempt to save as much intestine as possible. These premature infants are very ill and are at risk for mucocutaneous junction separation, leaving a large open wound around the stoma. Pouching is difficult because of the small abdominal area of infants. Caring for these infants is challenging for the staff. The basics of wound care must be applied along with a great deal of support for the staff and parents.

Hirschsprung's Disease is the absence of ganglion cells (parasympathetic nerves) in the intramural wall of the bowel. Ganglion cells are necessary for contraction of the bowel, which propels stool forward toward the rectum and eventually leads to defecation. In the absence of ganglionic cells, peristalsis is impaired and a functional obstruction results. Hirschsprung's Disease most often affects the rectosigmoid region but can involve greater lengths of the colon and small intestine. Most infants are diagnosed shortly after birth. They generally fail to pass meconium during the first 24 hours of life and have problems with constipation. Children with Hirschsprung's Disease will require a diverting ostomy (colostomy or ileostomy), removal of the aganglionic segment of bowel, anastomosis of the healthy bowel with the rectum, and closure of the ostomy. This is often a staged surgical procedure beginning with creation of a colostomy or ileostomy.

Anorectal malformation is a term used to describe the failure of the rectum to migrate in utero to connect with the anus. It includes a spectrum of congenital anomalies of the rectum and urinary and reproductive structures that vary significantly in complexity. Boys often have a rectourinary fistula, which is an abnormal communication between the rectum and the urinary tract. Girls generally have a fistula to the genitalia or perineum. A persistent cloaca is a more serious form of imperforate anus in girls that involves the fusion of the rectum, vagina, and urinary tract into a single common channel. The channel exits through one orifice located at the normal urethral site. Corrective surgery is necessary for all of these malformations. The operations are often staged, with the first stage being creating an ostomy (O'Connor Guardino, 2007).

Other congenital and acquired conditions that place the child at risk for skin and wound problems include feeding disorders, burns, obesity, and rare skin disorders.

Feeding disorders in children occur due to a variety of reasons. When feeding problems or supplemental nutritional needs are likely to last longer than a few months, placement of a gastrostomy tube may be necessary. Children may be born with anatomic defects of the mouth, esophagus, trachea, or stomach that prevent safe oral intake of food. Infants and children with neurologic deficits also have difficulty swallowing, or they may aspirate feedings. Children with human immunodeficiency virus or cystic fibrosis may require a gastrostomy tube to provide extra calories so that they can maintain a healthy weight or to administer medications. A variety of procedures are used to create a gastrostomy. Regardless of the technique used, children with a gastrostomy are at risk for skin breakdown from drainage, pressure, and balloon or mushroom displacement.

Epidermolysis bullosa (EB) is a skin condition involving various defects in the epidermal basement membrane. Manifestations include blisters and erosion in the skin and may affect the mucous membranes. EB precipitates significant caloric needs. Because children may have difficulty with oral intake due to oral lesions and esophageal strictures, a feeding tube may be necessary. Children with EB are often managed by physicians and nurses who specialize in their care. EB is described in greater detail in Chapter 30.

Burns, specifically scald and contact burns, most commonly occur in infants and toddlers. Toddlers are at high risk for sustaining burns as they begin to walk and grab onto tables, tablecloths, and radiators to pull themselves up to a standing position. Hot liquids pulled down from tables result in burns to the head, face, and chest. Radiator-type heaters are exposed in many homes and may be extremely hot, resulting in palm burns to infants as they begin exploring their environment. Hot water tanks set higher than 120°F put children at risk during bathing. Burns in children may also be associated with child abuse or neglect. The epidemiology, pathophysiology, and management of burns are discussed in detail in Chapter 32.

Obesity presents potential problems such as pressure ulcers, delayed wound healing, and wound dehiscence. Based on expert committee recommendations (Institute of Medicine and American Academy of Pediatrics), children with a body mass index percentile for age and sex in the 95th percentile or higher are considered obese (Chen and Escarce, 2010). As in the general population, the frequency of obesity in children has increased dramatically; the overall prevalence of obesity among children and adolescents aged 2-19 increased from 5.5% in 1980 to 16.9% in 2008 (Ogden and Carroll, 2010). The 2007 to 2008 National Health and Nutrition Examination Survey reported that 10.4% of 2- to 5-year-olds, 19.6% of 6- to 11-year-olds, and 18.1% of 12- to 19-year-olds were obese (Ogden and Carroll, 2010). The pathophysiology, prevention, and management of obesity-related skin problems are discussed in Chapter 35.

TOPICAL WOUND MANAGEMENT: DRESSINGS AND DRESSING CHANGES

Chapters 16 to 18 provide details on wound bed preparation and the principles of wound management, principles that guide the care of wounds in patients of any age. Considerations specific to the needs of children are addressed in this chapter.

Planning Wound Assessments and Dressing Changes

Providing assistance with skin care and wounds for infants and children requires planning. Premature infants need a great deal of undisturbed sleep for growth and development. The components of care of the premature infant, such as vital signs, blood draws, diaper changes, and feedings, are scheduled, when possible, to be done together at specific intervals so that the infant can sleep undisturbed for 3 to 6 hours at a time. Wound care, stoma pouch changes, and gastrostomy site care are best timed to occur during the infant's other care. This requires some advance planning with the nurse responsible for the infant.

Scheduled visits with the parent and/or the nurse when they are providing wound care for toddlers and older children are important to limit interruptions in the child's routine and to demonstrate respect for the needs of the child, the parent, and the nurse. Waking a sick irritable child who recently (or finally) fell asleep ignores the child's need for sleep and complicates the staff's workload by requiring them to settle the child again. On the other hand, the parent or nurse may be eager to have the child's wound or skin evaluated, and they may be quite willing to wake the child. Or the child may have already been asleep for several hours, and waking him or her will not pose a problem. Although nurse colleagues will be appreciative of assistance from an experienced wound/ostomy nurse, they also will be protective of the developmental needs of the child and will appreciate the effort of health care providers who respect the infant's needs for sleep. Coordinating schedules with the staff results in the best possible patient care.

Before making a decision on a dressing, it is advantageous to confer with any medical and surgical services involved with the patient's care. The most appropriate dressing may be one that remains in place for several days. However, if other services (e.g., infectious disease, orthopedics, or neurosurgery) need to assess the wound and will remove the dressing, it may be best, at least temporarily, to use a dressing that is easily removed with minimal discomfort. After everyone involved has evaluated the wound, a dressing that minimizes the frequency of dressing changes should be used.

Minimize Dressing Change Frequency

Dressing changes often are painful, and the experience can be quite traumatic for a child. Children endure many painful experiences during an illness or injury that cannot be mitigated. However, nurses can alter the pain experienced during dressing changes by choosing advanced wound care products that reduce the frequency of dressing changes and by selecting methods of securing dressings that eliminate or limit the use of adhesive tape. Box 36-2 lists a summary of issues to consider when selecting and securing dressings for pediatric use.

Although some colleagues will not appreciate the advantage of high-tech dressings over gauze for wound healing, most can be convinced of the advantage, to everyone involved, of minimizing the frequency of dressing changes. Alginates and fiber gel-forming dressings are safe and effective for wound care in children and significantly decrease the number of dressing changes. Decreasing the frequency of dressing changes from three times per day to once per day or every other day by using a hydrofiber instead of gauze reduces the stress on the child, parents, and staff. When dressings must be changed more often than once per day, dressings should be secured with wraps or flexible tube netting to reduce

BOX 36-2	Considerations when Selecting and Securing Dressings for Pediatric Use

- Choose products that will minimize the number of dressing changes.
- Eliminate or limit the use of tape.
- Use gauze wraps, elastic wraps, or flexible tube net dressing to secure dressings.
- Limit the use of adhesive removers; clean off skin after use.
- Use antibiotic ointments selectively and cautiously.
- Work with home care companies to carry the products you use in your practice.
- Know the number of dressings allowed per month by insurance carriers.
- Unless you are absolutely certain that the wound will heal in less than 1 month, order supplies for the entire month because some suppliers will ship only once every 30 days.

stress, pain, and the time associated with tape removal (Clinical Example 36-1).

Hydrocolloids do not require frequent dressing changes and are effectively used over eschar, intravenous infiltrates, pressure ulcers, and other small lesions that require protection and/or autolysis. Extra-thin hydrocolloid wafers conform to small body parts, such as heels, wrists, and elbows, and they can be left in place

for 5 to 7 days. The key to successful use of hydrocolloid dressings is education, as the tendency is to change this dressing too often (daily or twice daily). If the wound requires more frequent dressing changes, a different dressing should be selected.

Hydrocolloid dressings can be used to frame a wound that requires frequent dressing changes. By positioning hydrocolloid strips on two or all four sides of the wound, tape can be attached to the hydrocolloid and crossed over the dressing. During dressing changes the hydrocolloid is left in place; the hydrocolloid framing the wound changed every 4 to 5 days as it loosens (Clinical Example 36-2).

Limit or Eliminate Use of Adhesives

The method chosen to secure the dressing is extremely important. Children do not like having tape removed. Because skin irritation and tears can occur even when paper tape is used, dressings should be secured with

CLINICAL EXAMPLE 36-1

Premature infant in neonatal intensive care unit had a large abdominal wound draining copious amounts of fluid.

Subjective:
- Gauze dressing was in place and being changed every 15 minutes.
- Surgeon requests wound pouched with an ostomy pouch.

Objective:
- Large abdominal wound with copious drainage
- Insufficient periwound skin to secure a wafer

Assessment:
- Critically ill infant requires frequent dressing changes that prevent undisturbed rest which is critically important for infant growth and development
- Requires wound dressing to absorb fluid and minimize number of dressing changes

Plan:
- Replace gauze with hydrofiber dressing, which will absorb more drainage.
- Cover with foam dressing.
- Increase length of time between dressing changes.
- Use flexible tube net dressing to hold the dressings in place.

Outcome:
- Length of time between dressing changes increased from every 15 minutes to every 3 hours. Flexible net dressing conformed nicely to infant's abdomen and required little effort to move out of the way during dressing changes. Only the foam was changed every 3 hours and was weighed to document output. Within 48 hours, dressing changes were decreased to every 6 hours.

CLINICAL EXAMPLE 36-2

Five-year-old boy was hospitalized with meningococcemia. After discharge, his mother brought him to the wound clinic for assistance with wound care.

Subjective (Per Mother):
- I was told to change the hydrocolloid dressing twice a day.
- These dressing changes are very upsetting for both my son and me. It is too hard and painful. He has been through so much.
- The deeper wounds are covered with gauze and tape, which are changed three times daily.

Objective:
- Twelve lesions of various sizes and at various stages of healing are present on his back, buttocks, and legs.
- Some wounds were covered with a hydrocolloid; deeper wounds were packed with a hydrofiber, then covered with gauze and tape.
- The child began to cry as soon as he was approached for assessment.

Assessment:
- Both mother and child were upset by dressing changes.
- Frequency of dressing changes is unnecessary and painful.

Plan:
- Hydrocolloid to dry wounds; change every 5 days.
- Hydrofiber covered with gauze, secured with transparent film dressing applied to deeper wounds on legs and buttocks.
- Change every 2–3 days, more frequently only when gauze saturated.
- Instruct mother on correct technique for removing transparent film dressing that minimizes pain.

Outcome:
- At the next visit, mother and child were happy and grateful. The child did not cry when we entered the room. The wounds were healing nicely. Much of the child's discomfort could have been eliminated if a wound care nurse had been consulted early during his hospital stay.

gauze wraps, elastic wraps, self-adhesive wraps, or flexible tube net dressing whenever possible. Two- and three-inch wide conforming gauze is more effective than bulky loose weave gauze (e.g., Kerlix) on the extremities of smaller children. The conforming gauze can be taped to itself, thereby avoiding use of tape on the skin. Flexible tube net can be used to secure a dressing on the extremities of active children. It also performs well around the abdomen or chest of an infant or child to hold abdominal dressings, gastrostomy tubes, and central lines (Clinical Example 36-3).

Flexible net dressings need to be cut long enough to be effective; as they stretch, they decrease in length, roll, and fail to conform to the abdomen. For example, the distance on an infant's abdomen from below the nipples to several inches below the gastrostomy is about 4 to 6 inches. However, once stretched over the abdomen, a 4- to 6-inch piece will become 3 to 4 inches and will not cover the area adequately to secure the dressing. Flexible net dressing should be cut twice the length needed, so for this infant 8 to 10 inches is needed (Figure 36-1).

Elastic wraps and self-adhesive wraps are other options for securing dressings without tape. However, elastic wraps must be applied carefully when used to secure dressings to avoid applying unintended compression.

With the activity typical of infants and children, securing percutaneous tubes and drains is critical to maintain their proper position and to prevent peritubular skin breakdown. Again, flexible tube net dressing is

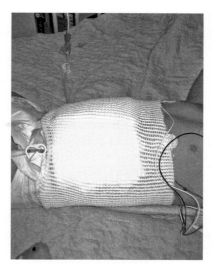

FIGURE 36-1 Flexible net dressing used to secure wound dressings.

invaluable for stabilizing central lines and gastrostomy tubes. The Hollister vertical drain/tube attachment device (Hollister, Inc., Libertyville, Ill., USA) can also be used to secure percutaneous tubes. This dressing encircles the tube site and has a locking ring that secures the tube perpendicular to the skin where the tube exits the tract. Because the percutaneous tube is kept erect at the skin level rather than lying against the skin, the risk of developing a device-related pressure ulcer along the tract is eliminated. For smaller abdomens the paper tape ring from the hydrocolloid portion of the attachment device can be removed. The vertical drain/tube attachment device can be left in place for 5 to 7 days.

The Grip-Lok (Zefon International, Ocala, Fla., USA) is another option for securing percutaneous tubes; however, it should be used cautiously because the tube often slips through the locking tape, creating traction on the tube. This problem can go unnoticed because the dressing of the locking system may not have moved. A pressure ulcer can develop along the tract, or the tube is at risk of being dislodged because it is no longer secured. Tubes are often stabilized more securely by applying a transparent film dressing to cover more of the tube. However, tubes secured by transparent film dressings must be moved every day to prevent development of a device-related pressure ulcer under the tape or along the tract.

Securing dressings in the burned child is particularly challenging because of the burn location and because children are so active. Toddlers are at high risk for sustaining burns to their chest, arms, face, hands, and abdomen as they begin exploring their environment. Burns to the hand are common, especially in cold climates and in homes with radiator heat. Toddlers need their hands to explore and are frustrated when their hands are wrapped. Application of a dressing that they cannot remove is challenging. Unaffected

---

CLINICAL EXAMPLE 36-3

Four-year-old girl was evaluated in the emergency room for a burn covering two thirds of her chest. She returned the following day to the wound clinic for her first dressing change.

Subjective:
- Large piece of gauze secured by bordering the gauze with cloth adhesive tape was used to cover the burn on her chest.

Objective:
- Removing the tape required a great deal of time and adhesive remover.
- The child cried during removal of the tape.
- She did not protest when the partial-thickness burn to her chest was cleaned.

Assessment:
- The method used to secure the dressing was more painful to the patient than the injury.

Plan:
- Apply silver sulfadiazine (Silvadene), then wrap the chest with 4-inch-wide conforming gauze dressing. Use flexible tube net dressing to keep the wrap from slipping.

Outcome:
- Child was very happy with her new "fishnet" shirt that held her dressing in place.

thumbs should be kept out of the dressing whenever possible. Gauze can be wrapped around the wrist to prevent the child from pulling off the dressing. Flexible tube net dressing or socks over the hand will help keep the dressing in place. Flexible net dressing is also useful for securing dressings on an extremity, the abdomen, and the chest. Although self-adhering wraps take more time to apply and remove, they are quite difficult for children to remove and therefore are very effective when the dressing does not need to be changed frequently (Clinical Example 36-3).

At times, use of tape or adhesive products may be unavoidable. Removing tape from a child's skin often proves challenging. Although adhesive removers are used in children's hospitals, they have not been tested for safety on children. When used, they should be washed off the child's skin as soon as possible to minimize the child's exposure to the chemicals in the product.

Adhesive removers can also be avoided by teaching nurses, caregivers, and patients a few key techniques for adhesive removal. This may seem unwarranted because nurses remove tape all the time. However, nurses often are not familiar with the techniques for tape removal that are less painful and damaging to the skin. A skin barrier wafer should be removed by pushing down gently on the skin just in front of the wafer. Tape should be rolled back while the same gentle pressure is applied on the skin just in front of the tape. Transparent film dressings can be removed by stretching them while keeping them horizontal to the skin. By about the age of 4 years, children can learn how to remove tape and ostomy pouch and may be more cooperative if they are allowed to help.

Prevent/Treat Wound Infections

The skin provides a physical barrier to the invasion of microorganisms. This physical barrier is compromised by surgery, trauma, percutaneous tubes, and chronic wounds. The first line of defense against bacterial invasion, infection, and antimicrobial resistance is to keep the wound clean and covered. Most small cuts, surgical incisions on healthy children, and gastrostomy tube sites require no more than routine washing and a cover dressing. Topical antibiotic ointments should not be used routinely because indiscriminate use of topical and systemic antibiotics contributes to the growth of antibiotic-resistant organisms and use of topical antibiotics can lead to delayed hypersensitivity reactions, superinfections, resistance, and contact allergies (White et al, 2006). Specifically, mupirocin or polymyxin may promote the growth of gram-negative bacteria, and polymyxin has an unacceptably high rate of contact sensitization (Darmstadt and Dinulos, 2000). Therefore, topical antibiotic ointments should be used sparingly or not at all on wounds that have limited risk for becoming infected. Topical antibiotics are not an appropriate

treatment option for colonized or infected wounds. Systemic antibiotics are warranted when bacterial infection or cellulitis is present.

Silver-based antimicrobial dressings can be used to inhibit bacterial growth and progression of bacterial penetration. As described in Chapter 16, silver binds to proteins in the cell wall (resulting in rupture of the wall), to bacterial enzymes and proteins (preventing them from performing their function and leading to cell death), and to bacterial cell DNA (interfering with cell division and preventing replication). This ability to bind to multiple sites results in an antimicrobial effect on a wide variety of microorganisms, including aerobic, anaerobic, gram-negative, and gram-positive bacteria, yeast, filamentous fungi, and viruses. This explains why resistance to silver is a rare occurrence (Ovington, 2004; Tomaselli, 2006). Silver is effective for treatment of mild wound infections. It is not indicted for cellulitis because it is effective only on superficial pathogens and not on those that have penetrated into the wound bed (Tomaselli, 2006). A variety of wound care products containing silver are available. Because some silver dressings cannot be mixed with normal saline, the wound should be cleaned with water and, if indicated, the dressing moistened with water. Evidence showing that silver dressings have no negative systemic or local effects is limited. Therefore, silver dressing should be used judiciously, for 2 to 4 weeks, until more research is available (Clinical Example 36-4) (Stotts, 2007).

Control Pain

Large pieces of dressings are often aggressively packed in a wound, particularly after an incision and drainage of an abscess is performed in the emergency room or

---

CLINICAL EXAMPLE 36-4

Healthy 15-year-old boy had undergone surgery to correct a rib deformity of his chest. Six months later, the top 2 cm of the midline incision had not healed.

Subjective:
- He is really healthy. I don't know why this will not heal.

Objective:
- Healthy 15-year-old is 6 months post pectus deformity repair.
- Incision has healed except for proximal 2 cm.
- Wound is clean and moist; wound bed is pink, with no signs of infection.

Assessment:
- Colonized wound in healthy 15-year-old boy

Plan:
- Cover with silver impregnated hydrogel dressing. Secure with island dressing.

Outcome:
- Wound healed in 7 days.

operating room. Removal of the packing when the child is awake is challenging. Packing often dries out and becomes adherent to the wound surface. Wetting the dressing before removing it will decrease discomfort. Wound packing is not well tolerated by children, is difficult for parents to do, and is generally not necessary. A dressing tucked in just far enough to keep the skin edges open and allow the wound to drain often is sufficient. A cotton-tipped applicator is helpful for gently tucking the dressing in the wound.

ELMA (eutectic mixture of local anesthetics) and cream for topical anesthesia can be used safely on neonates and children prior to painful procedures. The use of EMLA in premature infants of gestational age less than 37 weeks needs further study (Lillieborg, 2004). Features of development such as how a child of a particular age thinks, what they fear, and how they learn are pertinent to helping children cope with procedures like dressing changes (Table 36-1).

Safe Dressings for Preterm Infants

Transparent dressings have been evaluated extensively for use in preterm infants. They are versatile for securing wound dressings and catheters because they easily conform over wounds of various sizes and shapes, and they allow easy visualization of the site. Transparent, semipermeable film dressings provide an artificial epidermal layer for fragile, preterm skin and are effective at preventing trauma while providing a moist environment for reepithelialization of injured skin (Darmstadt and Dinulos, 2000). Transparent dressings allow some passage of water vapor, oxygen, and carbon dioxide, permitting the epidermal barrier to mature normally while resident and pathogenic bacteria and fungal populations are unchanged. The dressings can be left on for long periods, thus minimizing skin stripping when the dressings are removed. Hydrocolloids can also be used safely on preterm infants. The vertical drain/tube

TABLE 36-1	Features of Development that Are Pertinent to Helping Children Cope with Procedures			
	Birth–2 Years	**2–7 Years**	**7–12 Years**	**Adolescence**
How the child thinks and solves problems	Sensory motor experience develops schema (well-defined and repeated sequences of actions and perceptions) Memory is obvious by 3–4 months Begins using symbols for thought reasoning between 18 and 24 months	Thinking is dominated by perceptions rather than logic Verbal communication important for learning Exploratory manipulations helps child learn Child watches, listens, asks questions (Why? How?) Classifies similar things Perceptions limited to single salient feature, so difficult for child to differentiate unessential from essential properties of an experience Uses memory to reconstruct past events Uses imagination to cope Egocentric point of view	Learns from interacting with peers and own experiences Able to understand viewpoints of others Able to see relative nature of things (e.g., this hurts a little; that hurts a lot) Uses deductive logic with respect to tangible (concrete) experiences (if this, then that) Able to view things in context (e.g., "the shot hurt, but it will make me better") Evaluates painful intensive actions in terms of logical function rather than punishment Understands unseen body mechanics/functions Makes use of sensory and procedural information	Uses reason and logical thinking Interested in theoretically possible problems and questions Able to engage in self-reflection Learns from verbally presented ideas and arguments
Major fears and worries	Separation from parents Anything unfamiliar, especially when not with a parent	Separation from parents Harm to body Punishment for wrongdoing	Body injury Loss of body functions Loss of control	Uncertain about self as person Concerned if body, thoughts, feelings are "normal"
Understanding cause and effect	By about 3 months, may associate an action with a result In second year: magical thinking; believes that what is wished for happens	Everything happens by intention Misbehavior is followed by punishment Interprets unrelated events to be related	Prior to about 9 years, views illness as a consequence of transgressions of rules At about 9 years, begins to understand that illness may have multiple causes	Uses formal rules of logic and evidence to assess cause and effect

From Pridham K et al: Helping children deal with procedures in a clinic setting: a developmental approach, *J Pediatr Nurs* 2:13-22, 1987.

attachment device (Hollister, Inc.) can be used to secure tubes on newborn infants. If the umbilical cord is still intact, a small portion of the dressing should be trimmed away to allow the cord to remain uncovered so that it can dry out.

Safetac technology dressings (Molnlycke Health Care, Norcross, Ga., USA) are also safe for use on preterm infants and are excellent over wounds and under tubes to protect the skin. The silicone backing effectively holds the dressing in place without the use of tape and is easily removed from the skin without skin stripping.

INCONTINENCE-ASSOCIATED DERMATITIS

Incontinence-associated dermatitis or diaper rash is a common problem among children. Management is particularly challenging for children with Hirschsprung's Disease, imperforate anus, cloaca and cloacal extrophy, short bowel syndrome, inflammatory bowel disease, and other congenital anomalies or diseases that affect the digestive tract and require a corrective colorectal and/or urinary tract operation. After surgery, children often have frequent bowel movements that result in severe skin breakdown of the perineal area. Children undergoing chemotherapy may have diarrhea resulting in irritant-associated dermatitis.

Incontinence-associated dermatitis generally affects the skin in greatest contact with the diaper, including the convex areas of the buttocks, medial thighs, mons pubis, labia majora, and scrotum. The perianal area is not in contact with the diaper but also is affected because stool is held in the gluteal fold (Shin, 2005). As with the treatment of wounds, many misconceptions exist about the best method for treating incontinence-associated dermatitis. One common belief is that healing will occur by exposing the skin to air and letting the skin dry out. Caregivers will allow the child to crawl around without a diaper and may use a hair dryer to dry out the skin. This inappropriate practice is not surprising given that the same misconception about wounds is prevalent. When children are having frequent bowel movements, leaving the buttocks open to air exposes their skin to damage from the effluent of the next bowel movement.

Treatment of incontinence-associated dermatitis requires the same strategies used for treatment of wounds. The skin is cleansed gently no more than once or twice daily (to prevent mechanical damage from overly aggressive cleansing), followed by application of a barrier paste (a type of ointment designed specifically to adhere to moist surfaces) for protection from fecal incontinence (Box 36-3). Creams containing zinc oxide can be used on healthy children with mild irritation. However, children who have undergone colorectal or urinary tract procedures often suffer from severe perianal denudation and require aggressive management with a barrier paste.

BOX 36-3	Treatment of Incontinence-Associated Dermatitis

- Apply thick layer of barrier paste to all affected areas.
- Apply petrolatum or powder over paste so that it does not stick to the diaper.
- Change diapers frequently.
- Apply additional paste and petrolatum as necessary *without removing the paste that remains on the skin.*
- Gently remove all paste once or twice daily by soaking in a tub or with mineral oil or a commercial cleanser.

Product ingredients for a barrier paste includes emollients to protect and sooth the skin (almond oil, aloe vera, dimethicone copolyol, lanolin, glycerin, mineral oil, petrolatum), humectants to prevent drying by binding moisture to the skin (D-panthenol, propylene glycol, sodium pyrrolidone carbonic acid, glycerin), and surfactants to decrease the amount of friction necessary to remove stool and urine (poloxamer 188, potassium palmitate, polysorbate). Dimethicone, karaya powder, and carboxymethylcellulose are ingredients that aid in application to wet surfaces. Barrier pastes may also contain antimicrobials to decrease skin infections (Fiers, 1996; Foster, 2008; Nix, 2000).

The barrier paste is applied to the skin in a thick layer, similar to cake frosting, with each diaper change. Residual paste is not removed. A skin barrier powder can be used on very weepy skin before the paste is applied to help with application and adherence. (When powders are used, care must be taken to protect the infant's face in order to prevent him or her from inhaling the powder.) The last step is the application of a thin layer of petrolatum or a dusting with a skin barrier powder on top of the paste so that the paste does not stick to the diaper and remains on the skin during diaper changes.

Complete removal of all of the barrier paste must be limited to no more than once or twice daily. More frequent cleaning results in mechanical trauma to the skin and can delay healing. Caretakers struggle with the idea of leaving barrier paste that might contain stool on the skin and fail to recognize the significance of the mechanical damage that occurs with constant cleaning. If allowed, the child can soak in a bath tub to gently remove the paste. Mineral oil, baby oil, and commercial cleansers will also remove the paste without trauma. Commercial cleansing sprays are best applied to a wipe or washcloth instead of directly on the skin because the sprays are cold and can startle infants. Foam formulations are generally preferred. Constant education and reinforcement are necessary to prevent caregivers from removing all of the barrier paste with each diaper change.

A variety of barrier products are available. Products formulated with karaya or carboxymethylcellulose, which helps with application to wet or denuded skin, are generally more expensive and may be cost prohibitive, in which case a less expensive paste and skin barrier powder may be the only option. Barrier pastes may be covered by insurance, and in some states public assistance will pay for them, although a letter of medical necessity may be required. Box 36-4 lists over-the-counter products that often are effective. Familiarity with a few products is important because a product that works well for some children may not work well for others. Parents have reported that alternating products is helpful. Mixing products is not recommended outside of a pharmacy and in general is not necessary given the variety of commercially available barrier pastes.

Diapers must be changed frequently, preferably after each bowel movement and at least once during the night to limit the skin's exposure to urine and feces. Tight-fitting diapers hold irritants against the skin and should be avoided. Cloth diapers allow urine and feces to mix, activating the fecal proteases that may contribute to dermatitis. The airtight plastic pants used to cover cloth diapers prevent evaporation of water from the skin, thereby increasing hydration of the skin (Shin, 2005). Modern cloth diapers are designed with layers to increase absorbency. Disposable diapers have a synthetic material next to the skin that promotes passage of liquid through to the next layer, providing a dry surface next to the infant's skin. The core of some brands of diapers contains an absorbent gel material that can hold 80 times its weight in liquid. Urine is trapped in the gel, preventing further contact with the skin. However, the outer cover may contain an impenetrable film barrier that prevents urine leakage, and this occlusive layer can keep the skin under the diaper more hydrated. Some brands of diapers have a microporous membrane that is permeable to air and vapor but impervious to liquid, keeping the skin drier and aiding in treatment of diaper dermatitis (Akin et al, 2001).

Cotton washcloths may be recommended over disposable baby wipes for cleaning irritated perineal skin because of concerns that the components of the wipes will cause additional damage. However, several studies found that alcohol-free, scent-free disposable wipes may be superior to washcloths in terms of skin gentleness and preventing or minimizing mechanical trauma during wiping (Fiers, 1996; Odio et al, 2001). In addition, Fiers (1996) found no difference in the sensation of stinging between the two.

BOX 36-4	Common Over-the-Counter Skin Barrier Products

- Ilex Skin Protectant Paste (Medcon Bio Lab Technologies, Inc.)
- Sensi-Care Protective Barrier (ConvaTec)
- Calmoseptine Ointment (Calmoseptine, Inc.)
- Critic-Aid Anorectal Skin Paste (Coloplast Corporation)
- Boudreaux's Butt Paste (George Boudreaux PD; at local pharmacies)

Hydrocolloid wafers have been used in an attempt to protect the perianal skin from stool but are seldom effective. It is difficult to get even the thinnest wafer to conform well to an infant's bottom. Consequently, stool seeps unnoticed under the edges and is held against the skin, causing skin damage.

Candidiasis is frequently a component of severe irritant dermatitis. Candida presents as bright or beefy red erythema with satellite lesions. Unlike irritant dermatitis, it generally involves the skin folds. Nystatin, clotrimazole, and miconazole all are effective topical agents for treatment of candidal diaper dermatitis (Kazaks and Lane, 2000). The antifungal is applied to the skin before the barrier paste twice daily after the skin is cleaned completely. Some barrier pastes contain antifungals, but the amount of antifungal may not be sufficient to be effective.

GASTROSTOMY TUBES

Gastrostomy tubes are placed in children for a variety of feeding disorders. The most common type of gastrostomy tube used in pediatric facilities is the low-profile feeding tube with a balloon such as the MIC-key (Kimberly Clark Corp., Roswell, Ga., USA) or AMT Mini (Applied Medical Technology, Inc., Cleveland, Ohio, USA) or low-profile feeding tube with a mushroom such as the Bard Button (C.R. Bard, Tewksbury, Mass., USA) or AMT capsule (Applied Medical Technology). Complications include peristomal skin irritation, hyperplasia, cellulitis, wound dehiscence (Plate 69), and pressure ulcers.

The most common problems with use of a gastrostomy tube include peristomal skin irritation, denudement, and candidiasis caused by drainage from granulation tissue or leakage of formula. A small amount of drainage is not of great concern and can be easily managed with a 2×2 split gauze or thin foam such as Mepilex Transfer (Molnlycke Health Care). Larger amounts of drainage require investigation into the cause. An evaluation of the gastrostomy tube is important but the cause is often unrelated to the tube. Slow gastric emptying, poor motility, and feeding rates and volumes not tolerated by the child's gastrointestinal tract will result in leakage. Whatever the cause, the skin must be protected until the problem is resolved.

The first step is to evaluate the length of the tube, the volume of water in the balloon, and the length of time since the balloon was last changed. Low-profile tubes should sit gently on the skin and be easy to turn. Tubes that are too long move up and down in the tract, resulting in irritation and possibly leakage. Tubes that are too short compress the skin, causing moisture buildup under the tube that irritates the skin so that a pressure ulcer can develop. Balloons should be filled with the correct volume. Both overinflation and underinflation can create problems. An overinflated balloon may block the gastric outlet, resulting in poor emptying of the stomach. An underinflated balloon can be pulled out easily. The French size of the tube should never be increased to stop leakage. Although leakage may decrease for a day or two, the larger tube inevitably will create a larger stoma that leaks.

Excessive formula leakage will occur with dislodgment of the tube into the tract. This occurs when long gastrostomy tubes are used instead of low-profile tubes. Malecot and de Pezzer tubes can be placed during the initial operation and then changed to low-profile tubes after the tract is healed. The soft, small mushroom tip of these tubes can be pulled into the tract, causing leakage of formula, tissue breakdown similar to a pressure ulcer, and infection. A radiologic study can determine if the tube is located in the stomach or has been pulled into the tract. The tube must be replaced as soon as possible and then stabilized until healing occurs.

A less common gastrostomy tube–related reason for large amounts of formula leakage is blockage of the outlet of the stomach by the balloon, which decreases gastric emptying. The patient may vomit. This complication has occurred in very small infants with balloons that had appropriate volumes and in larger infants with balloons that were improperly overinflated. Although rare, this complication should be considered when evaluating leakage. A radiologic study can evaluate gastric emptying. For very tiny infants, the 5-ml balloon of a 14Fr low-profile tubes may be too large. Decreasing the volume in the balloon is not the best option because the balloon will not inflate to the correct shape, will be soft, and may be pulled out easily. Low-profile tubes that require only 2.5 ml of fluid to fully inflate the balloon are available.

The gastrostomy tube is universally blamed for large volumes of formula leakage. However, children often develop leakage of formula due to an inability to tolerate the volume or the rate of the feeding. Infants and children are generally fed by nasogastric tubes prior to gastrostomy placement. After surgery, children may return to their presurgical feeding rates within a few days. However, some children may take 2 to 3 weeks before they can tolerate the same presurgical rate without leaking. Generally these are children who have always had difficulty tolerating feedings, such as those with complex cardiac anomalies, gastroesophageal reflux, or short bowel syndrome. It is critically important to lengthen the time over which the feedings are given in order to allow the tract to heal and prevent peristomal skin breakdown. A child receiving feedings over 45 minutes may need to have feedings given over 1.5 hours. Some children need a period of continuous feedings.

Another typical scenario for leakage is a child who is doing well at home at a set rate and volume. With the onset of an acute illness such as an upper respiratory infection or virus, the child develops a cough or diarrhea. Depending on the diagnosis, antibiotics may be started. Formula begins to leak around the tube. In this situation,

it is best to slow the rate of feeding until the illness resolves. Critically ill children who are hospitalized and/or ventilated often do not tolerate their previous feeding schedules. Again it may be necessary to give continuous feedings or to stop feedings completely. When feedings are continued in spite of significant leakage, the peristomal skin breaks down from the constant moisture, compounding the problem. Because the child is not receiving any of the calories leaked around the tube, no harm is caused by slowing or discontinuing feedings and supporting the child with intravenous nutrition until feedings are tolerated.

Hyperplasia is the excessive growth of granulation tissue above the level of the skin (Plate 69). Drainage from granulation tissue is most often serosanguineous. The presence of green, yellow or brown drainage, often associated with infection, may occur with or without odor. A small amount of drainage is mostly annoying due to staining on clothes. Excessive granulation tissue may lead to peristomal irritation and candidiasis. Traditionally, hypergranulation tissue was treated with silver nitrate. However, many children cry when silver nitrate is applied despite claims that its use is painless. Kenalog or triamcinolone cream 0.1% and 0.5% applied two to three times daily effectively treats excessive granulation tissue in the majority of cases without the discomfort associated with silver nitrate. Because it is a steroid, triamcinolone cream should be limited to use when granulation tissue is visible. Crusty drainage on the skin may indicate granulation tissue in the tract but does not warrant use of triamcinolone cream. In cases of excessive leakage of formula or drainage from granulation tissue, the skin must be protected from the effluent. Solid wafer barriers are not recommended for these cases because they are not designed to absorb large amounts of fluid and tend to trap moisture around the stoma, causing additional skin damage. The same barrier paste products used for incontinence associated dermatitis can be used to protect the skin around a gastrostomy. An absorbent product such as a foam dressing will also be necessary to wick formula or drainage away from the skin. Foam dressings perform far better than gauze at wicking moisture off the skin. Fenestrated (precut) dressings are generally 3 × 4 inches, which is large for a child. A 4- × 4-inch foam pad cut in quarters is a good size for under skin-level devices. Molnlycke products (Molnlycke Health Care) have a backing that adheres to the skin without the need for tape and are easily removed. If additional dressings are necessary, an elastic wrap or flexible net dressing is an excellent option for securing and stabilizing tubes.

Cutaneous candidiasis can occur wherever the peristomal skin is moist from granulation tissue or leakage of formula. It may be mild, consisting of a few pustules, satellite lesions, and slight erythema, or more severe, with significant erythema and denuded peristomal skin. For mild cases, a topical antifungal ointment or cream is effective. For more severe cases, systemic treatment may be necessary.

Dehiscence of the incision can occur when the tube is placed through an abdominal incision. The wound can be packed with hydrofiber. A 2 × 2 piece of Mepilex transfer (Molnlycke Health Care) cut to fit under the tube and over the incision will hold the hydrofiber in the wound while protecting the peristomal skin by wicking off excess drainage. Stabilizing the tube also is critical with dehiscence of the incision. It may be necessary to stop feedings for 2 to 3 days and to support the patient with intravenous nutrition.

Pressure ulcers occur under any tube that is too tight. A low-profile tube must be changed to one with a longer length. On a long gastrostomy tube, the disk can be adjusted to relieve pressure. If a patient has a pressure ulcer without formula leakage, a solid wafer barrier can be used under the gastrostomy.

Gastrostomy tubes are removed when children can take all their nutrition by mouth. Most gastrostomies will close without intervention. In some cases a fistula may form, and require surgical closure. Until the operation is performed, the skin must be protected. Management of gastrocutaneous fistulas is the same as treatment of leakage: protect the skin with a barrier paste, use foam or gauze (foam is always preferred) to absorb drainage, and stabilize the foam over the site with flexible net dressing or an elastic wrap. Avoid taping these dressings because frequent changes are necessary.

PERISTOMAL WOUNDS AND SKIN BREAKDOWN

Fecal Ostomies

Infants and children with stomas can have stoma-related skin and wound problems (Box 36-5). Often the staff has limited experience with ostomies and wounds. They do their best to manage the wound/ostomy problems without the assistance of an experienced wound or ostomy nurse while they manage the other critical care needs of the infant. Nurses with knowledge of wound care can be invaluable in assisting with stomal wounds and peristomal skin breakdown.

Several factors contribute to peristomal skin irritation and stoma-related wounds. Ostomy surgery in children is rarely a planned event performed when the child's clinical status and nutrition have been optimized. The majority of infants and children undergo surgery when they are critically ill. Stomas are often brought out through the incision due to limited abdominal space and/or to minimize scarring. Infants with necrotizing enterocolitis can have multiple stomas brought through the incision. In addition, critically ill infants are at risk for mucocutaneous junction separation and wound dehiscence. Peristomal skin breakdown often occurs as a result of inappropriate use of products and inexperienced caretakers. Box 36-6 summarizes tips for pouching infant and pediatric stomas. Stoma wafers may not be cut appropriately to fit the stoma. Persons unfamiliar with the measuring guide will approximate the size of the stoma. The stoma may be an odd shape, and staff may have little experience with creating patterns. This is especially true when the patient has multiple stomas. Problems also occur when the same pattern is used without reassessing whether it still matches the shape of the stoma.

A common misconception is that a skin barrier should not be applied over irritated or denuded skin. This misconception most likely comes from the ingrained belief that injured skin should be left open to air. The wafer is cut larger than the stoma to prevent wafer contact with the irritated or denuded skin, resulting in additional skin damage from prolonged exposure to effluent. Providing education that skin barriers are designed to protect from damage and will heal injured skin is essential.

Skin breakdown also occurs when the skin barrier is left on too long. Infant and pediatric skin barriers are designed for delicate skin, but they are not formulated for extended wear. The barrier may appear intact but

---

BOX 36-5 | Problems with Infant/Pediatric Stomas and Stoma Pouching

- Stomas brought through incisions
- Smaller surface area for pouching with interference from monitor leads, umbilical cords, leg creases, gastrostomy tubes
- Rapid growth requiring changes in pouch sizes
- Skin exposed to effluent from wafers that are left on too long; wafer has melted around stoma but edges remain intact
- Paste used incorrectly over entire back of wafer

BOX 36-6 | Tips for Pouching Infant/Pediatric Stomas

- Avoid use of pastes that contain alcohol, which can irritate skin. A syringe can be filled with skin barrier paste to ease the application of a thin bead of paste to the wafer or skin.
- Barrier strips and rings have gentle adhesives and can be cut or molded to specific shape.
- Apply pouch to dry skin absent of wrinkles and creases.
- Change pouch on routine basis (do not wait for it to leak).
- Teach caregivers to assess skin barrier for signs of erosion upon removal.
- Inform parents that another pouch size may be necessary as child grows.
- Cotton balls can be put in pouch to wick effluent off wafer, extending wear time.
- Position pouch so that tail of pouch empties toward infant's side to facilitate emptying into diaper.
- Urinary pouch with antireflux will increase wear time when used to contain liquid output from ileostomy.
- Do not rinse pouch.

may have melted near the stoma, exposing the peristomal skin. The frequency of pouch changes may need to be increased in order to limit peristomal skin breakdown. Teaching nurses how to assess the integrity of the skin barrier and specifically to identify when the barrier is melting is important.

As an infant grows, he will outgrow the pouch initially used. A 5-lb premature infant will have a larger volume of stool by the time he weighs 10 lb. The continued use of premature pouches on a larger infant will result in frequent pouch changes and possible skin breakdown.

Traditional skin barrier pastes are an option for filling in healed incisions and extending the wear time of a pouch. However, they are often used incorrectly, causing additional problems. Because they are called *pastes*, caretakers often use them as they would any other paste, in large amounts over the entire wafer. These pastes contain alcohol, which may irritate the skin. When these pastes must be used, education on their use is essential. Putting a small amount in a syringe is a method for dispensing a bead of paste only where it is needed.

Strip pastes and barrier rings are a significantly better option. They are alcohol-free, can be cut or molded to the shape needed, are easier to remove from the skin, and are more likely to be used correctly. They can be used to increase wear time and to create convexity when needed. Caregivers will require detailed instructions on how to apply strip pastes and rings to the back of the wafer and how to mold the edge to the wafer (Clinical Example 36-5).

Mucocutaneous separation and wound dehiscence can be challenging to manage. An incision that dehisces can be packed with a strip of hydrofiber and then covered with a transparent film dressing and with gauze, if necessary. The goal is to create both a flat pouching surface and a healing environment for the wound. The skin barrier wafer is then applied over the transparent film. The dressing and pouch may need to be changed daily or twice daily depending on the amount of drainage from the wound and stool output.

Mucocutaneous separation also can be managed by packing strips of hydrofiber around the stoma(s). The wafer is applied in the usual manner. Use of a pouch may be difficult in patients with multiple stomas. In such cases, one option is use of a foam dressing over the stomas after packing around them with a hydrofiber. The foam absorbs the effluent, limiting the amount of stool entering the wound. It can be held in place with flexible net dressing. Another option is Molnlycke Mepilex Border and Mepilex Border Lite, which are absorbent soft silicone self-adhering foam dressings. They are cut similar to stoma wafers and are placed around the stomas to absorb drainage from the dehisced wound. The stoma pouch is secured on top of the Mepilex.

These wounds can be distressing to the staff. The staff may worry constantly about stool entering the wound and causing infection. Detailed instructions,

---

CLINICAL EXAMPLE 36-5

Three-year-old boy has short bowel syndrome and ileostomy.

Subjective:
- One-piece pouch is coming off three times per day.
- His skin is raw, and he is crying.
- Each time the pouch comes off, he is given a bath and the pouch is left off for 20 minutes to let the skin dry out.

Objective:
- Peristomal skin is denuded 3 cm around the stoma.
- He is currently living in a foster facility for children.
- He has multiple caretakers with a variety of ideas on stoma care and limited access to products.

Assessment:
- Ileostomy with serious peristomal skin breakdown
- No agreed upon plan for treating him
- Access to ostomy supplies limited

Plan:
- Apply skin barrier powder and skin sealant on denuded skin in multiple layers to form a crust.
- Use two-piece pouching system to allow visualization of stoma and skin when applying the wafer.
- Add barrier ring to wafer to increase wear time.
- Provide detailed instructions to caregivers.
- Provide supplies and a wafer already prepared with barrier ring.
- Return in 3 days.

Outcome:
- The child returned 3 days later. The wafer was intact when he arrived. The pouch and wafer were removed, and his peristomal skin had healed.

---

pictures, and frequent visits to assist with care and to reassure staff are vital.

PRESSURE ULCERS

Limited research exists on the incidence, risk factors, and assessment of pediatric pressure ulcers. As a result, health care providers may be unaware of the risk to children of skin breakdown from pressure. Although the extent of the problem is not completely understood, sufficient data warrant the education of pediatric nurses on the common risk factors, the tools available to assess risk, and the importance of routine skin assessments and interventions that help prevent pressure ulcers.

Chapters 7 through 9 present the epidemiology, pathophysiology, and prevention of pressure-related injury. Common locations for pressure ulcers in children are listed in Box 36-7.

Incidence and Prevalence

Prevalence. McLane et al (2004) conducted a multisite prevalence study, collecting data on 1,064 patients from nine pediatric hospitals in the United States. They reported

- Head (especially the occiput)
  - Heads of infants and children younger than 3 years comprise a disproportionately high amount of total body weight.
  - Children have less hair and less subcutaneous tissue.
  - Head movement may be restricted to prevent dislodgment of catheters or endotracheal tube.
  - When sedation and paralytic agents are stopped during weaning from a ventilator, the child's level of awareness increases even though he or she remains intubated. Side-to-side movement of the head that may occur during this agitated state increases the child's risk for shearing injury.
- Fingers and toes (under pulse oximetry probes)
- Coccyx and ileac crest
- Bridge of nose (under bilevel positive airway pressure mask)
- Ears (under oxygen tubing and cannula)
- Heels, ankles, and elbows from pressure on bed
- Skin under splinting devices and casts
- Any tubes in contact with skin (e.g., tracheostomy or gastrostomy)

Data from Butler, 2007; Curley et al, 2003; McLane et al, 2004; Neidig et al, 1989; Noonan et al 2006.

a pressure ulcer prevalence of 4%. Of those pressure ulcers, 92% were determined to be Stage I or II according to the National Pressure Ulcer Advisory Panel System. Sixty-six percent were considered facility acquired. Dixon and Ratliff (2005) reported a pressure ulcer prevalence of 4% from two prevalence studies completed 1 year apart in the same institution. Noonan et al (2006) reported a prevalence of 1.6% among 252 patients.

Incidence. Neidig et al (1989) reported the results of a retrospective chart audit of 59 infants and children who had undergone open heart surgery. Ten (16.9%) patients developed Stage I or II occipital pressure ulcers. A study by Curley et al (2003) included 322 patients from three pediatric intensive care units in one hospital. The incidence was 27%, with 70% Stage I, 27% Stage II, and 6% Stage III. The primary locations were the occiput, ear, heels, ankles, toes, elbows, coccyx, and ileac crest.

The results of the studies conducted vary and cannot be compared because the areas of practice and patient populations evaluated were very different. For example, the ages of patients varied significantly. The study by Dixon and Ratliff (2005) included premature infants through patients 21 years of age. The study by Noonan et al (2006) included neonates through patients 17 years of age. Including adult patients affects the data on pressure ulcers in pediatric patients. In their evaluation of the Braden Q Scale, Quigley and Curley (1996) only included children ranging in age from 21 days to 8 years. They limited the age to 8 years because the American Heart Association considers children older than 8 years to be adults in terms of cardiopulmonary resuscitation management.

A second difference among the studies is the patient populations. Patients included in the study by Curley et al (2003) had to have been on bed rest for 24 hours in the pediatric intensive care unit, could not have congenital heart disease, and could not have any preexisting pressure ulcers. The study by Neidig et al (1989) only included children who had undergone congenital heart surgery, had survived the postoperative period, and were discharged from the hospital. The prevalence study by McLane et al (2004) included all inpatients.

Another inconsistency among the studies is whether the data included information only on pressure ulcers or included information on all skin breakdown, including skin damage caused by something other than pressure, such as leakage from gastrostomy tubes or diaper dermatitis. Finally, the studies differed in how they reported pressure-related injury from medical devices such as oxygen saturation probes, intravenous catheter hubs, casts, and electroencephalographic electrodes. Noonan et al (2006) and Curley et al (2003) reported device related pressure ulcers separately.

Although these studies show great variability, they all demonstrate that pediatric patients are at risk for skin breakdown and pressure ulcers. Awareness of the risk factors allows for early intervention to prevent or mitigate skin breakdown.

Risk Factors

As mentioned earlier, pediatric nurses may be unaware that infants and children are at risk for pressure-related skin injury. According to Waterlow (1997), this knowledge deficit alone may represent a risk factor because skin condition may not be adequately assessed. The study by McLane et al (2004) highlights the problem. Of the 43 children reported to have pressure ulcers, 34% had no documentation of pressure ulcer in the 48 hours prior to the prevalence day.

The risk factors for critically ill children identified by Pasek et al (2008) include impaired perfusion, altered nutrition, unstable hemodynamic status, limited mobility, immunosuppression, and medications. The relative large size of the infant's head as well as the infant's undeveloped bowel and bladder control are additional risk factors.

Children with myelomeningocele, spina bifida, cerebral palsy, and other disorders that result in developmental delays and neurologic deficits are at higher risk for pressure ulcer development. These children are affected by decreased mobility, insensate areas (especially of the lower extremities), fecal and urinary incontinence, difficulty communicating, and feeding problems. Pressure ulcers may develop under plaster casts that are too tight, may create friction, or may have toys or other objects placed inside them (Samaniega, 2003). Orthotic devices for the lower extremities may rub on insensate areas or become moist from perspiration. These devices require frequent assessments for fit as children grow. Thoracolumbosacral orthoses, which are used for treatment of scoliosis, require ongoing assessment for correct fit, adjustments for growth, and monitoring of the skin, including the skin surrounding and under gastrostomy tubes. As children outgrow their wheelchairs, pressure can develop behind the knees and at the ankles. Medical equipment, such as the hubs of peripheral venous catheters, bilevel positive airway pressure masks, pulse oximeter probes, casts, gastrostomy tubes, and tracheostomy tubes, especially in infants with very short necks, are other causes of pressure ulcers (Clinical Example 36-6).

Pressure Ulcer Risk Assessment

Pressure ulcer prevention begins with timely and accurate assessment of the patient's risk. Quigley and Curley (1996) modified the Braden Scale to assess risk of pressure ulcers in pediatric patients. The modified pediatric version is called the *Braden Q Scale* (Table 36-2). Quigley and Curley modified the Braden Scale because it contained vivid categorical descriptions that had already been extensively tested on diverse groups of adult patients. The scale consists of seven subscales: mobility, activity, sensory perception, skin moisture, friction and shear, nutrition, and tissue perfusion. The subscales do not overlap. The scores for each subscale range from 1 (most risk) to 4 (least risk). The lower the total score, the higher the patient's risk for developing a pressure ulcer. The modified Braden Q Scale consists of three of the seven subscales: mobility, sensory perception, and tissue perfusion/oxygenation. The modified Braden Q Scale performed as well as the longer Braden Q Scale (Curley et al, 2003).

The sample of patients used to test the Braden Q Scale were infants at least 21 postnatal days of age to children up to 8 years of age. All were in the pediatric intensive care unit and were on bed rest; none had a congenital heart defect. Children with congenital heart disease were excluded because the "impact of chronic hypoxemia on pressure ulcer development is unclear and may be different from the general PICU population" (Curley et al, 2003, p. 285). Curley et al (2003) reported that a Braden Q Scale score of 16 or below indicates a considerable risk for development of a Stage II pressure ulcer.

Although research on the ability of the Braden Q Scale to predict risk of pressure ulcer development in pediatric patients is limited, it is a starting point that provides nurses with an awareness of possible risk and a guide for deciding which patients might benefit from the initiation of prevention strategies.

Prevention and Treatment

Regular and routine skin assessment is critical to identify pressure points and implement appropriate prevention measures. Box 36-7 lists important body sites that should be assessed frequently in the pediatric patient. Challenges to prevention occur when the patient's condition is not known prior to arrival, as in the case of trauma patients, transfers from outside facilities, and patients who are too unstable to move them to the best surface.

Gel-filled pillows (Spenco, Gel-E-Donut, Children's Medical Ventures, Norwell, Mass., USA) are versatile and easy to use with premature infants and older children. They can be used under heads, elbows, and heels. After observing scarring alopecia in five of their premature infants, Gershan and Esterly (1993) initiated the use of gel pads (Spenco) under the heads of their high-risk neonatal intensive care unit patients in conjunction with care plans stressing positioning. Over the next 6 months, no infants developed pressure ulcers or scarring alopecia. Neidig et al (1989) initiated the use of sheepskin under the heads of their patients after observing a significant incidence of occipital pressure ulcers in children after open heart surgery. They acknowledged that sheepskin has not been proven effective at reducing pressure ulcers but believed that it may have provided a reminder to the nurses of the importance of repositioning and skin assessment. During the 6 months following the initiation of this intervention, the incidence of occipital pressure ulcers dropped to 4.8%.

CLINICAL EXAMPLE 36-6

Eight-year-old girl has severe neurologic deficits and recent application of lower extremity casts.

Subjective (Per Mother):
- She started crying uncontrollably, which is not like her.
- The casts have been on for 48 hours.
- The only recent change in her care was application of the casts, so "I took them off."

Objective:
- Patient has severe and only partially controlled seizure disorder.
- She has severe alteration in mental status.
- She has no ability to communicate verbally.
- She usually is consolable.

Assessment:
- Stage III pressure ulcers on tops of both feet and on one heel with cellulitis

Plan:
- Admit to hospital for intravenous antibiotics and wound care.

Outcome:
- Cellulitis resolved, pressure ulcers healed after pressure from cast removed, and heels protected from pressure.

TABLE 36-2	Braden Q Scale			

Intensity and Duration of Pressure   Score

Scale	1	2	3	4
Mobility (ability to change and control body position)	Completely immobile: Does not make even slight changes in body or extremity position without assistance	Very limited: Makes occasional slight changes in body or extremity position without assistance	Slightly limited: Makes frequent though slight changes in body or extremity position independently	No limitations: Makes major and frequent changes in position without assistance
Activity (degree of physical mobility)	Bedfast: Confined to bed	Chairfast: Ability to walk severely limited or nonexistent; cannot bear own weight and/or must be assisted into chair/ wheelchair	Walks occasionally: Walks occasionally during day but for very short distances, with or without assistance; spends majority of each shift in bed or chair	All patients too young to ambulate *or* walks frequently: Walks outside room at least twice per day and inside room at least once every 2 hours during waking hours
Sensory perception (ability to respond in developmentally appropriate way to pressure-related discomfort)	Completely limited: Unresponsive (does not moan, flinch, grasp) to painful stimuli due to diminished level of consciousness or sedation *or* limited ability to feel pain over most body surfaces	Very limited: Responds only to painful stimuli; cannot communicate discomfort except by moaning or restlessness *or* has sensory impairment that limits ability to feel pain or discomfort over half of body	Slightly limited: Responds to verbal commands but cannot always communicate discomfort or need to be turned *or* has some sensory impairment that limits ability to feel pain or discomfort in one or two extremities	No impairment: Responds to verbal commands; has no sensory deficit that would limit ability to feel or communicate pain or discomfort

Tolerance of Skin and Supporting Structure

Moisture (degree to which skin is exposed to moisture)	Constantly moist: Skin is kept moist almost constantly by perspiration, urine, drainage; dampness is detected every time patient is moved or turned	Very moist: Skin is often but not always moist; linens must be changed at least once every 8 hours	Occasionally moist: Skin is occasionally moist; linens must be changed every 12 hours	Rarely moist: Skin usually is dry; routine diaper changes; linens require changing only every 24 hours
Friction (occurs when skin moves against support surfaces)/shear (occurs when skin and adjacent bony surface slide across one another)	Significant problem: Spasticity, contracture, itching, agitation lead to almost constant thrashing and friction	Problem: Requires moderate to maximum assistance in moving; complete lifting without sliding against sheets is impossible; frequently slides down in bed or chair, requiring frequent repositioning with maximum assistance	Potential problem: Moves feebly or requires minimum assistance; during a move, skin probably slides to some extent against sheets, chair, restraints, other devices; maintains relatively good position in chair or bed most of the time but occasionally slides down	No apparent problem: Able to completely lift patient during position change; moves in bed and chair independently and has sufficient muscle strength to lift up completely during move; maintains good position in bed or chair at all times

Continued

TABLE 36-2	Braden Q Scale—cont'd			
Intensity and Duration of Pressure				**Score**
Scale	*1*	*2*	*3*	*4*
Nutrition (usual food intake pattern)	Very poor: NPO and/or maintained on clear liquids or IVs for more than 5 days *or* albumin <2.5 mg/dl *or* never eats complete meal; rarely eats more than half of any food offered; protein intake includes only two servings of meat or dairy products per day; takes fluids poorly; does not take liquid dietary supplement	Inadequate: Is on liquid diet or tube feedings/ TPN that provide inadequate calories and minerals for age *or* albumin <3 mg/dl *or* rarely eats complete meal; generally eats only about half of any food offered; protein intake includes only three servings of meat or dairy products per day; occasionally takes dietary supplement	Adequate: Is on tube feedings or TPN, which provide adequate calories and minerals for age *or* eats over half of most meals; eats total of four servings of protein (meat, dairy products) each day; occasionally refuses a meal but usually takes a supplement if offered	Excellent: Is on a normal diet that provides adequate calories for age; eats most of every meal; never refuses a meal; usually eats total of four or more servings of meat and dairy products; occasionally eats between meals; does not require supplementation
Tissue perfusion and oxygenation	Extremely compromised: Hypotensive (MAP <50 mm Hg; <40 in newborn) or patient does not physiologically tolerate position changes	Compromised: Normotensive; oxygen saturation may be <95%; hemoglobin may be <10 mg/dl; capillary refill may be >2 seconds; serum pH <7.40	Adequate: Normotensive; oxygen saturation may be <95%; hemoglobin may be <10 mg/dl; capillary refill may be >2 seconds; serum pH is normal	Excellent: Normotensive; oxygen saturation >95%; normal hemoglobin; capillary refill <2 seconds
				Total

IV, Intravenous; *MAP,* mean arterial pressure; *NPO,* nothing by mouth; *TPN,* total parenteral nutrition.
From Curley M et al: Predicting pressure ulcer risk in pediatric patients: the Braden Q Scale, *Nurs Res* 52:22-33, 2003.

McLane et al (2002) evaluated the interface pressures under the occiput of infants and children younger than 6 years and under the occiput, coccyx, and heels of children 6 to 18 years old. Standard hospital mattress created the highest interface pressures in both groups. Their results showed that for children younger than 6 years, the Gel-E-Donut pillow alone did not consistently demonstrate lower interface pressures in the occipital area of the head. The foam overlay used alone or in conjunction with the Gel-E-Donut pillow resulted in the lowest interface occipital pressures for children 6 years and younger. The interface pressures of children 6 to 18 years old were measured under the occiput, coccyx, and heels. The highest pressures were under the heels when the feet were perpendicular to the support surface. Heel pressures decreased significantly when the feet were positioned with the outer sides of the feet and ankles on the bed, probably because the surface areas of the feet in contact with the bed were greatly increased. The Delta 120 foam overlay (Span America Medical Systems, Greenville, South Carolina, USA) and the Efica low air-loss bed (Hill Rom, Batesville, Ind., USA) had similar ability to decrease interface pressures.

Solis et al (1988) measured the interface pressure under the bony prominences of the occiput, scapula, and sacrococcygeal area of children between 10 weeks and 13.5 years of age. The 2-inch and 4-inch convoluted foam overlays were found to be effective at decreasing interface pressure and redistributing weight from bony prominences.

Low air-loss beds require input of the correct height and weight but do not have options for the weights of smaller pediatric patients. A child below the minimum weight may sink into the cushions, which could be dangerous.

Turning is important for altering interface pressures. Patients who are extremely unstable can benefit from slight position changes achieved using small rolled blankets. Education on correct use of support surfaces is important. Multiple layers of bedding and diapers (sheet, draw sheet, mattress protection pads, and multiple diapers) often are placed between the patient and the support surface, decreasing the performance of the support surface.

TABLE 36-3	Recommended Negative Pressure Settings for Children
Newborn (birth to 1 month)	50–75 mm Hg
Infants (>1 month to 2 years)	50–75 mm Hg
Children (>2 to 12 years)	75–125 mm Hg
Adolescents (>12 years)	75–125 mm Hg

Adapted from Baharestani MM : Use of negative pressure wound therapy in the treatment of neonatal and pediatric wounds: a retrospective examination of clinical outcomes, *Ostomy Wound Manage* 53:75-83, 2007.

NEGATIVE PRESSURE WOUND THERAPY

The use of negative pressure wound therapy (NPWT) is explained in Chapter 21. This chapter focuses on review of anecdotal articles describing the use of NPWT in infants and children. The principles of treatment are the same. The difference between adults and children treated with NPWT is that children may require sedation for dressing changes due to fear and pain. The dressing changes can be done in the operating room with anesthesia.

Negative pressure wound therapy has been used for treatment of acute and chronic wounds in children as young as 3 days. The treatment was successful in producing granulation tissue over exposed bone, tendon, joint, and/or hardware. Wounds treated included pressure ulcers, extremity wounds, dehisced surgical wounds, open sternal wounds, wounds with fistula, and complex abdominal wall defects (Mooney et al, 2000; Stone McCord, 2007). Fleck et al (2006) used negative pressure wound therapy for the treatment of neonates with infected sternal wounds. A setting of 50 mm Hg was sufficient for treatment of the wounds and did not affect the hemodynamics of the neonates, specifically ventricular filling and cardiac output.

Based on her experience and other published reports, Baharestani (2007) made recommendations for negative pressure settings for children (Table 36-3).

SUMMARY

Infants and children suffer from many skin-related problems. Research into all areas of pediatric wound care and prevention is needed. Ongoing education of staff and parents related to wound healing is essential. Nurses experienced in wound care can improve the lives of sick children through their knowledge of wound healing and expertise using advanced wound care products.

REFERENCES

Akin F et al: Effects of breathable disposable diapers: reduced prevalence of Candida and common diaper dermatitis, *Pediatr Dermatol* 18:282-290, 2001.

Baharestani MM: Use of negative pressure wound therapy in the treatment of neonatal and pediatric wounds: a retrospective examination of clinical outcomes, *Ostomy Wound Manage* 53:75-83, 2007.

Butler C: Pediatric skin care: guidelines for assessment, prevention, and treatment, *Dermatol Nurs* 9:471-485, 2007.

Chen AY, Escarce JJ: Family structure and childhood obesity, early childhood longitudinal study—kindergarten cohort. *Prev Chronic Dis* 7(3): 2010. Available at http://www.cdc.gov/pcd/issues/2010/may/09_0156.htm. Accessed July 7, 2010.

Curley M et al: Predicting pressure ulcer risk in pediatric patients: the Braden Q Scale, *Nurs Res* 52:22-33, 2003.

Darmstadt G, Dinulos J: Neonatal skin care, *Pediatr Dermatol* 47:757-780, 2000.

Dixon M, Ratliff C: Pediatric pressure ulcer prevalence—one hospital's experience, *Ostomy Wound Manage* 51:44-50, 2005.

Fiers SA: Breaking the cycle: the etiology of incontinence dermatitis and evaluating and using skin care products, *Ostomy Wound Manage* 42:32-40, 1996.

Fleck T et al: Vacuum assisted closure therapy for the treatment of sternal wound infections in neonates and small infants, *Interact Cardiovasc Thorac Surg* 5:285-288, 2006.

Foster E: Skin barrier paste, *Sutureline. Newsletter of the American Pediatric Surgical Nurses Association* 16:22-24, 2008.

Gershan LA, Esterly NB: Scarring alopecia in neonates as a consequence of hypoxaemia-hypoperfusion, *Arch Dis Child* 68:591-593, 1993.

Kazaks E, Lane A: Diaper dermatitis, *Pediatr Clin North Am* 47:909-919, 2000.

Lillieborg S et al: Topical anaesthesia in neonates, infants and children, *Br J Anaesth* 92:450-451, 2004.

McLane K et al: Comparison of interface pressures in the pediatric population among various support surfaces, *J Wound Ostomy Continence Nurs* 29:243-251, 2002.

McLane K et al: The 2003 national pediatric pressure ulcer and skin breakdown prevalence survey: a multisite study, *J Wound Ostomy Continence Nurs* 31:168-177, 2004.

Mooney JF et al: Treatment of soft tissue defects in pediatric patients using the V.A.C. system, *Clin Orthop Relat Res* 376:26-31, 2000.

Neidig J et al: Risk factors associated with pressure ulcers in the pediatric patient following open-heart surgery, *Prog Cardiovasc Nurs* 4:99-106, 1989.

Nix D: Factors to consider when selecting skin cleansing products, *J Wound Ostomy Continence Nurs* 27:260-268, 2000.

Noonan C et al: Skin integrity in hospitalized infants and children: a prevalence survey, *J Pediatr Nurs* 21:445-453, 2006.

O'Connor Guardino K: Anorectal malformations in children. In Tkacz Browne N et al, editors: *Nursing care of the pediatric surgical patient*, ed 2, Boston, 2007, Jones and Bartlett.

Odio M et al: Disposable baby wipes: efficacy and skin mildness, *Dermatol Nurs* 13:107-121, 2001.

Ogden C, Carroll M: Prevalence of obesity among children and adolescents: United States, trends 1963-1965 through 2007-2008, *NCHS health E-stat*, available at http://www.cdc.gov/nchs/data/hestat/obesity_child_07_08/obesity_child_07_08.htm. Accessed July 7, 2010.

Ovington L: The truth about silver, *Ostomy Wound Manage* 50(Suppl):1S-10S, 2004.

Pasek T et al: Skin care team in the pediatric intensive care unit: a model for excellence, *Crit Care Nurse* 28:125-134, 2008.

Quigley S, Curley M: Skin integrity in the pediatric population: preventing and managing pressure ulcers, *J Soc Pediatr Nurs* 1:7-18, 1996.

Samaniega I: A sore spot in pediatrics: risk factors for pressure ulcers, *Pediatr Nurs* 9:278-282, 2003.

Shin HT: Diaper dermatitis that does not quit, *Dermatol Ther* 18:124-135, 2005.

Solis I et al: Supine interface pressure in children, *Arch Phys Med Rehabil* 69:524-526, 1988.

Stone McCord S et al: Negative pressure wound therapy is effective to manage a variety of wounds in infants and children, *J Wound Ostomy Continence Nurs* 34:573, 2007.

Stotts N: Wound infection: diagnosis and management. In Bryant R, Nix D, editors: *Acute and chronic wounds: current management concepts*, ed 3, St. Louis, 2007, Elsevier.

Tomaselli N: The role of topical silver preparations in wound healing, *J Wound Ostomy Continence Nurs* 33:367-378, 2006.

Waterlow J: Pressure sore risk assessment in children, *Pediatr Nurs* 9:21-24, 1997.

White R et al: Topical antimicrobials in the control of wound bioburden, *Ostomy Wound Manage* 52:26-58, 2006.

PART II: THE NEONATE Annette B. Wysocki, Ruth A. Bryant, and Denise P. Nix

Infancy refers to the first year of life. During the first 28 days of life, an infant may be referred to as a *neonate*. An infant or neonate born prior to 37 weeks of gestational age is *premature*. A *micropreemie neonate* weighs less than 3 lb or is born prior to 28 to 29 weeks of gestational age. Additional definitions of terms for the infant and neonate are listed in Box 36-8. It is essential to appreciate developmental and structural differences of neonatal skin. Variations in neonatal skin that contribute to environmental influences and caregiving practices are listed in Tables 3-1 and 3-2. They include underdevelopment of the stratum corneum, diminished cohesion between the epidermis and dermis, dermal instability, and change in skin surface pH (Lund et al, 2007).

Micropreemie neonate skin is thin and poorly keratinized, and it functions weakly as a barrier. It is more suitable to an "aquatic environment" than to atmospheric conditions. Of interest, exposure of the premature infant's skin to air seems to accelerate skin maturation. Full maturation occurs about 2 weeks after birth. Infants born between 22 and 25 weeks' gestation may require up to 4 weeks to develop a functional stratum corneum (Kalia et al, 1998). Due to the greater ratio of surface area to volume in the premature infant compared to the full-term infant, percutaneous absorption of topically applied agents (soaps, lotions, antiseptics, alcohol) place the premature infant at greater risk for skin complications and systemic toxicities (Weston and Lane, 2008). Clinicians need to determine if wound and skin care products selected have been shown to be safe and effective for the intended indication and the neonatal patient population (Baharestani, 2007). Calcium

alginates are not recommended for use in neonates secondary to calcium absorption concerns (Irving, 2001). More specific complications associated with percutaneous absorption are addressed in Chapter 3.

The use of disinfectants and antiseptics to prevent colonization and infection of central venous catheters is considered "off label" for neonates (Lund et al, 2007). Povidone-iodine has been associated with skin injury and carries the risk of toxicity from iodine absorption leading to goiter and hypothyroidism (Lund et al, 2007; Rutter, 1996). Yet, studies continue to report the use of interventions considered to be harmful to wound healing such as hydrogen peroxide, povidone-iodine, and dry gauze in this patient population (Irving, 2001; Munson et al, 1999).

Bathing neonates with mild cleansers is equally effective as water alone in decreasing bacteria. A skin cleanser, if necessary, should have a neutral pH (5.5–7.0) and be used sparingly. The benefits of daily bathing have not been clearly justified. Bathing introduces changes to the stratum corneum that can lead to dry skin. Less frequent bathing and cold stress minimize behavioral and physiologic instability in infants. Heat loss during bathing must be minimized. Infants immersed in water at the correct temperature are calmer, quieter, and experience less heat loss than do infants receiving a sponge bath. The infant bath should be as brief as possible and should be followed by prompt drying and wrapping in warm blankets. Preterm infants younger than 32 weeks' gestation should be bathed with plain water or warm sterile water if breakdown is evident during the first week. A soft material should be used to squeeze water onto the skin; the skin should not be rubbed. Neonatal bathing equipment must be properly cleaned before and after each use (Lund et al, 2007).

If required, moisturizing creams or ointments can be applied to dry, flaking, or fissured skin. The best agents appear to be petrolatum based without preservatives, perfumes, or dyes (Weston and Lane, 2008). Every effort should be made to prevent contamination of the emollient container and surrounding treatment surfaces. An association between infection and use of petrolatum-based emollient in micropreemies has been noted (Lund et al, 2007). Therefore, the benefits of emollient use with

BOX 36-8	Definition of Terms
Premature infant	Infant born prior to 37 weeks of gestation
Neonate	Newborn infant less than 28 days of life (from birth to 4 weeks of age)
Infancy	First year of life
Micropreemie	Infant born before 28–29 weeks of gestation or weighing <3 lb

micropreemies should be weighed against the risk of infection.

SKIN INSPECTION AND RISK ASSESSMENT

AWHONN guidelines recommend conducting a head-to-toe skin inspection of the neonate at least daily (Lund et al, 2007). An assessment of risk for skin breakdown should occur in conjunction with the skin inspection. Box 36-9 gives an example of a validated tool for measuring neonatal skin condition (Lund and Osborne, 2004).

Many of the products commonly used for treatment of incontinence-associated dermatitis in adults and children are not appropriate for use in neonates. For example, A&D ointment can facilitate absorption and potential toxicity of vitamin A. Antifungal and pectin-based powders commonly used with incontinent skin care should not be used in nurseries. In fact, some hospitals are becoming powder free to protect the airways of their patients. Box 36-10 lists important considerations for selecting perineal skin care products for neonates (Lund et al, 2007).

Epidermal stripping is another common complication in the care of neonates because of diminished cohesion between epidermis and dermis. Epidermal stripping secondary to tape and adhesive removal is the primary cause of skin breakdown in children in neonatal intensive care units (Lund et al, 2007). Chapter 5 provides a comprehensive review of assessment and management of skin stripping. Tape or adhesive products should be avoided as much as possible. Box 5-3 lists strategies for preventing skin stripping by tapes and adhesives.

For the neonate older than 30 days, non–alcohol-based liquid barrier films can be applied to the skin prior to tape application to protect the epidermis from stripping when the tape is removed (Cavilon No Sting Barrier Film, 3M, St. Paul, Minn., USA). Staff should be taught to remove tape slowly, peeling the tape away from anchored skin or pulling one corner of the tape at an angle parallel with the skin while continuously wetting the adhesive–skin interface with a water-soaked cotton ball. Mineral oil or petrolatum can be used to loosen adhesive unless retaping at the same site is expected. Due to reports of toxicity and skin reaction with neonates, solvents and adhesive removers should not be used (Lund et al, 2007).

SUMMARY

Skin and wound care needs of the neonate and micropreemie are uniquely different from those of the full-term infant. Because the immature epidermis of the pre-term infant is an ineffective barrier to the environment the preterm infant experiences high transepidermal water loss, a risk of absorption of toxic substances through the skin and decreased resistance to skin trauma. With the increased loss of fluid and heat through the skin, the extremely preterm infant is vulnerable to hyperosmolar dehydration and hypothermia. Interventions such as highly humidified incubators and applying moisture retentive dressings and ointments reduce excessive water loss through the skin and improves temperature regulation. However, an unintended consequence of the decreased transepidermal water loss through humidification is a delay in the maturing of the epidermis (Agren et al, 2006). Thus, in contrast to the adult, leaving the skin "open to air" may in fact be a valid intervention for the extremely premature infant.

BOX 36-9	Neonatal Skin Condition Scale

Dryness
1 = Normal, no sign of dry skin
2 = Dry skin, visible scaling
3 = Very dry skin, cracking/fissures
Erythema
1 = No evidence of erythema
2 = Visible erythema, <50% body surface
3 = Visible erythema, ≥50% body surface
Breakdown
1 = None
2 = Small, localized areas
3 = Extensive

From the Association of Women's Health, Obstetric and Neonatal Nurses, 2007.

BOX 36-10	Considerations when Selecting Perineal Skin Care Products for Neonates

- Cleanse with water and soft cloths or with detergent-free, alcohol-free disposable wipes.
- Apply petrolatum-based or zinc-based barrier products with as few additives as possible to prevent topical absorption and toxicity (e.g., topical vitamin A).
- Treat candidiasis with *low*-concentration antifungal in zinc or petrolatum base.
- Do not use powders in hospital nurseries to prevent respiratory irritation from inhaled powder particles.
- Topical antibiotic ointments are not recommended for treatment of diaper dermatitis.

REFERENCES

Agren J et al; Ambient humidity influences the rate of skin barrier maturation in extremely preterm infants, *J Pediatr* 148:613-617, 2006.

Baharestani MM: An overview of neonatal and pediatric wound care knowledge and considerations, *Ostomy Wound Manage* 53(6):34-36, 38, 40, passim, 2007.

Irving V: Skin problems in the pre-term infant: avoiding ritualistic practice, *Prof Nurse* 17(1):63-66, 2001.

Kalia VN et al: Development of skin barrier function in premature infants, *J Invest Dermatol* 111:320, 1998.

Lund CH, Osborne JW: Validity and reliability of the neonatal skin condition score, *J Obstet Gynecol Neonatal Nurs* 33(3):320-327, 2004.

Lund CH et al: Neonatal skin care: evidence-based clinical practice guideline, ed 2, Washington, DC, 2007, Association of Women's Health, Obstetric and Neonatal Nurses.

Munson KA et al: A survey of skin care practices for premature low birth weight infants, *Neonatal Netw* 18(3):25–31, 1999.

Pridham K et al: Helping children deal with procedures in a clinic setting: a developmental approach, *J Pediatr Nurs* 2:13-22, 1987.

Rutter N: The immature skin, *Eur J Pediatr* 155:S18, 1996.

Weston WL, Lane AT: Neonatal, pediatric and adolescent dermatology. In Wolf K et al, editors: *Fitzpatrick's dermatology in general medicine,* ed 7, New York, 2008, McGraw-Hill.

37

Managing Wounds
in Palliative Care

Margaret T. Goldberg and Ruth A. Bryant

OBJECTIVES

1. Distinguish between palliative and hospice care.
2. List types of wounds common to palliative care
3. Describe the possible etiologies of a malignant cutaneous wound and clinical manifestations.
4. Define Marjolin ulcer.
5. List at least four goals in the management of a fungating wound in palliative care.

6. Describe at least four interventions used to achieve the goals associated with palliative wound care.
7. Explain the difference in debridement of a nonmalignant necrotic wound compared to debridement of a malignant cutaneous wound.
8. Identify at least four categories of dressings common in the care of the malignant cutaneous wound.

Palliative care is a concept associated with end of life and with goals such as relief from distressing symptoms, easing of pain, and enhanced quality of life. When healing the wound is not an appropriate or realistic goal, the most appropriate goal is palliation or maintenance. Many factors influence whether the goal is wound healing or palliation. This chapter describes the patient situations in which palliative wound care would be appropriate, the types of wounds that may be associated with palliation, and the principles of palliative wound care. Among the many challenges facing patients in palliative or hospice care are the issues surrounding skin and wound care. Because untreated wounds can lead to physical discomfort and impair quality of life, it is appropriate that they receive attention.

DEFINITION OF TERMS

Palliative care is an approach to care that is patient and family centered. Through the anticipation, prevention, and relief of suffering, palliative care optimizes quality of life. Physical, intellectual, psychosocial, and spiritual needs are addressed in palliative care to facilitate patient autonomy, informed decision making, and choice (National Quality Forum [NQF], 2006; World Health Organization [WHO], 2008). Palliative care is not synonymous with the abandonment of hope or treatment options. No specific therapies are excluded if they can improve the patient's quality of life (Alvarez et al, 2002; Stephen-Haynes, 2008). In fact, palliative care is ideally

a general approach to patient care that should be routinely integrated into primary care and should occur concurrently with other treatments. Specifically, palliative care is indicated for patients with a life-threatening *or* debilitating illness that encompasses a broad range of diagnoses, including people who are living with a persistent or recurring illness that adversely affects their daily functioning or will predictably reduce life expectancy (National Consensus Project for Quality Palliative Care, 2009). Palliative care focuses on the palliative journey from diagnosis onward rather than focusing on the last days of life (Morgan, 2009; Stephen-Haynes, 2008). Therefore, palliative care services are indicated across the trajectory of a patient's illness and are not restricted to the end-of-life phase (NQF, 2006). Specialists in palliative care, those who have received formal education in palliative care and are credentialed in the field, may be consulted to provide specialty-level palliative care when the complexity of the situation warrants (National Consensus Project for Quality Palliative Care, 2009).

Hospice care is similar to palliative care in that the goals are to alleviate symptoms and improve quality of life. However, hospice is appropriate when life expectancy is 6 months or less. When the patient enters the terminal stage of an illness or condition, curative treatments are no longer effective, and/or the patient no longer desires to continue them, hospice becomes the care of choice. Hospice provides comprehensive biomedical, psychosocial, and spiritual support as patients face the end of life (American Academy of Hospice and

Palliative Medicine [AAHPM] 2008; NQF, 2006). The key difference between palliative care and hospice is that palliative care is appropriate regardless of the stage of the disease or the need for other therapies and can be rendered along with life-prolonging treatment as the main focus of care (Malloy et al, 2008).

PALLIATIVE WOUND CARE

Palliative wound care has been defined as the "incorporation of strategies that prioritize symptomatic relief and wound improvement ahead of wound healing" (Alvarez et al, 2007). The focus of palliative wound care is the management of symptoms such as odor, exudate, bleeding, pain, and infection, and maintenance of skin integrity. Prevention of wound deterioration is desirable but is not always realistic, as with a fungating wound (Maund, 2008; Naylor, 2005; Stanley et al, 2008). Palliative care is elected care rather than care that is forced upon the patient; it focuses on physical, psychosocial, and spiritual issues during end of life (Hughes et al, 2005).

Indications

Palliative wound care as a goal of wound management is often related to end of life, when healing interventions are inconsistent with the patient's end-of-life goals. However, palliative wound care may also be indicated when the underlying etiology or existing cofactors cannot be overcome as a result of advanced illness and poor physical state. Although malignancies and metastases are commonly associated with palliative wound care, the patient's condition and situation will also dictate the need for palliative wound care. Palliation as a goal for wound management may be indicated in the following situations:

1. *The patient is terminally ill.* Most often this is a patient who has cancer, but it could just as well be a patient who has end-stage renal disease or significant congestive heart failure. The wound could be an open surgical wound, pressure ulcer, a burn, radiation dermatitis, etc.
2. *Overwhelming comorbidities are present.* As an example, a patient may have significant hypotension following a massive cardiac arrest and require high doses of a vasopressor medication to achieve an adequate blood pressure. The resulting vasoconstriction may be sufficient enough to cause a gradual transition in the finger tips or toes to cyanosis and then necrosis. Clearly the comorbidities dictate that the priority is sustaining adequate blood pressure.
3. *Patient choice.* This is the situation where a patient does not have overwhelming comorbidities or a terminal illness yet simply chooses palliation as a goal. Possible reasons may include a preference to

continue a certain lifestyle that jeopardizes wound healing, a realization that the modifications needed for treatment are not feasible or consistent with other priorities, a financial burden, or a decision based on the patient's age.

Types of Wounds Common to Palliative Care

The etiology of wounds in the patient receiving palliative care can be nonmalignancy or malignancy related. The nonmalignant wound common in palliative care is the wound that develops from mechanical trauma (e.g., unrelieved pressure, shear, friction, skin stripping), moisture and chemicals (e.g., urinary or fecal incontinence), or infection (e.g., candidiasis). These nonmalignant wounds are prevented and managed with the same interventions, resources, and tools as described throughout this textbook. Malignancy-related wounds may be a primary tumor, metastasis, or malignant transformation. Malignancy-related wounds have common wound characteristics that warrant unique kinds of care.

NONMALIGNANCY-RELATED WOUNDS

Any type of wound can be observed in a patient receiving palliative or hospice care. Some of the most common include pressure ulcers, skin stripping, and chemical dermatitis with co-existing pressure ulcers, which is perhaps the most common (Naylor 2005; Stephen-Haynes, 2008; Richards et al, 2007). Galvin (2002) reports that of all the ulcers that developed in the palliative care unit, 78.4% were sacral pressure ulcers.

The frequency of pressure ulcers in the patient receiving palliative care is varied, with an incidence reported as high as 43% (Walding, 2005). Galvin (2002) found 26.1% of patients admitted to a palliative care program over a 2-year time frame had a pressure ulcer, and 12% of all patients admitted to the palliative care setting developed a pressure ulcer during the stay. Within hospice programs, the literature reports an incidence of pressure ulcers ranging from 10% to 17.5%; prevalence is reported at 27% (Reifsnyder and Magee, 2005; Tippett, 2005). In a small study of a hospice program, a total of 35% of patients had some type of skin issue, 50% of them being pressure ulcers (Tippett, 2005).

Pressure Ulcer Prevention

Pressure ulcer prevention is an important component of palliative care (McGill and Chaplin, 2002). In a study of 980 home hospice patients, Reifsnyder and Magee (2005) reported 10% of patients developed a new pressure ulcer within the first 3 months of admission to the program. Of interest, however, in a survey of inpatient palliative care units, only 61% had a written policy for pressure ulcer prevention, 17.6% indicated their policy was under development, and 19.6% reported they did not have a policy. A pressure ulcer prevention program has been presented in detail in Chapters 8 and 9. In the palliative care setting, risk assessment and prevention have a few unique considerations.

Risk Assessment. International guidelines recommend pressure ulcer risk assessment for palliative care patients on a regular basis using a structured consistent approach (National Pressure Ulcer Advisory Panel [NPUAP] and European Pressure Ulcer Advisory Panel [EPUAP], 2009). Rather than assessing pressure ulcer risk solely by completing a risk assessment tool, they also recommend using a validated risk assessment tool, a comprehensive skin assessment, *and* clinical judgment with regard to key risk factors. Pressure ulcer risk assessment can be obtained using the Braden risk assessment form (Reifsnyder and Magee, 2005), the Hunters Hill pressure ulcer risk assessment tool specifically for the individual at or near the end of life (Chaplin, 2000; McGill and Chaplin, 2002), or the Waterloo risk assessment tool. In contrast, many experts suggest that *every* palliative care patient should be considered at "high risk" for pressure ulcer development (Richards et al, 2007; Walding, 2005).

Factors that contribute to pressure ulcer formation in palliative care patients include fragile skin condition, older age, decreasing food and fluid intake, altered sensation, poor general physical condition, and lean body constitution (Chaplin, 1999; Henoch and Gustaffson, 2003; Naylor and McGill, 2005). Of interest, Brink et al (2006) found that patients who used an indwelling urinary catheter or had an ostomy were more than four times more likely to develop one or more ulcers. Additional unique variables associated with pressure ulcer formation included new pain site, shortness of breath, and inability to lie flat (Brink et al, 2006). One fourth of all palliative home care patients experienced the inability to lie flat because of shortness of breath, which increased the patient's risk of pressure ulcer formation. Decreased mobility, unrelieved pain, lack of appetite, and muscle wasting are other risk factors for pressure ulcer development in the palliative care patient (Liao and Arnold, 2007; Morgan, 2009; Walding, 2005). Risk assessment should be obtained within 6 to 12 hours of admission and should be reassessed on a daily basis because of the speed with which the palliative patient's condition can change (McGill and Chaplin, 2002).

Prevention. Pressure ulcer prevention interventions are vital for the palliative care patient population, particularly because the development and resulting treatment often are painful (Eisenberger and Zeleznik, 2004). At the same time, the pressure ulcer prevention plan of care must be reflective of and consistent with the patient's clinical picture and end-of-life goals. Reducing or eliminating some risk factors may not be achievable or in accordance with the comfort-focused goals of palliative care (Reifsnyder and Magee, 2005). For example,

maintaining the head of bed lower than 30 degrees or turning the patient every 2 hours may not be realistic or consistent with the patient's wishes. In these instances, complete patient and family education becomes more critical than ever so that the patient and family are fully informed before they make decisions that may lead to pressure ulcer development. At the same time, it is the responsibility of the wound care provider to recommend the support surface that would best redistribute coccyx pressure while accommodating the patient's need for an elevated head of bed. The international pressure ulcer treatment guidelines (NPUAP-EPUAP, 2009) instruct the care provider to consider changing the support surface to improve pressure redistribution and comfort.

Prevention measures that are most universally appropriate in palliative care include (1) adequate and appropriate offloading with a support surface, (2) adequate pain control for optimal positioning, and (3) incontinence management (containment and skin protection). However, good pain management is critical to being able to provide these basic prevention interventions (Liao and Arnold, 2007). The NPUAP-EPUAP 2009 guidelines stipulate the patient should be premedicated 20 to 30 minutes prior to a scheduled position change when he or she experiences significant pain with movement.

Whether all pressure ulcers that occur in palliative care patients are preventable or whether some are inevitable is not clear (Chaplin, 2004). Debate is growing about the possibility that as death approaches the skin begins to fail, primarily because of altered perfusion, which puts the patient at risk for further breakdown (Stanley et al, 2008). Richards et al (2007) reported that among a group of 61 end-of-life patients in palliative care, 8 of 13 new ulcers developed within 2 weeks of the patient's death. In another study of palliative care wounds, nearly half of the pressure ulcers healed despite short treatment periods, underscoring the point that palliative wound care measures resulted in significant healing. However, regardless of the outcome of this debate, it is incumbent upon the wound specialist to provide care that is compliant with national guidelines for the prevention of pressure ulcers. Furthermore, documentation should record the implementation of assessments and interventions reflective of the guidelines as well as when interventions were withheld and why. A nosocomial pressure ulcer then can be considered inevitable when it develops even though the care provided met the standard of care for pressure ulcer prevention.

Pressure Ulcer Care

Pressure ulcer care in the palliative care patient should closely follow the international guidelines on pressure ulcer treatment and deviate from that standard only as needed and indicated in the 2009 Pressure Ulcer Management in Individuals Receiving Palliative Care section of the international guidelines (NPUAP-EPUAP,

2009). Overall, the palliative care guideline encourages comfort, prompt symptom management, consistency between care provided and the patient's goals, and change guided by the values and goals of the patient and family (NPUAP-EPUAP, 2009). Specific and unique issues relative to exudate control, pain control, odor control, debridement, assessment and monitoring of healing, and dressing selection are discussed later in this chapter.

MALIGNANCY-RELATED WOUNDS

Malignancy-related wounds can be a primary cutaneous tumor, a metastasis, or a malignant transformation of an existing ulcer. The common primary cutaneous tumors that can present as a wound are untreated basal cell cancer (Plate 71), squamous cell cancer, and malignant melanoma (Gerlach, 2005). A primary tumor also can invade up into the skin and erode through the skin to form a malignant wound (Hampton, 2008). Although any tumor left untreated can cause a malignant wound, the most common cancers are breast and soft tissue sarcoma (Naylor, 2002). A tumor can metastasize to the skin when it has invaded blood or lymph vessels; consequently, circulating malignant cells become trapped in the tiny skin capillaries. Seeding of malignant cells can occur during surgery to the abdominal wall, for example. Cancer of the ovary, cecum, and rectum can infiltrate the anterior wall of the abdomen (Grocott, 2007).

Malignant Cutaneous Wounds

Collectively, any wound that is a primary or metastatic skin lesion is referred to as a *malignant cutaneous wound*, also commonly known as a *fungating malignant wound* (Plate 70). These malignant cutaneous wounds usually are chronic, ulcerating, open, and draining (Bauer and Gerlach, 2000; Moore, 2002)

A malignant cutaneous wound begins as a small firm nodule under the surface of the skin that may be flesh colored, pink, red, violet, or brown (Gerlach, 2005; Naylor, 2002). As the malignant cells proliferate, they interfere with the capillaries and lymph vessels. While the tumor develops its own microcirculation, it is disorganized and has impaired blood clotting abilities (Naylor, 2002). These lesions can develop into necrotic "cauliflower-like" eruptions on the skin that progress to exudative and hemorrhagic wounds. Anaerobic organisms (usually *Bacteroides*) flourish on the necrotic tissue and produce volatile fatty acids as metabolic endproducts that are responsible for the characteristic pungent and penetrating odor; this odor is a source of great embarrassment and distress to the patient, family, and caregivers (Draper, 2005; Piggin, 2003). The patient with malignant cutaneous wound may have no symptoms or may experience pruritus, pain, stinging, exudate, odor, and thickening and hardening of the skin (Moore, 2002; Seaman, 2006).

Malignant cutaneous wounds have a poor outcome. Treatment options for these fungating malignant wounds are aimed at the underlying pathology and include radiotherapy, chemotherapy, hormone therapy, surgery, cryotherapy, or laser therapy. External beam radiation therapy may be used to control local metastases, which in turn may help control malignant cutaneous wound symptoms.

Malignant cutaneous wounds are often misinterpreted initially as an ulcer with an etiology of pressure, arterial insufficiency, or pyoderma. When the wound fails to progress despite appropriate topical therapy, cancer should be suspected and biopsies obtained from at least four different locations in the base of the wound. These kinds of wounds will appear abnormal (e.g., thickened, rolled wound edges) and should be thoroughly assessed (Gerlach, 2005).

Marjolin Ulcer

Malignant transformation of an existing ulcer occurs in approximately 2% of all chronic wounds (e.g., pressure ulcer, sinus tract, irradiated skin, burn wound, venous ulcer). The site of chronic irritation and inflammation is a common location for this malignant transformation, otherwise called a *Marjolin ulcer*, which tends to be an aggressive tumor. Treatment is based upon the size and extent of the wound and the condition of the patient (Gerlach, 2005).

OBJECTIVES IN THE CARE OF THE MALIGNANT CUTANEOUS WOUND

Wound management decisions are a balance of meeting the patient's priorities and achieving the identified aims arising from the comprehensive assessment (Chaplin, 2004). Goals of care and treatment priorities are negotiated with each patient based on the stage of the underlying disease process and the potential for available therapeutic options to be beneficial and meet personal preferences (Ferris et al, 2007). Above all, quality of life is the guiding principle when planning patient care (British Columbia Cancer Agency, 2001).

In most situations, the quality of care given to patients with malignant fungating wounds is the most important factor in determining their quality of life (Williams, 1997). The priorities of topical care address the common symptoms of a malignant wound: odor, exudate, pain, bleeding, and pruritus. Interventions include control of bioburden, debridement, exudate absorbent dressings, wound cleansing, and protection of the surrounding skin as summarized in Table 37-1 and described in the following sections.

TABLE 37-1	Interventions for Palliative Care Wound	
Pain Management	**Odor Management**	**Exudate Control**
Nontraumatic Dressing Changes Contact layer Gauzes, nonadherent, or coated Foam Protective barrier films Nontraumatic tapes	**Wound Cleansing** Ionic cleansers Sodium-impregnated gauze Antimicrobials	**Exudate Collection and Containment** Foam, alginates, hydrofiber dressings, absorptive powders Wound drainage pouch
Periwound Skin Management Nontraumatic tapes Skin sealants (alcohol-free) Barrier ointment/cream Hydrocolloid wafer	**Deodorizers** Charcoal dressings Chloromycetin solution Metronidazole gel	**Indicators for Dressing Changes** When pooling on intact skin occurs When strikethrough occurs

	Debridement
	Dry, hard, necrotic tissue (hydrogel,
	    enzymatic debriders)
	Wet sloughy tissue (polysaccharide
	    beads, starch, copolymer dressing)
		Control of Bleeding
		Hemostatic dressings
		Nonadherent gauze
		Alginates
		Sliver nitrate sticks
		Monsel solution

	Reduction of Bacterial Burden Irrigation with ionic cleansers Antimicrobial dressings and creams Absorptive dressings Sodium-impregnated gauze Oral antimicrobials	

Control Pain and Pruritus

Causes of pain in the malignant wound may be multiple and include emotional factors, neuropathic pain (due to nerve damage from the tumor), and procedural pain, as occurs with dressing removal (Grocott, 2007) (see Chapters 25 and 26 for detailed information related to pain assessment and management). When pain is related to underlying disease, practitioners including interventional radiologists, anesthesiology pain specialists, radiation oncologists, surgical oncologists, and pharmacists should be part of the team helping to manage complex pain issues (Krouse, 2008). In addition to systemic analgesia and rapid-onset, short-acting analgesics administered before beginning dressing changes, topical anesthetics can be used to control pain (Tice, 2006). Topical lidocaine or benzocaine or ice packs applied before or after wound care may be beneficial (Seaman, 2006). Daily application of a topical opioid-infused amorphous hydrogel (10 mg morphine sulfate in 8 g of hydrogel) has been used anecdotally to manage painful pressure ulcers and malignant wounds (Ashfield, 2005; Back and Findlay, 1995) as well as in randomized controlled studies (Zeppetella and Ribeiro, 2005; Zeppetella et al, 2003), with significantly improved pain control compared with pretreatment medications. Similar results have been reported with use of either crushed oxycodone or meperidine topically in two patients with sickle cell ulcers (Ballas, 2002). Clearly these options should be considered in conjunction with systemic pain control measures.

Although a malignant or fungating wound is characteristically painful, a key source of pain is the trauma associated with dressing changes. Consequently, controlling or minimizing pain requires attention to the reduction or elimination of mechanical trauma. Two primary interventions are (1) minimization of trauma associated with dressing changes by using nonadhesive dressings and (2) infrequent dressing changes. The malignant or fungating wound site has an increased tendency to bleed when disturbed, which may aggravate the presence of pain. Infrequent dressing changes reduce the potential for bleeding. When bleeding is a concern, appropriate dressings that reduce the potential for a bleeding episode must be selected.

The malignant wound often triggers pruritus at the wound site as the skin tissues stretch in response to the growing tumor. Diphenhydramine or hydroxyzine may be warranted to manage the pruritus and moisturizers applied to keep the periwound skin supple (Gerlach, 2005).

Atraumatic Dressing Changes

Nonadhesive but absorbent dressings are recommended to achieve atraumatic dressing removal. Dressing selection options include a contact-layer dressing, nonadherent gauze, impregnated gauze (e.g., hydrogel- or Vaseline-impregnated gauze), and semipermeable foam dressings. To eliminate unnecessary dressing changes, dressings that have a long wearing time should be selected and preferably changed no more often than every 3 days (Schim and Cullen, 2005). However, once-daily dressing changes may be necessary for the highly exudative wound. Protective barrier films, particularly those without alcohol, can be applied to the surrounding skin to further decrease trauma to periwound skin. Atraumatic tapes and mesh netting can be used to affix dressings, thereby avoiding trauma to the surrounding skin upon removal.

Control or Prevent Bleeding

Erosion of capillaries can lead to significant spontaneous bleeding. Atraumatic dressing removal is critical to avoid precipitating a bleeding episode. If bleeding occurs even with the use of atraumatic dressing removal techniques, direct pressure and an ice pack can be applied initially. If these are ineffective, many different types of dressings and products are available that assist in the control of bleeding (see Table 31-1). Monsel solution (ferrous subsulfate) has been shown to be an effective adjunct to compression for hemostasis (Alvarez et al, 2007). A comprehensive wound assessment should direct the choice of which dressing is most appropriate. Absorbable hemostatic dressings and silver nitrate cautery sticks can be used to specifically control small bleeding points. Alginates have been demonstrated to exhibit hemostatic effects and have been useful for heavily exudative wounds. Nonadherent gauze is an option that will absorb exudate without adhering to the wound bed. Significant bleeding events may require oral antifibrinolytics, radiotherapy, and embolization. Although vasoconstrictive effects can result in ischemia and consequently necrosis, gauze saturated with topical adrenaline 1:1,000 may be applied for emergent situations; however the patient should be monitored for systemic absorption of the medications (Grocott, 1999; Seaman, 2006). These more aggressive options are appropriate if they will improve the quality of life in patients with a malignant wound (Seaman, 2006).

Manage Periwound Skin

Stephen-Haynes (2008) states that the nature of wounds occurring in palliative care predispose toward maceration and denudement, and care should focus on their prevention to prevent complications. The skin surrounding the malignant or fungating wound is particularly fragile and therefore is vulnerable to epidermal stripping, maceration, contact dermatitis, and infection. Routine skin assessments should be obtained to monitor for signs and symptoms of bacterial infection (induration, localized erythema, heat, pain) and fungal infection (erythematous, papular rash). Interventions to protect the fragile periwound skin include nonadhesive dressings, alcohol-free skin sealants, and bracketing the wound bed with skin barrier strips to serve as a barrier to exudate and an anchor for adhesives. Additional measures to protect periwound skin are listed in Box 5-3.

Control Odor

Malodor is recognized as having a physical and psychological impact by reducing appetite, affecting well-being, causing social isolation, and distorting body image (Fletcher 2008; Piggin, 2003; West, 2007). Odor can be caused by necrotic tissue, bacterial burden, infection, or saturated dressings. Objective assessment for the presence of odor is difficult, so subjective reporting by the patient should guide interventions (Collier, 1997).

Interventions appropriate for control of odor include wound cleansing, use of wound deodorizers, debridement, and treatment of infection. Many of these interventions can be used simultaneously to aggressively attack the problem of odor. Grocott (2007) suggests three approaches for the management of odor: systemic antibiotics, topical antimicrobials, and charcoal dressings.

Wound Cleansing. Gentle removal of exudate and debris from the wound base can aid in odor management. Wound cleansing with gentle irrigations rather than swabbing of the surface is recommended. Normal saline, ionic irrigants, and commercial wound cleansers with surfactants can be used (Seaman, 2006). A daily shower with the water aimed slightly above the wound may be an effective method for cleansing the wound.

Deodorizers. Deodorizers can be used topically as well as within the room to control odor. Strategies such as use of aromatherapy oils, expensive aftershave lotions, room deodorizers, and scented candles tend to mask the odor of the malignant wound and overall yield unsatisfactory results (West, 2007; Wilson, 2005). Use of a "sugar paste" has been reported in the literature as an effective deodorizing preparation by reducing bioburden and necrotic tissue. However, the commercially available Manuka honey is preferred because its processing is standardized so that the product is sterilized, thus eliminating the risk of botulism, and is safe from toxins that are present in certain nectars (Wilson, 2005).

Although not appropriate when the objective is wound healing, Chloromycetin solution has been reported to be an effective wound deodorant. Gauze is moistened with the Chloromycetin solution and applied to the wound surface; it is generally changed twice daily so that the dressing will remain moist. Skin protection should be implemented to keep the solution from contacting the surrounding skin because Chloromycetin will cause an irritant reaction to intact skin. Puri-Clens (Coloplast Corp.) has also been applied to wounds for odor control.

Topical Antimicrobials. Antimicrobial creams and sodium-impregnated gauze both may assist in reducing bacterial numbers, thereby reducing odor. Dressings with an antimicrobial component that assist in controlling the wound bioburden include those that contain silver, iodine, or honey (White and Cutting, 2006). Exudate can increase and become viscous and malodorous when a wound becomes infected (Steven-Haynes, 2008). Infections are treated systemically, locally, or both.

Oral (systemic) metronidazole can be given as 200-mg tablets twice per day to reduce the anaerobic bacterial load in the wound. Although this treatment has been reported to be quite successful, notable adverse effects are metallic taste in mouth, furred tongue, nausea and vomiting, and intolerance to alcohol in addition to development of resistance to the bacteria (West, 2007).

In contrast, topical metronidazole decreases bacterial load at the wound site but without the nausea and vomiting that sometimes accompanies oral metronidazole (Finlay et al, 1996; Kalinski et al, 2005). Metronidazole has been applied directly to the wound or on petrolatum gauze and can be used in combination with calcium alginate, hydrofiber, or foam dressings (Alvarez et al, 2007). Seaman (2006) described crushing metronidazole tablets in sterile water and creating either a 0.5% solution (5 mg/1 cc) or a 1% solution (10 mg/1 cc). The solution can then be used as a wound irrigant or used to saturate gauze and pack on the wound bed, including any tunnels or undermining.

Metronidazole gel (0.75%) is commercially available and can be applied to the wound bed and then covered with a saline-soaked gauze or hydrogel. Topical metronidazole is changed daily, and odor should be eradicated or greatly diminished between 3 and 7 days.

Debridement. Necrotic tissue can be extremely pungent and malodorous, so removing nonviable tissue is beneficial to controlling odor. Only loose necrotic tissue should be removed by sharp debridement; it should be performed only by a clinician trained in sharp debridement and only if the process is not painful to the patient (Seaman, 2006). Surgical debridement of these wounds should be avoided because of the risk of bleeding (Wilson, 2005). However, when extensive necrotic tissue is present, surgical debridement may be warranted if it is compatible with the patient's palliative goals of care (Seaman, 2006). Similarly, mechanical debridement is not recommended because of the tendency for wounds to bleed and because of the pain that is triggered by wet-to-dry dressings (Young, 1997).

Conservative debridement (e.g., with autolysis or enzymes) is preferred. Hydrogel dressings are a gentle method of debridement because they soften the necrotic tissue (Plates 52-54) and facilitate its separation from the wound bed (Young, 1997) (see Chapters 17 and 18 for further discussion of debridement and contraindications). These dressings have the additional benefit of providing a soothing effect and providing pain control. Realistically, the malignant cutaneous wound is quite exudative, however, so a hydrogel dressing (a dressing designed to donate moisture, not absorb, moisture) often is inappropriate. Absorptive dressings (polysaccharide

beads, sodium-impregnated gauze, starch copolymer beads, alginates, hydrofibers) are most appropriate and can be combined with superabsorbent dressings to increase the absorptive capacity of the dressing and extend the time between dressing changes.

Charcoal Dressings. Charcoal dressings can reduce odor by filtering out the chemicals that cause the odor and by absorbing bacteria (Naylor, 2002). As an outer covering, charcoal-impregnated dressings can be used either as a primary dressing (when the wound is not exudative) or as a secondary dressing (over a primary absorptive dressing) to suppress odor. These dressings are changed when they become moist (moisture inactivates the charcoal) and when the charcoal is saturated so that it is no longer effective. Charcoal dressings are effective only when they are "sealed" around all four edges so that odor is forced to pass through the charcoal filter. Because some wounds are so irregularly shaped and the topography is so varied, securing the charcoal dressing may be too difficult to attain. Charcoal dressings may require changes ranging from daily to every 2 or 3 days depending on the extent of the odor. Charcoal dressings combined with an antimicrobial are available and serve the dual purpose of reducing bioburden and odor.

Collect and Contain Exudate

High levels of exudate from the malignant cutaneous wound are the result of abnormal capillary permeability within the wound (due to disorganized tumor vasculature), secretion of vascular permeability factor by tumor cells, and autolysis of necrotic tissue by bacterial proteases (Draper, 2005). The surrounding tissue of a malignant or fungating wound often is edematous such that even a small ulcer or nodule can produce prolific amounts of exudate. Interventions that aid in exudate control include (1) appropriate dressing selection and (2) appropriate dressing change frequency.

Moderately or highly exudative wounds require dressings that are capable of absorbing high volumes of exudate. Moderate to large amounts of exudate can be contained with semipermeable foam dressings and alginates. Very heavily exudative wounds may require a superabsorbent pad in conjunction with an alginate dressing, a hydrofiber dressing, or maltodextrin powder (see product formulary in Table 18-2).

A contact-layer dressing can be used to line the wound so that absorbent dressings can be applied and removed without traumatizing the wound bed. Two-layer permeable vented dressings also may be used. With these dressings, the perforated nonadherent layer protects the wound surface and permits passage of exudate to an absorbent and permeable layer (Grocott, 1999).

Wound drainage pouches are available from most ostomy manufacturers. These pouches are indicated when the volume of exudate produced exceeds the capabilities of the dressings. Pouching should be considered when dressings must be changed more often than two to three times daily, when the skin begins to show early signs of damage, when the patient's ability to ambulate is hampered, or when odor is uncontrolled. These products have various desirable features, such as attached skin barriers, flexible adhesive surfaces, and an access window over the wound site. Many wound pouches also have an attached tubular drain spout that facilitates connecting the pouch to a drainage container so that the fluid does not pool over the wound site.

Negative pressure wound therapy (NPWT) devices can help to contain wound fluids and decrease the number of painful dressing changes (Alvarez et al, 2007). NPWT has been used to contain odor and prevent the need for frequent painful dressing changes of a malignant wound (Ford-Dunn, 2006). While the treatment was reported to improve the patient's quality of life considerably, reimbursement for these devices when used in the palliative care wound are seldom approved and therefore not affordable. More information regarding the use of NPWT can be found in Chapter 21.

Dressing change frequency appears to be a function of the volume of exudate produced, the volume of necrotic tissue present, and the patient's hydration status and activity level. As with other wounds, dressings for malignant or fungating wounds should be changed when exudate is pooling over intact skin or when "strikethrough" occurs. Ideally, dressings should not require changing more often than once per day.

EVALUATION

Reviewing wound management decisions regularly is essential because the condition of any wound is dynamic, especially in palliative care (Chaplin, 2000). Toward this end, care is targeted to the areas of most concern to the patient and family while maximizing the effects of the intervention (Benbow, 2008). It is useful to begin the assessment by asking the patient what aspect of the wound or wound care interventions are of greatest concern. It may be surprising to learn that dressing changes as often as two to three times daily do not upset the patient as much as the odor from the wound or the constant drainage.

SUMMARY

The AAHPM (2008) position statement maintains that all seriously ill patients who have symptoms that are difficult to treat or who face challenging decisions about goals of care should have access to palliative care consultation and/or hospice. Efforts to enhance quality of life should be offered alongside curative and or restorative medical care, with palliative care a fundamental component of excellent medical care and not an alternative after other approaches have been pursued.

The potential skin complications associated with palliative wounds are amenable to the application of wound healing principles. As with other chronic wounds, the goals for these types of wounds range from healing to palliation and symptom management.

Practitioners must advocate for changes in policy, regulations, and reimbursement guidelines that may limit palliative wound care practice (Ferris et al, 2007). Furthermore, the wound care community should highlight nonclosure endpoints for wound care, such as wound stabilization and improvement (Alvarez, 2005).

REFERENCES

Alvarez OM et al: Chronic wounds: palliative management for the frail population—Part II–III, *Wounds* 14(8 Suppl):5S-27S, 2002.

Alvarez OM: Editors message, *Wounds* 17(4):2005.

Alvarez OM et al: Incorporating wound healing strategies to improve palliation (symptom management) in patients with chronic wounds, *J Palliat Med* 10(5):1161-1189, 2007.

American Academy of Hospice and Palliative Medicine (AAHPM): American Academy of Hospice and Palliative Medicine position statement: *Statement on access to palliative care and hospice*, Glenview Ill., 2008, AAHPM.

Ashfield T: The use of topical opioids to relieve pressure ulcer pain, *Nurs Stand* 19:45:90-92, 2005.

Back IN, Finlay I: Analgesic effects of topical opioids on painful skin ulcers, *J Pain Symptom Manage* 10(7):493, 1995.

Ballas SK: Treatment of painful sickle cell leg ulcers with topical opioids, *Blood* 99:1096:2002.

Bauer C, Gerlach MA: Care of metastatic skin lesions, *J Wound Ostomy Continence Nurs* 27(4):247-251, 2000.

Benbow M: Exuding wounds, *J Commun Nurs* 22(11):20:23-24, 26, 2008.

Brink P et al: Factors associated with pressure ulcers in palliative home care, *J Palliat Med* 9(6):1369-1375, 2006.

British Columbia Cancer Agency: Cancer management guidelines: supportive care: chronic ulcerating malignant skin lesions; care of malignant wounds, updated 2001. Available at http://www.bccancer.bc.ca/HPI/CancerManagementGuidelines/SupportiveCare/ChronicUlceratingMalignantSkinLesions/CareofMalignantWounds.htm. Accessed June 29, 2010.

Chaplin J, McGill M: Pressure sore prevention. *Palliative Care Today*, 8(3):38-39, 1999.

Chaplin J: Pressure sore risk assessment in palliative care, *J Tissue Viability* 10(1):27-31, 2000.

Chaplin J: Wound management in palliative care, *Nursing Standard* 19(1):39-42, 2004.

Collier M: The assessment of patients with malignant fungating wounds: a holistic approach, Part 1, *Nurs Times* 93(44 Suppl 1), 1997.

Draper C: The management of malodour and exudates in fungating wounds, *Br J Nurs* 14(11):S4-S12, 2005.

Eisenberger A, Zeleznik J: Care planning for pressure ulcers in hospice. The team effect, *Palliat Support Care* 2:283-289, 2004.

Ferris FD et al: Palliative wound care: managing chronic wounds across life's continuum: a consensus statement from the International Palliative Wound Care Initiative, *J Palliat Med* 10(1):37-39, 2007.

Finlay IG et al: The effect of topical 0.75% Metronidazole gel on malodorous cutaneous ulcers, *J Pain Symptom Manage* 11(3):158, 1996.

Fletcher J: Malodorous wounds, assessment and management, *Wound Essent* 3:14-17, 2008.

Ford-Dunn S: Use of vacuum assisted closure therapy in the palliation of a malignant wound, *Palliat Med* 20:477-478, 2006.

Galvin J: An audit of pressure ulcer incidence in a palliative care setting, *Int J Palliat Nurs* 8(5):214-221, 2002.

Gerlach MA: Wound care issues in the patient with cancer, *Nurs Clin North Am* 40(2):295-323, 2005.

Grocott P: The palliative management of fungating malignant wounds, *J Wound Care* 8(5):232, 1999.

Grocott P: Care of patients with fungating malignant wounds, *Nurs Stand* 21(24):57-66, 2007.

Hampton S: Malodorous fungating wounds: how dressing alleviate symptoms, *Br J Community Nurs* 13(6): Wound Care S31-32, S34, S36 passim, 2008.

Henoch I, Gustaffson M: Pressure ulcers in palliative care: development of a hospice pressure ulcer risk assessment scale, *Int J Palliat Nurs* 9(11):474–484, 2003.

Hughes RG et al: Palliative wound are at the end of life, *Home Health Care Manag Pract* 17(3):196-202, 2005.

Kalinski C et al: Effectiveness of a topical formulation containing metronidazole for wound odor and exudate control, *Wounds* 17:84-90, 2005.

Krouse RS: Palliative care for cancer patients: an interdisciplinary approach, *Cancer Chemother Rev* 3(4):152-160, 2008.

Liao S, Arnold RM: Wound care in advanced illness: application of palliative care principles, *J Palliat Med* 10(5):1159-1160 2007.

Malloy P et al: *End-of-life-care: improving communications skills to enhance palliative care*, Medscape.com continuing education program, 2008, available at http://cme.medscape.com/view-article/574420, accessed April 17, 2009.

Maund M: Use of an ionic sheet hydrogel dressing on fungating wounds: two case studies, *J Wound Care* 17(2):65-68, 2008.

McGill M, Chaplin J: Pressure ulcer prevention in palliative care 1: results of a UK survey, *Int J Palliat Nurs* 8(3):110-119, 2002.

Moore S: Cutaneous metastatic breast cancer, *Clin J Oncol Nurs* 6(5):255-260, 2002.

Morgan DY: *Improving quality of life for patients with life-limiting illnesses: the key role of nursing in palliative care*, 2009, available at http://www.nursingconsult.com/das/stat/view/135065113-2/cup?nid=204577&sid=836556303&SEQNO=3, accessed April 22, 2009.

National Consensus Project for Quality Palliative Care: *Clinical practice guidelines for quality palliative care*, ed 2, 2009, available at http://www.nationalconsensusproject.org.

National Pressure Ulcer Advisory Panel (NPUAP) and European Pressure Ulcer Advisory Panel (EPUAP): *Prevention and treatment of pressure ulcers*, Washington, DC, 2009, NPUAP.

National Quality Forum (NQF): *A national framework and preferred practices for palliative and hospice care*, 2006: Available at http://www.rwjf.org/pr/product.jsp?id=18736, accessed March 27, 2009.

Naylor W. *Part 1: symptom control in the management of fungating wounds*, 2005, available at http://www.worldwidewounds.com/2002/march/Naylor/Symptom-Control-Fungating-Wounds.html, accessed March 15, 2009.

Naylor WA: A guide to wound management in palliative care, *Int J Palliat Nurs* 11(11):572-579, 2005.

Piggin C: Malodorous fungating wounds: uncertain concepts underlying the management of social isolation, *Int J Palliat Nurs* 9(5):216-221, 2003.

Reifsnyder J, Magee HS: Development of pressure ulcers in patients receiving home hospice care, *Wounds* 17(4):74-79, 2005.

Richards A et al: Risk factors and wound management for palliative care patients, *J Hospice Palliat Nurs* 9(4):179-181, 2007.

Schim SM, Cullen B: Wound care at the end of life, *Nurs Clin North Am* 40(2):281-294, 2005.

Seaman S: Management of malignant fungating wounds in advanced cancer, *Sem Onc Nurs* 22(3):185-193, 2006.

Stanley KJ et al: Ethical issues and clinical expertise at the end of life, *Nurs Clin North Am* 43(2):259-275, 2008.

Stephen-Haynes J: An overview of caring for those with palliative wounds, *Br J Community Nurs* 13(12):S2-S4, 2008.

Tice M: Wound care in the face of life-limiting illness, *Home Health Nurse* 24(2):115-118, 2006.

Tippett A: Wounds at the end of life, *Wounds* 17(4):91-98, 2005.

Walding M: Pressure area care and the management of fungating wounds. In Faull C, Carter Y, Daniels L, editors: *Handbook of palliative care*, ed 2, Oxford, 2005, Blackwell Publishing.

West D: A palliative approach to the management of malodour from malignant fungating tumours, *Int J Palliat Nurs* 13(3): 137-142, 2007.

White R, Cutting K: *Modern exudate management: a review of wound treatments*, 2006. Available at http://www.worldwide-wounds.com/2006/september/White/Modern-Exudate-Mgt.html, accessed April 6, 2009.

Williams C: Management of fungating wounds, *Br J Community Nurs* 2(9):423, 1997.

Wilson V: Assessment and management of fungating wounds: a review, *Br J Community Nurs* 10(3):S28-S34, 2005.

World Health Organization (WHO): *WHO definition of palliative care*, 2008. Available at http://www.who.int/cancer/palliative/definition/en, accessed April 11, 2009.

Zeppetella G, Ribeiro MD: Morphine in intrasite gel applied topically to painful ulcers, *J Pain Symptom Manage* 29:118-119, 2005.

Zeppetella G et al: Analgesic efficacy of morphine applied topically to painful ulcers, *J Pain Symptom Manage* 25:555-558, 2003.

38

Management of Draining Wounds and Fistulas

Ruth A. Bryant and Bonnie Sue Rolstad

OBJECTIVES

1. Identify medical conditions associated with fistula formation.
2. List three complications that contribute to mortality from fistulas.
3. Describe three ways to classify fistulas.
4. List the risk factors for postoperative fistula development and for irradiation-induced fistulas.
5. Identify the six objectives of medical management for the patient with a fistula.
6. List factors known to correlate with spontaneous closure and known to impede spontaneous closure of fistula tracts.
7. Describe surgical procedures commonly used to close or bypass fistula tracts.
8. List eight nursing management goals for the patient with a fistula.
9. Describe four essential assessments that guide the management of the patient with a fistula.
10. Explain the role of four different types of skin barriers and their indications for use.
11. Identify features to be considered when selecting a fistula pouching system.
12. Briefly describe the "bridging" technique and identify indications for its use.
13. Identify options for odor control in a wound managed with dressings and in a wound managed with pouching.
14. Describe the role of NPWT and closed wound suction in the management of an enterocutaneous fistula.

The presence of a draining fistula can be a frustrating and disheartening experience for the patient and family because the fistula represents a major complication. It can also be a difficult experience for caregivers. However, management can be quite rewarding when effluent is successfully contained, odor is controlled, the patient is comfortable, and realistic resolution is attained. Management for this patient population requires astute assessment skills, knowledge of pathophysiology, competent technical skills, diligent follow-up, persistence, and knowledge of management alternatives.

Fistula management is more than skin protection and containment. In this chapter the pathophysiology of fistula formation, the medical and surgical aspects of managing a patient with a fistula and the nursing management (i.e., skin protection, odor control, containment techniques) of the patient with a fistula will be presented. The techniques discussed in this chapter also are applicable to other types of wounds and drain sites that are not adequately contained by dressings.

EPIDEMIOLOGY AND ETIOLOGY

Gastrointestinal fistulas are serious complications associated with high morbidity and high mortality (10%–20%), extended hospital stays, and increased costs (Kassis and Makary, 2008; Wong and Chang, 2008). Fistulas develop in a wide array of complex patient conditions and often are concentrated in large medical centers. Frequency data (i.e., incidence and prevalence) therefore tend to be skewed and difficult to interpret. Factors impacting on the prognosis of the patient with a fistula, however, are well known.

Medical conditions associated with fistula formation include technical difficulties with anastomosis, and coexisting disease such as inflammatory bowel disease, cancer, or diverticulitis. The following are risk factors that increase the likelihood of fistula formation when these medical conditions are present: severe malnutrition, sepsis, hypotension, vasopressor therapy, and steroid therapy. Enterocutaneous fistulas develop either spontaneously or postoperatively. In many reports, 75% to 85% of enterocutaneous fistulas are iatrogenic, occur postoperatively, and represent a leak in the anastomosis (Nussbaum and Fischer, 2006). Risk factors specific to developing a postoperative enterocutaneous fistula include reoperation requiring extensive lysis of adhesions, cancer, inflammatory bowel disease, emergency surgery where the bowel has not been adequately prepped, prior radiation therapy, and trauma surgery (Kassis and Makary, 2008; Nussbaum and Fischer, 2006). According to Wong et al (2004), postoperative fistulas caused by anastomotic breakdown are largely preventable by following basic surgical principles of anastomotic construction: (1) adequate blood supply, (2) lack of tension, and (3) good suture technique. Maykel and Fischer (2003) advocate specific prevention strategies when faced with emergency surgery: provide adequate intravenous fluids, ensure adequate circulatory support, keep the patient warm, and provide appropriately timed broad-spectrum antibiotics. In addition, when surgery is planned, they consider adequate nutritional preparation to be the most important step in preventing an anastomotic breakdown. The patients at highest risk for an anastomotic breakdown are the severely malnourished patients as manifested by a hydrated serum albumin level less than 3 g/dl and weight loss of 10% to 15% over a 4- to 6-month period (Kassis and Makary, 2008).

Approximately 25% of fistulas are acquired, that is, they develop spontaneously and are associated with an intrinsic intestinal disease (cancer, radiation, diverticulitis, inflammatory bowel disease, appendicitis) or external trauma. Spontaneous fistulas are generally resistant to spontaneous closure. Patients who have been treated for a pelvic malignancy are particularly vulnerable for fistula formation because of radiation damage to the rectum, anal canal, and gynecologic organs (Saclarides, 2002; Tran and Thorson, 2008). Irradiation triggers occlusive vasculitis, fibrosis, and impaired collagen synthesis, a process termed *radiation-induced endarteritis*. Because the endarteritis persists, complications may develop immediately after radiation or years later. Meissner (1999) reported that 17% of radiotherapy patients developed a fistula a mean of 3.4 years after receiving radiation therapy. Additional risk factors for irradiation-induced fistulas include coexisting processes such as atherosclerosis, hypertension, diabetes mellitus, advanced age, cigarette smoking, pelvic inflammatory disease, and previous pelvic surgery. Pelvic radiation doses exceeding 5000 cGy increase the incidence of bowel injury (Hollington et al, 2004; Saclarides, 2002; Tran and Thorson, 2008).

The three most common and highly significant complications associated with fistulas are sepsis, malnutrition, and fluid and electrolyte imbalance (Berry and Fischer, 1996). The loss of hypertonic protein-rich fistula effluent contributes to fluid and electrolyte depletion and malnutrition because of the loss of sodium bicarbonate and amino acids (Nussbaum and Fischer, 2006). Sepsis occurs as a result of abscess formation and compromised immune response due to poor nutritional status (Makhdoom et al, 2000). Uncontrolled sepsis and sepsis-associated malnutrition are primarily responsible for the mortality in patients with enterocutaneous fistulas, with mortality rates ranging from 6% to 20% (Hollington et al, 2004; Maykel and Fischer, 2003; Nussbaum and Fischer, 2006; Wong et al, 2004).

TERMINOLOGY

Definitions

Fistula is a Latin word meaning "pipe" or "flute." A fistula is an abnormal passage between two or more epithelialized surfaces so that a communication tract develops from one body cavity or hollow organ to another hollow organ or to the skin (Figures 38-1 to 38-3). Thus, a gastrointestinal fistula communicates between the lumen of the gastrointestinal tract and another organ. An enterocutaneous fistula communicates specifically between the lumen of the gastrointestinal tract and the skin. A draining wound, surgically placed drain site, or wound dehiscence should not be misinterpreted as a fistula.

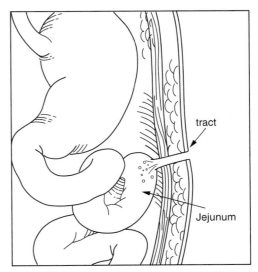

FIGURE 38-1 Simple enterocutaneous fistula.

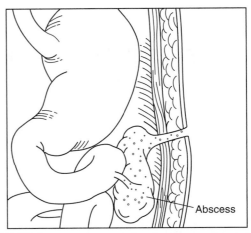

FIGURE 38-2 Complex type 1 fistula with associated abscess.

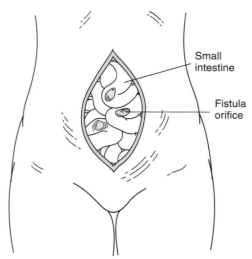

FIGURE 38-3 Complex type 2 fistula with multiple openings associated with large abdominal wall defect.

TABLE 38-1		Fistula Terminology	
From	**To**	**Name**	**Internal/External**
Pancreas	Colon	Pancreatico-colonic	Internal
Jejunum	Rectum	Jejunorectal	External
Intestine	Skin	Enterocutaneous	External
Intestine	Colon	Enterocolonic	Internal
Intestine	Bladder	Enterovesical	Internal
Intestine	Vagina	Enterovaginal	External
Colon	Skin	Colocutaneous	External
Colon	Colon	Colocolonic	Internal
Colon	Bladder	Colovesical	Internal
Rectum	Vagina	Rectovaginal	External
Bladder	Skin	Vesicocutaneous	External
Bladder	Vagina	Vesicovaginal	External

Modified from Irrgang S, Bryant R: Management of the enterocutaneous fistula, *J Enterostom Ther* 11:211, 1984.

Classification

Several methods are used to classify fistulas. These classification schemes are useful in predicting the morbidity rate, mortality rate, and potential for spontaneous closure (Wong et al, 2004).

From an anatomic perspective, the fistula may be simple or complex (Box 38-1). The simple fistula has a short, direct tract, no abscess, and no other organ involved, whereas the complex fistula is associated with an abscess, has multiple organ involvement, and may open into the base of a wound.

A fistula may be classified according to location. The internal fistula exists between internal structures, whereas the external fistula communicates between an internal organ and the skin, vagina, or rectum. This classification system is more specific in that the site of origin and site of termination are identified. Examples of such terminology are listed in Table 38-1.

A fistula may be classified according to volume of output (Table 38-2). A high-output fistula is most

commonly defined as producing more than 500 ml per 24 hours, a moderate-output fistula is associated with output of 200 to 500 ml per 24 hours, and a low-output fistula produces less than 200 ml per 24 hours (Maykel and Fischer, 2003; Nussbaum and Fischer, 2006). The frequencies of sepsis, malnutrition, and fluid and electrolyte imbalance are directly related to fistula output. Fistula output is a direct reflection of the fistula's site of origin. Distal large bowel fistulas typically have low output (<200 ml per 24 hours), whereas most proximal small bowel fistulas drain at least 1,000 to 1,500 ml per 24 hours initially and are considered high output. The high-output fistula is associated with severe malnutrition, significant fluid and electrolyte disturbance, higher morbidity and mortality rates, and lower spontaneous closure rate (Kassis and Makary, 2008; Wong et al, 2004).

BOX 38-1	Classification of Fistulas by Complexity

Simple
- Short, direct tract
- No associated abscess
- No other organ involvement

Complex
- Type 1
  - Associated with abscess
  - Multiple organ involvement
- Type 2
  - Opens into base of disrupted wound

TABLE 38-2	Fistula Classification		
	Designation	**Characteristics**
Location	Internal	Tract contained within body
	External	Tract exits through skin
Involved structures	Colon	Colon
	Entero-	Small bowel
	Vesico-	Bladder
	Vaginal	Vagina
	Cutaneous	Skin
	Recto-	Rectum
Volume	High-output	>500 ml per 24 hours
	Moderate-output	200–500 ml per 24 hours
	Low-output	<200 ml per 24 hours

Modified from Boarini J et al: Fistula management, *Semin Oncol Nurs* 2:287, 1986.

MANIFESTATIONS

Fever and abdominal pain are the initial indicators of a possible fistula (Nussbaum and Fischer, 2006). The passage of gastrointestinal secretions or urine through an unintentional opening onto the skin heralds the development of a cutaneous fistula. Manifestations of a fistula exiting through the vagina (i.e., rectovaginal or vesicovaginal) include passage of gas, feces, purulent material, or urine through the vagina, discharge that is extremely malodorous. Irradiation-induced rectovaginal fistulas often are preceded by diarrhea, passage of mucus and blood rectally, a sensation of rectal pressure, and a constant urge to defecate (Saclarides, 2002). Fistulas between the intestinal tract and the urinary bladder (e.g., colovesical fistula) present with passage of gas or stool-stained urine through the urethra.

MEDICAL MANAGEMENT

The desired endpoint of the medical management of a fistula is spontaneous closure. Approximately 19% to 40% of all fistulas will close spontaneously with conservative medical management, but only when sepsis is controlled and nutrition support is adequate and appropriate (Kassis and Makary, 2008). Of the fistulas that do heal spontaneously, 80% to 90% do so within 5 weeks, provided the patient is adequately nourished (Kassis and Makary, 2008; Maykel and Fischer, 2003). Factors known to correlate with spontaneous fistula closure include absence of sepsis, adequate nutritional support, low output, and classification as a postoperative fistula (Campos et al, 1999; Nussbaum and Fischer, 2006). Approximately 90% of simple type 1 fistulas close spontaneously, whereas less than 10% of complex type 2 fistulas close spontaneously (Wong et al, 2004).

Achievement of the medical management goals requires patience, astute assessment skills, and the cooperation of many health care specialists. Medical management can be divided into nonsurgical treatment and surgical treatment. A comprehensive and effective interdisciplinary and multidisciplinary team approach is vital to achieve closure and reduce mortality and morbidity.

Nonsurgical Treatment

The nonsurgical treatment of fistulas requires a comprehensive plan of care with attention to six specific objectives.

Objective 1: Fluid and Electrolyte Replacement. From 5 to 9 L of fluid rich in sodium, potassium, chloride, and bicarbonate is secreted into the gastrointestinal tract daily. The loss of fluid and electrolytes that accompanies the presentation of a high-output fistula may result in hypovolemia and circulatory failure. Such blood volume imbalances must be corrected before initiating nutritional support or definition of the fistula tract. Adequate tissue perfusion and urine output must be maintained. Potential electrolyte imbalances should be anticipated and can be inferred from an understanding of the usual electrolyte composition of gastrointestinal secretions.

Objective 2: Control of Infection. Sepsis is the major cause of death in patients with enteric fistulas. The bacteria proliferate rapidly in the poorly vascularized tissue typically surrounding a fistula tract (Kassis and Makary, 2008). Pooling of bowel contents as a result of the dehiscence of a suture line precipitates localized and then diffuse abdominal pain, ileus, fever, and, ultimately, septic shock. The presence of systemic or local sepsis must be evaluated, typically with computed tomographic scanning or ultrasound. Effective drainage can be accomplished by use of percutaneous radiographic techniques or surgery. The specific approach depends on abscess location, patient status, and available resources. Surgical laparotomy for control of sepsis should be limited to proximal diversion and drainage of the abscess. Definitive repair of the fistula is undertaken at a later time only after inflammation has receded and nutrition is restored. Abscess contents should be cultured (aerobic and anaerobic) and Gram stained to identify the causative organisms and sensitivities. Organisms are most commonly of bowel origin: coliform, bacteroides, and enterococci. Staphylococci also may be present. Antibiotics are only appropriate in the presence of an infection and in conjunction with adequate drainage of the abscess (Wong et al, 2004).

Objective 3: Control of Fistula Output and Skin Protection. Drainage of intestinal contents onto the skin will result in epidermal erosion and pain within only a few hours. Aggressive skin protection is essential and should be initiated at once. This is discussed specifically in the Nursing Management section.

Intestinal output must be minimized. Conventional methods for achieving this goal are giving the patient nothing by mouth (NPO) and administering histamine (H_2) receptor antagonists. NPO status decreases luminal contents, gastrointestinal stimulation, and pancreaticobiliary secretion. Administering H_2 antagonists (e.g., cimetidine) prevents stress ulcerations and decreases gastric, biliary, and pancreatic secretions. Despite reducing gastrointestinal secretions, H_2 receptors have not been shown to speed closing of the enterocutaneous fistula (Maykel and Fischer, 2003).

Although not a standard in routine fistula care, administration of somatostatin-14 has been shown to further decrease intestinal output in some situations. This naturally occurring hormone is present throughout the body; more than two thirds is derived from the gastrointestinal tract, especially the distal portion of the stomach, duodenum, jejunum, and pancreas. In the presence of fat, protein, and carbohydrates with a meal, somatostatin secretion significantly increases. Somatostatin release is inhibited by the release of acetylcholine from cholinergic neurons (Nussbaum and Fischer, 2006). It has extensive, well-known biologic effects that include inhibition of gastric, biliary, pancreatic, and salivary secretions and reduced gastrointestinal motility, gastric emptying, and gallbladder emptying. When used in combination with total parenteral nutrition (TPN), a synergistic effect on reduced gastrointestinal secretions can be expected. Fistula output reductions of at least 50% within 24 hours and a significant reduction in the time to spontaneous closure of the fistula have been reported (Fagniez and Yahchouchy, 1999; Hesse et al, 2001). The short half-life of 1 to 2 minutes requires that somatostatin-14 be administered through continuous intravenous infusion (250 mcg/hr). The analogue octreotide has a half-life of almost 2 hours, so it can be administered three times daily subcutaneously (300 mcg/day). Results from available prospective controlled studies and randomized controlled studies of octreotide have been mixed. Overall it appears to have similar but less dramatic reduction of output and closure rates (Makhdoom et al, 2000). The most encouraging results of octreotide are seen with postoperative, high-output small bowel fistulas in which fluid-, electrolyte-, and protein-store depletion is prevented. These medications are less effective with fistulas associated with intrinsic bowel diseases, such as ulcerative colitis or Crohn's Disease (Hild et al, 1986). Somatostatin or octreotide administration should be stopped if fistula output does not decrease in the first 48 hours of treatment or if no response is seen after 2 to 3 weeks of treatment, respectively.

Maykel and Fischer (2003) recommend caution when using somatostatin. They report that because use of somatostatin precipitates villous atrophy, interruption of intestinal adaptation, and acute cholecystitis, somatostatin should not be used routinely for treatment of the enterocutaneous fistula.

Objective 4: Nutritional Support. Malnutrition is a significant complication experienced by most patients with a fistula. Several factors contribute to the fistula patient's poor nutritional status. Often the patient is malnourished before the fistula develops. Additional factors contributing to negative nitrogen balance include reduced protein intake, inefficient nutrient use, excessive losses of protein-rich fluids (especially from pancreatic and proximal jejunal fistulas), and muscle protein breakdown (hypercatabolism) that occurs with sepsis.

Adequate nutritional support is achieved when the patient is maintained in a state of positive nitrogen balance and receives adequate vitamin and trace mineral replacement. The amount of calories and protein required will depend on the patient's preexisting status, sepsis, and fistula output. Caloric needs range from 30 to 40 kcal per kilogram per 24 hours; the goal should be a calorie-to-nitrogen ratio of 150:1. Protein requirements are estimated at 1.5 to 1.75 g per kilogram per 24 hours or 0.25 to 0.35 g of nitrogen per kilogram body weight per 24 hours (Wong et al, 2004). It is important to initiate nutritional support without delay because lean body mass is lost at a rate of 300 to 900 g per 24 hours depending upon the degree of stress (Maykel and Fischer, 2003). Trace elements (e.g., copper, zinc, magnesium), multivitamins, and vitamins (B, C, K) must be supplemented (Maykel and Fischer, 2003; Wong et al, 2004). González-Pinto and Moreno Gónzález (2001) recommend twice the recommended daily allowance (RDA) for vitamins and trace minerals and up to 10 times the RDA for vitamin C.

The route of nutritional support is contingent upon the patient's ability to ingest sufficient quantities, the location of the fistula tract, the absorptive capacity of the bowel mucosa, and the patient's tolerance. Historically, the preferred route of nutritional support has been parenteral nutrition accompanied by simultaneous "bowel rest," which has resulted in increased spontaneous closure rates and decreased mortality rates.

Interest in the use of enteral nutrition has resurfaced because of the recognition that even small amounts of enteral nutrition will maintain the normal structural, immunologic, and hormonal integrity of the gastrointestinal tract and prevent translocation of bacteria. However, enteral nutrition requires approximately 4 feet of small intestine (Knechtges and Zimmermann, 2009; Maykel and Fischer, 2003). Enteral nutrition is appropriate when fistulas are located in the most proximal or distal portion of the gastrointestinal tract; however, the gastrointestinal tract must be functional and the patient cooperative. Many types of enteral solutions are available, and a dietician should be consulted to recommend the most appropriate solution and administration procedure so that gastrointestinal intolerance (e.g., diarrhea, abdominal distention) can be avoided.

Objective 5: Definition of Fistula Tract. After the patient is stabilized (fluid and electrolytes balanced and infection controlled), the fistula must be examined to ascertain (1) the origin of the fistula tract, (2) the condition of adjacent bowel, (3) the presence of additional abscess pockets, and (4) the presence of distal obstruction or bowel discontinuity. Water-soluble contrast agents (e.g., Renografin, Hypaque, Gastrografin) are preferred to visualize the fistula tract and are administered through the fistula orifice using a soft-tip catheter. A computed tomographic scan is indicated only when the patient is not responding to conservative treatment. If other organs are involved, additional tests (e.g., cystoscopy or intravenous pyelogram) should be pursued (Wong et al, 2004).

Objective 6: Conservative Management. As already described, the majority of fistulas will heal spontaneously with patience, time, and conservative management (positive nitrogen balance with nutritional support, sepsis-free state). The challenge is trying to shorten the time to spontaneous healing as well as increasing the number of fistulas that heal spontaneously.

Fistula closure is sometimes successful with the insertion of clotting substances into the fistula tract. The concept of using fibrin for anastomosis of tissue was first used for hemostasis in 1909 (Migaly and Rolandelli,

2006). Fibrin sealants (also referred to as *fibrin glue*) are composed of a concentrated allotment of fibrinogen/factor XIII/fibronectin and thrombin that congeals to form an insoluble fibrin clot when mixed with calcium chloride, a process that essentially replicates the last step of the coagulation cascade (Kassis and Makary, 2008; Tran and Thorson, 2008). The mechanism of action consists of fibrin glue providing a "matrix" for the influx of various cells and collagen formation (Buchanan et al, 2003).

Fibrin sealant products can be created from the patient's own plasma (autologous) or from human plasma that has been collected and pooled from many donors (heterologous) after screening and viral testing. The fibrin glue is applied endoscopically at the origin of the fistula to seal the fistula (Migaly and Rolandelli, 2006). Although fibrin sealant products appear to have a role in the management of low-output fistulas (e.g., perirectal), the role of fibrin glue relative to the complexity of the fistula and timing of the procedure has yet to be determined.

Surgical Treatment

Immediate surgery is imperative when (1) a septic focus has been identified, (2) uncontrolled hemorrhage has developed, (3) bowel necrosis has developed, or (4) an evisceration is present. However, closure of the fistula or excision of the fistula tract should not be attempted under these circumstances.

Surgical intervention to close the fistula will be required when impediments to spontaneous closure have been identified. Factors known to prevent spontaneous closure are listed in Box 38-2 (Nussbaum and Fischer, 2006). If any of these factors are present and closure of the fistula is the ultimate goal for the patient, a surgical intervention will eventually be necessary. Surgical procedures may also be indicated for palliation.

The exact timing for surgical intervention is variable, depending on the patient's status. In general, operative interventions to close the fistula tract should be delayed until the patient is in optimum condition (i.e., positive nitrogen balance and control of infection are established). If the patient is nutritionally and metabolically stable,

---

BOX 38-2 | Factors that Prevent Spontaneous Fistula Closure

- Compromised distal suture line/anastomosis (i.e., tension on suture line, improper suturing technique, inadequate blood supply to anastomosis)
- Distal obstruction
- Foreign body in fistula tract or suture line
- Epithelium-lined tract contiguous with skin
- Presence of tumor or disease in site
- Previous irradiation to site
- Crohn's Disease
- Presence of abscess or hematoma

---

definitive surgery for a simple or complex type 1 fistula is appropriate when a persistently draining fistula is in a sepsis-free environment for 6 to 8 weeks. It is important that definitive surgery be delayed until the abdominal wall is soft and supple; tissues should return to a normal soft, pliable state, particularly in the presence of irradiated tissue (González-Pinto and Moreno Gónzález, 2001; Wong et al, 2004).

Complex type 2 fistulas invariably require definitive surgery; however, the timing of surgery is not well defined. Nutritional status, metabolic status, and immunocompetence should be normalized, and the obliterative peritonitis and inflammation associated with chronic peritoneal contamination should be resolved (Wong et al, 2004). Judicious timing of surgery for complex type 2 fistulas is warranted. The most often reported timing ranges from 3 to 6 months.

The surgical interventions available for management of enterocutaneous fistulas will either divert the gastrointestinal tract (without resection of the fistula) or provide definitive resection of the fistula tract (Nussbaum and Fischer, 2006). Factors such as location, size, and cause of the fistula, the patient's overall status, and the presence of irradiated tissue will influence the approach selected. However, Maykel and Fischer (2003) warn that the best results occur with resection of the fistula and end-to-end anastomosis and that other surgical procedures represent a compromise.

Diversion techniques divert the fecal stream away from the fistula site; removal of the fistula is not accomplished. Resection of the fistula is not always appropriate or possible in the presence of extensive or recurrent malignancy or when tissue perfusion is inadequate in the vicinity of the fistula (secondary to numerous surgical resections, scar formation, uncontrolled diabetes, or prior irradiation).

Diversion can be achieved by creating a stoma proximal to the fistula or by anastomosing (end-to-end or side-to-side) the two segments of bowel on both sides of the fistula (e.g., ileotransverse anastomosis when fistula communicates with right colon). This latter procedure may be referred to as an *intestinal bypass* in which the segment of bowel containing the fistula is completely isolated and separated from the fecal stream.

When closure of the fistula is the goal, resection of the fistula will be necessary. The advantage of this technique is that the diseased tissue is removed. An end-to-end anastomosis of the intestine with resection of the fistula tract is performed. To protect the anastomosis, diversion of the fecal stream through a temporary stoma may be indicated. If the distal part of the rectum is not suitable for anastomosis or the anal sphincters are not competent, a permanent stoma with a Hartmann's pouch may be the safest procedure.

Enteric fistulas communicating with the urinary tract will always require diversion of the fecal stream proximal to the fistula site to prevent urinary tract infections and pyelonephritis.

NURSING MANAGEMENT

The occurrence of a fistula lengthens recovery time, whether closure is spontaneous or occurs with surgical repair. This section focuses on the technical management of the patient with a fistula. The principles and techniques presented are applicable to all types of draining wounds and drain sites. Principles are presented so that management can be tailored to achieve effective solutions. However, the care plan must also include detailed attention to patient and family needs, involvement, education, and emotional support.

Technically, the patient with a fistula is one of the most challenging patients encountered by wound and ostomy care providers. Critical thinking skills are necessary to synthesize assessment data, product knowledge (advantages, disadvantages, effectiveness, and guidelines for use), patient needs, and physiology into realistic goals. Principles of wound care and principles of ostomy management are applied to the management of these clinical problems. There is also an art involved in the techniques presented in this chapter.

Goals

Effective nursing management of the enterocutaneous fistula strives to achieve the eight goals listed in Box 38-3. Optimally, all the goals are achieved simultaneously; however, that is not always possible, and prioritizing is frequently necessary. For example, a pouching system may effectively contain output and odor as well as provide significant skin protection. However, complete mobility may not be possible, or the pouching system may be expensive. Interventions to achieve the goals begin as soon as the patient is noted to have a fistula; they are not contingent upon medical diagnosis.

Four general principles should guide the care of the patient with a fistula (Rolstad and Wong, 2004):

1. Assess the pouching system and seal frequently; expect changes.
2. Build flexibility into the care plan.
3. Innovate, using the easiest, most practical approach first.
4. Recognize that care of the patient is frequently provided by inexperienced caregivers.

BOX 38-3	Nursing Goals for Fistula Management

- Perifistular skin protection
- Containment of effluent
- Odor control
- Patient comfort
- Accurate measurement of effluent
- Patient mobility
- Ease of care
- Cost containment

Assessment

The method selected to manage a fistula is guided by the assessment of the four key fistula characteristics outlined in Box 38-4. Because fistulas change in shape and contour over time, repeat assessment and monitoring are necessary. Modifications to the initial containment system are invariably necessary (Scardillo and Folkedahl, 1998; Wiltshire, 1996; Zwanziger, 1999).

Source. Initially, little information may be available regarding the origin of the fistula or the involved organs (if diagnostic studies have not yet been conducted). However, it may be possible to identify the probable origin of the fistula based on assessment of fistula output (volume, odor, consistency, composition) (Table 38-3). This information provides insight into the patient's risk for altered skin integrity and provides decision points for selection of the management approach. For example, a fistula producing semiformed, odorous effluent likely is communicating with the left transverse or descending colon. Effluent from the transverse or descending colon will be less damaging to the skin than the output from the ileum. Therefore, in this situation the primary goals of nursing management will be containment of effluent and odor control.

Characteristics of Effluent. Characteristics of effluent that must be considered in fistula management include volume, odor, consistency, and composition. In general, the fistula with output volumes greater than 100 ml over 24 hours requires containment using a pouch or suction.

BOX 38-4	Fistula Assessment and Documentation Guide

1. Source (e.g., small bowel, bladder, esophagus)
2. Characteristics of effluent
   A. Volume
   B. Odor? (If yes, describe)
   C. Consistency (e.g., liquid, semiformed, formed, gas)
   D. Composition
      I. Color (e.g., clear, yellow, green, brown)
      II. Active enzymes
      II. Extremes in pH
3. Topography and size
   A. Number of sites
   B. Location(s)
   C. Length and width of each (include patterns)
   D. Openings (e.g., below skin level, at skin level, above skin level)
   E. Proximity to bony prominences, scars, abdominal creases, incision, drain(s), stoma
   F. Muscle tone surrounding opening (e.g., firm, soft, flaccid)
   G. Contours at the fistula opening (e.g., flat, shallow depth [$<1/16$ inch], moderate depth [$1/16$–$1/4$ inch], or deep [$>1/4$ inch])
4. Perifistular skin integrity at each location (e.g., intact, macerated, erythematous, denuded or eroded, ulcerated, infected)

TABLE 38-3	Characteristics of Gastrointestinal Secretions							
					Electrolyte Concentration			
Source	Secretions	pH	24-Hour Volume (cc)	Color	Na (mg)	K (mEq)	Cl (mg)	HCO$_3$ (mg)
Saliva	Ptyalin, maltase	6–7	1,000–1,200	Clear	20–80	16–23	24–44	20–60
Gastric juice	Pepsin, rennin (chymosin) lipase, hydrochloric acid	1–3.5	2,000–3,000	Clear/green	20–100	4–12	52–124	0
Pancreatic juice	Amylase, trypsin, chymotrypsin, lipase, sodium bicarbonate	8–8.3	700–1,200	Clear/milky	120–150	2–7	54–95	70–110
Bile	Bile salts, phospholipids	7.8	500–700	Golden brown–greenish yellow	120–200	3–12	80–120	30–50
Duodenum, jejunum, ileum	Peptidase, trypsin, lipase, maltase, sucrase, lactase	7.8–8	2,000–3,000	Gold–dark gold	80–130	11–21	48–116	20–30
Colon		7.5–8.9	50–200	Brown	4	9	2	—

Cl, Chloride; *HCO$_3$,* bicarbonate; *Na,* sodium; *K,* potassium.

Odor is another factor when selecting a management method. The patient with a malodorous output of only 10 to 20 ml per 24 hours may require a pouching system, even if just to contain odor. Odor may originate from numerous sources, including exudate, necrotic or infected tissue, soiled dressings, dressing materials, and chemicals used during treatment.

Consistency of effluent is particularly important when pouching because it affects the type of drainage spout needed and subsequently the type of pouch selected. It also influences the need for additional skin barriers. Liquid effluent is much more corrosive than thick effluent and results in premature erosion of the skin barrier.

The color of effluent acts as an indicator of fistula source (see Table 38-3). In the presence of effluent with active enzymes or extremes in pH, the perifistular skin will require aggressive protection. However, all perifistular skin should be monitored and protected from moisture, even when effluent composition does not include active enzymes. Until radiographic studies are performed, the enzymatic and pH composition of the effluent can be inferred from the volume and consistency of the drainage.

Cutaneous Opening. The size of the opening is determined by measuring the length and width in centimeters. A pattern is always useful because a fistula is usually irregularly shaped. The pattern should be kept in the patient's room with supplies. The fistula opening may appear as a deep tunnel with the base not visible for assessment, or the base may be visible with the fistula exiting at a specific location. In some cases the fistula opening may exit above the skin level as mucosal or granulation tissue. Wound dressings may be warranted to pack the wound (e.g., alginates or foams) when the fistula is present in a deep wound base.

Abdominal Topography. Assessment is performed with the patient in a supine and semi-Fowler position. The cutaneous fistula locations are identified and documented. The area is assessed for the presence of irregular skin surfaces that are created by scars or creases. This assessment indicates how flexible the adhesive in contact with the skin must be and whether filling agents, such as skin barrier paste or strips, are needed to level irregular surfaces (see Color Plates 72 and 73). In addition, the number of cutaneous fistula openings, the location of each, and the proximity to bony prominence or other obstacles (e.g., retention sutures or stoma) are assessed and documented. These characteristics will help to determine the size and shape of adhesive surface needed to secure the sites but not impinge on the prominence or protrusion. If two cutaneous sites are too far apart to be pouched in one system, two pouches may be necessary.

Muscle tone in the area and skin contours should be assessed. Decreased abdominal muscle tone can be expected in the patient who lacks exercise or is overweight, in the elderly, and in the infant. Aging affects subcutaneous tissue support. Muscle tone may be characterized as firm, soft, or flaccid.

It is important to assess the level at which the fistula opening exits onto the skin. Contours of the skin surrounding the fistula opening may be classified as flat, shallow (<$\frac{1}{16}$ inch), moderate depth ($\frac{1}{16}$–$\frac{1}{4}$ inch), or deep (>$\frac{1}{4}$) (Rolstad and Boarini, 1996). Fistulas that empty into deep, open wounds require more pouch adaptations than do fistulas that empty flush with intact skin.

Perifistular Skin Integrity. Perifistular skin condition should be assessed and documented at each dressing or pouch change. Constant exposure of the epidermis to moisture, active enzymes, extremes in pH of fluids, and mechanical trauma frequently leads to breaks in skin integrity. Denudation of perifistular skin is a common complication in fistula patients and often is present when the patient is first seen with the fistula. Skin constantly bathed in fluid causes maceration, whereas effluent with enzymatic drainage or extremes in pH levels creates erythema and denuded or eroded perifistular skin. The perifistular skin may also develop an infection as a consequence of moisture entrapment against the skin and antibiotic precipitated changes in the normal skin flora. Candidiasis is a common secondary complication as depicted in Color Plate 16. Chapter 5 provides additional information to facilitate delineation of fungal infection from irritant, chemical or contact dermatitis.

Although visual inspection of the skin is best, data can also be obtained from the nursing staff and patient to aid assessment. For example, when frequent dressing changes (every 4 hours) are reported, skin will deteriorate quickly as a result of chemical and mechanical injury. Patient reports of burning or stinging sensations around the fistula or wound commonly indicate denudation of the epidermis.

Planning and Implementation

Four key questions should be asked when planning the technical management of a fistula:

1. Is the output volume more than 100 ml in 24 hours?
2. Is odor a problem?
3. Is the fistula opening less than 3 inches?
4. Is an access cap needed?

Figure 38-4 shows an algorithm that incorporates these four questions to guide decision making for managing a fistula.

Fistulas can be managed with pouches, dressings, suction, or all three. When planning the specific fistula

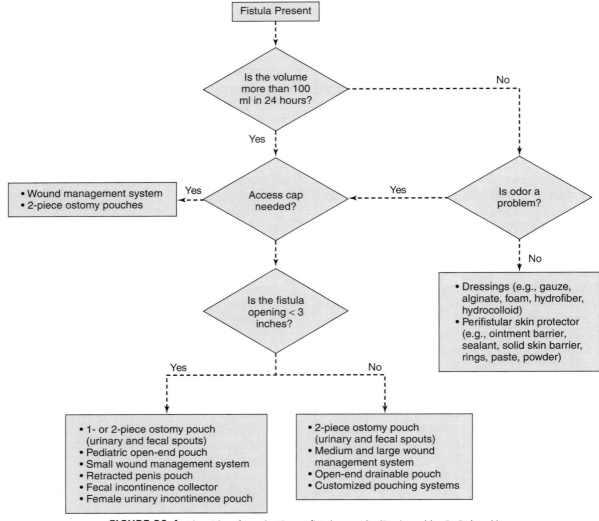

FIGURE 38-4 Algorithm for selecting a fistula pouch. (Designed by B. Rolstad.)

management approach, the four key questions and the goals that have been identified by the health care team and patient must be considered. In most situations, the priority goals are containment of effluent, odor control, and perifistular skin protection. Initially some goals may be compromised, such as ease of care, patient mobility, and cost containment, because of the acuteness of the situation. This section presents nursing interventions that facilitate attainment of each goal for the nursing management of fistulas.

Perifistular Skin Protection. The potential for skin breakdown is always present when a fistula exists, regardless of the management option selected. Preventive strategies should be implemented early and be accompanied by frequent monitoring. Protective strategies include atraumatic adhesive removal and protection of the skin from exposure to effluent. Dressings alone do not offer skin protection, so concurrent use of a skin barrier often is necessary. Skin barriers are available in various forms (Figure 38-5). Table 38-4 summarizes the characteristics and indications of each type of skin barrier.

If pouching is selected as the management approach, solid-wafer skin barriers usually are integrated into the pouching system during manufacturing. However, additional skin barrier products may be required to caulk edges, fill creases, and/or add convexity.

At times, skin barrier wafers and pastes need to be applied over an intact incision as part of the management system. This is done to secure the system and prevent leakage of effluent from the fistula onto the incision.

Skin barrier powders are used to absorb moisture from denuded skin and to create a dry surface. Adhesives or ointments then can be applied to the dry surface. Severely denuded skin may require the creation of an "artificial scab" with the skin barrier powder by alternating layers of the skin barrier powder and a skin sealant or skin cement. The pouching system then may be applied

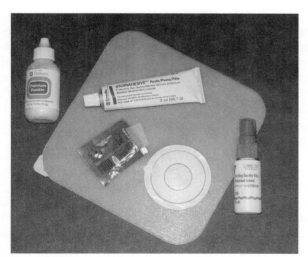

FIGURE 38-5 Examples of skin barriers: wafer, paste, ring, powder, sealant.

directly over the artificial scab. Applying either skin cement or spray adhesive to the artificial scab and pouch adhesive surface is often needed to enhance adherence. Skin barrier powders should not be confused with talc or cornstarch, which do not provide skin protection.

In nonpouching management approaches, petroleum, dimethicone, or zinc-based ointments are used to provide skin protection. These products are particularly useful for low-volume, odorless fistulas and usually are inexpensive. They are applied to perifistular skin, particularly the edges, and covered with dressings. Ointments are not intended for use under adhesives. Frequency of application is indicated on the product and may differ depending on the product formulation and use.

Containment of Effluent. Containment of effluent is accomplished with nonpouching and pouching approaches. The volume of effluent, presence of odor, abdominal contours, and care setting influence which approach is most effective.

Nonpouching Options. Nonpouching options include dressings and barriers, drains, and suction techniques. The method chosen is greatly influenced by the volume of output.

Dressings and Barriers. Nonpouching options are indicated when (1) fistula output is low (<100 ml per 24 hours), (2) odor is not present, and (3) skin contours or location of the fistula makes pouching impossible. Containment of effluent can be achieved with dressings intended for absorption, which include gauze (sponges or strip packing), alginates, foam, and combinations of dressings. Packing should be done only with dressing materials that can be retrieved from the wound. For example, a strip packing material may be gently packed into a low-volume drain site. A 2-inch tail of dressing material is left outside the wound and is used to retrieve the packing at dressing changes. Entrapment of effluent against the skin may cause maceration and breakdown; therefore, skin barriers must be used in conjunction with the dressings to protect the perifistular skin (see Table 38-4).

If, despite best efforts, perifistular skin becomes compromised or output volume exceeds 100 ml in 24 hours, dressings become less effective and more time intensive to manage. The application of additional dressings will not increase the absorbency of the dressing or lengthen the time between dressing changes. As a rule, a pouching system should be used when dressings must be changed more often than every 4 hours. Conversely, when a fistula site has low volume, a small pouching system may be used so that the patient does not have to change the pouch more than once every 7 days. This approach provides convenience and protects perifistular skin.

Vaginal Fistula Drain Device. Vaginal fistulas (Fig. 38-6) occasionally develop secondary to pelvic irradiation or obstetrical trauma; and as a result the patient is incontinent of feces or urine through the vagina. The uncontrolled passage of feces or urine

TABLE 38-4	Guide to Use of Skin Barriers in Fistula Management	
Type of Skin Barrier	**Characteristics**	**Indications**
Solid wafers (4 inch × 4 inch or 8 inch × 8 inch)	• Pectin-based wafers with adhesive surface • Available as wafers or rings • Have moist tack • Have varied flexibility • May be cut into wedges, rings, or strips • Have varied durability to effluent • Changed only when they loosen from perifistular edges or once every 7 days	• Provide skin protection, referred to as laying down a protective platform • Level irregular skin surfaces • Protect perifistular skin from effluent when dressings are used or skin is exposed • Gauze dressings are applied over the skin barrier wafer and taped to wafer rather to skin
Skin barrier rings	• Available in hydrocolloid and karaya formulations • Have moist tack • Have varied flexibility • Have varied durability to effluent • Hydrocolloid formulations • Recommended for fistula management	• Level irregular skin surfaces • Protect perifistular skin from effluent when dressings are used or skin is exposed
Paste (tube or strip)	• Commercial preparations contain alcohol, which can create burning sensation if skin is denuded • Extremely tacky; should be applied as thin bead and smoothed into place with damp gloved finger or tongue blade • Contains solvents; allow to dry briefly so that solvents can escape before other products are applied	• Level irregular skin surfaces • Protect exposed skin from effluent (i.e., with pouching) • Extend duration of solid-wafer barrier when pouching
Powder	• Must be used lightly; can be used in combination with sealants to create artificial scab • Residual powder alters adhesion	• Absorb moisture from superficial denudement before applying ointments or adhesives
Skin sealants	• Liquid, nonalcohol, and alcohol preparations • Nonalcohol skin sealants are indicated for use on denuded skin • Must be allowed to dry to permit solvents to dissipate • Available in various forms (wipes, gel, wands, roll-ons, pump spray)	• Can be used under adhesives to protect fragile skin during adhesive removal • Improve adherence of adhesives to skin (particularly oily skin) • Protect perifistular skin from effluent or maceration when dressings are used • Used in combination with skin barrier powders; creates artificial scab

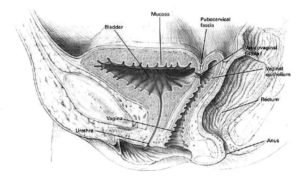

FIGURE 38-6 Vaginal fistula between vagina and bladder.

vaginally results in severe perivaginal skin denudation and discomfort. Aggressive nursing care is essential to prevent these complications.

Skin protection can be achieved with ointments and pads. Frequent dressing changes are necessary to prevent entrapment of caustic drainage contents against the skin. Ointments and pads for vaginal fistulas are less than optimal because they are labor intensive, do not promote patient mobility, do not adequately contain the fecal contents, and fail to control odor. A female urinary incontinence pouch may be useful in these situations and may be connected to straight drainage. However, the difficult location and moist surface surrounding the vaginal orifice make application of an adhesive pouching system challenging.

A vaginal fistula drain device is another method for managing a vaginal fistula and does not require adhesives. This type of system can be constructed with a Davol breast shield, Evenflo nipple shield, or vaginal diaphragm and large Malecot catheter (O'Connor, 1983). A cruciate incision is made through the nipple shield or diaphragm, through which the catheter is threaded. The shield or diaphragm occludes the vagina so that the drainage is directed down the catheter.

The soft, cone-shaped device, shield, or diaphragm is inserted a short distance into the vagina. The discomfort to the patient created by such manipulation of the labia and vagina can be minimized by lubricating the device with lidocaine (Xylocaine). Tubing is attached to the device to channel the fistula contents into a straight drainage collection bag. The drainage tubing can be anchored to the patient's inner thigh.

A vaginal fistula drain device will remain in place effectively while the patient is reclining. As the patient becomes more ambulatory, the device may have a tendency to become dislodged; however, because the procedure is so easy, the patient can reinsert the vaginal drain as needed. Gentle irrigation of the tubing may be indicated if the tubing becomes occluded by fistula material. A vaginal fistula drain device may be a temporary or permanent management technique depending on the patient's status.

Closed Suction Systems. Closed suction systems continue to be a viable, reliable, and cost-effective method for managing high-output fistulas, especially when the fistulas are located in a dehisced abdominal wound (Davis et al, 2000; Jones and Harbit, 2003; Kordasiewicz, 2004). Catheters attached to low intermittent suction may be used when routine pouching is ineffective or overwhelmed by the volume of output (Beitz and Caldwell, 1998; Lange et al, 1989). However, suction does not provide complete containment of effluent; dressings and skin protection still are necessary. Effluent must be liquid if suction is to be effective; thick or particulate drainage will occlude the catheter. The wound is cleansed, and a layer of saline-moistened gauze is placed in the wound bed. The catheter is laid in the wound and directed toward the bottom of the setup. Another layer of moist gauze may be applied over the catheter, and a large transparent dressing may be applied as a secondary dressing (Hollis and Reyna, 1985; Jeter et al, 1990). Skin barrier paste or strips are sometimes necessary to fill in irregular skin surfaces and to seal around the catheter as it exits from the transparent dressing. Suction tubing is then attached to the suction catheter and set at a low level of continuous suction. A Hemovac can provide the suction for short periods to increase the patient's mobility. This dressing usually is changed every 1 to 2 days.

A catheter that is inserted into the fistula tract will act as a foreign body and may interfere with healing and even increase fistula output (Welch, 1997). On the other hand, a catheter coiled in a defect above the orifice or in the open wound surrounding the fistula opening will not inhibit closure. Because firm tubes can injure fragile tissue, only soft, flexible suction catheters should be used with fistulas (Welch, 1997). Suction catheters should be considered a short-term intervention because of the limitations placed on patient mobility and the time-intensive nature of the care.

Negative Pressure Wound Therapy. The evolution of the closed suction system is negative pressure wound therapy (NPWT). This technique has demonstrated clinical wound healing benefits. The system incorporates a sponge and subatmospheric pressure, which results in reduced periwound edema and mechanical stretching of cells. Mechanical stretching of cells is believed to stimulate the wound repair process. The use of NPWT is contraindicated for nonenteric (e.g., biliary and pancreatic) fistulas and for fistulas that have not been explored for involved organs, abscesses, and distal obstruction. NPWT has built-in sensors to alert caregivers to potential and actual breaches in the integrity of the system. Further information about the application and use of NPWT is presented in Chapter 21

Pouching System Options and Features. Volume and odor are the primary indications for pouching. Dressings are contraindicated when odor is problematic or the volume of effluent exceeds 100 ml in 24 hours. However, patients with low-volume, nonodorous output may choose a pouch for convenience. The pouch may be changed once per week and is less expensive than dressings.

Numerous techniques for managing fistulas have been reported in the literature (Boarini et al, 1986; Davis et al, 2000; Irrgang and Bryant, 1984; Jones and Harbit, 2003; Kordasiewicz, 2004; O'Brien et al, 1998; Rolstad and Wong, 2004; Skingley, 1998; Smith, 1982, 1986). Ostomy pouches (fecal or urinary; adult or pediatric) can be used, as well as pouches specifically designed for managing complex wounds. Pouching preserves patient dignity by containing embarrassing odor and drainage. Pouching is an effective strategy for pain control because it requires less manipulation of the wound and protects the surrounding skin from painful denudement caused by caustic drainage. An effective pouching system also offers a sense of control to the nursing staff because effluent is contained and emptied at specific intervals. Pouch changes are scheduled at convenient times before leakage occurs. By preventing the embarrassment of odor and leaking dressings, the patient's dignity is supported. A routine pouch change procedure and fistula pouching tips are listed in Boxes 38-5 and 38-6, respectively.

Historically, frequent modifications of skin barriers, adhesives, and/or pouches were required to effectively manage the complicated fistula. Few alternatives were available to manage the fistula with a large cutaneous opening, irregular contours of the skin, and other unique situations. Materials used for pouches included garbage bags, colostomy irrigation sleeves, and sandwich bags. Today, manufactured wound management systems are designed for the difficult-to-manage site. Solid-wafer skin barriers with durable formulations that provide longer wear time are integrated into most pouching systems. Cutting surfaces of the skin barriers are available to manage a broad range of fistula opening sizes, ranging from the small opening of a starter hole to

---

BOX 38-5 | **Sizable Pouch Change Procedure: Fistula**

1. Assemble equipment: pouch with attached skin barrier, pattern, skin barrier paste, scissors, paper tape, closure clip, water, gauze, or tissue.
2. Prepare pouch.
   A. Trace pattern onto skin barrier surface of pouch.
   B. Cut skin barrier pouch to size of pattern.
   C. Remove protective backing(s) from pouch.
3. Remove and apply pouch.
   A. Remove pouch, using one hand to gently push skin away from adhesive.
   B. Discard pouch and save closure clip.
   C. Control any discharge with gauze or tissue.
   D. Clean skin with water and dry thoroughly.
   E. Apply paste around fistula or stoma. Fill in any uneven skin surfaces with paste or skin barrier strips. Use damp finger or tongue blade to apply paste.
   F. Apply new pouch, centering wound site in opening.
   G. Tape edges of adhesive surface in picture frame effect with paper tape.
   H. Close bottom of pouch with clip.

BOX 38-6 | **Fistula Pouching Tips**

1. Schedule the procedure, if possible, to allow education and participation from nursing staff and other caregivers.
2. Set up all equipment before starting procedure. Fistula function is unpredictable and may otherwise occur when adhesives are not completely set up.
3. Cut opening in pouch adhesive approximately 1/8 inch larger than fistula cutaneous opening.
4. Protect exposed periwound skin with skin barrier paste (see Color Plate 73).
5. Apertures much larger than actual fistula opening may be necessary with severe, deep depressions that create irregular skin surfaces.
6. Follow universal precautions with clean technique during procedures. Sterile products are an unnecessary expense and are not shown to control infection.
7. To remove adhesives from skin, gently roll off adherent material with dry gauze. Solvents may be used but must be cleansed thoroughly from skin before adhesive application. Do not scrub or abrade skin. It may be necessary to leave small amounts of residual paste or cement on skin but should not hinder pouch adhesion.
8. Cleanse skin with tap water or commercially available skin cleanser and gauze. Cleansers will emulsify fecal material and are primarily indicated when fistula drainage is adherent to surrounding skin. Cleansers should be nongreasy and rinsed thoroughly; use on denuded skin is discouraged. Dry thoroughly.
9. Minimize pooling of corrosive effluent over skin barrier by angling tail of pouch off to reclining patient's side, or attach drainage tubing to enable continuous drainage.
10. Empty pouch when one third to half full. Encourage patient to monitor.

9½ × 6 inches. However, it remains essential to fill irregular skin surfaces so that a flat, stable surface is attained for the pouching system.

Selecting a pouching system that supports the perifistular tissue and stabilizes soft skin may be necessary. In general, if the skin is soft or flaccid, a firm skin barrier adhesive and possibly a belt may be indicated. In contrast, firm skin surrounding the fistula site is best managed with a flexible, soft adhesive surface. Examples of soft, pliable materials include powder, skin barrier paste, wafers, strips, and rings. Methods for achieving firm support include firm rings, convexity in ostomy pouching systems, and belts.

Knowledge of available features of products is essential to make appropriate choices. Features include adhesive skin barrier surface, pouch capacity, pouch material (film and outlet), and wound access (Box 38-7 and Figure 38-7).

Adhesive Skin Barrier Surface. When the cutaneous opening is less than 3 inches, a one- or two-piece ostomy pouch may be used. For fistulas larger than 3 inches, commercially available wound management systems or modifications of larger pouches are warranted. In either case, the adhesive skin barrier surface must be large enough to accommodate the fistula opening and generally allow for 1 to 2 inches of adhesive contact around the fistula. The adhesive surface should be applied in such a fashion as to avoid obstacles in the perifistular skin area, such as a bony prominence or drain site. If this is not possible, a pouch with a smaller adhesive surface may be needed.

Conversely, a large amount of adhesive contact (over 4 to 5 inches) with the surrounding skin is generally not necessary and may be detrimental. Movement-induced

---

BOX 38-7 | **Features of Fistula Pouch**

Adhesive Surface
- Integrated skin barrier
- Size and shape of cutting surface
- Sizable versus presized adhesive surface
- Presence or absence of starter hole
- Degree of flexibility of skin barrier wafer

Pouch Capacity
- Volume (3- to 4-hour capacity preferred)

Pouch Material
- Odorproof or odor-resistant pouch film
- Transparent versus opaque film
- Fecal outlet (clamp closure)
- Spout for liquids (urinary outlet)
- Wide drain for viscous material
- Wide tubular outlet can be converted to open-end drain

Wound Access
- Two-piece pouch
- Access window on wound management system
- Wide tubular outlet can be converted to open-end drain

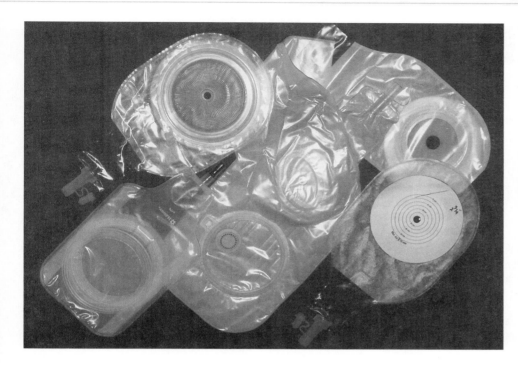

FIGURE 38-7 Examples of pouches. Note variety of sizes of the adhesive surface, outlet spouts, and access windows.

skin changes under the adhesive surface will precipitate leakage and disruption of the pouch seal.

Pouching systems may have a starter hole for cutting the opening into irregular shapes or may be presized (e.g., for round, regular shapes). Although starter holes are convenient for cutting, they restrict the positioning of the opening in the adhesive because the opening includes the starter hole. In some situations, the opening may have to be covered with a skin barrier so that other locations on the adhesive may be cut to fit the size of the fistula.

A few pouches are available without an integrated skin barrier wafer. In these situations, the fistula pattern must be used to cut a hole in the skin barrier wafer and the pouch. The skin barrier is then attached to the pouch, and the system is applied directly to the skin.

Pouch Capacity. The capacity of the pouch is predetermined by the size of the adhesive surface; typically pouches with larger adhesive surfaces have larger pouch capacities. Generally, a pouch with the capacity to contain 3 to 4 hours' worth of effluent is recommended so that the risk of leakage is minimized. A smaller-capacity pouch may be used if the caregiver or patient is willing to empty the pouch more frequently or if the pouch can be connected to straight drainage. Small-volume closed-end pouches may also be indicated for the patient with minimal malodorous output. This pouch can be changed and discarded once or twice per week.

Pouch Outlet. Effluent consistency and volume dictate the best type of outlet spout for pouch management. Pouches are designed with either urinary (or liquid) outlets or fecal outlets (see Figure 38-7). The urinary outlet is indicated for liquid effluent. It is convenient because it may be connected to straight drainage. When a urinary pouch is used for fistula care, the antireflux mechanism will obstruct flow; therefore, the antireflux mechanism must be pulled apart. Fecal outlets (or open-end drains) are appropriate for thick, mushy effluent and are secured with a clamp.

The two-piece ostomy system, fecal incontinence collectors, and wound management systems offer the benefit of having a urinary outlet that can be attached to a bedside bag. As the effluent thickens, the outlet can be trimmed off and secured with a clamp, transforming the pouch from a urinary to a fecal pouch without having to remove the pouch from the skin.

Two-piece high-output pouching systems are available that combine the desirable features of an ostomy system (e.g., presized adhesive surface and convexity) with outlets than can accommodate the varying consistency of effluent typical of a fistula.

Adaptations can be made to pouches to accommodate fistula consistency. For example, when formed output becomes liquid, urinary pouch–adapter latex drainage tubing can be attached to a fecal pouch. If the output begins to thicken or form particulate matter, wider respiratory tubing can be attached to the tail of an open-end drain (Box 38-8).

Wound Access. At times, access to the fistula site may be desirable so that tubes can be advanced, the fistula can be assessed easily, or skin barrier pastes can be reinforced. Access to the site without disruption of the pouch adhesive can be achieved with a two-piece pouch or with a pouch that has an attached "access window." When such access features are not available or have an inadequate adhesive surface size, wide open-end drains can be used. Cuffing the pouch film back can facilitate limited access to the fistula site.

BOX 38-8 | **Addition of Continuous Drainage Tube to Fecal Outlet Pouch**

Equipment
- Fecal pouch or open-end drain
- Connector to fit tubing and bedside system
- 5 inches of wide-lumen tubing or respiratory tubing
- Rubber band
- Bedside drainage system

Procedure
1. Cut desired size for fistula in skin barrier adhesive of fecal pouch or open-end drain.
2. Insert wide-lumen tubing or respiratory tubing into drain spout.
3. Working at adhesive surface, reach inside pouch and pull drain spout and tubing through opening cut in skin barrier adhesive.
4. Wrap rubber band securely around tubing to secure.
5. From bottom of pouch, pull tubing through so that outlet spout is in its normal location. Tail of pouch now is cuffed around tubing inside pouch.
6. Attach to bedside drainage system.

Note: If wide respiratory tubing is used, a condom catheter can be used to connect the pouch to bedside drainage.

BOX 38-9 | **Procedure for Adding Adhesive Sheets to Enlarge Pouch Adhesive Surface**

Equipment
- Pouch without floating collar
- Double-faced adhesive sheet or disk

Procedure
1. Remove protective paper from one side of adhesive sheet.
2. Attach this adhesive sheet adjacent to existing adhesive on pouch (edges may overlap slightly).
3. Trace desired opening size on protective paper, covering adhesive surface.
4. Cut to desired size.
5. Prepare solid-wafer skin barrier (usually 8 × 8 inches), attach to adhesive surface on pouch, and continue in usual fashion.

BOX 38-10 | **Procedure for Making Temporary Fistula Pouch**

Equipment
- Plastic bag
- Skin barrier wafer
- Double-faced adhesive sheet or double-faced tape

Procedure
1. Remove protective paper from one side of adhesive sheet and apply to area of pouch where adhesive and barrier are intended to be (in absence of adhesive sheets, substitute with overlapping strips of double-sided tape).
2. Remove other side of adhesive sheet or tape.
3. Attach skin barrier wafer (top side toward exposed adhesive on pouch).
4. Cut barrier of pouch to desired size.
5. Remove skin barrier wafer protective paper backing.
6. Continue in usual fashion.

Pouch Film. Urinary drainage equipment and some fecal pouches may be more odor resistant than odor-proof. More frequent pouch changes may be necessary to prevent the odor from permeating the pouch film, or more aggressive odor management techniques (e.g., oral deodorizers) may be required. Pouching systems marketed as wound management systems are transparent to allow for visual inspection. Ostomy pouches adapted for fistula care provide choices in film color (transparent, opaque, beige tone).

Pouching System Adaptations

Adhesives. Additional adhesive is available as cement, medical adhesive spray forms, and sheet form. Cements and sprays are applied according to the manufacturer's instructions; most require time to become tacky. They are used to enhance the tack of an existing adhesive and to extend the adhesive surface on a pouch. Adhesives may also be warranted to improve the tack when several applications of skin barrier powder are required in the presence of severe denudation. Occasionally, liquid adhesive is used in combination with skin barrier powders to protect exposed skin from caustic effluent. This procedure is similar to the artificial scab discussed previously.

Because fistulas vary in size and shape and abdominal contours can be dramatic, large and unusually shaped pouch apertures may be necessary. Sheets of adhesives (or double-faced adhesive disks) can be used to increase the adhesive surface on a pouch. Box 38-9 describes the procedure for adding an adhesive sheet to a pouch.

Another option is simply to create a pouch (Box 38-10). The advantage to this technique is that it offers immediate skin protection and containment of affluent using readily available supplies. Although this is a temporary intervention, it allows the care provider time to design a management system and to obtain commercially available products with the desirable features identified in the plan of care.

Another method that can be used to acquire a large adhesive surface is to attach two open-end drainable pouches, a technique called *saddlebagging* (Figure 38-8). Pouch features that facilitate saddlebagging include no attached solid-wafer skin barrier, no floating collar, and no starter hole. A large solid-wafer skin barrier is then attached to the new combined adhesive surface, and the pouch is prepared in the usual fashion. Box 38-11 describes the saddlebagging technique.

Bridging Technique. The bridging technique is a procedure that can be used to isolate one area of a wound from another part of the wound. It has two primary indications for use:

1. Wounds may present with two distinct areas of "needs": one area of the wound has drainage and requires containment, whereas another area requires moist wound healing or packing.

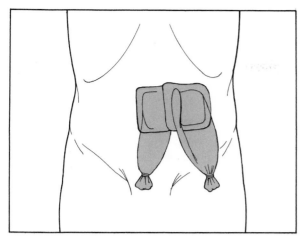

FIGURE 38-8 Saddlebagging technique in which two open-ended drainable pouches are connected along the adhesive surface to create a large adhesive surface.

2. Very large wounds may be more manageable if the wound is "divided." Solid-wafer skin barriers are cut into small pieces to fill the wound at the selected bridge location and layered into place (Figure 38-9). A routine pouch or more complicated pouching system can then be applied over the bridge that now exists in the wound. Box 38-12 describes the steps involved in the bridging technique.

Catheter Ports. When a catheter or tube is in place at a fistula site, leakage onto perifistular skin may occur. A pouching system with an attached catheter port may be used to collect the drainage. A catheter port is a nipple-shaped device that attaches to the external wall of a

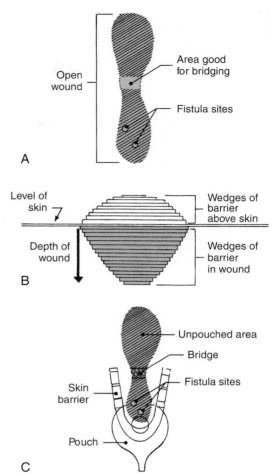

FIGURE 38-9 Bridging technique. **A,** Area of wound where fistula sites are located and identified can be separated from remainder of wound. **B,** Cross-sectional view of tapered skin barrier wedges used to fill wound defect and to extend slightly above level of skin. **C,** Demonstration of how a pouch is applied over a bridge and fistula, leaving the area of the wound that is not draining available for more appropriate wound care.

pouch. The catheter is disconnected, threaded through the pouch opening on the adhesive surface, and then threaded through the catheter port itself so that the catheter can be reconnected to drainage. The pouch is then secured to the skin in the usual fashion. Detailed instructions from the manufacturer accompany the catheter port. With this technique, drainage around the catheter is collected in the pouch while the catheter continues to drain by suction or gravity (see Figure 39-16).

Silicone Molding. A silicone molding technique using a dental mold material to fashion an impression of the fistula opening and perifistular area in an attempt to create a smooth surface to which a pouch can be applied has been reported (Laing, 1977). When used, this procedure was reserved for the recessed fistula located in an open wound or the fistula surrounded by numerous irregular skin surfaces. However, the silicone mold procedure is less commonly used now because of the advances in wound management products (Box 38-13).

BOX 38-11 | Saddlebagging Technique

Equipment
- Two open-end drains (without floating collar or attached skin barrier or starter hole)
- Solid-wafer skin barrier (8 × 8 inches)
- Skin barrier paste

Procedure
1. Align pouches as final product is intended to appear on abdomen.
2. Peel protective backing away from adhesive along common edges of pouches approximately ½ to 1 inch.
3. Attach two pouches along this ½- to 1-inch margin only.
4. Trace pattern of wound onto new adhesive surface (combined pouch adhesive surfaces).
5. Cut out pouch opening; do not cut into "seam" created by combining pouches.
6. Trace pattern onto solid-wafer skin barrier and cut out.
7. Remove protective paper backing from pouch adhesive surface and attach to solid-wafer skin barrier.
8. Prepare skin as indicated by wound contours and continue pouching procedure.

Note: Both pouches will fill with drainage and will require emptying.

BOX 38-12 | **Bridging Technique**

1. Assess wound and determine most appropriate location for "bridge." Be sure all sites from which drainage is produced are included on side of wound to be pouched. For simplification of bridging procedure, areas that are narrower or shallower should be selected.
2. Apply layered wedges of solid-wafer skin barrier and paste to create bridge. Wedges must be custom cut to fit dimensions of wound at that level; usually the bottom wedge is narrowest because the deepest part of the wound typically is the narrowest area. Each successive wedge is a little wider until the skin barrier wafer wedges reach skin level.
3. Continue to layer solid-wafer barrier wedges above skin level, using progressively smaller and narrower wedges (to create pressure dressing effect).
4. Apply solid-wafer skin barrier to cover newly created bridge and extend onto intact skin. Paste may be needed to smooth "seams."
5. Continue with routine or complex pouching procedure as indicated.

Note: Skin barrier paste, adhesive spray, or cement can be used between wedges but is not routinely necessary.

BOX 38-13 | **Silicone Mold**

Equipment
- Emesis basin
- Tongue blade
- Dow Corning medical grade elastomer 382
- Dow Corning Catalyst M and eye dropper
- Red rubber catheter (optional)
- Skin barrier paste
- Ostomy pouch with belt
- Adhesives (silicone spray necessary to adhere to mold)

Preparation
1. Cleanse skin around wound with water and pat dry.
2. Pour elastomer into dry emesis basin; usually 1 or 1½ ounces is enough for moderate-sized cast.
3. Add 10 to 12 drops of Catalyst M for each ounce of elastomer.
4. Stir thoroughly with tongue blade.
5. If necessary, place suction catheter into fistula opening to contain drainage while cast is setting.
6. When elastomer has slightly thickened, pour on patient's abdomen or in open wound around fistula orifice to a ¼-inch thickness.
7. Allow mold to harden for 3–5 minutes in wound.
8. Gently lift mold out of wound.
9. Remove catheter from cast.
10. Trim edges of cast to form gently rounded surfaces.
11. Trim fistula opening in cast to be sure opening is adequate.

Application
1. Spread smooth layer of skin barrier paste on back of mold using tongue blade and allow to set until it is firm to touch. *Note:* Silicone spray can be applied to the surface to increase adherence with or without the paste.
2. Place mold into wound. Seal edges with skin barrier paste.
3. Apply tape on all edges of mold.
4. Apply ostomy pouch with belt tabs over opening in the mold; attach belt.

Trough Procedure. When fistulas are contained within the depressions of a wound such that a routine pouching system fails, the trough procedure may be useful. With this procedure, one or several strips of a transparent dressing are used to occlude the wound and trap effluent in the wound depression (Figure 38-10). A small opening is made in the transparent dressing at the most dependent aspect of the wound, and an ostomy pouch is applied over this opening. No pattern is required.

To enhance adherence of the transparent dressing to the skin peripheral to the fistula or wound (and to protect perifistular skin), strips of a solid-wafer skin barrier should be applied. Directions for the trough procedure are given in Box 38-14.

Odor Control. In general, odor control measures are indicated any time the patient and/or family perceives an odor to be objectionable, even if the odor seems almost imperceptible.

The method of odor control depends on whether dressings or pouches are being used. Gauze dressings do not control odor; therefore, charcoal-impregnated dressings may be needed over the gauze dressings. However, charcoal becomes inactivated with moisture, so these dressings should not come into contact with wound drainage. Charcoal dressings are most cost effective with low-output fistulas, for which the dressings remain intact for 24 to 48 hours. These dressings are effective only when all edges of the dressing are taped to the skin. Pouches provide odor control. However, when the pouch is emptied, odor may be noticeable. Therefore, odor management must be a component of the care plan.

Odor is best controlled by use of a pouch to contain the effluent. A pouch may be the preferred management technique simply to contain the odor, regardless of the volume of output. Although most pouches have an odorproof film, the film's ability to contain odor varies. For example, many urinary pouches and urinary drainable systems are not odorproof and may become saturated with odor quickly.

To control odor, you should (1) dispose of soiled linens and dressings from the room promptly, (2) use care in emptying pouches to prevent splashing effluent on the patient or on linens, (3) cleanse the tail of drainable fecal pouches after emptying, and (4) use deodorants appropriately.

Deodorants can be taken internally (orally) or used externally (in the pouch or as a room spray). Internal deodorants are available in tablet form but are generally discouraged in the presence of a pathologic condition such as a fistula. External deodorants are available in liquids, powders, and tablets and are placed in the pouch after each emptying. Room deodorants are particularly useful when emptying the pouch, changing the pouch, or

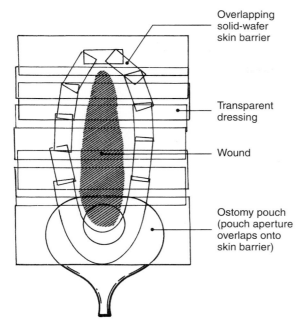

Overlapping
solid-wafer
skin barrier

Transparent
dressing

Wound

Ostomy pouch
(pouch aperture
overlaps onto
skin barrier)

FIGURE 38-10 Trough procedure. Note overlapping skin barrier wafers and transparent dressing strips. Pouch opening must overlap onto skin barrier wafer at inferior aspect of wound.

changing dressings. The room deodorant selected should eliminate rather than mask odor. With the many types of deodorants now available, patients, families, and caregivers should not have to tolerate the odor that often accompanies fistulas.

Patient Comfort. Areas to address to promote patient comfort include prevention and early treatment of

perifistular skin irritation, pain control, and education to decrease anxiety. Leaking pouches, wet dressings on the skin, and odor in the patient's room all negatively affect morale. Medicating the patient before dressing or pouch changes may be indicated. Factors contributing to skin irritation include damp dressings, presence of caustic effluent in contact with the skin, and frequent tape application and removal. When selecting and evaluating a management technique, interventions appropriate to prevent unnecessary patient discomfort should be considered.

Accurate Measurement of Effluent. Accurate measurement of effluent from a fistula or drain site is critical to the success of fluid and electrolyte resuscitation and nutritional support. As the patient becomes stabilized, accurate measurement of the effluent is less important. Pouching offers the most objective method for monitoring output, and suction is accurate only if the effluent does not leak around the catheters. Dressings can provide an estimate of volume if the dressings are weighed; however, this method is time consuming, messy, and inconsistent from caregiver to caregiver.

Patient Mobility. Consideration for optimizing the patient's activity should be of paramount importance when a fistula management method is being selected. Restrictions on physical activity predispose the patient to physical complications such as pneumonia, pressure ulcers, and thrombophlebitis, as well as to psychosocial complications such as depression and withdrawal. Because limitations on a patient's physical activity are sometimes necessary when suction or dressings are used to contain effluent, these interventions should be used only on a temporary basis. Pouches are less likely to restrict mobility.

Ease of Use. Complex patient situations may necessitate unique pouching systems that may be expensive and labor intensive. These unique adaptations often set up hurdles to the successful participation of care providers. These complicated systems increase the chance of error in application and the time required of the caregiver. Therefore, management may be complex initially and require the expertise of a certified ostomy care nurse (COCN). As care progresses, the method of pouching should be simplified as much as possible to a more user-friendly system so that its care can be delegated. Several conveniences are available and should be considered as long as effectiveness is not compromised (Box 38-15).

Cost Containment. Accountable, appropriate fistula management requires selection of treatment options that are cost effective. For example, a fistula pouch with a wound access window is more costly than a sizable ostomy pouch, which probably would yield the same wear time. However, if use of a pouch with an access window prolongs wear time by providing access for wound care and paste application, it may be the most cost-effective option, even if the pouch is changed every other day. Cost containment implies attention not only to products and materials but also to labor and time.

BOX 38-14   Trough Procedure

1. Prepare skin and fill irregular skin surface as usual.
2. Apply overlapping strips of solid-wafer barrier along wound edges.
3. Apply skin barrier paste to smooth "seams" (between barrier edges and along skin edges). *Note:* Inferior aspect of wound should be bordered with solid piece of barrier instead of overlapping strips to prevent leakage.
4. Cut strips of transparent dressing wide enough to cover wound and skin barrier strips. Calculate length of strips so that strips overlap intact skin with 1- to 2-inch margins.
5. Reserve one strip of transparent dressing to be applied to most inferior aspect of wound.
6. Attach a drainable pouch (can be urinary or fecal) to this one strip of transparent dressing.
7. Cut hole in pouch or transparent dressing adhesive surface so that it is lower than inferior wound margins (should clear wound edges to provide adequate drainage).
8. Beginning at top of wound, apply transparent dressing in overlapping strips.
9. Attach final strip of transparent dressing (with attached pouch) so that bottom of pouch opening is secured onto skin barrier wafer.

BOX 38-15**User-Friendly Considerations in Fistula Care**

1. Use presized pouch rather than sizable pouch whenever possible.
2. Avoid suction when pouching is effective.
3. Fill skin defects with strip paste rather than tube paste in patients with manual dexterity problems.
4. Use pouching systems with convexity rather than creating convexity with layers of skin barriers.
5. Use one-piece rather than two-piece pouches.
6. Select equipment that is easy to access in the community. Mail order of products is a convenience as long as orders are placed before patient's supplies are depleted.

Evaluation

Accomplishment of Goals. The nurse should take time to reflect on the eight nursing management goals and evaluate how well they have been accomplished. Can steps be omitted? Is the skin intact? Is odor controlled? As the fistula stabilizes, the technical approach should be reevaluated and simplified as much as possible. One management system is seldom effective from the onset of the fistula until closure. For example, one fistula may be managed over its course with a pouch, dressings, suction, or all three. While the patient in the hospital, suction may be a workable option; however, mobility is compromised, and plans for home care are complicated. Therefore, developing a pouching system that does not require suction would be an important simplification. Similarly, using products that are difficult to obtain is a complicating step and may be expensive. Planning to use an effective system that is easy and readily available is essential to facilitate the delivery of care.

Making Changes. It is important to expect change in fistula care and to modify interventions as needed. Seldom will the first pouch applied to a complex fistula be effective. Generally, modifications are necessary in the pouch pattern, size of adhesive surface, and use of skin barrier pastes or wafer strips. Changes are best made one at a time so that the effect of each modification can be accurately assessed. The addition of a belt may be warranted to add security to the pouch system, particularly on obese patients, or when the perifistular skin is mobile.

The nurse must provide close monitoring for the duration of the fistula regardless of the health care setting. An inquisitive, analytic approach will facilitate identifying steps to improve the duration of the pouching system. For example, if the pouch leaks, is the leak between the skin and the barrier or the barrier and the pouch? Is the pouch being emptied when it is one third to one half full to prevent overfilling?

SUMMARY

Successful management of a patient with a fistula requires close monitoring and a plan of care that addresses the technical, educational, and emotional needs of the patient. Care often crosses many health care settings with varying levels of expertise in the unique containment and skin protection vital to the patient's well-being. In these situations, special arrangements must be made for appropriate follow-up of these complex patients.

REFERENCES

Beitz JM, Caldwell D: Abdominal wound with enterocutaneous fistula: a case study, *J Wound Ostomy Continence Nurs* 25(2):102, 1998.

Berry SM, Fischer JE: Classification and pathophysiology of enterocutaneous fistulas, *Surg Clin North Am* 76(5):1009, 1996.

Boarini J et al: Fistula management, *Semin Oncol Nurs* 2:287, 1986.

Buchanan GN et al: Efficacy of fibrin sealant in the management of complex anal fistula, a prospective trial, *Dis Colon Rectum* 46:1167, 2003.

Campos ACL et al: A multivariate model to determine prognostic factors in gastrointestinal fistulas, *J Am Coll Surg* 188:483, 1999.

Davis M et al: Options for managing an open wound with draining enterocutaneous fistula, *J Wound Ostomy Continence Nurs* 27(2):118-123, 2000.

Fagniez PL, Yahchouchy E: Use of somatostatin in the treatment of digestive fistulas, *Digestion* 60(Suppl 3):65, 1999.

González-Pinto I, Moreno Gónzález E: Optimizing the treatment of upper gastrointestinal fistula, *Gut* 49(Suppl IV):iv22, 2001.

Hesse U et al: Role of somatostatin-14 and its analogues in the management of gastrointestinal fistulae: clinical data, *Gut* 49(Suppl IV):iv11, 2001.

Hild P et al: Treatment of enterocutaneous fistulas and somatostatin, *Lancet* 2:626, 1986.

Hollington P et al: An 11-year experience of enterocutaneous fistulas, *Br J Surg* 91:1646, 2004.

Hollis HW, Reyna TM: A practical approach to wound care in patients with complex enterocutaneous fistulas, *Surg Gynecol Obstet* 161:179, 1985.

Irrgang S, Bryant R: Management of the enterocutaneous fistula, *J Enterostom Ther* 11:211, 1984.

Jeter KF et al: Managing draining wounds and fistulae: new and established methods. In Krasner D, editor: *Chronic wound care: a clinical source book for healthcare professionals*, King of Prussia, Penn., 1990, Health Management.

Jones EG, Harbit M: Management of an ileostomy and mucous fistula located in a dehisced wound in a patient with morbid obesity, *J Wound Ostomy Continence Nurs* 30(6):351, 2003.

Kassis ES, Makary MA: Enterocutaneous fistula. In Cameron JS, editor: *Current surgical therapy*, ed 9, St. Louis, 2008, Mosby.

Knechtges P, Zimmermann EM: Intra-abdominal abscesses and fistulae. In Yamada T et al, editors: *Textbook of gastroenterology*, vol II, ed 6, Philadelphia, 2009, Lippincott Williams & Wilkins.

Kordasiewicz LM: Abdominal wound with fistula and large amount of drainage status after incarcerated hernia repair, *J Wound Ostomy Continence Nurs* 31(3):150, 2004.

Laing BJ: Making silicone casts for enterocutaneous fistulas, *ET J* Fall:11, 1977.

Lange MP et al: Management of multiple enterocutaneous fistulas, *Heart Lung* 18:386, 1989.

Makhdoom ZA et al: Nutrition and enterocutaneous fistulas, *J Clin Gastroenterol* 31(3):195, 2000.

Maykel JA, Fischer JE: Current management of intestinal fistulas. In Cameron JL, editor: *Advances in surgery*, St. Louis, 2003, Mosby.

Meissner K: Late radiogenic small bowel damage: guidelines for the general surgeon, *Dig Surg* 16:169, 1999.

Migaly J, Rolandelli RH: Suturing stapling and tissue adhesives. In Yeo CJ et al, editors: *Shackelford's surgery of the alimentary tract*, ed 6, St. Louis, 2006, Saunders.

Nussbaum MS, Fischer DR: Gastric, duodenal and small intestinal fistulas. In Yeo CJ et al, editors: *Shackelford's surgery of the alimentary tract*, ed 6, St. Louis, 2006, Saunders.

O'Brien B et al: Nursing management of multiple enterocutaneous fistulae located in the center of a large open abdominal wound: a case study, *Ostomy Wound Manage* 44(1):20, 1998.

O'Connor E: Vaginal fistulas: adaptation of management method for patients with radiation damage, *J Enterostom Ther* 10(6):229, 1983.

Rolstad B, Boarini J: Principles and techniques in the use of convexity, *Ostomy Wound Manage* 42(1):24, 1996.

Rolstad B, Wong WD: Nursing considerations in intestinal fistulas. In Cataldo PA, MacKeigan JM, editors: *Intestinal stomas: principles, techniques and management*, ed 2, New York, 2004, Marcel Dekker.

Saclarides TJ: Rectovaginal fistula, *Surg Clin N Am* 82:1261, 2002.

Scardillo J, Folkedahl B: Management of a complex high-output fistula, *J Wound Ostomy Continence Nurs* 25:217, 1998.

Skingley S: The management of a faecal fistula, *Nurs Times* 94(16):64, 1998.

Smith DB: Fistulas of the head and neck, *J Enterostom Ther* 9(5):20, 1982.

Smith DB: Multiple stomas, fistulas and draining wounds. In Smith DB, Johnson DR, editors: *Ostomy care and the cancer patient: surgical and clinical considerations*, New York, 1986, Grune & Stratton.

Tran NA, Thorson AG: Rectovaginal fistula. In Cameron JL, editor: *Current surgical therapy*, ed 9, St. Louis, 2008, Mosby.

Welch JP: Duodenal, gastric, and biliary fistulas. In Zinner MJ et al, editors: *Maingot's abdominal operations*, vol 1, ed 10, Stamford, Conn., 1997, Appleton and Lange.

Wiltshire BL: Challenging enterocutaneous fistula: a case presentation, *J Wound Ostomy Continence Nurs* 23(6):297, 1996.

Wong SL, Chang AE: Acute abdomen, bowel obstruction, and fistula. In Abeloff MD et al, editors: *Abeloff's clinical oncology*, ed 4, Oxford, 2008, Churchill Livingstone.

Wong WD et al: Management of intestinal fistulas. In Cataldo PA, MacKeigan JM, editors: *Intestinal stomas: principles, techniques, and management*, ed 2, New York, 2004, Marcel Dekker.

Zwanziger PJ: Pouching a draining duodenal cutaneous fistula: a case study, *J Wound Ostomy Continence Nurs* 26(1):25, 1999.

39

Percutaneous Tube Management

Ruth A. Bryant

OBJECTIVES

1. Identify two primary reasons for using percutaneous tubes.
2. Distinguish among the placement approaches for gastrostomy and jejunostomy, including indications and overview of technique.
3. Explain why tube stabilization is a priority in the management of the patient with a percutaneous tube.
4. Describe at least two options for stabilizing gastrostomy or jejunostomy tubes.

5. For each complication listed, identify a prevention and management approach: peritubular leakage, tube migration, candidiasis, and tube occlusion.
6. Identify percutaneous tubes that can be irrigated and those that cannot be irrigated.
7. Describe routine site care for the patient with a percutaneous tube.

Although described in the thirteenth century, planned surgical gastrostomy as a procedure was first proposed in 1837 and performed 12 years later in 1849, with the first reported survival of the procedure performed by S. Jones in 1876 (Wu and Soper, 2004). Today the use of tubes is commonplace within the gastrointestinal (GI) tract, as well as other organs and spaces, on a temporary or a long-term basis. Percutaneous tubes are placed for a variety of purposes, including feeding, decompression, and drainage. The tubes are inserted into the desired body part by an interventional radiologist using computed tomographic or fluoroscopic guidance.

Malfunction of these tubes can result in skin erosion, denudement, inflammation, and pain such that referral to the wound care nurse becomes necessary. This chapter reviews the different types of percutaneous tubes, their purpose, procedures for placement, nursing management, and potential complications.

Effective nursing management of the patient with a percutaneous tube requires an understanding of the anatomy and physiology of the affected body system, the pathology involved, the rationale for tube placement, the method of tube insertion, and the anticipated length of time that the tube will be necessary. Although specific care procedures vary depending on the body system involved and the purpose of tube placement, management should always include routine care designed to maintain tube function and prevent peritubular complications, patient/caregiver education, and routine surveillance for tube dysfunction or complications. Comprehensive care is best provided with a collaborative team approach

involving, but not limited to, the interventional radiologist, interventional radiology nurse, gastroenterologist, surgeon or internist, and nurse.

GASTROSTOMY AND JEJUNOSTOMY DEVICES

A *gastrostomy* is an opening into the stomach, and a *jejunostomy* is an opening into the jejunum. Such procedures may be used to provide decompression or enteral support for a patient unable to ingest adequate nutrients orally (DeChicco and Matarese, 2003). Enteral nutrition offers many potential advantages over parenteral nutrition, including lower rates of infectious and metabolic complications, decreased hospital length of stay, and reduced cost. Many of the benefits of enteral feeding are in part due to preservation of gut integrity (histologic structure and physical viability) better than parenteral feeding (Fish and Seidner, 2003; Harbison, 2007). Enteral support is generally appropriate through a nasogastric or nasoenteric feeding tube for short-term access (i.e., less than 3 to 4 weeks) in the patient who is at low risk for aspiration (Bloch and Mueller, 2004; DeChicco and Matarese, 2003; Wu and Soper, 2004). When the risk of aspiration exists, postpyloric placement of a tube is preferred. The patient's history and results of physical examination, barium studies, fluoroscopy, and manometry are useful when evaluating the patient's risk for aspiration. Consultation with the neurologist and speech pathologist also is beneficial. Box 39-1 lists the risk factors for aspiration.

- Altered mental status
- Swallowing dysfunction
- History of aspiration
- Severe gastroesophageal reflux
- Gastric outlet obstruction
- Gastroparesis

From Gorman RC, Nance ML, Morris JB: Enteral feeding techniques. In Torosian MH: *Nutrition for the hospitalized patient: basic science and principles of practice,* New York, 1995, Marcel Dekker.

PLACEMENT APPROACHES

For more than a century, gastrostomy placement required surgical intervention involving anesthesia and the traditional preoperative preparation for abdominal surgery. Historically, a suture was placed around the base of the tube at skin level and then through the skin to immobilize the gastrostomy tube. Gastrostomy tubes usually were connected to suction for 12 to 24 hours to reduce tension on the suture line. Feedings were delayed until bowel sounds, tube patency, and proper placement of the tube were confirmed.

Today, a gastrostomy or jejunostomy is created by one of three approaches: surgical, endoscopic, or interventional radiologic. Open laparotomy is rarely performed due to the success of the much less invasive endoscopic and laparoscopic techniques (Duh and McQuaid, 2000). Figure 39-1 presents an algorithm for determining the most appropriate means of enteral access.

Surgical Approaches

A surgically placed gastrostomy or jejunostomy tube can be accomplished through an open surgical procedure or a laparoscopic procedure. Surgical placement is relatively expensive, requires anesthesia and the use of sterile dressings, and exposes the patient to many potential complications. The surgical approach is reserved for the patient with pharyngeal, esophageal, or gastric obstructions or upper GI tumors, or for the patient in whom abdominal surgery is already being performed for other purposes. Surgical placement is also performed when endoscopic placement has failed (Beyers, 2003).

Open Surgical Procedure. The most common open surgical procedures for gastrostomy tube placement are the Stamm, the Witzel, and the Janeway. The Stamm and the Witzel are the simplest procedures and are considered temporary; the Janeway is more of a long-term or permanent procedure (Bloch and Mueller, 2004; Gincherman and Torosian, 1996).

Stamm Gastrostomy. Stamm gastrostomy is the standard open gastrostomy, the gold standard for transabdominal gastric access (Harbison, 2007). Creation of a Stamm gastrostomy begins by making a small incision in the left upper quadrant of the abdomen. Another small incision is made over and through the body of the stomach, through which a catheter (Foley, mushroom, Malecot, or gastrostomy replacement tube) is inserted (Figure 39-2). Several pursestring sutures are used to invaginate the stomach around the tube. The stomach is then fixed to the abdominal wall at the catheter site, and traditionally a nonabsorbable suture is used to secure the catheter to the skin. Although the Stamm gastrostomy is

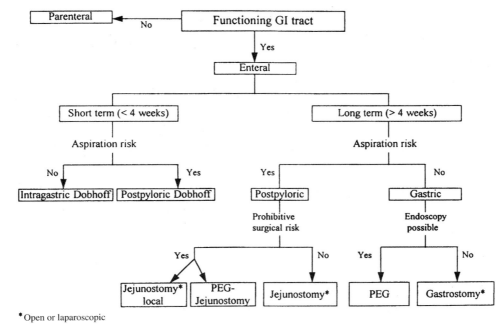

FIGURE 39-1 Enteral access algorithm for selecting the most appropriate technique for an individual patient. (From Gorman RC, Morris JB: Minimally invasive access to the gastrointestinal tract. In Rombeau JL, Rolandelli RH: *Clinical nutrition: enteral and tube feeding,* ed 3, Philadelphia, 1997, WB Saunders.)

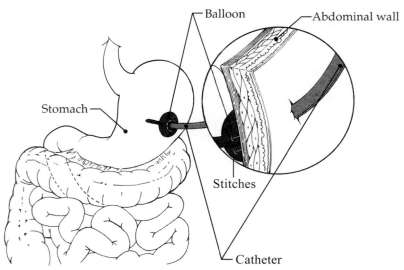

FIGURE 39-2 Stamm gastrostomy tube technique, oblique view. An incision is placed through the abdominal wall into the stomach, through which a catheter is passed.

the simplest surgical technique to perform and remove, it is frequently difficult to manage and is plagued with complications such as peritubular leakage, wound infection, peritonitis, and tube dislodgment (Beyers, 2003).

Witzel Gastrostomy. Witzel gastrostomy is created similarly to the Stamm gastrostomy, with the additional construction of a 4- to 6-cm seromuscular tunnel of the stomach wall through which the gastrostomy tube is placed (Figure 39-3). The seromuscular tunnel is designed to reduce the risk of peritubular leakage, particularly when the stomach is distended or the tube is removed.

Janeway Gastrostomy. Janeway gastrostomy is a surgically constructed, mucosa-lined gastric passageway that is brought out onto the abdominal surface as a permanent mucocutaneous stoma. Figure 39-4 illustrates

how the Janeway gastrostomy is constructed. Postoperatively, an inflated balloon-tip catheter is placed in the tract. Once the tract has matured (7–10 days), the tube is removed. A tube is inserted into the Janeway gastrostomy during each feeding and then removed. This type of permanent gastrostomy requires more operative time than the Stamm gastrostomy and results in many similar complications (Gorman et al, 1995).

Witzel Jejunostomy. The Witzel technique is the most common technique for surgically placed jejunostomy. The Witzel technique can be used to create a jejunostomy either at the conclusion of a surgical procedure or as an isolated procedure. The usual site is the left upper quadrant. A loop of jejunum 15 to 20 cm from the ligament of Treitz is brought up to the wound, and a circular pursestring suture is placed in the antimesenteric

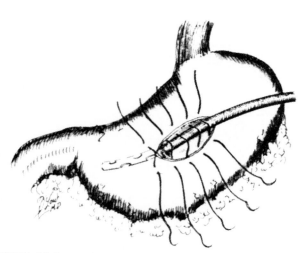

FIGURE 39-3 Witzel gastrostomy. This is similar to the Stamm gastrostomy with the addition of a 4- to 6-cm seromuscular tunnel of the stomach wall, through which the gastrostomy tube is placed. (From Patterson RS: Enteral nutrition delivery systems. In Grant JA, Kennedy-Caldwell C, editors: *Nutritional support nursing,* Philadelphia, 1988, Grune & Stratton.)

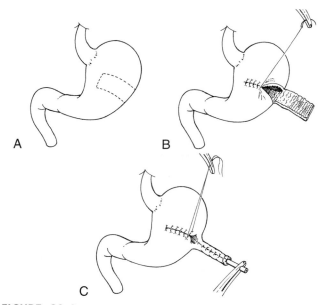

FIGURE 39-4 Janeway gastrostomy. A surgically constructed, mucosa-lined gastric passageway is brought out onto the abdominal surface as a permanent mucocutaneous stoma.

border. An incision through the center of the pursestring suture is made, and a 14-French (14Fr) feeding catheter is inserted into the jejunal lumen and advanced. A serosal tunnel is constructed at the exit site in the jejunal wall, extending approximately 5 to 6 cm proximally. The catheter is brought to the skin through a separate incision and secured, typically with sutures. The loop of intestine is anchored to the anterior abdominal wall (Wu and Soper, 2004).

Needle Catheter Jejunostomy. The needle jejunostomy is a simple procedure that is most often done at the conclusion of a surgical procedure when prolonged enteral support is anticipated. At approximately 30 to 40 cm distal to the ligament of Treitz, a 14- to 16-gauge needle is inserted into the jejunal wall. A feeding catheter is advanced through the needle 30 to 40 cm distally, and the needle is withdrawn. A pursestring suture is made around the tube to close the jejunal opening around the catheter. The loop of bowel is anchored to the anterior abdominal wall, and the catheter is secured to the skin (Figure 39-5) (Harbison, 2007).

Laparoscopic Surgical Approach. The laparoscopic approach for insertion of the gastrostomy or jejunostomy has been possible since the introduction of high-resolution video cameras and has the advantages of minimal invasion and few surgical side effects (Georgeson, 1997). This approach also provides the opportunity to selectively determine the site of the tube within the stomach (e.g., lesser-curvature gastrostomy rather than the more commonly selected greater-curvature), which may be im-

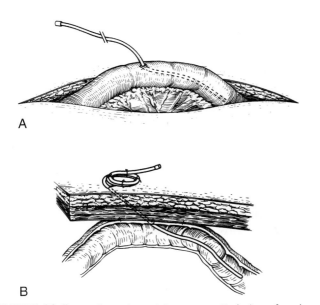

FIGURE 39-5 Needle catheter jejunostomy. Technique for placement of a needle catheter jejunostomy. **A,** The catheter is inserted into the lumen of the jejunum for a distance of 40 to 50 cm and secured into place with a pursestring suture. **B,** The jejunum is secured to the anterior abdominal wall. The feeding catheter is removed postoperatively when the patient can tolerate oral feedings. (From Bland KI et al: *Atlas of surgical oncology,* Philadelphia, 1995, WB Saunders.)

portant in the patient who is at high risk for reflux or aspiration. A key advantage to a laparoscopic approach is that the abdomen can be examined under direct vision without the need for a large surgical incision so that biopsy specimens can be obtained if necessary or malignancy staging can be conducted (Coates and MacFadyen, 1996). This technique requires a smaller incision than the open surgical approach, but local or general anesthesia is still needed.

Laparoscopic Gastrostomy. The indication for laparoscopic gastrostomy for feeding is the inability to perform percutaneous endoscopic gastrostomy, such as with a morbidly obese patient. A small supraumbilical incision is made through which the camera port is placed, and a 5-mm port is placed in the epigastrium. An atraumatic instrument is used to grasp the stomach, and the site for the proposed gastrostomy is identified. An 18-gauge angiocatheter is passed through the anterior abdomen, at the site chosen for the gastrostomy, and into the stomach. The needle is removed, and a soft J-wire is passed into the stomach. Dilators (12Fr and 14Fr) are placed over this J-wire. A 16Fr peel-away catheter is placed over the dilator, and a 16-Fr catheter is inserted through the sheath. The catheter is positioned against the stomach wall by inflating the balloon or securing the internal bumper. This particular type of gastrostomy is less commonly used than the Stamm due to technical requirements and pneumoperitoneum (Harbison, 2007).

Laparoscopic Jejunostomy. Specific indications for laparoscopic jejunostomy include concomitant laparoscopy for other problems and difficult laparoscopic gastrostomy. It is a minimally invasive procedure with desirable advantages of reduced postoperative pain and shortened recuperative time; general anesthesia is required. The procedure is more expensive than percutaneous or surgical placement. Two methods described by Wu and Soper (2004) are briefly discussed in this section.

The laparoscope is inserted through a small incision above the umbilicus. The proximal small bowel is identified and traced 25 cm distal to the ligament of Treitz, and the antimesenteric border is withdrawn into the umbilical wound. At this location in the small bowel, a Witzel tunnel is created or concentric pursestring sutures are placed, and a 12Fr catheter is inserted into the bowel. The bowel is secured to the fascia around the tube and returned to the abdominal cavity, and the fascia and skin are closed. The catheter is tunneled subcutaneously to exit the skin at the site previously selected on the abdomen.

In another technique, T-fasteners (or tacks) are inserted through the skin into the bowel lumen to anchor and retract the bowel against the abdominal wall (Duh and McQuaid, 2000; Wu and Soper 2004). Once the bowel is anchored, a percutaneous jejunostomy tube can be placed directly through the abdominal wall (Figure 39-6).

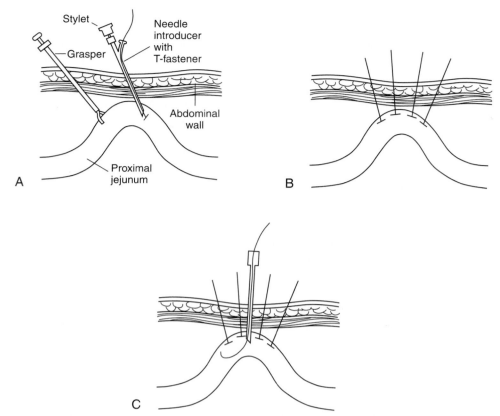

FIGURE 39-6 Laparoscopic jejunostomy with T-fasteners, which are inserted through the skin into the bowel lumen to anchor and retract the bowel against the abdominal wall before a percutaneous jejunostomy tube is inserted directly through the abdominal wall.

Endoscopic Approach

The endoscopic approach to gastrostomy tube placement, known as *percutaneous endoscopic gastrostomy* (PEG), was first described by Gauderer and Ponsky (1980) and has quickly become the procedure of choice. These devices can be placed under local anesthesia and conscious sedation outside the operating room, thus avoiding the complications associated with surgical procedures.

Contraindications to PEG include inability to perform upper endoscopy, inability to illuminate the abdominal wall, ascites, esophageal obstruction, hepatomegaly, previous gastric resection, and uncorrectable coagulopathy (Bankhead and Rolandell, 2005).

Variations to the original technique exist; all involve a complete esophagogastroduodenoscopy, insufflation of air into the stomach, and transillumination of the stomach. After application of a topical pharyngeal anesthetic and sedation, an endoscope is passed into the stomach. Air is insufflated into the stomach, which distends the stomach against the anterior abdominal wall. The proposed gastrostomy site is then transilluminated. The endoscopy assistant indents the abdomen at the proposed gastrostomy site, which should be at least 2 cm below costal margin. At this point, several different techniques have been described to insert the PEG.

"Pull" (Ponsky) Technique. A small incision is made over the illuminated site, and a large-gauge angiocatheter is inserted into the stomach. The needle is withdrawn, and 60 inches of suture is passed through the catheter into the stomach. With a biopsy snare, the endoscopist grasps the suture and pulls so that the endoscope is removed with the suture attached (Figure 39-7). The gastrostomy tube is attached to the suture. By pulling on the suture at the abdominal gastrostomy site, the endoscopist draws the tube through the esophagus into the stomach and positions it snugly against the anterior stomach wall. To verify proper position of the PEG, an endoscope is passed again. Once placement is confirmed, the endoscope is removed, and the PEG secured at the skin level (Harbison, 2007).

"Over the Wire" (Sachs-Vine) Technique. With this technique, a long, flexible guidewire is inserted through the angiocatheter into the stomach. With use of the biopsy snare and endoscope, the wire is snared and pulled up through the esophagus and out the patient's mouth (Figure 39-8). The PEG tube is pushed over the guidewire and advanced through the esophagus to the stomach and positioned against the anterior stomach wall. As with the "pull" technique, PEG placement is checked with the endoscope, which is then removed, and the PEG is secured.

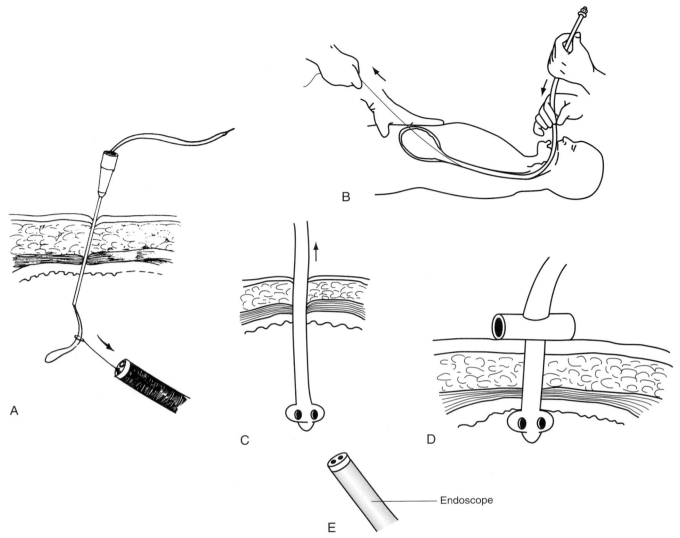

FIGURE 39-7 Ponsky (pull) percutaneous endoscopic gastrostomy (PEG) technique. **A,** After local anesthesia is instilled, a 10-mm transverse incision is made, through which a tapered cannula needle is introduced under direct endoscopic vision. A looped heavy suture is directed through the catheter into the stomach, secured with a polypectomy snare, and withdrawn from the patient's mouth. **B,** The well-lubricated PEG catheter is now secured to the suture, and steady traction is directed down the posterior pharynx into the esophagus. **C,** The endoscope is reintroduced (see **E**), and under direct vision the catheter is pulled across the gastroesophageal junction and then approximated to the anterior gastric wall. It is imperative that the inner cross-bar gently approximates the mucosa without excess tension to avoid ischemic necrosis. The stomach is decompressed by aspiration, and the gastroscope is withdrawn. **D,** The outer cross-bar is gently approximated to the skin level and secured with two 0-0 Prolene sutures. (From Gorman RC, Morris JB: Minimally invasive access to the gastrointestinal tract. In Rombeau JL, Rolandelli RH: *Clinical nutrition: enteral and tube feeding,* ed 3, Philadelphia, 1997, WB Saunders.)

"Push" (Russel) Technique. Modifications to the Ponsky or Sachs-Vine technique in which the second passage of the endoscope is obviated have been described. Another technique is a modification of the push technique that involves passing a dilator with a peel-away introducer over the guidewire. The endoscopist confirms the position of the dilator, the dilator is removed, and a well-lubricated catheter is placed through the introducer as the introducer is peeled away. The endoscopist verifies adequate placement of the catheter against the anterior stomach wall, and the endoscope is removed (Bankhead and Rolandell, 2005).

Percutaneous Endoscopic Jejunostomy. Several innovative techniques to obtain postpyloric enteral access through endoscopic placement of the percutaneous endoscopic jejunostomy (PEJ) have been described. The two basic approaches—transpyloric PEJ and directed PEJ—are briefly described.

Transpyloric PEJ. A small feeding tube with a weighted tip and an attached heavy suture tie are passed through a previously established gastrostomy. Under endoscopic visualization, the suture is grasped with a biopsy forceps, and the suture and attached feeding tube are guided into the duodenum (Figure 39-9). The endoscope is withdrawn. An excess amount of tubing is left within the stomach to allow peristalsis to pull the weighted tip past the ligament of Treitz.

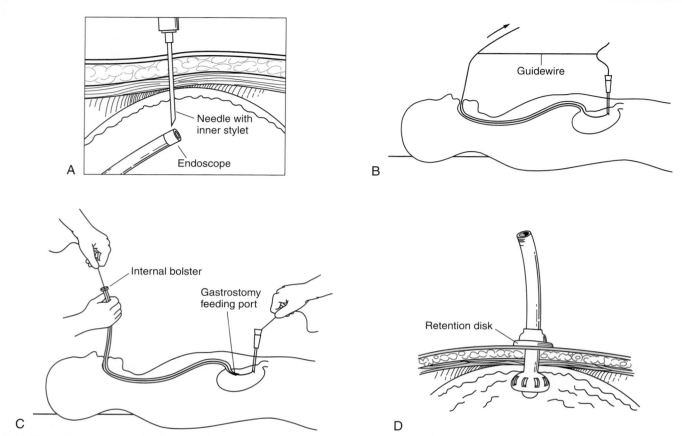

FIGURE 39-8 Sachs-Vine technique for percutaneous endoscopic gastrostomy (PEG) insertion. **A,** Needle is inserted through abdomen into stomach under visualization by endoscopist. **B,** Endoscope is withdrawn, pulling guidewire up through the esophagus, out the patient's mouth. **C,** PEG tube is pushed over the guidewire and advanced through the esophagus to the stomach. **D,** PEG is positioned against the anterior stomach wall.

Transpyloric PEJ is associated with considerable long-term complications, including (1) separation of the inner PEJ tube from the outer gastrostomy tube, (2) clogging of the small-diameter PEJ, and (3) kinking of the PEJ. Furthermore, the goal of reduced aspiration pneumonia has not been achieved, possibly as a result of retrograde migration of the tube back into the stomach or impaired pyloric sphincter function triggered by the presence of the tube (Gorman and Morris, 1997).

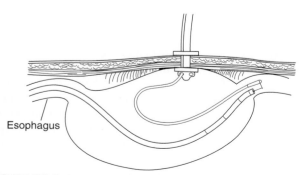

FIGURE 39-9 Transpyloric percutaneous endoscopic jejunostomy. Endoscopist guides the weighted tip of the feeding tube into the duodenum.

Directed PEJ. A PEJ can be placed directly through the abdominal wall into the jejunum using a modification of the Ponsky PEG procedure. In this approach, the endoscope is advanced past the pylorus approximately 20 cm distal to the ligament of Treitz, and the abdominal wall is transilluminated. Using a small-gauge needle, the jejunum is cannulated through the abdominal wall, a heavy thread is inserted, a biopsy forceps is used to grasp the thread, and the thread is withdrawn through the mouth. The thread is tied to a feeding tube (typically mushroom-tipped), which is pulled into position under endoscopic observation.

Another directed PEJ technique involves a small incision in the upper quadrant. The endoscope is inserted beyond the ligament of Treitz. and the proximal end of the jejunum is clamped. In the small incision, a short segment of jejunum is eviscerated using the Witzel technique. The feeding tube is placed into the jejunum, the jejunum is returned to the abdominal cavity, and the proximal and distal ends of the jejunum are secured to the abdominal wall. The directed PEJ seems to alleviate the problems associated with transpyloric placement (tube migration, clogging, and aspiration). Evidence for the long-term benefits, efficacy, and use of this procedure is inconclusive.

Interventional Radiologic Approach

Percutaneous Gastrostomy via Radiologic Intervention. Recent advances have led to the development of a radiographic approach to percutaneous gastrostomy tube placement. Percutaneous tubes placed by the interventional radiologist are an alternative when surgical or endoscopic procedures are not feasible. In many hospitals, it is the preferred method of tube placement. The interventional radiology nurse takes the lead in preparing the patient for the procedure, providing patient education, and monitoring the patient's recovery.

In the radiographic approach, the stomach is dilated with air, and a needle is percutaneously inserted into the stomach. A J-wire is threaded into the stomach under fluoroscopic guidance, and the needle is withdrawn. A 1-cm-long incision is made into the skin at the exit site of the wire. When entry into the stomach has been determined, the tract is slowly dilated and the permanent catheter inserted. These catheters usually have a balloon that is inflated and positioned snugly against the gastric wall. Stabilization at the skin surface is achieved using a suture or a tube stabilization device.

- T-tacks are small anchors that are deployed into the stomach during the beginning phase of gastrostomy or gastrostomy-jejunostomy tube placement.
- T-tacks pull and hold the stomach firmly against the abdominal wall. This helps the radiologists so that they do not have to work through "dead" space when placing the tube into the stomach.
- T-tacks *must* be cut within 7 to 10 days of placement to prevent reverse crater ulcerations in the stomach mucosal lining.
- Metal "T"s simply pass through the patient's GI tract.

Percutaneous Jejunostomy via Radiologic Intervention. This technique first requires radiologic access to the stomach as is done for percutaneous gastrostomy placement via radiology. A guidewire is passed through the duodenum and into the jejunum. A balloon occluder catheter is inserted over the guidewire and placed in the jejunum. The balloon is inflated with air and water-soluble contrast so that the position can be checked by fluoroscopy. Still under fluoroscopic surveillance, an 18-gauge needle is inserted into the jejunum, and the balloon is punctured. A guidewire is passed into the tract, and the tract is dilated to approximately 10 Fr size so that a feeding catheter can be inserted. The balloon occluder catheter is removed, and the feeding catheter is secured to the skin.

Conversion of Gastrostomy to Gastrostomy-Jejunostomy Tube. Repeat aspirations may necessitate conversion of an existing gastrostomy tube to a gastrostomy-jejunostomy tube. This can be done using endoscopy or radiology with a combined gastrostomy-jejunostomy tube, or by inserting a smaller-diameter feeding tube through the gastrostomy tube. When a combined gastrostomy-jejunostomy tube is used, the gastrostomy tube is removed, and an angiocatheter and guidewire are inserted and advanced through the pylorus. The guidewire is further advanced distal to the ligament of Treitz and the angiocatheter is removed. A gastrostomy-jejunostomy tube is inserted over the guidewire and advanced into the jejunum, and the guidewire is removed. The gastrostomy internal bumper or balloon is secured snugly against the stomach mucosa. An external securing device (bumper, flange, or commercial device) is used to secure the tube against the skin. Three ports will be apparent: gastric (proximal) port, duodenal or jejunal (distal) port, and balloon port (Figure 39-10).

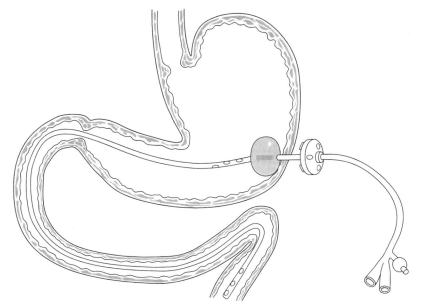

FIGURE 39-10 Transgastric jejunal tube. This dual-lumen tube is placed surgically and allows for jejunal feedings while providing gastric decompression. (From Rombeau JL, Rolandelli RH: *Clinical nutrition: enteral and tube feeding*, ed 3, Philadelphia, 1997, WB Saunders.)

When a combined gastrostomy-jejunostomy tube is not available, a jejunal tube can be placed, and the external end of the jejunal tube can be threaded into a gastrostomy tube. The gastrostomy tube is advanced over the jejunal tube, and the internal gastrostomy bumper is positioned against the anterior stomach wall. External stabilization of the tube to the skin is necessary.

Summary of Placement Techniques

The type of patient who typically requires these tubes is a major reason for the high morbidity rate. Patients commonly have multiple medical problems and are malnourished. For these reasons, the surgical approach to tube placement is quickly being replaced by the endoscopic or radiographic approach. Endoscopic techniques for enteral tube placement have a lower complication rate, are more cost effective than surgical methods, and can be performed on an outpatient basis. Performance of these techniques requires the ability to insert an endoscope. Laparoscopic and radiologic techniques are used less frequently but are options when endoscopy is not anatomically feasible or when surgery is too risky.

A key consideration for the type of tube placed is whether prepyloric or postpyloric delivery of enteral feedings is preferred (Harbison, 2007). In the presence of significant gastroesophageal reflux, increased risk of aspiration, impaired gastric emptying, or primary disease of the stomach, a jejunostomy is preferred.

FEEDING TUBE FEATURES

The type of tube used for gastrostomy or jejunostomy depends in part on the anatomic site in which the tube is placed and the reason for tube placement. Features of the tube to consider include material composition, tube diameter, tip configurations, and number of ports.

Material Composition

Historically, gastrostomy and jejunostomy tubes were made from rubber, polyvinyl chloride, and latex, which are very stiff and uncomfortable. The softer and more pliable polyurethane and silicone tubes have been used most frequently because these materials are associated with less soft tissue reaction and longer wear time. These features are particularly advantageous in older patients because of the increased fragility of the GI mucosa in this population (Lysen, 2003). However, aspiration of intestinal or gastric contents from silicone tubes is difficult because the walls of the tube collapse (Lysen, 2003).

Tube Diameter

The outer diameter (OD) of the lumen is referred to in French (Fr) units. A 1Fr tube is 0.33 mm across. However, the internal diameter (ID) can vary for any OD

French size depending on the material used. For example, silicone tubes have thicker walls than polyurethane tubes, so their internal diameter will be smaller even though they are labeled with the same French size.

The risk of the tube becoming clogged decreases as ID increases. However, for the patient's comfort, the smallest ID nasogastric tube possible that allows unimpeded flow of formula should be used. When enteral formulas containing fiber or viscous formulas will be administered, an 8 Fr or larger tube is recommended. Gastrostomy tubes most often are 12 Fr, jejunostomy tubes should be 6 Fr, and needle catheter jejunostomy tubes should be smaller than 8 Fr (Lysen, 2003).

Tip Configurations

Several tip configurations are illustrated in Figure 39-11. Foley catheters are not designed for use as gastrostomy tubes and should not be used because the balloon of the Foley catheter is subject to decay from gastric acid, necessitating periodic and regular replacement. In addition, Foley catheters do not have an external bumper and will migrate if an external tube stabilization device is not applied. Migration can cause gastric outlet obstruction by blocking the pylorus. Silicone-based replacement gastrostomy tubes are preferable.

Another tip configuration (and one used to a great extent on the PEG) is the disk. This tip cannot be removed by simple extraction through the skin; it must be cut off. The tip is passed through the GI tract or retrieved endoscopically. The PEG tip may also have a cross-bar or bulb tip, which cannot be extracted through the skin.

Tubes may have a type of mushroom catheter known as a *Pezzer tip*. These rubber tubes have stiff, round, pointed tips. The Pezzer tip has only minimal tiny holes and becomes easily plugged. This type of tip cannot be removed easily. The Malecot tube, also considered a mushroom catheter, has a bulbous tip with much larger openings. This type of tube can be removed more easily and is less likely to become obstructed than the Pezzer tip.

Ports

Tubes with multiple ports are available. Some gastrostomy tubes have three ports: balloon, feeding, and medication. A triple-lumen tube may be used when patients require both proximal decompression and enteral feeding. This tube has four outlets or ports: a gastric lumen for gastric suction, a proximal duodenal lumen for duodenal suction, a distal duodenal lumen for feeding, and a gastric balloon. To maintain proper tube placement, the gastric balloon is inflated with sterile water or air (depending on the manufacturer's specific recommendation), and a retaining disk or tube stabilization device is applied at skin level. These tubes may be confusing to the staff because the tubes are placed in the anticipated location for a gastrostomy tube but deliver feedings to

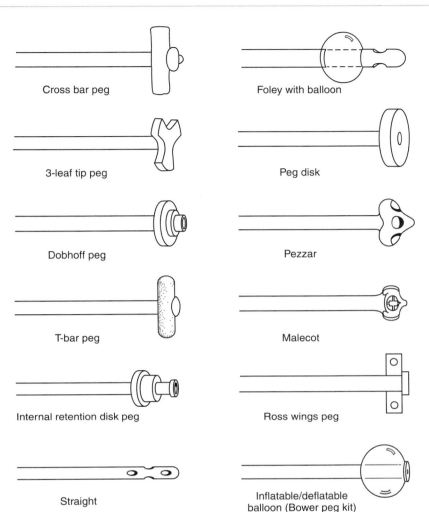

Cross bar peg

3-leaf tip peg

Dobhoff peg

T-bar peg

Internal retention disk peg

Straight

Foley with balloon

Peg disk

Pezzar

Malecot

Ross wings peg

Inflatable/deflatable balloon (Bower peg kit)

FIGURE 39-11 Tip configuration of enteral tubes. Note that the Foley with balloon tip is included to provide comparison in tip designs; it is not an appropriate tube for enteral feedings.

the jejunum. Ports should be clearly labeled, and a diagram of the tube should be available in the patient's care plan to provide clarity.

LOW-PROFILE GASTROSTOMY DEVICE (BUTTON)

A skin-level gastric conduit that is flush with the abdominal surface is known as a *gastrostomy button* (Foutch et al, 1989; Gauderer and Stellato, 1986; Gauderer et al, 1988). The button was first developed for use in children who require long-term gastrostomy feedings. It is a short silicone tube with a flip-top opening, a one-way antireflux valve (to prevent leakage of stomach contents around the tube), and a radiopaque dome that fits snugly against the stomach wall (Figure 39-12). Some devices have special tubing that opens the reflux valve to permit decompression of the stomach.

To administer feedings, an adapter is passed through the one-way valve and connected to a feeding catheter. When the feeding is completed, the tube is flushed with water, the adapter is removed, and the flip-top opening is closed.

A button can be inserted in a clinic setting in an established gastrostomy tract and does not require patient anesthesia. It may also be placed as the initial device in a one-step procedure (Georgeson, 1999). The device is available in different shaft lengths and diameters. Correct shaft length is critical to ensure proper positioning of the dome of the button against the anterior stomach wall and prevent gastric reflux around the button. The appropriate shaft length is determined by inserting a special measuring device into the tract. An obturator is inserted into the button to straighten the dome of the button, making insertion of the button into the tract possible. The button should be lubricated to facilitate insertion. Once the button is in place, the obturator is removed and the flip-top opening closed. The device may have to be resized if the patient's weight changes.

Disadvantages of the button include the potential for dysfunction of the antireflux valve with subsequent leakage and the need for replacement every 3 to 4 months. Studies and refinements of the device are ongoing. Current reports demonstrate good success, few complications, and high user satisfaction.

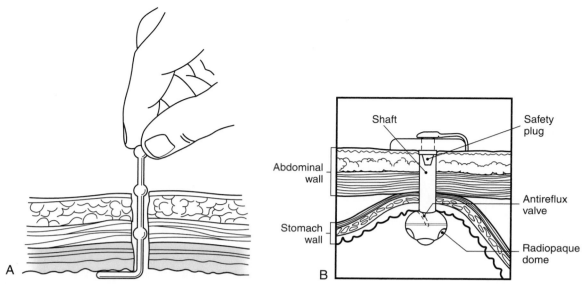

FIGURE 39-12 Gastrostomy button. **A,** Correct gastrostomy button size is determined by using a device to measure the width of the abdominal wall. **B,** Gastrostomy feeding button in place.

NURSING MANAGEMENT OF ENTERIC TUBES

Any patient who is malnourished or expected to have inadequate oral intake for 5 to 7 days should be considered for enteral access for nutritional support. The GI tract should be used whenever possible when nutritional supplementation is required (Harbison, 2007). Short-term support can be delivered through a small-bore nasoenteric tube such as the Dobhoff. When supplementation for more than 7 to 14 days is anticipated, GI intubation through a gastrostomy or jejunostomy should be considered. The patient with moderate to severe malnourishment who is undergoing an open laparotomy should be considered for a low jejunostomy or gastrostomy placed at the same time (Harbison, 2007).

Optimal management of patients requiring long-term gastrostomy or jejunostomy tubes begins in the preplacement phase. Assessment of each patient should include the reason for each tube alternative, the risks and benefits associated with various treatment options, and the commitment of the patient or caregiver to long-term management. Preplacement information and instructions are critical to adequately prepare the patient and family for what they will be expected to do.

Nursing staff must be prepared to care for the patient with an enteric tube. Much of the success of these tubes depends on proper care. Topics that must be addressed include preplacement site selection, site care, tube patency, tube stabilization, and management of complications. It is advisable to develop a competency checklist for the nursing staff who care for a significant number of patients with feeding tubes.

Preplacement Site Selection

Tube exit sites should be selected preoperatively to reduce the potential for complications and to facilitate self-care. Site selection is commonly based on vague guidelines such as "3 to 5 cm below the costal margin" and "avoidance of the costal margin." However, in the patient who has a protuberant hernia or is malnourished or confined to a wheelchair, this location may present a substantial problem such that it affects the integrity of the skin. Two techniques can be used to select a site preplacement, depending on whether the tube will be placed endoscopically or surgically (Hanlon, 1998).

Endoscopic Placement. When the tube is placed by the endoscopic approach, the location of the tube depends on transillumination. Therefore, the specific site for the tube cannot be determined before the procedure. Nonetheless, by marking important abdominal landmarks (e.g., skin crease, fold, or scar; costal margin; belt line; prosthetic equipment; hernia), the endoscopist can attempt to place the tube in a site that will avoid these landmarks. An indelible marker should be sufficient for these markings.

Surgical Placement. When the tube will be placed surgically, the technique used for preplacement site selection is the same as that used to mark a stoma site. The patient should be assessed while he or she is standing, sitting, bending, and in the supine position. The objective is to find 1 inch of smooth skin surface that is free of creases, folds, and scars and avoids the belt line and bony structures. Again, a surgical marking pen can be used to place an "X" at the desired location. A transparent dressing can be applied over the marking when surgery is not scheduled for several days.

Site Care

Daily site care should include gentle cleansing with water. If desired, a mild soap can be used but should also be rinsed off. A cotton-tipped applicator may be necessary to clean under an external bumper or disk. Diluted hydrogen peroxide is used to clean accumulated crusty drainage at the insertion site only when soap and water are ineffective. Routine and regular use of hydrogen peroxide should be avoided because hyperplasia (Plate 69A) at the tube site is associated with frequent use of hydrogen peroxide. A moisture barrier may be used after cleansing around the tube to protect skin from drainage. Dressings under the external button should be avoided because they can trap moisture and allow movement of the tube (Box 39-2).

Daily assessments should include the condition of the peritubular site and proper positioning of the stabilization device. The insertion site and surrounding tissue should be monitored for signs and symptoms of infection (e.g., erythema, induration, pain). The external bumper should rest lightly against the skin. Soft tissue infections should be managed with culture-based antibiotics (Plate 69B). Occlusive dressings for the tube site are generally unnecessary.

Tube Stabilization

The most common complications related to gastrostomy or jejunostomy placement are (1) leakage of gastric or jejunal contents around the tube onto the skin and (2) tube dislodgment. As many as half of all feeding tubes are dislodged by patients and their caregivers (O'Brien and Erwin-Toth, 1999). These complications are frequently attributed to the failure to adequately stabilize the tube. Therefore, postplacement nursing management must include measures to stabilize the tube.

Adequate tube stabilization requires proper internal positioning and proper external (skin-level) positioning. To achieve proper internal positioning, a tube that has a balloon, bumper, mushroom, or disk tip is used. These devices are snugly positioned against the anterior wall of the stomach (Figure 39-13). When a balloon tip is used, it must be inflated with an adequate volume of sterile water or air (in accordance with the manufacturer's guidelines) to work properly (Lord, 1997). Although saline may be readily available, it should not be used for balloon inflation because saline can crystallize and cause the balloon to rupture. Because water and air will diffuse through the walls of the balloon, adequacy of inflation should be checked weekly and whenever peritubular leakage is noted. Tubes with balloon tips should not be used as jejunal tubes because an inflated balloon within the jejunum is sufficient to obstruct the jejunum.

Adequate skin-level stabilization of the tube is necessary to prevent (1) lateral movement in the tube at skin level and (2) tube migration (in-and-out movements). Lateral movement of the tube contributes to leakage of gastric or intestinal contents onto the skin by eroding the tissue along the tract. Inflammation of the site can also develop from the presence of this chronic irritant. A stabilized tube should not allow lateral movement of the tube (Lord, 1997).

To maintain proper tube positioning in the stomach or small bowel, migration of the tube in and out of the tract must be prevented. Nonstabilized tubes are subject to migration as a result of gastric and intestinal motility and abdominal wall motion. The tube can migrate and obstruct the gastric outlet (causing gastric distention, nausea, and vomiting) and compromise tube function.

Historically, sutures have been used to stabilize tubes. However, sutures can cause tearing of the skin, with subsequent inflammation and significant pain at the suture site. In addition, sutures prevent tube migration but they do not eliminate lateral tube movement. When sutures are used, an external tube stabilization device, such as the drain tube attachment device, should be applied to provide more secure stabilization and comfort to the patient.

Baby-bottle nipples have been used to secure gastrostomy tubes. Typically the nipple is cut along one edge, wrapped around the tube, and secured with tape where

---

BOX 39-2 | Site Care for Drainage Tubes

- Change dressing every 1–2 days.
- Remove dressing from site.
- Use a clean washcloth to cleanse the area around the tube with soap and water.
- Use a dry washcloth to pat dry skin around tube.
- If necessary, reposition tube so that it does not kink or twist sharply.
- Secure fresh, sterile gauze (split 4 × 4) around tube site and over the retention disk using tape.
- Covering the tube site is not necessary while showering. These steps can be done in the shower or after the shower.

Note: Never submerge the tube site under water. No tub baths or swimming is permitted.

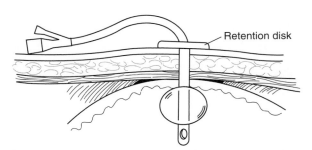

FIGURE 39-13 Proper stabilization of gastrostomy tube. Tube is secured between anterior wall of stomach and abdomen by a properly inflated internal balloon and externally with a tube stabilization device. Side-to-side mobility of the tube and tube migration are thus prevented.

the tube exits from the nipple. Although these nipples are popular and readily available, the technique in isolation is not completely effective at preventing lateral movement or tube migration. Effective tube stabilization with a nipple can be accomplished only when it is used with tape to secure the nipple to the abdomen or with a skin barrier flange. However, with the variety of external tube stabilization devices available, this technique is no longer needed.

Commercial external tube stabilization devices should be readily available and used to secure percutaneous tubes (Figure 39-14). The commercial tube stabilization device is changed as needed; frequency is determined by the need to assess the tube site or provide site care. When frequent site care is required (as with newly placed tubes), a stabilization system that allows easy visualization of the site without removal of adhesives is desirable. The Hollister vertical drain/tube attachment device (Hollister, Inc., Libertyville, IL) effectively holds tubes. The dressing is designed so that the tube comes straight out of the tract and is secured by the strap. Because the tube does not lay against the skin, there is no concern for development of a pressure ulcer along the tract. For smaller abdomens the tape ring can be removed. The vertical drain/tube attachment device can be left in place for 5 to 7 days.

Many tubes are being created specifically as gastrostomy tubes complete with stabilization features inherent in the design, thereby eliminating the need for commercial external stabilization devices. For example, the button has an internal dome, limited shaft length, and a flip-top cap to ensure stabilization of the tube. PEG tubes are designed with an internal bolster and an external bolster. The internal bolster can be a bumper, disk, or balloon that, when properly positioned, lies against the anterior stomach wall. Exteriorly, on the abdominal surface, the bolster is a bumper or disk that can be adjusted to lie snugly against the abdominal wall. This stabilization is critical to prevent dislodgment of the tube, mobility, obstruction, and peritubular leakage. A few Silastic catheter feeding tubes (with a balloon to secure the tube against the anterior stomach wall) have an adjustable external flange (Figure 39-15). Once the Silastic catheter is in position and the balloon is inflated, the flange is slid down against the skin, stabilizing the catheter without the use of adhesives.

Regardless of the type of stabilization device or bolster used, adequate stabilization is critical to the success of the tubes. The devices secure the tube against the abdominal wall and against the anterior stomach wall. The tension between the internal and external securing devices should allow slight leeway from the skin to prevent necrosis of the skin or gastric mucosa (Lord, 1997). This leeway should be monitored daily because changes in abdominal girth, as occurs with ascites, can develop, which predisposes the patient to a pressure point under the external stabilization device. Modifications should be made as necessary.

Tube Patency

All enteral feeding tubes require routine flushing. This easy procedure is key to the prevention of tube clogging (Bowers, 2000; Fish and Seidner, 2003; Lysen, 2003). In adults, the tube should be flushed three times per day with 60 ml of warm tap water; this is in addition to the 60-ml flushes before and after each tube feeding and medication administration. Tubes should always be flushed between each medication and after all medications are instilled. Only liquid medications should be administered.

COMPLICATIONS

Although the placement and care of gastric or jejunal tubes may appear to be relatively simple, they are associated with numerous significant complications. Complications may be related to the surgical technique or the tube. Examples include tube dislodgment, skin erosion at the exit site, skin-site wound infection, bleeding, peritonitis, and bowel obstruction. The wound specialist may see a patient with an intestinal tube for the first time when a skin complication develops. Although the skin problem must be addressed, investigation and correction of the

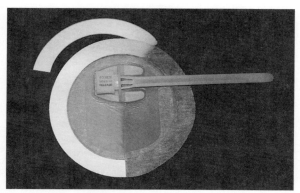

FIGURE 39-14 Commercial external tube stabilization device.

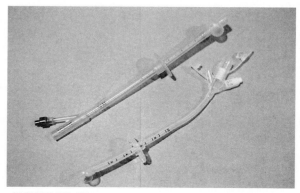

FIGURE 39-15 Sample replacement gastrostomy tubes.

underlying problem precipitating the skin irritation also are necessary.

Leakage

Leakage around the tube site warrants a thorough evaluation. Steps must be taken to correct any possible cause of the leakage. Replacing the tube with a larger size will not correct the problem. First check the adequacy of tube stabilization, appropriate balloon placement, adequate inflation of the balloon, and tube patency. The balloon should be deflated and reinflated with the amount of air or sterile water recommended by the manufacturer. Medications to reduce stomach acid may be warranted. Leakage may occur as a result of bolus feedings and may resolve with slower delivery or continuous delivery. When all attempts to halt the leakage fail, replacement of the tube may be necessary.

Skin Irritation

Skin irritation surrounding a tube most commonly results from chemical irritation (exposure to gastric or intestinal contents) or fungal infection. If all attempts to halt leakage fail and tube replacement is not an option, methods to contain the drainage and protect the skin must be implemented. Hydrocolloids and absorbent dressings are not appropriate because they will trap drainage against the skin and cause chemical irritation.

To contain drainage around a tube site, an ostomy pouch and catheter port can be applied. By attaching a catheter port to the pouch, the tube can exit the wall of the pouch through the port, which allows for feeding, suction, or gravity drainage to continue. The ostomy pouch then contains peritubular drainage (Figure 39-16). Such a pouching system is cost effective and allows collection, identification, and measurement of the drainage as well as skin protection. Instructions for containing peritubular leakage are outlined in Box 39-3. The frequency of pouch changes is determined by the duration of the pouch seal, but on average the pouch is changed every 4 to 7 days. If a urinary pouch is selected, it may be necessary to "pop" the antireflux mechanism within the pouch, particularly when drainage is thick or contains particulate matter.

BOX 39-3	Pouching Procedure for Leakage around Tube

1. Assemble pouch and catheter access device:
   A. Cut opening in barrier and pouch to accommodate tube site.
   B. Make small slit in anterior surface of pouch.
   C. Attach access device to anterior surface of the pouch.
   D. Tear paper backing on pouch or wafer but leave in place.
2. Prepare skin.
   A. Cleanse and dry skin.
   B. Treat any denuded skin (skin barrier powder to denuded area; skin sealant if needed).
   C. Apply thin layer of skin barrier paste to skin around insertion site, if needed.
3. Disconnect and plug tube.
4. Feed catheter through opening in pouch. Use water-soluble lubricant to pass tube, and use hemostat to pull tube through the pouch or barrier opening, anterior wall of the pouch, and access device.
5. Reconnect tube.
6. Ensure skin is dry. Remove paper backing from wafer and secure pouch to skin.
7. Secure tube to stabilization device with tape.

Fungal infections (e.g., candidiasis) can result when moisture is trapped at the insertion site. Corrective measures include protecting the skin from moisture with skin sealants or ointments, or containing the moisture with appropriate dressings. Antifungal medications (e.g., powders) may be necessary when extensive candidiasis is present.

Allergic contact dermatitis can occur when a patient's skin is sensitive to anchoring devices, tapes, soaps, or other commercial products. Mechanical trauma and folliculitis can result from traumatic removal of tape or other products used to anchor the tube (O'Brien and Erwin-Toth, 1999). These issues are discussed further in Chapter 5.

Peristomal Hyperplasia. An overgrowth of granulation tissue at the tube exit site can develop and is commonly referred to as *hyperplasia*. This overgrowth of granulation tissue seems to occur in response to chronic irritation of the tissue lining the tract. The source of the chronic irritation can be the type of tube material used

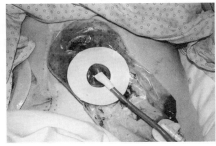
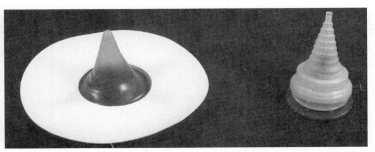

FIGURE 39-16 Catheter access port attached to drainable ostomy pouch *(left)*. Two examples of a catheter access port *(right)*. (Courtesy NuHope and Hollister.)

(latex is more irritating than Silastic material), tube mobility (particularly in-and-out movements of the tube), and the chronic presence of excessive moisture. Hyperplasia may or may not be uncomfortable. However, when hyperplasia is allowed to persist, seepage from the overgrowth will develop and compromise the integrity of the external stabilization and skin integrity. Treatment should address the underlying causative factor for the hyperplasia. Once the cause is corrected, the hyperplasia should resolve. Occasionally debridement and cautery with silver nitrate sticks are warranted. Because it can be painful for the patient, cautery with silver nitrate sticks should be done infrequently and only by an experienced care provider.

Tube Occlusion

The care plan should incorporate measures to prevent or manage tube obstruction. Occlusion can result from administration of powdered or crushed medications in the feeding tube, viscous formulas, poor or inadequate flushing techniques, partially digested proteins, yeast, and aspiration of gastric or intestinal contents into the tube (Beyers, 2003; Frankel et al, 1998). Water should be used initially to dislodge an occlusion. This process can also assist in distinguishing a kinked tube from a clogged tube. Kinked tubes allow slow passage of water, whereas clogged tubes do not allow any passage of water (Frankel et al, 1998). When irrigation with water fails, activated pancreatic enzymes should be instilled (Fish and Seidner, 2003). The use of cranberry juice, chymotrypsin, carbonated drinks, and meat tenderizers is discouraged because they tend to precipitate in the feeding solution within the tube or cause adverse effects in patients with severe hepatic, renal, or coagulation abnormalities (Frankel et al, 1998; Metheny et al, 1988).

Declogging Devices. Some devices consist of a catheter that can be inserted into the feeding tube to which a syringe can be attached and a solution delivered to the occlusion site. Some of these devices can be used to instill a mixture of pancreatic enzymes and sodium bicarbonate near the site of the clog. Devices that actually bore through the clog or brush the walls of the feeding tube also are available (Frankel et al, 1998). Box 39-4 provides a sample protocol for managing tube occlusion.

TUBE REMOVAL

Enteral tubes are removed when the patient is able to resume adequate oral nutrition and may need to be removed when they are hopelessly occluded, kinked, or malpositioned. The method of removal will depend on the type of tube, the technique used to insert the tube, and the type of tube tip (Boxes 39-5 to 39-7). PEG tubes can be removed by external traction, endoscopy, or "cut and push" (Kejariwal et al, 2009). With the "cut and push" method, the outer bumper is loosened, the tube is

---

BOX 39-4	Sample Protocol for Enteral Tube Occlusion

Method A
1. Attach 5-ml Luer-Lok syringe and attempt to flush tube with warm water and moderate pressure.
2. If irrigation is unsuccessful, attach an Intro-Reducer (Health Improvement Associates, Freeland, MI) and attempt to irrigate with warm water using a 20- to 60-ml syringe.
3. If unsuccessful, instill activated pancreatic enzyme mixture through the Intro-Reducer.

Method B
1. Attach a 30- to 60-ml syringe to the end of the enteral tube and aspirate as much fluid as possible. Discard the fluid.
2. Fill the syringe with 5 ml of warm water and attach the syringe to the end of the enteral device. Instill the water under manual pressure for 1 minute, using a back-and-forth motion with the plunger to loosen the clot/obstruction.
3. Clamp the tube for 5–15 minutes.
4. Try to aspirate or flush the tube with warm water.
5. If the tube remains clogged, repeat this procedure with a pancrease and sodium bicarbonate solution (one crushed Viokase tablet or 1 teaspoon Viokase powder mixed with one non–enteric-coated sodium bicarbonate tablet, or ⅛ teaspoon baking soda dissolved in 5 ml of warm water).

Data from Frankel EH et al: Methods of restoring patency to occluded feeding tubes, *Nutr Clin Pract* 13:129, 1998; Lord LM: Enteral access devices, *Nurs Clin North Am* 32(4):685, 1997.

---

rotated and advanced slightly into the stomach (to ensure the internal bumper is mobile and not attached to the gastric mucosa), and, while external traction is applied on the tube, the tube is severed at skin level. The internal portion of the tube will be expelled in the stool.

BOX 39-5	Instructions for Removal of Original PEG Tube

Equipment Needed
- Nonsterile gloves
- Gauze (4 × 4)

Procedure
1. Obtain permission from physician.
2. Using dominant hand, grasp PEG tubing above bumper and rotate it 360 degrees. If it does not rotate freely, stop and call physician. If it rotates freely, wrap it around your hand to maintain a firm grip.
3. Use other hand to stabilize the patient's abdomen around the site.
4. While exerting moderate force, pull on PEG tube until inner bumper comes through skin opening. Slight bleeding may occur. If resistance is too great, stop and call physician.
5. Cover opening with gauze until ready to insert replacement gastrostomy tube. Insert tube immediately to prevent closure of the tract.
6. *Note:* Original PEG tube must be at least 2 weeks past time of insertion before nurse performs this procedure.

PEG, Percutaneous endoscopic gastrostomy.
Courtesy Karen Huskey.

BOX 39-6	Instructions for Removal of Balloon Replacement Gastrostomy Tube

Equipment
- 20-ml Luer-Lok syringe
- Gauze (4 × 4)
- Nonsterile gloves

Procedure
1. Connect 20-ml syringe to balloon port of tube and aspirate all water out of balloon. *(Note:* Less than 20 ml may be present as a result of evaporation.)
2. Slowly withdraw tube from abdominal site.
3. Cover opening with gauze until ready to reinsert replacement tube. Insert tube immediately to prevent closure of the tract.

BOX 39-7	Instructions for Insertion of Balloon Replacement Gastrostomy

Equipment
- Replacement gastrostomy tube of correct size
- 60-ml syringe with male tip
- Lubricant (e.g., K-Y jelly)
- Stethoscope
- Nonsterile gloves
- 20-ml Luer-Lok syringe
- 20 ml of sterile water

Procedure
1. Choose replacement gastrostomy tube that is the same size as the previously used tube unless otherwise indicated.
2. Draw up 20 ml of sterile water into syringe. Do not use saline.
3. Insert syringe into balloon port; fill balloon to ensure proper inflation.
4. Withdraw water out of balloon and lubricate distal end of gastrostomy tube.
5. Gently insert gastrostomy tube into existing opening in abdomen. Tube should go in without resistance. If resistance is detected, pull back and attempt to insert again at a slightly different angle. If resistance is met again, stop and call physician.
6. Once gastrostomy tube is inserted into existing tract, gastric contents should return into the tube. To confirm proper placement, instill 30 ml of air into gastrostomy tube and auscultate for sound, which should be heard in the stomach (not the abdomen).
7. Once placement is confirmed, fill balloon with 20-ml water-filled syringe. (Check balloon port to determine exact amount of water needed to fill balloon.)
8. After balloon is inflated, gently pull back on tube until resistance is felt, then slide down external bumper or disk until it rests lightly on the skin.
9. Rotate the catheter 360 degrees to confirm that tube has free rotation.
10. Cleanse skin around tube with soap and water; no dressing is necessary.

Courtesy Karen Huskey.

A dressing is applied over the percutaneous tube site and replaced daily. Patients are NPO for 6 hours before the procedure and for 2 hours after the procedure. Performance of these PEG tube removals should be reserved for nurses who have successfully completed a formal competency check, such as nutritional therapist nurses and interventional radiology nurses.

PATIENT EDUCATION

Patient education is a key nursing responsibility and is absolutely critical to the patient with a gastrostomy or jejunostomy tube. Because the hospitalization period after tube placement may be brief to nonexistent, detailed caregiver education is essential, and outpatient follow-up care is imperative. In some situations, percutaneous tube placement may be performed strictly on an outpatient basis. In either case, home health care will be important to facilitate patient and caregiver independence in the process, safety with the procedure, and monitoring for complications. Key content areas to be included in a patient teaching plan are listed in Box 39-8.

MISCELLANEOUS DRAIN TUBES

A drainage tube can be placed to drain an abscess or fluid collection that will not resolve on its own and antibiotics are ineffective. Although surgery may be performed to manage a fluid collection, surgery may not be appropriate due to local inflammation, the severity or location of the abscess, or the patient's comorbidities. With the assistance of computed tomography or fluoroscopy, a catheter can be placed anywhere in the body where pus accumulates. Once the drain is in place, the abscess may require a few weeks to a few months to resolve. The drain tube will facilitate resolution of inflammation so that a patient who does require surgical intervention will be in a more stable overall condition and therefore at decreased risk for complications associated with surgery. Each drain tube should be labeled so that documentation is clear and consistent among the

BOX 39-8	Key Content for Patient Education

1. Name of procedure
2. Purpose for tube insertion
3. Characteristics of normal tube function
4. Type of tube placed
5. Size of balloon (if present)
6. Tube stabilization (why it is important, how it is achieved)
7. Routine site care (daily)
8. Weekly balloon inflation checks (if present)
9. Signs and symptoms of complications, and appropriate response
10. Tube feeding schedule and procedure (when applicable)
11. Name of person to call with questions or problems
12. What to do if tube falls out

physicians, nurses, and interventional radiologists. Drain tubes should be irrigated only when specific instructions to do so are given by the physician who inserted the catheter. Orders to irrigate drainage tube should specify use of sterile saline, the amount of solution to use, and the frequency of irrigations. Slight force is used to irrigate the drain tube so that "debris" that has lodged in the lateral holes of the catheter can be dislodged.

SUMMARY

Percutaneous tubes contribute to both quantity and quality of life for many patients. Nurses play a vital role in providing tube stabilization, maintaining tube patency, providing surveillance for complications, and teaching the patient self-care.

REFERENCES

Bankhead R, Rolandell R: Access to gastrointestinal tract. In Rolandelli RH, editor: *Enteral and tube feeding*, Philadelphia 2005, Elsevier Saunders.

Beyers PL: Complications of enteral nutrition. In DeChicco LE, Matarese MM, editors: *Nutrition support practice: a clinical guide*, Philadelphia, 2003, Saunders.

Bland KI et al: *Atlas of surgical oncology*, Philadelphia, 1995, WB Saunders.

Bloch AS, Mueller C: Enteral and parenteral nutrition support. In Mahan LK, Escott-Stump S, editors: *Krause's food, nutrition, and diet therapy*, ed 11, Philadelphia, 2004, Elsevier.

Bowers S: All about tubes, *Nursing* 30(12):41, 2000.

Coates NE, MacFadyen BV Jr: Laparoscopic placement of enteral feeding tubes. In Latifi R, Dudrick SJ, editors: *Medical intelligence unit: current surgical nutrition*, Austin, Tex., 1996, RG Landes.

DeChicco RS, Matarese MM: Determining the nutrition support regimen. In DeChicco LE, Matarese MM, editors: *Nutrition support practice: a clinical guide*, Philadelphia, 2003, Saunders.

Duh QY, McQuaid K: Flexible endoscopy and enteral access. In Eubanks WS et al, editors: *Mastery of endoscopic and laparoscopic surgery*, Philadelphia, 2000, Lippincott Williams & Wilkins.

Fish J, Seidner DL: Enteral nutrition support. In Hark L, Morrison G, editors: *Medical nutrition and disease: a case based approach*, Malden, Mass., 2003, Blackwell Science.

Foutch PG et al: The gastrostomy button: a prospective assessment of safety, success and spectrum of use, *Gastrointest Endosc* 35(1):41, 1989.

Frankel EH et al: Methods of restoring patency to occluded feeding tubes, *Nutr Clin Pract* 13:129, 1998.

Gauderer MWL, Ponsky JL: Gastrostomy without laparotomy: a percutaneous technique, *J Pediatr Surg* 15:872, 1980.

Gauderer MWL, Stellato TA: Gastrostomies: evolution, techniques, indications and implications, *Curr Probl Surg* 23:657, 1986.

Gauderer MWL et al: Feeding gastrostomy button: experience and recommendations, *J Pediatr Surg* 23(1):24, 1988.

Georgeson KE: Laparoscopic versus open procedures for long-term enteral access, *Nutr Clin Pract* 12(1 Suppl):S7, 1997.

Georgeson KE: Laparoscopic gastrostomy. In Bax NMA et al, editors: *Endoscopic surgery in children*, New York, 1999, Springer.

Gincherman Y, Torosian M: Enteral nutrition: indications, methods of delivery and complications. In Latifi R, Dudrick SJ, editors: *Current surgical nutrition*, New York, 1996, Chapman and Hall.

Gorman RC, Morris JB: Minimally invasive access to the gastrointestinal tract. In Rombeau JL, Rolandelli RH, et al: *Clinical nutrition: enteral and tube feeding*, ed 3, Philadelphia, 1997, WB Saunders.

Gorman RC et al: Enteral feeding techniques. In Torosian MH editor: *Nutrition for the hospitalized patient: basic science and principles of practice*, New York, 1995, Marcel Dekker.

Hanlon MD: Preplacement marking for optional gastrointestinal and jejunostomy tube site locations to decrease complications and promote self-care, *Nutr Clin Pract* 13:167, 1998.

Harbison SP: Intubation of the stomach and small intestine. In Yeo CJ et al: *Shackelford's surgery of the alimentary tract*, ed 6, Philadelphia, 2007, Saunders.

Kejariwal D et al: The "cut and push" method of percutaneous endoscopic gastrostomy tube removal in adult patients: the Ipswich experience, *Nutr Clin Pract* 24(2):281-283, 2009.

Lord LM: Enteral access devices, *Nurs Clin North Am* 32(4):685, 1997.

Lysen L: Enteral equipment. In DeChicco LE, Matarese MM, editors: *Nutrition support practice: a clinical guide*, Philadelphia, 2003, Saunders.

Metheny N et al: Effect of feeding tube properties and three irrigants on clogging rates, *Nurs Res* 37(3):165, 1988.

O'Brien B, Erwin-Toth P: G-tube site care: a practical guide, *RN* 62(2):52, 1999.

Patterson RS: Enteral nutrition delivery systems. In Grant JA, Kennedy-Caldwell C, editors: *Nutritional support nursing*, Philadelphia, 1988, Grune & Stratton.

Rombeau JL, Rolandelli RH: *Clinical nutrition: enteral and tube feeding*, ed 3, Philadelphia, 1997, WB Saunders.

Wu JS, Soper NJ: Gastrostomy and jejunostomy. In Jones DB et al, editors: *Laparoscopic surgery: principles and procedures*, ed 2, New York, 2004, Marcel Dekker.

Self-Assessment Exercises

QUESTIONS

A. General Principles of Assessment

1. Distinguish between assessment and evaluation of healing.
2. Which of the following methods is an example of categorizing a wound by classification?
   a. Linear measurements
   b. Photographs
   c. Staging
   d. Wound molds
3. A full-thickness wound is one that
   a. involves the muscle layer
   b. extends into the dermis
   c. is limited to the epidermis
   d. contains necrotic tissue
4. List 10 indices of wound healing that should be assessed and recorded.
5. Eschar can also be described as which of the following?
   a. Viable tissue
   b. Necrotic tissue
   c. Fibrin
   d. Granulation tissue
6. Describe eschar.
7. Describe slough.
8. List six factors known to damage the skin.
9. Which of the following is described as a lesion that is raised, solid, and less than 1 cm in diameter?
   a. Macule
   b. Papule
   c. Pustule
   d. Nodule
10. A blister that measures 1.5 cm in diameter may also be called which of the following?
    a. Bulla
    b. Pustule
    c. Vesicle
    d. Wheal
11. Which of the following statements about an erosion is *true*?
    a. Erosion involves the loss of epidermis and dermis.
    b. Erosion heals by scar formation.
    c. Erosion involves partial loss of epidermis.
    d. Erosion extends into subcutaneous tissue.

12. Which of the following accurately characterizes chemical skin irritation?
    a. Erythema with satellite lesions
    b. Erythema and erosion of skin
    c. Ulcerations with necrotic tissue in wound bed
    d. Ulcerations with pustules
13. Which of the following characterizes varicella-zoster virus?
    a. It requires prior exposure to genital herpes.
    b. It is reactivated by mechanical trauma.
    c. It consists of a bilateral vesicular rash.
    d. It develops along one or two dermatomes.
14. State the two phases of an allergic contact dermatitis.
15. Candidiasis can be described as which of the following?
    a. Pustular or macular papular rash with erythema
    b. Papular rash within the hair follicle
    c. Pustular rash in clusters
    d. Vesicular rash with plaque formation
16. Which of the following statements about herpes simplex virus is *true?*
    a. It initially develops as papules.
    b. Secondary lesions consist of necrotic plaques.
    c. Erythema signifies a secondary infection.
    d. Vesicles are uniformly shaped and grouped.
17. Which of the following is a usual result of severe traumatic injury with associated wounds?
    a. Increased metabolic rate for 10 to 14 days after injury
    b. Decreased metabolic rate to help conserve energy for the first 2 to 5 days after injury
    c. Decreased metabolic rate for 48 hours, then increased for the following 10 to 14 days
    d. Unknown metabolic consequences (cannot be determined without more information)
18. Which of the following permits definitive diagnosis of malnutrition?
    a. Weight loss of 10 pounds in 1 year
    b. Body mass index of 16
    c. Albumin level of 4.0 g/dl
    d. Petechiae

19. FD is a 65-year-old man who is retired and lives alone. He is healthy except for a venous ulcer on his right leg, and he needs a "water pill for his high blood pressure." He does not eat breakfast or lunch, but he goes to the local restaurant every evening for dinner. Over the past 3 months he has lost 15 pounds. Your initial suspicion is that he has which of the following?
    a. Protein-calorie malnutrition
    b. Protein malnutrition
    c. Depression
    d. Chronic dehydration

20. Which of the following explains why obesity is a risk factor for poor healing?
    a. Fat is more poorly perfused than lean tissue.
    b. Many obese people are dehydrated.
    c. Obese persons often are hypotensive.
    d. Skin is pulled tight by obesity.

21. Which of the following are symptoms of brief starvation with hypermetabolism?
    a. Slow weight loss and low albumin
    b. Slow weight loss and normal albumin
    c. Rapid weight loss and low albumin
    d. Rapid weight loss and normal albumin

22. Which of the following findings in the patient's history indicates risk of malnutrition?
    a. Eating alone
    b. Inability to prepare his or her own food
    c. Low income
    d. All of the above

23. Vitamin C is essential to which of the following?
    a. White blood cell synthesis
    b. Capillary wall integrity
    c. Angiogenesis
    d. Cell wall formation

24. Which of the following describes protein needs for repair after injury?
    a. They decrease because of reduced basal metabolic rate.
    b. They decrease to conserve losses.
    c. They increase to provide energy for basal functions.
    d. They increase to support anabolism.

25. What is the ideal way to feed a person with a healing wound?
    a. Enterally with a nasogastric tube because it is the least time consuming
    b. Parenterally because it is associated with a low infection rate and reduced risk of aspiration
    c. Orally because it maintains gut function and enhances independence
    d. It doesn't matter—there is no ideal way to feed a person with a wound.

26. Anabolism over the last 2 to 3 days of feeding with either enteral or parenteral nutrition is most accurately evaluated with which of the following?
    a. Weight change
    b. Serum albumin
    c. Blood urea nitrogen (BUN)–creatinine level
    d. Prealbumin

27. Which of the following best describes the pain associated with conservative sharp debridement?
    a. Noncyclic acute wound pain
    b. Cyclic acute wound pain
    c. Chronic wound pain
    d. All of the above

28. Which of the following pain assessment scales would be *most* appropriate for a nonverbal nursing home resident with severe Alzheimer disease and a Stage IV sacral pressure ulcer?
    a. McGill Pain Questionnaire
    b. Pain Assessment in Advanced Dementia (PAINAD) scale
    c. Visual analogue scale
    d. Wong-Baker faces scale

29. Explain why wounds confined to the epidermal and dermal layers heal by regeneration, whereas wounds that extend through the dermal layer into the subcutaneous tissue or fascia or muscle layer must heal by scar formation.

30. Explain what is meant by primary-, secondary-, and tertiary-intention wound healing.

31. Identify the major components of partial-thickness repair.

32. Explain why epidermal resurfacing and dermal repair proceed more rapidly when the wound surface is kept moist.

33. Summarize the activities that occur in the three key phases of repair for full-thickness wounds healing by primary intention (in order).

34. Which of the following cells are responsible for collagen synthesis?
    a. Macrophages
    b. Neutrophils
    c. Fibroblasts
    d. Platelets

35. The process of contraction is important for wound healing in which of the following?
    a. Wounds healing by primary intention
    b. Wounds healing by secondary intention
    c. Superficial abrasions
    d. Partial-thickness wounds

36. Explain why large wounds healing by secondary intention may require skin grafting, whereas large, partial-thickness wounds will epithelialize.

37. Summarize the differences between acute and chronic wound healing.

38. List at least six factors that affect wound healing.

39. Which of the following characterizes the molecular environment of a chronic wound?
    a. High levels of growth factors
    b. Increased levels of proteases (matrix metalloproteinases)
    c. Increased levels of protease inhibitors (tissue inhibitors of metalloproteinase)
    d. Excessive collagen synthesis

B. General Principles of Management

1. What are the three principles of wound management?
    a. Debridement, control of infection, and exudate management
    b. Establishment of a treatment goal, wound cleansing, and physiologic local wound care
    c. Assessment of the host, debridement, and physiologic local wound care
    d. Address the wound etiology, support the host, and maintain a physiologic local wound environment
2. Which of the following interventions indicates an attempt to control or eliminate the etiology of a venous ulcer?
    a. Resizing of shoe to include orthotics
    b. Applying an alginate and foam cover dressing
    c. Monitoring blood glucose levels
    d. Encouraging elevation of the leg three times daily
3. Which of the following statements about semiocclusive dressings is *true*?
    a. They are occlusive to liquids and gases.
    b. They are occlusive to liquids but transmit moisture vapor and gases.
    c. They are occlusive to gases and vapors but transmit liquids.
    d. They are inconsistent in their nonocclusive properties.
4. In the patient with a new approximated surgical wound, the primary wound care objective is
    a. autolysis
    b. hydration
    c. cleansing
    d. protection
5. Dressing selection is primarily based on which of the following?
    a. Forms of the dressing
    b. Characteristics of the wound
    c. Product availability and cost
    d. Number of dressing changes required daily
6. In the patient with a highly exudative pressure ulcer, which category of dressings should be considered?
    a. Hydrocolloids
    b. Collagens
    c. Transparent dressings
    d. Alginates

7. Which of the following statements about wound care products is *true*?
    a. Hydrocolloids absorb more exudate than alginate dressings.
    b. Transparent dressings are contraindicated for Stage II pressure ulcers.
    c. Wound fillers can be used to fill undermining and tunnels.
    d. Silver-impregnated dressings are indicated when critical colonization is suspected.
8. List seven objectives for local wound management.
9. Which of the following methods of debridement is nonselective?
    a. Autolysis
    b. High-pressure irrigation
    c. Enzymatic
    d. Surgical sharp
10. High-pressure wound irrigation requires which of the following?
    a. Bulb syringe
    b. Daily dressing changes
    c. Personal protective gear
    d. Expensive equipment
11. List three considerations in the use of enzymatic debridement.
12. Selection of debridement approach is guided by all of the following *except*
    a. patient's age
    b. presence of wound infection
    c. extent and type of necrotic tissue
    d. clinician experience
13. The risk of transient bacteremia is associated with which of the following debridement techniques?
    a. Autolysis
    b. Conservative sharp
    c. Enzymes
    d. Wet-to-dry dressings
14. Infection occurs when microorganisms
    a. reside on the surface of the wound
    b. invade the tissue
    c. multiply on the wound
    d. reside on the surface and multiply there
15. Which of the following statements accurately characterizes wound colonization?
    a. Colonization is associated with a fever and local inflammation of the wound.
    b. Colonization is manifested when the wound has stalled in the healing process.
    c. Colonization is diagnosed with a culture result of 10^5 or more organisms per gram of tissue.
    d. Colonization is often present and is not indicative of an infection.

16. Mr. H is a 35-year-old man with an open wound of his foot caused when he was dragged by a tractor in a farm accident 3 days ago. He does not have insurance, so he did not seek medical assistance at the time of the injury. He comes today because he has shaking chills. By history he is a healthy, active adult. On physical examination you find that he has abrasions over his legs, but x-ray examination shows no fracture. The wound involves the plantar surface of his foot, where a full-thickness triangular flap is visible, but the wound is filled with eschar and its depth cannot be evaluated. The entire foot is reddened, swollen, and hot. He is alert, oriented, and concerned. Which of the following is the major risk factor for infection in this man?
    a. Local wound environment because of the contamination
    b. Malnutrition because he has not eaten well as a result of his fever
    c. Ischemia resulting from trauma to the foot and leg
    d. Immunosuppression resulting from the stress of the injury
17. All of the following features define surgical site infection *except*
    a. less than 10^5 CFU per gram of tissue
    b. redness, induration, and local warmth surrounding a wound
    c. purulent drainage
    d. increased white blood cell count
18. Which of the following should cause suspicion of infection in a 63-year-old man with diabetes who has been coming to the clinic routinely for care of his left foot, plantar surface neuropathic ulcer?
    a. Presence of granulation tissue in wound bed
    b. Sudden low glucose level
    c. 10^3 or more organisms per gram of tissue
    d. Absence of any improvement over past 3 weeks
19. You inadvertently contaminated a culture when you were obtaining it. How should the findings be interpreted?
    a. False-positive. The laboratory work shows infection when it really is not present.
    b. False-negative. The laboratory work shows no infection when in fact it is present.
    c. False. You cannot know if the patient had infection because of the contamination.
    d. Accurate. A little contamination is expected because the skin is always contaminated.
20. In a culture obtained by aspiration, what would you expect the number of organisms to be?
    a. More than by swab culture
    b. More than by tissue biopsy
    c. The same as by swab culture
    d. Fewer than on tissue biopsy
21. To get the most accurate culture, it is important that the specimen be taken from
    a. pus
    b. necrotic tissue or slough
    c. exudate
    d. healthy wound tissue
22. Which of the following must be included in the comprehensive wound treatment of a 47-year-old patient with an open wound of the abdomen secondary to a retroperitoneal abscess?
    a. Wet-to-dry dressings
    b. Pain control
    c. Debridement of granulation tissue
    d. Treatment for depression
23. Which of the following is *not* a *primary* mechanism of action of negative pressure wound therapy (NPWT)?
    a. Wound edge contraction
    b. Wound environment stabilization
    c. Reduction of bioburden
    d. Wound surface microdeformations
24. Bioburden reduction with use of NPWT is believed to occur through which of the following?
    a. Removal of growth factors
    b. Increased perfusion
    c. Irrigation daily with normal saline
    d. Creation hypoxic environment for bacteria with suction
25. Which of the following describes appropriate use of NPWT in the care of enteric fistulas?
    a. It can only be used after exploration of the enteric fistula
    b. It is only used to contain effluent.
    c. It is never indicated with enteric fistulas.
    d. The wound should be covered with a wound liner instead of porous foam filler dressing.
26. Serious complications associated with NPWT including death are related to which of the following?
    a. Hemorrhage
    b. Retrograde migration of bacteria from canister to wound surface
    c. Fluid and electrolyte depletion
    d. Excess wound moisture
27. Contraindications to NPWT include which of the following?
    a. Patient taking anticoagulants
    b. Treated osteomyelitis
    c. Nonenteric or unexplored fistulas
    d. Postsurgical dehiscence

28. Which of the following statements about hyperoxygenation that occurs with hyperbaric treatment is *true?*
    a. Hyperoxygenation occurs because the hemoglobin molecule is saturated with oxygen molecules.
    b. Hyperoxygenation results from increasing the oxygen-carrying capacity of the plasma.
    c. Several treatments are needed to achieve hyperoxygenation.
    d. Hyperoxygenation may be sustained for 8 to 10 hours after exposure.
29. All of the following personal care items are contraindicated during hyperbaric treatment *except*
    a. hairspray
    b. hearing aids
    c. contact lenses
    d. perfume
30. True or False: Wound care dressings with a petrolatum base should be removed during hyperbaric treatment.
31. True or False: Hyperbaric oxygen is a definitive treatment of hard to heal wounds.
32. List three types of adhesion molecules or adhesion receptors that participate in inflammation.
33. True or False: Growth factors are proteases.
34. All of the following growth factors have shown significant benefit in healing acute or chronic wounds in clinical trials *except*
    a. fibroblast growth factor
    b. epidermal growth factor
    c. transforming growth factor-β
    d. insulin-like growth factor
35. Differentiate between cellular and acellular skin or dermal replacement products.
36. Describe the sources of skin substitutes and extracellular matrix (ECM) scaffolds used in wound care.
37. Define cell therapy and discuss how it relates to skin substitutes used in chronic wound care.
38. Name an epidermal, dermal, and bilayer product currently on the market in the United States.
39. In the future, cell therapy may include which of the following?
    a. Melanocytes, endothelial cells, and stem cells
    b. The release of certain growth factors depending on wound requirements
    c. Cells that are engineered to release antimicrobial compounds
    d. All of the above
40. Name at least two ECM scaffolds currently available in the United States.
41. Identify which skin substitutes have strong evidence for their use.
42. List the keys to success when using skin substitutes and ECM scaffolds in chronic wound care.

43. Which of the following frequently causes procedural wound pain?
    a. Adhesive dressings
    b. Wet-to-moist gauze
    c. Debridement
    d. All of the above
44. Which of the following is included among best practices for managing wound pain?
    a. Assuming that the pain is bearable
    b. Medicating for pain after the procedure
    c. Using a combination of strategies
    d. Addressing nonprocedural pain before procedural pain
45. True or False: Decreasing swelling by compression in patients with a venous ulcer has been shown in several recent studies to reduce venous ulcer pain.
46. List five interventions for pain reduction during dressing changes.

C. Pressure Ulcers

1. Define pressure ulcer.
2. What is the role of muscle in preventing pressure ulcers?
    a. Muscle redistributes pressure load.
    b. Muscle provides the blood supply to the skin.
    c. Muscle enables blood vessels to resist shear injury.
    d. Muscle concentrates pressure over the bony prominence.
3. Describe how intensity of pressure and duration of pressure affect tissue ischemia.
4. Which of the following are major factors that contribute to pressure ulcer development?
    a. Shear, smoking, and friction
    b. Age, smoking, and blood pressure
    c. Nutrition and stress
    d. Shear, friction, and nutritional debilitation
5. Which of the following statements about blanching erythema is *false?*
    a. It resolves once pressure is removed.
    b. It indicates deep tissue damage.
    c. It is an area of erythema that turns white when compressed.
    d. It implies that pressure is not adequately relieved or reduced.
6. The undermining that is commonly observed with pressure ulcers may be the result of which of the following?
    a. Shear
    b. Friction
    c. Maceration
    d. Advanced age

7. Nonblanchable erythema of intact skin describes which classification of pressure ulcer?
   a. Suspected deep tissue injury
   b. Stage I
   c. Stage II
   d. Stage III

8. Exposed tendon describes which classification of pressure ulcer?
   a. Stage III
   b. Stage IV
   c. Unstageable
   d. Partial thickness

9. A brown dry wound base on the right trochanter describes which classification of pressure ulcer?
   a. Suspected deep tissue injury
   b. Stage III
   c. Stage IV
   d. Unstageable

10. A blood-filled blister on the heel describes which classification of pressure ulcer?
    a. Suspected deep tissue injury
    b. Stage I
    c. Unstageable
    d. Iatrogenic

11. Intact, nonblanchable, persistant purple discoloration over the coccyx describes which classification of pressure ulcer?
    a. Suspected deep tissue injury
    b. Stage I
    c. Unstageable
    d. None of the above

12. An intact serous-filled blister on the heel describes which classification of pressure ulcer?
    a. Suspected deep tissue injury
    b. Stage I
    c. Stage II
    d. Stage III

13. Application of a skin barrier oinment to the perineal skin addresses which pressure ulcer risk factor?
    a. Impaired mobility
    b. Impaired activity
    c. Moisture
    d. Nutrition

14. Keeping the head of the bed less that 30 degrees addresses which pressure ulcer risk factor?
    a. Impaired mobility
    b. Friction/shear
    c. Moisture
    d. Nutrition

15. Repositioning the patient every 2 hours helps to address which pressure ulcer risk factor?
    a. Impaired mobility
    b. Nutrition
    c. Altered sensory perception
    d. Both a and c

16. Which is the best rationale for obtaining a pressure redistribution mattress?
    a. The patient has a pressure ulcer on both trochanters and sacrum.
    b. A nurse requests a lateral rotation low air loss bed because he does not have enough time to turn his patient every 2 hours.
    c. The patient is on a ventilator.
    d. Both a and c.

17. Which of the following is the most appropriate intervention for a Stage II ischial tuberosity pressure ulcer?
    a. Pressure redistribution mattress
    b. Pressure redistribution chair cushion
    c. Bed rest
    d. Wound culture

18. Which of the following is an appropriate treatment option for the adult to prevent chemical skin irritation due to acute diarrheal consistency fecal incontinence?
    a. Apply skin sealant twice per day.
    b. Remove all skin barrier ointment when cleansing perianal area after incontinent stool.
    c. Apply skin barrier paste.
    d. Apply transparent dressing over perianal skin.

19. According to the WOCN Society, pressure ulcer risk reassessment in acute care should be conducted:
    a. Every 48 hours
    b. Only by an RN
    c. Twice weekly
    d. Upon discharge

20. Friction damage to the skin is characterized by which of the following statements?
    a. It is commonly seen in the periwound field under adhesives.
    b. It results from prolonged elevation of the head of bed.
    c. Tissue necrosis can be present.
    d. Injury typically is very shallow and limited to epidermis.

21. Prolonged moisture on the skin due to urinary incontinence has which of the following effects?
    a. Thickening and strengthening of collagen bonds
    b. Decreased resistance to mechanical trauma
    c. Ulceration due to caustic nature of urine
    d. Stabilization of skin normal flora

D. Lower Extremity Ulcers

1. Rest pain is indicative of which of the following?
   a. Mild occlusive disease, as occurs with 25% occlusion
   b. Moderate occlusive disease, as occurs with 50% occlusion
   c. Advanced occlusive disease, as occurs with 90% occlusion
   d. Need for amputation

2. Risk factors for lower extremity arterial disease include which of the following?
   a. Alcoholism
   b. Hypertension
   c. Elevated high-density lipoprotein levels
   d. Diabetes insipidus
3. What type of pain is claudication?
   a. Pain that exists without precipitating activity
   b. Pain that develops when the patient elevates the legs
   c. Pain that is triggered by moderate to heavy activity
   d. Pain that worsens with rest
4. Which of the following ankle–brachial index (ABI) values is indicative of calcification of vessel wall in a person with diabetes?
   a. 0.95–1.1
   b. 0.5–0.95
   c. 0.5
   d. >1.3
5. Which of the following descriptions is classic for an arterial ulcer?
   a. Highly exudative
   b. Presence of red granulation tissue
   c. Common location above medial malleolus
   d. Dry wound bed
6. Which of the following describes the situation in which maintenance of an eschar-covered arterial ulcer is preferred?
   a. The involved limb can be revascularized.
   b. The TcP0$_2$ is 20 mm Hg.
   c. The wound is infected.
   d. Indications of infection are absent and potential for healing is limited.
7. Describe how a competent venous system and the calf muscle pump work together to prevent venous hypertension.
8. Which of the following levels of pressure would be considered therapeutic for graduated compression when a patient has an ABI of 0.95 in the lower extremity?
   a. 20 mm Hg compression at the ankle
   b. 25 mm Hg compression at the ankle
   c. 30 mm Hg compression at the ankle
   d. 50 mm Hg compression at the ankle
9. Which of the following management options would be *best* for the patient with a venous ulcer complicated by arterial disease, as evidenced by an ABI of 0.5?
   a. Use leg elevation to control edema and 20 mm Hg graduated compression wrap.
   b. Use pneumatic compression or graduated compression to provide pressures in the 25–30 mm Hg range.
   c. Recommend Trental (pentoxifylline) as an alternative to compression.
   d. Delay any treatment until patient undergoes revascularization.
10. Distinguish between elastic and nonelastic static compression products, and explain which is best for the sedentary patient.
11. Which of the following symptoms would indicate venous dermatitis instead of cellulitis?
    a. Erythema, elevated temperature
    b. Erythema, crusting, and itching
    c. Pain, fever, and bullae
    d. Inflammation, pain, and exudate
12. Venous contact dermatitis can be best managed with which of the following treatments?
    a. Antibiotic cream daily
    b. Lanolin cream bid
    c. Topical corticosteroid daily for 1 week
    d. Antifungal powder twice per day
13. Instructions to the patient being fitted for compression stockings for venous insufficiency include which of the following?
    a. Apply stockings first thing in the morning.
    b. Do not remove stockings at bedtime, only when bathing.
    c. Launder the stockings once per week.
    d. Do not perform ankle exercises while wearing the stockings.
14. Lipedema occurs
    a. in both sexes equally
    b. in the feet as well as the legs
    c. in both legs
    d. often in conjunction with cellulitis
15. Which of the following is the gold standard for diagnosing lymphedema?
    a. Isotopic lymphoscintigraphy
    b. Magnetic resonance imaging
    c. Computed tomographic scan
    d. Lymphangiogram
16. Comorbid conditions associated with lymphedema may include which of the following?
    a. Venous ulcer disease
    b. Obesity
    c. Hepatic disease
    d. All of the above
17. The Kaposi-Stemmer's sign is the ability to pinch the skin
    a. at the base of the second and third toes
    b. on the dorsal surface of the foot
    c. between the third and fourth fingers
    d. of the great toe
18. Identify the types of neuropathy and the effects of each on skin integrity.
19. Which of the following is the primary cause of diabetic foot ulcers?
    a. Peripheral neuropathy
    b. Infection
    c. Edema
    d. Peripheral arterial disease

20. Which of the following findings is suggestive of osteomyelitis in the patient with a diabetic foot ulcer?
    a. Abnormal bone scan
    b. Nonhealing ulcer
    c. Abnormal x-ray study findings
    d. All of the above
21. Identify factors other than topical therapy that must be addressed in the management plan of a patient with a diabetic foot ulcer.
22. Identify routine precautions that should be included in the teaching of the patient with lower-extremity neuropathic disease.
23. Which of the following is *not* important information in gathering the patient's pertinent health history?
    a. Arthritis status
    b. Smoking habits
    c. Vision problems
    d. Nasal polyps
24. In assessing the anatomic level in the lower extremity at which arterial insufficiency becomes apparent, which of the following is diagnostically most useful?
    a. Segmental pressures
    b. Femoral bruit
    c. Venous refill time
    d. Ankle-brachial index
25. When instructing the patient and caregiver on proper shoe fit, which of the following is important to emphasize?
    a. Shoes should be selected based on the printed shoe size provided by the manufacturer.
    b. Shoes should be tested for fit early in the morning before the patient is too fatigued to adequately assess how it feels.
    c. Shoes should be fitted while the patient is sitting with the foot elevated on a slanted shoe-fitting stool.
    d. Shoes with heavy rubber soles that curl over the top of the toe area should be avoided.
26. Which of the following is *not* recommended when treating warts on the foot, particularly in younger individuals?
    a. Electrocautery
    b. Liquid nitrogen (cryotherapy)
    c. Salicylic acid
    d. Capsaicin ointment
27. Onychomycosis is
    a. a bacterial infection
    b. commonly painful
    c. a fungal infection
    d. treatable with bleach solution soakings in persons with weak or frail skin

28. Options for toenail debridement should include the use of all of the following *except*
    a. manual nippers
    b. mechanical rotary tools fitted with tungsten carbide burs
    c. salicylate solutions
    d. personal protective equipment to reduce exposure to dust
29. Which of the following causes foot odor?
    a. Fungi
    b. Isovaleric acid
    c. Foot powders
    d. Acetic acid
30. Natural, age-specific changes of the foot include which of the following?
    a. Bunions
    b. Narrowing of the foot
    c. Thickening of fat pad over calcaneous
    d. Decreased range of motion
31. The patient should notify his or her physician when any of the following develop *except*
    a. foot pain that persists for more than 72 hours
    b. foot pain that increases with elevation of the legs
    c. swelling of one leg or foot that persists less than 8 hours
    d. any sudden progression of a foot deformity
32. What causes maceration between the toes?
    a. Inflammation
    b. Allergy
    c. Excessively dry skin
    d. Excessively moist skin

E. Other Types of Wounds

1. Which of the following descriptions is representative of a skin tear classified as category III using the Payne-Martin scale?
    a. Partial-thickness wound with epidermal flap that can be approximated
    b. Both epidermis and dermis are pulled apart as if incisions were made
    c. Partial-thickness wound with no epidermal flap
    d. Full-thickness wound that occurs in skin wrinkle
2. Which of the following terms refers to a tinea infection of the nails?
    a. Tinea pedis
    b. Tinea cruris
    c. Tinea corporis
    d. Onychomycosis
3. Suggestions to prevent tinea infections include which of the following?
    a. Wash hair daily.
    b. Avoid wearing socks.
    c. Wear flip-flops or sandals in public places instead of going barefoot.
    d. Use antideodorant rather than antiperspirant.

4. Which of the following medication histories places the patient with fecal or urinary incontinence at risk for candidiasis?
   a. Prophylactic use of an antifungal agent
   b. History of recent antibiotic use
   c. Current use of anticoagulants
   d. Current use of antiseizure medications
5. Which of the following characteristics is distinctive for perianal herpes simplex?
   a. Common location is inner thighs or groin
   b. Associated with history of moisture and antibiotics
   c. Initial manifestations are painful clusters of vesicles
   d. Commonly has a pathergy response
6. Which of the following is *not* appropriate for a sutured postoperative incision?
   a. Keep moist with a topical antibiotic ointment.
   b. Maintain original postoperative dressing for 48–72 hours.
   c. Begin showering 48–72 hours postoperatively.
   d. Protect surgical incision from exposure to sun.
7. Which of the following hygiene practices is *not* recommended in the presence of radiation skin damage?
   a. Warm showers
   b. Antimicrobial soap to prevent infection
   c. Washing hair with baby shampoo
   d. Shaving with a straight edge razor
8. Which of the following interventions to promote comfort is *not* recommended in the presence of radiation skin damage?
   a. Gently apply (do not rub) a petrolatum-based product to dry irritated skin.
   b. Use aloe vera to sooth and cool the skin.
   c. For burning and itching, apply normal saline compresses as needed.
   d. Wear loose, soft, breathable, nonbinding clothing that protects skin from sun and wind.
9. The surgical procedure used to relieve compartment syndrome and nerve damage from tissue edema is known as
   a. grafting
   b. fasciotomy
   c. escharotomy
   d. incision and drain
10. Which of the following interventions is recommended when the traumatic wound is heavily colonized?
    a. Surgically debride daily.
    b. Pack with Silvadene-coated gauze dressings twice daily.
    c. Surgically close the wound by approximation of wound edges within 36 hours.
    d. Pack the wound with one-quarter strength Dakin solution twice daily temporarily.
11. The wound that undergoes malignant transformation is known as a
    a. Marjolin ulcer
    b. fungating wound
    c. fistula
    d. draining wound
12. Odor control in a malignant cutaneous wound includes applying:
    a. TNF (tumor necrosis factor) topically every day
    b. gentamycin powder topically every day
    c. metronidazole powder topically with every dressing change
    d. either b or c to the wound every day
13. A condition in which the skin develops superficial blistering and a sandpaper feel and exfoliates after exposure to bacterial toxins is known as
    a. toxic epidermis necrosis (TEN)
    b. epidermolysis bullosa
    c. staphylococcal scalded skin syndrome (SSSS)
    d. calciphylaxis
14. General signs and symptoms of vasculitis include which of the following?
    a. Sandpaper feel to skin
    b. Severe pruritus
    c. Fever and arthralgias
    d. Mental confusion and imbalance
15. The extent of irreversible tissue damage due to frostbite is primarily influenced by which of the following?
    a. Lowest tissue temperature achieved
    b. Rewarming process
    c. Body part that is involved
    d. Speed with which skin froze

ANSWERS

A. General Principles of Assessment

1. Assessment includes verification and interpretation of observations made. Evaluation of healing involves monitoring and assessment documented over time to reveal patterns and trends that indicate improvement or deterioration in the wound. (Chapter 6)
2. c (Chapter 6)
3. a (Chapter 4)
4. Indices of wound healing (Chapter 6)
   - Etiology/type of skin damage
   - Factors that impede healing
   - Duration of wound
   - Anatomic location of wound
   - Extent of tissue loss (stage)
   - Characteristics of wound base
   - Type of tissue
   - Percentage of wound containing each type of tissue observed
   - Dimensions of wound in cm (length, width, tunneling, undermining)
   - Exudate (amount, type, odor)
   - Wound edges
   - Periwound skin
   - Presence or absence of signs of infection
   - Pain
5. b (Chapter 6)
6. Eschar is black or brown necrotic, devitalized tissue that commonly has leathery necrotic; tissue can be loose or firm adherent, hard, soft, or boggy. (Chapter 6)
7. Slough is soft, moist, avascular (necrotic/devitalized) tissue; it may be white, yellow or tan; it may be loose or firmly adherent. (Chapter 6)
8. Factors known to damage the skin include mechanical, chemical, vascular, allergic, infectious, immunologic, burn, and disease-related types. (Chapter 5)
9. b (Chapter 5)
10. a (Chapter 5)
11. c (Chapter 5)
12. b (Chapter 5)
13. d (Chapter 5)
14. The two phases of an allergic contact dermatitis are the sensitization phase and the elicitation phase. (Chapter 5)
15. a (Chapter 5)
16. d (Chapter 5)
17. a (Chapter 27)
18. b (Chapter 27)
19. a (Chapter 27)
20. a (Chapter 27)
21. d (Chapter 27)
22. d (Chapter 27)
23. b (Chapter 27)
24. d (Chapter 27)
25. c (Chapter 27)
26. d (Chapter 27)
27. a (Chapter 25)
28. b (Chapter 25)
29. Wounds involving only the epidermis and dermis heal relatively quickly because epithelial, endothelial, and connective tissue can be reproduced. Wounds extending through the dermis and involving deeper structures must heal by scar formation because the deep dermal structures, subcutaneous tissue, and muscle do not regenerate. (Chapter 4)
30. Wounds that are well approximated with minimal tissue defect are said to heal by primary intention. Wounds that are left open and allowed to heal by production of granulation tissue are said to heal by secondary intention. Wounds are described as healing by tertiary intention when there is a delay between injury and reapproximation of the wound edges. (Chapter 4)
31. The major components of partial-thickness repair are inflammatory response, epithelial proliferation and migration, and reestablishment and differentiation of epidermal layers. If dermis is involved, connective tissue repair proceeds concurrently with reepithelialization. (Chapter 4)
32. A moist wound surface facilitates epidermal migration because epidermal cells can migrate only across a moist surface. In a dry wound, epidermal cells must tunnel down to a moist level and secrete collagenase to lift the scab away from the wound surface in order to migrate. Connective tissue repair begins earlier when the wound surface is kept moist because new connective tissue forms only in the presence of suitable exudate. (Chapter 4)
33. *Inflammatory phase:* hemostasis and inflammation. *Proliferative phase:* neoangiogenesis, matrix deposition/collagen synthesis, epithelialization, and, when a full-thickness wound is left to heal by secondary intention, contraction of wound edges. *Maturation phase:* matrix deposition and collagen lysis. (Chapter 4)
34. c (Chapter 4)
35. b (Chapter 4)
36. There is a limit to epidermal cell migration. In full-thickness wounds, epidermal cells are present only at the wound margins. In partial-thickness wounds, epidermal cells are present in the lining of hair follicles and sweat glands as well as at the wound periphery. (Chapter 4)
37. Chronic wounds are likely to begin with circulatory compromise as opposed to injury. Injury initiates hemostasis, which triggers the wound healing cascade; circulatory compromise does not trigger the wound healing cascade. Chronic wounds contain higher levels of proteases (i.e., neutrophil elastase and matrix metalloproteases ([MMPs]) resulting in the prolonged presence and increased volume of proinflammatory cells (cytokines). (Chapter 4)

38. Factors that affect wound healing include tissue perfusion and oxygenation, nutritional status, infection, diabetes mellitus, corticosteroid administration, immunosuppression, and aging. Systemic factors include renal or hepatic disease, malignancy, sepsis, hematopoietic abnormalities, and stress. (Chapter 4)
39. b (Chapter 4)

B. General Principles of Management

1. d (Chapter 18)
2. d (Chapter 12)
3. b (Chapter 18)
4. d (Chapter 34)
5. b (Chapter 18)
6. d (Chapter 18)
7. d (Chapter 18)
8. Objectives for local wound management are to prevent and manage infection, cleanse the wound, remove nonviable tissue (debridement), maintain an appropriate level of moisture, eliminate dead space, control odor, eliminate or minimize pain, and protect the wound and periwound skin. (Chapter 18)
9. d (Chapter 17)
10. c (Chapter 17)
11. Considerations in the use of enzymatic debridement include the following (Chapter 17):
    * Enzymes are inactivated by heavy metal ions (chlorine, silver, mercury).
    * Enzymes may be used to debride an infected wound.
    * Enzymatic debridement necessitates dressing changes one to three times daily.
    * Selection of debriding enzyme is primarily based on clinician preference, cost, availability, and ease of use.
12. a (Chapter 17)
13. b (Chapter 17)
14. b (Chapter 16)
15. d (Chapter 16)
16. a (Chapter 16)
17. a (Chapter 16)
18. d (Chapter 16)
19. c (Chapter 16)
20. d (Chapter 16)
21. d (Chapter 16)
22. b (Chapter 16)
23. c (Chapter 21)
24. b (Chapter 21)
25. a (Chapter 21)
26. a (Chapter 21)
27. c (Chapter 21)
28. b (Chapter 22)
29. c (Chapter 22)
30. True (Chapter 22)
31. False (Chapter 22)
32. Selectins, integrins, cell adhesion molecules (Chapter 20)
33. False (Chapter 20)
34. d (Chapter 20)
35. Cellular products contain living cells, either autologous or allogeneic, whereas acellular products do not contain cells but usually have the extracellular matrix proteins produced by cells. Some acellular products are synthetic and function as either a matrix or an epidermal skin substitute. (Chapter 19)
36. Sources include autologous (derived from the patient's own body), allogeneic (derived from humans other than the patient, also called *homografts*), xenographic (derived from nonhuman sources, e.g., porcine, bovine, equine, avian, etc., also called *heterografts*), biosynthetic (biologic and man-made materials), and synthetic (man-made materials). (Chapter 19)
37. Cell therapy is the administration of cells to the body to the benefit of the recipient. When living cells are delivered to the wound as a skin substitute, they manufacture and release growth factors that speed wound healing, and they produce extracellular matrix proteins that provide scaffolding for cell attachment and migration. (Chapter 19)
38. Epicel, Dermagraft, Apligraf (Chapter 19)
39. d (Chapter 19)
40. Alloderm, Cymetra, GraftJacket, GraftJacket Xpress, DermaMatrix, Oasis, MatriStem, Unite Biomatrix, PriMatrix, Mediskin, E-Z Derm, Biobrane, Integra (all forms) (Chapter 19)
41. Dermagraft, Apligraf (Chapter 19)
42. Address underlying pathology; correct systemic factors interfering with wound healing; identify and treat clinical infection; debride all necrotic tissue, fibrinous slough, and surrounding callus; ensure complete contact of product with wound bed; fenestrate product; keep products without synthetic backings moist; follow package insert for directions specific to individual products. (Chapter 19)
43. d (Chapter 26)
44. c (Chapter 26)
45. True (Chapter 26)
46. Minimize the degree of sensory stimulus (e.g., drafts from open windows, or prodding and poking); allow patient to perform his or her own dressing change; allow time-outs during painful procedures; schedule dressing changes when the patient is feeling best; give an analgesic and then schedule the dressing change when its peak effect occurs; soak dried dressings before removal; avoid use of cytotoxic cleansers; avoid aggressive packing; minimize number of dressing changes; prevent periwound trauma; position and support wounded area for comfort; consider using low-adhesive or nonadhesive dressings; and offer and use distraction techniques (e.g., headphones, television, music, warm blanket). (Chapter 26)

C. Pressure Ulcers

1. A pressure ulcer is a localized area of tissue necrosis that develops when soft tissue is compressed between a bony prominence and an external surface for a period of time. (Chapter 7)
2. a (Chapter 7)
3. Amount and duration of pressure share an inverse relationship in producing tissue ischemia. A long time is needed for low pressure to create ischemia, whereas a short time is needed for high pressure to cause tissue ischemia. (Chapter 7)
4. d (Chapter 8)
5. b (Chapter 7)
6. a (Chapters 7 and 8)
7. b (Chapter 7)
8. b (Chapter 7)
9. d (Chapter 7)
10. a (Chapter 7)
11. a (Chapter 7)
12. c (Chapter 7)
13. c (Chapter 8)
14. b (Chapter 8)
15. d (Chapter 8)
16. a (Chapter 9)
17. b (Chapter 9)
18. c (Chapter 5)
19. b (Chapter 5)
20. d (Chapter 5)
21. b (Chapter 5)

D. Lower Extremity Ulcers

1. c (Chapter 11)
2. b (Chapter 11)
3. c (Chapter 11)
4. d (Chapter 11)
5. d (Chapter 11)
6. d (Chapter 11)
7. Competent venous system includes deep veins, superficial veins, and perforator veins. The perforator veins (communicating veins) connect the deep and superficial veins to transport blood. Veins function by one-way valves to prevent backflow. The calf muscle pump and one-way valves work together to propel venous blood back to the heart. During ambulation, the calf muscle contracts and pumps the blood out of the deep veins, and the one-way valves in the perforator system close to prevent backflow into superficial veins. When the calf muscle relaxes, the valves in the perforator veins open to permit blood flow into the deep veins. (Chapter 12)
8. c (Chapter 12). 30–40 mm Hg is considered a therapeutic level. 20–25 mm Hg compression is considered a light compression, whereas 50 mm Hg is a very high compression usually indicated for lymphedema.
9. d (Chapter 12). An ABI of 0.5 indicates ischemia, and any additional compression to a leg with compromised arterial circulation could increase claudication and put the patient at risk for ischemic damage. In addition, the wound will not heal unless revascularization is performed.
10. Elastic compression devices deliver a sustained pressure regardless of the patient's activity level. Nonelastic compression devices compress the calf muscle during ambulation. The constant compression increases interstitial tissue pressure to reduce leakage of fluid from capillaries. The sedentary patient should be managed with elastic compression devices because he or she has decreased calf muscle pump action. (Chapter 12)
11. b (Chapter 12)
12. c (Chapter 12). Lanolin skin products and topical antibiotic creams should not be used because of sensitivities to topical creams/lotions that develop in the patient with chronic venous insufficiency.
13. a (Chapter 12). Compression stockings need to be applied in the morning before the patient gets out of bed to prevent the return of ankle edema which can occur as soon as the patient dangles their foot over the edge of the bed. Ankle exercise can be performed while the stockings are worn.
14. c (Chapter 13)
15. a (Chapter 13)
16. d (Chapter 13)
17. a (Chapter 13)
18. *Autonomic:* Results in decreased sweating and oil production, loss of skin temperature regulation, and abnormal blood flow in the soles of the feet. Resultant xerosis can precipitate fissures, cracks, callus, and finally ulceration. *Sensory:* Loss of protective sensation leads to lack of awareness of pain and temperature change, resulting in increased susceptibility to injury. Minor trauma caused by poor-fitting shoes or an acute injury can precipitate a chronic ulcer. *Motor:* Affects the muscles required for normal foot movement and can result in muscle atrophy, resulting in collapse of the arch, cocked-up or claw toes, hammer toes, and weight redistribution from the toes to the metatarsal heads, which leads to increased pressures and subsequent ulceration. (Chapter 14)
19. a (Chapter 14)
20. d (Chapter 14)
21. Glycemic control, offloading, callus management, pain control, education (Chapter 14)

22. Routine precautions in the teaching of the patient with lower-extremity neuropathic disease include the following (Chapter 14):
    - Wash feet daily; dry carefully, including between the toes.
    - Test the water with hands or elbow.
    - Do not soak feet.
    - Apply moisturizing cream to feet, but not between toes.
    - Do not use heating pad or hot water bottle to warm feet.
    - Do not use chemical corn or callus removers or corn pads.
    - File away calluses with pumice stone.
    - Do not walk barefoot; wear slippers with rubber sole; no open toes or heels; avoid pointed-toe shoes or boots; do not wear sandals with strap between toes.
    - Buy shoes later in the day when feet are their largest.
    - Inspect shoes for objects inside before putting them on.
    - Wear clean socks every day; avoid nylon socks; no tight elastic or seams.
    - Do not smoke; exercise regularly.
23. d (Chapter 15)
24. a (Chapter 15)
25. d (Chapter 15)
26. d (Chapter 15)
27. c (Chapter 15)
28. c (Chapter 15)
29. b (Chapter 15)
30. d (Chapter 15)
31. c (Chapter 15)
32. d (Chapter 15)

E. Other Types of Wounds

1. c (Chapter 5)
2. d (Chapter 15)
3. c (Chapter 15)
4. b (Chapter 5)
5. c (Chapter 5)
6. a (Chapter 34)
7. d (Chapter 5)
8. a (Chapter 5)
9. b (Chapters 31 and 32)
10. d (Chapter 31)
11. a (Chapter 37)
12. c (Chapter 37)
13. c (Chapter 30)
14. c (Chapter 30)
15. b (Chapter 30)

B

Documentation Tools

NORTON RISK ASSESSMENT SCALE

		Physical Condition		Mental Condition		Activity		Mobility		Incontinent		TOTAL SCORE
		Good	4	Alert	4	Ambulant	4	Full	4	Not	4	
		Fair	3	Apathetic	3	Walk/help	3	Sl. limited	3	Occasional	3	
		Poor	2	Confused	2	Chairbound	2	V. limited	2	Usually/Urine	2	
		Very Bad	1	Stupor	1	Bed	1	Immobile	1	Doubly	1	
Name	Date											

From Norton D, McLaren R, Exton-Smith AN: *An investigation of geriatric nursing problems in hospital*, Churchill Livingstone, 1975, Edinburgh.

Waterlow Scale

Build/Weight for Height		Mobility		Special Risks	
Average	0	Fully	0	Tissue Malnutrition	8
Above Average	1	Restless/Fidgety	1	e.g. Terminal cachexia	
Obese	2	Apathetic	2	Cardiac Failure	5
Below Average	3	Restricted	3	Peripheral Vascular Disease	5
		Inert/Traction	4	Anemia	2
		Chairbound	5	Smoking	1
Continence		**Sex/Age**		**Neurological Deficit**	
Complete/Catheterized	0	Male	1	e.g. Diabetes, MS, CVA,	4-6
Occasional	1	Female	2	Motor/Sensory, Paraplegic	
Cath/Incontinence of Feces	2	14-49	1		
Doubly Incontinent	3	50-49	2		
		65-74	3		
		75-80	4		
		81+	5		
Skin Type **Visual Risk Areas**		**Appetite**		**Major Surgery/Trauma**	
Healthy	0	Average	0	Orthopaedic – below waist, spinal	5
Tissue Paper	1	Poor	1	On Table – 2 Hours	5
Dry	1	NG Tube/Fluids Only	2		
Oedematous	1	NBM/Anorexic			
Clammy (temp)	1				
Discolored	2				
Broken/Spot	3			**Medication**	
				Steroids, Cytotoxics, High Dose Anti-Inflam.	4

SCORE	10+ AT RISK	15+ HIGH RISK	20+ V. HIGH RISK

SEVERAL SCORES PER CATEGORY CAN BE USED; ADD TOTAL

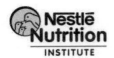

Mini Nutritional Assessment
MNA®

Last name:		First name:	
Sex:	Age:	Weight, kg:	Height, cm:	Date:

Complete the screen by filling in the boxes with the appropriate numbers. Total the numbers for the final screening score.

Screening

A **Has food intake declined over the past 3 months due to loss of appetite, digestive problems, chewing or swallowing difficulties?**
0 = severe decrease in food intake
1 = moderate decrease in food intake
2 = no decrease in food intake ☐

B **Weight loss during the last 3 months**
0 = weight loss greater than 3 kg (6.6 lbs)
1 = does not know
2 = weight loss between 1 and 3 kg (2.2 and 6.6 lbs)
3 = no weight loss ☐

C **Mobility**
0 = bed or chair bound
1 = able to get out of bed / chair but does not go out
2 = goes out ☐

D **Has suffered psychological stress or acute disease in the past 3 months?**
0 = yes   2 = no ☐

E **Neuropsychological problems**
0 = severe dementia or depression
1 = mild dementia
2 = no psychological problems ☐

F1 Body Mass Index (BMI) (weight in kg) / (height in m^2)
0 = BMI less than 19
1 = BMI 19 to less than 21
2 = BMI 21 to less than 23
3 = BMI 23 or greater ☐

IF BMI IS NOT AVAILABLE, REPLACE QUESTION F1 WITH QUESTION F2.
DO NOT ANSWER QUESTION F2 IF QUESTION F1 IS ALREADY COMPLETED.

F2 Calf circumference (CC) in cm
0 = CC less than 31
3 = CC 31 or greater ☐

Screening score ☐☐
(max. 14 points)

12-14 points: Normal nutritional status
8-11 points: At risk of malnutrition
0-7 points: Malnourished

For a more in-depth assessment, complete the full MNA® which is available at **www.mna-elderly.com**

Ref.   Vellas B, Villars H, Abellan G, et al. *Overview of the MNA® - Its History and Challenges.* J Nutr Health Aging 2006;10:456-465.
Rubenstein LZ, Harker JO, Salva A, Guigoz Y, Vellas B. *Screening for Undernutrition in Geriatric Practice: Developing the Short-Form Mini Nutritional Assessment (MNA-SF).* J. Geront 2001;56A: M366-377.
Guigoz Y. *The Mini-Nutritional Assessment (MNA®) Review of the Literature - What does it tell us?* J Nutr Health Aging 2006; 10:466-487.
® Société des Produits Nestlé, S.A., Vevey, Switzerland, Trademark Owners
© Nestlé, 1994, Revision 2009. N67200 12/99 10M
For more information: www.mna-elderly.com

Malnutrition Screening Tool (MST)

Please circle appropriate answer to each question.

Have you lost weight recently without trying?	If No	0
	If unsure	2
If Yes, how much weight have you lost?	1–5 kg (2-11 lb)	1
	6–10 kg (1-1 ½ st)	2
	11–15 kg (1 ¾ - 2 ⅓ st)	3
	>15 kg (>2 ⅓ st)	4
	Unsure	2
Have you been eating poorly because of a decreased appetite?	If No	0
	If Yes	1
TOTAL SCORE (If the score is 2 or more please refer to the dietitian.)		

Source: Ferguson M, Capra S, Bauer J, Banks M: Development of a valid and reliable malnutrition screening tool for adult acute hospital patients. *Nutrition* 1999;15(6):458–464.

Subjective Global Assessment (SGA) Scoring Sheet

Patient Name:_____ Patient ID:_____ Date:_____

Part 1: Medical History

SGA Score

A	B	C

1. Weight Change

   A. Overall change in past 6 months: _____ kg

   B. Percent change: _____ gain <5% loss

                          _____ 5%–10% loss

                          _____ >10% loss

   C. Change in past 2 weeks: _____ increase

                          _____ no change

                          _____ decrease

2. Dietary Intake

   A. Overall change: _____ no change

                          _____ change

   B. Duration: _____ weeks

   C. Type of change:

       _____ suboptimal solid diet _____ full liquid diet

       _____ hypocaloric liquid   _____ starvation

3. Gastrointestinal Symptoms (persisting for >2 weeks)

    _____ none _____ nausea   diarrhea _____ anorexia

          _____ vomiting _____

4. Functional Impairment   (nutritionally related)

   A. Overall impairment: _____ none

                          _____ moderate

                          _____ severe

   B. Change in past 2 weeks: _____ improved

                          _____ no change

                          _____ regressed

Part 2: Physical Examination

5. Evidence of: Loss of subcutaneous fat
                     Muscle wasting
                     Edema
                     Ascites (hemo only)

SGA Score

Normal	Mild	Moderate	Severe

Part 3: SGA Rating (Check One)

A. ☐ Well-nourished   B. ☐ Mildly–moderately malnourished   C. ☐ Severely malnourished

Reproduced from Covinsky KE et al: The relationship between clinical assessments of nutritional status and adverse outcomes in older hospitalized medical patients, *J Am Geriatr Soc* 47:432-538, 1999.

Short Nutritional Assessment Questionnaire (SNAQ) Assessment Tool

My appetite is

    a. very poor

    b. poor

    c. average

    d. good

    e. very good

When I eat

    a. I feel full after eating only a few mouthfuls

    b. I feel full after eating about a third of a meal

    c. I feel full after eating over half a meal

    d. I feel full after eating most of the meal

    e. I hardly ever feel full

Food tastes

    a. very bad

    b. bad

    c. average

    d. good

    e. very good

Normally I eat

    a. less than one meal a day

    b. one meal a day

    c. two meals a day

    d. three meals a day

    e. more than three meals a day

Directions

Tally the results based on the following numerical scale: a = 1, b = 2, c = 3, d = 4, e = 5. The sum of the scores for the individual items constitutes the SNAQ score. SNAQ score ≤14 indicates significant risk of at least 5% weight loss within six months.

From Kruizenga H, Seidell J, de Vet H et al: Development and validation of a hospital screening tool for malnutrition: the short nutritional assessment questionnaire (SNAQ), *Clin Nutr* 24(1):75-82, 2005.

Skin Inspection and Prevention Form

POA = Present on Admission   sDTI = Suspected Deep Tissue Injury

---

Date: _____ **Time:** _____

	Skin Intact				**3**	Wound or lesion	☐ New	☐ POA
1	Edema	☐ New	☐ POA		**4**	At-risk area	☐ New	☐ POA
2	Bruising	☐ New	☐ POA		**5**	Incision	☐ New	☐ POA

6	Pressure ulcer	☐ New	☐ POA	**Circle Stage:**	I	II	III	IV	Unstageable	sDTI
7	Pressure ulcer	☐ New	☐ POA	**Circle Stage:**	I	II	III	IV	Unstageable	sDTI
8	Pressure ulcer	☐ New	☐ POA	**Circle Stage:**	I	II	III	IV	Unstageable	sDTI
9	Pressure ulcer	☐ New	☐ POA	**Circle Stage:**	I	II	III	IV	Unstageable	sDTI

☐ Float heels w/pillow   ☐ Lift-sheet   ☐ Float Heels w/_____   ☐ Skin Barrier Product_____

☐ HOB<30°   ☐ Pillow betw knees   ☐ Trapeze   ☐ Elbow protectors   ☐ Mattress_____

Turn Q2H: Time: _____ _____ _____ _____ _____ _____

(Circle: right,left,back)   R L B   R L B   R L B   R L B   R L B   R L B

Use numeric key to indicate location

☐ See Ns Notes   Nsg Signature:

Date: _____ **Time:** _____

	Skin Intact				**3**	Wound or lesion	☐ New	☐ POA
1	Edema	☐ New	☐ POA		**4**	At-risk area	☐ New	☐ POA
2	Bruising	☐ New	☐ POA		**5**	Incision	☐ New	☐ POA

6	Pressure ulcer	☐ New	☐ POA	**Circle Stage:**	I	II	III	IV	Unstageable	sDTI
7	Pressure ulcer	☐ New	☐ POA	**Circle Stage:**	I	II	III	IV	Unstageable	sDTI
8	Pressure ulcer	☐ New	☐ POA	**Circle Stage:**	I	II	III	IV	Unstageable	sDTI
9	Pressure ulcer	☐ New	☐ POA	**Circle Stage:**	I	II	III	IV	Unstageable	sDTI

☐ Float heels w/pillow   ☐ Lift-sheet   ☐ Float Heels w/_____   ☐ Skin Barrier Product_____

☐ HOB<30°   ☐ Pillow betw knees   ☐ Trapeze   ☐ Elbow protectors   ☐ Mattress_____

Turn Q2H: Time: _____ _____ _____ _____ _____ _____

(Circle: right,left,back)   R L B   R L B   R L B   R L B   R L B   R L B

Use numeric key to indicate location

☐ See Ns Notes   Nsg Signature:

Date: _____ **Time:** _____

	Skin Intact				**3**	Wound or lesion	☐ New	☐ POA
1	Edema	☐ New	☐ POA		**4**	At-risk area	☐ New	☐ POA
2	Bruising	☐ New	☐ POA		**5**	Incision	☐ New	☐ POA

6	Pressure ulcer	☐ New	☐ POA	**Circle Stage:**	I	II	III	IV	Unstageable	sDTI
7	Pressure ulcer	☐ New	☐ POA	**Circle Stage:**	I	II	III	IV	Unstageable	sDTI
8	Pressure ulcer	☐ New	☐ POA	**Circle Stage:**	I	II	III	IV	Unstageable	sDTI
9	Pressure ulcer	☐ New	☐ POA	**Circle Stage:**	I	II	III	IV	Unstageable	sDTI

☐ Float heels w/pillow   ☐ Lift-sheet   ☐ Float Heels w/_____   ☐ Skin Barrier Product_____

☐ HOB<30°   ☐ Pillow betw knees   ☐ Trapeze   ☐ Elbow protectors   ☐ Mattress_____

Turn Q2H: Time: _____ _____ _____ _____ _____ _____

(Circle: right,left,back)   R L B   R L B   R L B   R L B   R L B   R L B

Use numeric key to indicate location

☐ See Ns Notes   Nsg Signature:

Date: _____ **Time:** _____

	Skin Intact				**3**	Wound or lesion	☐ New	☐ POA
1	Edema	☐ New	☐ POA		**4**	At-risk area	☐ New	☐ POA
2	Bruising	☐ New	☐ POA		**5**	Incision	☐ New	☐ POA

6	Pressure ulcer	☐ New	☐ POA	**Circle Stage:**	I	II	III	IV	Unstageable	sDTI
7	Pressure ulcer	☐ New	☐ POA	**Circle Stage:**	I	II	III	IV	Unstageable	sDTI
8	Pressure ulcer	☐ New	☐ POA	**Circle Stage:**	I	II	III	IV	Unstageable	sDTI
9	Pressure ulcer	☐ New	☐ POA	**Circle Stage:**	I	II	III	IV	Unstageable	sDTI

☐ Float heels w/pillow   ☐ Lift-sheet   ☐ Float Heels w/_____   ☐ Skin Barrier Product_____

☐ HOB<30°   ☐ Pillow betw knees   ☐ Trapeze   ☐ Elbow protectors   ☐ Mattress_____

Turn Q2H: Time: _____ _____ _____ _____ _____ _____

(Circle: right,left,back)   R L B   R L B   R L B   R L B   R L B   R L B

Use numeric key to indicate location

☐ See Ns Notes   Nsg Signature:

Patient Label

Wound Assessment Flow Sheet

Patient information

Date			
Location			
L x W x D in cm Undermining Tunneling	_____ x _____ x _____ cm □No □Yes _____cm @ _____ □No □Yes _____cm @ _____	_____ x _____ x _____ cm □No □Yes _____cm @ _____ □No □Yes _____cm @ _____	_____ x _____ x _____ cm □No □Yes _____cm @ _____ □No □Yes _____cm @ _____
Stage (Pressure Wounds)	□I □II □III □IV□ Unstageable □ sDTI	□I □II □III □IV□ Unstageable □ sDTI	□I □II □III □IV□ Unstageable □ sDTI
Visible depth	□Intact □PT □FT □N/A	□Intact □ PT □FT □N/A	□Intact □ PT □FT □N/A
Eschar	□No □Yes_____ %	□No □Yes_____ %	□No □Yes_____%
Necrotic tissue	□No □Yellow Black _____%	□No □Yellow Black ____ %	□No □Yellow Black _____ %
Granulation tissue /wound base	□Red □Pink □Pale □None	□Red □Pink □Pale □None	□Red □Pink □Pale □None
Drainage amount	□Small □Mod □Large □None	□Small □Mod □Large □None	□Small □Mod □Large □None
Drainage color	□Clear □Yellow □Sero-sang □Blood □Purulent □Green	□Clear □Yellow □Sero-sang □Blood □Purulent □Green	□Clear □Yellow □Sero-sang □Blood □Purulent □Green
Wound edge	□Flat □Rolled □N/A	□Flat □Rolled □N/A	□Flat □Rolled □N/A
Induration	□No □Yes	□No □Yes	□No □Yes
Peri-wound skin	□Intact □Macerated □Red □Callus □Ecchymotic □Dermatitis □Fungal	□Intact □Macerated □Red □Callus □Ecchymotic □Dermatitis □Fungal	□Intact □Macerated □Red □Callus □Ecchymotic □Dermatitis □Fungal
Structure exposed	□No □Tendon □Muscle □Bone	□No □Tendon □Muscle □Bone	□No □Tendon □Muscle □Bone
Sign of infection	□None □Red ring □Red streak □Warm □>Pain □>Drainage □Purulent drainage □Odor	□None □Red ring □Red streak □Warm □>Pain □>Drainage □Purulent drainage □Odor	□None □Red ring □Red streak □Warm □>Pain □>Drainage □Purulent drainage □Odor
Dressing	□Xeroform □Hydrogel □Alginate □Hydrocolloid □Mesalt □ NPWT □Barrier □Multilayer Compression □Other_____	□Xeroform □ Hydrogel □Alginate □Hydrocolloid □Mesalt □ NPWT □Barrier □Multilayer Compression □Other_____	□Xeroform □ Hydrogel □Alginate □Hydrocolloid □Mesalt □ NPWT □Barrier □Multilayer Compression □Other_____

Teaching record

Date	Topic	To whom	Method	Tools	Comments	Staff Signature

1 Dressing change	9 Venous disease	**To Whom:** P- Patient F – Family C- Caregiver
2 Keep dressing clean and dry	10 Arterial disease	**Method:** E- Explanation D- Demonstration V - Video
3 When to call physician	11 Nutrition	**Tools:** H – Handout W – Written instructions
4 Signs / symptoms of infection	12 Smoking cessation	**Evaluation:** V – Verbalized understanding
5 Medications	13 Diabetes	D – Demonstrated understanding
6 Skin care	14 Offloading	NR – Needs reinforcement
7 Foot care	15 Follow up needed	
8 Edema control	16 other – write in topic	

Home Care Wound Trending Record

KAISER PERMANENTE.
HOMECARE SERVICES
WOUND TRENDING RECORD

a. SURGICAL	d. DIABETIC / NEUROPATHIC	g. FISTULA
b PRESSURE	e. VENOUS / STASIS	h. DRAIN / TUBE
c. TRAUMA	f. ARTERIAL	i. OTHER

MED. REC.#

_____

PATIENT NAME:

Document at least 1 x week	Document on initial assessment, deterioration and recert

Document all other parameters with each dressing change.

Location: Check corresponding box

1. ☐ Sacrum	16. ☐ (L) Ear
2. ☐ Coccyx	17. ☐ (R) Foot
3. ☐ (R) Heel	18. ☐ (L) Foot
4. ☐ (L) Heel	19. ☐ (R) Leg
5. ☐ (R) Ischium	20. ☐ (L) Leg
6. ☐ (L) Ischium	21. ☐ (R) Arm
7. ☐ (R) Trochanter	22. ☐ (L) Arm
8. ☐ (L) Trochanter	23. ☐ (R) Hand
9. ☐ (R) Malleolus	24. ☐ (L) Hand
10. ☐ (L) Malleolus	25. ☐ Chest
11. ☐ Back	26. ☐ Abdomen
12. ☐ Occipital	27. ☐ Perineum
13. ☐ (R) Shoulder	28. ☐ Nose
14. ☐ (L) Shoulder	29. ☐ Other
15. ☐ (R) Ear	

USE CORRESPONDING NUMBER(S) FROM LIST TO IDENTIFY LOCATION OF WOUND(S) ON FIGURE

Right Left   Left Right

Right Left   Left Right

SKILLED CARE COMPLETED		Wnd ____Location:____ Type: _____	Wnd ____Location:____ Type: _____
Wound #_____	**BRADEN PER POLICY**	Risk for pressure ulcers per Braden Scale: ☐ Mild (15-18 pts) ☐ Moderate (13-14 pts) ☐ High (10-12 pts) ☐ Very High (9 or below)	Risk for pressure ulcers per Braden Scale: ☐ Mild (15-18 pts) ☐ Moderate (13-14 pts) ☐ High (10-12 pts) ☐ Very High (9 or below)
Cleansed: _____	**SIZE**	L_____ cm x W_____ cm x D_____ cm	L_____ cm x W_____ cm x D_____ cm
	STAGE Do not reverse stage	ONLY STAGE PRESSURE ULCERS ☐ I ☐ II ☐ III ☐ IV ☐ Unstageable	ONLY STAGE PRESSURE ULCERS ☐ I ☐ II ☐ III ☐ IV ☐ Unstageable
Applied/packed: _____	**HEALING OUTCOMES**	☐ Improved ☐ Healed ☐ Not Healed	☐ Improved ☐ Healed ☐ Not Healed
Covered: _____ Secured: _____ Protected periwound skin: _____ _____ _____	**WOUND PRODUCTS REMOVED**	☐ Transparent dressing ☐ Nu-gauze_____ ☐ Hydrocolloid ☐ 2x2's_____ ☐ Hydrogel ☐ 4x4's_____ ☐ Alginate ☐ Kerlix roll_____ ☐ Foam ☐ ABD_____ ☐ Silver dressing ☐ Other: _____ ☐ Enzyme ☐ N/A ☐ Antibiotic Ointment ☐ Impregnated gauze ☐ Unna boot	☐ Transparent dressing ☐ Nu-gauze_____ ☐ Hydrocolloid ☐ 2x2's_____ ☐ Hydrogel ☐ 4x4's_____ ☐ Alginate ☐ Kerlix roll_____ ☐ Foam ☐ ABD_____ ☐ Silver dressing ☐ Other: _____ ☐ Enzyme ☐ N/A ☐ Antibiotic Ointment ☐ Impregnated gauze ☐ Unna boot
Wound #_____	**TRACTS/ UNDERMINING**	☐ None ☐ Tracts ☐ Undermining Location _____ Size :_____	☐ None ☐ Tracts ☐ Undermining Location _____ Size :_____
Cleansed: _____	**EXUDATE AMOUNT**	☐ N/A ☐ 0% ☐ 25% ☐ 50% ☐ 75% ☐ 100%	☐ N/A ☐ 0% ☐ 25% ☐ 50% ☐ 75% ☐ 100%
Applied/packed: _____	**EXUDATE TYPE & COLOR**	☐ Serous ☐ Creamy ☐ Beige, Tan ☐ Sanguineous ☐ Yellow ☐ Green ☐ Serosanguineous ☐ N/A	☐ Serous ☐ Creamy ☐ Beige, Tan ☐ Sanguineous ☐ Yellow ☐ Green ☐ Serosanguineous ☐ N/A
Covered: _____	**EXUDATE ODOR**	☐ None ☐ Mild ☐ Foul ☐ N/A	☐ None ☐ Mild ☐ Foul ☐ N/A
Secured: _____ Protected periwound skin: _____ _____ _____	**WOUND BED APPEARANCE**	☐ Granular (Red): ☐ 0 ☐ 25 ☐ 50 ☐ 75 ☐ 100 ☐ Slough (Yellow): ☐ 0 ☐ 25 ☐ 50 ☐ 75 ☐ 100 ☐ Eschar (Black): ☐ 0 ☐ 25 ☐ 50 ☐ 75 ☐ 100	☐ Granular (Red): ☐ 0 ☐ 25 ☐ 50 ☐ 75 ☐ 100 ☐ Slough (Yellow): ☐ 0 ☐ 25 ☐ 50 ☐ 75 ☐ 100 ☐ Eschar (Black): ☐ 0 ☐ 25 ☐ 50 ☐ 75 ☐ 100

	PERIWOUND / SURROUNDING SKIN	☐ Clear/Intact ☐ Erythema ☐ Discoloration
		        ☐ Maceration ☐ Callous
		        ☐ Induration ☐ Edema ____
		        ☐ Denuded
			☐ Clear/Intact ☐ Erythema ☐ Discoloration
			        ☐ Maceration ☐ Callous
			        ☐ Induration ☐ Edema ____
			        ☐ Denuded

PT / CGR Teaching ☐ N/A ☐ Pt ☐ Cgr verbalized understanding re: ☐ S/S of infection ☐ Universal precautions ☐ Pt ☐ Cgr returned demo wnd care of: _____	**WOUND PAIN**	☐ No ☐ Yes ☐ with w/c only ☐ **See VPR**	☐ No ☐ Yes ☐ with w/c only ☐ **See VPR**

	PRESSURE REDUCING SURFACE DEVICE	☐ Heel protection ☐ Alternating air overlay/
		☐ Elbow protection mattress
		☐ Static air overlay / ☐ Low air loss,
		  mattress zoned bed
		☐ Foam overlay / ☐ Air fluidized bed
		  mattress ☐ Gel overlay /
		☐ Low air loss mattress
		  overlay mattress ☐ N/A
			☐ Heel protection ☐ Alternating air overlay/
			☐ Elbow protection mattress
			☐ Static air overlay / ☐ Low air loss,
			  mattress zoned bed
			☐ Foam overlay / ☐ Air fluidized bed
			  mattress ☐ Gel overlay /
			☐ Low air loss mattress
			  overlay mattress ☐ N/A

Pt. Tolerated care:	**REFERRAL DIAGNOSTIC**	☐ Nutrition consult ☐ Lab / blood work ☐ N/A	☐ Nutrition consult ☐ Lab / blood work ☐ N/A

Signature / Title	Date	Time

Courtesy of Kaiser Permanente.

Structured Assessment Form for Lower Extremity Ulcers

Reason for visit _____

_____

Ulcer History
Onset and duration
Prior treatment/response

Pain History
Severity
Description
Exacerbating and relieving factors
Location

Risk Factors for Neuropathic Disease
_____ Diabetes mellitus
_____ Alcoholism
_____ Vitamin B_{12} deficiency

Risk Factors for Venous Disease
_____ Deep vein thrombosis
_____ Obesity
_____ Multiple pregnancies
_____ Limited range of motion in ankle joint
_____ Sedentary lifestyle
_____ Thrombophilia

Risk Factors for Arterial Disease
_____ Atherosclerotic heart disease
_____ History of myocardial infarction or cerebrovascular accident
_____ Hyperlipidemia
_____ Diabetes mellitus (type, duration, last hemoglobin A_{1C}, management)
_____ Tobacco use (pack-years, any attempts to quit, willingness to consider quitting)
_____ Hypertension (duration, management)

Vascular Assessment
Compare affected limb to contralateral limb
Color/response to elevation and dependency
Temperature/warmth
Status of skin/hair/nails

Pulses: R (DP) _____ (PT) _____ L (DP) _____ (PT) _____
Venous refill: R: _____ seconds L: _____ seconds
Capillary refill: R: _____ seconds L: _____ seconds
ABI: R _____ L _____
Edema: R _____ L _____

Sensorimotor Assessment
Response to 5.07 monofilament:
    R: /10 L: /10
Response to 6.10 monofilament:
    R: /10 L: /10

Vibratory response: R: _____ L: _____
Position sense: R: _____ L: _____
Toe/foot deformities: R: _____ L: _____
Gait/wear patterns of footwear _____

Ulcer Assessment
Location:
Dimensions and depth:
Appearance/color of wound bed:
Status of wound edges:
Volume of exudate:
Status of surrounding tissue:

Guidelines for Differential Assessment of Leg Ulcers

Arterial Ulcers: Usually located distally (on toes) or in areas exposed to pressure/trauma. Ulcer bed typically pale or necrotic with very little exudate. Additional indicators: thin skin, pallor, or ashen tone; absence of hair; weak or nonpalpable pulses; ankle-brachial index (ABI) <0.9. Rule out coexisting edema.

Venous Ulcers: Usually located around malleoli. Ulcer bed typically either dark red or covered with slough; generally large amount of exudates. Additional indicators: edema, hemosiderosis, dermatitis. Rule out coexisting ischemia (ABI <0.9) or symptomatic heart failure. Modify compression for ABI >0.5 and <0.8. Avoid compression for any patient with symptoms of heart failure.

Neuropathic Ulcers: Usually located on feet in areas exposed to chronic trauma (tips of toes, plantar surface, sides of feet). Ulcer bed usually red (unless coexisting ischemia); usually moderate to large amounts of exudates. Rule out coexisting ischemia (if present, needs vascular workup).

Wound, Ostomy, and Continence Nurses Society Guidance on OASIS-C* Integumentary Items

Overview and Background

OASIS-C is a modification of the Outcome and Assessment Information Set (OASIS) that home health agencies must collect in order to participate in the Medicare program. This is the first major update of the OASIS since it was implemented in 2000.

It includes removing items not used for payment or quality, adding items to address clinical domains not covered, modified wording for selected items, and adding process items that support measurement of evidence-based practices. The system for wound classification uses terms that lack universal definition, and clinicians have verbalized concerns that they may be interpreting these terms incorrectly. The Wound, Ostomy and Continence Nurses (WOCN) Society has therefore developed the following guidelines for the classification of wounds. These items were developed by consensus among the WOCN Society panel of content experts.

(M1300) Pressure ulcer assessment: Was this patient assessed for risk of developing pressure ulcers?

(M1302) Does this patient have a risk of developing pressure ulcers?

(M1306) Does this patient have at least one unhealed pressure ulcer at stage II or higher or designated as "unstageable"?

Definitions

- **Unhealed:** Absence of the skin's original integrity
- **Nonepithelialized:** Absence of regenerated epidermis across a wound surface
- **Pressure Ulcer:** A pressure ulcer is localized injury to the skin and/or underlying tissue, usually over a bony prominence, as a result of pressure or pressure in combination with shear and/or friction. A number of contributing or confounding factors are also associated with pressure ulcers; the significance of these factors is yet to be elucidated.

Pressure Ulcer Stages (NPUAP 2007)

Stage I: A stage I pressure ulcer presents as intact skin with nonblanchable redness of a localized area, usually over a bony prominence. Darkly pigmented skin may not have visible blanching; its color may differ from the surrounding area.

Further Description: The area may be painful, firm, soft, and warmer or cooler compared to adjacent tissue. Stage I ulcers may be difficult to detect in individuals with dark skin tones and may indicate "at-risk" persons (heralding sign of risk).

Stage II: A stage II pressure ulcer is characterized by partial-thickness loss of dermis presenting as a shallow open ulcer with a red-pink wound bed without slough. It also may present as an intact or open/ruptured serum-filled blister.

Further Description: A stage II ulcer also may present as a shiny or dry shallow ulcer without slough or bruising (bruising indicates suspected deep tissue injury). This stage should not be used to describe skin tears, tape burns, perineal dermatitis, maceration, or excoriation.

Stage III: A stage III pressure ulcer is characterized by full-thickness tissue loss. Subcutaneous fat may be visible, but bone, tendon, or muscle is not exposed. Slough may be present but does not obscure the depth of tissue loss. Stage III ulcers may include undermining and tunneling.

Further Description: The depth of a stage III pressure ulcer varies by anatomic location. The bridge of the nose, ear, occiput, and malleolus do not have subcutaneous tissue; stage III ulcers in these locations can be shallow. In contrast, areas of significant adiposity can develop extremely deep stage III pressure ulcers. Bone/tendon is not visible or directly palpable.

Stage IV: A stage IV pressure ulcer presents with full-thickness tissue loss with exposed bone, tendon, or muscle. Slough or eschar may be present on some parts of the wound bed. Stage IV ulcers often include undermining and tunneling.

Further Description: The depth of a stage IV pressure ulcer varies by anatomic location. The bridge of the nose, ear, occiput, and malleolus do not have subcutaneous tissue; stage IV ulcers in these locations can be shallow. Stage IV ulcers can extend into muscle and/or supporting structures (e.g., fascia, tendon, or joint capsule); osteomyelitis is possible. Exposed bone/tendon is visible or directly palpable.

Unstageable: Full-thickness tissue loss in which the base of the ulcer is covered by slough (yellow, tan, gray, green, or brown) and/or eschar (tan, brown, or black) in the wound bed may render a wound unstageable.

Further Description: Until enough slough and/or eschar is removed to expose the base of the wound, the true depth (and, therefore, the stage) cannot be determined. Stable (dry, adherent, intact without erythema or fluctuance) eschar on the heels serves as "the body's natural (biologic) cover" and should not be removed.

Suspected Deep Tissue Injury: Deep tissue injury may be characterized by a purple or maroon localized area of discolored intact skin or a blood-filled blister due to damage of underlying soft tissue from pressure and/or shear. Presentation may be preceded by tissue that is painful, firm, mushy, boggy, and warmer or cooler compared to adjacent tissue.

Further Description: Deep tissue injury may be difficult to detect in individuals with dark skin tones. Evolution may include a thin blister over a dark wound bed. The wound may further evolve and become covered by thin eschar. Evolution may be rapid, exposing additional layers of tissue even with optimal treatment.

(M1307) The oldest nonepithelialized stage II pressure ulcer that is present at discharge

(M1308) Current number of unhealed (nonepithelialized) pressure ulcers at each stage

(M1310) Pressure ulcer length: longest length "head-to-toe"

(M1312) Pressure ulcer width: width of the same pressure ulcer; greatest width perpendicular to the length

(M1314) Pressure ulcer depth: depth of the same pressure ulcer; from visible surface to the deepest area

(M1320) Status of most problematic (observable) pressure ulcer

    0 Newly epithelialized

    1 Fully granulating

    2 Early/partial granulation

    3 Not healing

    NA No observable pressure ulcer

    (NOTE: Definitions for these terms at end of document)

(M1322) Current number of stage I pressure ulcers

(M1324) Stage of MOST PROBLEMATIC UNHEALED (OBSERVABLE) PRESSURE ULCER

(M1330) Does this patient have a stasis ulcer?

(M1332) Current number of (observable) stasis ulcer(s)

(M1334) Status of most problematic (observable) stasis ulcer

    0 Newly epithelialized

    1 Fully granulating

    2 Early/partial granulation

    3 Not healing

    NA No observable stasis ulcer

(M1340) Does this patient have a surgical wound?

(M1342) Status of most problematic (observable) surgical wound

    0 Newly epithelialized

    1 Fully granulating

    2 Early/partial granulation

    3 Not healing

    NA No observable surgical wound

This guidance applies to surgical wounds closed by either primary intention (i.e., approximated incisions) or secondary intention (i.e., open surgical wounds).

(M1350) Does this patient have a skin lesion or open wound, excluding bowel ostomy, other than those described above that is receiving intervention by the home health agency?

Definitions

- Newly epithelialized
  - wound bed completely covered with new epithelium
  - no exudate
  - no avascular tissue (eschar and/or slough)
  - no signs or symptoms of infection
- Fully granulating
  - wound bed filled with granulation tissue to level of surrounding skin
  - no dead space
  - no avascular tissue (eschar and/or slough)
  - no signs or symptoms of infection
  - wound edges are open
- Early/partial granulation
  - ≥25% of wound bed is covered with granulation tissue
  - <25% of wound bed is covered with avascular tissue (eschar and/or slough)
  - no signs or symptoms of infection
  - wound edges open
- Not healing
  - wound with ≥25% avascular tissue (eschar and/or slough) *or*
  - signs/symptoms of infection *or*
  - clean but nongranulating wound bed *or*
  - closed/hyperkeratotic wound edges *or* persistent failure to improve despite appropriate comprehensive wound management

Glossary-OASIS glossary terms are listed in the textbook glossary, pages 606-608.

---

*This is an abbreviated document. The complete document is available at www.WOCN.org

BATES-JENSEN WOUND ASSESSMENT TOOL
Instructions for use

General Guidelines:

Fill out the attached rating sheet to assess a wound's status after reading the definitions and methods of assessment described below. Evaluate once a week and whenever a change occurs in the wound. Rate according to each item by picking the response that best describes the wound and entering that score in the item score column for the appropriate date. When you have rated the wound on all items, determine the total score by adding together the 13-item scores. The HIGHER the total score, the more severe the wound status. Plot total score on the Wound Status Continuum to determine progress.

Specific Instructions:

1.   **Size**: Use ruler to measure the longest and widest aspect of the wound surface in centimeters; multiply length x width.

2.   **Depth**: Pick the depth, thickness, most appropriate to the wound using these additional descriptions:
       1 =   tissues damaged but no break in skin surface.
       2 =   superficial, abrasion, blister or shallow crater. Even with, &/or elevated above skin surface (e.g., hyperplasia).
       3 =   deep crater with or without undermining of adjacent tissue.
       4 =   visualization of tissue layers not possible due to necrosis.
       5 =   supporting structures include tendon, joint capsule.

3.   **Edges**: Use this guide:

Indistinct, diffuse	=	unable to clearly distinguish wound outline.
Attached	=	even or flush with wound base, <u>no</u> sides or walls present; flat.
Not attached	=	sides or walls <u>are</u> present; floor or base of wound is deeper than edge.
Rolled under, thickened	=	soft to firm and flexible to touch.
Hyperkeratosis	=	callous-like tissue formation around wound & at edges.
Fibrotic, scarred	=	hard, rigid to touch.

4.   **Undermining**: Assess by inserting a cotton tipped applicator under the wound edge; advance it as far as it will go without using undue force; raise the tip of the applicator so it may be seen or felt on the surface of the skin; mark the surface with a pen; measure the distance from the mark on the skin to the edge of the wound. Continue process around the wound. Then use a transparent metric measuring guide with concentric circles divided into 4 (25%) pie-shaped quadrants to help determine percent of wound involved.

5.   **Necrotic Tissue Type**: Pick the type of necrotic tissue that is <u>predominant</u> in the wound according to color, consistency and adherence using this guide:

White/gray non-viable tissue	=	may appear prior to wound opening; skin surface is white or gray.
Non-adherent, yellow slough	=	thin, mucinous substance; scattered throughout wound bed; easily separated from wound tissue.
Loosely adherent, yellow slough	=	thick, stringy, clumps of debris; attached to wound tissue.
Adherent, soft, black eschar	=	soggy tissue; strongly attached to tissue in center or base of wound.
Firmly adherent, hard/black eschar	=	firm, crusty tissue; strongly attached to wound base <u>and</u> edges (like a hard scab).

6.   **Necrotic Tissue Amount**: Use a transparent metric measuring guide with concentric circles divided into 4 (25%) pie-shaped quadrants to help determine percent of wound involved.

7.   **Exudate Type**: Some dressings interact with wound drainage to produce a gel or trap liquid. Before assessing exudate type, gently cleanse wound with normal saline or water. Pick the exudate type that is <u>predominant</u> in the wound according to color and consistency, using this guide:

Bloody	=	thin, bright red
Serosanguineous	=	thin, watery pale red to pink
Serous	=	thin, watery, clear
Purulent	=	thin or thick, opaque tan to yellow
Foul purulent	=	thick, opaque yellow to green with offensive odor

8.   **Exudate Amount**: Use a transparent metric measuring guide with concentric circles divided into 4 (25%) pie-shaped quadrants to determine percent of dressing involved with exudate. Use this guide:

None	=	wound tissues dry.
Scant	=	wound tissues moist; no measurable exudate.
Small	=	wound tissues wet; moisture evenly distributed in wound; drainage involves $\leq 25\%$ dressing.
Moderate	=	wound tissues saturated; drainage may or may not be evenly distributed in wound; drainage involves $> 25\%$ to $\leq 75\%$ dressing.
Large	=	wound tissues bathed in fluid; drainage freely expressed; may or may not be evenly distributed in wound; drainage involves $> 75\%$ of dressing.

9.   **Skin Color Surrounding Wound**: Assess tissues within 4 cm of wound edge. Dark-skinned persons show the colors "bright red" and "dark red" as a deepening of normal ethnic skin color or a purple hue. As healing occurs in dark-skinned persons, the new skin is pink and may never darken.

10.   **Peripheral Tissue Edema & Induration**: Assess tissues within 4 cm of wound edge. Non-pitting edema appears as skin that is shiny and taut. Identify pitting edema by firmly pressing a finger down into the tissues and waiting for 5 seconds, on release of pressure, tissues fail to resume previous position and an indentation appears. Induration is abnormal firmness of tissues with margins. Assess by gently pinching the tissues. Induration results in an inability to pinch the tissues. Use a transparent metric measuring guide to determine how far edema or induration extends beyond wound.

11.   **Granulation Tissue**: Granulation tissue is the growth of small blood vessels and connective tissue to fill in full thickness wounds. Tissue is healthy when bright, beefy red, shiny and granular with a velvety appearance. Poor vascular supply appears as pale pink or blanched to dull, dusky red color.

12.   **Epithelialization**: Epithelialization is the process of epidermal resurfacing and appears as pink or red skin. In partial thickness wounds it can occur throughout the wound bed as well as from the wound edges. In full thickness wounds it occurs from the edges only. Use a transparent metric measuring guide with concentric circles divided into 4 (25%) pie-shaped quadrants to help determine percent of wound involved and to measure the distance the epithelial tissue extends into the wound.

BATES-JENSEN WOUND ASSESSMENT TOOL   NAME

Complete the rating sheet to assess wound status. Evaluate each item by picking the response that best describes the wound and entering the score in the item score column for the appropriate date.

Location: Anatomic site. Circle, identify right **(R)** or left **(L)** and use **"X"** to mark site on body diagrams:

____	Sacrum & coccyx	____	Lateral ankle
____	Trochanter	____	Medial ankle
____	Ischial tuberosity	____	Heel Other Site

Shape: Overall wound pattern; assess by observing perimeter and depth.

Circle and <u>date</u> appropriate description:

____	Irregular	____	Linear or elongated
____	Round/oval	____	Bowl/boat
____	Square/rectangle	____	Butterfly Other Shape

Item	Assessment	Date Score	Date Score	Date Score
1. Size	1 = Length × width <4 sq cm 2 = Length × width 4—<16 sq cm 3 = Length × width 16.1—<36 sq cm 4 = Length × width 36.1—<80 sq cm 5 = Length × width >80 sq cm			

2. Depth	1 = Non-blanchable erythema on intact skin
	2 = Partial thickness skin loss involving epidermis &/or dermis
	3 = Full thickness skin loss involving damage or necrosis of subcutaneous
	      tissue; may extend down to but not through underlying fascia; &/or
	      mixed partial & full thickness &/or tissue layers obscured by
	      granulation tissue
	4 = Obscured by necrosis
	5 = Full thickness skin loss with extensive destruction, tissue necrosis or
	      damage to muscle, bone or supporting structures			

3. Edges	1 = Indistinct, diffuse, none clearly visible 2 = Distinct, outline clearly visible, attached, even with wound base 3 = Well-defined, not attached to wound base 4 = Well-defined, not attached to base, rolled under, thickened 5 = Well-defined, fibrotic, scarred or hyperkeratotic			
4. Under-mining	1 = None present 2 =Undermining < 2 cm in any area 3 = Undermining 2-4 cm involving < 50% wound margins 4 = Undermining 2-4 cm involving > 50% wound margins 5 = Undermining > 4 cm or Tunneling in any area			
5. Necrotic Tissue Type	1 = None visible 2 = White/grey non-viable tissue &/or non-adherent yellow slough 3 = Loosely adherent yellow slough 4 = Adherent, soft, black eschar 5 = Firmly adherent, hard, black eschar			
6. Necrotic Tissue Amount	1 = None visible 2 = < 25% of wound bed covered 3 = 25% to 50% of wound covered 4 = > 50% and < 75% of wound covered 5 = 75% to 100% of wound covered			
7. Exudate Type	1 = None			

Item	Assessment	Date Score	Date Score	Date Score
	2 = Bloody 3 = Serosanguineous: thin, watery, pale red/pink 4 = Serous: thin, watery, clear 5 = Purulent: thin or thick, opaque, tan/yellow, with or without odor			
8. Exudate Amount	1 = None, dry wound 2 = Scant, wound moist but no observable exudate 3 = Small 4 = Moderate 5 = Large			
9. Skin Color Surrounding Wound	1 = Pink or normal for ethnic group 2 = Bright red &/or blanches to touch 3 = White or grey pallor or hypopigmented 4 = Dark red or purple &/or non-blanchable 5 = Black or hyperpigmented			
10. Peripheral Tissue Edema	1 = No swelling or edema 2 = Non-pitting edema extends <4 cm around wound 3 = Non-pitting edema extends ≥4 cm around wound 4 = Pitting edema extends < 4 cm around wound 5 = Crepitus and/or pitting edema extends ≥4 cm around wound			
11. Peripheral Tissue Induration	1 = None present 2 = Induration, < 2 cm around wound 3 = Induration 2-4 cm extending < 50% around wound 4 = Induration 2-4 cm extending ≥ 50% around wound 5 = Induration > 4 cm in any area around wound			
12. Granulation Tissue	1 = Skin intact or partial thickness wound 2 = Bright, beefy red; 75% to 100% of wound filled &/or tissue overgrowth 3 = Bright, beefy red; < 75% & > 25% of wound filled 4 = Pink, &/or dull, dusky red &/or fills ≤ 25% of wound 5 = No granulation tissue present			
13. Epithelialization	1 = 100% wound covered, surface intact 2 = 75% to <100% wound covered &/or epithelial tissue extends >0.5cm into wound bed 3 = 50% to <75% wound covered &/or epithelial tissue extends to <0.5cm into wound bed 4 = 25% to < 50% wound covered 5 = < 25% wound covered			
	TOTAL SCORE			
	SIGNATURE			

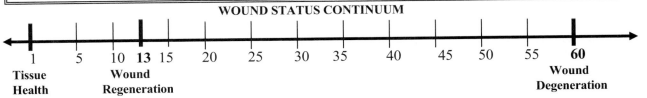

WOUND STATUS CONTINUUM

1   5   10 **13** 15   20   25   30   35   40   45   50   55   **60**

Tissue Health   Wound Regeneration   Wound Degeneration

Plot the total score on the Wound Status Continuum by putting an **"X"** on the line and the date beneath the line. Plot multiple scores with their dates to see-at-a-glance regeneration or degeneration of the wound.

Pressure Ulcer Scale for Healing (PUSH)

PUSH Tool 3.0

Patient Name: _____ Patient ID#: _____

Ulcer Location: _____ Date: _____

DIRECTIONS:
Observe and measure the pressure ulcer. Categorize the ulcer with respect to surface area, exudate, and type of wound tissue. Record a sub-score for each of these ulcer characteristics. Add the sub-scores to obtain the total score. A comparison of total scores measured over time provides an indication of the improvement or deterioration in pressure ulcer healing.

	0	1	2	3	4	5	
Length	0 cm²	<0.3 cm²	0.3-0.6 cm²	0.7-1.0 cm²	1.1-2.0 cm²	2.1-3.0 cm²	
× Width		6	7	8	9	10	**Sub-score**
		3.1-4.0 cm²	4.1-8.0 cm²	8.1-12.0 cm²	12.1-24.0 cm²	>24.0 cm²	
Exudate Amount	0	1	2	3			**Sub-score**
	None	Light	Moderate	Heavy			
Tissue Type	0	1	2	3	4		**Sub-score**
	Closed	Epithelial Tissue	Granulation Tissue	Slough	Necrotic Tissue		
							Total Score

Length × Width: Measure the greatest length (head to toe) and the greatest width (side to side) using a centimeter ruler. Multiply these two measurements (length × width) to obtain an estimate of surface area in square centimeters (cm²). Caveat: Do not guess! Always use a centimeter ruler and always use the same method each time the ulcer is measured.

Exudate Amount: Estimate the amount of exudate (drainage) present after removal of the dressing and before applying any topical agent to the ulcer. Estimate the exudate (drainage) as none, light, moderate, or heavy.

Tissue Type: This refers to the types of tissue that are present in the wound (ulcer) bed. Score as a "4" if there is any necrotic tissue present. Score as a "3" if there is any amount of slough present and necrotic tissue is absent. Score as a "2" if the wound is clean and contains granulation tissue. A superficial wound that is reepithelializing is scored as a "1". When the wound is closed, score as a "0".

　　4 - Necrotic Tissue (Eschar): black, brown, or tan tissue that adheres firmly to the wound bed or ulcer edges and may be either firmer or softer than surrounding skin.
　　3 - Slough: yellow or white tissue that adheres to the ulcer bed in strings or thick clumps, or is mucinous.
　　2 - Granulation Tissue: pink or beefy red tissue with a shiny, moist, granular appearance.
　　1 - Epithelial Tissue: for superficial ulcers, new pink or shiny tissue (skin) that grows in from the edges or as islands on the ulcer surface.
　　0 - Closed/Resurfaced: the wound is completely covered with epithelium (new skin).

PRESSURE ULCER HEALING CHART
(use a separate page for each pressure ulcer)

Patient Name: _____ Patient ID#: _____

Ulcer Location: _____ Date: _____

Directions: Observe and measure pressure ulcers at regular intervals using the PUSH Tool. Date and record PUSH Sub-scale and Total Scores on the Pressure Ulcer Healing Record below.

	PRESSURE ULCER HEALING RECORD												
DATE													
Length× Width													
Exudate Amount													
Tissue Type													
Total Score													

Graph the PUSH Total Score on the Pressure Ulcer Healing Graph below.

PUSH Total Score	PRESSURE ULCER HEALING GRAPH											
17												
16												
15												
14												
13												
12												
11												
10												
9												
8												
7												
6												
5												
4												
3												
2												
1												
Healed 0												
DATE												

Tinetti Balance Assessment Tool

BALANCE TESTS: Subject is seated on hard, armless chair				
DATE:				
SITTING BALANCE Leans or slides in chair = 0; Steady, safe =1				
ARISES Unable without help = 0; Able, uses arms to help = 1; Able without using arms = 2				
ATTEMPTS TO RISE Unable without help = 0; Able, requires > 1 attempt = 1; Able on first attempt = 2				
IMMEDIATE STANDING BALANCE (first 5 seconds) Unsteady (moves feet, sway, swaggers) = 0; Steady but uses support = 1; Steady without support = 2				
STANDING BALANCE Unsteady = 0; Steady but > 4 inch BOS and requires support = 1; Narrow stance without support = 2				
STERNAL NUDGE (feet close together) Begins to fall = 0; Staggers, grabs, catches self = 1; Steady = 2				
EYES CLOSED (feet close together) Unsteady = 0; Steady = 1				
TURNING 360° Discontinuous steps = 0; Continuous steps = 1				
TURNING 360° Unsteady (grabs, staggers) = 0; Steady = 1				
SITTING DOWN Unsafe (misjudges distance, falls) = 0; Uses arms or not a smooth motion = 1; Safe, smooth motion = 2				
BALANCE SCORE TOTAL	/16	/16	/16	/16
GAIT TESTS: Subject walks at normal pace				
GAIT INITIATION (immediate after told "go") Any hesitancy, multiple attempts to start = 0; No hesitancy = 1				
STEP LENGTH R swing foot passes L stance leg = 1; L swing foot passes R stance leg = 1				
FOOT CLEARANCE R foot completely clears floor = 1; L foot completely clears floor = 1				
STEP SYMMETRY R and L step length unequal = 0; R and L step length equal = 1				
STEP CONTINUITY Stopping or discontinuity between steps = 0; Steps appear continuous = 1				
PATH (excursion) Marked deviation = 0; Mild/moderate deviation or uses device = 1; Straight without assistive device = 2				

TRUNK   Marked sway or uses assistive device = 0;
            No sway, but knee or trunk flexion or spreads arms out while walking = 1;
            None of above deviations = 2				

BASE OF SUPPORT Heels apart = 0; Heels almost touching with gait = 1				
GAIT SCORE TOTAL	/12	/12	/12	/12
Assistive Device				
COMBINED BALANCE AND GAIT SCORE	/28	/28	/28	/28
THERAPIST INITIALS				

From Tinetti ME: Performance-oriented assessment of mobility problems in elderly patients, *J Am Geriatric Soc* 34:119-126, 1986.

ADMINISTRATION OF THE TINETTI GAIT & BALANCE INSTRUMENT

The Tinetti Gait and Balance Instrument is designed to determine an elder's risk for falls within the next year. It takes about 8–10 minutes to complete. The evaluator should review the questions prior to evaluation of the patient and ask any questions regarding the Instrument prior to beginning. The patient is asked to complete the gait portion first with the evaluator walking close behind the elder and evaluating gait steppage and drift. The patient is then asked to complete the balance portion with the evaluator again standing close by the patient (towards the right and in front). The patient is then asked to sit and the score is then totaled.

Scoring— The higher the score, the better the performance. Scoring is done on a three point scale with a range on each item of 0–2 with 0 representing the most impairment. Individual scores are then combined to form three scales: a Gait Scale, a Balance Scale and an overall Gait and Balance score. The maximum score for gait is 12 points while the maximum for Balance is 16 points with a total maximum for the overall Tinetti Instrument of 28 points.

Interpretation—Risk for falling:

< 19:	High risk of falling
19 to 23:	Increased risk of falling
> 24:	Low risk of falling

Also available at: *www.bhps.org.uk/falls/documents/TinettiBalanceAssessment.pdf*

Infrastructure Support Examples: Policies, Procedures, Protocols, and Decision-Making Tools

POLICY AND PROCEDURE: PREVENTION OF PRESSURE ULCERS

Policy:

All patients will be assessed for risk of pressure ulcers on admission, daily, and with significant change in condition. Appropriate preventive interventions will be implemented.

Risk Assessment Procedure:

Risk assessment includes determining a person's risk for pressure ulcer development using the appropriate Braden Scale. Pressure ulcer preventive interventions will target risk factors as determined by the pressure ulcer risk assessment. For patient older than 16 years, the Braden Scale will be used. For patient younger than 16 years, the Braden Q Scale will be used

Note: Braden Scale for Predicting Pressure Score Risk (Braden Scale) is a standardized tool for determining level of risk for pressure ulcer development in adult patients. Level of risk is determined by the following scores:

15–18 = Mild risk
13–14 = Moderate risk
10–12 = High risk
≤9 = Very high risk

Skin Inspection:

A head-to-toe skin inspection will include palpation. During inspection, pressure points are examined closely for any of the following conditions:

- Alteration in skin moisture
- Change in texture, turgor
- Change in temperature compared to surrounding skin (warmer or cooler)
- Color changes (e.g., red, blue, purplish hues)
- Nonblanchable erythema
- Consistency (e.g., bogginess [soft] or induration [hard])
- Edema
- Open areas, blisters, rash, drainage
- Pain

Note: Blanching erythema is an early indicator of the need to redistribute pressure. Nonblanching erythema is suggestive that tissue damage has already occurred or is imminent. Indurated or boggy skin is a sign that tissue damage may have occurred.

Preventive Interventions

1. Minimize or Eliminate Friction and Shear

One or more of the following interventions and observations will be used to minimize or eliminate shear if it is identified as a risk factor:

- Lift rather than drag patient's body when moving patient up in bed or chair.
- Avoid elevating head of the bed more than 30 degrees unless contraindicated.
- Decrease shear/friction by having patient sit in chair at 90-degree angle rather than reclining.
- Use transfer methods that minimize sliding (mechanical lifts, HoverMatt, trapeze, surgical slip sheets).
- Place a pad between skin surfaces that may rub together.
- Apply heel and elbow pads to reduce friction (they do not reduce pressure).
- Apply creams or lotions frequently to lower surface tension on skin and reduce friction.
- Apply transparent film dressing, hydrocolloid dressing, or skin sealant to bony prominences (e.g., elbows) to decrease friction.
- Keep skin well hydrated and moisturized.
- Lubricate bedpan before placing under patient. Position bedpan by rolling patient on and off rather than pushing and pulling bedpan in and out.

- Apply skin protectants and ointments to protect skin from moisture. Excessive moisture weakens dermal integrity and destroys the outer lipid layer, so less mechanical force is needed to wound the skin and cause a physical opening.

2. Minimize Pressure

Immobility is the most significant risk factor for pressure ulcer development. Patients who have any degree of immobility should be closely monitored for pressure ulcer development. One or more of the following interventions will be used if immobility is identified as a risk factor:

Patients in Bed
- Make frequent, small position changes.
- Use pillows or wedges to reduce pressure on bony prominences.
- Turn patient a minimum of every 2 hours.
- Do not position patient lying on side directly on trochanter (hip).
- Use pressure redistribution mattresses/surfaces.
- Free-float heels by placing a pillow under calf muscle and keeping heels off all surfaces.
- Avoid elevating head of the bed more than 30 degrees unless contraindicated.

Patients in Chair
- Encourage patient to shift weight every 15 minutes (e.g., perform chair pushups if able to reposition self; stand and reseat self if able; make small shift changes, such as elevating legs).
- Reposition patient every hour if he or she is unable to reposition self.
- Use chair cushions for pressure redistribution.

3. Minimize/Eliminate Pressure From Medical Devices

- Follow manufacturers instructions for appropriate use of medical devices (e.g., oxygen masks and tubing, catheters, cervical collars, casts, intravenous tubing, restraints),
- Routinely remove or reposition devices as needed for skin inspection, pressure relief and pressure redistribution.

4. Manage Moisture

Management of moisture from perspiration, wound drainage, and incontinence is an important aspect of pressure ulcer prevention. Moisture from incontinence may be a precursor to pressure ulcer development because of skin maceration and increased friction. Fecal incontinence is a greater risk factor than urinary incontinence for pressure ulcer development because the stool contains bacteria and enzymes that are caustic to the skin. In the presence of both urinary and fecal incontinence, fecal enzymes convert urea to ammonia, raising the skin pH. With a more alkaline skin pH, the skin becomes more permeable to other irritants. One or more of the following interventions will be used to minimize or eliminate moisture when it is identified as a risk factor:
- Contain wound drainage.
- Keep skin folds dry.
- Evaluate type of incontinence (urinary, fecal, or both).
- Implement toileting schedule or bowel/bladder program as appropriate.
- Check for incontinence a minimum of every 2 hours, and as needed.
- Cleanse skin gently with pH-balanced cleanser at each soiling. Avoid excessive friction and scrubbing, which can further traumatize the skin. Cleansers with nonionic surfactants are more gentle on the skin than are anionic surfactants in typical soaps.
- Use incontinence skin barriers (e.g., creams, ointments, pastes, film-forming skin protectants) as needed to protect and maintain intact skin, or to treat nonintact skin.
- Consider use of stool containment devices. Rectal tubes not approved by the U.S. Food and Drug Administration will not be used.
- Assess for candidiasis and treat as appropriate.

5. Maintain Adequate Nutrition/Hydration

The patient who is malnourished and/or dehydrated is at increased risk for pressure ulcer development. One or more of the following interventions will be used when nutrition is identified as a risk factor:

- Provide nutrition compatible with individual's wishes or condition.
- Encourage hydration as well as high-protein and high-calorie supplements for the patient with multiple risk factors for pressure ulcer development.

6. Address Sustainability of Plan of Care and Goals

The patient's ability to participate in pressure ulcer prevention interventions may be affected by physical and behavioral factors. Noncompliance may be related to inability to participate, lifestyle issues, cultural differences, medical condition, physical condition, lack of trust, or knowledge gaps. Possible activities to address include the following:

- Provide education that increases patient/family knowledge of pressure ulcer risk and appropriate interventions.
- Identify barriers to patient participation and develop strategies to address those barriers.

7. Documentation

- All assessments and skin inspection findings will be documented within 24 hours of admission. A plan of care for prevention of skin breakdown, patient response to interventions and informed refusals will be described and documented.

8. Patient/Family Education

The patient, family, and/or caregivers will be educated on risk assessment and skin inspection technique. They will be informed of current status of risk assessment and skin inspection findings and will be involved in planning interventions.

POLICY AND PROCEDURE: WOUND ASSESSMENT, DOCUMENTATION, AND QUALITY TRACKING

Policy:

All wounds will be assessed upon admission or occurrence, weekly, within 24 hours of discharge, and with significant changes.

Procedure.

The following parameters will be documented:

A. Anatomic location of skin breakdown
B. Etiology (type) of skin breakdown
C. Classification of skin breakdown
- Pressure ulcers will be classified according to the National Pressure Ulcer Advisory Panel (NPUAP) staging system.
- All other wounds will be classified as either "partial thickness" or "full thickness."
  ○ *Partial thickness:* Wounds extend through the first layer of skin (the epidermis) and into, but not through, the second layer of skin (the dermis).
  ○ *Full-thickness:* Wounds extend through both the epidermis and dermis and may involve subcutaneous tissue, muscle, and possibly bone.
  ○ *Approximated incisions:* Staples, sutures, or Steri-strips are present.
D. Wound measurements in centimeters

Length and Width: To ensure consistency, use the clock method for wound measurement. Visualize the wound as if it were the face of a clock. The top of the wound (12 o'clock position) is always toward the patient's head. Conversely, the bottom of the wound (6 o'clock position) is in the direction of the patient's feet. Therefore, length will be measured from the 12 o'clock to the 6 o'clock position, using the head and feet as guides. Width will be measured from side to side, or from the 3 o'clock to the 9 o'clock position.

Depth: The depth of the wound can be described as the distance from the visible surface to the deepest point in the wound, perpendicular to the skin surface. To measure the depth of the wound, use a sterile, flexible, cotton-tipped applicator.
- Put on gloves and gently insert the applicator into the deepest portion of the wound.
- Grasp the applicator with the thumb and forefinger at the point level to the skin surface.
- Withdraw the applicator while maintaining the position of the thumb and forefinger.
- Measure (with a ruler marked in centimeters) from the tip of the applicator to that position.

Tunneling (also known as *sinus tracts*): This is a passageway under the surface of the skin that is generally open at the skin level. However, most of the tunneling is not visible.

- Put on gloves and gently insert the sterile cotton-tipped applicator into the deepest extent of the tunnel.
- Pinch the applicator at the point where it meets the wound edge.
- Hold the pinched length of applicator next to a centimeter ruler to determine the depth of tunneling.
- Document the length and location of the tunnel using the clock method.

Undermining: Tissue destruction underlies intact skin. Both the direction and extent of undermining should be documented.
- Put on gloves and gently insert the sterile cotton-tipped applicator into the sites where undermining occurs.
- View the wound as though it were the face of a clock (as previously described). The 12 o'clock position corresponds to the wound edge that aligns toward the patient's head.
- Progressing in a clockwise direction, gently probe to determine the extent of undermining (e.g., 2 o'clock to 5 o'clock position).
- Insert the cotton-tipped applicator into the deepest area of the undermining. Grasp the applicator with thumb and forefinger at the point where it is level to the skin surface.
- Withdraw the applicator while maintaining the position of thumb and forefinger. Measure (using a ruler marked in centimeters) from the tip of the applicator to that position.
- Document the extent and deepest measurement of undermining in a manner similar to the following example: "Undermining from 2 o'clock to 5 o'clock position. Deepest point is 2.5 cm at 3 o'clock position."

E. Wound bed appearance (type and percentage of tissue in the wound bed)
F. Exudate/drainage
- Color
- Amount (percentage saturating dressing and type of dressing)
G. Periwound
- *All Wounds:* Assess and document condition of periwound skin condition (maceration, induration, erythema)
- *Lower-Extremity Wounds:* Assess and document edema and dorsalis pedis and posterior tibial pulses and sensation
H. Presence or absence of local signs of infection/overcolonization
- New/increased slough
- Drainage excess, change in color/consistency
- Poor granulation tissue (friable, bright red, exuberant)
- Redness, warmth, induration around wound
- Suddenly high glucose level in patient with diabetes
- Pain or tenderness

- Unusual odor
- Lack of improvement after 2 weeks of optimal management (including elimination or reduction of pressure ulcer risk factors as well as cofactors to impaired wound healing)

I. Pain
- Assess pain using a visual analogue scale or a faces rating scale

J. Patient/family education
- Signs and symptoms of infection
- Status or assessment of wound

K. Pressure ulcer reporting
- Pressure ulcers that are present on admission will be reported to the physician/provider for evaluation and documentation in the physician's notes.
- Nosocomial pressure ulcers will be reported to the physician/provider and a quality tracking report will be sent to quality management.

POLICY AND PROCEDURE: WOUND MANAGEMENT

Policy: A wound treatment plan will be initiated for a patient at the time of admission or upon development of a wound. The patient's treatment plan will be evaluated at least every week thereafter and revised as necessary. The treatment plan will be based on the principles outlined below.

Procedure:

A. Establish realistic goals related to wound management in collaboration with the patient, family, caregivers, and physician.
   - If wound healing is *not* a realistic goal, create a plan of care that will minimize pain, odor, and infection while optimizing quality of life.
   - If wound healing *is* a realistic goal, the following interventions should be incorporated into the care plan.

B. Control/eliminate causative factors.
C. Optimize nutrition.
   - Complete a nutritional screening on admission per nutritional assessment policy and procedure,
   - Consult registered dietician (RD) per nutritional assessment policy and procedure.
   - Reassess and consider RD consult if wound does not improve within 1 week of optimal wound management.

D. Assess, prevent, or manage pain.
E. Remove devitalized tissue when appropriate.
   - In the presence of adequate perfusion, remove devitalized tissue through mechanical, autolytic, or enzymatic debridement.
   - Heel ulcers with dry eschar need not be debrided if no signs of infection are present.
   - Sharp debridement by a qualified professional should be conducted when indicated.

F. Cleanse wound.
   - Cleanse wound initially and at each dressing change.
   - Use minimal mechanical force while cleaning a wound.
   - Avoid cleaning wounds using abrasive or antiseptic agents. (Normal saline is most often appropriate.)

G. Provide a physiologic wound environment with appropriate dressings.
   - If blood supply to the wound site is adequate, keep the wound bed moist.
   - If blood supply to wound site is *not* adequate, keep the wound clean and dry.
   - Keep periwound skin dry and intact.
   - Control exudate.
   - Consider caregiver time.
   - Eliminate dead space.
   - Avoid overpacking the wound.

H. Manage bacterial colonization and infection.
   - When treating multiple wounds on the same patient, attend to the most contaminated wound last.
   - Clean technique may be used for chronic wounds and pressure ulcers.
   - Perform cleansing and debridement of wounds as appropriate.
   - Consider a 2-week trial of topical antimicrobials as a course of treatment of wounds that are not healing after 2 weeks of optimal care.
   - Protect wounds from exogenous sources of contamination (e.g., feces).
   - Immediately report signs of infection to the physician.

I. Provide patient/family education.

The patient, family, and/or caregivers will be educated regarding the following:
   - Signs and symptoms of infection
   - Status or assessment of wound
   - Skin inspection and preventive interventions for skin breakdown (see policy on prevention of skin breakdown)
   - Pressure ulcer risk assessment findings (see policy on prevention of skin breakdown)
   - Dressing changes (if applicable)

POLICY: NAIL CARE

Purpose. To identify patients who need expert nail clipping from a certified or trained specialist after discharge.

Responsibility

MD (referral for expert nail care)
Nursing (basic nail trimming)

Policy

- *Expert nail clipping* is required for patients with nail disorders and conditions with risk factors known to lead to significant infection, poor wound healing, excessive bleeding, or limb loss. Expert nail care is *not* within the scope of nursing and requires an MD referral upon discharge to a podiatrist or trained/certified professional.
- *Basic nail clipping* is considered part of patient hygiene and within the scope of nursing practice.

Process

A. The need for nail clipping is identified by the patient, family, hospital personnel, or MD.
B. The MD evaluates risk factors and determines if patient requires any of the following:
  - *Basic nail trimming by staff nurse* as specified in the *Nursing Procedure Manual*
  - *Expert nail clipping by a trained expert* due to nail disorders and conditions with risk factors known to lead to significant infection, poor wound healing, excessive bleeding, or limb loss. Examples include but are not limited to the following:
    1. Onychophosis (incurvated or involuted nails)
    2. Onychogryposis (deformed, hypertrophic nails)
    3. Diabetes
    4. Rheumatoid arthritis
    5. Pernicious anemia
    6. Peripheral vascular disease
    7. Conditions that require warfarin (Coumadin)
    8. Neutropenia (absolute neutrophil count ≤1,000).
    9. Thrombocytopenia (platelet count ≤60,000).
C. The MD orders *basic* nail trimming by nurse or generates a podiatry referral upon discharge if *expert nail clipping* is indicated. (*Note:* Inpatient podiatry consultations remain available for acute needs such as surgical procedures and debridement.)

Related Resources

Howes-Trammel S et al: Foot and nail care. In Bryant R, Nix D: *Acute and chronic wounds: current management concepts,* ed 4, St. Louis, 2011, Mosby/Elsevier.

Itano JK, Taoka KN: *Oncology Nursing Society core curriculum for oncology nursing,* ed 4, St. Louis, 2005, Saunders/Elsevier.

POLICY: ANTIEMBOLISM STOCKINGS

Purpose:

To assist health care providers in the appropriate assessment and use of antiembolism stockings (AES) and to delineate patient care requirements to minimize/eliminate risks associated with AES use.

Policy:

Use of AES may be indicated in the immobile/bedridden patient as a mechanical means of deep vein thrombosis (DVT)/pulmonary embolus (PE) prophylaxis in patient who is at risk.

Procedure:

Adherence to the following assessment, use, and maintenance requirements is required. By definition, AES are elastic stockings that provide between 18 and 25 mm Hg gradient pressure. Medical center use is limited to knee-high stockings.

A. Indications for Use:
1. An order by a licensed independent practitioner
2. For DVT/PE prophylaxis in the immobile/bedridden patient
3. *Contraindications* for use (listed below):
   a. __ Arterial insufficiency (including symptoms of claudication, lower-extremity pain with elevation)
   b. __ Absent peripheral pulses
   c. __ Anatomic abnormality
   d. __ Dermatitis
   e. __ Loss of skin integrity
   f. __ Massive edema of legs or pulmonary edema from congestive heart failure
   g. __ Suspected or actual acute DVT
   h. __ Lower-extremity ischemia or gangrene
   i. __ Recent vein ligation
   j. __ Recent skin graft
   k. __ Ambulatory patient

B. Assessment, Care, and Maintenance:
1. Initial assessment as noted above in A, no. 1 through 3.
2. Provide patient education, emphasizing the stocking is to be used only while the patient is immobile or bedridden. Once he or she is ambulatory, the stocking should be discarded.
3. Measure the patient for knee-high AES only after he or she has been supine for at least 30 minutes.
4. Measure the extremity(ies) for the appropriate size according to the manufacturer's directions and brand being used. (The ankle is the most important measurement.)
5. Ensure the patient's leg is clean and completely dry prior to initial application of the stocking.

6. *Safety Check:* Apply the stockings according to nursing procedure and complete a safety check, including the following:
   a. __ Heel is located in the center of the heel pocket.
   b. __ Toes are freely mobile and patient reports no cramping.
   c. __ Fit is smooth over sensitive areas (toes, heel, anterior foot, ankle).
   d. __ Knit change at the knee is just below popliteal fossa.
7. Reassess lower-extremity circulation within 1 to 2 hours after initial application. If circulation is diminished (i.e., toes discolored, patient reports numbness, burning sensation), remove the stockings and notify the ordering practitioner.
8. Remove the stockings for 30 to 60 minutes every shift and conduct a reassessment. Particular at-risk areas include the patient's toes, heels, malleolus, anterior ankle, and top of stocking (possible tourniquet effect). Once daily, wash the lower extremities and lubricate the skin. Allow the lubricant to absorb before reapplying the stockings. Powder can be used if the extremity is thoroughly dried prior to application.
9. Discontinue and discard the stockings when the patient is ambulatory.

C. Documentation:
1. *Stocking Note:* Document as a progress note the initial assessment (including peripheral pulse assessment), measurements, size applied, and education provided.
2. Ongoing q.s. removal, assessment, and hygiene is recorded on the treatment record. Discontinuation of AES is also recorded on the treatment record.
3. Additional progress notes are required only when stockings require discontinuation due to impaired circulation, potential loss of skin integrity, or patient intolerance. Such progress notes will include provider notification.
4. Skin breakdown associated with use of the stockings requires an incident report to be initiated.

D. Special Notes:
1. Alternative interventions effective for prevention of DVT/PE:
   a. Dorsal and plantar flexion of the foot at least 10 times every hour while the patient is awake. Such interventions should be documented on the treatment sheet.
   b. Progressing patients to an ambulatory status as soon as clinically and physically indicated is one of the most effective measures for DVT/PE prevention.

c. AES are not recommended for use with sequential compression devices (SCDs). Rather, absorbent cotton stockings or stockinette is recommended for use.

d. Mechanical foot pumps or compression therapy increase lower-extremity peripheral blood flow

2. Pharmacologic agents effective for prevention of DVT/PE:
   a. Low-molecular-weight heparin
   b. Warfarin
   c. Subcutaneous heparin

3. Little-known facts:
   a. AES *are not* effective in treating lower-extremity edema in the upright patient. Ambulatory compression stockings (Jobst) can be ordered for this purpose. A variety of gradient pressure models (range 20–50 mm Hg) are available from prosthetics department.
   b. Treatment of orthostatic hypotension may include ambulatory compression stockings (Jobst).

c. Ankle-brachial index (ABI) is a noninvasive test that measures the patency of lower-extremity arteries. ABI <0.8 indicates arterial occlusion. Normal ABI is 1.0–1.2. Although no data suggest a critical level for not using AES stockings, vascular devices should not be used if ABI is <0.8, which is the level where critical limb ischemia becomes a serious concern.

E. Patient/Family Education: Describe the purpose of the stockings before application and instruct the patient to notify the nurse immediately of any burning, tingling, numbness, or pain following application. In rare situations where patients are discharged with AES, provide a written handout and review application, maintenance, laundering, and problem reporting with the patient.

From Department of Veterans Affairs, VHA, VA Upper Midwest Healthcare Network 13, Minneapolis, MN, Network Policy Memo V13-18, September 20, 1999.

Interdepartmental Handoff
Fairview Southdale Hospital
Communication Tool

Hospital Handoff Information

Date:_____ Time:_____

Discharge/Transport from:

_____

Patient Sticker Here

Primary Patient Problem(s):

Allergies:	**None**	**See Arm Band**	**Latex**

Safety Risks:
- ☐ **Full CODE**
- ☐ **DNR/DNI**
- ☐ **Fall Risk: Mental Status (orientation/confusion):**
- ☐ **Fall Risk: Functional Status (indep/limited Mobility):**
- ☐ **Infection Risk: MRSA   VRE   Other:**
- ☐ **Pressure Ulcer Risk (Braden $\leq$18)** – See back of sheet for interventions (excluding OR)
   - ○ **Existing Pressure Ulcer   Location:** _____ See back for interventions (excluding OR)
- ☐ **Restraints**
- ☐ **Suicide or Elopement Precautions–72 Hours HOLD** (Security w/Patient)

   Special Alert Care Plan: _____

Sensory Risk(s):
- ☐ **HOH   (R)   (L)   Both**
- ☐ **Vision Aids:**_____
- ☐ **Speech/Language difficulties:**_____
   _____
- ☐ **Interpreter Needed: Yes   No**
   Contacted:_____

Equipment & Special Needs:
- ☐ **Needs assistance to transfer X**_____
   people (more than 2, please send on cart)
- ☐ **Only guidance needed**
- ☐ **Uses cane/walker/other:**_____
- ☐ **Special Needs:**
   _____

   Able to have water: Yes   No

RN Signature:_____   **Ext:**_____

Note Patient Belongings:
____Glasses   ____Dentures   ____Hearing aide   ____Clothing   ____Other (list)
Sending Department: _____ Initial
Receiving Department: _____ Initial
Discharging Department: _____ Initial

Return from procedural department:

Test #1   *Test #2*
Signature:_____ ext:_____   **Signature:**_____ ext:_____

ATTENTION NURSING:_____
_____
_____
_____

The chart should remain with patient whenever possible.
Completion of this form is expected for patient safety, employee safety, tracking of patient belongings and
communication between inpatient and procedural areas.
A new form is needed each day or anytime greater than 2 procedures have occurred in one day.
This is not a permanent chart copy.

FSH Communication Tool
Hospital Handoff Information

Suggested (but not limited to) Action Steps for Pressure Ulcer Prevention Related to Procedure Areas:

- Add padding to boney body areas when appropriate
- Elevate the heels of supine and immobile patients
- Keep the head elevation of the cart/bed less than 30 degrees
- Turn the patient on their side, and off their back pre and post procedure during waiting and transport times
- Take a break to reposition the patient during long procedures when clinically appropriate
- Change or shorten long procedures when clinically appropriate
- Use AirMatt for lateral transfers of patient to and from carts/tables

DOCUMENTATION REQUIRED

Postprocedure, procedural staff will document the following in the permanent chart:

- Patient was a known Braden Risk, if applicable
- What procedures or interventions were taken for pressure prevention
- How long and in what position the patient experienced skin pressure risk
- Any early sign of change in skin redness or open skin noted after the procedure

Pressure Ulcer Prevention[1]
Algorithm

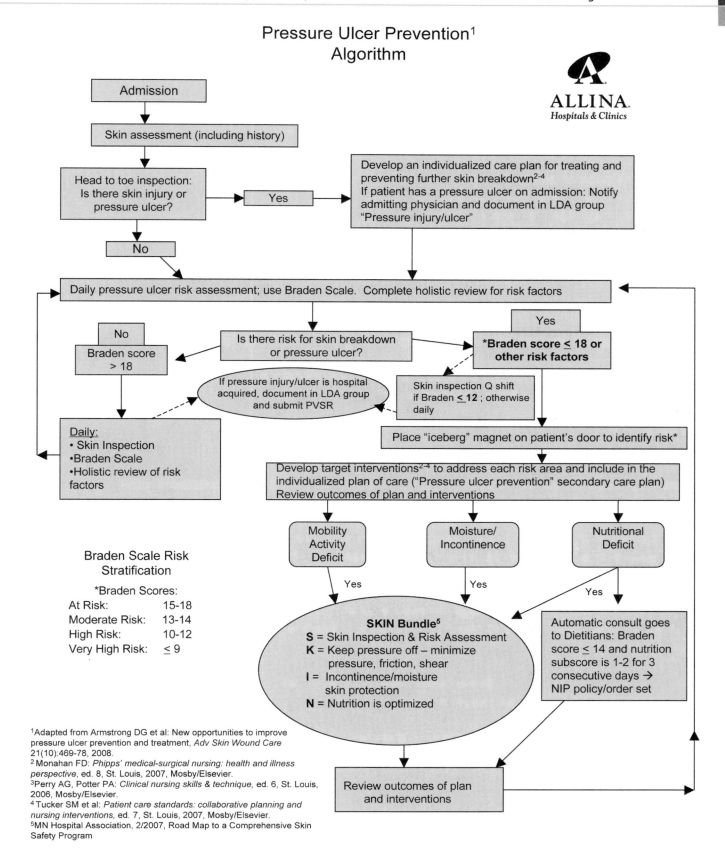

ALLINA.
Hospitals & Clinics

Admission

↓

Skin assessment (including history)

↓

Head to toe inspection: Is there skin injury or pressure ulcer? → **Yes** → **Develop an individualized care plan for treating and preventing further skin breakdown[2-4]. If patient has a pressure ulcer on admission: Notify admitting physician and document in LDA group "Pressure injury/ulcer"**

↓ **No**

Daily pressure ulcer risk assessment; use Braden Scale. Complete holistic review for risk factors

Is there risk for skin breakdown or pressure ulcer?

No — **Braden score > 18**

Yes — ***Braden score ≤ 18 or other risk factors***

If pressure injury/ulcer is hospital acquired, document in LDA group and submit PVSR

Skin inspection Q shift if Braden ≤ 12 ; otherwise daily

Daily:
- Skin Inspection
- Braden Scale
- Holistic review of risk factors

Place "iceberg" magnet on patient's door to identify risk*

Develop target interventions[2-4] to address each risk area and include in the individualized plan of care ("Pressure ulcer prevention" secondary care plan) Review outcomes of plan and interventions

Mobility Activity Deficit — Yes

Moisture/ Incontinence — Yes

Nutritional Deficit — Yes

SKIN Bundle[5]
S = Skin Inspection & Risk Assessment
K = Keep pressure off – minimize pressure, friction, shear
I = Incontinence/moisture skin protection
N = Nutrition is optimized

Automatic consult goes to Dietitians: Braden score ≤ 14 and nutrition subscore is 1-2 for 3 consecutive days → NIP policy/order set

Review outcomes of plan and interventions

Braden Scale Risk Stratification

*Braden Scores:
At Risk: 15-18
Moderate Risk: 13-14
High Risk: 10-12
Very High Risk: ≤ 9

[1]Adapted from Armstrong DG et al: New opportunities to improve pressure ulcer prevention and treatment, *Adv Skin Wound Care* 21(10):469-78, 2008.
[2] Monahan FD: *Phipps' medical-surgical nursing: health and illness perspective*, ed. 8, St. Louis, 2007, Mosby/Elsevier.
[3]Perry AG, Potter PA: *Clinical nursing skills & technique*, ed. 6, St. Louis, 2006, Mosby/Elsevier.
[4] Tucker SM et al: *Patient care standards: collaborative planning and nursing interventions*, ed. 7, St. Louis, 2007, Mosby/Elsevier.
[5]MN Hospital Association, 2/2007, Road Map to a Comprehensive Skin Safety Program

* Magnets optional on high-risk patient care areas

Courtesy of M. Zink and S. Sendelbach, Allina Hospitals & Clinics.

Skin Care Instructions

Patient identification

Pressure Ulcer Prevention

☐ Turn and position every 2 hours
☐ Pressure ulcer prevention mattress (i.e., group 1)
☐ Specialty mattress (i.e., low air loss)
☐ Float Heels/heels off bed
☐ Chair cushion
☐ HOB no more than 30°
☐ Other _____

Care of moisture related skin issues (perineal, groin, buttocks, skin folds)

☐ Antifungal cream to affected area, BID and after incontinence
☐ Perineal cleanser (i.e., Baza Cleanse and Protect) and barrier paste (i.e., Criticaid) BID and after incontinence
☐ Other _____

Care of pressure related suspected deep tissue injury or Stage I pressure ulcer

☐ _____ Suspected deep tissue injury (Intact-pressure related nonblanchable, dark discoloration or blood blister) keep clean, dry and free from pressure/injury, discoloration may resolve or slough to reveal extent of skin breakdown. No dressings needed as long as tissue is intact

☐ _____ Stage I pressure ulcer (Intact pressure related nonblanchable erythema) keep clean, dry and free from pressure breakdown. No dressings needed as long as tissue is intact

☐ _____ Blister keep clean, dry and free from pressure breakdown. No dressings needed as long as tissue is intact

☐ _____ ointment to shallow _____ wound twice daily

☐ Other _____
_____
_____
_____
_____

Alginate Dressing Change Procedure

Purpose: Promote autolysis of necrotic tissue and absorb exudate.

Wound Location: _____   Dressing Change Frequency: _____

Supplies (Circle all that apply):

a. Calcium alginate

b. Normal saline or hospital-approved wound cleanser to clean wounds

c. Tape

d. Gauze to dry periwound skin

e. Secondary dressing (ABD transparent dressing, border gauze)

f. Barrier ointment (zinc, Vaseline) or skin sealant

g. Sterile cotton-tipped applicators (Q-tips)

h. Other: _____

Procedure:

1. Wash hands and apply gloves.

2. Remove and discard dressing. Remove gloves and wash hands thoroughly per hand washing policy. Apply new gloves and put on appropriate personal protective equipment.

3. Cleanse with normal saline or hospital-approved wound cleanser.

4. Apply skin barrier to protect periwound skin from exudate.

5. Apply calcium alginate. If the wound has depth, gently fill wound space with alginate.

6. Cover with secondary dressings and secure as needed.

Gel/Ointment/Enzyme Dressing Change Procedure

Purpose: Enzymes promote enzymatic debridement in a moist environment. Ointments and gels facilitate autolysis.

Wound Location: _____   Dressing Change Frequency: _____

Supplies (Circle all that apply):

a. Gel/ointment/enzyme as applicable.
   (*Note:* Most ointments and enzymes come from pharmacy.)

b. Normal saline or hospital-approved wound cleanser

c. Secondary dressing (4 × 4 cover sponge, ABD, border gauze)

d. Tape

e. Sterile gauze

f. Barrier ointment or skin sealant

g. Sterile cotton-tipped applicators (Q-tips)

h. Other: _____

Procedure:

1. Wash hands and apply gloves.

2. Remove and discard dressing per facility policy. Remove gloves, wash hands, apply new gloves, and put on appropriate personal protective equipment.

3. Cleanse with normal saline or wound cleanser.

4. If needed, apply skin barrier around wound to protect patient's surrounding, intact periwound skin from moisture.

5. Apply thin layer of ointment to wound base or saturate into moist sterile gauze for packing into wounds with depth.

6. Cover with secondary dressings and secure as needed.

Note: Most enzymes require a moist environment to be effective

Hydrocolloid Dressing Change Procedure

Indication: Noninfected, minimally exudative wound
Purpose: Promote autolysis of nonviable tissue and provide a moist wound healing environment.

Wound Location: _____   Dressing Change Frequency: _____

Supplies (Circle all that apply):

- Hydrocolloid

- Normal saline or hospital-approved wound cleanser

- Gauze to dry around wound

Procedure:

1. Wash hands and apply gloves.

2. Carefully remove and discard dressing per facility policy. Carefully remove gloves, wash hands, apply new gloves, and put on appropriate personal protective equipment.

3. Cleanse with normal saline or hospital-approved wound cleanser.

4. Apply hydrocolloid to wound base. Allow 1 additional inch of product to cover and protect surrounding, intact periwound skin.

5. Apply paper tape if needed to prevent dressing edges from rolling up.

Hydrogel-Saturated Gauze Dressing Change Procedure

Indication: Dry to minimally exudative wound
Purpose: Donate moisture to prevent tissue dehydration, promote autolysis of nonviable tissue, and provide a moist wound healing environment.

Wound Location: _____   Dressing Change Frequency: _____

Supplies (Circle all that apply):

a. Hydrogel product

b. Normal saline or hospital-approved wound cleanser to clean wounds

c. Tape

d. Gauze to dry around wound

e. Secondary dressing (ABD, 4 × 4 cover sponge, foam, border gauze)

f. Barrier ointment or skin sealant

g. Sterile cotton-tipped applicators (Q-tips)

h. Other: _____

Procedure:

1. Wash hands and apply gloves.

2. Remove and discard dressing. Remove gloves, wash hands, apply new gloves, and put on appropriate personal protective equipment.

3. Cleanse with normal saline or wound cleanser.

4. Apply skin barrier to protect periwound skin from exudate.

5. Spread apart gel-impregnated sterile gauze and gently place or pack in wound base (or saturate gauze with hydrogel from a tube).

6. Follow with additional sterile gauze only if needed to fill depth of wound.

7. Cover with secondary dressing and secure as needed.

WOUND AND SKIN CARE COMPETENCIES

Learner Name:_____

Learner: It is your responsibility to get the individual competencies in front of your preceptor for observation, checking off, and signatures.

Preceptor: It is your responsibility to observe, initial, and date each item *only* if learner is deemed competent by meeting each criterion.

Pressure Ulcer Prevention Competency Criteria	Preceptor's Signature/Date
1. Performs head to toe skin inspection	
2. Documents accurate Braden assessment	
3. Develops and documents skin safety care plan; links risk assessment to interventions	
4. Places patient *and all tubes* in proper position	
5. Prevents shear injury by keeping head of bed at 30 degrees or less	
6. Uses draw sheet and gets assistance to minimize dragging patient against mattress while moving in bed	
7. Keeps heels off of bed with use of pillows under legs	
8. Shifts weight every hour while in the chair	
9. Describes strategies for managing moisture and incontinence, identifies and finds relevant supplies	
Wound Assessment Competency Criteria	**Preceptor's Signature/Date**
1. Identifies self and explains procedure to patient	
2. Washes hands	
3. Gathers necessary supplies *prior* to beginning the procedure (measuring guide, cotton-tipped applicators, method for recording measurements and dressing change supplies)	
4. Follows infection control guidelines for discarding dressings into the red container	
5. Cleans wound prior to assessment using appropriate infection control technique	
6. Notes correct anatomic location of wound	
7. Measures the wound's (in cm) height, width, depth, tunneling, and undermining	
8. Notes tissue type (red, granular, yellow, necrotic)	
9. Notes condition of periwound skin	
10. Notes presence or absence of signs of infection	
11. Applies new dressing according to step-by-step instructions	
12. Documents accurate wound assessment	
Wound Care Competency Criteria	**Preceptor's Signature/Date**
1. Washes hands	
2. Reviews step-by-step instructions for dressing change	
3. Gathers necessary supplies *prior* to beginning the procedure	
4. Follows infection control guidelines for discarding dressings	
5. Washes hands again after removing the dressing and applies new gloves	
6. Follows step-by-step instructions during dressing change, including a strategy for protecting the periwound skin	
7. Places patient in proper position	
Pouch Change Competency Criteria	**Preceptor's Signature/Date**
1. Empties ostomy pouch when 1/3 full of gas or stool	
2. Changes pouch *immediately* if leaking occurs and verbalizes why leakage can and should be prevented	
3. Reviews step-by-step instructions for ostomy pouch change procedure	
4. Gathers necessary supplies	
5. Follows infection control guidelines for discarding pouch	
6. Positions patient flat (or ensures no abdominal wrinkles) during procedure	

7. Dries the skin completely before applying a new pouch	
8. Follows step-by-step instructions during pouch change	
Support Surface Competency Criteria	**Preceptor's Signature/Date**
1. Demonstrates use of CPR controls on a low air-loss surface	
2. Explains rationale for using the least amount of linen possible under the patient	
3. Demonstrates use of max inflate button on a low air-loss surface	
4. Explains why max inflate should be used during repositioning on a low air-loss surface	
5. Demonstrates appropriate selection of under pads (air permeable for air beds only)	
6. Identifies process for selecting and obtaining pressure redistribution support surfaces for beds, chairs, and heels	
Negative Pressure Wound Therapy (NPWT) Competency Criteria	**Preceptor's Signature/Date**
1. Locates and views video in resource room	
2. Reviews step-by-step instructions	
3. Identifies self and explains procedure to patient	
4. Washes hands	
5. Gathers necessary supplies *prior* to beginning the procedure	
6. Follows infection control guidelines for discarding dressings into the red container	
7. Washes hands again after removing the dressing and applies new gloves	
8. Cuts the sponge to fit the wound so that the sponge does not overlap onto intact skin	
9. Ensures that tubing is positioned so that the patient does not lay or sit on the tubing	
10. Applies transparent dressing to ensure adequate seal	
11. Verbalizes or demonstrates how to change the canister	
12. Verbalizes or demonstrates ability to interpret alarms and operate machine	

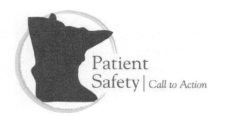

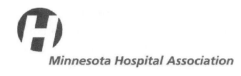

Pressure Ulcer Prevention in the O.R.
Recommendations and Guidance

These recommendations are intended to provide guidance to improve the consistency of pressure ulcer prevention in operating rooms and other invasive procedure areas across Minnesota hospitals and to address issues identified through the reporting of pressure ulcer events. The recommendations are not intended to address all of the AORN Perioperative Standards and Recommended Practices or other regulatory surgical requirements.

Risk Assessment, Skin Inspection and Communication — Prior to Handoff to Perioperative Team

- A thorough preoperative skin inspection should be performed the day of the procedure prior to handoff to the perioperative team.

- *Sample scripting for staff conducting skin inspection*
  "Because we know that being in one position for a period of time such as in surgery can put you at risk for getting a bedsore or what we call a pressure ulcer, I am going to take just a couple of minutes and check your skin from head to toe now before you go into surgery."

Hand-off Communication:
- Upon transfer of patient care to perioperative staff, staff transferring care should communicate:
  - o Most recent Braden Assessment information (this information will be communicated to postoperative staff)
  - o Any history of previous pressure ulcers
  - o Location of any existing pressure ulcers

Risk Assessment — Perioperative Staff

- All surgical patients should be considered at risk for pressure ulcer development and standard pressure ulcer prevention precautions should be followed.

- Perioperative staff should assess the patient's surgical risk factors for pressure ulcer development. Patients with the following risk factors should be considered high-risk for pressure ulcer development:
    - Any procedure lasting longer than four hours
    - Cardiac, vascular, trauma, transplants, bariatric surgeries or procedures involving at-risk positioning such as those requiring patient to be in a sitting position.
    - Patient with weight or nutritional extremes — obese or thin, small in stature

Intraoperative Surface Selection

- If a patient is assessed to be at high-risk for pressure ulcer development, it is strongly recommended that an OR table mattress pad with pressure redistributing properties greater than the standard* OR mattress pad be used during the procedure.

A standard OR mattress usually is constructed of one to two inches of foam covered with a vinyl or nylon fabric. Research studies have found that foam overlays or replacement pads do not have effective pressure redistribution capabilities.

Additional Considerations:

- The number of pads, blankets and warming blankets placed **beneath** the patient between the patient and the OR table mattress interferes with the pressure redistribution properties of the mattress.
- If a cooling blanket is placed between the patient and the OR table mattress, a higher grade surface should be considered to account for the change in pressure redistribution.
    - Suggestion: Explore using Bair Hugger warming system vs. water-filled warming blanket.

Lateral Transfers — preventing lateral shear during patient transfer

- Facilities should have a policy addressing patient transfer processes to prevent shearing of patient's skin during transfers. The policy should address, at minimum:
    - The number of staff required during transfer based on patient's weight
    - Appropriate transfer devices
    - Repositioning of patient after transfer
- Examples of transfer devices: Samarit Rollboard, HoverMatt, AirMatt, Z-Slider

Patient Positioning

- Perioperative team should anticipate any positioning equipment needed for the procedure specific to pressure redistribution.
- Patient's pressure ulcer risk, correct patient position and related equipment should be communicated and verified during the preoperative/pre-procedure briefing or during the time-out.
- The perioperative team should implement general positioning safety measures as defined in positioning standards.
- Responsibility for positioning and repositioning the patient should be assigned and well defined.
- When patient is in a supine position, the patient's heels should be suspended off the surface.
- Other areas of increased risk for pressure ulcers, based on patient position include:

Position	Areas of increased risk for pressure ulcer development
Supine/Lithotomy	Scapula, occiput, elbows, sacrum, coccyx, heels
Lateral	Ear, acromion process, trochanter, medial and lateral condyles of the knee, malleolus, foot edge on involved side
Prone/Jackknife	Nose, forehead, chest, acromion process, genitalia, breasts, iliac crests, patella, foot edge and toes

Additional Considerations:

- Pillows and molded-foam devices may produce only a minimum amount of pressure redistribution and are less effective during long procedures.
- Blankets, towels and sheet rolls do <u>not</u> reduce pressure injury and may contribute to friction injuries.
- When using positioning devices, the positioning devices should be placed underneath the patient and **not** beneath the mattress or overlay.

Patient Repositioning

- The perioperative team should communicate planned strategies for repositioning the patient during lengthy procedures (>4 hours). Examples of repositioning, *if not medically contraindicated*:
    - Anesthesia care provider moves patient's head when in a supine position to prevent pressure ulcers on the occiput.
    - Circulating nurse performs range of motion of patient extremities on patient in a lateral position.

Postoperative Surface Selection

- Patients meeting the following criteria should be considered for a Group II* pressure redistribution surface for postoperative care:
    - Expected postoperative hemodynamic instability, e.g., IABP, dissection case, ALVAD procedure or trauma
    - Medical contraindications to turning patient
    - Surgeon/RN discretion

*Examples of Group II pressure redistribution surface include: low air loss, alternating pressure and fluid air.

- Patient should be transferred from OR table to Group II surface

Following surgery, patients often remain immobile for extended periods of time, e.g., time in PACU + time getting settled in back on the floor. Effective postoperative communication and appropriate surface selection are vital to preventing pressure ulcer development during this postoperative time period.

Postoperative Handoff Communication, Surface Selection and Positioning

- The perioperative nurse should communicate to the postoperative nurse the following information related to pressure ulcers:
    - Patient positioning in the OR, e.g., lateral, prone
    - Any existing pressure ulcers
    - Patient's preoperative Braden Score
- Suspend heels off the bed/surface
- If not medically contraindicated, reposition patient from alternate position than OR position
- Consider upgrading surface for patient at-risk for pressure ulcer development, e.g., gurney with upgraded pressure redistribution surface

PACU Handoff Communication

- The postoperative nurse should communicate to the floor nurse the following information:
    - Patient positioning in the PACU, e.g., lateral, prone, with suggestion to place patient in alternate position if not medically contraindicated
    - Any existing pressure ulcers
    - Patient's preoperative Braden Score

MEDICARE COVERAGE OF SUPPORT SURFACES

For all three support surface groups, patients should have a care plan established by their physician or home care nurse, which is documented in their medical records. This plan generally should include, among other things, education of the patient and regular assessment by a healthcare practitioner. Coverage for all three groups continues until the patient's pressure ulcer is healed. In addition to the above common requirements, coverage for specific groups of support surfaces varies as follows:

GROUP 1 Support Surface

A group 1 support surface is generally designed to either replace a standard hospital or home mattress or as an overlay placed on top of a standard hospital or home mattress. Products in this category include mattresses, pressure pads, and mattress overlays (foam, air, water, or gel).

Coverage criteria (must meet 1 of the following):
- The patient is completely immobile.
  OR
- The patient is partially immobile with one of the following:
  - impaired nutritional status
  - incontinence
  - altered sensory perception
  - compromised circulatory status
- The patient has a pressure ulcer with one of the following:
  - impaired nutritional status
  - incontinence
  - altered sensory perception
  - compromised circulatory status

GROUP 2 Support Surface

A group 2 support surface is generally designed to either replace a standard hospital or home mattress or as an overlay placed on top of a standard hospital or home mattress. Products in this category include powered air flotation beds, powered pressure-reducing air mattresses, and non-powered advanced pressure-reducing mattresses.

Coverage criteria (must meet 1 of the following):
- The patient has large or multiple stage III or IV pressure sores on the trunk or pelvis
  OR
- The patient had a myocutaneous flap or skin graft for a pressure sore on the trunk or pelvis and has been on a group 2 or 3 support surface.
  OR
- The patient has a stage II pressure sore located on the trunk or pelvis AND has been on a comprehensive pressure sore treatment program (which has included the use of an appropriate group 1 support surface for at least one month)

GROUP 3 Support Surface

A group 3 support surface is a complete bed system known as air-fluidized.

Coverage criteria (must meet ALL of the following):
- The patient has a stage III or stage IV pressure ulcer AND
- Is bedridden or chair-bound AND
- Would be institutionalized without the use of the group 3 support surface AND
- Is under the close supervision of the patient's treating physician AND
- At least one (1) month of conservative treatment has been administered (including the use of a group 2 support surface) AND
- A caregiver is available and willing to assist with patient care AND
- All other alternative equipment has been considered and ruled out.

Support Surface Examples Using CMS Criteria for Reimbursement	
Category, Description, and Medicare Codes	Product Examples*
Group 1 Mattresses, pressure pads and mattress overlays; foam, air, water, or gel Medicare Codes: E0181-E0189, E0196-E0199, A4640	EHOB -WAFFLE® Mattress Overlay Gaymar - Sof.Care II SpanAmerica- Geo Matt MAX KCI- TheraRest® SMS Hill-Rom Tempur-Pedic
Group 2 Powered air flotation beds, powered pressure reducing air mattresses, and non-powered advanced pressure reducing mattresses Medicare Codes: E0193, E0277, E0371, E0372, E0373	Gaymar Plexus Air Express LAL Sizewise- Sunflower Pulse, True Low Air Loss SpanAmerica- Pressure Guard CFT KCI- First Step® HillRom-VersaCare Talley Medical Quattro Overlay™
Group 3 Complete bed systems known as air-fluidized Medicare Code: E0194	Hilrom -Clinitron At•Home® AFT KCI- KCI's FluidAir ® EliteTM

Reference: Centers for Medicare and Medicaid Services (CMS) Medicare Policy Regarding Pressure Reducing Support Surfaces Information for Medicare Fee for Services Health Care Professionals MLN Matters Number: SE1014 August 17, 2010. Available at https://www.cms.gov/MLNMattersArticles/downloads/SE1014.pdf accessed 9-13-2010

*Note: product examples and group classification came from the manufacturer's website and are not inclusive. Websites accessed September 13, 2010.

Satisfaction Survey

Wound, Ostomy, Continence, Foot Care Nursing Program

Riverwood HEALTHCARE CENTER

Recently, you have received services of our Wound, Ostomy, Continence, Foot Care Nursing Program. Please take a moment to give us your assessment of the program to aid us in evaluating our services.

Please indicate below the service you received (check only one)

☐ Wound Care   ☐ Ostomy Care   ☐ Continence Care   ☐ Foot & Nail Care

Please indicate the most recent date of service ....

Response Definition: P=Poor   F=Fair   G=Good   VG=Very Good   E=Excellent

	P	F	G	VG	E
1. Procedures, treatment and care practices were thoroughly explained by staff	☐	☐	☐	☐	☐
2. Professionalism of staff	☐	☐	☐	☐	☐
3. Staff members were friendly and encouraging	☐	☐	☐	☐	☐
4. The space provided for care and education was adequate	☐	☐	☐	☐	☐
5. Comfort and pain issues were addressed appropriately and in a timely manner	☐	☐	☐	☐	☐
6. How would you rate the Wound, Ostomy, Continence, Foot Care Nursing Program?	☐	☐	☐	☐	☐

	Y	N
7. Were your questions regarding your condition answered to your satisfaction?	☐	☐
8. Have you continued with the home instructions regarding care and prevention?	☐	☐
9. Has this program assisted you in changing your self-care habits?	☐	☐
10. Were you provided with appropriate education regarding your condition?	☐	☐
11. Would you recommend the Wound, Ostomy, Continence, Foot Care Nursing program to others?	☐	☐

Is there anything in the program that could be added or changed that would be helpful to you?

Please feel free to make any comments regarding the program inside the box below. Include your name and telephone if you would like someone to contact you regarding the services you received.

Please make no marks below this line

Activity Log

WOUND/SKIN CARE SERVICES

Daily Activity, Patient Case Mix, and Time Summary (1 unit =15 minutes)

1. Pressure Ulcer (PU) nosocomial 2. PU-present on admission 3. Skin Tear 4. Surgical wound 5. Incontinence 6. Venous 7. Arterial 8. Neuropathic 9. Mixed 10. Tube 11. Colostomy 12. Ileostomy 13. Urostomy 14. Committee work 15. Quality Management 16. Staff Education 17. Research/Trials 18. _____ 19. _____

Month _____

Patient	Unit #	1	2	3	4	5	6	7	8	9	10	11	12	13	14	15	16	17	18	19	20	21	22	23	24	25	26	27	28	29	30

abrasion Wearing away of the skin through some mechanical process (friction or trauma).

abscess Localized and encapsulated or walled off collection of pus in any part of the body.

aerobe Microorganism that lives and grows in the presence of free oxygen.

allodynia Pain due to a stimulus that does not normally provoke pain.

anaerobe Microorganism that lives and grows in the absence of free oxygen.

antibacterial Agent that inhibits the growth of bacteria.

antibiotic Pharmacologic agent that can destroy or inhibit organisms; has a single target and therefore is vulnerable to resistance.

antimicrobial Agent that inhibits the growth of microbes; general term for a substance that destroys or inhibits growth and replication of microorganisms.

antiseptic Chemical agent that prevents or inhibits microorganism growth; *topical substance* (also known as *antibacterial*) that inhibits growth and reproduction of microorganisms.

apoptosis Programmed cell death initiated when activating molecules bind to their specific receptors on target cells; mechanism to delete unwanted cells from the body.

arterial Pertaining to one or more arteries, which are vessels that carry oxygenated blood to the tissue.

arteriosclerosis Term applied to several pathologic conditions in which there is thickening, hardening, and loss of elasticity of the walls of blood vessels, especially arteries.

atrophie blanche Dermal sclerosis with dilated abnormal vasculature with ivory-white plaques on the ankle or foot and hemosiderin-pigmented borders.

autocrine stimulation Process of one cell acting on or stimulating specific cellular activities within itself.

autologous skin graft Graft of patient's own skin; also known as *autograft*.

autolysis Disintegration or liquefaction of tissue or cells by the body's own mechanisms, such as leukocytes and enzymes.

avascular* Lacking in blood supply; synonyms are dead, devitalized, necrotic, and nonviable. Specific types include slough and eschar.

bactericidal Agent that destroys bacteria.

bacteriostatic Agent that is capable of inhibiting the growth or multiplication of bacteria.

biofilm Polysaccharide matrix that microorganisms produce and live in. Bacteria within biofilm respond to signals from other bacteria in the community to change their phenotype. Highly resistant to and poorly penetrated by antimicrobials. Must be removed with debridement. Reformation is prevented with antimicrobials and maintenance debridement (including autolysis).

blanching Becoming white; maximum pallor.

callus Common, usually painless, thickening of the skin at locations of pressure, friction, or repetitive stress.

cell migration Movement of cells in the repair process.

cellulitis Inflammation of tissue around a lesion characterized by redness, swelling, and tenderness; signifies a spreading infectious process.

claudication Inadequate blood supply that produces severe pain in calf muscles during walking; subsides with rest.

clean wound* Wound free of devitalized tissue, purulent drainage, foreign material, or debris.

closed wound edges* Edges of top layers of epidermis have rolled down to cover lower edge of epidermis, including basement membrane, so epithelial cells cannot migrate from wound edges. *Also described as epibole or hyperkeratotic.* Presents clinically as sealed edge of mature epithelium. Wound edge may present clinically as hard/thickened and/or discolored (e.g., yellowish, gray, white).

collagen Main supportive protein of skin, tendon, bone, cartilage, and connective tissue.

colonization Replicating microorganisms on the wound surface without a host reaction.

contamination *Non*replicating microorganisms *on* the wound surface without a host reaction. All open wounds are contaminated by normal skin flora.

contraction Pulling together of wound edges in the healing process.

crater Tissue defect extending at least to the subcutaneous layer.

critical colonization Replicating microorganisms present on the wound and attaching to the cells and structures in the wound.

crusted Dried secretions.

cytokine Substances other than growth factors that contribute to regulation of cellular function and wound repair; examples include tumor necrosis factor-β and interferons.

dead space* Defect or cavity.

debridement Removal of devitalized tissue.

debris Remains of broken-down or damaged cells or tissue.

decubitus Latin word referring to the reclining position; misnomer for a pressure sore.

dehisced/dehiscence* Separation of surgical incision; loss of approximation of wound edges.

demarcation Line of separation between viable and nonviable tissue.

denude Loss of epidermis.

dependent rubor, or edema A change in the condition of the extremity when positioned lower than the heart; dependent rubor is a change in the color such that the extremity becomes dusky red; dependent edema is swelling of the extremity when placed in dependent position.

dermatomes Specific skin surface areas innervated by a single spinal nerve or group of spinal nerves.

disinfectant Topical liquid chemical that destroys or inhibits growth of microorganisms.

endocrine stimulation Process of one cell acting on or stimulating specific cellular activities in distant cells.

---

*indicates definition from CMS Outcome and Assessment Information Set (OASIS) data collection toll for home health agencies.

608

envelopment Ability of a support surface to conform so as to fit or mold around irregularities in the body.

enzymes Biochemical substances that are capable of breaking down necrotic tissue.

epibole* See *closed wound edges.*

epidermal stripping Remove epidermis by mechanical means; denude.

epidermis* Outer most layer of skin; new epidermis appears pink and dry and may look shiny.

epithelialization* Regeneration of the epidermis across a wound surface.

erosion* Wearing away or gradual destruction of a surface caused by inflammation, injury, or other cause.

erythema Redness of the skin surface produced by vasodilation.

eschar* Black or brown necrotic, devitalized tissue; tissue can be loose or firmly adherent, hard or soft, dry or wet.

excoriation Linear scratches on skin.

exudate Accumulation of fluid in a wound; may contain serum, cellular debris, bacteria, and leukocytes.

fibroblast Cell or corpuscle from which connective tissue is developed.

filariasis Disease of the tropics caused by an infection with any of several round, thread-like parasitic worms; most common is an infection with a parasite that lives in the lymph system.

fistula Abnormal passage from an internal organ to the body surface or between two internal organs.

friction Surface damage caused by skin rubbing against another surface.

full thickness* Tissue damage involving total loss of epidermis and dermis and extending into the subcutaneous tissue and possibly into the muscle or bone.

granulation Formation or growth of small blood vessels and connective tissue in a full-thickness wound.

granulation tissue* Pink/red, moist tissue composed of new blood vessels, connective tissue, fibroblasts, and inflammatory cells, which fills an open wound when it starts to heal. Typically appears deep pink or red with an irregular, "berry-like" surface.

growth factors Polypeptides that control growth and differentiation of cells (e.g., platelet-derived growth factor [PDGF], fibroblast growth factor [FGF], epidermal growth factor [EGF]).

healing* Dynamic process involving synthesis of new tissue for repair of skin and soft tissue defects.

hydrophilic Attracting moisture.

hydrophobic Repelling moisture.

hyperemia Presence of excess blood in the vessels; engorgement.

hyperkeratosis* Hard, white/gray tissue surrounding a wound.

immersion Depth of penetration (sinking) into a support surface.

induration Abnormal firmness of tissue with a definite margin.

infection* Presence of bacteria or other microorganisms in sufficient quantity to damage tissue or impair healing. Wound can be classified as infected when the wound tissue contains $\geq 100,000$ microorganisms per gram of tissue. Typical signs and symptoms of infection include

purulent exudate, odor, erythema, induration, warmth, tenderness, edema, pain, fever, and elevated white cell count. However, clinical signs of infection may not be present, especially in a patient who is immunocompromised or has poor perfusion.

inflammation Defensive reaction to harmful stimuli (pathogens, tissue injury or irritants); involves complex biological response including increased blood flow, increased capillary permeability and accumulation of leukocytes; facilitates physiologic cleanup of the wound; accompanied by increased heat, redness, swelling, and pain in the affected area.

insulation Maintenance of wound temperature close to body temperature.

intertriginous Area where apposing skin surfaces are in prolonged contact, such as groin, axilla, and under breasts; common complications are friction and moisture entrapment.

intertrigo Mild inflammatory condition that occurs on opposing skin surfaces precipitated by heat, moisture, friction and lack of air circulation; ; may be complicated by infection, most often fungal but may also be bacterial or viral; characterized by erythema, superficial linear erosion at the base of the skin fold, or circular erosion between the buttocks.

ischemia Deficiency of blood caused by functional constriction or obstruction of a blood vessel.

lesion Broad term referring to any abnormal tissue found on or in an organism; on the skin a lesion may be a wound or growth.

leukocytosis Increase in number of leukocytes (>10,000/ mm^3) in the blood.

maceration Softening of tissue by soaking in fluids.

macrophage Type of white blood cell that regulates wound repair through the ability to destroy bacteria and devitalized tissue and produce a variety of growth factors.

MMP Matrix metalloproteinase; enzymatic compound capable of protein and connective tissue degradation; classified as collagenase, gelatinase, and stromelysin.

moisture-retentive wound dressings General term that refers to any dressing that is capable of consistently retaining moisture at the wound site by interfering with the natural evaporative loss of moisture vapor.

MVTR Moisture-vapor transmission rate; measured in units of weight of moisture vapor per area of material per time period (e.g., g/m^2/day).

necrotic Dead; avascular, nonviable.

neuralgia Pain in distribution of nerve or nerves.

neuropathy Neuropathic progression from functional to structural to nerve death.

newly epithelialized* Process of regeneration of epidermis across a wound surface or (the presence of) regeneration of epidermis across a wound surface.

nociceptor Receptor preferentially sensitive to a noxious stimulus or to a stimulus that would become noxious if prolonged.

nonepithelialized* Absence of regenerated epidermis across a wound surface.

nongranulating* Absence of granulation tissue; wound surface appears smooth as opposed to granular. For example, in a wound that is clean but nongranulating, the wound surface appears smooth and red as opposed to cobblestone or berry-like.

occlusive wound dressings No liquids or gases can be transmitted through the dressing material.

osteomyelitis Inflammation of bone and marrow, usually caused by pathogens that enter the bone during an injury or surgery. Bone infection characterized by a mixture of inflammatory cells, fibrosis, bone necrosis, and new bone formation.

pallor Lack of natural color, paleness.

paracrine stimulation Process of one cell acting on or stimulating specific cellular activities within a neighboring cell.

paresthesia Abnormal neurologic sensations described as "pins and needles," "electric-like," "numb, aching feet," "as if my feet have been in ice water," "knifelike," or shooting pains.

partial thickness* Confined to the skin layers; skin damage that does not penetrate below the dermis and may be limited to the epidermal layers only.

periwound Area immediately around the wound.

physiologic wound environment Presence of physical, chemical, and biotic (living) factors in a wound that are characteristic of healthy intact skin; desirable to facilitate the natural process of wound healing.

planktonic bacteria Free-floating (not anchored) bacteria, as seen with contamination and colonization.

pliable Supple, flexible.

pressure redistribution Ability of the support surface to distribute load over the contact areas of the human body; this term replaces prior terminology *pressure reduction* and *pressure relief.*

pressure ulcer Area of localized tissue damage caused by ischemia because of pressure.

purpura Bleeding beneath the skin or mucous membranes; causes black and blue spots (ecchymosis) or pinpoint bleeding.

pus Thick fluid indicative of infection containing leukocytes, bacteria, and cellular debris.

pyogenic Producing pus.

reactive hyperemia Extra blood in vessels occurring in response to a period of blocked blood flow.

scab* Crust of dried blood and serum.

semiocclusive wound dressings No liquids are transmitted through dressing naturally; variable levels of gases can be transmitted through dressing material; most dressings are semiocclusive.

senescent cells Age-related decrease in proliferation potential of dermal fibroblasts; occurrence observed in chronic wounds in which fibroblasts have impaired responsiveness to growth hormone; response that may be due to increased number of senescent cells.

shear Trauma caused by tissue layers sliding against each other; results in disruption or angulation of blood vessels.

sinus tract* Course or path of tissue destruction occurring in any direction from the surface or edge of the wound; results in dead space with potential for abscess formation. Sometimes called *tunneling* (which can be distinguished from undermining in that the sinus tract involves a small portion of the wound edge, whereas undermining involves a significant portion of the wound edge).

slough* Soft moist avascular (devitalized) tissue; may be white, yellow, tan, or gray, may be loose or firmly adherent.

stasis Stagnation of blood caused by venous congestion.

Stemmer sign Thickened skin fold at base of second toe or second finger that is an early diagnostic sign for lymphedema. In a positive result, this tissue cannot be lifted but only grasped as lump of tissue. In a negative result, the tissue can be lifted normally.

support surface Specialized device for pressure redistribution designed for management of tissue loads.

synthetic wound dressings Dressings that are composed of man-made materials, such as polymers, as opposed to naturally occurring materials, such as cotton.

telangiectasia tortuous, spidery, distended superficial blood vessels; commonly located on face around nose, cheeks, and chin but also develop on upper thigh, around ankles, and below knee joint; will blanch when palpated.

TIMP Tissue inhibitor of matrix metalloproteinases; binds to matrix metalloproteinase and renders it inactive.

trophic Changes that occur as a result of inadequate circulation, such as loss of hair, thinning of skin, ridging of nails.

tunneling* See *sinus tract.*

ulcer Open sore.

undermining* Area of tissue destruction extending under intact skin along the periphery of a wound; commonly seen in shear injuries. Can be distinguished from tunneling or sinus tract in that undermining involves a significant portion of the wound edge, whereas tunneling involves only a small portion of the wound edge.

unhealed* absence of skin's original integrity.

unstageable pressure ulcer Covered with eschar or slough, which prohibits complete assessment of the wound.

varicosities Dilated tortuous superficial veins.

vasoconstriction Constriction of the blood vessels.

vasodilation Dilation of blood vessels, especially small arteries and arterioles; also called *vasodilatation.*

venous Pertaining to the veins.

venous insufficiency Deep or superficial veins become incompetent, permitting reverse flow and resulting in increased pressure in the superficial veins during ambulation.

wound bioburden Presence of microorganisms on or in a wound. Continuum of bioburden ranges from contamination, colonization, critical colonization, biofilm and infection. Bioburden includes quantity of microorganisms present, as well as their diversity, virulence, and interaction of the organisms with each other and the body (synergism).

wound margin Rim or border of wound.

wound repair Healing process; partial-thickness healing involves epithelialization; full-thickness healing involves contraction, granulation, and epithelialization.

xenograft Tissue from another species (e.g., pig) used as a temporary graft.